Davidson's P...

Medicine

D0489351

The Editors

Christopher R.W. Edwards

Professor of Clinical Medicine, University of Edinburgh; Honorary Consultant Physician, Western General Hospital; Chairman, Department of Medicine, Western General Hospital, Edinburgh, UK

Ian A.D. Bouchier

Professor of Medicine, University of Edinburgh; Honorary Consultant Physician, Royal Infirmary of Edinburgh, Edinburgh, UK

Illustrated by Robert Britton

For Churchill Livingstone:

Publishers: Joan Morrison, Laurence Hunter
Project Editor: Thérèse Duriez
House Editor: Wendy Lee
Production: I. Macaulay Hunter
Design: Design Resources Unit
Sales Promotion Executive: Marion Pollock

SIXTEENTH EDITION

Davidson's Principles & Practice of Medicine

Edited by CHRISTOPHER R.W. EDWARDS & IAN A.D. BOUCHIER

CHURCHILL LIVINGSTONE
EDINBURGH LONDON MELBOURNE NEW YORK AND TOKYO 1991

CHURCHILL LIVINGSTONE
Medical Division of Longman Group UK Limited

Distributed in the United States of America by Churchill Livingstone Inc.,
1560 Broadway, New York, N.Y. 10036, and associated companies, branches
and representatives throughout the world.

© E. & S. Livingstone 1956, 1958, 1960, 1962, 1964, 1966, 1968
© Longman Group Limited 1971, 1974, 1977, 1981, 1984
© Longman Group UK Limited 1987, 1991

All rights reserved. No part of this publication may be reproduced, stored in a
retrieval system, or transmitted in any form or by any means, electronic,
mechanical, photocopying, recording or otherwise, without either the prior
written permission of the publishers (Churchill Livingstone, Robert Stevenson
House, 1–3 Baxter's Place, Leith Walk, Edinburgh EH1 3AF) or a licence
permitting restricted copying in the United Kingdom issued by the Copyright
Licensing Agency Ltd, 33–34 Alfred Place, London WC1E 7DP.

First Edition 1952
Second Edition 1954
Third Edition 1956
Fourth Edition 1958
Fifth Edition 1960
Sixth Edition 1962
Seventh Edition 1964
Eighth Edition 1966
Ninth Edition 1968
Tenth Edition 1971
Eleventh Edition 1974
Twelfth Edition 1977
Thirteenth Edition 1981
Fourteenth Edition 1984
Fifteenth Edition 1987
Sixteenth Edition 1991

ISBN 0-443-04092-3

British Library Cataloguing in Publication Data
Davidson, Sir Stanley 1894–1981
    Davidson's principles and practice of medicine – 16th ed.
    1. Man. Diseases
    I. Title   II. Edwards, Christopher R.W. (Christopher Richard Watkin)
    1942–   III. Bouchier, Ian A.D. (Ian Arthur Dennis) 1932–
    616

Library of Congress Cataloging in Publication Data
Davidson's principles and practice of medicine/edited by
    Christopher R.W. Edwards, Ian A.D. Bouchier – 16th ed.
        p.   cm.
    Includes bibliographical references.
    Includes index.
    1. Internal medicine.   I. Davidson, Leybourne Stanley Patrick,
    Sir, 1894–1981.   II. Edwards, C.R.W. (Christopher Richard Watkin)
    III. Bouchier, Ian A.D. (Ian Arthur Dennis)   IV. Title: Principles
    and practice of medicine.
    [DNLM: 1. Medicine.   WB 100 D253]
    RC46.D24   1991
    616 – dc20
    DNLM/DLC
    for Library of Congress   90-2695
                                                                CIP

Produced by Longman Group (FE) Limited
Printed in Hong Kong

Preface

The Sixteenth Edition of *Davidson's Principles and Practice of Medicine* has undergone a number of major changes. After many years as Editor, Dr John MacLeod has retired. John MacLeod was associated with the *Principles and Practice of Medicine* from its very beginning. He worked closely with Sir Stanley Davidson and was responsible for ensuring the particular presentation and balance of information which has made the book so respected throughout the medical world. In a very real sense, therefore, the book enters a new phase of its long history and we are very aware of our responsibility as Editors to maintain the tradition of excellence in medical knowledge and communication which has been the hallmark of *Davidson's Principles and Practice of Medicine*.

There have been a number of changes in our contributors and our thanks go to Dr W J Irvine, Dr D G Julian, Professor J A Simpson and Professor H Walton who have made some valuable contributions to previous editions. At the same time we welcome a number of new members to our team: Dr N Boon, Professor Anne Ferguson, Professor J A A Hunter, Dr G Lloyd, Dr C A Ludlam, Dr C Soutar, Dr A D Toft and Dr R G Will. Major changes have been made in the presentation and content of the Sixteenth Edition of the book, perhaps more than in any of the preceding fifteen editions. The text has been almost entirely re-written and a considerable update has been undertaken. A great deal of effort has been taken to ensure that this new edition reflects the practice of medicine in Britain but at the same time carries an account of the experience of medicine in tropical and developing countries. Major alterations have been made in the chapter layout and content with new sections on disorders of the skin, climatic and environmental factors in disease and re-organisation of the material on infection and antimicrobial therapy. We have attempted to ensure that the textbook will be of practical use to the reader, with an emphasis not only on the clinical features and investigations used to achieve a diagnosis, but also by providing much more information on the management of the various diseases. To offset the effects of these changes on the size of the book, we have reduced the amount of space given to descriptions of anatomy, physiology and the techniques of clinical examination.

Those familiar with previous editions of *Davidson's Principles and Practice of Medicine* will appreciate how radical has been the transformation of the Sixteenth Edition. Much thought and effort has gone into the presentation of the book with an improved layout of the text, a greater use of illustrations and tables and the introduction of information boxes. In making these changes, however, we have made every attempt to ensure that academic quality, which has been the essential basis of the continuing success of this Edinburgh textbook, has not declined. It is our hope that *Davidson's Principles and Practice of Medicine* will continue to instruct and stimulate undergraduates and postgraduates around the world.

Edinburgh   C.R.W.E.
1991   I.A.D.B.

Acknowledgements

We are grateful to Dr Simon Walker, Department of Clinical Chemistry, University of Edinburgh for revising the tables on biochemical values.

It gives us great pleasure to acknowledge the many letters we have received with comments on content, suggestions for inclusion and improvement, and, on occasion, errors in the text. Wherever appropriate, these suggestions have been incorporated into the new edition. It is our pleasure to record our gratitude to our contributors who have undertaken willingly all the many demands placed upon them. The many pressures experienced by busy clinicians today leave little time for medical writing but we have been fortunate in working with a team who have taken their tasks seriously and never permitted a slackening of standards.

Finally, and by no means least, we are most grateful to the staff of Churchill Livingstone for their support during the preparation of the Sixteenth Edition. They have handled the great deal of work with both efficiency and good humour.

Edinburgh
1991

C.R.W.E.
I.A.D.B.

Contributors

N C Allan FRCP(Edin) FRCPath
Consultant Haematologist, Western General Hospital;
Part-time Senior Lecturer, Department of Medicine,
University of Edinburgh, Edinburgh, UK

Joyce D Baird MA FRCPath
Reader in Medicine, Department of Medicine,
University of Edinburgh; Honorary Consultant
Physician, Western General Hospital, Edinburgh, UK

N A Boon MD FRCP(Edin)
Consultant Cardiologist, Royal Infirmary of
Edinburgh; Honorary Senior Lecturer, Department of
Medicine, University of Edinburgh, Edinburgh, UK

Ian A D Bouchier CBE MD FRCP FRCP(Edin) FIBiol FRSE
Professor of Medicine, University of Edinburgh;
Honorary Consultant Physician, Royal Infirmary of
Edinburgh, Edinburgh, UK

A D M Bryceson MD FRCP(Edin) FRCP DTM&H
Senior Lecturer, London School of Hygiene &
Tropical Medicine; Consultant Physician, Hospital for
Tropical Diseases; Consultant in Tropical
Dermatology, St John's Hospital for Diseases of the
Skin, London, UK

Gerard P Crean PhD FRCP(Edin) FRCP(Glas) FRCP(I)
Honorary Lecturer in Medicine, University of
Glasgow, Western Infirmary; Consultant Physician,
Southern General Hospital; Physician-in-Charge,
Gastrointestinal Centre, Southern General Hospital,
Glasgow; Director, Diagnostic Methodology, Research
Unit, Southern General Hospital, Glasgow, UK

G K Crompton FRCP(Edin)
Consultant Physician, Respiratory Unit, Northern
General Hospital; Part-time Senior Lecturer,
Departments of Medicine and Respiratory Medicine,
Western General Hospital, City Hospital,
Edinburgh, UK

R E Cull BSc PhD FRCP(Edin)
Consultant Neurologist, Royal Infirmary of
Edinburgh; Part-time Senior Lecturer in Neurology,
University of Edinburgh, Edinburgh, UK

A M Davison BSc MD FRCP(Edin) FRCP
Consultant Renal Physician, St James's University

Hospital; Senior Clinical Lecturer, University of
Leeds, Leeds, UK

David DeBono MA MD FRCP(Edin)
British Heart Foundation Professor of Cardiology,
University of Leicester, Leicester, UK

Christopher R W Edwards MA MD FRCP FRCP(Edin)
FRSE
Professor of Clinical Medicine, University of
Edinburgh; Honorary Consultant Physician, Western
General Hospital; Chairman, Department of Medicine,
Western General Hospital, Edinburgh, UK

A E H Emery MD PhD DSc FRCP(Edin) FLS FRSE
Emeritus Professor of Human Genetics and Honorary
Fellow, University of Edinburgh, Edinburgh; Visiting
Fellow, Green College, Oxford, UK; Research
Director, European Alliance of Muscular Dystrophy
Associations, European Centre for Euromuscular
Diseases, Baarn, The Netherlands

A Ferguson PhD FRCP FRCPath
Professor of Gastroenterology, University of
Edinburgh; Honorary Consultant Physician, Gastro-
intestinal Unit, Western General Hospital, Edinburgh,
UK

N D C Finlayson FRCP(Edin) FRCP
Consultant Physician, Royal Infirmary of Edinburgh;
Honorary Senior Lecturer, Department of Medicine,
University of Edinburgh, Edinburgh, UK

A M Geddes FRCP FRCP(Edin)
Senior Consultant in Infectious Diseases, West
Midlands Regional Health Authority; Professor of
Infectious Diseases, University of Birmingham,
Birmingham, UK

J A A Hunter BA MD FRCP(Edin)
Professor of Dermatology, University of Edinburgh;
Honorary Consultant Dermatologist, Royal Infirmary
of Edinburgh, Edinburgh, UK

Anne T Lambie FRCP(Edin) FRCP
Honorary Fellow, University of Edinburgh; Former
Senior Lecturer, University of Edinburgh; Former
Consultant Physician, Renal Unit, Royal Infirmary of
Edinburgh, Edinburgh, UK

Alexander A H Lawson MD FRCP(Edin)
Consultant Physician, Milesmark Hospital,
Dunfermline; Honorary Senior Lecturer, Department
of Medicine, University of Edinburgh, Edinburgh,
UK

G Lloyd MA MD MPhil FRCP(Edin) FRCP FRCPsych
Consultant Psychiatrist, Royal Free Hospital, London,
UK

Christopher A Ludlam BSc PhD FRCP FRCPath
Consultant Haematologist; Director, Haemophilia
Centre; Part-time Senior Lecturer, Department of
Medicine, University of Edinburgh, Edinburgh, UK

G J R McHardy MA MSc BM(Oxon) FRCP FRCP(Edin)
Consultant Clinical Respiratory Physiologist, Lothian
Health Board; Part-time Senior Lecturer,
Departments of Respiratory Medicine and Medicine,
Western General Hospital, University of Edinburgh,
Edinburgh, UK

G Nuki FRCP FRCP(Edin)
Professor of Rheumatology, University of Edinburgh;
Honorary Consultant Physician, Northern General
Hospital, Edinburgh, UK

J Richmond MD FRCP(Edin) FRCP(Glas) PRCP
Former Professor of Medicine, University of Sheffield,
Sheffield; President, Royal College of Physicians,
Edinburgh, UK

D J C Shearman PhD FRCP(Edin) FRACP
Professor of Medicine, Chairman, Department of
Medicine, University of Adelaide; Head of the
Professorial Medical Unit and Senior Visiting
Physician, Royal Adelaide Hospital, Adelaide,
Australia

J F Smyth MA MD(Cantab) MSc(Lond) FRCP(Edin) FRCP
Imperial Cancer Research Fund Professor of Medical
Oncology, University of Edinburgh; Honorary
Consultant Physician, Western General Hospital and
Royal Infirmary of Edinburgh, Edinburgh; Director of
the Imperial Cancer Research Fund Medical Oncology
Unit, Edinburgh, UK

Colin A Soutar MD FRCP(Edin) MFOM
Director, Institute of Occupational Medicine;
Honorary Senior Lecturer, Department of Respiratory
Medicine, University of Edinburgh, Edinburgh, UK

R N Thin MD FRCP(Edin) FRCP
Consultant Physician, Department of Genito-Urinary
Medicine, St Thomas' Hospital, London, UK

A D Toft BSc MD FRCP(Edin)
Consultant Physician, Royal Infirmary of Edinburgh,
Edinburgh; Honorary Senior Lecturer, Department of
Medicine, University of Edinburgh, Edinburgh, UK

A S Truswell MD FRCP FRACP FFCM
Boden Professor of Human Nutrition, University of
Sydney; Honorary Consultant in Nutrition, Royal
Prince Alfred Hospital, Sydney, Australia; Vice
President, International Union of Nutritional Sciences

R G Will MA MD MRCP FRCP(Edin)
Consultant Neurologist, Western General Hospital;
Part-time Senior Lecturer, University of Edinburgh,
Edinburgh, UK

Contents

Contents

1

Genetic Factors in Disease

Nowadays there is an increasing awareness of the importance of genetic factors in the aetiology and pathogenesis of many disorders affecting man. Perhaps of more importance is that this knowledge has also led to possible means of prevention of such disorders through genetic counselling and antenatal diagnosis.

At the turn of the century morbidity and mortality in infancy and childhood could largely be attributed to environmental factors such as infections and nutritional deficiencies. With advances in medicine these problems are decreasing, at least in the developed countries, while others, in which genetic factors are largely or even entirely responsible, are becoming more obvious. In a survey carried out in Edinburgh a few years ago, no less than 50% of childhood deaths could be attributed to genetic diseases. The contribution of genetic factors to mortality and morbidity in adults is more difficult to assess but is also increasing.

It is useful to consider human disease as forming a spectrum at one end of which we have those diseases which are entirely genetic in origin and in which environmental factors play little if any part. This group of disorders includes *chromosomal abnormalities* and so-called *unifactorial disorders*.

UNIFACTORIAL DISORDERS

These are due to single gene defects (Mendelian factors); though individually rare there are over 4000 of them. They are usually serious disorders which often present at birth or in childhood, though notable exceptions are Huntington's chorea, myotonic dystrophy and polyposis coli. The mode of inheritance is straight-forward and follows Mendelian principles, and the risks of occurrence in relatives are high. For the vast majority of these unifactorial disorders there is as yet no effective treatment and prevention is the main approach to the problem.

MULTIFACTORIAL DISORDERS

At the other end of the spectrum are those diseases such as infections and nutritional deficiencies which are entirely environmental in aetiology. In the middle of the spectrum are many common conditions which are partly genetic and partly environmental in causation, so-called *multifactorial disorders* (Table 1.1). In multifactorial disorders the genetic component is complex, probably involving in each case many genes. The risks to relatives are usually low.

In this chapter, after a review of the chemical basis of inheritance, an outline is given of chromosomal abnormalities, unifactorial and multifactorial disorders and the prevention of genetic disease.

Table 1.1   Multifactorial disorders

Congenital	Dislocation of hip
	Club foot
	Pyloric stenosis
	Heart disease
	Anencephaly/spina bifida
Late onset	Diabetes mellitus
	Essential hypertension
	Coronary artery disease
	Schizophrenia
	Manic depressive psychosis

CHEMICAL BASIS OF INHERITANCE

In the nucleus of every cell are the chromosomes containing the genes composed of segments of deoxyribonucleic acid within which genetic information is stored. Molecular studies have now shown that genes can no longer be considered as being arranged like contiguous beads on a string. They are separated by long stretches of DNA, sometimes referred to as 'junk DNA', the function of which is as yet largely unknown.

DNA STRUCTURE

DNA is made up of two polynucleotide chains, twisted together to form a double helix (Fig. 1.1). Each nucleotide is composed of a nitrogenous base, a sugar molecule (deoxyribose) and a phosphate molecule. The nitrogenous bases in DNA are adenine and guanine (purines) and cytosine and thymine (pyrimidines). A purine in one chain always pairs with a pyrimidine on the other chain. There is also specific base pairing: guanine in one chain always pairs with cytosine in the other chain and adenine always pairs with thymine. At nuclear division the two strands of the DNA molecule separate and as a result of specific base pairing each chain then builds its complement. In this way, when a cell divides, genetic information is conserved and transmitted to each daughter cell.

The primary action of the gene is to synthesise protein by various combinations of 20 different amino acids. Genetic information is stored within the DNA molecule in the form of a triplet code such that a sequence of three bases specifies the structure of one amino acid.

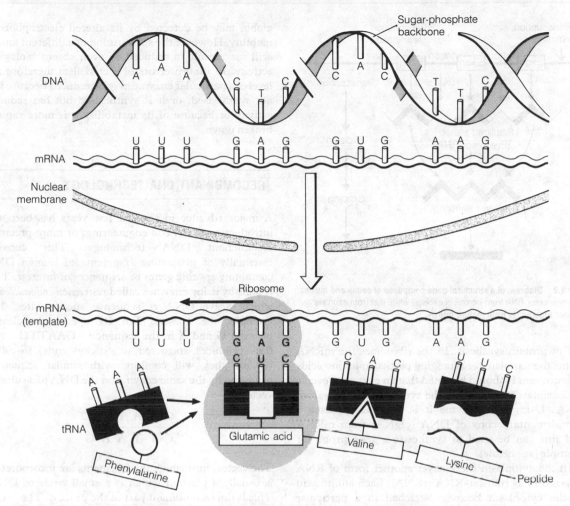

Fig. 1.1   Protein synthesis. Sequences of bases in nuclear DNA (genes) send instructions via messenger RNA (mRNA), to transfer RNA (tRNA) on ribosomes in the cytoplasm, whereby amino acids are linked to form polypeptides. In these processes guanine (G) pairs with cytosine (C) and adenine (A) with thymine (T) or uracil (U).

RNA STRUCTURE

Whereas DNA is found mainly in the chromosomes, ribonucleic acid (RNA) is found mainly in the nucleolus and the cytoplasm. RNA has a structure similar to DNA (Fig. 1.1): both nucleic acids contain adenine, guanine and cytosine but thymine is replaced by uracil in RNA and the latter contains the sugar ribose.

Transcription

The information stored in the DNA code of the gene is transcribed from one strand to a particular type of RNA, so-called messenger RNA (mRNA). Each mRNA is formed by a particular gene, such that every base in the mRNA molecule is complementary to a corresponding base in the DNA of the gene: cytosine with guanine, thymine with adenine but adenine with uracil since the latter replaces thymine in RNA. However recent studies have shown that genes are composed of *exons* and *introns* and that the latter generate a precursor RNA which is excised, while the precursor RNA from exons is spliced together to form the mRNA (Fig. 1.2). Defects in this splicing process can significantly affect the gene product and are now recognised as the cause of some genetic disorders (e.g. certain types of thalassaemia).

Translation

The mRNA now migrates into the cytoplasm where it becomes associated with the ribosomes which are the

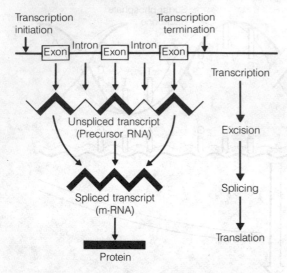

Fig. 1.2 Diagram of a structural gene composed of exons and introns. The precursor RNA from introns is excised while that from exons is spliced together to form mature mRNA.

site of protein synthesis. In the ribosomes the mRNA forms the template for arranging particular amino acids in sequence. It should be noted that an enzyme (reverse transcriptase) can catalyse the synthesis of DNA from RNA. Using this enzyme it is possible to make a complementary copy of DNA (cDNA) from mRNA and this can be used to synthesise a gene probe for example (see below).

In the cytoplasm there is yet another form of RNA referred to as transfer-RNA (tRNA). Each amino acid in the cytoplasm becomes attached to a particular tRNA. The other end of the tRNA molecule consists of three bases which combine with complementary bases on the mRNA. Thus a particular triplet in the mRNA is related through tRNA to a specific amino acid. The ribosome moves along the mRNA in a zipper-like fashion, the assembled amino acids linking up to form a polypeptide chain.

A change (mutation) of a base pair of the DNA molecule may result in any one of a number of possible effects. If the altered triplet codes for the same amino acid then of course the change will go undetected. Possibly 20 to 25% of all possible single base changes are of this type. Alternatively a single base mutation may result in a triplet which codes for a different amino acid resulting in an altered protein. The latter may retain its biological activity (e.g. enzyme activity) but have altered physico-chemical properties such as electrophoretic mobility or stability so that it is more rapidly broken down. This is the case in many of the haemoglobinopathies in which the aberrant haemo-

globin may be detected by its altered electrophoretic mobility. However the substitution of a different amino acid may result in reduced or even absent biological activity. In inborn errors of metabolism therefore the level of a particular enzyme may be reduced because it is not synthesised, or it is synthesised but has reduced activity or because of its instability it is more rapidly broken down.

RECOMBINANT DNA TECHNOLOGY

A major advance in the last few years has been the introduction of genetic engineering, or more precisely recombinant DNA technology. This consists essentially of generating fragments of human DNA containing specific genes or sequences of interest. This is done by using enzymes called *restriction endonucleases* which cleave DNA at sequence specific sites. For example, the enzyme *Eco* RI specifically cleaves between G and A in the sequence – GAATTC – and thus produces staggered or 'sticky' ends, so-called because they will combine with similar sequences produced by the same enzyme on the DNA of a suitable vector

$$\text{G\,A\,A\,T\,T\,C}$$
$$\text{C\,T\,T\,A\,A\,G}$$

The vector, into which the fragments are incorporated, is usually a plasmid which is a small circle of DNA. This is the recombinant part of the process. The vector is then introduced into a microbial host, usually *Escherichia coli*, which is grown in culture to produce *clones* with multiple copies of the incorporated human DNA. The cloned DNA may be labelled with ^{32}P and can then be used as a *probe*. A probe is a labelled, single stranded DNA fragment which will hybridise with, and thereby detect and locate (by autoradiography), complementary sequences among DNA fragments on a *Southern blot* (Fig. 1.3). The latter is a technique of transferring DNA fragments, which have been separated by electrophoresis on an agarose gel, to a nitrocellulose filter where they can hybridise with the probe (fusion of 2 single strands of DNA by complementary base pairing).

MEDICAL APPLICATIONS

These techniques have wide applications in medicine, the most important being the synthesis of biologically important molecules (such as human insulin, growth hormone, blood clotting factors) and the diagnosis of

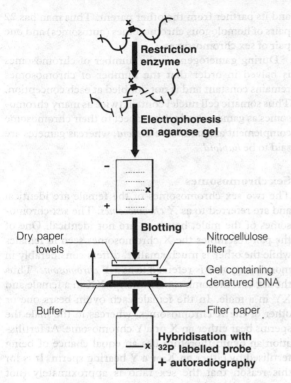

Fig. 1.3 The Southern blot technique. 'X' indicates the gene or sequence of interest. (From *An Introduction to Recombinant DNA* by A.E.H. Emery (1985), John Wiley Publishers, with permission.)

genetic disease. The latter is possible by using a gene specific probe which is a cloned and labelled DNA sequence complementary to at least part of the gene responsible for a particular disorder. The technique is illustrated in Figure 1.4 with regard to the antenatal diagnosis of haemoglobinopathies.

Restriction fragment length polymorphism
The use of a gene specific probe requires that details of the disease gene are known. But in many disorders this is not so and gene specific probes are not available. In this case diagnosis depends on demonstrating that the disease gene is linked to (on the same chromosome and close to) a DNA marker or so-called restriction fragment length polymorphism (RFLP). RFLPs result from variations in DNA sequences which occur throughout the entire genome and are without any effects on the individual. They are due to either the loss of an existing restriction site or the acquisition of a new site so that the fragments produced by a particular restriction enzyme are of different sizes in different people and can be recognised by their different mobilities on a Southern blot. RFLPs are inherited as simple genetic traits (Fig. 1.5). If a disease-producing

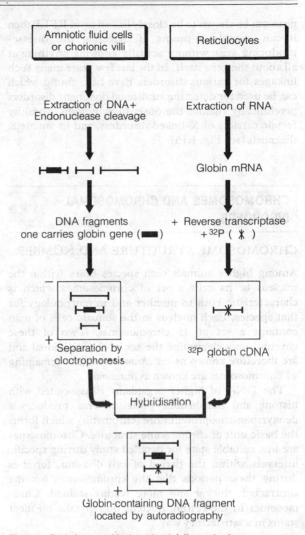

Fig. 1.4 Technique used in the antenatal diagnosis of haemoglobinopathies. The probe used here is a complementary DNA copy (cDNA) produced from mRNA using RNA-dependent DNA polymerase (reverse transcriptase) and labelled with ^{32}P (*).

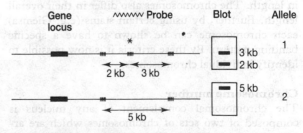

Fig. 1.5 Diagrammatic representation of an autosomal RFLP. On one chromosome (allele 1) two DNA fragments are produced, whereas on the homologous chromosome (allele 2) only one DNA fragment is produced by a particular restriction enzyme.
* Indicates the site of the RFLP (kb = kilobase = 1000 base pairs).

gene can be shown to be closely linked to an RFLP then it can provide a means of detecting the disease-producing gene without actually knowing anything at all about the gene itself. In the last few years many such linkages for various disorders have been found which can be used for detecting autosomal dominant disorders preclinically (before the onset of symptoms), healthy female carriers of X-linked disorders, and in antenatal diagnosis (see Fig. 1.15).

CHROMOSOMES AND CHROMOSOMAL DISORDERS

CHROMOSOME STRUCTURE AND NUMBER

Among higher animals each species bears within the nucleus of its cells a set of chromosomes which is characteristic both in number and in morphology for that species. Each nucleus in the somatic cells of man contains a set of 46 chromosomes. Two of these chromosomes determine the sex of the individual and are therefore known as *sex chromosomes*; the remaining 44 chromosomes are known as *autosomes*.

The DNA of higher organisms is associated with histone and non-histone proteins. This produces a deoxyribonucleoprotein fibre (chromatin) which forms the basic unit of chromosome structure. Chromosomes are in a suitable state for detailed study during specific intervals within the period of cell division, for it is during these periods that the chromosomes become contracted, thicker and more readily stained. Chromosomes in the resting nucleus do not take up most stains in a satisfactory way.

Chromosome identification
Each chromosome has a point along its length, a constriction, known as the *centromere* which divides the chromosomes into two arms which are usually unequal in length. The chromosomes also differ in their overall length. Further, by using certain stains (e.g. Giemsa) each chromosome can be shown to have a specific banding pattern. By these criteria it is now possible to identify individual chromosomes.

Chromosome number
The chromosomal complement of any nucleus is composed of two sets of chromosomes which are arranged in pairs. Because the two members of any given pair (with the exception of the sex chromosomes) resemble one another they are said to be *homologous*. One homologue of any pair is derived from one parent

and its partner from the other parent. Thus man has 22 pairs of homologous chromosomes (autosomes) and one pair of sex chromosomes.

During gametogenesis the number of chromosomes is halved in order that the number of chromosomes remains constant and is not doubled at each conception. Thus somatic cell nuclei contain twice as many chromosomes as gametes and with respect to their chromosome complement are said to be *diploid*, whereas gametes are said to be *haploid*.

Sex chromosomes
The two sex chromosomes of the female are identical and are referred to as *X chromosomes*. The sex chromosomes of the male, however, are not identical. One of the pair resembles the X chromosomes seen in females while the other is much smaller, differs considerably in morphology and is referred to as a *Y chromosome*. Thus the sex chromosome constitution is XX in a female and XY in a male. In the female each ovum bears one or other of the X chromosomes, whereas in the male the sperms bear either an X or a Y chromosome. At fertilisation an ovum therefore has an equal chance of being fertilised by either an X or a Y bearing sperm. It is for this reason that the sex ratio is approximately (not exactly) unity at birth.

MITOSIS

Unlike highly differentiated cells such as neurones, the cells of many tissues in the body repeatedly undergo division. In fact some cells, such as those of the intestinal tract and bone marrow, continue to divide throughout the life of an individual. For the error rate in cell division to remain as low as it is, nuclear division must be extremely well regulated. The process by which nuclei divide to produce two identical daughter nuclei is known as mitosis.

During mitosis each chromosome divides into two so that the number of chromosomes in each daughter nucleus is the same as in the parent cell. Though mitosis is a continuous process, one step merging imperceptibly into the next, it can be divided into stages for ease of description. These stages are known as interphase, prophase, metaphase, anaphase and telophase (Fig. 1.6).

Interphase. This is the resting stage between nuclear divisions when the chromosomes are loosely coiled and difficult to visualise. By the end of interphase each chromosome has divided longitudinally into two daughter chromosomes, or *chromatids*, which remain attached to each other at the centromere.

Prophase. In this phase the chromosomes take up stains more readily and therefore become easier to visualise. By the end of prophase the nucleoli are no longer visible and each chromatid is a tightly coiled structure which is closely aligned to its partner.

Metaphase. This begins with the disappearance of the nuclear membrane and the formation of the spindle apparatus, which consists of a number of minute 'threads' which run from one pole (centriole) of the spindle to the other. The chromosomes become orientated around the centre of the cell in the equatorial plane. Each chromosome is attached to the spindle by

means of its centromere. The spindle is responsible for the movement of the chromosomes during mitosis.

Anaphase. During this phase the centromere of each chromosome divides into two, each half 'repels' the other and the chromatids move apart towards opposite poles of the spindle. When the chromatids reach the poles they form two separate but identical groups.

Telophase. This begins as the daughter chromosomes arrive at the poles of the spindle. The two groups of chromosomes become surrounded by a new nuclear

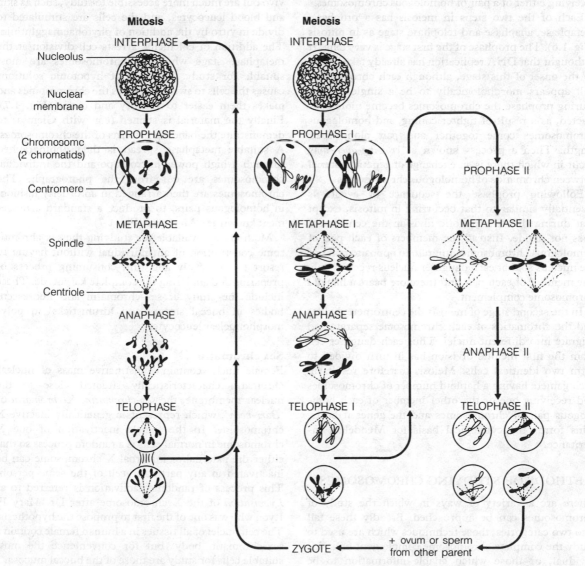

Fig. 1.6   Stages of mitosis and meiosis.

membrane and gradually become less visible. Cell division is completed by cleavage of the cytoplasm. New cell membranes develop and the nuclei of the two daughter cells re-enter the interphase stage. Thus at the end of mitosis a cell has divided into two daughter cells with an identical genetic constitution.

MEIOSIS

The process by which the chromosome number is halved during gametogenesis is known as meiosis. Although meiosis involves two division stages, the chromosomes divide only once, each gamete normally receiving either of a pair of homologous chromosomes.

Each of the two steps in meiosis has a prophase, metaphase, anaphase and telophase stage as in mitosis (Fig. 1.6). The prophase of the first stage is very long. It is thought that DNA replication has already taken place by the onset of this stage, although each chromosome still appears morphologically to be a single thread. During prophase the chromosomes become more contracted, as a result of tighter coiling, and homologous chromosomes come together and pair along their length. Then a process known as *crossing-over* may occur in which there is an exchange of genetic material between chromatids of homologous chromosomes.

Following prophase the sequence of events is essentially similar to that occurring in mitosis, except that during this first meiotic division the centromere does not divide. Instead the members of each pair of homologous chromosomes migrate to opposite poles of the nucleus so that each daughter nucleus receives only one member of each pair and therefore bears a haploid chromosome complement.

In the second stage of meiosis the centromere divides and the chromatids of each chromosome separate and migrate into different nuclei. Thus each daughter cell from the first meiotic division has in turn divided to form two identical cells. Meiosis therefore results in each gamete having a haploid number of chromosomes and receiving one or the other member of each homologous pair of chromosomes and the genes it bears. This forms the cytological basis for Mendelian inheritance.

METHODS OF STUDYING CHROMOSOMES

There are a variety of ways in which the study of chromosomes can be approached. Broadly these fall into two categories: those techniques which are used to study the complete chromosome complement of an individual, or those which enable information to be gained about the sex chromosome constitution of a person without having to do a complete chromosome analysis.

Since it is only during critical stages of the mitotic or meiotic cycle that the chromosomes are in a suitable state to study, chromosome analysis requires the provision of a large number of cells which are actively dividing. Meiotic studies can of course be done only on specimens of tissue obtained from the gonads. Mitotic studies, on the other hand, can be made on a variety of different and more easily available tissues, e.g. directly from cells which are rapidly dividing in vivo, as in bone marrow. More commonly, however, specimens are obtained from tissues which are not rapidly dividing in vivo but are much more accessible to study, such as skin and blood leucocytes, and the cells are stimulated to divide in vitro by the addition of phytohaemagglutinin. The addition of colchicine arrests cell division at the metaphase stage when the chromosomes are most suitable for study. The use of hypotonic solutions causes the cells to swell, disperses the chromosomes and makes them easier to identify and count (Fig. 1.7). Finally the material is stained (e.g. with Giemsa) to demonstrate the banding patterns of the chromosomes. A suitable metaphase spread is then photographed through a high power microscope and the individual chromosomes are cut from the photograph. The chromosomes are then arranged in an orderly fashion, in homologous pairs, to produce a standard arrangement known as a *karyotype* (Fig. 1.7).

Methods are available for studying the sex chromosome constitution of an individual without having to resort to the costly and time-consuming process of preparing and analysing the complete karyotype. These include the study of sex-chromatin and fluorescent bodies in buccal smears and 'drumsticks' in polymorphonuclear leucocytes.

Sex chromatin

Female nuclei contain a distinctive mass of nuclear chromatin characteristically situated close to the nuclear membrane, the *sex-chromatin, X-chromatin* or '*Barr-body*', which represents a genetically inactive X chromosome. In the female inactivation of one X chromosome in normal cells is a random process so that either the paternal or maternal X chromosome can be inactivated in any particular cell of the same person. This process of random inactivation is referred to as *Lyonisation* of the X chromosome after Dr. Mary F. Lyon who was one of the first to propose the hypothesis. The cell nuclei of all tissues in a human female contain a sex-chromatin body, but for convenience the most suitable cells for study are those of the buccal mucosa.

The inside of the cheek is gently scraped with a

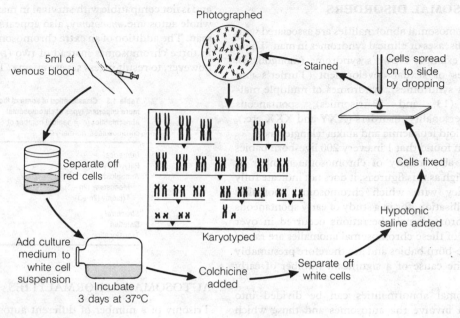

Fig. 1.7 Preparation of a karyotype.

spatula and the cells obtained spread onto a glass slide (*buccal smear*). These cells are then fixed and stained and can be examined for the presence of sex-chromatin bodies which are seen in 30 to 60% of nuclei of a normal female. Since only one X chromosome is active per cell, then the number of sex-chromatin bodies (inactivated X chromosomes) is one less than the total number of X chromosomes (Table 1.2).

Table 1.2 Incidence of sex chromatin bodies

Karyotype		Number of sex chromatin bodies
XX	Normal female	1
XY	Normal male	0
XO	Turner's syndrome	0
XXY	Klinefelter's syndrome	1
XXXY	Klinefelter's syndrome	2

In suitably stained smears of peripheral blood about 3% of the polymorphonuclear leucocytes of females show a small accessory nuclear lobule, which resembles a drumstick and projects from the main mass of the nuclear lobes. This is not seen in polymorphs from normal males, or females with an XO sex-chromosome constitution. The number of drumsticks is not, however, related to the number of X chromosomes.

Interphase nuclei of cells from males exhibit a fluorescent spot called the *F body* (or Y chromatin); the number of F bodies represents the number of Y chromo-somes. The technique can be adapted for use with buccal smears and so provides a method of assessing the number of Y chromosomes comparable with the sex-chromatin method of studying X chromosomes.

It can be seen, therefore, that these techniques are complementary and by combining them the sex chromosome constitution of an individual can be determined with ease, speed and accuracy. This is extremely useful clinically in the investigation of patients with abnormalities of sexual development or infertility, or for use in large-scale population surveys.

CHROMOSOME NOMENCLATURE

A shorthand notation is used to describe a karyotype in the simplest way. This consists first of the total number of chromosomes (in numerals), followed by the sex chromosome constitution, and finally by any abnor-malities that are present. Thus a normal male is 46,XY; a normal female is 46,XX. A girl with Turner's syndrome may be 45,XO and a boy with Klinefelter's syndrome, 47,XXY. The short and long arms of any chromosome are designated 'p' and 'q' respectively. A (+) or (−) sign is placed before an appropriate symbol where it means an additional or missing whole chromo-some, but after a symbol when it refers only to part of a chromosome. Thus a boy with Down's syndrome is 47,XY,+21 and a boy with part of the short arm of chromosome 5 missing is 46,XY,5p−.

CHROMOSOMAL DISORDERS

Specific chromosomal abnormalities are associated with recognised diseases or clinical syndromes in man. These include for example Down's syndrome (mongolism), abnormalities of sexual development (Turner's and Klinefelter's syndromes), syndromes of multiple malformations (13- and 18-trisomies), spontaneous abortions, personality disorders (XXY and XXX etc.), chronic myeloid leukaemia and ataxia telangiectasia.

It has been found that 1 in every 200 live-born babies has a gross abnormality of chromosome number or structure. High as this figure is, it does not indicate fully the frequency with which chromosomal anomalies occur at fertilisation, for in a study of early spontaneous abortions chromosomal aberrations occurred in over 50%. Many of these chromosomal anomalies are rarely found in live-born babies and are therefore presumably lethal and the cause of a significant number of early abortions.

Chromosomal abnormalities can be divided into those which involve the autosomes and those which involve the sex chromosomes. These can be further divided into abnormalities of number and of structure. Numerical abnormalities arise when one or more chromosomes are either lost or gained, a phenomenon referred to as *aneuploidy*. When a whole set of chromosomes is gained the phenomenon is known as *polyploidy*

and is not compatible with survival in man. The loss of a whole autosome, *monosomy*, also appears to be lethal in man. The addition of an extra chromosome, so resulting in three chromosomes instead of two (*trisomy*), seems, however, to result in less severe effects (Table 1.3).

Table 1.3   Classification of some of the more important types of chromosomal abnormalities (n = haploid number of chromosomes, normally 23)

Numerical
Polyploidy (3n, 4n . . .)
Aneuploidy
    Monosomy (2n − 1)
    Trisomy (2n + 1)

Structural
Deletion
Translocation

AUTOSOMAL ABNORMALITIES

Trisomy of a number of different autosomes has now been reported in man; the most common is trisomy-21 which results in Down's syndrome (Fig. 1.8). The two other well-recognised syndromes (trisomy-13 and trisomy-18) occur far less frequently than Down's syndrome. They are both more severe in effect and usually result in death within the infant period.

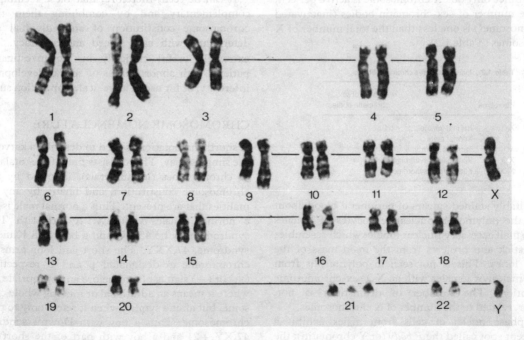

Fig. 1.8   Karyotype of a boy with Down's syndrome (trisomy 21).

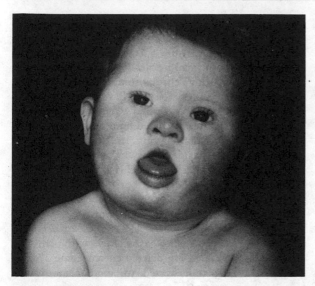

Fig. 1.9   Down's syndrome.

Down's syndrome

This occurs in about 1 in 700 live-births and is characterised by a flat face with widely spaced and upward
slanting eyes, epicanthic folds, brachycephaly, mal-
formed ears, broad and/or short neck, and a single,
transverse palmar crease (Fig. 1.9). Patients with
Down's syndrome are invariably mentally retarded, but
have a pleasant, quiet personality and show a great
fondness for music. The condition is also associated
with an increased frequency of both congenital heart
disease, and acute leukaemia. Although the mortality
rate of these patients is high within the first year of life,
many now survive into adulthood and there are several
reports of women with Down's syndrome having
children; on average half their offspring are normal and
half have Down's syndrome.

Cytogenetics of Down's syndrome. About 95%
of cases of Down's syndrome are due to regular
trisomy-21 which arises as a result of non-disjunction
during meiosis. Normally during meiosis the two
homologous chromosomes of any pair separate and pass
into different gametes. Occasionally an accident occurs
and the chromosomes fail to separate, both members of
the pair passing into the same gamete. If such a gamete
is then fertilised by a normal gamete the resulting
zygote will possess an additional chromosome.

All the trisomy syndromes are found to have a significant relationship to maternal age, the frequency of
trisomic births increasing with increasing maternal age.
It is thought that perhaps some effect of ageing in the
ova of older mothers makes them more prone to non-
disjunction. There have been reports, however, of

trisomy-21 recurring in some families, which suggests
that the phenomenon of non-disjunction may be under
genetic control at least in these rare families.

About 1% of cases of Down's syndrome are *mosaics*,
that is, they possess two different cell lines, one of which
has a normal chromosome constitution, the other an
extra chromosome 21. This arises as a result of non-
disjunction occurring at or after the first zygotic
division and is very rarely inherited. The clinical
picture may often be considerably modified in some of
these cases.

About 4% of cases of Down's syndrome result from a
phenomenon known as *translocation*, in which there is
an exchange of segments between different chromosomes (Fig. 1.10). The mechanism is thought to be that
two chromosomes lying close to one another suffer
simultaneous breaks followed by an exchange of
chromosomal material. For example, in Down's
syndrome a large part of chromosome 21 may be united
with part of chromosome 14. A carrier of such a translocation (who has only 45 chromosomes) produces four
types of gametes. A gamete may contain a normal
chromosome 14 and a normal chromosome 21, in which
case the resulting offspring will be normal. Or a gamete

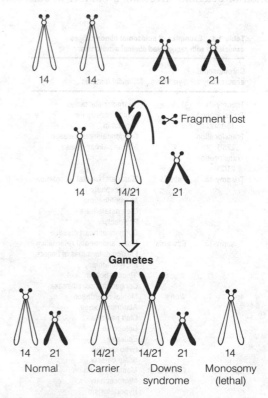

Fig. 1.10   Translocation mechanism in Down's syndrome.

may contain a translocation (14/21), in which case the resulting offspring will have only 45 chromosomes and will be a carrier like the parent. Or a gamete may contain the translocation and a normal chromosome 21, in which case the offspring will have 46 chromosomes but in effect will be trisomic for chromosome 21 and will therefore have Down's syndrome. Finally a gamete may contain a chromosome 14 but no chromosome 21; this would produce a zygote monosomic for chromosome 21 which is lethal and would presumably result in an abortion. Theoretically, therefore, a carrier of such a translocation has a 1 in 3 chance of having a child with Down's syndrome, but for reasons which are not clear, the actual risk is much less. In Down's syndrome the translocation usually involves an exchange of material between chromosomes 13, 14 or 15 and chromosome 21. Rarely there may be an exchange between chromosomes 21 and 22 or even between two 21s. In the case of a parent who carries a translocation involving two 21s, all the offspring will have Down's syndrome.

Other autosomal abnormalities

Deletions arise when a segment of a chromosome has been lost. New techniques have led to the demonstration of deletions involving a number of autosomes

Table 1.4   Examples of autosomal abnormalities associated with recognised clinical syndromes

Chromosome abnormality	Syndrome	Clinical features
Trisomy-21	Down's	Characteristic facies
Translocation 13-15/21		Mental retardation
		Hypotonia
Translocation 22/21		Congenital heart disease
		Simian palmar crease
Translocation 21/21		
Trisomy-13	Patau's	Motor and mental retardation
		Microcephaly
		Microphthalmia
		Cleft palate/hare lip
		Polydactyly
		Congenital heart disease
Trisomy-18	Edwards'	Motor and mental retardation
		Flexion deformities of fingers
		Micrognathia
		'Rocker-bottom' feet
		Congenital heart disease
4p-	Wolf's	Mental retardation
		Abnormal facies
		Cleft palate
		Coloboma
		Epilepsy
		Hypospadias
		Scalp defects
5p-	Cri du chat	Mental retardation
		Microcephaly
		Hypertelorism
		Characteristic cry

and an increasing number of these are being associated with clinically recognisable syndromes, examples of which are given in Table 1.4. Other rarer forms of chromosomal abnormalities are *ring chromosomes* and *isochromosomes*. Ring chromosomes involving both autosomes and sex chromosomes have been described; they are thought to be formed when two ends of a chromosome have been deleted and the broken (more 'sticky') ends fuse to form a ring. In effect ring chromosomes are manifest as deletions and in shorthand they are represented as an 'r'. An isochromosome is formed when the centromere divides horizontally instead of longitudinally resulting in a chromosome consisting of either two long arms or of two short arms.

The *Philadelphia chromosome* (Ph^1) is an *acquired* chromosomal abnormality associated with chronic myeloid leukaemia. It is a deleted chromosome 22, the long arm being translocated to another autosome, usually chromosome 9.

SEX CHROMOSOME ABNORMALITIES

Numerical abnormalities of the sex chromosomes are more common than with the autosomes, and in general they produce less severe effects. They are brought about by the same phenomenon of non-disjunction. As with the autosomes, abnormalities of structure also occur although they are far less common than the numerical anomalies.

Klinefelter's syndrome

This was the first sex chromosome aneuploidy to be demonstrated in man. Affected males have an extra X chromosome resulting in an XXY sex chromosome constitution or as many as four X chromosomes may be present; an extra Y chromosome may also be present on occasions resulting in an XXYY sex chromosome constitution. The main clinical features are eunuchoid body proportions (Fig. 1.11), sterility (due to azoospermia), hypogonadism, gynaecomastia and often mental retardation.

There appears to be a relationship between mental retardation and the number of X chromosomes in both males and females. In Klinefelter's syndrome all individuals with an XXXY sex chromosome constitution are mentally retarded, whereas this is so in only about one-quarter of those with XXY sex chromosome constitution. Like the autosomal trisomies, Klinefelter's syndrome is found to occur more frequently in the sons of older mothers.

The XYY constitution

This is another sex chromosome aneuploidy in the

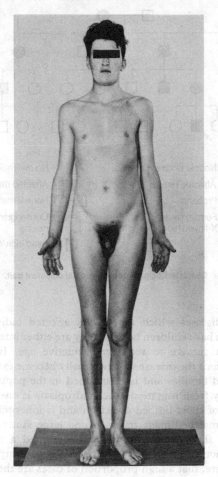

Fig. 1.11 Klinefelter's syndrome.

CLINICAL FEATURES OF KLINEFELTER'S AND TURNER'S SYNDROMES

Klinefelter's Syndrome
Sterility
Small testes
Eunuchoid body proportions
Gynaecomastia
Mental retardation

Turner's Syndrome
Primary amenorrhoea
Sterility
Lack of secondary sexual characteristics
Short stature
Various congenital abnormalities (note coarctation of the aorta)
(See Fig. 1.12)

The main clinical features of Klinefelter's and Turner's syndromes are listed in the information box above. Although, overall, patients with Turner's syndrome have a significantly lower IQ than normal, marked retardation is uncommon and the discrepancy is mainly in the performance aspect of their IQ.

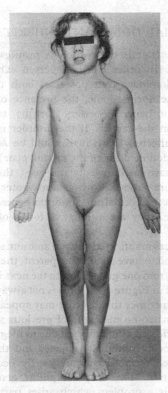

Fig. 1.12 Turner's syndrome; note the increased carrying angle at the elbows and webbing of the neck.

male. Such men are reported to occur with increased frequency amongst inmates of institutions for the mentally retarded with criminal tendencies. It has been shown by various surveys that between 2 and 5% of such populations may be XYY. However, the exact relationship of this chromosomal anomaly with either mental retardation or criminal tendencies is uncertain especially as XYY individuals have been found amongst the normal general population.

Turner's syndrome
This was the first sex chromosome aneuploidy to be described in females. An XO sex chromosome constitution is the commonest abnormality and also arises by non-disjunction, but unlike Klinefelter's syndrome, Turner's syndrome does not show a relationship with maternal age. Turner's syndrome may also result from isochromosomes, deletions, and rings involving the X chromosome.

Females have also been described with three or even four X chromosomes (XXX, XXXX); they may occasionally be mentally subnormal or have psychiatric disorders, but in all other respects appear to be healthy. Usually children born to XXX females are normal.

UNIFACTORIAL INHERITANCE

These disorders are due to defects of a single gene, i.e. to a primary error in the DNA code. They are inherited in a simple fashion, following Mendelian laws. The risk of their recurring in a family may therefore be accurately predicted on theoretical grounds making genetic counselling more straightforward.

These disorders may be subdivided according to the chromosome on which the abnormal (or mutant) gene is situated and also by the nature of the trait itself. Thus a trait which is determined by a gene situated on an autosome is said to be inherited as an *autosomal* trait, and this may be either *dominant* or *recessive*. A trait determined by a gene situated on one of the sex chromosomes is said to be *sex-linked* and may also be either dominant or recessive.

AUTOSOMAL DOMINANT INHERITANCE

A dominant trait is one which is manifested in the *heterozygote*. In other words a person exhibiting an autosomal dominant trait possesses both the mutant gene and the normal gene, the presence of only one mutant gene being necessary for the trait to be manifested in the carrier. If the disorder is common, then some affected individuals could be *homozygotes* (i.e. have a 'double dose' of the mutant gene), but if the disorder is rare (as is usually the case), then affected individuals are almost always heterozygotes. It should be noted that the normal and abnormal genes are known as *alleles*, i.e. they are alternative forms of the same gene.

Usually persons affected with an autosomal dominant trait are found to have an affected parent, the trait being transmitted from one generation to the next in a family, as illustrated in Figure 1.13. This is not always the case, however; sometimes the disorder may appear suddenly in a family when no members of previous generations have been affected. This may be due to illegitimacy, to one parent being minimally affected and the disorder not recognised, or more commonly to the occurrence of a new mutation. This may complicate genetic counselling and is a problem which arises particularly in conditions inherited in a dominant fashion.

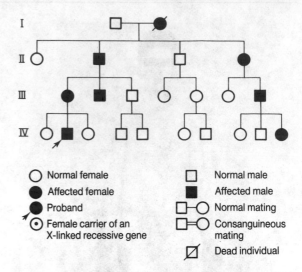

Fig. 1.13   Characteristic pedigree: autosomal dominant trait.

In diseases which are severe, affected individuals seldom have children because they are either infertile or do not survive to reach reproductive age. In such conditions the disease will eventually become extinct in affected families and is maintained in the populations only by fresh mutations. Achondroplasia is one of the forms of short-limbed dwarfism and is inherited as an autosomal dominant trait. In one large study it was shown that affected individuals exhibited a marked reduction in reproductive fitness. It is not surprising, therefore, that a high proportion of cases are the result of new mutations.

In conditions which do not have much effect on survival it is often possible to trace the conditions through many generations of a family. Such a condition is the adult form of polycystic disease of the kidneys. Although affected individuals may eventually die from chronic renal failure, they often show no symptoms or signs of the disease until early middle life when they have already had their family and run the risk of transmitting the trait to their children.

In autosomal dominant conditions, if an affected individual marries a normal person, then on average half their children will be similarly affected. This arises because the affected individual produces gametes, half of which contain the normal gene and the other half contain the mutant gene. The normal partner produces gametes all of which contain the normal gene. Thus at fertilisation the normal partner's gametes have an equal chance of uniting with a gamete carrying either a normal (a) or abnormal (A) gene with the result that at conception there is a 1 in 2 chance of producing an

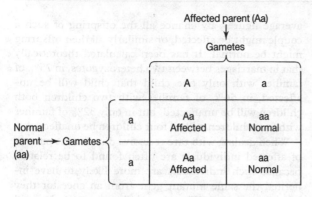

Fig. 1.14 Possible gametic combinations when one parent is normal (aa) and the other heterozygous (Aa) for a dominant gene (A).

affected individual. Because of the smaller size of modern families, by chance all the children of an affected individual may be normal, or similarly by chance again all his children may be affected. It is on average that half the offspring of an affected individual will be affected (Fig. 1.14).

Some autosomal dominant traits are extremely variable in severity, this variability in clinical manifestation being referred to as *expressivity*. Osteogenesis imperfecta, for example, is an autosomal dominant condition in which affected individuals may have only blue sclerae, whereas others may exhibit the full syndrome of blue sclerae, deafness and multiple fractures.

Penetrance

Occasionally an individual may carry a mutant gene and yet not exhibit any of its effects; the gene is then said to be non-penetrant, *penetrance* being the probability that an individual with the genetic predisposition will express clinical disease. This phenomenon explains situations where dominant mutant traits appear to have 'skipped' generations in certain families. This variation in expression of a mutant gene results both from the modifying influence of other genes and from environmental factors. The degree of penetrance of a gene is that proportion of heterozygotes who express the gene in any degree, however mild. For a gene to be *fully penetrant* its effects must be manifest to some degree in all individuals who carry the gene.

The phenomenon of varying penetrance can give rise to problems when estimating recurrence risks in order to give genetic advice. For example, tuberous sclerosis (epiloia) is inherited as a dominant trait but is not always penetrant. This condition is characterised by adenoma sebaceum (small papules over the cheeks and nose), epilepsy and mental retardation of varying

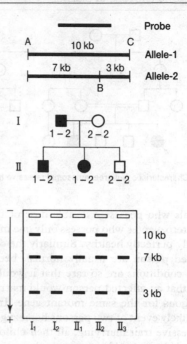

Fig. 1.15 Diagrammatic representation of an autosomal RFLP (above), its inheritance within a family in which 3 members are affected with an autosomal dominant disorder (middle), and the appearance of the resultant DNA fragments on a Southern blot (below).

severity. Some individuals carrying the gene may be so mildly affected as to pass as normal and so produce an apparently 'skipped' generation. However, it is unusual to find a proven carrier (e.g. with an affected child and an affected parent) who does not show at least some evidence of the disease, such as a few typical papules on the face.

The use of linked restriction fragment length polymorphisms (RFLPs) is important in detecting autosomal disorders before symptoms and signs are evident, and in antenatal diagnosis. For example in Figure 1.15 there is an RFLP at site B such that there is no recognition site on one chromosome (allele-1) but one is present on the homologous chromosome at site B (allele-2). The father and two of his children are affected and the disease in the family is co-inherited with allele-1 (10 kilobase (kb) fragment, 1 kb = 1000 base pairs). Any subsequent child which inherits allele-1 from father will thus also inherit the disease gene.

AUTOSOMAL RECESSIVE INHERITANCE

Autosomal recessive traits also affect both males and females. Unlike dominant traits, recessive traits are manifest only in the homozygous state, that is, in those

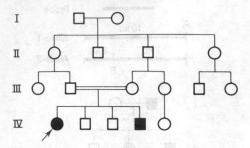

Fig. 1.16   Characteristic pedigree: autosomal recessive trait.

individuals who possess a double dose of the mutant gene. Heterozygotes who possess only one mutant gene are usually perfectly healthy. Similarly the offspring of an affected person are usually normal, because most recessive conditions are so rare that it would be most unlikely that an affected person would marry a person heterozygous for the same mutant gene. In the even more unlikely event of two persons homozygous for the same recessive trait marrying, all their children would be affected. In general, however, both parents and offspring of a person homozygous for a rare recessive gene will be healthy. Characteristically in recessive traits, affected individuals cannot be traced from one generation to the next and if more than one member of a family is affected they are usually sibs, i.e. brothers and sisters. The pedigree of an autosomal recessive trait (Fig. 1.16), therefore, differs from that of a dominant trait.

At conception there is a 1 in 4 chance that any child of two heterozygous parents will be affected. Each parent produces gametes of two types, one bearing the normal gene (A) and the other bearing the mutant gene (a). At conception, therefore, one-quarter of the offspring will be normal, one-half will be healthy heterozygotes and one-quarter will be affected (Fig. 1.17). These are average figures; by chance all the offspring of such a couple might be affected, or similarly all their offspring might be normal. It has been calculated theoretically that in marriages between two heterozygotes, in 75% of families with only one child that child will be unaffected, in 56% of families with two children both children will be unaffected, but in only 32% of families with four children will all four children be unaffected.

When dealing with rare recessive diseases the parents of affected individuals are often found to be related, because such individuals are more likely to have inherited the same mutant gene from an ancestor they have in common. The chance that first cousins will carry the same recessive gene is 1 in 8, but the chance that two unrelated individuals will carry the same recessive gene is very much lower and depends on the frequency of the particular gene in the population. In general the rarer the gene the greater the frequency of consanguinity amongst the parents of affected individuals.

At present roughly 1 in 200 marriages in Britain is between first cousins, so that giving advice on the genetic consequences of cousin marriages is a problem with which geneticists are frequently faced. Several extensive studies have shown that among the offspring of consanguineous matings there is an increased perinatal mortality rate together with an increased frequency of both congenital abnormalities and mental retardation, but the actual risks are small and in fact only slightly greater than in the general population. The situation is quite different, however, if there is a family history of a recessive disorder, when the risks will be greatly increased.

Many conditions show an autosomal recessive mode of inheritance and include, for example, many inborn errors of metabolism, some types of deaf-mutism and some types of congenital blindness. The commonest autosomal recessive trait known in Western Europe is cystic fibrosis which affects one in every 2000 births.

SEX-LINKED INHERITANCE

Conditions determined by genes situated on either of the sex chromosomes are said to be inherited as sex-linked traits. Genes carried on the X chromosome are said to be X-linked, those on the Y chromosomes being Y-linked. Y-linkage of a gene implies that only males would be affected and that all the sons of an affected male would inherit the gene. There are no proven examples of Y-linked single gene disorders in man. Thus all known sex-linked conditions are due to genes on the X chromosome. As with autosomal traits these conditions may be either dominant or recessive.

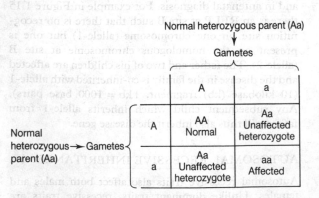

Fig. 1.17   Possible gametic combinations when both parents are heterozygous (Aa) for a recessive gene (a).

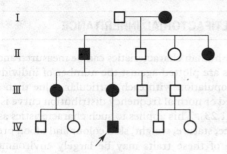

Fig. 1.18 Characteristic pedigree: X-linked dominant trait.

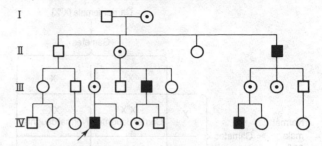

Fig. 1.20 Characteristic pedigree: X-linked recessive trait – when affected males do reproduce (e.g. haemophilia).

X-linked dominant conditions

These are manifest both in females who are heterozygous for the mutant gene and in males who carry the mutant gene on their single X chromosome. The pedigree of an X-linked dominant trait (Fig. 1.18) can superficially resemble that of an autosomal dominant trait, but there is fundamental difference. Although an affected female will transmit the trait to half her offspring of either sex, an affected male will transmit the trait to all of his daughters but to none of his sons. There will therefore be an excess of affected females in families exhibiting such conditions. There are few X-linked dominant disorders but a notable example is one form of vitamin D resistant rickets.

X-linked recessive conditions

These are caused by genes carried on the X chromosome and are manifest in females only when the gene is in the homozygous state. In males, a mutant gene present on the single X chromosome is always manifest because it is unopposed by the modifying effect of a normal gene on the second X chromosome, as happens in females. As with autosomal recessive conditions, the heterozygous carrier is usually healthy. Conditions inherited in this way therefore predominantly affect males and are transmitted by healthy female carriers (Fig. 1.19). In those conditions where affected males may

survive to have children, the condition will also be transmitted by affected males (Fig. 1.20).

Haemophilia is the best known example of an X-linked recessive trait. Whereas in the past most boys with this disease died at an early age, with improvements in treatment most now survive. If an affected man (X^hY) marries a normal woman, then all his daughters will be carriers but none of his sons will be affected. An X-linked trait is never transmitted from father to son. This is because a man transmits his only X chromosome (which if he is affected bears the mutant gene) to each of his daughters but his Y chromosome to each of his sons (Fig. 1.21).

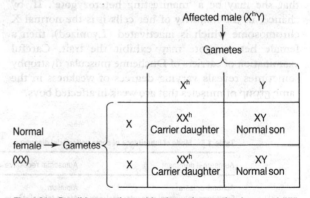

Fig. 1.21 Possible gametic combinations when mother is normal (XX) but father is affected by an X-linked recessive gene, in this case haemophilia (X^hY).

If a woman carrying an X-linked recessive trait (X^hX) marries a normal man, then half of her sons will be affected and half of her daughters will be carriers because each of her children has an equal chance of inheriting from her either the normal X chromosome or the one bearing the mutant gene (Fig. 1.22).

Duchenne muscular dystrophy is inherited as an X-linked recessive trait and because affected boys die young, it is transmitted solely by healthy female carriers.

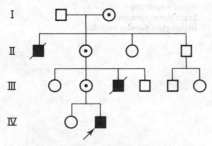

Fig. 1.19 Characteristic pedigree: X-linked recessive trait – when affected males do not reproduce (e.g. Duchenne muscular dystrophy).

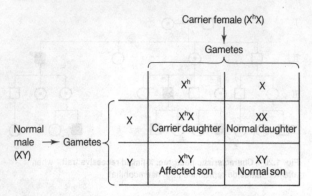

Fig. 1.22   Possible gametic combinations when father is normal (XY) but mother is a heterozygous carrier for an X-linked recessive gene, in this case haemophilia (XʰX).

Very rarely a female may exhibit an X-linked recessive trait. This situation may arise in several different ways. Firstly, she may have an abnormal chromosomal constitution resulting in her having only one X chromosome, such as in Turner's syndrome (XO). Secondly, she may be homozygous for the mutant gene, but this is very unlikely with rare recessive disorders because she would have to have inherited the disorder from both her parents. The third possibility is that she may be a 'manifesting heterozygote'. If, by chance, in the majority of her cells it is the normal X chromosome which is inactivated (Lyonized), then a female heterozygote may exhibit the trait. Careful examination of carriers of Duchenne muscular dystrophy sometimes reveals varying degrees of weakness in the same group of muscles that are weak in affected boys.

MULTIFACTORIAL INHERITANCE

Many human characteristics can be measured and if the values are plotted against the number of individuals in the population with each particular value then a bell-shaped or normal frequency distribution curve is found (Fig. 1.23). This applies to such characteristics as intelligence, stature, weight, skin colour and blood pressure. Some of these traits may be largely environmentally determined, whereas others are largely genetically determined, such as stature and intelligence. In each case many genes are probably involved. Characteristics which are due to many genes plus the effects of environment are said to be inherited on a multifactorial basis.

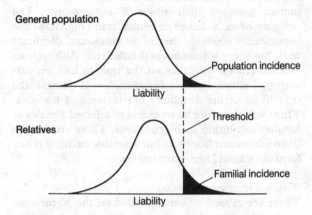

Fig. 1.23   Liability. Hypothetical curve of liability in the general population and in relatives for a hereditary disorder in which the genetic predisposition is multifactorial.

Table 1.5   Mode of inheritance of some unifactorial disorders

Autosomal dominant	Autosomal recessive	X-linked recessive
Achondroplasia	Albinism	Christmas disease
Facioscapulohumeral muscular dystrophy	Ataxia telangiectasia	Duchenne muscular dystrophy
Gilbert's syndrome	Congenital adrenal hyperplasia	Glucose-6-phosphate dehydrogenase deficiency
Hereditary spherocytosis	Congenital goitrous cretinism	Haemophilia
Huntington's chorea	Crigler-Najjar syndrome	Hunter's syndrome
Hyperlipoproteinaemia Type II	Cystic fibrosis	Lesch-Nyhan syndrome
Marfan's syndrome	Dubin-Johnson syndrome	Nephrogenic diabetes insipidus
Myotonic dystrophy	Fanconi's syndrome	
Neurofibromatosis	Friedrich's ataxia	
Osteogenesis imperfecta	Galactosaemia	
Polycystic disease of kidneys (adult form)	Gaucher's disease	
Polyposis of colon	Glycogen storage diseases	
Porphyria, acute intermittent	Hurler's syndrome	
Tuberous sclerosis	Limb girdle muscular dystrophy (Erb)	
von Willebrand's disease	Niemann-Pick disease	
	Phenylketonuria	
	Pendred's syndrome	
	Tay-Sachs disease	
	Wilson's disease	

It is now believed that many common disorders are inherited in this way. In such conditions it is assumed that there is some underlying graded attribute which is related to causation. This is referred to as the individuals' *liability*, which includes not only their genetic predisposition but also the environmental factors which render them more or less likely to develop the disease. It is assumed that the curve of liability has a normal distribution in the general population.

Threshold model

In one simple model (Fig. 1.23), it is believed that there is a *threshold* value such that all affected individuals have a liability above this value and all unaffected individuals have a liability below this value. Relatives of affected individuals have a higher average liability than the population average so the curve of liability for relatives is shifted to the right. In the general population the proportion above the threshold is the population incidence and among relatives the proportion above the threshold is the familial incidence. Such a model can be used to explain the familial incidence of such disorders as essential hypertension, coronary artery disease, peptic ulceration and many of the commoner congenital malformations.

There are several consequences of such a model. Familial incidence will be greater among the relatives of more severely affected individuals because presumably they are more extreme deviants along the curve of liability and the number of abnormal genes segregating in such families is greater than in families in which individuals are less severely affected. Thus in hare lip with or without cleft palate the proportion of affected sibs and children is roughly 6% when the index patient has double hare lip and cleft palate, but only 2.5% if the index patient has a single hare lip. By similar reasoning it would be expected that the incidence among sibs born subsequent to the index patient would be greater the more affected relatives there were in the family. In spina bifida, for example, the incidence of this condition, or the related disorder anencephaly, in sibs born after one affected child is roughly 5%, but the incidence rises to 10% after the birth of two affected children. This is quite different from the situation in unifactorial disorders where the risk to subsequent sibs remains constant irrespective of the number of affected individuals in the family (e.g. 1 in 4 for an autosomal recessive trait). Finally as a consequence of this model it might be expected that when there is a sex difference in the population incidence, the relatives of the less frequently affected sex would be more often affected. The reason for this is that in the less frequently affected sex, when individuals are affected they are presumably more

extreme deviants along the curve of liability and possess more abnormal genes. Thus in congenital pyloric stenosis, which is 5 times commoner in boys than girls, the proportions of affected relatives of male index patients are roughly 5.5% for sons and 2.4% for daughters, but 19.4% for sons and 7.3% for daughters when the index patient is a female.

Heritability

Though it is not possible to measure liability to a particular disease it is possible to estimate how much of the aetiology can be ascribed to genetic factors as opposed to environmental factors. This is referred to as the *heritability* which is calculated from the known incidences of the disorder in the general population and in relatives. Some estimates of heritability are given in Table 1.6. The values, though approximate, do indicate that genetic factors are of more importance in aetiology in asthma and schizophrenia than in, for example, peptic ulcer

Table 1.6   Estimates for heritability for various multifactorial disorders

Disorder	Incidence (%)	Heritability (%)
Schizophrenia	1	85
Asthma	4	80
Cleft lip ± cleft palate	0.1	76
Pyloric stenosis (congenital)	0.3	75
Ankylosing spondylitis	0.2	70
Club foot (congenital)	0.1	68
Coronary artery disease	3	65
Hypertension (essential)	5	62
Dislocation of hip (congenital)	0.1	60
Anencephaly and spina bifida	0.5	60
Peptic ulcer	4	37
Congenital heart disease (all types)	0.5	35

PREVENTION OF GENETIC DISEASE

Since there is at present no effective treatment for most genetic disorders the role of the medical practitioner lies mainly in the prevention of such conditions through genetic counselling. This involves providing advice on the chances of recurrence of a genetic disorder in the children of either healthy parents who already have an affected child, or when one of the parents or a near relative is affected with a disease which is known to be inherited.

Chromosomal disorders

If the parents with chromosomal disorders have normal karyotypes, i.e. do not carry a translocation which in the unbalanced state would cause abnormality, then the

Table 1.7   Recurrence risks of Down's syndrome (C = Carrier, N = Normal)

	Karyotypes		
	Father	Mother	Recurrence risk (%)
Translocation			
21/13-15	N	C	10–15
	C	N	5
21/22	N	C	10–15
	C	N	5
21/21	N	C	100
	C	N	100
Trisomy 21	N	N	1
Translocation or mosaic	N	N	1

chances of recurrence are usually low. The most important chromosomal disorder from this point of view is Down's syndrome. The risk of having a child with Down's syndrome is about 1 in 100 in women who have previously had an affected child, and at least 1 in 50 in women over the age of 40. However, the risks are higher if one of the parents carries a chromosome translocation (Table 1.7).

Unifactorial disorders

The chances of recurrence in unifactorial disorders are based on Mendelian principles. As we have seen, for example, for a fully penetrant autosomal dominant disorder there is a 1 in 2 chance of recurrence in any child of an affected parent. However, if both parents are healthy an affected child is most likely to be the result of a new mutation and the chances of recurrence in subsequent children are negligible. If parents have had a child with an autosomal recessive disorder the chance of recurrence in subsequent children is 1 in 4. Should such a child survive there is very little chance of its having affected children. Finally, with X-linked recessive disorders there is a 1 in 2 chance that any son of a known carrier will be affected and a 1 in 2 chance that any daughter will be a carrier. All the daughters of an affected male will be carriers.

Developments in recombinant DNA technology have led to the generation of gene specific probes and linked DNA markers which can now be used to detect pre-clinical cases of many autosomal dominant disorders (such as Huntington's chorea), and female carriers of X-linked disorders (such as haemophilia and Duchenne muscular dystrophy).

Multifactorial disorders

The risk of recurrence of multifactorial disorders cannot be predicted from Mendelian principles but has to be determined by studying the frequency of the condition among the relatives of affected individuals. Examples of risk figures, derived in this way (*empiric risks*), are given in Table 1.8.

GENETIC COUNSELLING

The procedure for giving genetic counselling is listed in the information box. Without a precise diagnosis it is not possible to give reliable genetic counselling since certain disorders though superficially similar may be inherited differently. For example Hunter's syndrome and Hurler's syndrome (Fig. 1.24) both present similar clinical features of 'gargoylism' but whereas clouding of

---

ESSENTIAL FEATURES OF GENETIC COUNSELLING

Establish
An accurate diagnosis
Mode of inheritance
Reliable pedigree

Recognise the psychological effects of the disorder on the family
Coping process

Consider the options available
Family limitation
Antenatal diagnosis, etc.

Table 1.8   Examples of empiric risks (in percent)

Disorder	Incidence	Sex ratio M:F	Normal parent having a second affected child	Affected parent having an affected child	Affected parent having a second affected child
Asthma	3–4	1:1	10	26	–
Congenital heart disease (all types)	0.50	1:1	1–4	1–4	10
Diabetes mellitus (juvenile, insulin-dependent)	0.20	1:1	6	1–2	–
Epilepsy ('idiopathic')	0.50	1:1	5	5	10
Manic-depressive psychosis	0.40	2:3	10–15	10–15	–
Mental retardation ('idiopathic')	0.30–0.50	1:1	3–5	10	20
Schizophrenia	1–2	1:1	10	16	–
Tracheo-oesophageal fistula	0.03	1:1	1	1	–

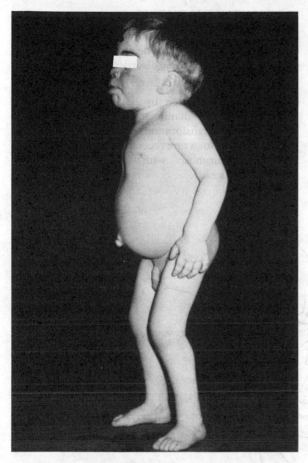

Fig. 1.24 Hurler's syndrome. The protuberant abdomen is due to enlargement of the liver and spleen.

the cornea does not occur in the former condition it is present in the latter. Further, Hunter's syndrome is an X-linked recessive trait and therefore the unaffected sister of an affected boy may be at risk of having affected children. Hurler's syndrome on the other hand is an autosomal recessive disorder and only affects sibs. In this latter condition there is therefore no chance of an unaffected sister having affected children, provided she does not marry a near relative who might also carry the mutant gene.

Phenocopies

It is always advisable to check that the disease in question is in fact genetic and not due to some environmental factor (i.e. a *phenocopy*). For example congenital deafness is often due to a rare recessive gene but it may also result from intrauterine infection with rubella during the first three months of pregnancy which may also cause abnormalities in the fetus such as congenital heart disease and eye defects. If it can be shown in a particular case that congenital deafness was due to maternal rubella then there would be no chance of recurrence in subsequent children. It is therefore important before giving genetic advice to ask about the possibility of maternal exposure to radiation, drugs or infections during pregnancy and details of any birth trauma which might possibly account for the disorder in question.

Decision making

Factors which influence the parents' decision whether or not they will accept a risk of having an affected child include the severity of the abnormality, whether or not there is an effective treatment, the actual risk, their religious attitude and possibly their socio-economic status. In general, however, parents usually accept the risk of having an affected child if this is less than 1 in 20 but do not accept a risk of greater than 1 in 10 if the disease is serious.

PSYCHOLOGICAL ASPECTS

It is very important to recognise the psychological effects serious genetic disease may have on the parents following the initial diagnosis in an affected child. The sequence of events is referred to as the *coping process* which is similar in other emotionally traumatic experiences such as bereavement. The five sequential stages involved are listed in the information box below.

THE COPING PROCESS

- Shock and denial
- Anger and guilt
- Anxiety
- Depression
- Homeostasis

Each stage requires that counselling should be tailored accordingly if it is to be at all effective and if the parents are going to be helped to make a rational decision. Thus at the beginning the parent may be unable to accept that the child is affected and at this stage sympathy and compassion are essential until acceptance occurs. Later hostility may develop against the counsellor himself and this requires tolerance and possibly temporary withdrawal until the resentment has tempered. Feelings of guilt and recrimination have to be dispelled. Anxiety impairs judgement and reason and here emotional support is required. At this stage information may have to be repeated on several occasions if it is to be fully understood and appreciated. It is probably at the stage of depression that genetic counselling can begin more earnestly and should not be postponed until homeostasis is reached. Finally the decision to accept or not the risks involved must be the individual's and not the counsellor's. Genetic counselling should never be directive.

In summary, genetic counselling must be based on an accurate diagnosis, it should be tailored according to the stage reached in the coping process, it should be compassionate and sympathetic yet truthful, and must be non-directive. Genetic counselling, like many other aspects of medicine, is as much an art as a science.

ANTENATAL DIAGNOSIS

Family limitation is not the only course of action open to parents who are found to be at high risk of having a child with a serious genetic disorder. Other possibilities include:

1. Artificial insemination by donor (if the father is affected with a dominant disorder or carries a chromosome translocation or if both parents are heterozygous for a rare recessive gene).
2. Antenatal diagnosis with selective abortion of affected fetuses.

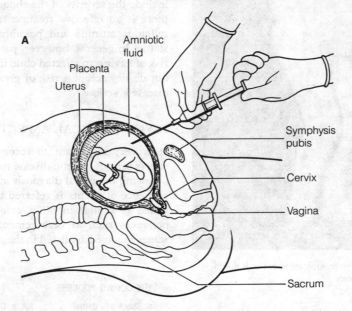

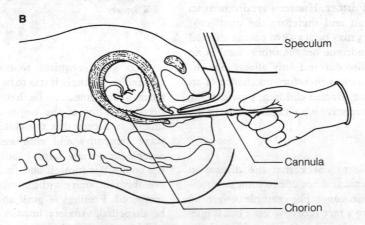

Fig. 1.25   Technique of A. transabdominal amniocentesis, and B. chorion biopsy. (From *An Introduction to Recombinant DNA* by A.E.H. Emery (1985) John Wiley Publishers, with permission.)

The second procedure is possible by studying cells present in amniotic fluid or the amniotic fluid itself. About 5–10 ml of fluid is removed by transabdominal amniocentesis around the 16th week of gestation. The specimen is centrifuged and the fluid can be used, for example, to measure the level of alpha-fetoprotein which is significantly raised in anencephaly and open spina bifida, disorders which can therefore be diagnosed in utero in this way. The contained cells are of fetal origin and can be cultured and used for biochemical, cytogenetic and DNA studies. Some 60 inborn errors of metabolism can be diagnosed from enzyme and other studies on cultured amniotic fluid cells. However the main application of such studies is in the cytogenetic diagnosis of Down's syndrome and many centres now offer amniocentesis to all pregnant women over the age of around 37 because of their increased risk of having a child with this disorder. DNA can also be extracted from the cultured cells and relevant disorders diagnosed prenatally either using gene specific probes or linked RFLPs.

Recently the technique of transcervical chorionic villus biopsy has been introduced and this tissue can also be used for biochemical, cytogenetic and DNA studies. The technique has the advantage that it can be carried out as early as 8–10 weeks' gestation and therefore if pregnancy termination is indicated this can be done earlier and is therefore less traumatic and more acceptable to most mothers (Fig. 1.25).

PREIMPLANTATION DIAGNOSIS

Recent studies indicate that preimplantation diagnosis of genetic disease is now technically possible and might one day provide an alternative to antenatal diagnosis. Here an ovulated egg is removed and artificially fertilised with the husband's sperm (in vitro fertilisation) and then cultured up to the 8-cell stage. A cell (blastomere) is carefully removed and a particular DNA sequence of interest amplified by the so-called polymerase chain reaction (PCR). This powerful and sensitive technique provides millions of copies of a specific DNA sequence or gene within a few hours. The resultant amplified DNA is then studied (using an appropriate gene probe) to see if the embryo carries a particular genetic disorder. If not, the blastula is implanted in the mother's uterus and pregnancy allowed to continue to term.

FURTHER READING

Emery A E H, Pullen I M 1984 Psychological aspects of genetic counselling. Academic Press, London & New York. Psychological problems involved in counselling and antenatal diagnosis and in various common disabilities.

Emery A E H 1985 An introduction to recombinant DNA. Wiley, Chichester. Basics of genetic engineering and its applications in medicine.

Emery A E H 1986 Methodology in medical genetics, 2nd Edn. Churchill Livingstone, Edinburgh. A textbook concerned with the more statistical aspects of medical genetics.

Emery A E H, Mueller R F 1988 Elements of medical genetics, 7th Edn. Churchill Livingstone, Edinburgh. An introductory textbook.

Emery A E H, Rimoin D 1990 Principles and practice of medical genetics, 2 vols, 2nd Edn. Churchill Livingstone, Edinburgh. A detailed and comprehensive textbook of medical genetics.

2

Immunological Factors in Disease

The science of immunology arose from the study of man's resistance to infection. It was appreciated that, after recovery from a particular infectious disease the same disease rarely occurred again. This altered reactivity is what we now call *specific immunity*. Immunology also encompasses a number of entirely *non-specific* antimicrobial protective mechanisms, innate in that they are not affected by prior contact with the infectious agent although their activity can be up and down regulated by a number of factors.

Resistance to infection is not an essential feature of immunity. Bacteria may induce antibodies which have no obvious protective value and immune responses are evoked by injection of intrinsically harmless non-living organic substances, such as serum protein from another individual or species.

A distinction must be made between the induction phase of immunity in which, at the first encounter with antigen, a pattern is established of altered reactivity, involving T and B cells and the production of antibody, and expression of one or more types of immune response upon subsequent re-encounter with the same antigen. Specific immune responses can also produce hypersensitivity, which has unpleasant and sometimes dangerous effects, upon subsequent exposure to the provoking antigen. There are also circumstances where antigen encounter leads to down-regulation of specific reactivity. This is called tolerance, and occurs when antigen is fed, and in some species when antigen is encountered early in life.

Thus immunology encompasses molecular and cellular biology of antigen recognition and of immune reactions, specific and non-specific.

LYMPHOID ORGANS

Cells and tissues involved in immunity comprise about 2% of the body weight. Many of the cells migrate throughout the body but there are also organs where cells which participate in immune responses are collected together in an environment where they can perform their functions more effectively.

PRIMARY AND SECONDARY LYMPHOID ORGANS

Primary lymphoid organs
The *bone marrow, thymus* and *fetal liver* are the major sites of *production of lymphocytes*, and the environments where lymphocytes undergo differentiation and proliferation so that they leave as functional effector cells.

Secondary lymphoid organs
Lymph nodes, spleen, tonsils and *Peyer's patches* provide an environment in which *lymphocytes can interact* with each other and with antigens because there are phagocytic macrophages, antigen presenting cells, mature T and B lymphocytes collected together.

Dispersed immune cells
In addition to the organised lymphoid tissues, there are other sites, particularly the mucosae, where many immunocytes are dispersed between other cells, for example within the gut epithelium and lamina propria.

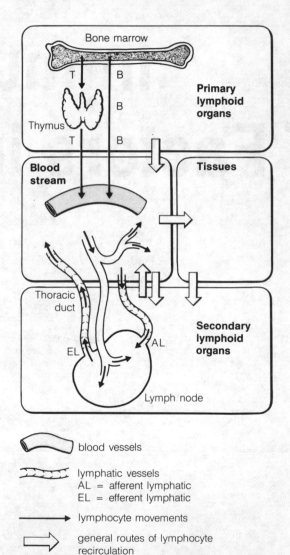

Fig. 2.1 Organisation of the lymphoid system. There is one-way traffic of T and B cells from the primary lymphoid organs into the blood stream, and continuous recirculation of cells between the secondary lymphoid organs, tissues and blood stream.

Migration of lymphocytes

Migration of cells between lymphoid organs is illustrated in Figure 2.1.

The exit route for lymphocytes from the blood stream is through a specialised section of the post capillary venules, high endothelial venule. In the spleen it is via the marginal zone of the peri-arteriolar lymphoid sheath and there are similar specialised blood vessels in the lamina propria of the gut, and some other sites, to allow emigration of particular populations of lymphocytes into these parts of the body. Matching of receptors on lymphocytes to molecules on these specialised blood vessels explains the apparent selection of only certain types of cells for migration into the tissues.

Within the lymphoid tissues there are areas mainly populated by T cells (T dependent areas) and B areas which also contain germinal centres.

There are also routes of return of lymphocytes, e.g. from the mucous membranes back to lymph nodes via afferent lymphatics, and via the thoracic duct into the venous system.

Clinical relevance of the organisation of lymphoid tissues

An appreciation of the organisation of primary and secondary lymphoid organs, and movement of cells between them, has been critical to the development of specific immunotherapy for some immunodeficiency diseases; also the characteristics of a number of malignancies of the lymphoid tissues (lymphomas) relate to where, within the general developmental and migration sequences, the malignant clone has occurred.

CELLS INVOLVED IN IMMUNITY

A wide range of cells participate in non-specific and specific immunity, and many of these, such as macrophages and T cells, fulfil several different functions.

Identification of cell types

There are characteristic cytological features of the various cells, but it must be appreciated that, particularly within the population of lymphocytes, cells which appear morphologically identical may be functionally very different.

Many techniques are now available to detect cell membrane molecules which indicate the stage of differentiation and activation of lymphocytes, macrophages and other cells, and thus allow subdivision of the main morphological categories. Formerly called T1, T3, etc. they have been renamed CD1, CD3 etc. (CD = cluster of differentiation) (Table 2.1). Identi-

Table 2.1 Lymphocyte and macrophage surface markers (cluster of differentiation, CD)

CD nomenclature	Terminology previously used	Significance of the marker
CD2	T1	All T cells are positive
CD3	T3	Present on all mature peripheral T lymphocytes, 25% of human thymocytes
CD4	T4	60% of circulating T cells, helper/inducer T cell subset
CD8	T8	Approximately 35% of circulating peripheral human T cells, suppressor/cytotoxic T cell subset
CD20	B1	Present on all human B cells from peripheral blood, lymph node, spleen, tonsil and bone marrow
CD21	B2	Similar pattern to CD20, but expression varies. This marker is useful in classifying B cell malignancies

Other markers including CD21, 19, 11, 13, 14 are used in classification of myeloid and lymphoid malignancies.

fication of CD and other surface markers on lymphocytes is valuable in clinical diagnosis (e.g. of immunodeficiency syndromes) and in the classification of lymphomas, as well as in research.

CD testing is usually done with monoclonal antibodies, and new determinants and antibodies are described each year. However there remain some functionally distinct groups of cells and, so far, no antibody can distinguish between them, for example T suppressor and T cytotoxic cells, which can only be identified by their functional characteristics.

T lymphocytes

The majority of normal human blood and recirculating T cells are small lymphocytes with a high nuclear to cytoplasmic ratio. They are derived from precursor stem cells of the bone marrow, which have matured under the influence of a hormone or factor produced by the epithelial cells of the thymus.

T cells perform important immunoregulatory functions via their secreted products, and also act as effector cells, capable of killing other cells (Table 2.2). Given appropriate stimulation they proliferate and differentiate into a range of subsets with differing functions – immunoregulatory helper (T_H), suppressor (T_S); and effector cytotoxic (T_C), capable of cell killing, and the T cells that mediate delayed-type hypersensitivity reactions (T_{DTH}), by virtue of the properties of lymphokines which they secrete. The lymphokines produce local inflammation, and attract and then activate macrophages.

Many immunological diseases, both immunode-

Table 2.2   Functional classification of T cells

Cell type	Abbreviation	Marker	Properties
Immunoregulatory			
Helper	T$_H$	CD4	Recognise antigen in association with Class 2 HLA; provide help signals for B cells (e.g. IL-4)
Suppressor	T$_S$	CD8	Recognise antigen in association with Class I HLA. Precise mode of suppression unknown
Effector			
Cytotoxic	T$_C$	CD8	Recognise antigen in association with Class I HLA; this is potentially on the surface of any nucleated cell
Mediators of delayed hypersensitivity	T$_{DTH}$	CD4	Recognise antigen in association with Class 2 HLA; this antigen usually will have been processed in endosomes and then presented at the surface of an antigen presenting cell. Since the tissue distribution of Class 2 is restricted, only in special circumstances are T$_{DTH}$ cells provided with activation signals by other cells

ficiency and abnormally enhanced reactivity, can ultimately be attributed to defects of T cell regulatory function. In terms of protective immunity, T cells are particularly important in defence against intracellular bacterial and protozoal pathogens, viruses and fungi.

B lymphocytes
B lymphocytes are independent of the thymus and in man probably complete their early maturation within the bone marrow. They are called B cells because they mature within the Bursa of Fabricius in birds.

When appropriately stimulated, B lymphocytes undergo proliferation, maturation and differentiation to form plasma cells, responsible for the synthesis of antibodies (immunoglobulins) in their abundant endoplasmic reticulum. Eventually there are many identical daughters derived from a single B cell, forming a clone. The enormous diversity of antibodies which an individual can produce is explained partly by re-arrangements of nucleic acid within precursor B cells and partly by random mutation.

ANTIGEN PRESENTING CELLS

These are found mainly in the lymphoid organs and the skin and their main role is to present antigen in a particular way to lymphocytes so as to start off the antigen specific immune responses. They include interdigitating cells in the thymus, the Langerhans cells of the skin, veiled cells in afferent lymph, interdigitating cells in the T areas of lymph nodes, and follicular dendritic cells in B areas of lymph nodes. Some macrophages probably also act as antigen presenting cells and other non-immune cells, including epithelial cells, can also perform this function.

Neutrophil polymorphs
Polymorphonuclear granulocytes are derived from haemopoetic stem cells in the bone marrow. They are short-lived cells, normally concentrated in the blood stream but can respond to chemotactic signals in the presence of tissue injury or infection. They marginate in the capillaries and move into the tissues where they can phagocytose and kill bacteria or other foreign materials which are adherent to their surface. Although they are intrinsically capable of these functions the properties of polymorphs are made much more efficient if the bacterium is coated with antibody and/or complement, and they are also influenced by a variety of cytokines released by other lymphocytes and other cells.

The importance of polymorphs is emphasised by the greatly increased susceptibility to infection found in patients with neutropenia.

Macrophages
Macrophages are derived from bone marrow precursors which differentiate to blood monocytes and finally settle in the tissues as mature, mononuclear phagocytes. Many organs contain characteristic populations of the phagocytic series, e.g. lung alveolar macrophages, liver Kupffer cells, resident and recirculating macrophages in lymph nodes, brain microglial cells, and kidney mesangial cells. Macrophages, like polymorphs, are capable of phagocytosis and killing of microorganisms. They also secrete a number of important cytokines and are influenced by, as well as themselves influencing T lymphocytes and other important cells. Their main functions are listed in the information box (p. 29).

Aggregates of macrophages, granulomas, are characteristic of many chronic infectious and idiopathic inflammatory diseases such as tuberculosis, leprosy, sarcoidosis and Crohn's disease.

Natural killer cells
Natural killer (NK) cells are large granular cells, morphologically quite similar to lymphocytes. They are thought to be important in resistance to virus infections and probably also malignancy. When a cell becomes infected by a virus, or transforms into a cancerous cell its surface molecules are altered. These alterations can sometimes be recognised by NK cells which engage the infected or altered cell and kill it. NK cells bear receptors which recognise high molecular weight glycoproteins on the surface of virally infected cells, at an

MAIN FUNCTIONS OF MACROPHAGE

Secretory functions
Monocytes and macrophages secrete around 100 substances whose actions range from induction of cell growth to cell death. Furthermore, single factors, such as IL-1 and tumour necrosis factor (TNF), can have many different actions.

Acute phase response
This is a systemic inflammatory action to an infection or injury comprising fever, tachycardia, shock, changes in the serum concentration of proteins such as C reactive protein and fibrinogen. IL-1, TNF and IL-6 mediate these effects.

Regulation of haemopoiesis
Peripheral blood leucocytes are influenced indirectly via the effects of IL-1 and TNF on T cells, and directly via factors such as macrophage colony stimulating factor which induces a peripheral blood leucocytosis.

Haemostasis
The host response to injury may activate the coagulation system which occasionally results in disseminated intravascular coagulation. In response to stimuli such as bacterial endotoxin and immune complexes, cells of the mononuclear phagocyte system synthesise thromboplastin, a potent activator of the coagulation pathway.

Lymphocyte activation
Mononuclear phagocytes are central to induction of the immune response via antigen presentation.

Killing of microorganisms
Mononuclear phagocytes can migrate to and stay in the vicinity of a focus of infection and phagocytose the agents concerned. Mechanisms by which microorganisms are recognised are ill understood. Organisms are killed by oxygen-dependent and oxygen-independent mechanisms.

Killing of tumour cells
Lysis of tumour cells by monocytes and macrophages is probably one of the main mechanisms of host defence against tumours, for example via TNF and gamma interferon.

Tissue repair and remodelling
These important functions are produced by collagenase, elastase, and substances that induce fibroblast proliferation and osteoclast bone resorption.

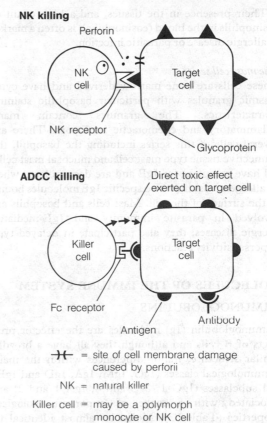

Fig 2.2   Direct mechanisms of cell killing. NK cells have receptors which recognise a cell membrane glycoprotein on the target cell and toxic molecules are secreted in close proximity to the target cell. In antibody dependent cellular cytotoxicity (ADCC), a variety of types of cell can act as killer cells. They are attached to the target cell by immunoglobulin molecules. Specific antibody combines with antigen on the surface of the target cell, and the heavy chains of the immunoglobulin molecules concerned link to Fc receptors as shown.

early stage, before the virus has had a chance to reproduce. They are activated by interferons (produced by virally infected cells and sometimes by other cells such as T lymphocytes). When activated they release their granule contents into the space between the target and NK cell (Fig. 2.2), including a molecule called perforin which acts, as its name implies, by producing a hole in the cell membrane of the target cell leading to cell death.

NK cells also have receptors for immunoglobulin and thus have enhanced cell killing activity in the presence of specific antibody to virus. The antibody links host and target cell closely (Fig. 2.2). This phenomenon is called antibody dependent cell mediated cytotoxicity (ADCC), and is not confined to NK cells, but can be performed by polymorphs and macrophages.

Eosinophils
Eosinophils are granulated blood leucocytes which can migrate into the tissues. They appear to be metabolically very active and among their granule mediators are the toxic protein eosinophilic major basic protein, and the anti-inflammatory histaminases and other substances which inactivate mast cell products. They are attracted by factors released by T cells, mast cells and basophils, for example eosinophilic chemotactic factor of anaphylaxis.

Their presence in the tissues, and a high count of eosinophils in the blood (eosinophilia), is often a marker of allergic disease or parasitic infection.

The mast cell series

These cells are bone marrow derived and have cytoplasmic granules with particular basophilic staining characteristics. The granules contain many inflammatory and chemotactic mediators. There are several cells of this series including the basophil, the connective tissue type mast cell and mucosal mast cells. All have receptors for IgE and are degranulated when an allergen cross links two specific IgE molecules bound to the surface of the cell. Mast cells and basophils are involved in parasite immunity and IgE-mediated allergic diseases; they also participate in delayed-type hypersensitivity reactions.

MOLECULES OF THE IMMUNE SYSTEM

IMMUNOGLOBULINS

Immunoglobulin (Ig) molecules are the effector products of B cells and although they all have a broadly similar structure, minor differences within the main immunological classes (IgG, IgM, IgA, IgD and IgE) and subclasses (IgG 1, 2, 3 and 4; IgA 1 and 2) are associated with a range of important biological properties (Table 2.3). Molecules almost identical to secreted immunoglobulins are incorporated in the cell membranes of B cells (surface Ig), and there are many related molecules concerned with antigen recognition and cell–cell communication.

Structure of immunoglobulin molecules

An immunoglobulin molecule is made up of distinct sub-units held together by disulphide (S–S) bonds, which can be broken by reducing agents, so that the molecule falls apart into pairs of polypeptide chains

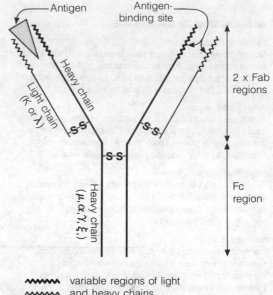

variable regions of light and heavy chains

-S-S-   disulphide bond

Fig. 2.3   The typical structure of an immunoglobulin molecule, illustrating the two heavy and two light chains linked by disulfide bonds; the antigen-binding sites comprise variable regions of light and heavy chains; the Fc region, which possesses isotype specific properties such as complement binding and capacity to attach to mast cells.

called light and heavy chains. Two types of light chain exist, kappa and lambda, of which individual immunoglobulins have only one type, and there are several different heavy chains which confer on the Ig molecule its class-specific properties.

A typical immunoglobulin molecule such as IgG (Fig. 2.3) has two antigen-binding regions (Fab) and one Fc component which is the part of the molecule which performs the class-related functions such as

Table 2.3   Properties of immunoglobulins

	Sedimentation coefficient	Number of basic 4 chain units	Approximate range of concentration in normal serum	Other properties	Subclasses
IgG	7S	1	8–16 g/l	Complement fixing activity (IgG1, G3) placental transfer	IgG1, IgG2, IgG3, IgG4,
IgA	7S, 10S, 11S	1 or 2	1.5–4 g/l	Present in external secretions	IgA1, IgA2
IgM	19S	5	0.5–2 g/l	Complement fixing activity, small amounts in external secretions	
IgD	7S	1	0.003–0.04 g/l		
IgE	8S	1	17–450 ng/ml	Binds to mast cells and basophils	

complement fixation. The section of the heavy chain contained in the Fc component is responsible for the antigenic differences between the classes of immunoglobulin which enable their laboratory measurement by the use of heavy-chain-specific antisera.

The molecular basis of diversity of antigen-binding function (i.e. antibody activity) resides in the so-called variable regions of the Fab components. The antigen-combining site of an immunoglobulin molecule (the idiotype) can itself be recognised and reacted to by other immunocompetent cells, with the production of anti-idiotype antibodies which can influence the magnitude and duration of antibody production to a given antigen.

Immunoglobulin G (IgG)

In healthy adults, IgG accounts for more than 70% of the immunoglobulins in normal serum and is distributed equally between the blood and extracellular fluids. About a quarter of all the body's IgG passes out of the blood stream each day and the same amount returns via the thoracic duct. In man, IgG is the only immunoglobulin that is transported across the placenta to reach the fetus and provide the newborn baby with passively acquired antibody during its early life.

IgG antibodies are very important in anti-bacterial immunity. They readily neutralise soluble toxins such as those responsible for many of the clinical manifestations of diphtheria or tetanus. IgG also has an opsonic effect on bacteria, coating them so that their ingestion by phagocytes is facilitated. IgG antibodies also can produce disease, e.g. by forming immune complexes, or as autoantibodies.

Immunoglobulin M (IgM)

The macro-molecular IgM is predominantly intravascular. It is made up of five immunoglobulin units linked with disulphide bonds to provide ten identical antigen combining-sites, together with a J (joining) chain. IgM is especially effective in activating complement to produce immune lysis of foreign cells. IgM antibodies are also much more efficient than IgG antibodies in linking particulate antigens together for agglutination and phagocytosis and would seem to be specially adapted for dealing with cell debris or bacteria in the blood stream.

Immunoglobulin A (IgA)

IgA accounts for about 20% of the total serum immunoglobulins. However its function, if any, within the blood stream and tissues is thought to be much less important than its role as a secretory antibody. The major sites of IgA synthesis are the laminae propriae

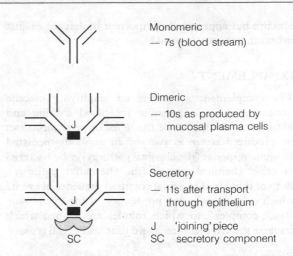

Monomeric
— 7s (blood stream)

Dimeric
— 10s as produced by mucosal plasma cells

Secretory
— 11s after transport through epithelium

J   'joining' piece
SC   secretory component

Fig. 2.4 Forms of IgA which are present in man. J chain is synthesised by plasma cells. 10S IgA attaches to secretory component on the basolateral membrane of epithelial cells. The composite molecule is then internalised and finally expelled at the luminal surface as secretory 11S IgA, containing four light chains, four heavy chains, J chain and secretory component.

underlying the respiratory tract, the gut and other mucosae. IgA is found in three main molecular forms (Fig. 2.4). In blood it is 7S, monomeric, similar in size to IgG. Dimeric 10S IgA (also containing J chain) is produced by plasma cells in the mucosae and is transported across epithelia into colostrum, saliva, intestinal juice, respiratory secretions, tears and several other body fluids. During trans-epithelial transport, another polypeptide, secretory component, is incorporated to form secretory 11S IgA, relatively resistant to digestive enzymes.

Secretory IgA confers immunity to infection by enteric bacterial and viral pathogens, and may also be involved in the regulation of the commensal gut flora. Oral immunisation is now being used to try to induce protective immunity to intestinal infections such as cholera and rotavirus.

Immunoglobulin D (IgD)

IgD is almost exclusively found on the surface of immature B lymphocytes and may be involved in their maturation and regulation.

Immunoglobulin E (IgE)

IgE concentration in serum is very low. This is in part because it has a considerable affinity for cell surfaces and binds firmly to mast cells and basophils. IgE antibodies are necessary for immediate hypersensitivity reactions, such as occur in atopic individuals, e.g. in hay fever. The physiological function of IgE antibodies is obscure but appear to be important in defence against helminth parasites (worms).

COMPLEMENT

The complement system is an amplifying cascade similar to those responsible for blood clotting and fibrinolysis. Activation of this effector mechanism can be produced *either* as part of an antibody-mediated immune response (the classical pathway) *or* by bacterial or other chemical stimuli (the alternative pathway). Both of these lead to a final common sequence of events which culminates in the production of the 'membrane attack complex', in which tubules are formed which traverse the cell membrane and thus lead to cell lysis.

Complement components

There is an agreed nomenclature for the many components, e.g. C2, C3 but they do not act in the same sequence as their identification numbers. A full account of complement will be found in any textbook of immunology, and this description concentrates on the general principles of the reactions and their clinical significance. Most complement components are proteins (beta globulins) made in the liver, and have proteinase activity when activated. The exception is C1q which is a strange molecule, shaped rather like a bunch of six tulips. Inhibitors are also involved at various points in the cascades and feedback loops.

Sequence of events in complement activation

Complement is usually associated with a membrane or immune complex and there is sequential activation of complement enzymes (Fig. 2.5). By virtue of its mem-

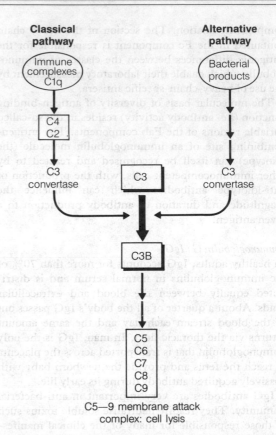

Fig. 2.6   **Diagrammatic illustration of complement and its components.** The conversion of C3 to C3B is central, and the final result is produced when the membrane attack complex causes tiny holes to appear in the cell membrane and cell death ensues.

brane effects and release of active peptides, the complement system fulfils a number of functions, including cell activation, cell lysis, inflammation and opsonisation.

An outline of the important stages of complement activation is shown in Figure 2.6. The activation of C3 by the enzyme C3 convertase is the central event of the complement sequence. The classical pathway is triggered when immune complexes combine with C1q. In the alternative pathway, a C3 convertase is generated by a process that starts with activation of complement components by materials such as bacterial cell walls and endotoxin. The alternative pathway may therefore be particularly relevant before a primary immune response has been mounted.

Biological activities and control

Some of the important biological activities of complement are listed in Table 2.4. Clinically, if the complement sequence is involved in disease, C3 may be

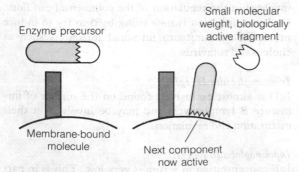

Fig. 2.5   **Principles of the complement cascade.** An active molecule (produced by an earlier part of the cascade and already fixed to the cell membrane) acts on an enzyme precursor breaking it into a large component which adheres to the cell membrane and is now active, and a low molecular weight fragment released into the extracellular fluid, which may have any of a variety of biological activities.

Table 2.4 Important, biologically active molecules generated during complement activation

Component	Effect
C3a	Smooth muscle contraction
	Vascular permeability increased
	Eosinophil, basophil and mast cell degranulation
	Platelet aggregation
C3b	Opsonisation and phagocytosis
C4a	Smooth muscle contraction
	Vascular permeability increased
C5a	Smooth muscle contraction
	Vascular permeability increased
	Eosinophil, basophil and mast cell degranulation
	Platelet aggregation
	Polymorph and monocyte chemotaxis
	Neutrophil hydrolytic enzymes released
C5a-des-arg	Neutrophil chemotaxis and hydrolytic enzymes released

Table 2.5 Important cytokines

Cytokine	Abbreviation	Main cellular source
α interferon	IFN α	Monocytes
		Macrophages
β interferon	IFN β	Fibroblasts
γ interferon	IFN γ	T cells
Interleukin 1	IL-1	Macrophages
		Fibroblasts
		T cells
Interleukin 2	IL-2	T cells
Interleukin 3	IL-3	T cells
Interleukin 4	IL-4	T cells
Interleukin 5	IL-5	T cells
Interleukin 6	IL-6	T cells, monocytes
Tumour necrosis factor	TNF	Macrophages
		Monocytes
		T cells

used up in large amounts and so the finding of low blood levels of this protein is of some diagnostic value.

The complement pathway is controlled by two mechanisms. A number of the activated components are inherently unstable; if the next protein in the cascade is not immediately available, the active substance decays. There are also a number of specific inhibitors, e.g. C1 inhibitor.

CYTOKINES

Some of these are often still called lymphokines; others are being renamed as Interleukins.

In the late 1960s it was recognised that lymphocyte mediated effects were sometimes produced by soluble factors. Many such factors were described and various tests of antigen-specific cell-mediated immunity were developed, based on the presumed secretion of these factors by T cells. A good example is the leucocyte migration inhibition test. Now many secreted products of T and other cells have been studied in great detail, their biochemistry and even their coding genes identified. It has become clear that many of the properties of lymphokines are possessed by only a few molecules. The most important are Interleukin 1 (IL1)

made by macrophages; IL2 made by T cells, and the interferons. Some further information on these and other cytokines is given in Table 2.5.

THE MAJOR HISTOCOMPATIBILITY COMPLEX

Although the major histocompatibility complex (MHC) was originally identified by its role in transplant rejection it is now recognised that proteins encoded by this region of the genome are involved in many aspects of immunological recognition. These include interactions between different lymphoid cells as well as between lymphocytes and antigen presenting cells.

The MHC gene cluster is located on chromosome 6 (Fig. 2.7). It contains genes coding for the 'Human Leucocyte Antigens' (HLA), cell surface glycoproteins which are found on many cells, not only leucocytes. It also contains the genes for some important complement proteins. An individual inherits one HLA haplotype from each parent and since there are several gene loci, and a large number of different specificities at each locus, this makes for a very large number of HLA genotypes within a population.

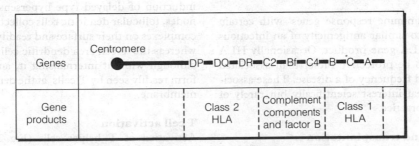

Fig. 2.7 Structure of the major histocompatibility complex on chromosome 6.

Of the MHC encoded proteins, Class 1 antigens HLA-A and HLA-B are present on all nucleated cells and platelets. They comprise one peptide chain encoded by the MHC associated with a different polypeptide, beta-2 microglobulin, encoded elsewhere in the genome. Class 2 antigens, the HLA-D series, have more limited tissue distribution, including B lymphocytes, macrophages and activated T cells.

There are several important clinical applications of knowledge of the MHC.

Antigen recognition by T cells

Immunoglobulin (antibody) molecules recognise the general contour of an antigenic determinant. The T cell antigen receptor, a small chain related to the immunoglobulin family, can only 'see' its particular antigen when that antigen is held at the surface of another cell in close relationship to HLA. T cytotoxic cells only recognise antigens (such as a virus) in association with HLA class 1 molecules on the surface of a cell. It is as if HLA is a signpost, guiding the T cytotoxic cell to its target. On the other hand, T helper cells recognise antigen on macrophages and B cells (antigen presenting cells) in association with the HLA-D, class 2 antigens. This antigen will usually have been previously internalised and 'processed' by the antigen presenting cell.

Diseases associated with HLA

There are a number of diseases associated with particular HLA types (Table 2.6). This may partly relate to

Table 2.6 Diseases associated with particular HLA antigens

Ankylosing spondylitis	B27
Reiter's syndrome	B27
Addison's disease	B8 DR3
Thyrotoxicosis	B8 DR3
Myasthenia gravis	B8 DR3
Coeliac disease	B8 DR3
Insulin dependent diabetes	B8 DR3 DR4
Multiple sclerosis	DR2
Haemochromatosis	A3
Psoriasis	B13

the linkage of 'immune response genes' with certain HLA genes, or to similar antigenicity of an infectious agent and the HLA gene product. Occasionally HLA status appears to be protective rather than associated with an increased frequency of a disease. These associations are of great interest scientifically but rarely of value in clinical practice.

Tissue typing and transplantation

It has been known for many years that grafts of skin and other organs between HLA identical siblings or identical twins have prolonged survival whereas in unrelated individuals, transplantation when donor and host have been matched for HLA improves transplant survival for some organs (e.g. kidney) but not others (e.g. liver). Tissue type details of patients awaiting transplants are collected nationally, and in difficult cases, even internationally, to enable matching with suitable donors. HLA typing is also important (along with blood grouping) in the selection of live donors, e.g. of kidney or bone marrow.

PRESENTATION OF ANTIGEN AND INITIATION OF THE IMMUNE RESPONSE

Antigen distribution

Antigen which has penetrated the tissue reaches the draining lymph nodes. If it arrives via the respiratory tract or the gut it concentrates in the organised tissues of the mucosa-associated lymphoid tissues. Antigen from the blood stream is removed in the spleen. All of these above routes lead to the induction of a specific immune response, usually active immunity but occasionally immunological tolerance. On the other hand particulate antigen is removed from the blood stream without induction of immunity by some macrophages in the liver and lung.

Antigen presentation

Macrophages which have phagocytosed antigen digest and process it, express it on their surface and signal B cells for activation. Antigen complexed with MHC products can switch on T cells.

The fact that T cells require antigen to be presented to them along with MHC class 1 or class 2 antigens on the surface of an antigen presenting cell means that T cells ignore antigens in the free state and are not swamped by them, for example by virus or bacteria in the blood stream.

Antigen presenting cells in different sites appear to have slightly different properties so that the Langerhans cells of the skin seem particularly adapted towards induction of delayed type hypersensitivity. In lymph nodes, follicular dendritic cells collect antigen-antibody complexes on their surface and readily stimulate B cells whereas the T cell area dendritic cells process antigen, although without internalising it, and present it in a form readily seen by T cells, at the dendritic cell surface membrane.

T cell activation

Activation of T helper cells (Fig. 2.8) requires two signals, antigen and IL-1. When both of these signals

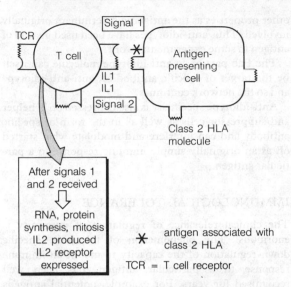

Fig. 2.8 **Signals necessary for T helper cell activation.** Signal one is provided by the combination of antigen and Class 2 HLA on the surface of an antigen-presenting cell. Signal two is IL-1 which will have been released in the vicinity of the T cell by macrophages.

are received there is RNA and protein synthesis, including production of the important protein IL-2. The cell moves from G0 to G1 of the mitotic cycle.

As well as synthesis of IL-2 the activated T blast cell also expresses surface receptors for IL-2 and this leads to a burst of proliferative activity of cells, and they secrete a wide variety of biologically active lymphokines.

B cell activation

Activation of B cells can occur in two ways. There are a small number of physico-chemically unusual antigens (for example pneumococcus polysaccharide) which can stimulate B cells directly without the need for T cell involvement. Such thymus independent antigens usually induce an IgM response with little or no memory.

Most antigens are thymus dependent. Events which eventually lead to antibody production by B cells require messages to be delivered by the antigen both directly to a B cell and, after intracellular processing, to a T cell (Fig. 2.9). This explains why the antigenic determinant to which antibody is being produced is not necessarily the same as the antigenic determinant recognised by T cells (in the so-called hapten carrier system). Both these determinants must be present on the same molecule for T help to be given to B cells.

B cell activation also requires two signals, first the binding of an antigenic determinant to the B cell

receptor; second, an activating signal produced by the T cell, probably the B cell stimulatory factor IL-4, since this is capable of bringing resting B cells to the activated G1 state. Once activated the stimulated B cell acquires a number of new surface receptors for growth factors and continues to proliferate and mature. The newly active B cells express surface receptors for IL-4. Further clonal expansion of B cells is engineered by a second B cell growth factor and other lymphokines may be synergistic.

Other signals then lead to the generation of memory B cells, final differentiation of the B cells into IgM producing plasma cells, and also switching of the immunoglobulin produced by the stimulated cells from IgM to IgG, IgA or IgE (class switch). This is achieved by transfer of a particular gene segment for the variable segment of the heavy chain, to an alternative constant region gene so that the antibodies produced are of exactly the same specificity but of a different class.

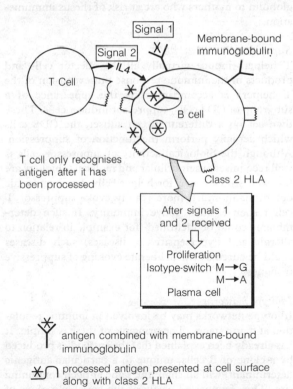

Fig. 2.9 **B cell activation.** The first signal is the simple combination of antigen with membrane-bound immunoglobulin on the surface of the B cell. The second signal requires a fairly complex series of events. Antigen is internalised by the B cell, processed and re-presented at the cell surface together with Class 2 HLA. The T cells recognise this processed antigen, and secrete a stimulatory interleukin which acts as the second signal for B cell activation.

REGULATION OF IMMUNE RESPONSES

It is inappropriate for a specific immune response to progress and expand indefinitely, and so there have evolved several immunological factors which inhibit rather than potentiate specific immunity.

MECHANISMS OF IMMUNOREGULATION

Loss of antigen

Antigen is a very important drive to B and T cell proliferation and as the concentration of antigen in the body drops so the intensity of the drive falls off in parallel.

Presence of antibody

Antibody itself exerts negative feedback control, partly by simply neutralising the available antigen but also probably by other mechanisms. An important clinical example of this is the administration of anti-D immunoglobulin to mothers who are at risk of rhesus immunisation.

Suppressor T cells

T helpers induce virtually all the effector cells and products of the immune response but expansion of the T helpers is accompanied by the appearance of a subgroup of CD4 cells, suppressor inducer cells. These then act on a different T cell subset, the CD8 cells which actually perform the function of suppression. Although the biological activity of suppressor cells is well recognised, their cellular and molecular biology are less well studied than for helper cells. Some antigenic determinants much more readily evoke suppressor T cell responses than active immunity. If such determinants could be identified (for example in relation to allergic and hypersensitivity diseases) such diseases could be cured by the deliberate evoking of suppressive responses.

Idiotype networks

Idiotype networks may be involved in immune regulation at many stages. The principle of these is simple. It has already been explained that the antibodies produced by a clone of B cells, unique to a particular antigenic determinant, will all share the same antigen combining site. This, comprised partly of the variable regions of the light and heavy immunoglobulin chains, is called an idiotype. Since the idiotype is a protein it can itself, of course, act as an antigen and antibodies to this are called anti-idiotypes.

The antigen-combining-site of the anti-idiotype antibody is often almost exactly the same in contours and other properties as the antigenic determinant originally involved. Thus anti-idiotypes have been used instead of antigen in some experimental work.

The Fab part of an anti-idiotype molecule can itself be the target of specific antibodies, anti-anti-idiotype and so the network continues.

Anti-idiotype specificity is also expressed on T helper and suppressor cells as well as in the form of specific antibody and can interfere and modulate what started off as an originally simple immune response to a particular antigen.

IMMUNOLOGICAL TOLERANCE

The clinical relevance of regulation of immunity is enormous. The phenomenon of tolerance, specific down-regulation of the capacity to mount an immune response to a particular antigen, has been well recognised for years. For example, potential antigens which reach the lymphoid cells of the fetus, during their immunological development, specifically suppress any future response to that antigen when the individual is immunologically mature. This is a means whereby unresponsiveness develops to the body's own constituents (self) and enables the lymphoid cells to distinguish potentially harmful non-self. Thus, immunological tolerance is what protects us against overwhelming auto (anti-self) immunity.

A state of tolerance can sometimes be induced in adult life by giving particularly large or small doses of antigen, or chemically modified antigen. Additionally, antigens which are normally encountered via the gut usually induce a state of oral tolerance. Thus food allergic diseases such as coeliac disease can be envisaged as due to a breakdown in the physiological down-regulation of immunity to dietary and other gut antigens.

Successful transplantation requires the induction of tolerance, or at least the suppression of active immunity, to the transplanted organ.

ALLERGY AND HYPERSENSITIVITY

The terms allergy and hypersensitivity are synonomous although allergy is often used to describe immediate hypersensitivity reactions and atopic diseases. Hypersensitivity can be defined as tissue damage resulting from an immune response.

Traditionally hypersensitivity has been classified according to the immune mechanism predominantly involved. This remains a useful approach reminding us that the original disease process relates to a defect in the regulation of a particular component of the immune response. This also provides a basis for rational treatment.

CAUSES OF HYPERSENSITIVITY

Hypersensitivity may result from the induction of an inappropriate pattern of immunity, for example to an environmental agent which is totally harmless. This occurs in many people who readily make IgE antibodies (atopics). Sometimes T cell mediated immunity is involved, for example in cows' milk protein sensitive enteropathy in infants.

Hypersensitivity may also occur when the immune response to an antigen such as a virus not only damages or destroys the offending agent, but incidentally produces damage to adjacent tissue. 'Innocent bystanders' are damaged by an immune response which has to be vigorous in order to kill the pathogen. A good example of this is the fibrosis and cavity formation of pulmonary tuberculosis.

There is a range of conditions in which the clinical manifestations are virtually identical to those of immune mediated hypersensitivity, but these occur when non-specific immune effector mechanisms are triggered directly by agents other than antigen, for example when drugs or physical factors lead to mast cell degranulation.

Immediate (anaphylactic) hypersensitivity

This is due to IgE antibodies and most if not all manifestations are produced by mast cell degranulation (Table 2.7). The pattern and severity of reaction

Table 2.7 Products of mast cell degranulation

Mediator	Biological effects
Pre-formed, stored within granules	
Histamine	Vasodilation, increased capillary permeability, chemokinesis, bronchoconstriction
Heparin	Anti-coagulant
Tryptase	Activates C3
β-glucosaminidase	Splits off glucosamine
ECF	Eosinophil chemotaxis
NCF	Neutrophil chemotaxis
Platelet activating factor	Mediator release
Newly synthesised	
By the lipoxygenase pathway	
Leukotrienes C_4 and D_4 (SRS-A) Leukotriene B_4	Vasoactive, bronchoconstriction, chemotaxis and/or chemokinesis
By the cyclo-oxygenase pathway	
Prostaglandins Thromboxanes	Affect bronchial muscle, platelet aggregation and vasodilation

depend on the amount and route of exposure to antigen, the density of tissue mast cells, and the amounts of IgE antibody that they bear on the surface.

Respiratory tract allergies

Relatively mild although inconvenient symptoms may occur when antigen-IgE reactions take place in the upper respiratory tract or on other epithelial surfaces. For example, reactions to pollens or animal dander may cause rhinorrhoea, sneezing, conjunctivitis. On the other hand, inhalation of the antigen can lead to intense bronchospasm in atopic asthma. Skin prick tests with common inhalant allergens can give the clinician a reasonably good indication of a patient's likely sensitivities.

Anaphylaxis

Systemic anaphylaxis consists of a group of much more severe reactions which may occur rapidly if the antigen is injected, as in the case of a drug such as penicillin, or the sting of an insect. Rarely, anaphylaxis can be produced by ingested food, in a highly sensitised individual.

The features are bronchospasm, laryngeal oedema with extreme dyspnoea and cyanosis, and a marked fall in blood pressure (anaphylactic shock). There may also be nausea, vomiting and diarrhoea.

Systemic anaphylaxis is a potentially fatal condition if not treated promptly with adrenaline (500–1000 µg i.m.) and an antihistamine (e.g. chlorpheniramine 10–20 mg slowly i.v.) followed, in severely ill patients, by intravenous corticosteroids.

Urticaria

Urticaria, the formation of weal and flare lesions in the skin, is an anaphylactic phenomenon which can develop as a result of absorption of antigen (some foods and food additives) from the intestinal tract. Not all urticaria is caused by immune reactions. The mediators that cause urticaria can be released by other means, especially physical agents such as trauma or cold.

Other atopic diseases

There are a number of other, less well-characterised diseases in which IgE is certainly involved, although other immune effector mechanisms are also implicated. These include atopic eczema, and some acute reactions to foods, particularly in infants.

Immune complex reactions

Immune complex reactions are induced by the deposition of antigen and antibody in blood-vessel walls. Complement, platelets, mast cells, basophil and polymorph leucocytes are all involved in the subsequent inflammatory processes. Factors that determine the deposition of immune complexes in tissues also include the size of the immune complexes, the ratio of antigen to antibody, the nature of the antigen, and local haemodynamics. There are several situations in which a disease is caused by immune complex formation.

Persistent infection
In some cases a chronic infection (e.g. infective endocarditis, malaria or viral hepatitis) together with a weak antibody response leads to the chronic formation of immune complexes and their deposition in the tissues.

Extrinsic allergic alveolitis
Immune complexes may be formed in the lungs, in response to repeated inhalation of antigenic materials from moulds, plants or animals. In farmer's lung and bird fancier's lung there are circulating IgG antibodies to fungi which have been induced by repeated exposure to mouldy hay or to avian antigens. When antigen enters the body again by inhalation, local immune complexes are formed in the alveoli and local inflammation then interferes with pulmonary function.

Arthus reactions
An Arthus reaction may occur when an antigen is injected into the skin of a subject who has previously encountered that antigen and has high titres of serum antibody. The reaction of preformed antibody with this antigen results in a high concentration of local immune complexes. The reaction develops in some 6–24 hours with oedema, haemorrhage and necrosis at the injection site.

Serum sickness
In serum sickness IgG antibody is produced in response to the injection of foreign antigen in large quantity, as when horse serum is used to confer passive immunity. The antibody reacts with remaining antigen to form circulating, soluble immune complexes. Local swelling at the injection site, urticaria, fever, enlargement of the lymph nodes, arthralgia and sometimes glomerulonephritis occur about 10 days after initial exposure to the antigen. As the immune complexes are formed, the antigen concentration is rapidly lowered. Since the process continues only as long as the antigen persists, the disease is usually self-limiting.

Autoimmunity
In autoimmune diseases, immune complexes may be deposited in the kidneys, joints, arteries, skin and elsewhere.

Delayed-type hypersensitivity
In the classification of hypersensitivity suggested by Gell and Coombs in 1963 delayed-type hypersensitivity (cell-mediated or type IV) was used as a general category to describe all those hypersensitivity reactions that took more than 12 hours to develop. It is now evident that several different reactions can produce delayed hypersensitivity, and that although T_{DTH} cells are implicated they act by recruiting other cell types to the site of the reaction, particularly macrophages.

Chronic infections
Reactions effected by T_{DTH} lymphocytes are characteristically induced by infectious agents which are predominantly intracellular in the infected host, e.g. many viral infections and some bacterial infections such as tuberculosis and syphilis. The classical example of this reaction is the tuberculin test. The normal tissues of the host, as well as infected cells, are damaged by the reaction.

Granulomatous diseases
Granulomatous hypersensitivity is an important form of delayed hypersensitivity, causing many of the pathological effects in diseases which involve T cell mediated immunity. It results from the presence of a persistent antigen within macrophages which the cell is unable to destroy.

Contact hypersensitivity
Contact hypersensitivity, producing local eczema usually maximal at 48 hours, is most commonly caused by haptens such as nickel, chemicals found in rubber, and poison ivy. Contact hypersensitivity is predominantly epidermal and the antigen is presented by the Langerhans cell.

Food-related intestinal diseases
T cell mediated hypersensitivity is also involved in some chronic forms of immune mediated food intolerance, such as cows' milk protein sensitive enteropathy with malabsorption, and coeliac disease (Fig. 2.10).

AUTOIMMUNITY AND AUTOIMMUNE DISEASES

Normally a person or animal does not mount a significant immune response against its own body constituents because intricate controlling and suppressor mechanisms exist to prevent this happening. A defect in immunological tolerance may either occur spontaneously or be induced by some exogenous factor such

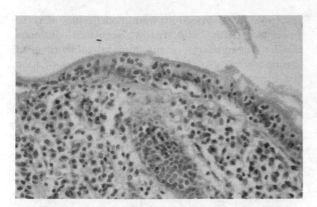

Fig. 2.10 Histology of part of a jejunal biopsy taken from a patient with coeliac disease. The surface epithelium contains large numbers of intraepithelial lymphocytes, which signal the presence of a local delayed type hypersensitivity (DTH) reaction.

as virus infection, often in a genetically predisposed individual.

In general autoimmune reactions occur in related groups reflecting the spectrum of autoimmune disease, ranging from the organ-specific to the non-organ-specific. Thus there are a number of autoantibodies formed to different thyroid antigens in autoimmune thyroid disease, and patients with one of the diseases in the organ-specific group tend to have an increased prevalence of autoantibodies to the target organs of other diseases in the group. Some important autoimmune diseases are listed in the information box below.

IMPORTANT AUTOIMMUNE DISEASES

Organ specific
Hashimoto's thyroiditis
Primary myxoedema
Thyrotoxicosis
Pernicious anaemia
Autoimmune atrophic gastritis
Autoimmune Addison's disease
Type I diabetes mellitus
Goodpasture's syndrome
Myasthenia gravis
Sympathetic ophthalmia
Autoimmune haemolytic anaemia
Idiopathic thrombocytopenic purpura
Primary biliary cirrhosis
Chronic active hepatitis
Sjögren's syndrome

Non-organ specific
Rheumatoid arthritis
Dermatomyositis
Systemic sclerosis
Systemic lupus erythematosus (SLE)

THEORIES OF AETIOLOGY OF AUTOIMMUNITY

Loss of suppressor functions

There is some evidence to suggest that in the autoimmune diseases there is a loss of suppressor T cell (T_S) control of the T helper (T_H) cells. The observation that T_S cell function diminishes with age provides an attractive explanation for the rising incidence of subclinical and clinical organ-specific autoimmune disease with advancing years.

Sequestrated antigen

There are some antigens that do not normally come into contact with the immunological system so that there has been no opportunity for immunological tolerance or self-recognition to develop. For example, sperm, if extravasated following unilateral blockage of the vas deferens, may induce antibody formation and contribute to sterility. Sperm antibodies may also be produced following vasectomy in normal men.

Infection

Invading microorganisms may have antigens that also occur in host tissues; a microbial antigen may thus induce the formation of antibodies which cross-react with these tissues. For example the sharing of antigen between some Group A haemolytic streptococci and the heart is thought to be the reason why rheumatic carditis is an occasional late complication of streptococcal tonsillitis.

Drugs

Occasionally the development of auto-antibodies is a side-effect of drug treatment. Some patients treated with methyldopa develop a haemolytic anaemia due to red blood cell auto-antibodies; the anaemia resolves when treatment with the drug is stopped. Other drugs may be associated with the production of antinuclear antibodies.

Genetic factors

Genetic factors are important in autoimmune disease as can be seen from experimental animal models, from family studies and from the association of many autoimmune diseases with the MHC system. In some autoimmune diseases, such as insulin-dependent diabetes, cells of the target organ express MHC class 2 antigens on their surfaces. This facilitates sensitisation and activation of the T_H cells. It may be that viruses are implicated in the abnormal expression of MHC antigens.

AUTO-ANTIBODIES

While some antibodies may play a crucial role in the pathogenesis of autoimmune disease, others seem to have little pathological function but may be useful evidence of an autoimmune diathesis. The antibody that is most readily detectable and useful as a marker in the serum may or may not be implicated as a damaging agent.

In the organ-specific group of disorders, antibody in the serum may indicate that immunological damage of some degree is occurring even though there is at that time no clinical evidence of organ failure. This can be explained by the fact that most tissues have a substantial reserve of function that must be eroded before clinical disease is manifest (e.g. only 10% of pancreatic islets are required to maintain normal glucose homeostasis). The rate of progression of the disease process may be over many years or more rapid; so far, the genetic factors in an individual patient that determine the rate of progression have not been identified.

IMMUNODEFICIENCY DISORDERS

Virtually any component of the immune system, specific or non-specific, can be absent or abnormal; the consequent immunodeficiency states vary in severity from trivial to fatal. There are many genetically determined conditions, but immunodeficiency can also result from acquired disease. This is well illustrated in severe form in the acquired immune deficiency syndrome (Chapter 5), but it is also part of common experience of many infections including influenza, infectious mononucleosis and measles. Acquired immunodeficiency may also be iatrogenic, for example as a result of treatment with corticosteroids or other immunosuppressive drugs (Fig. 2.11). In addition to causing

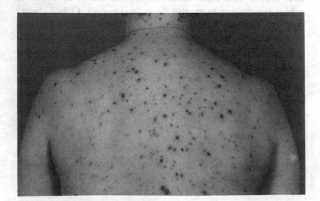

Fig. 2.11   Very severe chickenpox in a patient receiving the immunosuppressive drug, cyclosporin A, to treat Crohn's disease.

susceptibility to infection, immunodeficiency may be associated with abnormally regulated immune reactions, as in allergy or autoimmunity. The range of immunodeficiency diseases is shown in the information box below. Treatment is discussed in the section on immunotherapy.

CLASSIFICATION OF PRIMARY IMMUNODEFICIENCY DISEASES

Humoral immunodeficiencies
X-linked hypogammaglobulinaemia
Transient hypogammaglobulinaemia of infancy
Common, variable, unclassifiable immunodeficiency
Selective IgA deficiency

Cellular (T-cell) immunodeficiencies
Congenital thymic aplasia (DiGeorge syndrome)

Combined immunodeficiencies
Severe combined immunodeficiency
Cellular immunodeficiency with abnormal immunoglobulin synthesis (Nezelof's syndrome)
Immunodeficiency with ataxia-telangiectasia
Immunodeficiency with eczema and thrombocytopenia (Wiskott–Aldrich syndrome)
Immunodeficiency with lymphotoxins

Phagocytic deficiencies
Chronic granulomatous disease
Myeloperoxidase deficiency
Chediak–Higashi syndrome
Job's syndrome

Complement deficiencies

Abnormalities of polymorph function, and deficiencies of complement components or antibodies, all result in susceptibility to bacterial infection. Deficiencies of the humoral and cellular components of the specific immunological system may occur separately or together. The information box indicates the probable sites of the primary defects in the immune system for a number of clinical patterns that have been recognised. The more precise analysis of these immunodeficiencies is being greatly aided by the development of monoclonal antibody markers for the different T cell subsets, for the different stages of maturity of B cells, and for monocytes.

Severe combined immunodeficiency syndrome

This condition, which can be caused by several different gene defects, autosomal or X-linked, is characterised by a defect of stem cells that leads to deficiency in both the T and B lymphocyte systems and therefore to impairment of cell-mediated immunity and of synthesis of humoral antibody. Failure of stem-cell development at an early stage of development gives the additional feature of agranulocytosis although the red cells and platelets are normal. About half the infants with the autosomal recessive form of severe combined immunodeficiency have a concomitant deficiency of adenosine deaminase which has enabled prenatal diagnosis by finding the enzyme deficiency in cultured amnion cells. The affected infants are susceptible to even the most benign viral infections, and may die from generalised chickenpox, measles, cytomegalovirus or other viral infections. When smallpox vaccination is inadvertently given to affected infants, this results in progressive, ultimately fatal vaccinia infection; similarly they are at risk of severe disease if given BCG.

Deficiency of immunoglobulins

Primary hypogammaglobulinaemia
Selective deficiency of the B lymphocyte system occurs in X-linked recessive hypo- or agammaglobulinaemia. The lack of immunoglobulins is not absolute but the patient fails to respond to antigenic stimuli. However, cell mediated immunity is normal. This disorder is compatible with survival for many years, though the patient is very susceptible to bacterial infections.

Common variable immunodeficiency
Most patients with immunoglobulin deficiency have 'acquired' or 'late onset' hypogammaglobulinaemia known as 'common, variable immunodeficiency'. This is associated with an unusually high incidence of auto-immune disease, such as pernicious anaemia and haemolytic anaemia. An occasional complication is a malabsorption syndrome which may be due to *Giardia lamblia* infection.

Isolated immunoglobulin deficiencies
IgM deficiency renders the patient susceptible to blood-borne infection such as that due to the meningo-coccus. Lack of IgA may be associated with gastro-intestinal or respiratory tract infections.

Hypogammaglobulinaemia of prematurity
Maternal IgG is transferred across the placenta during the third trimester of pregnancy. Premature babies may thus have some degree of hypogammaglobulinaemia; for them, prophylactic IgG treatment may reduce the incidence of infections.

Other causes of immunoglobulin deficiency
Immunoglobulin deficiency may result from abnormal losses of serum proteins, for example in lymphangi-ectasia. Drugs may also depress the immune system; for example phenytoin or penicillamine may induce IgA deficiency.

Deficiency of cellular immunity

Thymic aplasia
In this disease there is a selective deficiency of T lymphocytes, with severe lymphocytopenia and a pre-dominance of reticulum cells in the lymphoid tissue. Because T cell mediated immunity is deficient, affected children do not respond in the normal way to antigens such as candida and tuberculin on skin testing. Infants with thymic aplasia are highly susceptible to viral infections, which usually prove fatal.

Secondary T cell deficiency
Secondary T cell defects may occur in Hodgkin's disease or sarcoidosis, and following infections such as leprosy, miliary tuberculosis or measles. It may also result from loss of lymphocytes from the gut in protein-losing enteropathy, or due to thoracic duct fistula, and may be caused by treatment with cytotoxic drugs.

Diseases of complement

Deficiencies of complement components
In the inherited complement deficiencies there is usually a total absence of the complement protein and this implies the lack of a functional gene. The associ-ation of C1, 4 and 2 deficiencies with immune complex-like or lupus-like disorders is probably due to the failure to eliminate immune complexes.

Deficiency of a complement inhibitor
The interactions between the complement system and the clotting, fibrinolytic and kinin pathways are illustrated in the condition of hereditary angio-oedema resulting from a deficiency of C1 inhibitor. This auto-somal dominant condition causes sporadic attacks of tissue oedema often affecting the face and gut. Blood levels of C1 inhibitor are well below normal and the angio-oedema is probably produced by excessive action of C1 leading to high levels of an active peptide derived from C2, C2 kinin. The disease is treated either by the drug danazol which increases the level of C1 inhibitor, or by decreasing the activity of plasmin with epsilon aminocaproic acid.

PRINCIPLES OF IMMUNOTHERAPY

The immune response to antigens and other extrinsic agents is mounted by B and T cells and their subsets to produce specific antibodies and T cells and embraces many non-antigen specific humoral and cellular reactions and host tissue reactions to immune signals. Accordingly, there is enormous potential for preventive and therapeutic manipulation of immunity. There are promising indications that the clinical application of our knowledge and technology in this field will develop rapidly.

IMMUNISATION

Active immunisation

Induction of protective immunity to many infectious diseases is the most successful and most widely applied example of immunotherapy. For active immunisation it is necessary to administer several doses of material which will induce a host-protective immune response in the form of serum antibodies, secretory antibodies or T cell mediated reactivity. In developing further strategies for immunisation against diseases not currently covered, knowledge of the natural history of the disease is essential. For example if some of the clinical manifestations are due to the host immune response rather than the pathogen itself, as in some parasite infections, care must be taken to induce mainly protective (e.g. IgG, IgA), rather than immunopathological (e.g. IgE, T cell) immunity.

Passive immunisation

Administration of immunoglobulin (preferably human) of known high antibacterial or antiviral titre is of proven clinical value in the prevention and treatment of specific infections. This is particularly so in immuno-compromised individuals, for example when immunoglobulin of high titre anti-cytomegalovirus activity is used in bone marrow transplant recipients.

SPECIFIC TREATMENT OF IMMUNODEFICIENCY SYNDROMES

Knowledge of the precise mechanism and natural history of the condition is essential for the proper use of immunotherapy, either to cure by transplantation, or to treat by more temporary means such as giving immunoglobulin on a regular basis. Specific drugs to enhance immune responses are used in immunology research, as 'adjuvants' given along with antigen to stimulate immune responsiveness to antigen given at the same time. Immune modulatory agents are also used in some vaccines, e.g. alum salts given with diphtheria toxoid and tetanus toxoid as adjuvants.

With increasing experience of the use of interleukins and new techniques to enable their production in bulk, specific molecular immunotherapy of immunodeficiency states may become a reality.

The stem cell deficiency in the severe combined immunodeficiency syndrome can be replaced by bone marrow transplantation, and 10-year survivals with maintenance of normal T and B cell function have been recorded in a few children. In thymic aplasia, transplantation of fragments of human fetal thymus provides the necessary educative environment for host stem cells to develop into normal T cells, and this corrects the cellular immune deficiency.

Hypogammaglobulinaemia is treated by immunoglobulin injections (i.m. or i.v.). These consist mainly of IgG and can provide effective protection against severe, recurrent pyogenic infections. Since the half-life of the gammaglobulin injected is approximately four weeks, patients are usually given a monthly injection of 100 mg/kg.

TREATMENT OF HYPERSENSITIVITY BY MANIPULATION OF ANTIGEN EXPOSURE

Reduction of antigen load

The classical example of this is the use of an elimination diet to treat a food allergy. For example withdrawal of cows' milk in infants with enteropathy, colitis or eczema associated with cows' milk allergy; the use of a gluten-free diet in coeliac disease; and the strict avoidance of a food such as fish, egg, peanut, to which anaphylactic reaction has previously occurred.

Reduction of the antigen load is also important in inhalant allergies, for example the use of a mask by farmers with farmer's lung, bird breeders with bird fancier's lung; changes in bedding, curtains, etc. in children with asthma and house dust mite sensitivity.

Hyposensitisation

Anaphylactic individuals can be made less sensitive by multiple subcutaneous injections of antigen in gradually increasing dosage. Pollen antigens can be used to prevent the development of hay fever and asthma in some patients. The patient develops IgG antibodies against the antigen; these antibodies have a higher avidity for the antigen than do IgE antibodies and are able to compete successfully for the antigenic sites on the pollen or other allergen. These IgG antibodies are referred to as blocking antibodies. Hyposensitisation regimens may also induce other suppressor mechanisms that ultimately down-regulate IgE biosynthesis.

DRUGS USED TO TREAT ALLERGY AND ALLERGIC REACTIONS

Most of these act on the mast cell and block the effects of mast cell mediators, or have an antagonistic effect.

Sodium cromoglycate

This drug inhibits the release of the mediators from mast cells after the interaction of antigens with IgE antibodies. It is partially effective in preventing the induction of asthma by specific antigens. If inhaled by an asthmatic subject before exposure to the antigen, protection may last for several hours, but if given after exposure to the antigen it has little effect. The drug is also beneficial in exercise-induced asthma.

Antihistamines

The antihistamines occupy the same tissue receptors as histamine without providing any stimulus to the effector cells. The intravenous injection of an antihistamine quickly produces adequate tissue concentrations. The weal, the erythema and the itch of acute urticaria are reduced but there is no consistent improvement in lung function in acute bronchial asthma.

The failure of the antihistamines to relieve airway obstruction caused by an anaphylactic reaction has been attributed to high concentrations of histamine close to the smooth muscle cells. It may also be due to the presence of other mediators of the anaphylactic response. For example, bradykinin is rapidly inactivated in plasma by a kininase but its effects are not inhibited by antihistamines.

Adrenaline and related drugs

These act by producing effects which oppose the mediators and are more effective in emergencies than the antihistamines. Adrenaline, isoprenaline and aminophylline are efficient bronchodilators in bronchial asthma and in anaphylaxis. Urticaria is relieved and where oedema threatens the airway, the risk of asphyxia is lessened.

Despite their effectiveness these non-specific antagonists have serious disadvantages. They act on receptors that differ from those occupied by the mediators, and their effects never precisely counteract those of the mediators. The dose of a sympathomimetic amine which relieves airflow obstruction may produce tachycardia and palpitations even when the amine is administered as an aerosol. Salbutamol does not have these disadvantages as it is more specific in its actions on β-adrenergic receptors in the bronchi.

Corticosteroids

Corticosteroids such as prednisolone interfere at many points in the immune response, affecting lymphocyte recirculation and cytotoxic effector cells. The anti-inflammatory effect of steroids is due to their inhibition of neutrophil adherence to vascular endothelium in an inflammatory area and suppression of monocyte/macrophage functions such as microbicidal activity and response to lymphokines.

Immunosuppressive drugs

The production of immunoglobulins and the cellular immune response are dependent upon the division of lymphoid cells. Drugs that interfere with dividing cells are therefore all potentially immunosuppressive and were originally developed as anti-tumour agents. Of these, azathioprine, cyclophosphamide and methotrexate have been used for immunosuppression. Such drugs may have serious adverse effects, including bone marrow suppression and recrudescence of latent tuberculous, viral or fungal infection. A further possible hazard is an increased incidence of malignant tumours, such as lymphomas, possibly on account of the suppression of immunological surveillance of the body tissues in relation to infection with oncogenic viruses.

Cyclosporin A

This is a naturally occurring fungal metabolite. It suppresses both humoral and cell mediated immunity, and has been shown to have a direct suppressive (but non-cytotoxic) effect on B cells and T helper cells. Resting cells which carry the vital memory of immunity to microbial infections are spared and there is little toxicity for dividing cells in the gut and bone marrow. Cyclosporin must be used at doses below those causing nephrotoxicity so that blood levels have to be monitored regularly.

PLASMAPHERESIS

Apheresis is the generic term for removal of a component from the blood; a prefix indicates whether this is plasma, leucocytes, etc. Plasmapheresis (plasma exchange) has been used beneficially in myasthenia gravis and Goodpasture's syndrome, removing acetylcholine-receptor and glomerular basement membrane antibodies respectively. It is sometimes used in conjunction with cytotoxic drugs and corticosteroids in order to retard the resynthesis of antibody.

FURTHER READING

Male DK, Champion B, Cooke A, (eds.) Advanced
  Immunology. J B Lippincott Company, Philadelphia 1987.
Roitt IM, (ed.) Essential Immunology 1988 Blackwell

Scientific Publications, Oxford.
Roitt IM, Brostoff J, Male DK, (eds.) Immunology 1987
  Churchill Livingstone, Edinburgh.

3

Nutritional Factors in Disease

No medical history is complete without enquiring about the patient's food and drink intake. What people eat is one of the major environmental influences that affects health and can sooner or later contribute to disease. Lack of food or of essential nutrients in food also leads to disease. The word nutrition comes from the Latin *'nutrire'* which means to breast feed or nurse and from the time of Hippocrates diet has been a primary part of the management of sick people. Modern physicians can in addition use purified nutrients and parenteral formulas and they advise healthy people about prudent eating to suit the individual.

STUDY AND CLINICAL APPLICATIONS OF NUTRITION

Origins of specific knowledge about nutrition
For at least 99% of the time *homo sapiens* has been evolving from his primate precursors he has been a hunter-gatherer (Table 3.1). Agriculture started only 10 000 years ago, so that our bodies have presumably evolved well adapted for eating hunter-gatherers' food. We have information from archaeological records and from studies of the few fast-disappearing groups of contemporary hunter-gatherers.

From peoples who eat different foods from us, under stable conditions or during a disaster, we can form hypotheses about the physiological effects of different food patterns. For example we have learnt about the role of very long chain polyunsaturated fatty acids from the Eskimos and about deficiency diseases from nutritional observations by medical prisoners of war.

Knowledge has also been derived from controlled

experiments in humans and animals and from food analysis. A list of human experiments and trials is shown in the information box below.

HUMAN EXPERIMENTS AND TRIALS

- Absorption and uptake studies e.g. Glycaemic index
- Metabolic balance studies e.g. Nitrogen or sterol
- Energy expenditure
- Single nutrient depletion studies
- Dietary intervention trials e.g. Reduced saturated fat diet
- Long-term testing on value and safety of novel protein foods
- Pharmacokinetic studies of food additives
- Trials of vitamin C for prevention of colds

Some clinical records. These have been informative about the role of diet in disease, including some of the inborn errors of metabolism. Information about requirements for trace elements has come recently from experiences with total parenteral nutrition.

Epidemiological studies. These range in the power of their design. Associations and correlations of disease characteristics and dietary variables do not prove cause and effect, but prospective (cohort) studies, especially if repeated in different groups, give valuable information on the relation between usual diets and chronic diseases, e.g. dietary fat and coronary heart disease.

Food analysis. Food constituents are the independent variables in nutritional epidemiology and in the

Table 3.1   Nutrition at 5 stages of technical development

Stage	People and their food	Characteristic nutritional disorders
Hunter-gatherers (HG)	Our ancestors till 10 000 years ago or less. Few contemporary HGs left, e.g. !Kung Bushmen. Collect wide range of veg foods; also eat meat (lean if terrestrial) and fish. No salt, alcohol, milk (other than mother's), little cereal or sugar (wild honey)	Lean (no obesity) Malnutrition unlikely No coronary disease, hypertension, no dental caries or alcoholism
Pastoralists	Follow their grazing animals where adequate pasture, e.g. Lapps, Tibetans, Mongols, Tuareg, Fulani, Masai. Diet high in animal foods and milk	Least studied of all groups Some groups are tall Persistence of adult lactase
Peasant agriculturalists	Nearly all rural people in Third World and in industrial countries till this century. Tend to rely on one crop which yields best. Vulnerable to crop disease, crop toxin and to drought. Seasonal shortages. Milling and refining cereals increases risk of malnutrition.	Famine in areas with unreliable rainfall Malnutrition from lack of some nutrient(s) in staple food, e.g. kwashiorkor, pellagra, beriberi Mycotoxins. Hypertension but no coronary disease
Urban slum and periurban shanty	The poor masses in and round the rapidly growing cities of today's Third World. Similar situation in London, New York, etc. in 19th century. Loss of food traditions, no home gardens, mothers often have to work, poor food hygiene, food expensive	Children most vulnerable; not breast fed; gastroenteritis and marasmus Rickets in high latitudes Alcoholism. Adults may be obese Hypertension but not coronary disease
Affluent societies	Favourite food year round. High fat diet. Processed, convenience and take-away food. Tower of Babel of nutritional breakthroughs, scares and advice. Alternative and unorthodox advice. 'Health foods.' Many take vitamin tablets	Malnutrition confined to hospital patients and the elderly disabled. Coronary heart disease common 'Nutritional hypochondriasis' Hypersensitivity to foods apparently common Obesity unfashionable but difficult to avoid – Anorexia nervosa

dietetic treatment of disease. Food analysis is work that is never finished; foods keep changing and demand develops for constituents not measured before such as certain fatty acids, trace elements or natural toxicants.

Animal experiments. These were the principal technique for working out the vitamins. The right animal model has to be used, for example the guinea pig in the study of vitamin C (p. 65).

Nutrition and disease

Like immune reactions and infections, nutrition can affect any organ of the body or several at once. Different parts of the whole field of human nutrition are used regularly by different specialists. Cardiologists are interested in dietary fats and plasma cholesterol, nephrologists in protein deficiency and in potassium excess, gastroenterologists in multiple deficiencies from malabsorption, in dietary fibre and in hypersensitivity to whear and milk, neurologists are interested in alcohol excess and thiamin deficiency, haematologists in deficiencies of iron, folate and vitamin B_{12}, psychiatrists in anorexia nervosa, geriatricians in the effects of drugs on nutritional status and general practitioners in dietary advice for pregnancy and middle age and in infant feeding. Consequently some nutritional disorders are dealt with in this chapter; others have their main description elsewhere in the book.

There are differences also between Third World and industrial countries in the nutritional knowledge used in everyday practice. Which nutritional disorders are common depends on where and with whom one is working (Table 3.1), but the study of human nutrition has grown because some workers have taken a global view. Our understanding of protein deficiency and of dietary fibre originated in Africa; human zinc deficiency was first described in the Middle East and selenium deficiency in China. On the other hand some 'Western diseases' like diabetes mellitus are now increasingly occurring in tropical countries.

Uses of nutritional knowledge in clinical medicine

Primary nutritional diseases. Some diseases result primarily from disturbed nutrition – the major deficiency diseases and obesity. These are described in this chapter.

Deficiency diseases seldom present in pure form. More often than not they are secondary to some other illness. Even where food is short all the members of a community are not equally affected. Individuals with some physical or mental abnormality usually show clinical manifestations first.

When malnutrition occurs it is unlikely to involve only one nutrient. Even if the clinical features suggest a single deficiency, biochemical tests usually reveal depletion of other nutrients. Treatment should therefore not be confined to large intakes of the nutrient whose deficiency is indicated by the clinical signs. Furthermore, malnourished patients are liable to complications, especially certain infections which may be the presenting illness or may occur in modified form because malnutrition has suppressed some of their characteristic signs. Thus complications of malnutrition must be looked for and treated. Much of the skill in diagnosing patients with malnutrition is being aware of and disentangling predisposing illnesses, other associated malnutrition and complicating diseases.

Secondary nutritional depletion. In developed countries, patients in hospital for long periods with a serious illness are very likely to develop some degree of nutritional depletion such as protein-calorie malnutrition and/or other deficiencies, e.g. of folate, potassium or iron. It is important to monitor patients' nutrition and provide appropriate support because nutritionally-depleted patients are weaker and have impaired wound healing and reduced resistance to infection. The principles of nutritional diagnosis and management for hospital patients are summarised in this chapter (pp. 70–74).

Dietary modification as treatment. Some diseases, notably coeliac disease, hepatic encephalopathy and phenylketonuria are not caused by disturbed nutrition, but for each of them a specific modification of the usual diet is the principal treatment, which may be life saving. In other conditions, e.g. diabetes mellitus and mild hypertension, the appropriate diet is useful treatment, alternative or complementary to drugs. In other chapters therapeutic diets are outlined under the diseases concerned. Examples of diet sheets for obesity, diabetes and hypercholesterolaemia appear in the Appendix. Space does not allow inclusion of others; the reader is referred to a textbook of nutrition and dietetics (p. 78).

Chronic degenerative diseases. Evidence is accumulating that the habitual diet is one of the multiple causative factors in many chronic degenerative diseases (e.g. coronary heart disease, hypertension, diabetes mellitus, dental caries and diverticular disease) and even in some carcinomas (e.g. stomach, liver and large bowel). These diseases take a long time to develop; exactly which dietary components are involved, and how closely, needs discussion and is often controversial.

Elsewhere in this book the role of diet is mentioned briefly in the paragraphs on aetiology of the different diseases.

CLASSIFICATION OF NUTRITIONAL DISORDERS

These disorders are listed in the information box.

CLASSIFICATION OF NUTRITIONAL DISORDERS

Undernutrition	Insufficient food energy and causing starvation (adults), marasmus (children)
Malnutrition	Deficiency of protein or other essential nutrients (Table 3.2)
Obesity	From prolonged positive energy balance
Nutrient excess	Harmful in short or long-term, e.g. iron overload, alcohol, vitamin D, saturated fat
Effect of toxicants	e.g. in coeliac disease, urticaria, favism, migraine

Nutrients can be subdivided into four groups as shown in the information box below.

SUBDIVISION OF NUTRIENTS

- Energy-yielding, e.g. carbohydrates, fats, proteins, alcohol
- Water, electrolytes and other essential (inorganic) elements
- Vitamins
- Fibre

Table 3.2 Size of adult requirements for different nutrients

Adult daily requirement in foods	Essential nutrients for man
2–10 µg	Vit B$_{12}$, vit D, vit K, Cr
c.100 µg	Biotin, I, Se
200 µg	Folate, Mo
1–2 mg	Vit A, thiamin, riboflavin, vit B$_6$, F, Cu
5–10 mg	Pantothenate, Mn
c.15 mg	Niacin, vit E, Fe, Zn
c.50 mg	Vit C
300 mg	Mg
c.1 g	Ca, P
1–5 g	Na, Cl, K, essential fatty acids
c.50 g	Protein (8–10 essential amino acids)
50–100 g	Available carbohydrate
1 kg (l)	Water

Figures are approximate, in places rounded to fit with others on a line. The range of requirements for different nutrients is about 10^9. In addition sulphur is required in the form of the amino acids, methionine and cysteine. Cobalt is required in the form of vitamin B$_{12}$.

In this chapter the nutritional diseases will be described under these headings and obesity will be considered on p. 74.

ENERGY-YIELDING NUTRIENTS

Carbohydrates (4 kcal/g). These usually provide a major part of the energy in a normal diet. No individual carbohydrate is an essential nutrient in the sense that the body needs it but cannot make it for itself from other nutrients. If the carbohydrate intake is less than 100 g per day ketosis is likely to occur. Sugars are found in fruits, milk (lactose) and some vegetables. Starches are mostly found in cereals and root vegetables and legumes. Most forms of dietary fibre are poly-saccharides too but these cannot be digested in the small intestine. The major carbohydrates in food are listed in the information box below.

SOURCES OF CARBOHYDRATES IN FOOD

Available sugars
Monosaccharides – ribose, glucose, fructose
Disaccharides – sucrose, lactose, maltose

Available polysaccharides
Starch, glycogen, synthetic glucose polymers

Unavailable polysaccharides
Most forms of dietary fibre (p. 70)

Fats. With their high calorie value (9 kcal/g) fats are useful to people with a large energy expenditure. On the other hand they are an insidious cause of obesity for sedentary people. Saturated fats, especially those containing palmitic (16:0) and myristic (14:0) acids increase plasma low-density lipoproteins and total cholesterol. Monounsaturated fatty acids contain one double bond, e.g. oleic acid (18:1 ω9); polyunsaturated fatty acids, with two or more double bonds are in two main groups, depending on the distance of their first double bond, counting from the methyl (ω) end of the molecule. The principal fatty acid in plant seed oils is linoleic acid (18:2 ω6). This and its elongated ω6 derivatives linoleic acid (18:3 ω6) and arachidonic acid (20:4 ω6) are the essential fatty acids (EFAs), precursors of the prostaglandins and part of the structure of lipid membranes in all cells.

Essential fatty acid deficiency is rare in man but it has been reported in patients fed solely by vein for long periods without fat emulsions. If sufficient glucose and amino acids are given they inhibit free fatty acid mobilisation from adipose tissue (where there is usually a moderate store of linoleic acid) and tissues in the rest of the body become depleted. There is a scaly dermatitis and the diagnosis can be confirmed biochemically by an increased ratio of eicosatrienoic acid ($20:3 \omega 9$) to arachidonic in plasma lipids.

The $\omega 3$ series of polyunsaturated fatty acids, e.g. eicosapentaenoic ($20:5 \omega 3$) and docosahexaenoic ($22:6 \omega 3$) occur in fish oils. Though not essential they are inhibitors of thrombosis and appear to act by competitively antagonising thromboxane A2 formation (p. 50). Purified fish body oils, e.g. 'Maxepa' are one of the treatment options which may reduce the tendency to thrombosis, e.g. in people with coronary heart disease.

Proteins. These provide some 20 amino acids, of which eight are essential for normal synthesis of the different proteins in the body and for maintaining nitrogen balance in adults. These *essential amino acids* are listed in the information box below.

ESSENTIAL AMINO ACIDS

- Methionine
- Lysine
- Tryptophan
- Phenylalanine
- Leucine
- Isoleucine
- Threonine
- Valine

Histidine and perhaps arginine are also needed for growth in infants.

The 'biological value' of different proteins depends on the relative proportions of essential amino acids they contain. Proteins of animal origin, particularly from eggs, milk and meat, are generally of higher biological value than the proteins of vegetable origin which are deficient in one or more of the essential amino acids. However it is possible to have a diet of mixed vegetable proteins with high biological value if the principle of *complementation* is used. For example cereals, e.g. wheat, contain about 10% protein and are relatively deficient in lysine. Legumes contain around 20% of protein which is relatively deficient in methionine. If two parts of wheat are mixed (or eaten) with one part of legume, a food results which contains 13% protein of high biological value. This happens because cereals contain enough methionine and legumes enough lysine to supplement the other component of the mixture.

The usual recommended allowance for an adequate protein intake is 10% of the total calories, i.e. about 65 g

Table 3.3 Potentially toxic substances in foods

Natural	
Inherent, naturally occurring	Usually present in the food and affects everyone if they eat enough, e.g. solanine in potatoes (green sprouts); tropical spinal ataxia from cassava
Toxin resulting from abnormal conditions of animal or plant used for food	e.g. Neurotoxic mussel poisoning; ergotism
Consumer abnormally sensitive	e.g. Coeliac disease from wheat gluten; allergy to particular food; or drug-induced, e.g. cheese reaction
Contamination by pathogenic bacteria	Acute illness, usually gastrointestinal, e.g. toxins produced by *Staphylococcus aureus* or *Clostridium botulinum*
Mycotoxins	Food mouldy or spoiled, e.g. aflatoxin B, from *Aspergillus flavus* is a liver carcinogen
Man made	
Unintentional additives – man-made chemical used in agriculture and animal husbandry	e.g. Fungicides on grain, insecticides on fruit, antibiotics or hormones given to animals
Environmental pollution	e.g. Organic mercury, cadmium, lead, PCB and radioactive fall-out can affect any stage of food chain
Intentional food additives – preservatives, emulsifiers, flavours, colours, etc.	The most thoroughly tested and monitored of all chemicals in foods. Occasional individuals hypersensitive, e.g. to some azo colours

per day for the average adult. The minimum requirement is around 40 g of protein of good biological value.

Energy requirements. The largest component of energy expenditure is the basal metabolic rate (BMR). This increases with lean body mass (which is related to weight and height); it declines with age and is less in women than men. Extra energy is required for growth, pregnancy and lactation, for muscular activity and for pyrexia. There is considerable variation of energy expended between individuals of the same size, age, sex and activity. Adaptation occurs to an inadequate energy intake and to a lesser degree to superfluous energy intake. Approximate daily energy requirements are listed in the information box below.

DAILY ENERGY REQUIREMENTS

- Apyrexial males in bed in industrial countries — 2000 kcal
- Male office workers in industrial countries — 2700 kcal
- Subsistence farmers in developing countries — 2800 kcal
- Men doing heavy work — 3500 kcal
- Apyrexial females in bed in industrial countries — 1600 kcal
- Healthy housewives in industrial countries — 2000 kcal
- Rural women in developing countries — 2250 kcal

Individuals in Britain, including children, need somewhere around 2500 kcal per day. The food moving into consumption has to provide more to allow for wastage, pets, tourists, etc. This gross value, around 3000 kcal, is easier to estimate. It is this higher figure that is discussed in the press and parliament and often confused with average physiological requirements.

There are two units in use for energy: kilocalories and kilo-joules (1 kcal = 4.184 kJ). Though both are metric, joules are SI units and are preferred in Europe for scientific usage.

STARVATION

Starvation is severe undernutrition from a prolonged negative energy balance. What follows here describes the features seen in adults and older children. In infants and pre-school children a similar process (marasmus) is described on page 51.

Aetiology
The main causes of undernutrition and starvation are listed in the information box below.

CAUSES OF UNDERNUTRITION

- Insufficient food
- Persistent regurgitation or vomiting
- Anorexia
- Malabsorption, e.g. small intestine disease
- Increased BMR, e.g. thyrotoxicosis, prolonged infections
- Loss of calories, e.g. glycosuria in diabetes mellitus
- Cachexia

Clinical features
Children stop growing and adults lose weight. The symptoms include craving for food, thirst, weakness, feeling cold, nocturia, amenorrhoea and impotence.

The face at first looks younger but later becomes old, withered and expressionless. The skin is lax, pale and dry and may show pigmented patches. Hair becomes thinned or lost except in adolescents. The extremities are cold and cyanosed and there may be pressure sores. Subcutaneous fat disappears, skin turgor is lost, and muscles waste. The arm circumference is subnormal. Oedema may be present in famine victims without hypoalbuminaemia ('famine oedema'). Body temperature is subnormal. The pulse is slow, blood pressure low and the heart small. The abdomen is distended and diarrhoea is common. Tendon jerks are diminished. Psychologically, starving people lose initiative; they are apathetic, depressed and introverted but become aggressive if food is nearby.

Under-nourished individuals are susceptible to infections. With respiratory muscles weakened by wasting, bronchopneumonia carries an increased mortality. Starving groups in famines have often had high mortalities from epidemics, e.g. typhus or cholera. The usual signs of infection may not appear. In advanced starvation patients become completely inactive and may assume a flexed, fetal position. Death comes quietly and often quite suddenly in the last stage of starvation. The very old are most vulnerable. All the organs are atrophied at necropsy except the brain which tends to maintain its weight.

Investigation
The investigations into starvation are listed in the information box below.

INVESTIGATIONS IN STARVATION

- Plasma free fatty acids – increased
- Ketosis – mild metabolic acidosis
- Hypoglycaemia
- Diminished insulin secretion
- Increased plasma glucagon concentrations
- Increased plasma cortisol concentrations
- Reverse T_3 replaces normal triiodothyronine
- Reduced resting metabolic rate
- Fixed SG in urine
- Low urinary creatinine
- Mild anaemia, leucopenia, thrombocytopenia
- Tests of delayed skin sensitivity gives false negative
- ECG shows sinus bradycardia and low voltages

Management
Whether in a famine or dealing with wasting secondary to disease, people or patients need to be graded (Table 3.4).

People with mild starvation are in no danger; those with moderate starvation need extra feeding. People who are severely underweight need hospital type care. 1500 to 2000 kcal/day will prevent the downward progress of undernutrition.

In severe starvation there is atrophy of the intestinal epithelium and of the exocrine pancreas and bile is dilute. When food becomes available the extra should be given in small amounts at first. Food should be bland

Table 3.4 Grades of undernutrition

1. Mild undernutrition (starvation) = weight for height from 90% down to 81% of standard* (BMI 20–18).
2. Moderate undernutrition (starvation) = weight for height from 80% down to 71% of standard* (BMI 18–16)
3. Severe undernutrition (starvation) = weight for height 70% of standard* or less (BMI less than 16).

* See Table 3.6.

and preferably similar to the usual staple meal, for example a cereal with some sugar, milk powder and oil. Salt should be restricted and a multivitamin preparation is desirable. A refeeding schedule of 1 month to replace every 5% loss of body weight is a good guide.

Circumstances and resources are different in every famine. The problems are mainly non-medical, e.g. organising transport and repair of trucks and shelters or co-ordinating relief from different organisations, reconciling international workers with local politicians and administrators, arranging security of food stores, ensuring that food is distributed on the basis of need and trying to procure the right food and appropriate medical supplies. Civil disturbances do not occur during severe famine. They may happen at an early stage (food riots) or afterwards (revolution). Lastly, plans must be made for the future; for example, agricultural workers will be needed with enough strength to plough and plant the next crop when the rains return.

PROTEIN-ENERGY MALNUTRITION (IN YOUNG CHILDREN)

Classification and epidemiology

Severe protein-energy malnutrition (PEM or protein-calorie malnutrition) in early childhood is a spectrum of disease. At one end there is *kwashiorkor* in which the essential feature is deficiency of protein with relatively adequate energy intake. At the other end is *nutritional marasmus* which is total inanition of the infant, usually under one year of age, and which is due to a severe and prolonged restriction of all food, i.e. energy sources and other nutrients in addition to protein. In the middle of the spectrum is *marasmic kwashiorkor* in which there are clinical features of both disorders.

Some children adapt to prolonged energy and/or protein shortage by *nutritional dwarfism*. The most prevalent of all the varieties is *mild to moderate PEM* or the underweight child (Table 3.5). Children with one form of PEM often shift to another form. Thus a child with mild to moderate PEM may develop kwashiorkor

Table 3.5 Classification of PEM in young children

	Body weight as percentage of international standard	Oedema	Deficit in weight for height
Kwashiorkor	80–60	+	+
Marasmic kwashiorkor	< 60	+	+ +
Marasmus	< 60	0	+ +
Nutritional dwarfing	< 60	0	minimal
Underweight child	80–60	0	+

For international standard weights see Table 3.6.

after an infection. Such a child, when treated, loses oedema and may look marasmic. In marasmus there is a major loss of muscle, the body's main mass of protein as well as the loss of fat; in kwashiorkor anorexia is characteristic and leads to inadequate secondary energy intake. For reasons like these, marasmus, kwashiorkor and milder forms are grouped together as protein-energy malnutrition.

The incidence of PEM in its various forms is high in India and S.E. Asia, in most parts of Africa and the Middle East, in the Caribbean islands and in South and Central America. PEM is the most important dietary deficiency disease in the world. Severe forms affect around 2% and mild to moderate PEM affects around 20% (and in many places more) of young children in the Third World.

NUTRITIONAL MARASMUS

Aetiology

This is the commoner form of severe protein-energy malnutrition. It is the childhood version of starvation. It usually occurs in the second six months of life. The cause is a diet very low in calories and incidentally in protein and other essential nutrients. Typically the child was weaned early and fed with dilute cows' milk formulae. This is a disease of infants of poor mothers in the cities of developing countries. The mother may have to go out to work and leave her baby with its grandmother, older sister or a neighbour. She has difficulty paying for the feeds and has neither the kitchen equipment nor the knowledge to prepare them without bacterial contamination. Poor hygiene leads to gastroenteritis and a vicious cycle starts. Diarrhoea leads to poor appetite and the decision to give more dilute feeds. In turn further depletion leads to intestinal atrophy and more susceptibility to diarrhoea.

Clinical features

The child is very thin with no subcutaneous fat, and looks wizened and shrunken; its muscles are severely wasted (Fig. 3.1). The head is large for the body, the ribs stand out, the abdomen may be distended (with gas), the limbs look like sticks and the buttocks are baggy. Diarrhoea is usual. In contrast to kwashiorkor, there is no oedema and skin and hair changes are mild or absent. The child is not usually anorexic but the weight is reduced below 60% of standard (Table 3.6). Although the child has not been growing, weight is reduced more than length.

A search must be made for chronic infection like tuberculosis or other major disease (cardiac, renal, intestinal) that could produce secondary marasmus.

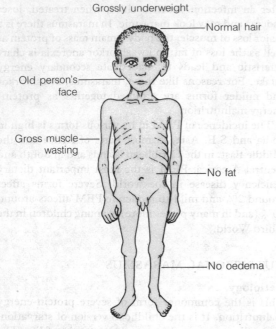

Grossly underweight

Normal hair

Old person's face

Gross muscle wasting

No fat

No oedema

Fig. 3.1   Marasmus.

Table 3.6   Reference or standard weights
Weight for age: birth to 5 years.[1] Sexes combined[2]

Weight (kg)				Weight (kg)			
Age (months)	Standard	80% Std	60% Std	Age (months)	Standard	80% Std	60% Std
0	3.25	2.6	1.95	31	13.45	10.8	8.1
1	4.15	3.3	2.5	32	13.65	10.9	8.2
2	4.95	4.0	3.0	33	13.85	11.1	8.3
3	5.7	4.6	3.4	34	14.05	11.2	8.4
4	6.35	5.1	3.8	35	14.15	11.3	8.5
5	7.0	5.6	4.2	36	14.35	11.5	8.6
6	7.5	6.0	4.5	37	14.55	11.6	8.7
7	8.0	6.4	4.8	38	14.7	11.8	8.8
8	8.5	6.8	5.1	39	14.9	11.9	8.9
9	8.9	7.1	5.3	40	15.05	12.0	9.0
10	9.2	7.4	5.5	41	15.2	12.2	9.1
11	9.55	7.6	5.7	42	15.4	12.3	9.2
12	9.85	7.9	5.9	43	15.5	12.4	9.3
13	10.1	8.1	6.1	44	15.7	12.6	9.4
14	10.35	8.3	6.2	45	15.85	12.7	9.5
15	10.55	8.4	6.3	46	16.05	12.8	9.6
16	10.75	8.6	6.45	47	16.15	12.9	9.7
17	10.95	8.8	6.6	48	16.35	31.1	9.8
18	11.15	8.9	6.7	49	16.5	13.2	9.9
19	11.35	9.1	6.8	50	16.6	13.3	10.0
20	11.5	9.2	6.9	51	16.8	13.4	10.1
21	11.7	9.4	7.0	52	16.95	13.6	10.2
22	11.85	9.5	7.1	53	17.1	13.7	10.3
23	12.05	9.6	7.2	54	17.25	13.8	10.4
24	12.25	9.8	7.35	55	17.45	14.0	10.5
25	12.25	9.8	7.35	56	17.55	14.1	10.5
26	12.45	10.0	7.47	57	17.7	14.2	10.6
27	12.65	10.1	7.6	58	17.85	14.3	10.7
28	12.85	10.3	7.7	59	18.0	14.4	10.8
29	13.05	10.4	7.8	60	18.2	14.6	10.9
30	13.25	10.6	7.95				

[1] Based on: A growth chart for international use in maternal and child health care 1978. WHO, Geneva.
[2] On average boys are 0.3 kg heavier and girls 0.3 kg lighter than the mean standard but the differences are smaller than this in the first 2 months and 0.4–0.5 kg from 50–60 months.

Dehydration frequently occurs from diarrhoea or vomiting. There may be associated deficiencies of vitamins, such as vitamin A causing keratomalacia and of inorganic nutrients such as potassium and magnesium. Associated infections are shown in the information box below.

INFECTIONS ASSOCIATED WITH PEM

Patients with marasmus, kwashiorkor and starvation have increased susceptibility to:
- Gastroenteritis and Gram-negative bacteraemia
- Respiratory infections
- Certain viral diseases, especially measles and herpes simplex
- Tuberculosis
- Streptococcal and staphylococcal skin infections
- Helminthic infestations

Management
Management of marasmus is *substantially* the same as for kwashiorkor (p. 53).

KWASHIORKOR

Aetiology
The name comes from Ghana where the condition was first described by Cicely Williams in 1933. This form of malnutrition occurs most often in the second year of life when the child is weaned from the breast on to a diet low in protein such as cassava, plantain or yam or to a cereal that has been refined and diluted. There is little milk and custom, sometimes reinforced by taboos, determines that the limited foods of animal origin are given to the men of the family, or the small amount of protein-rich food is in a sauce made with hot peppers or spices and unsuitable for young children. If the customary diet of a population is limited in protein and in calories to around the levels of minimum requirements, a child may be in moderate health until the protein requirements are increased by an infection. Gastroenteritis, measles and malaria are all notorious precipitants of kwashiorkor.

Pathogenesis
This is summarised in the information box (p. 53).

PATHOGENESIS OF KWASHIORKOR

- Low dietary protein + adequate carbohydrate
  ↓
- Insulin secretion maintained
- Insulin spares muscle protein at expense of liver protein
  ↓
- Fall in albumin
  ↓
- Oedema
- Free fatty acids from adipose tissue → liver → fatty liver

Clinical features

The child is not very thin. There is oedema which tends to be generalised. The child is miserable and apathetic and has a characteristic mewing cry. The skin shows symmetrical changes, maximally in the napkin (diaper) area. At first it is pigmented and thickened as if varnished, then it cracks and leads to denuded areas of shallow ulceration (Fig. 3.2). In moderate cases the areas of dermatosis resemble crazy paving; when severe the desquamated area can look as if the child has been

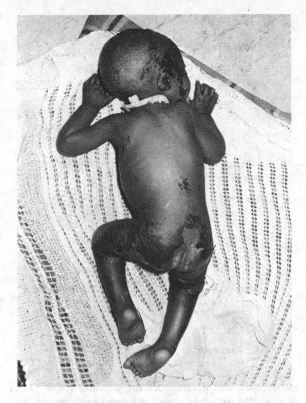

Fig. 3.3 A child with kwashiorkor, showing pigmented lesions especially over the buttocks, thighs, side of head and backs of hands. (By courtesy of Professor Walter Gordon.)

burnt (Fig. 3.3). The hair alters in colour from black to blond, reddish or grey; it becomes thin and sparse. Mucosal changes, such as angular stomatitis, may be seen. Anorexia is present and diarrhoea is common. The liver may be palpable (Fig. 3.4). The characteristic laboratory finding is a very low plasma albumin concentration.

Management

Severe PEM whether kwashiorkor or marasmus, is dealt with in three phases.

Resuscitation. This consists of correction of dehydration, electrolyte disturbances, acidosis, hypoglycaemia and hypothermia and also treatment for infections (p. 52).

Start of the cure. This consists of refeeding, gradually working up the calories to 150 kcal/kg with protein about 1.5 g/kg. The major units with research experience of PEM have each evolved somewhat different dietary formulas, depending on local

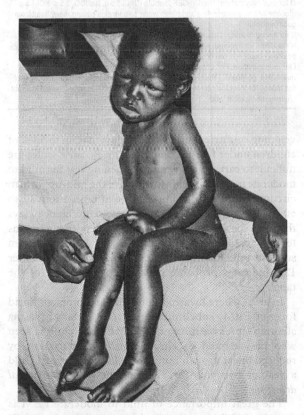

Fig. 3.2 A child with kwashiorkor, showing oedema of face, feet and hands, and skin lesions. (Photo by Dr. R.G. Whitehead.)

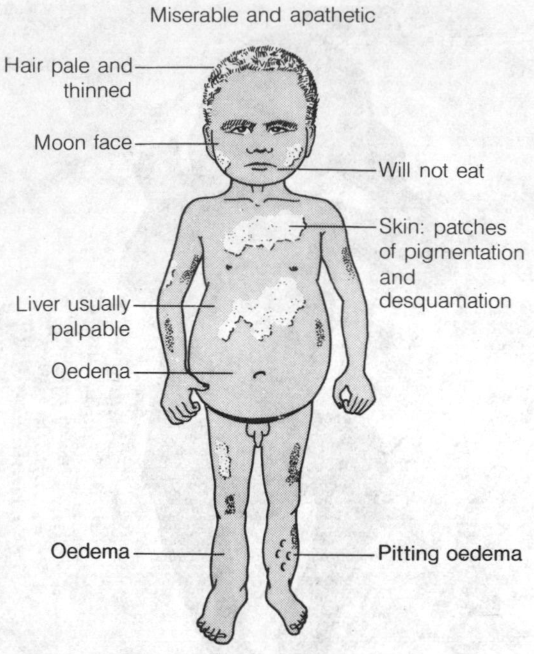

Miserable and apathetic

Hair pale and thinned

Moon face

Will not eat

Skin: patches of pigmentation and desquamation

Liver usually palpable

Oedema

Oedema

Pitting oedema

Fig. 3.4   Kwashiorkor.

availability and preferences for weaning foods. They are usually based on dried skimmed milk mixed with some flour or sugar and some oil and given 5–6 times a day. Because of anorexia, children often have to be handfed, preferably in the lap of their mother or a nurse they know. Potassium, magnesium and a multi-vitamin mixture are also needed.

Nutritional rehabilitation. After about 3 weeks the child should be obviously better. If there was oedema this will have cleared, any skin lesions are healing and diarrhoea has ceased. The child is stronger, mentally bright and has a good appetite but is still underweight for his or her age. During this stage of rehabilitation and catch-up growth, the child should be looked after in a convalescent home or by the mother who should have been educated about nutrition and helped to obtain extra food. The diet should be based on nutritious combinations of local, familiar foods.

Prognosis
Severe PEM has a mortality around 20% even in well-equipped hospitals. Most deaths occur in the first 10 days. Follow-up studies have shown that the fatty liver of acute kwashiorkor resolves quickly and does not go on to cirrhosis. Physical growth of the brain is retarded in children who suffer severe PEM in the first two years of life (usually marasmus). There is circumstantial

evidence that intelligence may be impaired, particularly if the child goes home to a poor environment.

MILD TO MODERATE PEM (THE UNDERWEIGHT CHILD)

For every florid case of kwashiorkor or marasmus there are likely to be 7 or 10 in the community with mild to moderate PEM. The situation is like an iceberg; there is more malnutrition below the surface than is recognisable on clinical inspection. Even the mothers themselves do not notice most of these cases because their children are similar in size and vitality to many others of the same age in the neighbourhood. Most children with subclinical PEM can, however, be detected by their weight for age, which is less than 80% of the international standard (Table 3.6). In parts of many de-

Table 3.7   UNICEF's inexpensive measures to prevent PEM

Mnemonic GOBI

G for *growth monitoring*. The mother keeps the simple growth chart – the Road to Health card – in a cellophane envelope and brings the child to a clinic regularly for weighing and advice

O for *oral rehydration*. The UNICEF formula (NaCl 3.5 g, NaHCO$_3$ 2.5 g, KCl 1.5 g, glucose 20 g or sucrose 40 g and clean water to a litre) is saving many lives from gastroenteritis

B for *breast feeding*. This is a matter of life and death in a poor community with no facilities for hygiene. Additional food – which should be prepared from locally available foods – is not usually needed until 6 months of age

I for *immunisation*. For a few dollars a child can be protected against measles, diphtheria, pertussis, tetanus, tuberculosis and poliomyletis. In a rational world the money for this could be taken from a small part of the $1 000 000 000 000 spent on armaments each year

veloping countries surveys may show that up to 50% of children under five are underweight. Because scales are difficult to carry, a convenient screening test for mild to moderate malnutrition is to measure the mid-upper arm circumference with a simple piece of tape. From 12 to 60 months of age the normal arm circumference stays the same for 4 years. Over 13.5 cm is a normal circumference (coloured green on the tape), 12.5 to 13.5 cm suggests mild malnutrition (coloured amber) and under 12.5 indicates probable malnutrition (red part of the tape).

In areas where kwashiorkor is the predominant florid form of PEM, subclinical cases have reduced plasma albumin ('prekwashiorkor'). Sometimes a child is seen who has adapted to chronic inadequate feeding by reduced linear growth but who looks like a normal child a year or two younger. This is known as *nutritional dwarfism*.

The great importance of mild to moderate PEM is that these children are growing up smaller than their potential and they are very susceptible to gastroenteritis and respiratory infections, which in turn can precipitate frank malnutrition. Mild to moderate PEM is probably the major underlying reason why the 1 to 4-year mortality in a developing country can be 30 to 40 times higher than in Europe or North America. Official statistics record most of these deaths as due simply to infections.

Prevention

Preventive measures for kwashiorkor and marasmus are listed in the information boxes below.

PREVENTION OF KWASHIORKOR

- Educate mothers
- Advice to farmers
- Provide food supplements in clinics
- Legumes, nuts and seeds (locally produced)

PREVENTION OF MARASMUS

- Family planning
- Immunisation programme
- Encourage breastfeeding
- Maternity and child health clinics

WATER, ELECTROLYTES AND MINERALS

Sixteen or more inorganic elements are essential for man, as they are for other animals; deficiency disease is known for each due to inadequate diet or from excessive losses. The elements are sodium (p. 205), potassium (p. 216), chloride magnesium (p. 221), calcium, phosphorus, iron, iodine, zinc, copper, chromium, selenium, manganese and molybdenum. Fluoride appears to be essential for rats and optimal intakes reduce dental caries in a man. Cobalt is physiologically active only in the form of vitamin B_{12} and sulphur is required in the form of the amino acids methionine and cysteine.

In addition tin, vanadium, nickel and silicon have been shown, by artificial isolator systems, to be essential for animals. Human deficiency disease is not known for any of these minor trace elements.

The normal distribution of water and electrolytes, sodium, potassium and chloride in the body and the disturbances which result when their intake or output is diminished or increased are discussed in detail on pages 204 to 221.

ELEMENTS OF IMPORTANCE IN HUMAN NUTRITION

Calcium

The body of an adult normally contains about 1200 g of calcium. At least 99% of this is present in the skeleton, where calcium salts (chiefly hydroxyapatite), held in a cellular matrix, provide the hard structure of the bones and teeth. The dietary sources are listed below.

DIETARY SOURCES OF CALCIUM

- Cheeses, milks, yoghurt and their products
- Fish eaten with bone, e.g., sardines, pilchards
- Some shellfish
- Some nuts, e.g., almonds, peanuts
- Some vegetables, e.g., chick peas, beans
- Egg and bread (fortified)

Absorption. In adults around 70% of the calcium in food is excreted in faeces; during growth the efficiency of absorption is greater. Calcium absorption may be impaired either by lack of vitamin D, by any condition causing small intestinal hurry, by the combination of calcium with excess fatty acids to form insoluble soaps in steatorrhoea, or by certain substances in the diet which can form insoluble salts with calcium. These include foods rich in oxalic acid (e.g. spinach) and phytic acid which is present in the outer layers of cereal grains. Hence 'wholemeal' bread contains more phytic acid than white.

Recommended intakes of calcium. The amount of calcium which has to be added to the bones to produce the final adult amount averages 180 mg/day from 0 to 18 years but reaches 400 mg/day at the peak of adolescent growth. Since calcium absorption is inefficient the recommended intake in Britain is 600 mg for children and 700 mg in adolescents. Expert opinion is divided on the safe minimum intake in adults. WHO recommended 500 mg/day because in many parts of Africa and Asia children develop and adults maintain healthy bones on this intake or lower. The USA recommends 800 mg for adults and 1000 mg have been advised for post-menopausal women. These figures are based on calcium balances. It appears that calcium is handled less economically by people in developed countries. Possible explanations include less skin synthesis of vitamin D from sunshine and increased obligatory urinary calcium because of high animal protein and sodium intakes. In pregnancy and lactation extra calcium is needed – 1200 mg per day.

Calcium is the most obvious and persistent of the

micro-nutrients, the fifth most abundant element, and the most abundant cation, in the body, yet it is more difficult to measure adequacy of intake for calcium than for other nutrients. Any reduction of absorbed calcium does not show in the plasma concentration, which is immediately reset by increased parathyroid secretion and formation of 1,25 dihydroxy-vitamin D, probably because any change of ionised plasma concentration would disturb neuromuscular irritability and blood co-agulation. Likewise intracellular plasma concentration, which affects activities of many enzymes, is also tightly controlled. If calcium intake is inadequate, therefore a little less will go into the bones in children or a little will be removed from the bones in adults. Small changes in total bone calcium can be measured only as research procedures at present.

The two major questions about calcium nutrition are:

1. Will a high intake during the growing phase of life contribute to taller adult height or heavier bones. If so, how much is optimal?
2. Will a high intake from about 45 years onwards delay the onset of osteoporosis (p. 804).

Phosphorus
This is used by the body in the form of phosphate which is present in all cells and so in all unrefined plant and animal foods and in milk. Dietary deficiency is rare. Usual dietary intakes are rather higher than for calcium, about 1.5 g/day. Total body phosphorus is about 700 g, most being in the bones.

Phosphate deficiency occurs in premature infants fed on human milk, in patients with Fanconi's syndrome and other forms of renal tubular phosphate loss, from prolonged high dosage of aluminium hydroxide antacids, sometimes when alcoholics are re-fed with high carbohydrate foods and in patients on total parenteral nutrition if not enough phosphate is pro-vided. The features of deficiency are hypophos-phataemia (subnormal plasma inorganic phosphorus) and muscle weakness.

Iron
A good mixed diet with average amounts of meat and vegetable contains about 12–15 mg of iron. Cheap, monotonous high carbohydrate diets based on refined wheat flour contain much less. Foods rich in iron are listed in the information box below.

DIETARY SOURCES OF IRON

- Meat, liver
- White meal cereals, oatmeal, peas, beans and lentils

There is no physiological mechanism for secretion of iron so maintenance of its homeostasis depends on iron absorption. Normally body iron loss from desquamated surface cells adds up to about 1 mg daily. Assuming 10% absorption, about 10 mg are therefore required in the diet daily in men, but if there is any bleeding this brings with it much more loss of iron. Blood is the tissue richest in iron; 1 ml contains 0.5 mg of iron so that a regular blood loss of only 2 ml/day doubles the iron requirement. At menstruation 30 mg of iron can be lost and considerably more in a few women.

An account of iron metabolism and of the measures for the prevention and treatment of iron deficiency anaemia is given on page 708. This is one of the most important nutritional causes of ill-health in Britain and other prosperous countries.

Siderosis. Dietary iron overload is seen in South African black men who cook and brew beer in iron pots. They may ingest as much as 100 mg of iron per day. Iron accumulates in the liver and when severe can lead to cirrhosis. A similar condition has been described in other countries following excessive indulgence in cheap wines which can contain 30 mg of iron per litre.

Iodine
This has the heaviest atomic weight of the essential elements. It is present in the sea, in seafoods and in trace amounts in soil and water over most of the land and in foods grown there. Iodine is lacking in the major mountainous areas of the world, e.g. the Alps, Himalayas, Rockies, Andes and the mountains of central America and Papua New Guinea. About 400 million people living in these areas are estimated to have an inadequate iodine intake and they show endemic goitre and other iodine deficiency disorders.

When visible goitres are found in 5% or more of the adolescents this indicates that the whole community has very low urinary iodine, e.g. <30 µg/per 1 g creatinine. Where most women have endemic goitre, 1% or more of the babies are born with cretinism and the other 'normal' people in the community show a higher pre-valence than usual of deafness, slowed reflexes and poor learning.

Endemic goitre has now almost disappeared from most of the low iodine regions of Europe and North America due to the use of iodised salt and inter-regional trade of foods. In remote mountainous parts of the Third World without roads, shops and a cash economy, iodised salt will not reach enough people and the best way of preventing cretinism is by injecting all women of child-bearing age with 1–2 ml of iodised poppyseed oil every 5 years.

Fluoride

The regular presence of fluoride in minute amounts in human bones and teeth and its influence on the prevention of dental caries justifies its inclusion as an element of importance in human nutrition.

Fluoride sources. Most adults ingest between 1 and 3 mg of fluoride daily. The chief source is usually drinking water, which, if it contains 1 part per million (p.p.m.) of fluoride, will supply 1–2 mg/day. Soft waters usually contain no fluoride, whilst very hard waters may contain over 10 p.p.m.

Compared with that in water, the fluoride in foodstuffs is of little importance. Very few contain more than 1 p.p.m.; the exceptions are sea-fish which may contain 5–10 p.p.m. and tea. In Britain, Australia and China, where people drink tea frequently, the adult intake from this source may be as much as 3 mg daily.

Use of fluoride in the prevention of dental caries. Epidemiological studies in many parts of the world have established that where the natural water supply contains fluoride in amounts of 1 p.p.m. or more, the incidence of dental caries is lower than in comparable areas where the water contains only traces of the element.

The benefit of fluoride is greatest when it is taken before the permanent teeth erupt, while their enamel is being laid down. Traces of fluoride incorporated in the surface enamel increase its resistance to acid attack.

The deliberate addition of traces of fluoride (at 1 p.p.m.) to those public water supplies which are deficient is now a widespread practice throughout North America where about 100 million people are now drinking fluoridated water. In at least 30 other countries similar projects have been started. In Britain regrettably some local authorities are not yet adding fluoride to their water supplies in those areas in which the element is lacking. But even here some fluoride reaches people's mouths in toothpaste.

Fluorosis. In parts of the world where the water fluoride is high (over 3–5 p.p.m.) mottling of the teeth is common. The enamel loses its lustre and becomes rough, pigmented and pitted. The effect is purely cosmetic; fluorotic teeth are resistant to caries and not usually associated with any evidence of skeletal fluorosis, or impairment of health.

Chronic fluoride poisoning. This occurs in several localities in India, China, Argentina, East and South Africa, where the water supply contains over 10 p.p.m. fluoride. Fluorine poisoning has also occurred as an industrial hazard among workers handling fluorine-containing minerals such as cryolite, used in smelting aluminium. The main clinical features are in the skeleton which shows sclerosis of bone, especially of the spine, pelvis and limbs, and calcification of ligaments and tendinous insertions of muscles.

Zinc

Although human deficiency was not clearly established before 1972, zinc is emerging as a nutrient of clinical importance. In PEM, associated zinc deficiency causes thymic atrophy and zinc supplements may accelerate the healing of skin lesions. Causes of low plasma zinc are listed in the information box below.

> **CAUSES FOR NEGATIVE ZINC BALANCE AND LOW PLASMA ZINC IN ADULTS**
>
> - Intestinal disease
> - Chronic alcoholism
> - Anorexia nervosa
> - Diabetes mellitus
> - Nephrotic syndrome
> - Burns
> - Haemodialysis
> - Chronic febrile illnesses

Acute zinc deficiency has been reported in patients receiving prolonged intravenous alimentation without added zinc. Diarrhoea, mental apathy, a moist eczematoid dermatitis especially round the mouth and loss of hair were accompanied by a very low plasma zinc concentration and all responded to administration of zinc.

Chronic deficiency has been described in association with dwarfism and hypogonadism.

The recommended intake in adults is 15 mg/day. The best dietary sources are listed in the information box below.

> **DIETARY SOURCES OF ZINC**
>
> - Oysters (very high), wheat bran
> - Liver, beef, lamb, other meats
> - Wholemeal wheat flour and bread, oatmeal
> - Sardines, crab, breakfast cereals
> - Nuts, legumes

Selenium

The content of selenium in soil varies. In some areas farm animals develop disease from too much selenium, in others they will thrive only when given a selenium supplement. In Keshan in N.E. China a cardiomyopathy was described in children in 1979. Soil and blood seleniums are very low and Keshan disease can be prevented by giving small selenium supplements. In the rest of the world a little selenium should be included in the fluid for long-term total parenteral nutrition; myopathy has occurred when it was not. Selenium is part of the enzyme glutathione peroxidase which helps prevent hydroperoxides accumulate in lipids of cell membranes. Some of the functions of selenium and vitamin E overlap.

Other minerals
Sulphur is mainly supplied by the S-containing amino acids in the diet – methionine and cysteine; effects of its deficiency are therefore inseparable from those of protein. *Copper* metabolism is abnormal in Wilson's disease (p. 533). Deficiency occasionally occurs in young children, the main features are anaemia, retarded growth and skeletal rarefaction. *Chromium* facilitates the action of insulin. Deficiency has been reported in some children with PEM and as a rare complication of prolonged parenteral nutrition, presenting as hyperglycaemia.

The roles of *sodium*, *potassium* and *magnesium* are discussed in the next chapter.

THE VITAMINS

Deficiencies of vitamins still occur in affluent countries, e.g. of folate, thiamin and vitamins D and C. Some of these are induced by diseases or drugs. In the Third World deficiency diseases are more prevalent, e.g. vitamin A deficiency (xerophthalmia) is a major cause of blindness.

Table 3.8 Names of vitamins

	Recommended name[1]	Alternative name(s)	Usual pharmaceutical preparation
	Vitamin A	Retinol	Retinol
	Thiamin	Vitamin B₁	Thiamin HCl
	Riboflavin	Vitamin B₂	Riboflavin
	Niacin	Nicotonic acid and nicotinamide	Nicotinamide
Vitamin B complex	Vitamin B₆	Pyridoxine	Pyridoxine HCl
	Pantothenic acid		Calcium pantothenate
	Biotin		Biotin
	Folate	Folacin	Folic acid
	Vitamin B₁₂	Cobalamin	Cyanocobalamin or hydroxocobalamin
	Vitamin C	Ascorbic acid	Ascorbic acid
	Vitamin D	D₂ and D₃	(Ergo)calciferol
	Vitamin E		α-Tocopherol
	Vitamin K		Vitamin K₁

[1] Where there is only one substance with vitamin activity (e.g. thiamin, riboflavin) the International Union of Nutritional Sciences recommends that the chemical name be used. Where there are several compounds with vitamin activity, names like vitamin A, vitamin E, cover them all.

Some vitamins have pharmacological actions above the intake that prevents classic deficiency disease, e.g. vitamins A, C and B₆; nicotinic acid is a standard treatment for some types of hyperlipidaemia.

Taking vitamin tablets is fashionable in affluent countries and a few unorthodox practitioners recommend 'megavitamin therapy'. Doctors therefore need to know the features of both deficiency and of overdosage of the major vitamins.

Vitamins are organic substances in food which are required in small amounts but which cannot be synthesised in adequate quantities. Twelve vitamins have, so far, been demonstrated to have clinical effects in man.

Pantothenic acid, a major component of coenzyme A, also appears to be essential, but human deficiency disease has not been reported, perhaps because the vitamin is widely distributed in foods, as its name implies.

Factors influencing the utilisation of vitamins are listed in the information box below.

FACTORS INFLUENCING UTILISATION OF VITAMINS

- Availability
- Antivitamins, e.g. thiaminase in raw fish; drugs
- Provitamins, e.g. carotenes
- Bacteria in gut – may synthesise (e.g. vit K) or extract vitamins
- Biosynthesis in skin – vitamin D
- Interactions of nutrients, e.g. more thiamin needed if diet rich in carbohydrate or alcohol

VITAMIN A (RETINOL)

Retinol has a place in the function of the retina and of epithelial and probably other cells. It may be a protective factor against cancer of the lung and possibly other epithelial sites. On the world scale vitamin A deficiency is one of the seven most common causes of blindness. WHO estimates that 250 thousand children become blind every year from keratomalacia.

Dietary sources
Retinol is found only in foods of animal origin. Herbivores obtain the vitamin from its precursors or provitamins – some of the carotenoid pigments in plants. The conversion of even the best of these, beta carotene, into retinol in the human small intestinal wall is only 30% efficient. The absorption of both retinol and carotene is facilitated by fats in the diet and bile salts in the duodenum. The sources of retinol and carotene are listed in the information boxes on page 59.

DIETARY SOURCES OF RETINOL

- Milk
- Butter
- Cheese
- Egg yolk
- Liver (richest natural source)
  (Retinol or carotene is added to margarine in Britain and other countries)

DIETARY SOURCES OF CAROTENE

- Dark green leafy vegetables
- Yellow and red fruits
- Red palm oil

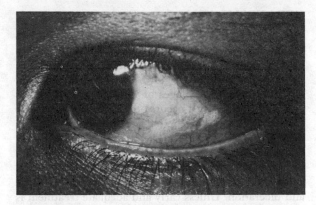

Fig. 3.6 Bitôts spots, showing the white triangular plaques. (By courtesy of the Institute of Ophthalmology.)

Healthy adults in Britain have large stores of retinol in their livers (pp. 489 and 491).

In many parts of the world most or all of the requirements are obtained from carotenoids in vegetable foods. Because only approximately $\frac{1}{3}$ of beta carotene is absorbed into the intestinal wall and then only $\frac{1}{2}$ of this is converted into retinol, 1 µg retinol equivalent ($= 1$ µg retinol) is now taken as $= 6$ µg beta carotene (Fig. 3.5).

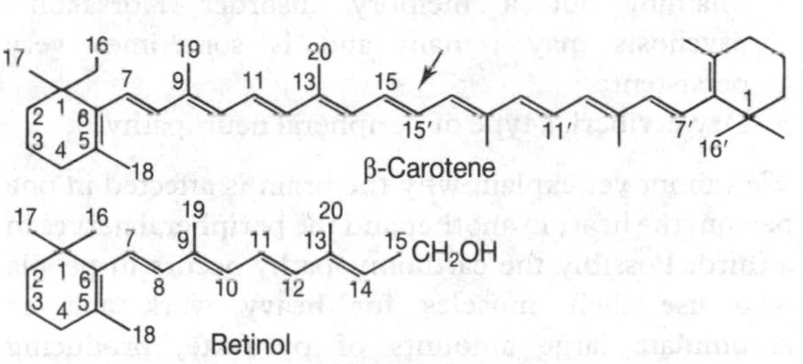

β-Carotene

Retinol

Fig. 3.5 Formation of retinol from Beta-carotene.

NIGHT BLINDNESS

Retin*al* (the aldehyde form) is an essential component of the pigment rhodopsin on which rod vision in dim light depends. Hence lack of retinol may result in impairment of dark adaptation. Night blindness is common, as also is vitamin A deficiency, in poor people living in underdeveloped countries; it can occur in the malabsorption syndrome in affluent countries. The diagnosis of vitamin A deficiency is supported by low plasma vitamin A concentration and is confirmed by marked improvement in dark adaptation following therapeutic doses of retinol.

XEROPHTHALMIA

The earliest sign is xerosis conjunctivae – a dry,

thickened and pigmented bulbar conjunctiva with a peculiar smoky appearance. Bitôt's spots are glistening white plaques of desquamated thickened conjunctival epithelium, usually triangular in shape and firmly adherent to the underlying conjunctiva (Fig. 3.6). When dryness spreads to the cornea it takes on a dull, hazy, lacklustre appearance due to keratinisation, and xerophthalmia is said to be present.

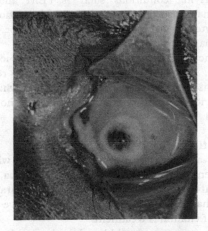

Fig. 3.7 Keratomalacia. (By courtesy of the Institute of Ophthalmology.)

In young children, xerophthalmia is almost always attributed to recent vitamin A deficiency and is usually associated with PEM. In older children and in adults its interpretation is less simple. Exposure to dust and glare may produce similar changes. They should, however, always call attention to the diet. Recognition of xerophthalmia is very important in young children because once the cornea is involved the process can rapidly progress to keratomalacia.

KERATOMALACIA

This disease causes blindness among Indians, Indonesians and other rice-eating people of Asia; it also occurs in parts of Africa, the Middle East and Latin America. In Europe and North America it is very rare. Children between the ages of 1 and 5 years are most commonly affected. It occurs only in persons who have been living for a long period on diets almost entirely devoid of vitamin A. The disease is frequently associated with PEM.

The earliest manifestations are night blindness and xerophthalmia. Later the cornea undergoes necrosis and ulceration. Unless early and adequate treatment is given, there is a grave risk of blindness or death from associated diseases. Evidently vitamin A deficiency affects epithelia beyond the eye and these children have a high mortality from infections.

Management

Immediately on diagnosis 60 mg retinol as palmitate or acetate (200 000 i.u.) should be given orally, or, if there is vomiting or severe diarrhoea 55 mg retinol palmitate by intramuscular injection. The oral dose should be repeated the next day and again prior to discharge or at a follow-up visit.

Underlying conditions such as PEM and other nutritional disorders, diarrhoea, dehydration and electrolyte imbalance and infections must be treated appropriately.

For the secondary bacterial infection, antibiotics are of value. Local treatment of the eye will be required only if disorganisation is already present, in which case the services of an ophthalmic surgeon should be obtained.

Prevention

Doctors and nurses working in the tropics, who may have been trained in Europe or North America, should make sure they are familiar with the appearances of xerophthalmia. If in doubt it is better to give a short course of vitamin A treatment.

Pregnant women should be advised to eat dark green leafy vegetables. This helps to build up stores of retinol in the fetal liver. They should also be taught to give such vegetables or locally available carotene-rich fruits to their babies. In some countries where keratomalacia is a major cause of blindness, e.g. in India, single prophylactic oral doses of 60 mg retinol (200 000 i.u.) are being tried in young children.

THIAMIN (VITAMIN B$_1$)

Thiamin pyrophosphate (TPP) is an essential co-enzyme for the decarboxylation of pyruvate to acetyl coenzyme A. This is the bridge between anaerobic glycolysis and the tricarboxylic acid (Krebs) cycle. TPP is also the coenzyme for transketolase in the hexose monophosphate shunt pathway and for decarboxylation of α-ketoglutarate to succinate in the Krebs cycle. Consequently when thiamin is deficient:

1. the cells cannot utilise glucose aerobically; this is likely to affect the nervous system first, since it depends entirely on glucose for its energy requirements
2. there is accumulation of pyruvic acid and of lactic acid derived from it, which produce vasodilatation and increase cardiac output.

Thiamin deficiency can produce high output cardiac failure and/or peripheral neuropathy and/or encephalopathy. These occur in various combinations in wet and dry beriberi, infantile beriberi and Wernicke's encephalopathy.

1. Wet beriberi: a high output cardiac failure with few ECG changes and prompt response to thiamin;
2. Wernicke's encephalopathy: quiet confusion, ophthalmoplegia and ataxia. These respond to thiamin, but a memory disorder Korsakoff's psychosis may remain and is sometimes very persistent;
3. Dry beriberi: a type of peripheral neuropathy.

We cannot yet explain why the brain is affected in one person, the heart in another and the peripheral nerves in a third. Possibly the cardiomyopathy occurs in people who use their muscles for heavy work and so accumulate large amounts of pyruvate, producing intense vasodilation and increasing cardiac work, while encephalopathy is the first manifestation in less active people.

High carbohydrate diets, heavy alcohol intake or intravenous glucose infusions predispose to and aggravate thiamin deficiency. The body contains only 30 mg of thiamin – 30 times the adult daily requirement – and deficiency starts after about a month on a thiamin-free diet, sooner than for any other vitamin.

Dietary sources of thiamin are listed in the information box (p. 61).

WET BERIBERI

Aetiology

Beriberi is a nutritional disorder formerly widespread in South and East Asia. The word comes from the Singhalese language and means 'I cannot' (said twice),

---

DIETARY SOURCES OF THIAMIN

- Wheat germ, wholemeal wheat flour and bread
- Yeast, legumes, nuts
- Pork, duck, Marmite
- Oatmeal, fortified breakfast cereals
- White bread if flour enriched
- Cod's roe, other meats

---

signifying that the patient is too ill to do anything. Beriberi has almost disappeared from prosperous Asian countries such as Japan, Taiwan and Malaysia and from big cities such as Hong Kong, Manila and Singapore.

Oriental beriberi is usually caused by eating diets in which most of the calories are derived from polished, i.e. highly milled, rice. The disorder is often precipitated by infections, hard physical labour or pregnancy and lactation. In Britain and North America occasional cases of beriberi heart disease are seen, usually in alcoholics who have been consuming little but alcohol for some weeks.

Owing to a lack of thiamin, glucose is incompletely metabolised and pyruvic and lactic acids accumulate in the tissues and body fluids. These metabolites cause dilatation of peripheral blood vessels, as in normal exercise. In beriberi this vasodilatation may be extreme, so that fluid leaks out through the capillaries, producing oedema. At the same time the blood flows rapidly through the dilated peripheral circulation. There is a high cardiac output and as the disease progresses the heart dilates because the myocardium is both overworked and unable to use glucose efficiently as an energy substrate. Cardiac failure accentuates the oedema. Sudden death may result. Microscopic examination usually shows loss of striation of myocardial fibres, which are also finely vacuolated and often fragmented and separated by oedema.

Clinical features

Oedema is the most notable feature and may develop rapidly to involve not only the legs but also the face, trunk and serous cavities. Palpitations are marked and there may be pain in the legs after walking, probably due to the accumulation of lactic acid. There is usually tachycardia and an increase in pulse pressure. The heart is enlarged and the jugular venous pressure rises.

While the circulation is well maintained, the skin is typically warm owing to the vasodilatation; as heart failure advances, the skin of the extremities can become cold and cyanotic. The mind is usually clear. Electrocardiograms often show no changes except sinus

tachycardia but in some cases there are inverted T waves or conduction defects.

The best laboratory test is measurement of transketolase activity in red cells with and without added thiamin pyrophosphate (TPP) in vitro. The test requires fresh heparinised whole blood and this must be taken before thiamin treatment is started. A TPP effect above 30% is to be expected in beriberi or Wernicke's encephalopathy. Plasma pyruvate and lactic acids are elevated in acute forms of thiamin deficiency but not in the more chronic forms and if they are increased this is not specific.

Management

Treatment must be started as soon as the diagnosis is made because fatal heart failure may occur suddenly. Complete rest is essential and 50 mg thiamin should be given intramuscularly for 3 days. Thereafter 10 mg 3 times a day should be continued by mouth until convalescence is established.

The response of a patient with beriberi to thiamin is one of the most dramatic therapeutic events. Within a few hours the breathing is easier, the pulse rate slower, the extremities cooler and a rapid diuresis begins to dispose of the oedema. In a few days the size of the heart is restored to normal. Muscular pain and tenderness are also dramatically improved.

DRY BERIBERI

This is essentially a peripheral neuropathy, formerly common in South-East Asia. The nutritional background is similar to that of wet beriberi. In longstanding cases there is degeneration and demyelination of both sensory and motor nerves, resulting in severe wasting of muscles. The vagus and other autonomic nerves can also be affected. In dry beriberi the blood pyruvate level is usually normal and the transketolase test (TPP effect) may be too. The management is that of a nutritional polyneuropathy, as described on p. 903.

WERNICKE'S ENCEPHALOPATHY AND KORSAKOFF'S PSYCHOSIS

Aetiology

This cerebral form of thiamin deficiency occurs in Europe and North America. It often presents acutely, usually in an alcoholic but it is sometimes seen in people with malnutrition, e.g. persistent vomiting; it occurred in prisoners of war on small rations of polished rice.

Clinical features

In *Wernicke's encephalopathy* the patient is quietly confused and the most valuable clinical sign is some form of bilateral, symmetrical ophthalmoplegia. This may be in one or more than one direction and accompanied by abnormal pupillary reflexes and/or nystagmus. Ataxia is also present. The confusion is liable soon to progress to stupor or death if treatment is delayed. There are foci of congestion and petechial haemorrhage in the upper part of the mid-brain, the hypothalamus, and the wall of the third ventricle. Involvement of the mamillary bodies is a pathognomonic finding at postmortem.

Korsakoff's psychosis. In some cases the predominant change in mental function is a memory defect, the characteristic bedside feature of which is confabulation. Psychological tests show a severe defect in storing new information.

Wernicke's encephalopathy and Korsakoff's psychosis are sometimes associated with polyneuropathy and/or with superior midline cerebellar degeneration (p. 903) but it is surprising how uncommon these cerebral forms are in S.E. Asia and that beriberi cardiomyopathy is seldom seen with Wernicke/Korsakoff disease.

Management
Wernicke's encephalopathy should be treated without delay with 50 mg thiamin hydrochloride by slow intravenous injection followed by 50 mg intramuscularly daily for a week. Confusion, disorientation and ophthalmoplegia should respond within 2 to 3 days. Indeed this response to thiamin helps to confirm the diagnosis. The memory disorder (Korsakoff's psychosis) takes longer to improve; it may become more obvious as confusion clears and the patient's general condition improves. Some degree of memory impairment often persists.

Prevention
In Western countries the prevention of beriberi and Wernicke's encephalopathy is related to the control of alcoholism. In a chronic alcoholic vitamin B complex tablets can at least prevent the complications of thiamin deficiency. Beriberi is much less common in Asia than it used to be.

NIACIN (nicotinic acid and nicotinamide)
Nicotinamide is an essential part of the two important pyridine nucleotides, NAD and NADP which are hydrogen-accepting coenzymes for dehydrogenases at many steps in the pathways of glucose oxidation. NAD is also the coenzyme for alcohol dehydrogenase. Nicotinic acid is readily converted in the body into the amide. For nutritional purposes the two have equal biological activity and are considered together in foods under the generic term 'niacin'. Both are water-soluble and resistant to heat. The dietary sources are listed in the information box below.

DIETARY SOURCES OF NIACIN

- Liver, kidney
- Meat, fish
- Yeast (brewer's), Marmite
- Peanuts, bran, legumes
- Wholemeal wheat
- Coffee

A special feature of this vitamin is that it is normally synthesised in the body in limited amounts from the amino acid tryptophan; 60 mg of tryptophan yields 1 mg of nicotinamide. For this reason niacin equivalents in a diet are calculated by adding together the niacin plus 1/60 of the tryptophan intake (in mg). As a rule of thumb it can be assumed that tryptophan is about 1/100th of the protein intake. Therefore a protein intake of 60 g provides 10 mg ($60\,000 \times 1/100 \times 1/60$ mg) of the adult daily requirement of 18 mg niacin equivalents (pre-formed niacin + that from tryptophan).

PELLAGRA

Aetiology
Pellagra is a nutritional disease formerly endemic among poor peasants who subsisted chiefly on maize (American corn). The greater part of the niacin in maize is in a bound form, niacytin, which is unavailable to the consumer. In areas where pellagra remains, e.g. in parts of Africa, the incidence is much less than formerly. In developed countries it is occasionally seen in alcoholics and in the malabsorption syndrome. In the rare inborn error of metabolism, *Hartnup disease*, tryptophan absorption is impaired and there is a pellagrous dermatitis with neurological abnormalities which respond to nicotinamide.

Clinical features
Pellagra can develop in only 8 weeks on diets very deficient in niacin and tryptophan. It has been called the disease of the three Ds: dermatitis, diarrhoea and dementia.

Skin. The diagnosis is usually first suggested by the appearance of the skin. Characteristically, there is an erythema resembling severe sunburn, appearing symmetrically over the parts of the body exposed to sunlight and especially on the neck (Fig. 3.8). Local trauma or irritation of the skin may also determine the site of the

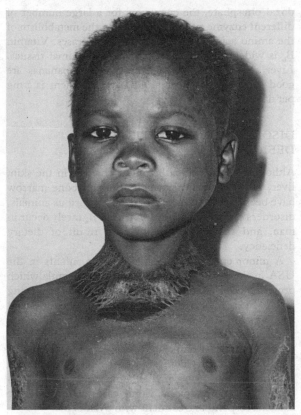

Fig. 3.8 Pellagra in a girl of 5 years. Skin lesion on the neck (Casel's collar) is pathognomonic.

lesion. The affected areas are well demarcated from normal skin. In acute cases the skin lesions may progress to vesiculation, cracking, exudation and crusting with ulceration and sometimes secondary infection. In chronic cases the dermatitis occurs as a roughening and thickening of the skin with a brown pigmentation. Dermatitis of the vulva, perineum and perianal area is usually present.

Alimentary tract. There may be anorexia, nausea and dysphagia. Glossitis is an early symptom and may precede the skin lesions. The mouth is sore and often shows angular stomatitis and cheilosis (p. 64). It is probable that a non-infective inflammation extends throughout the gastrointestinal tract and accounts for the diarrhoea which is usually present.

Nervous system. In severe cases delirium is the most common mental disturbance in the acute form of the disease and dementia in the chronic form. Because of these changes, chronic pellagrins have in the past been admitted to mental hospitals.

Management

Nicotinamide is given in a dose of 100 mg every 6 hours by mouth, although a smaller dose is likely to be effective. The vitamin is well absorbed but can be given parenterally. The response is usually rapid; within 24 hours the erythema of the skin diminishes and the diarrhoea ceases. Often there is also striking improvement in the patient's behaviour and mental attitude.

Nicotinamide alone is usually insufficient to restore health. There are likely to be associated nutritional deficiencies. A relatively low intake of protein including tryptophan is an essential condition for development of the disease, and hypoalbuminaemia is common. Deficiencies of other B complex vitamins (riboflavin and vitamin B_6) are likely. Nicotinamide treatment should therefore be supplemented with a nutritious diet, high in protein. Vitamin B complex tablets should be given and iron, folic acid and vitamin B_{12} may be necessary in addition for some cases. Alcohol should be forbidden.

Prevention

The disappearance of pellagra from the southern States of the USA since 1938 must have been partly due to the enrichment of bread and maize meal with niacin. But the overall improvement in the economic state, education and general nutrition of the poor people in the south probably had an important effect as well.

In Central America the peasants eat a staple diet of maize but pellagra is unusual. This is because the traditional method of boiling the maize in lime water (dilute calcium hydroxide) before they make tortillas hydrolyses the indigestible bound niacin to free niacin.

RIBOFLAVIN

Riboflavin is a constituent of the flavoproteins which are concerned with tissue oxidation. It is a yellow-green fluorescent compound soluble in water. Though stable to boiling in acid solution, in alkaline solution it is decomposed by heat. It is also destroyed by exposure to UV light.

The dietary sources are listed in the information box below.

DIETARY SOURCES OF RIBOFLAVIN

- Liver, kidney
- Milk, yoghurt, cheese
- Marmite, eggs, wheat germ
- Wheat bran, mushrooms, meats
- Forfitied white flour and breakfast cereals

DISORDERS DUE TO RIBOFLAVIN DEFICIENCY

When human volunteers have been given diets very low in riboflavin, the most consistent clinical manifestations were angular stomatitis, cheilosis and nasolabial dyssebacea; these responded to the addition of pure riboflavin in the deficient diet

Angular stomatitis. This is not specific for lack of riboflavin. Deficiencies of niacin, pyridoxine and iron can all produce it. It can follow herpes febrilis at the angle of the mouth. A common cause is ill-fitting dentures, associated with candidiasis.

Cheilosis. This is a zone of red, denuded epithelium at the line of closure of the lips. It has also occurred in experimental pure niacin deficiency. It is often associated with angular stomatitis and frequently seen in pellagra.

Nasolabial dyssebacia. This consists of enlarged follicles around the sides of the nose which are plugged with dry sebaceous material. This occurs in primates on a diet deficient only in riboflavin. It is seen in some patients with pellagra.

Other abnormalities. Vascularisation of the cornea, scrotal dermatitis, a magenta-coloured tongue and anaemia have been attributed to riboflavin deficiency but they may have alternative explanations.

Riboflavin clearly plays a vital role in cellular oxidation and there are communities and individuals who have both low dietary intakes and very low concentrations in urine or blood. Yet it is surprising that the clinical effects of riboflavin deficiency are superficial and mainly non-specific. Features of riboflavin deficiency are most likely to be found in pellagrins and in malnourished rice-eaters in S.E. Asia. In the first situation they are overshadowed by niacin deficiency and in the second by thiamin or protein deficiency.

Management

The therapeutic dose of riboflavin is 5 mg 3 times a day by mouth. It gives the patient's urine a green fluorescence. As discussed above, other B complex vitamins should also be given.

PYRIDOXINE (VITAMIN B₆)

Pyridoxine, pyridoxal and pyridoxamine are three closely related compounds with similar physiological actions. The active form of the vitamin in man is pyridoxal phosphate, the coenzyme for a large number of different enzyme systems involved in the metabolism of the amino acids including aminotransferases. Vitamin B_6 is widely distributed in plants and animal tissues. Liver, whole grain cereals, peanuts and bananas are good sources. The normal adult requirement is 2 mg per day.

DISORDERS DUE TO VITAMIN B₆ DEFICIENCY

Although a series of pathological changes in the skin, liver, blood vessels, nervous tissue and bone marrow have been produced experimentally in various animals, disorders due to deficiency of vitamin B_6 rarely occur in man, and then very seldom as a result of dietary deficiency.

A minor epidemic of convulsions in infants in the USA in the 1950s was traced to a milk formula which provided little vitamin B_6 because of a manufacturing error. In adults dermatitis, cheilosis, glossitis and angular stomatitis have been produced by means of the pyridoxine inhibitor, 4-desoxy-pyridoxine. The peripheral neuropathy associated with isoniazid therapy is due to a secondary vitamin B_6 deficiency. Certain drugs such as isoniazid and penicillamine, act as chemical antagonists to pyridoxine. Some cases of sideroblastic anaemia respond to treatment with pyridoxine.

Biochemical features suggesting vitamin B_6 deficiency can occur in women taking oral contraceptives, and the mild depression which affects a small proportion of such women may be relieved by pyridoxine.

Megavitamin doses of vitamin B_6 (200 mg/day or more) taken for some weeks cause a sensory polyneuropathy.

BIOTIN

Biotin functions as coenzyme for several carboxylases. It is present in a number of different foods; the requirement is small (about 100 µg/day) and it can be synthesised by intestinal bacteria. Human deficiency is rare; it has occurred in adults who have taken for long periods large amounts of raw egg-white which contain the biotin antagonist avidin, and an otherwise poor diet. The clinical features include dermatitis and hypercholesterolaemia. A form of seborrhoeic dermatitis of infants responds to biotin.

VITAMIN B₁₂ AND FOLATE

These vitamins and disorders due to their deficiency are discussed on page 711 and page 713.

VITAMIN C (ASCORBIC ACID)

Ascorbic acid is a modified simple sugar. It is the most active reducing agent in the aqueous phase of living tissues and is easily and reversibly oxidised to dehydro-ascorbic acid. Its highest concentrations are in the adrenal cortex and in the eye. Stress and corticotrophin secretion lead to a loss of ascorbic acid from the adrenal cortex. The presumption. therefore, is that ascorbic acid is somehow concerned in bodily reactions to stress.

Dietary sources of vitamin C are listed in the information box below.

DIETARY SOURCES OF VITAMIN C

- Blackcurrants, guavas
- Green peppers, broccoli, cauliflower (raw)
- Oranges and other citrus fruits
- Brussels sprouts, cabbage
- Potatoes
- (Liver)

Ascorbic acid is very easily destroyed by heat, alkalies such as sodium bicarbonate, traces of copper or by an oxidase liberated by damage to plant tissues. Ascorbic acid is very soluble in water. For these reasons many traditional methods of cooking reduce or eliminate it from the diet. The recommended intake is 30 60 mg in different countries. Body stores last for about $2\frac{1}{2}$ to 3 months on a deficient diet.

SCURVY

Aetiology

In 1497 when Vasco da Gama sailed round the Cape of Good Hope 100 out of his 160 men died of scurvy. For the next 300 years scurvy was a major factor determining the success or failure of all sea ventures even after it was recognised by Lind (1753) and by Cook (1755) that it results from the prolonged consumption of a diet devoid of fresh fruit and vegetables. Final proof and isolation of vitamin C were not possible until the guinea pig was found (1907) to provide a suitable animal model because, like man and unlike most animals, it cannot synthesise ascorbic acid from glucose.

Sporadic cases of scurvy continue to arise in infants as a result of ignorance, poverty and maternal neglect and also amongst old people, especially men living alone who are not feeding themselves properly. Scurvy appears to be rare in most tropical countries but is more likely to occur in arid regions in times of drought.

Pathology

Ascorbic acid deficiency results in defective formation of collagen in connective tissue because of failure of hydroxylation of proline to hydroxyproline, the characteristic amino acid of collagen. There is in consequence delayed healing of wounds. There are also capillary haemorrhages and subnormal platelet stickiness.

Clinical features

Adult scurvy

The pathognomic sign is the swollen and spongy gums particularly of the papillae between the teeth, sometimes producing the appearance of 'scurvy buds'. These bleed easily. The teeth may become loose and even fall out. There is always some infection; indeed this seems necessary for the production of the scorbutic gingival appearances because volunteers suffering from experimental deficiency did not develop it if their gums were previously healthy. In patients without teeth the gums appear normal.

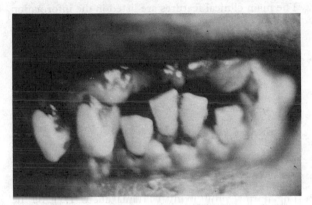

Fig. 3.9   The gums in scurvy.

The first sign of cutaneous bleeding is often found on the lower thighs. These are perifollicular haemorrhages – tiny points of bleeding around the orifice of a hair follicle. There is a heaping-up of keratin-like material on the surface around the mouth of the follicle, through which a deformed 'corkscrew' hair characteristically projects. Perifollicular haemorrhages are often followed by petechial haemorrhages, developing independently of the hair follicles, which are usually first seen on the feet and ankles. Thereafter large spontaneous bruises (ecchymoses) may arise almost anywhere in the body, but usually first in the lower extremities, producing the characteristic 'woody leg'. Haemorrhage may occur into joints, into a nerve sheath, under the nails or conjunctiva or into the gastrointestinal tract; there may be epistaxis. Scurvy can present with any of these features. By the time the disease is fully developed the patient is usually anaemic.

Before the changes in the gums and skin appear, the patient has usually felt feeble and listless for some weeks. Another characteristic of scurvy is that fresh wounds fail to heal – a possibility that the surgeon has to bear in mind. A patient with scurvy may die suddenly without warning, apparently from cardiac failure.

The dietary and social history is helpful in doubtful cases. Old, solitary people may insist that they fend very well for themselves, but careful questioning will reveal that they do not buy fresh fruit or vegetables. In other instances vegetables may be purchased but they are overcooked and lose all vitamin C.

Plasma ascorbate is very low or absent (Table 20.1, p. 989); a fresh sample of plasma should be analysed because the vitamin can decompose in a few hours at warm room temperatures. If this test is done it should be *before* any vitamin C is given.

Infantile scurvy
The main clinical features are listed in the information box below.

CLINICAL FEATURES OF INFANTILE SCURVY

- Lassitude
- Anorexia
- Painful limbs
- Enlargement of costochondral junctions
- Subperiosteal haemorrhage
- Gingivitis once teeth have erupted

Management
The normal adult body contains about 1.5 g of the vitamin, so that a dose of 250 mg by mouth 4 times daily should saturate the tissues quickly. Attention should be paid to correcting the general deficiencies of the patient's former diet. A liberal mixed diet should be given. If the patient is anaemic iron and sometimes folic acid are indicated. With adequate treatment no patient dies of scurvy and recovery is usually rapid and complete.

Prevention
In breast milk the vitamin C content responds to maternal intake. Fruit juice should be given to bottle-fed infants.

No simple administrative means has been found of preventing scurvy among the old and solitary. Should the physician be unable to persuade such a person to eat fruit or vegetables, 50 mg synthetic ascorbic acid should be taken daily.

Trauma, surgery and burns, infections, smoking and certain drugs – adrenocortical steroids, aspirin, indo-methacin and tetracycline – all increase the requirement for vitamin C. Consequently such persons require more than the recommended intake of 30–60 mg/d.

Ascorbic acid and the common cold
It has been claimed that ascorbic acid in doses of 1–2 g daily, or even more, will prevent the common cold. If it does, this is a pharmacological and not a vitamin effect as coryza is not a manifestation of scurvy. In the largest controlled trial, in Toronto, two placebo groups were included. One of these had fewer colds than those taking 0.25, 1 or 2 g vitamin C per day prophylactically. Another 14 double-blind controlled trials found no significant preventive effect. The trials that did report benefit were smaller and less rigorously controlled. It is inadvisable for people to dose themselves with large quantities of ascorbic acid as this favours the formation of oxalate stones in the urinary tract.

VITAMIN D

There are two chemical forms. *Cholecalciferol* is the natural form of the vitamin which occurs in man and other animals. It is formed in the skin by the action of ultraviolet light on 7-dehydrocholesterol. *Ergocalciferol* is manufactured by the action of ultraviolet light on ergosterol, a sterol found in fungi and yeasts. Although used in therapeutics, it occurs very rarely in nature.

Cholecalciferol is converted in the liver to 25-hydroxycholecalciferol (25-OH-D) which is further hydroxylated in the kidney, mainly to 1,25 dihydroxy-cholecalciferol (1,25(OH)$_2$D). Most of the hydroxylated forms of vitamin D in human plasma are based on cholecalciferol derived from synthesis in the skin or from fish liver oils. A smaller proportion is based on ergocalciferol from calciferol tablets or fortified milk (e.g. in USA). They and their corresponding derivatives appear to have identical activities.

1,25(OH)$_2$D is many times more potent than chole-calciferol and can be regarded as a hormone. It is transported in the blood to target organs, notably gut and bone and is regulated by a complex feedback system. The most important function of 1,25(OH)$_2$D is, by inducing a specific transport protein in the enterocyte, to increase calcium absorption. An adequate concentration of calcium is thus ensured for the formation of calcium phosphate in bone where calcium comes in contact with inorganic phosphates, liberated from organic phosphates under the influence of phos-phatase produced by osteoblasts.

Alfacalcidol, 1α-hydroxycholecalciferol (1αOH-D), is a synthetic analogue which is converted into 1,25 (OH)$_2$D in the liver without the need for hydroxy-

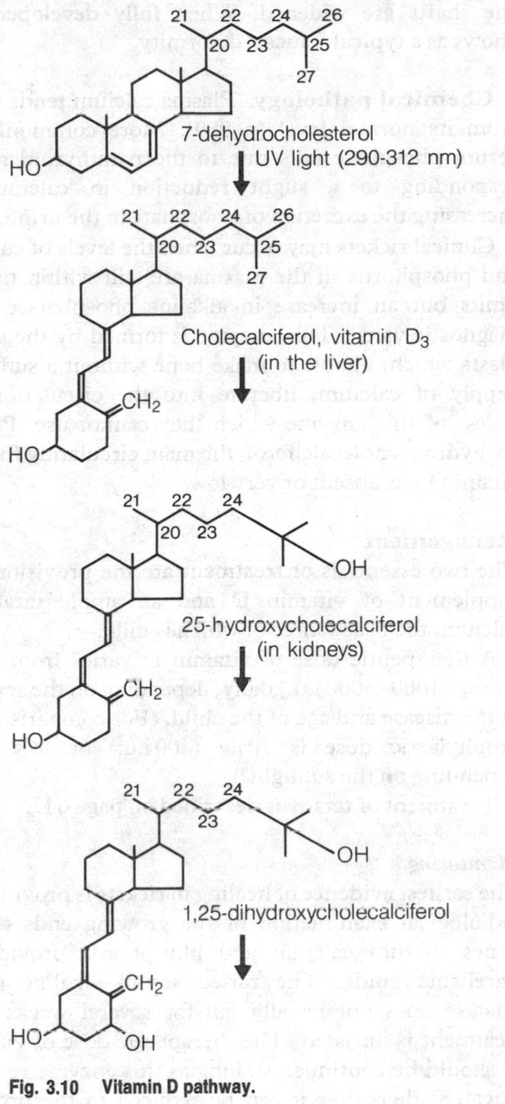

7-dehydrocholesterol

UV light (290-312 nm)

Cholecalciferol, vitamin D₃
(in the liver)

25-hydroxycholecalciferol
(in kidneys)

1,25-dihydroxycholecalciferol

Fig. 3.10   Vitamin D pathway.

lation in the kidney. It is used in treating hypocalcaemia and osteomalacia due to renal disease.

The main reasons for impaired production of 1,25 $(OH)_2D$ are:

1. deficiency of 25-OH-D due to lack of sunlight, an inadequate diet or malabsorption
2. disturbed metabolism in liver or renal disease, notably chronic renal failure
3. depression of the feedback system as in hypoparathyroidism.

Dietary sources of vitamin D
These are listed in the information box above.

DIETARY SOURCES OF VITAMIN D

- Fish liver oils, e.g., cod liver oil
- Fatty fish (herring, mackerel, salmon, sardines, pilchards, tuna)
- Fortified margarine
- Infant milk formulas
- Eggs, liver

People who regularly have adequate exposure of their skin to sunlight do not normally need vitamin D in their diet. Otherwise the recommended daily intake (WHO) for infants and children up to 5 years of age and for pregnant or lactating women is 10 µg. For older children and adults about 2.5 µg is adequate (1 µg = 40 i.u.).

RICKETS

Rickets is the characteristic result of deficiency of vitamin D in children. When the epiphyses have fused the corresponding deficiency disease is osteomalacia. Both mainly affect the bones but they differ in details.

Infants in their first year are susceptible to rickets because of the inadequate vitamin D in cows' milk. If they are always kept indoors or completely covered whenever they are taken outside they are never exposed to sunlight. By the second year the infant is able to crawl about in the sunshine and spontaneous healing usually occurs.

The disease is now uncommon in countries where vitamin D is freely available. In Britain clinical rickets occurs in Asian immigrant children, often of school-going age, from a combination of little exposure of the skin to sunlight and very low dietary intakes of vitamin D. High phytate intake in chapatti flour may contribute by inhibiting calcium absorption. The disease is also liable to occur in premature babies.

Clinical features
The infant with rickets has often received sufficient calories and may appear well nourished, but is restless, fretful and pale, with flabby muscles and is prone to respiratory and gastrointestinal infections. Development is delayed; the teeth often erupt late and there is failure to sit, stand, crawl and walk at the normal ages.

The bony changes are the most characteristic signs of rickets. The earliest lesion is often craniotabes – small round unossified areas in the membranous bones of the skull, yielding to the pressure of the finger, with a crackling feeling. This sign suggests the possibility of rickets in an infant under one year of age but it is not pathognomonic. It is not found over this age.

Two other early signs are enlargement of the epiphyses at the lower end of the radius and swelling of the costochondral junctions of the ribs ('rickety rosary'). Later there may be 'bossing' of the frontal and parietal bones and delayed closure of the anterior fontanelle. Later still, there may be deformities of the chest. In the second or third year of life, deformities such as kyphosis develop as a result of the new gravitational and muscular strains caused by sitting up and standing. At the same time there may be enlargement of the epiphyses at the lower ends of the femur, tibia and fibula. When the rachitic child begins to walk, deformities of the shafts of the leg bones develop, so that 'knock knees' or 'bow legs' are seen. Pelvic deformities can follow severe rickets in later childhood and lead later to serious difficulties at childbirth.

When there is a reduction in ionised plasma calcium, infantile tetany may result, with spasm of the hands and feet and of the vocal cords. The latter causes a high-pitched distressing cry and difficulty in breathing. Epileptic fits may also occur.

Investigation

X-ray examination. Examination of the wrist will show characteristic changes in the epiphyses at the lower ends of the radius (Fig. 3.11). The zones of epiphyseal cartilages are thickened and the distal ends of

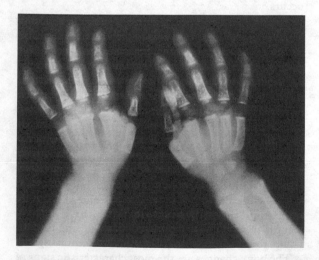

Fig. 3.11   Wrist X-ray showing the effects of rickets. The lower ends of the shafts of radius and ulna become splayed and epiphyseal surfaces appear fuzzy and ill-defined. Unossified zone (cartilage) between shaft and radial epiphysis is widened. (By courtesy of the Institute of Ophthalmology.)

the shafts are widened. When fully developed this shows as a typical 'saucer' deformity.

Chemical pathology. Plasma calcium tends to fall from its normal level (p. 989). More commonly the serum phosphate falls due to the parathyroid glands responding to a slight reduction in calcium by increasing the excretion of phosphate in the urine.

Clinical rickets may occur when the levels of calcium and phosphorus in the plasma are still within normal limits but an increase in alkaline phosphatase is of diagnostic value. This enzyme is formed by the osteoblasts which, unable to make bone without a sufficient supply of calcium, liberate into the circulation the excess of this enzyme which they cannot use. Plasma 25-hydroxycholecalciferol, the main circulating form of vitamin D, is absent or very low.

Management

The two essentials of treatment are the provision of a supplement of vitamin D and an ample intake of calcium, the best source of which is milk.

A therapeutic dose of vitamin D varies from 25 to 125 µg (1000–5000 i.u.) daily, depending on the severity of the disease and age of the child. (For comparison the prophylactic dose is 10 µg (400 i.u.) or less daily depending on the sunlight.)

Treatment of tetany is described on page 642.

Monitoring

The earliest evidence of healing in rickets is provided by radiological examination of the growing ends of the bones. Serum calcium and phosphorus provide an unreliable guide. The raised serum alkaline phosphatase does not usually fall for several weeks after treatment is initiated. The therapeutic dose of vitamin D should be continued so long as this enzyme remains elevated; thereafter it can be reduced to the prophylactic dose of 10 µg daily.

Rickets is not a fatal disease per se, but the untreated rachitic child is always at risk of infections, notably bronchopneumonia. The skeletal changes, if mild in degree, usually tend to heal spontaneously as the child gets older, but in severe cases pigeon chest, spinal curvature, knock knees, bow legs or contracted pelvis persist.

Secondary and resistant rickets

In malabsorption, e.g. in coeliac disease, rickets is common. Children on long-term anti-epileptic drugs are liable to develop rickets; these drugs induce changes in liver microsomal enzymes which convert vitamin D to inactive metabolites.

Occasional cases of rickets are resistant to ordinary therapeutic doses of vitamin D. The commonest type of vitamin D resistant rickets is familial hypophosphataemic rickets, an X-linked dominant condition in which there is renal tubular loss of phosphate. There are also two types of 'vitamin D dependent rickets', in one of which 1α hydroxylation of 25 OH vitamin D is impaired; in the other form there appears to be end-organ resistance to the active metabolite. Alfacalcidol is useful in these conditions.

Hypervitaminosis D

In the case of vitamin D it is possible to have too much of a good thing. Large doses are toxic and cause hypercalcaemia. The symptoms include nausea, vomiting, constipation, drowsiness and signs of renal failure; metastatic calcification in the arteries, kidneys and other tissues may occur.

Since renal damage may occur before clinical signs of toxicity appear, all patients on large doses of vitamin D should have their serum calcium level checked regularly at 3-monthly intervals and if this is found to be above 2.6 mmol/l (10.5 mg/100 ml) it is an early indication of overdosage.

Prevention

The natural means of prevention is regular exposure to the sun's UV light. There is no need for oral intake of vitamin D in tropical and subtropical countries except in the elderly housebound and chronic sick (see p. 70). In high latitude northern countries very little UV light gets through the atmosphere in winter. Modern infant milk-based formulae include adequate vitamin D and there appears to be enough in breast milk for full-term infants for the first few months of life. After infancy North American children and adults are protected by added vitamin D in liquid milk. In Britain, however, none of the common foods is a good source of vitamin D. Growing children may benefit from a daily supplement of 10 µg/day during the winter months. There are many suitable and inexpensive preparations. Cod liver oil is still effective but unpopular because of its taste.

OSTEOMALACIA

Osteomalacia, which means softening of bone, is primarily due to a deficiency of vitamin D. This results in a failure to replace the turnover of calcium and phosphorus in the organic matrix of bone. Hence the bone content is demineralised and bony substance becomes replaced by soft osteoid tissue. It contains less calcium and phosphate per 100 g than normal bone.

Osteoporosis is atrophy of bone. It is believed to be due to predominance of resorption over formation of the cellular matrix of bone which leads to a reduction in the total mass of bone. In other words osteoporosis is too little bone of normal mineral content. In contrast to osteomalacia the calcium phosphate per 100 g bone is normal. Osteoporosis is described on page 808.

Aetiology

Osteomalacia is the adult counterpart of rickets. It was formerly common in women in purdah in oriental countries, living on poor cereal diets devoid of milk, kept indoors and seldom seeing the sun. Symptoms occurred with pregnancy.

The disease may be due to malabsorption from any cause, including operations like partial gastrectomy, and in countries like the UK which do not have the insurance of fortification of milk with vitamin D it can occur in people who are housebound and never sit in the sun. Chronic renal disorders are a less important cause. Adults who have to take antiepileptic drugs for years are likely to develop osteomalacia.

Clinical features

Skeletal discomfort is usually present and persistent and ranges from backache to severe pain. Bone tenderness on pressure is common. Muscular weakness is often present and the patient may find difficulty in climbing stairs or getting out of a chair. A waddling gait is not unusual. Tetany may be manifested by carpopedal spasm and facial twitching. Spontaneous fractures may occur, independent of the pseudo-fractures described below. The biochemical changes in the blood are the same as in rickets.

Radiological examination shows rarefaction of bone and commonly translucent bands (pseudo-fractures or Looser's zones), often symmetrical, at points submitted to stress. Common sites are the ribs, the axillary border of the scapula, the pubic rami and the medial cortex of the upper femur. Pseudo-fractures are pathognomonic when well developed.

Histological examination of stained undecalcified sections of bone obtained by biopsy shows the presence of excess osteoid tissue.

Management

When osteomalacia is primarily due to defective intake, treatment is essentially the same as for rickets, namely 25 to 125 µg vitamin D daily. The response is usually dramatic. If there is evidence of malabsorption the dose should be increased or given intramuscularly at weekly intervals. If the disease is secondary to renal disorders alfacalcidol (p. 66) should be used.

Maintenance treatment with vitamin D will be required for all cases of osteomalacia in which the cause cannot be removed. In addition a good diet should be given which includes milk, cheese or yoghurt

Prevention

Free access to sunshine and an adequate intake of dairy produce, supplemented when necessary with prophylactic vitamin D (10 µg/day), will prevent nutritional osteomalacia. Particular attention to these prophylactic measures should be given to inmates of geriatric and mental hospitals and to old people living alone whose exposure to sunshine is limited and also to those who have had gastric surgery. Patients on long-term anti-epileptic therapy should be given prophylactic doses of vitamin D.

VITAMIN E

Alpha-tocopherol is the most potent of eight related substances with vitamin E activity. Good sources include vegetable oils, wholegrain cereals and nuts.

Vitamin E prevents oxidation of polyunsaturated fatty acids in cell membranes. The first feature of human deficiency is a mild haemolytic anaemia which has been described only in premature infants and in a few cases of malabsorption. Early oral administration reduces the severity of retrolental fibroplasia in premature infants given oxygen. In chronic deficiency, e.g. in cystic fibrosis, ataxia and visual scotomas occur which respond to vitamin E.

There is no scientific justification for self-medication with vitamin E in the belief that this will increase energy or virility. Pharmacological doses of vitamin E have produced surprisingly few side-effects but they do appear to interfere with thyroid function and potentiate the action of coumarin anticoagulants.

VITAMIN K

Vitamin K is required for the formation in the liver of factors necessary for the normal clotting of blood (p. 759). It exists in nature in two forms, vitamin K_1 and vitamin K_2. Vitamin K_1 (phytomenadione) is found in leafy vegetables. Adequate amounts are normally supplied in the average diet and absorbed with other lipids. Bacterial synthesis of vitamin K_2 occurs within the colon.

Primary vitamin K deficiency is not uncommon in the (unsupplemented) newborn when there is no formation of vitamin K in the gut and hypoprothrombinaemia occurs. 1 mg vitamin K_1 at birth is a safe prophylactic measure against the development of haemorrhagic disease of the newborn.

Secondary vitamin K deficiency and its clinical features and treatment are discussed on page 759.

DIETARY FIBRE

Dietary fibre is the natural packing of plant foods. It can be defined as those parts of food which are not digested by human enzymes. The principal classes of dietary fibre are cellulose, hemicelluloses, lignins, pectins and gums. These are all polysaccharides (i.e. carbohydrates) except lignin, which occurs with cellulose in the structure of plants. Pectins and gums are viscous, not fibrous.

Some types of dietary fibre, notably the hemicellulose of wheat, increase the water-holding capacity of colonic contents and the bulk of the faeces. They relieve simple constipation, appear to prevent diverticulosis and may reduce the risk of cancer of the colon. Other, viscous indigestible polysaccharides like pectin and guar gum have more effect in the upper gastrointestinal tract. They tend to slow gastric emptying, contribute to satiety, may flatten the glucose tolerance curve and reduce plasma cholesterol concentration.

Dietary fibre is in fact partly digested in the large intestine, by resident bacterial flora, not endogenous enzymes, with flatus formation, and a small quantity of volatile fatty acids is absorbed through the colonic mucosa. There are as yet no official recommended intakes for fibre because analyses for the different types in foods are not complete, but the present average intakes of about 15 to 20 g/day in affluent countries are thought to be too low.

NUTRITION OF PATIENTS IN HOSPITAL

Malnutrition does not occur only in poor children in developing countries. It affects a substantial proportion of seriously ill people in the hospitals of affluent countries. This was fully recognised only after the deficiency diseases in the Third World had been well delineated and approaches established to their management. During the 1970s it was realised that:

1. some degree of malnutrition affects an important minority of patients in hospital; it may be obscured by the primary illness;
2. malnourished patients have a worse prognosis;

3. with modern technology something can be done to maintain or improve patients' nutrition even when the gastrointestinal tract is not functioning.

Disease leads to nutritional depletion

A few patients are admitted to hospital in a malnourished state but more become nutritionally depleted in hospital. Serious illness, major operations and long stay are all associated with a greater chance of depletion partly because patients may be unable to ingest, digest or absorb their food but also because nutritional requirements and/or losses are increased in a number of diseases. The causes of nutritional depletion are listed in the information box below.

CAUSES OF NUTRITIONAL DEPLETION

- Anorexia
- Unfamiliar food
- 'Nil per mouth' for hospital tests
- Failure to feed, e.g. neurological or psychological illness
- Vomiting
- Malabsorption
- Increased protein catabolism (trauma, infections)
- Increased metabolic rate (fever)
- Antagonism of nutrients by drugs
- Losses, e.g. burns, bleeding, diarrhoea, in urine

Functional consequences of nutritional depletion

These depend on the degree and type of depletion, but sooner or later malnutrition will have some or even all the following effects:

1. reduced cellular or humoral responses to infections
2. muscular weakness, reduced ability to cough and susceptibility to bronchopneumonia
3. impaired healing of wounds (whether traumatic or surgical)
4. atrophic surface epithelium with reduced protective secretions is more easily penetrated by bacteria
5. bedsores and ulcers
6. reduced haemopoiesis
7. reduced ability to metabolise drugs
8. mental impairment
9. dehydration and its consequences
10. specific types of malnutrition, e.g. Wernicke's encephalopathy.

Controlled prospective studies show that patients with features of malnutrition have more postoperative complications, more infections, longer stay in hospital and a higher mortality. In some diseases nutritional support has been demonstrated in controlled trials to improve the outcome significantly, e.g. in inflammatory bowel disease, in burns and in patients with enterocutaneous fistulae. In other conditions clinical trials are insufficient to allow generalisations and it is sensible to assess each patient's status and if this is subnormal, to consider the indications for the different types of nutritional support.

Patients at increased nutritional risk

Before using technical methods to work out a detailed nutritional profile, the first step is to recognise the high-risk patient. A patient in any of the categories in Table 3.9 is at increased risk of malnutrition though it may not yet have developed:

Table 3.9 Patients at increased risk of hospital malnutrition

- Severely underweight; weight for height < 80% of standard (Table 3.6)
- Recent weight loss of 10% or more of usual body weight
- Alcoholism
- Malabsorption syndromes
- Increased metabolic rate: burns, trauma, severe infections, prolonged fever
- Increased losses, e.g. fistulae, draining wounds, renal dialysis, haemorrhage
- No food by mouth for over a week while receiving simple intravenous nutrition (glucose/electrolyte/water)
- Antinutrients or catabolic drugs, e.g. immunosuppressants, cancer chemotherapy, adrenocortical steroids
- Course of radiotherapy

Systematic nutritional assessment

This consists of four components:

The history

In medical use this is usually qualitative; has the patient been eating too little food, or omitted any major foods? Is an unusual diet being taken? Quantitative nutrient intake first elicits estimates of weights of all foods eaten by one of four methods – dietary history, 24 hour recall, food diary or food frequency questionnaire. By using food tables, usually in computer form, the daily intake of the major nutrients is obtained. These can then be compared against the recommended dietary allowance (RDA), a more detailed version of Table 3.2. An intake just below the RDA shows there is a risk of malnutrition but does not establish it because:

1. the days on which food intake was estimated may have been unrepresentative,
2. the physiological requirements between individuals for different nutrients range by a factor of about 2 and the RDAs are set to cover the requirements of nearly all healthy people,
3. for some nutrients, e.g. vitamins A and B_{12}, there are considerable reserves in the body.

Clinical examination

Thinness, oedema, pallor, weakness and other signs described in this chapter may be found, but one should not wait for the classic features of deficiency disease before intervening with nutritional support in a seriously ill patient in hospital. The primary illness may obscure or confuse signs of malnutrition.

Anthropometry

Changes of body weight reflect the water and/or energy (calorie) balance. If there is no unusual loss of water, each kilogram lost corresponds to 6000 to 7000 kcal of energy (i.e. mostly adipose tissue), unless there is increased protein catabolism when the energy values of weight lost is less. Regular weighing of patients in hospital is valuable in management but it is difficult in paralysed, deformed, and very sick patients, those nursed at strict bed rest, or with splints, fluid lines, catheters and drains. Weighing beds are scarce in most hospitals. The patient should in addition be watched for wasting of both subcutaneous fat and of muscles. If weighing is impractical these observations are more critical. Clinical estimation can be made more objective by measuring mid-arm circumference with a tape (Table 3.10). The relative contributions of fat and

Table 3.10   Reference standards for mid-arm circumference (mm)

	Men			Women		
		Centiles			Centiles	
Age	50th	10th	5th	50th	10th	5th
19–24	308	272	262	265	230	221
25–34	319	282	271	277	240	233
35–44	326	287	278	290	251	241
45–54	322	281	267	299	256	242
55–64	317	273	258	303	254	243
65–74	307	263	248	299	252	240

Figures based on a large sample of healthy US citizens from Frisancho AR. *Am J Clin Nutr* 1981; 34: 2540–5, and Bishop CW, *et al. Am J Clin Nutr* 1981; 34: 2530–9.

muscle can be calculated (mid-arm muscle circumference = arm circumference $- \pi \times$ triceps skinfold), but accurate measurement of skinfold thickness requires special calipers.

Laboratory investigations

These consist of:

1. those that indicate the protein status
2. biochemical tests for micronutrient deficiencies.

Plasma albumin concentration is the most reliable method to assess visceral protein depletion but it is also reduced (moderately) as part of the 'acute phase' reaction to trauma. Urinary nitrogen (or urea nitrogen) shows the degree of protein catabolism. A reduced total lymphocyte count indicates the possibility of impaired cell-mediated immunity of which protein depletion is one cause. Biochemical tests for vitamins and some other essential nutrients are listed in Table 3.11. As with other tests in chemical pathology there can be both false positives and negatives. Each result needs to be evaluated with critical understanding; for example serum vitamin B_{12} is increased in acute hepatitis and alkaline phosphatase may not be elevated if rickets is accompanied by PEM.

In general when the dietary intake of a nutrient is inadequate (less than obligatory losses) the individual goes through three stages. The first stage is that of adaptation to the low intake. For example, urine excretion falls but there is no evidence of abnormal function or of depletion of the cells. In the second stage there are in addition biochemical changes indicating either impaired function, e.g. reduced red cell transketolase activity in thiamin deficiency, or cellular depletion, e.g. reduced red cell folate. But clinical manifestations of deficiency are absent or non-specific. The third stage is that of clinical deficiency disease.

Most clinical biochemistry laboratories provide only some of the methods as a routine but others could be set up in special circumstances or, alternatively, a laboratory specialising in nutrition research could be asked to help.

Types of nutritional depletion in hospital patients

Protein-energy malnutrition (PEM) is the most important but is not always obvious and tends to be overshadowed by the primary disease. Calories and protein cannot be given as capsules or an injection and providing enough of them parenterally is expensive.

As in poorly fed children, there are different forms of PEM in hospital patients. At one end of the range is *semi-starvation* seen, for example, in anorexia nervosa or obstruction of the oesophagus. There is depletion of food energy but neither increased catabolism nor increased losses of body protein. There is loss of weight, decrease of arm circumference and skinfolds and normal plasma albumin.

At the other end of the range is *hypoalbuminaemic malnutrition*, which is sometimes called 'adult kwashiorkor'. This form is to be expected in a patient with increased protein catabolism, e.g. after burns or severe trauma, who has been receiving only intravenous glucose and water. This stimulates insulin which causes disproportional loss of visceral protein. Plasma albumin

Table 3.11 Biochemical methods used in diagnosing nutritional deficiencies

| Nutrient | Principal methods | | Supplementary methods |
	Indicating reduced intake	Indicating impaired function (IF) or cell depletion (CD)	
Protein	Urinary nitrogen	Plasma albumin (IF)	Fasting plasma amino acid pattern
Vitamin A	Plasma carotene	Plasma retinol	
Thiamin	Urinary thiamin	Red blood cell transketolase and TPP effect (IF)	
Riboflavin	Urinary riboflavin	Red blood cell glutathione reductase and FAD effect (IF)	
Niacin	Urinary N'methyl-nicotinamide		Fasting plasma tryptophan
Vitamin B$_6$	Urinary 4 pyridoxic acid and/or plasma pyridoxal phosphate	Red blood glutamic oxalacetic transaminase and PP effect (IF)	Urinary xanthurenic acid after tryptophan load
Folate	Plasma folate	Red blood cell folate (CD) (haemoglobin, packed cell volume, and bone marrow)	Urinary FIGLU after histidine load
Vitamin B$_{12}$	Plasma vitamin B$_{12}$	Reduced vitamin B$_{12}$ or transcobalamin II (haemoglobin, packed cell volume, and bone marrow)	Schilling test
Vitamin C	Plasma ascorbate	Leucocyte ascorbate (CD)	Urinary ascorbate
Vitamin D	Plasma 25-hydroxy-cholecalciferol	Raised plasma alkaline phosphatase (bone isoenzyme) (IF)	
Vitamin E	Plasma tocopherol	Red cell haemolysis with H$_2$O$_2$ in vitro (IF)	
Vitamin K	PIVKA II	Plasma prothrombin	
Sodium	Urinary sodium	Plasma sodium	
Potassium	Urinary potassium	Plasma potassium	Total body potassium by counting ^{40}K
Iron	Plasma iron and transferrin	Plasma ferritin (CD) (haemoglobin, packed cell volume, and smear)	Stainable iron in bone marrow
Magnesium	Plasma magnesium		
Iodine	Urinary (stable) iodide	Plasma protein-bound iodide (IF), plasma thyroxine (IF)	Radioactive iodine uptake by thyroid gland
Zinc	Plasma zinc	White blood cell zinc	Hair zinc

FAD = flavine adenine dinucleotide. There are no reliable simple methods for assessing calcium status.

is low, there can be oedema and cell-mediated immunity is impaired so resistance to infection is reduced.

Types of *micronutrient deficiency* likely to occur in hospitals are included in the information box below.

MICRONUTRIENT DEFICIENCY IN HOSPITAL

- Thiamin – patient starving or vomiting 3 wks if given IV glucose may develop Wernicke's encephalopathy
- Folate
- Vitamin B$_{12}$
- Vitamin C – losses increased by stress, wound healing requires increased supply
- Vitamin K – from biliary obstruction, antibiotics
- Iron – from bleeding
- Zinc

Nutritional support

Intake of vitamins and other micronutrients can be boosted by giving these in one or other pharmaceutical preparation, by mouth or by injection. When a multi-vitamin preparation is given it is important to check that it contains all the major vitamins (e.g. some omit folic acid).

As micronutrients can be provided fairly easily in hospital the main problem of nutritional support is to get water, calories and protein into the patient. There are four principal routes and more than one can be used together:

Oral feeding. The ordinary diet can be reinforced with calorie-dense or protein-rich supplements.

Tube (enteral) feeding. This is usually given by fine bore plastic nasogastric tubes but sometimes a gastrostomy or jejunostomy is used. Feeding can be continuous or intermittent and there is a wide range of enteral preparations. The 'polymeric' ones are mixtures, for example, of casein, maltodextrin, oils and micronutrients. Chemically-defined, 'monomeric' or 'elemental' preparations (amino acids, glucose, oil and micronutrients) are intended for patients who cannot take whole foods, e.g. for those with inflammatory bowel disease.

Parenteral feeding by a peripheral vein. This is easily established and is used for supplementary calorie and/or fluid support. Glucose infusions must be at not more than 10% concentration. Higher concentrations will cause phlebitis. Since 10% glucose in 2.5 l water is 250 g glucose and provides only 1000 kcal, energy requirements cannot be achieved unless intravenous lipid emulsion is given daily.

Parenteral feeding by central venous alimentation. This allows more concentrated glucose infusions (25–35%). Although it is possible to provide all a patient's calorie needs in this way, there are disadvantages to such a high carbohydrate intake such as high insulin levels and essential fatty acid deficiency. It is probably best to give about 30% of energy as intravenous fat emulsion, along with glucose, amino acids and micronutrients. The day's prescription can be made up sterile in the pharmacy in a 3-litre bag container. A stable patient with intestinal failure usually requires about 2500 kcal of energy, partly from glucose/electrolyte solutions, partly from an intravenous lipid preparation, e.g. 'Intralipid' (which contains essential fatty acids) and partly from an intravenous preparation of mixed crystalline L-amino acids, e.g. 'Aminoplex', 'Synthamin' or 'Vamin N'. The amino acid infusion usually provides 10–12 g nitrogen per day. This (× 6.25) is equivalent to 63–75 g of protein/day. Its pattern of essential amino acids is similar to that in egg albumin, i.e. it has a high biological value. In patients on total parenteral nutrition the minor nutrients, which are taken for granted in a diet of mixed foods by mouth, all have to be provided, i.e., all the nutrients in Table 3.2. Total parenteral nutrition costs considerably more than enteral feeding.

Indications

Total enteral nutrition is indicated in patients who cannot eat or drink because of unconsciousness, dysphagia, oesophageal obstruction, head and neck surgery and general weakness. Total parenteral nutrition is life-saving in patients with major disease of the small intestine. A number of patients have been nourished for years entirely by the intravenous route.

OBESITY

Obesity is the most common nutritional disorder in affluent societies. Its significance requires constant emphasis because it is associated with increased mortality, predisposes to the development of important diseases and diminishes the efficiency and happiness of those affected.

Obesity may be defined as a condition in which there is an excessive amount of body fat. This simple definition gives rise to two questions: how can body fat be measured, and what is 'excessive'?

All methods of measuring the fat content in the living subject are, to a greater or lesser degree, indirect. The simplest, but also the least direct, is the measurement of body weight and this is the method almost exclusively used in clinical practice. In the clinical context the 'desirable' or 'ideal' weight for height (p. 75) is that associated with the lowest mortality in actuarial terms and excessive weight that associated with increased mortality.

Aetiology

Excess fat accumulates because there is imbalance between energy intake and expenditure. This can arise in different ways and obesity is a clinical sign with several possible causes. There is no satisfactory aetiological classification of obesity, but a number of factors are known to be associated with its development.

Age. Obesity is most prevalent in middle-age, but can occur at any stage of life. Obesity in childhood and adolescence is likely to be followed by obesity in adult life.

Socio-economic. In affluent countries obesity is more common in the lower socio-economic groups. In developing countries it can occur only in the prosperous elite. Some occupations predispose to obesity, e.g. cooks and barmen, whilst jockeys, fashion models and airline pilots have to keep themselves slim. In some societies fat men are respected and fat women considered beautiful; in others they are not.

Heredity. A familial tendency exists in many cases, but it is difficult to disentangle environmental and genetic components. Patterns of eating and activity are influenced by social, cultural and economic factors which may be handed on from one generation to another. However, studies involving twins and adopted children indicate the importance of genetic factors in influencing both total body fat and its distribution. There is no evidence in man of obesity produced by a single gene, as in the genetically obese strains of rodents.

Endocrine factors. An endocrine influence on body fat is seen both in normal physiological situations and in pathological states. The normal fat content of young adult women is about twice that of young men and pregnancy is characterised by an increase in body fat. Obesity in women commonly begins at puberty, during pregnancy or at the menopause. Obesity frequently, but not invariably, accompanies hypothyroidism, hypogonadism, hypopituitarism and Cushing's syndrome. However, the overwhelming majority of obese patients show no clinical evidence of an endocrine disorder. The plasma concentration of insulin and cortisol is commonly raised and that of growth hormone reduced in obese subjects, but these changes probably result from, rather than cause the obesity, since they disappear when weight is lost.

Energy balance. A very small excess of calories, if habitual, can lead eventually to a large accumulation of fat. If a person eats a slice (28 g) of bread that is not needed each day or goes by car instead of walking for 15 minutes, the daily extra 60 kcal (250 kJ) will build up over 4 years to 10 kg of fat deposited.

Social factors, such as advertising and business lunches, may contribute to overeating and some people overeat because they are unhappy. There is some evidence that in obese people eating is determined less by 'internal cues', i.e. hunger and satiety, than by external influences like the availability, appearance and taste of food or the environment in which the food is served.

Physical inactivity has an important role in the development of obesity. Affluence is commonly associated with reduced energy expenditure. It is well recognised that physical activity is less in the obese than in the lean, but this may result from, rather than cause, the obesity. Moreover, the amount of energy expended by an obese person on most tasks is likely to be more because of the extra weight to be moved.

Many obese people believe that they do not eat more than their lean counterparts and frequently report an inability to lose weight on a low energy diet. These claims together with the failure of most dietary surveys to demonstrate a significant difference in the daily energy intake of obese and non-obese subjects have led to the hypothesis that in many instances the development of obesity is due to a metabolic defect causing reduced energy expenditure. The recent development of a new non-invasive technique (the doubly labelled water method) in conjunction with whole body calorimetry to measure total energy expenditure has made it possible to study, for the first time, unrestricted living subjects over an extended period. Such studies have shown that not only the basal metabolic rate but also the thermic response to food and the energy cost of activity are approximately the same in lean and obese subjects when corrected for differences in fat-free mass and total body mass. Moreover while self-recorded monitoring of energy intake reflected energy expenditure for lean subjects, those who were obese reported lower energy intakes than their energy expenditure. Thus it is clear that relatively mild but significant overeating may remain undetected in surveys employing standard techniques.

Drugs. The use of steroids, oral contraceptives, phenothiazines and insulin is commonly followed by obesity, mainly because appetite is stimulated.

Clinical features

In most cases the diagnosis will be apparent from the patient's appearance but the degree of obesity should also be assessed, usually by measurement of height and weight and reference to a table such as Table 3.12. In

Table 3.12 Guidelines for body weight in adults (men and women)

Height without shoes m	Approx. ft in	Weight (kg) without clothes			
		Significantly underweight (80% of lower end of Acceptable)	Acceptable	Obese	Grossly obese
1.45	4 9	34	42–53	63	84
1.48	4 10	35	44–55	66	88
1.50	4 11	36	45–56	68	90
1.52	5 0	37	46–58	69	92
1.54	5 1	38	47–59	71	95
1.56	5 1	39	49–61	73	97
1.58	5 2	40	50–62	75	100
1.60	5 3	41	51–64	77	102
1.62	5 4	42	52–66	79	105
1.64	5 5	43	54–67	81	108
1.66	5 5	44	55–69	83	110
1.68	5 6	45	56–71	85	113
1.70	5 7	46	58–72	87	116
1.72	5 8	47	59–74	89	118
1.74	5 9	48	61–76	91	121
1.76	5 9	50	62–77.5	93	124
1.78	5 10	51	63–79	95	127
1.80	5 11	52	65–81	97	130
1.82	6 0	53	66 83	99	132
1.84	6 0	54	68 85	102	136
1.86	6 1	55	69–86	104	138
1.88	6 2	57	71–88	106	141
1.90	6 3	58	72–90	108	144
1.92	6 4	59	74–92	111	147
BMI		< 16	20–25	> 30	> 40

The body mass index (BMI) is used to define nutritional status. It is derived from the formula, $weight(kg)/height(m)^2$. The acceptable (normal) range is 20–25. Obesity is taken to start at a BMI of 30 and gross obesity at 40. The grading of starvation is given on page 50. The standards are the same for men and women.

addition, the skinfold thickness over the triceps muscle can be measured using special spring-loaded calipers. Obesity is indicated by a reading above 20 mm in a man, and above 28 mm in a woman.

This very common disorder is frequently overlooked because the doctor is preoccupied by one of its many complications or ignores it because it is so familiar.

Obesity must be distinguished from a gain in weight due to fluid retention associated with cardiac, renal or hepatic disease, bearing in mind the fact that oedema does not become manifest clinically until the extracellular fluid has increased by about 15%

Complications

Psychological. Obese patients often have psychological difficulties, but it is difficult to distinguish between cause and effect. Depressed or anxious patients or the emotionally deprived may seek solace in food. Many obese people, especially younger adult females, are ashamed of their unattractive appearance and develop psychological and sexual problems.

Mechanical disabilities. These are listed in the information box below.

MECHANICAL DISABILITIES ASSOCIATED WITH OBESITY

- Flat feet
- Osteoarthrosis of knees, hips, lumbar spine
- Abdominal hernias
- Diaphragmatic hernias
- Varicose veins
- Exertional dyspnoea
- Respiratory infections
- Accidents

Metabolic disorders. Non-insulin dependent diabetes mellitus, hyperlipidaemia (elevation of cholesterol and triglyceride), gallstones, hyperuricaemia and gout are all more common among the obese than in the general population.

Cardiovascular disorders. Obesity increases the work done by the heart, which enlarges with rising body weight. Cardiac output, stroke volume, and blood volume all increase. Hypertension is common but, in the obese, blood pressure recorded with a standard sphygmomanometer cuff may be higher than direct intra-arterial measurements. The major source of error is failure of the cuff completely to encircle the arm.

The contribution which obesity alone makes to the aetiology of ischaemic heart disease is controversial. There is little doubt that obesity is associated with this disease, but it is difficult to separate the contribution of obesity from that of other risk factors which may be causally associated, such as diabetes, hypertension and hyperlipidaemia. In some prospective studies a direct association has been reported between central (abdominal) obesity, with a high waist/hip ratio and coronary disease. Special mention should also be made of physical inactivity, which may be both a cause and an effect of obesity and also plays an important role in the genesis of ischaemic heart disease.

Life expectancy. Overweight is associated with an increased rate of mortality at all ages. The level of excess mortality varies more or less in proportion to the degree of obesity.

There is also evidence that a substantial reduction of the body weight of obese people is alone sufficient to diminish the greater death rate. In the Society of Actuaries Build and Blood Pressure Study of 1979, the mortality was reduced to near normal in those who successfully lost and maintained weight within the desirable range. Thus the diagnosis and effective treatment of obesity is of vital importance, and recording the patient's weight and height must be just as much a routine part of clinical examination as taking the blood pressure or testing the urine.

Management

Whatever the ultimate cause of obesity in the individual case the immediate cause is energy imbalance, and weight reduction can be achieved only by reducing energy intake or by increasing output, or by a combination of the two. This involves change in the individual's way of life. Thus treatment is difficult and the patient needs motivation. Rewards must be seen ahead and psychological understanding and behavioural advice are essential weapons. It is most important for success that patients should be educated and informed about their disorder and misconceptions corrected. There are no 'slimming foods' or 'slimming tablets', which do not depend on a reduced energy intake.

Long-term results are best where patients are well motivated and educated, follow structured diets designed to provide 800 to 1600 kcal daily (p. 986) and are being seen and weighed regularly, every 1 to 2 weeks initially, by the same person. The number of patients requiring supervision is so great, the need for support is so prolonged and the success of some lay organisations such as 'Weight Watchers' compares so favourably with conventional medical methods, that it is justifiable to take advantage of the facilities provided by these groups. Most refer members to their own doctors at the first suggestion of any untoward developments.

However supervision is arranged, it is important that obese patients should be given precise advice as to how they should reorganise their dietary and other habits, an agreed target weight to aim for and an indication of the rate of weight loss expected.

Success does not depend upon operations, drugs, injections or other manipulations undertaken by the therapist but rather on the ability of the patient to manage the disorder himself or herself and to persist indefinitely with some restriction on dietary freedom.

The physician's role is to provide advice and continuing support. Many doctors find obese people unattractive, have difficulty in sympathising with their problems and fail to establish satisfactory rapport with them. Such attitudes contribute to the frequent lack of success in treatment.

The construction of a weight reducing diet

A weekly weight loss of 0.5 to 1 kg should be the general aim. An obese middle-aged housewife will usually lose weight satisfactorily on a diet providing 800 to 1000 kcal per day, such as the example on page 986. An obese man engaged in active physical work will not tolerate a diet as low as 1000 kcal per day but a satisfactory weight loss can be expected from a diet containing about 1500 kcal per day.

Obese people seldom develop more than a trace of ketosis and never sufficient to cause symptoms as long as they consume small amounts of carbohydrate. In a diet of 1000 kcal/day, 100 g of carbohydrate is a suitable allowance, taken as foods providing complex carbohydrates and dietary fibre (such as fruits and vegetables and whole grain cereals).

Fat. A 1000 kcal diet containing 100 g of carbohydrate and 50 g of protein, cannot include more than 40–45 g of fat. This allowance of fat, though small, is sufficient to make the diet palatable.

Vitamins. The diet should contain plenty of green vegetables and fruits, since they contain few calories, while their bulk helps to fill the stomach and relieve hunger; they also help to minimise the constipation common with a low food intake. Their vitamin A activity and vitamin C content will be sufficient to meet the body's needs. With meat, fish and eggs and fruit and vegetables in the diet there should be enough of the other vitamins.

Minerals. The only minerals that need serious consideration are calcium and iron. Provided the diet includes 300 ml of skimmed milk (100 kcal), there is little likelihood of a negative calcium balance developing in an adult. The supply of iron is less sure and may call for the prescription of iron supplements.

Alcoholic drinks. These are also a source of calories without essential nutrients and tend to stimulate appetite. They are best avoided, but if taken, a corresponding reduction in the diet is necessary. A 100 ml glass of dry wine or 30 ml whisky and water provide 70 kcal and half a pint of lager 80 kcal.

General. This diet is suitable for treatment of obese persons in Britain but it may be unsuitable in other cultures. Dietitians with knowledge of local eating customs can devise socially acceptable diets which provide about 1000 kcal made up from about 100 g carbohydrate, 50–60 g protein and 40–45 g fat.

Failure to respond to such a diet nearly always indicates non-compliance, despite protestations to the contrary! In such cases, treatment in hospital under strict supervision for 1 to 2 weeks may be beneficial to demonstrate that the prescribed regimen is effective if carefully followed and to allow a period of intensive education.

Therapeutic starvation

A period of several weeks of starvation in hospital with only water, non-caloric drinks with vitamin, mineral and protein supplements being allowed, has been recommended for very obese patients who have failed to respond to orthodox treatment.

Although the initial loss of weight may be marked, the long-term results are no more satisfactory than with other systems since many patients regain most of the weight lost when strict measures are discontinued. Such a regimen is contraindicated for older patients, especially if they have cardiovascular complications, since deaths have occasionally occurred. Ketosis may be troublesome in the early stages and hyperuricaemia, sometimes accompanied by gout, can develop.

Exercise

Most obese people lead sedentary lives and benefit from physical activity such as walking, swimming and gardening, provided it does not exceed their cardiovascular capacity. Regular daily exercise is much more valuable than episodic activity.

An hour's walk at 3 miles per hour will expend about 240 kcal above basal (or more for a heavy person). This may seem a small amount, equivalent to about 30 g of body fat, but if the daily walk becomes a habit it will add up, other things being equal, to a weight loss of 10 kg in a year. Doctors should suggest, discuss and work out with each patient an increasing programme of exercise which is within the physical capacity and which will add to the quality of life of the individual (see Table 3.13).

Table 3.13 Energy used in exercise (rounded approximate figures)

At rest	
(Men + 10%, women − 10%)	1 kcal/min
Moderate exercise	
For example, walking, gardening, golf	5 kcal/min
Intermediate	
For example, cycling, swimming, tennis	7 kcal/min
Strenuous	
For example, squash, jogging, hill climbing, heavy work	10 kcal/min

In SI units
1 kcal/min = 4.2 kJ/min = 70 watts

Drug therapy

This is no substitute for a dietary regimen but has a limited use as an adjunct in carefully selected patients with refractory obesity. Some of the more effective drugs used in the past, notably amphetamine, are addictive and have been so widely abused that they should not be prescribed for the treatment of obesity.

Amphetamine-like drugs with similar anorectic properties but causing less central nervous stimulation include diethylpropion (75 mg in a single dose daily) and phentermine (15–30 mg before breakfast). They may be given intermittently for periods of about a month to help attain a short-term goal. They should not be used in patients with hypertension or coronary heart disease.

Fenfluramine, which increases release of serotonin in the brain, probably acts by stimulating satiety rather than inducing anorexia. It may cause nausea, diarrhoea, lethargy, breathlessness due to pulmonary hypertension, excessive dreaming and, particularly on abrupt withdrawal, depression. It must be given only under medical supervision in a dose of 20 mg b.d., gradually increased to not more than 120 mg daily, unless adverse effects intervene. Treatment can be continued as long as weight is being lost.

These drugs must not be given to a patient with a history of psychiatric illness. Diuretics must be used with care and only if there is oedema because potassium depletion is more likely than usual while patients are on a restricted diet.

The administration of thyroxine to euthyroid patients is not only useless but is potentially dangerous, especially if heart disease is present. It should be prescribed only if hypothyroidism coexists with obesity.

Surgical treatment

Wiring the jaws together to prevent eating has been used to treat those who have found it impossible to adhere to a low-energy diet. Although this usually results in marked loss of weight, many patients regain weight when the procedure is reversed. An alternative and fairly safe operation (though a major one) is to reduce the size of the stomach, for example by stapling, which can be undone. Small intestine bypass, aimed at inducing malabsorption, has been undertaken in some centres for the treatment of severe 'morbid' obesity but complications can be severe and sometimes fatal. It should be emphasised that surgery should be considered only for those with gross, intractable obesity.

Prognosis

It is easy for an obese person to lose up to 5 kg in weight. This accounts for the temporary success of numerous popular 'slimming cures'. How difficult it is to achieve further losses is not generally realised. The published records of seven obesity clinics in the USA showed that satisfactory results ranged only from 12 to 28% if the index of success was the loss of 12 kg or more.

Experience in many clinics has also shown that it is difficult for patients to maintain their reduced weight since this requires some restriction of energy intake on a long-term basis.

Prevention

This must depend in part on the doctor who notices when patients, be they infants, children or adults, are gaining too much weight. For this purpose alone, among the most useful information that a doctor can keep about patients is a record of body weight, measured at regular intervals. The doctor's responsibility with an overweight patient, at any time, is advisory and educational; the attention of patients must be drawn to the dangers of obesity and to the appropriate methods of correcting it.

All the health agencies available should be mustered to support a steady campaign of education and persuasion of patients and potential patients on the need to avoid obesity. The antenatal services, infant welfare clinics, school health authorities, health visitors and many others to whom the public look for advice should contribute to this educational programme. The media also play an increasingly important role.

FURTHER READING

General nutrition

Truswell A S 1990 ABC of nutrition 2nd Edn. Originally British Medical Journal. A series of 20 articles that appeared in the BMJ in the second half of 1985.
Passmore R, Eastwood M A 1986 Davidson's Human nutrition and dietetics, 8th Edn. Churchill Livingstone, Edinburgh. A well-established standard textbook.
Paul A A, Southgate D A T 1978 McCance & Widdowson's

The composition of foods, 4th Edn. HMSO, London. British food tables but used in other countries because there is so much data in a single volume.
Shils M E, Young V R 1988 Modern Nutrition in Health and Disease, 7th Edn. Lea & Febiger, Philadelphia. The major American textbook (1694 pages).
Silk D B A 1983 Nutritional support in hospital practice. Blackwell Scientific Publications, Oxford.

Cameron M, Hofvander Y 1983 Manual on feeding infants and young children (for application in the developing areas of the world with special reference to home-made weaning foods), 3rd Edn. Oxford University Press, Delhi.

Obesity
Garrow J S 1981 Treat obesity seriously. A clinical manual. Churchill Livingstone, Edinburgh. The author has translated his research and clinical practice on obesity into a book with emphasis on management.
Royal College of Physicians 1983 Obesity. Royal College of Physicians, London. A comprehensive report.
Burton B T, Foster W R 1985 Health implications of obesity: an NIH consensus development conference. Journal of the American Dietetics Association 85: 1117–1120.

4

Climatic and Environmental Factors in Disease

Many factors affect the patterns of disease around the world. Climate makes physiological demands on the body which, if not met, may lead to ill health. Climate helps determine the range of pathogenic microbes in the environment and the pattern of diseases that they cause (Table 4.1, Fig. 4.1). Climate helps determine the crops that are grown, the animals tended and what foodstuffs are eaten. Thus wealth, nutrition, education and development, and their interaction with health, depend to a large extent on climate.

The majority of tropical countries are hot, humid and poor. They cannot feed themselves and have rudimentary health services that cannot educate or protect their exploding populations.

EXPOSURE TO ULTRAVIOLET LIGHT

Shortwave ultraviolet (U/V) light (290–320 nm) causes more direct damage than long wave (320–400 nm). Ultrashort waves < 290 nm are filtered out by the earth's ozone layer. As this layer is becoming thinner, more skin cancers are to be expected (Table 4.2).

SUNBURN

Clinical features

Sunburn is a complex type of acute inflammation that proceeds through erythema, itching, oedema, and bullae, to malaise, nausea, prostration and circulatory collapse.

Management

It may be prevented by the use of UV barrier creams or lotions (5–10% para-amino benzoic acid), and gradual exposure which encourages production of melanin. Treatment is by cooling, simple analgesics, for example aspirin or paracetamol, calamine lotion and fluid replacement which may be either oral or intravenously administered dextrose saline until volume depletion is corrected.

Prevention

People should not expose their skin to direct sunlight and should use barrier creams against reflected sunlight which is rich in shortwave. Those with ginger hair, green eyes, fair skin and large freckles, do not tan normally and are at special risk.

CHRONIC SOLAR DAMAGE

Clinical features

Chronic solar damage causes premature ageing of skin, dyspigmentation, atrophy and hyperkeratotic patches (solar keratoses) and skin cancers.

Table 4.1 Effects of climate and geography on the distribution of some important infectious diseases of the tropics (see Fig. 4.1)

Disease	Africa					Asia and Pacific				America			Europe
	A1	A2	A3	A4	A5	B1	B2	B3	C	D	E	F	G
Malaria	+++	+++	+	++	+	++	+++	+++	++	++	+		
Schistosomiasis	++	++	+	+++	+	++	1	++		++	+		
Trypanosomiasis 2	++	++		+	+					++			
Leishmaniasis	+	3,++	++	++	+	++	++	+		++	++		+
Cholera 4	+	+	+	+		+	+++	++				+	
Amoebiasis	++	++	++	++	++	++	+++	+++	++	+++	++	+	+
Typhoid fever	++	++	++	++	+	+++	+++	+++	+	++	++	+	+
Leprosy	+++	+++	++	+++	+	+	+++	+++	++	++	+	5	5
Onchocerciasis	+++	++		++		6,+				6,+			
Lymphatic filariasis	+++	+++		++		+	++	+++	+++	++	+		
Paragonimiasis	+						7,+	+++	7,+				
Clonorchiasis								+++					

+ Endemic
++ Highly endemic
+++ Very highly endemic
1. Small foci in B2, near Bombay and Madras.
2. Sleeping sickness in A, Chagas' disease in D.

3. Visceral in A2, both in other areas.
4. Situation varies with gradual spread of seventh pandemic.
5. Only a few small residual foci in F and G.
6. Yemen only in B1, north of equator in D.
7. Nepal and Sri Lanka in B2, Korea in C.

Table 4.2 The effects of ultraviolet light on the body

Shortwave 290–320 nm	Longwave 320–400 nm
Vasodilation, erythema, exudation, increased pigment (tanning) Changes in DNA: cell death, burning, ageing, keratoses, basal and squamous cell carcinoma, ? melanoma	*Direct* burning and tanning *Indirect* 1. Photoallergy to plants, chemicals and drugs 2. Photosensitivity in e.g. porphyria, SLE, pellagra

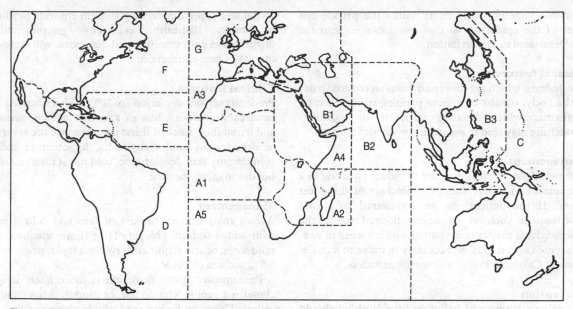

Fig. 4.1 Geographical distribution of disease due to infection. (Based on information supplied by the Ross Institute of Tropical Hygiene, London.)

Management

Solar keratoses may be treated with 5% fluoruracil ointment, applied for one week. Australia has the highest incidence of skin cancer in the world.

DISORDERS RELATED TO HEAT

In cool climates heat production in the body is balanced by loss from the surface chiefly by radiation and convection. When the environmental temperature approaches that of the body, evaporation of sweat becomes the most important mechanism in maintaining body temperature

Acclimatisation to heat (Table 4.3) is an essential preparation for workers exposed to excessive heat in certain industries in cool climates as well as for people who go to the tropics. This can be achieved by exercising daily under artificially produced or natural hot weather conditions for 10 to 14 days. With these

Table 4.3 Physiological changes of acclimatisation to heat

Circulatory volume	↑
Cardiac output	↑
Heart rate	↕
Aldosterone production	↑
Renal sodium retention	↑
Sweating	
responsiveness	↑
volume	↑
Demand for salt water	↑

adjustments the individual is able to work and remain well in a hot environment, provided an adequate intake of water and salt is maintained. In desert people renal retention of salt and water is so efficient that sweating is reduced to under 500 ml/day.

HEAT SYNCOPE

This occurs in people dressed in unsuitable clothes in a warm atmosphere with poor air circulation. It can occur in both physically active and sedentary individuals. The syndrome represents a failure of cardiovascular responses.

Clinical features

The onset is usually sudden and may be preceded by weakness or vertigo or headache. The patient has a brief period of collapse during which he appears ashen, the skin is cold and clammy and the blood pressure is low. Temperature is normal or sub-normal.

Management

This requires removal of the patient to a cool area. The patient is placed recumbent and intravenous administration of saline is rarely required. Recovery is usually rapid.

PRICKLY HEAT (MILIARIA RUBRA)

Many Europeans living in the tropics, especially when humidity is high, suffer from prickly heat. This arises from blockage of sweat ducts within the prickle cell layer of the epidermis so that sweat escapes into the epidermis and causes irritation.

Clinical features
The lesions, which are most numerous on covered parts of the body, consist of minute papules, surrounded by erythema, which become vesicular or pustular. Scratching may lead to secondary pyogenic infection.

Management
The principles of treatment are to reduce sweating to a minimum and to overcome the blockage of the sweat ducts. If the patient can be transferred to a cool environment such as an air-conditioned room, the blocked ducts may become patent within a week or two. In severe cases it may be necessary to move to a cooler climate. Calamine lotion relieves the irritation.

Prevention
Excessive washing and irritation from clothing should be avoided and a bland soap containing hexochlorophane used if prickly heat is to be prevented. Clothing must be loose fitting, changed frequently and thoroughly rinsed after washing. Obese patients must lose weight. Spices and alcohol, which cause sweating, should be avoided.

TROPICAL ANHIDROTIC ASTHENIA

Patients with this disorder cannot sweat properly. The defect may be congenital or secondary to prickly heat.

Clinical features
The condition develops insidiously, with headache, giddiness, lethargy, diminished sweating and often marked polyuria. Fever is common and hyperpyrexia (rectal temperature greater than 41°C, 106°F) may develop.

Management
The patient must live in a cool climate for several months until the skin has recovered and sweating has returned to normal.

HEAT EXHAUSTION

This is brought on by a period of great heat or by extra effort in hot weather, when the patient has not taken enough fluid and salt to balance the increased loss by sweating. The amount of fluid lost as sweat during a working spell in a hot environment may be as much as 6–8 litres especially in unacclimatised people,

containing approximately 2 g sodium chloride per litre of water. Ill-health, especially gastrointestinal disturbances with vomiting and diarrhoea, will increase the risk of heat exhaustion.

Clinical features
Predominant salt depletion (p. 205) is characterised by headache, giddiness, loss of appetite, nausea, cramps and irritability. Lack of thirst may disguise the severity of dehydration until tachycardia, hypotension and a cold clammy skin develop (the 'cold moist man', c.f. the hot dry man, see below).

Management
A cool environment, the use of fans and cold drinks with added sodium chloride (10 g/l) are adequate for mild cases; others require intravenous replacement with 0.9% sodium chloride.

Predominant water depletion is more likely in acclimatised people who do not, or cannot, drink enough water. Thirst and signs of dehydration (p. 206) are present. Treatment is by giving water by mouth or 5% glucose intravenously. As much as 5–10 litres may be needed in the first 24 hours. The patient may develop heat hyperpyrexia when heat exhaustion is not recognised and treated.

HEAT HYPERPYREXIA (HEATSTROKE)

Heatstroke is a syndrome due to overheating the body core. It is often a complication of heat exhaustion, tropical anhidrosis or prickly heat. It can also occur, especially in unacclimatised people or in those with congenital lack of sweat glands, in response to exertion in a hot humid environment. In exceptional weather even local inhabitants may suffer. Unsuitable clothing and poor ventilation increase the risk. The disorder is always associated with cessation of sweating and the rectal temperature may reach 42°C to 43°C or even higher.

The most important pathological changes are in the central nervous system. There is general congestion of the brain with increased pressure of the cerebrospinal fluid. Microscopic examination may show degeneration of nerve cells, particularly in the hypothalamic region and base of the brain.

Clinical features
The onset is usually dramatic with no warning in a person who appears to be neither dehydrated nor deficient in salt, but who may have noticed that perspiration has diminished. Loss of consciousness is rapid and may be preceded by prodromal signs of cerebral irri-

tation. On examination a dry burning skin is found (the 'hot dry man'). When the temperature reaches 41° and 42°C the patient loses consciousness and dies, unless treated. Hyperpyrexia may be complicated by acute circulatory failure, hypokalaemia, acute renal or hepatic failure and hamorrhage.

Management
The aim is to reduce the temperature as quickly as possible. In the field, the patient is moved into the shade, the clothing removed and the skin kept wet and fanned vigorously. In hospital this is done by spraying the naked patient with water or loosely wrapping the individual in a cool, wet sheet and promoting evaporation by fanning. Ideally the water should be at 15°C and the airstream at 30–35°C. The use of iced water, or immersion in cold water causes vaso-constriction and hinders heat loss. Cooling should be stopped when the rectal temperature has fallen to 39°C. The airway must be maintained and oxygen given. Potassium deficiency should be corrected and severe haemorrhage controlled by blood transfusion. Acute circulatory failure (p. 281), acute renal failure (p. 588) or hepatic failure (p. 512) may require treatment. Parenteral antimalarial therapy (p. 154) should be given concurrently if malaria is a possibility. With energetic treatment 90% of patients recover.

Prevention (Table 4.4)
Heavy work in a hot, humid climate may require a daily intake of up to 15 litres of water and 30 g of sodium chloride. The extra salt is taken with food and in drinking water or in enteric coated tablets.

Table 4.4   Prevention of heat related disorders

Pre employment selection	Predisposing factors	Practical measures
Physically fit	Fever	Acclimatisation
Mentally stable	Gastrointestinal disease	Adequate water intake
Healthy skin	Obesity	Adequate salt intake
Healthy bowels	Alcoholism	Light loose clothing
	Defective sweating	Air conditioning
	Over exertion in hot humid conditions	Early treatment

DISORDERS RELATED TO COLD

FROSTBITE

Dry cold, below 0°C, freezes poorly-insulated tissues such as fingers especially in people exercising at altitudes where oxygen demand is high and availability low.

Clinical features
The warning sign is intense pain in fingers or feet. Superficial frostbite causes blistering of skin; in deep frostbite there is necrosis of tissue leading to gangrene.

Management
Frostbite is treated by rapidly rewarming the whole patient with good insulation and hot drinks, and by warming the affected part in water at 40°C.

HYPOTHERMIA

Hypothermia is less common than hyperthermia but it is an important condition as it represents a medical emergency which requires urgent therapy.

Hypothermia can occur either from accidental causes when an individual has been exposed to low temperatures and secondarily as a complication of acute illness.

Accidental hypothermia may occur in babies, the elderly, the drunk and the sick, who have been exposed to low temperatures. It is associated with various diseases, notably Addison's disease, myxoedema, cerebro-vascular accidents and sepsis, and may arise as a complication of hypoglycaemia, uraemia, hepatic failure, starvation, muscular paralysis and certain drugs, especially phenothiazines which inhibit shivering. Hypothermia can also occur as a result of immersion in cold water or evaporation and is a particular problem in North Sea oil-rig workers, long-distance swimmers, sailors and hill walkers.

Clinical features
The body temperature is, by definition, below 34°C and may be as low as 25°C. It is important that a true temperature is recorded using a thermocouple or an incubation thermometer. The patient is cold, pale and there may be stiffness of the muscles. When the temperature falls below 26.7°C the patient becomes unconscious and may develop general oedema. Pupillary and tendon reflexes disappear.

Investigations
Haemoconcentration will be present and mild uraemia and a metabolic acidosis due to lactacidaemia which is in part due to hypoxia of peripheral tissues. Hypoglycaemia may be present, but some patients are hyperglycaemic. Pancreatitis develops in a few patients and this may cause a rise in serum amylase. The electrocardiogram (ECG) is characteristic, showing a J-wave which occurs at the junction of QRS complex and the ST segment. Abnormalities of cardiac rhythms including ventricular fibrillation are common. A bradycardia is present. The ECG may be distorted by muscular tremor.

Management

The patient is rewarmed gradually using a space blanket. Too rapid rewarming may result in shock and will not cause sufficient elevation of the core temperature to warm the myocardium. Particular attention must be paid to the development of arrhythmia. Intravenous sodium bicarbonate should be given if pH is less than 7.25. It is important to monitor the serum potassium and blood gases. Warmed oxygen may be used. Careful attention to the lungs is necessary as there is a high prevalence of pneumonia which should be treated with appropriate antibiotic therapy. Maintenance of blood volume is essential and this can be achieved using glucose and saline or albumen or low molecular weight dextran which may be warmed to 37°C.

Prognosis

There is a particularly high mortality rate in people over the age of 75. Care must be exercised in pronouncing hypothermic individuals dead. No certification of death should be issued until patients have been rewarmed to 36°C and have been unresponsive at that temperature. This applies particularly to younger patients who are capable of surviving hypothermia for suprisingly long periods.

DISORDERS RELATED TO ALTITUDE

The partial pressure of atmospheric oxyen decreases with altitude so that oxygen tension in the lungs falls from 149 m Hg at sea level to 43 m Hg at the top of Mount Everest (8848 m). Physiological acclimatisation (Table 4.5) starts at about 1500 m and most people feel

Table 4.5 Physiological changes of acclimatisation to altitude

↑ Ventilation: respiratory alkalosis
↑ Urinary bicarbonate excretion
↑ Pulmonary diffusion
↑ Red blood cell mass
↑ Cardiac output

Altered distribution of blood to tissues
↑ Tissue capillarity

the need to acclimatise by about 3500 m. Physically fit young people acclimatise best and do better with each ascent. Lowlanders, however, never attain the performance of highlanders. Lack of acclimatisation is shown by increased respiration, Cheyne-Stokes respiration, mild headache and irritability, easy fatiguability and sleeplessness.

Acclimatisation continues successfully up to 5330 m above which maximal heart rate and cardiac output start to fall, pulmonary diffusion becomes impaired, arterial oxygen saturation falls and physical performance declines. Short bursts of work can be undertaken, but at the risk of production of an exaggerated lactic acidosis. Prolonged residence above this height causes anorexia, weight loss, decreasing mental and physical capacity and increasing susceptibility to infection. There are no permanent human habitations above 4575 m.

ACUTE MOUNTAIN SICKNESS

This is experienced by people who go up too high too quickly; some suffer at 2500 m, others reach 5500 m without trouble. The cause of the syndrome is unknown.

Clinical features

The earliest symptoms are headache, nausea and vomiting, followed by lassitude, muscle weakness, breathlessness, dizziness, rapid pulse and insomnia. Retinal haemorrhages may ocurr.

Acute mountain sickness may herald the onset of two severe, possibly fatal, complications: pulmonary oedema (p. 250) and, less commonly, cerebral oedema. Youth, speed of ascent, reascent, exertion and absolute altitude are associated with pulmonary oedema. Cerebral oedema causes drowsiness, irritability, confusion, fits and coma. Its presence may be confirmed by the detection of papilloedema.

Venous thromboses, which may lead to pulmonary embolism, may afflict the partially acclimatised; they are due to increased viscosity of blood and are prevented by adequate hydration and exercise.

Management

The complications are prevented by time spent acclimatising, ascending gradually, adequate hydration and by acetazolamide which probably acts by causing metabolic acidosis and an increased drive to ventilation. They are treated by descending 500–1000 m rapidly and by giving oxygen. Frusemide 40–120 mg daily and morphine 15 mg as required is the treatment for pulmonary oedema, and dexamethasone (p. 848) for cerebral oedema.

CHRONIC MOUNTAIN SICKNESS

This is due to alveolar hypoventilation and chronic hypoxia brought about by inappropriate polycythaemia, and may affect highlanders as well as acclimatised lowlanders. People with sickle cell disease (homozygous Hb S, p. 719), are at risk of infarction at 2000 m, which is equivalent to the pressure in a commercial airliner flying at 11 000 m. Heterozygotes can normally tolerate altitudes of 3000 m or more. Patients with myocardial disease should not ascend rapidly above 2000 m.

Clinical features
These include cyanosis, cardiac failure, pulmonary hypertension and neuropsychiatric symptoms.

Management
Chronic mountain sickness is treated by taking the patient down to sea level.

DISORDERS RELATED TO INCREASED BAROMETRIC PRESSURE

At sea level the barometric pressure is 760 mm Hg, or one atmosphere. Under water, pressure rises by one atmosphere for every 10 m of depth. Following Boyle's law, the volume of enclosed gas varies inversely with the surrounding pressure. This pressure/volume effect accounts for most diving pathology. As the greatest *changes* in pressure happen at shallow depths many of the problems associated with diving occur at shallow depths.

MIDDLE EAR 'SQUEEZE'

Middle ear 'squeeze' is the commonest injury of divers. *Sinus squeeze* is less common.

Clinical features
Unless air is allowed into the middle ear to equalise pressure, the lining becomes oedematous, then haemorrhagic and the tympanic membrane may rupture at depths of 1–2 m below. Rarely the round or oval window may rupture, causing severe vertigo, tinnitus and deafness. Both forms of squeeze, and reverse squeezes during decompression, also occur during air travel, especially in babies and in those with upper respiratory tract disease.

Management
Middle ear squeeze is prevented by Valsalva manoeuvre, or by ascending in response to pain, and is treated with decongestants such as 1% ephedrine nasal drops.

SHALLOW WATER BLACKOUT
Swimmers and free divers (snorkling without compressed air) may hyperventilate before submerging in order to drive off CO_2 and so reduce the stimulus to breathe. The raised ambient pressure maintains a high arterial O_2 tension, but this falls profoundly when the diver is eventually forced to surface. The resulting cerebral hypoxia is made worse by cerebral vasoconstruction induced by the low PCO_2, and can result in unconsciousness and drowning.

PULMONARY OVERINFLATION

This occurs in scuba divers breathing compressed air. On ascending from 10 m to the surface the lung volume doubles. Unless air is driven off by repeated exhalation, the alveoli become over-pressurised and rupture. This can happen in dives of no more than 2 m.

Clinical features
Air from ruptured alveoli may escape in one of three ways and cause:

1. interstitial emphysema in the chest, neck or retroperitoneal space with the production of pain, crepitus, impaired venous return and characteristic radiographic appearances;
2. pneumothorax (p. 414);
3. air embolism where air leaks into the pulmonary capillaries, reaches the coronary or cerebral arteries, impairs local circulation, increases capillary permeability and precipitates intravascular coagulation.

The clinical condition is usually evident within minutes of surfacing, and varies from minor changes of mood to apnoea, coma and cardiac arrhythmia.

Management
Treatment requires recompression, but while transporting the patient supine to the treatment centre it is important to maintain a good airway, administer 100% oxygen, treat any dysrhythmia, treat hypotension with fluids and dopamine, 2–5 µg/kg/min by i.v. infusion and control seizures with diazepam (p. 859). Air embolism is one of the commonest causes of death among divers.

DECOMPRESSION SICKNESS

This is also known as 'the bends'. The amount of gas dissolved in tissue depends upon the partial pressure of that gas in a mixture of gases, the ambient pressure and the duration under pressure. Tissue metabolism removes oxygen from dissolved inhaled air. Therefore, during a long deep dive, dissolved nitrogen accumulates in tissues, especially fatty tissues, a process known as 'on-gassing'. When that tissue is saturated, bubbles form. As pressures fall during ascent saturation levels are easily reached. Gas bubbles are released ('off-gassing') and cause decompression sickness.

Clinical features

Symptoms are usually evident within an hour of surfacing and rarely start after 4 hours.

Type 1, or musculoskeletal decompression sickness

This is limited to the effects of gas released into muscle, skin or lymphatics. It is characterised by pain in the limbs, pruritis, marbling of skin, painful lymph nodes and lymphoedema.

Type 2, or neurologic decompression illness/sickness

This is associated with gas released into the central nervous system and viscera, and causes pain in head, neck and abdomen, paraesthesiae, dermatomal numbness and pain, paraplegia, bowel and bladder disturbances and a wide range of signs of cerebral damage including visual disturbances, seizures and hemiplegia. Gas bubbles in the inner ear causes vestibular damage 'the staggers'. Pulmonary decompression causes pain and dyspnoea 'the chokes' and may be rapidly fatal.

Management

Treatment of decompression sickness is by recompression. Prompt treatment usually leads to complete recovery, but delayed treatment may result in permanent disability. Those with type 2 sickness benefit from the emergency measures described for gas embolism, plus generous intravenous fluid replacement, during transport to the treatment centre.

INDIRECT EFFECTS OF CLIMATE ON HEALTH AND DISEASE

Climate chiefly determines the distribution, type and density of vegetation and crops, of microbes, insects and larger animals including man. Thus climate has diverse effects on human behaviour, nutrition, and opportunities for transmission of infection, and indirect effects on health and disease. Some examples are given Table 4.6. Climate also determines the distribution of some natural toxins, such as aflatoxin, a fungal contaminant of stored grains causing hepatoma, and angemone poisoning of crops in India causing epidemic dropsy (p. 981).

Table 4.6 Indirect effects of climate on disease: some examples

Climate	Effect	Disease
Cold/dry	Crowding, extra clothing, little washing	Louse-borne disease
	Damage to upper respiratory mucosa	Respiratory tract infection
Hot/dry	Cyclical drought	Starvation
	Production of concentrated urine	Urolithiasis
	Sandflies live in rodent burrows	Zoonotic cutaneous leishmaniasis
Hot/moist	Sweaty skin	Pyoderma, nephritis
	Seasonal rivers	Onchocerciasis, seasonal malaria
	Man meets tse-tse fly at rivers	Trypanosomiasis
Hot/wet	Soil rich in microorganisms	Tropical and Buruli ulcers
	Interaction of two microbes	Burkitt's lymphoma
	Precise requirement met for vector	Loa loa infection
	Crowding, riverine festivals	Ganges delta is the home of cholera
	Filarial infections cause eosinophilia	Endomyocardial fibrosis

Table 4.7 Characteristics of extreme climatic zones

Characteristic	Rain forest	Tropical savanna	Tropical deserts	Mountains	Tundra
Climate	Hot/wet	Hot/moist	Hot/dry	Cold/moist	Cold/dry
Water	Plenty	Seasonal	Scarce, local	Variable	Variable
Leaf crops	Plenty	Seasonal	Oases only	∝ rainfall	Scarce
Grains	Scarce	Plenty	Scarce	Grown	Grown
Herds, flocks	Scarce	Plenty	Tended	Plenty	Tended
Diet	↓ protein	↓ seasonally	↓ vitamins	∝ rainfall	↓ seasonally
Insects	+++	++	+	∝ temperature	+(summer)
Microbes	+++	++	+	∝ temperature	+
People	Gatherers	Nomads	Nomads	Farmers	Nomads
	Farmers	Farmers	Settlements	Towns	Farmers
		Towns			

+Occasional
++Common
+++Frequent

MICROCLIMATES

Most people live in the temperate zones which are warm and moist. The effects of climate are best seen by examining the zones of extreme climate (Table 4.7). It is important, however, not to overgeneralise. Within the broad ranges of gross climate, there are micro-climates which further affect the distribution of disease. For example, mosquitoes breed on surface water and rest above ground, so the distribution of malaria is an absolute reflection of peak annual temperature; whereas phlebotomine sandflies find their very precise require-ments for temperature and moisture in burrows, tree-holes, cracks and crevices (p. 158) where the microbes that they carry can also find vertebrate reservoirs; so they transmit disease over a wide climatic and geo-graphical range.

SEASON

Within any climatic zone, season is also an important determinant of disease. In semi-arid zones food is scarce before the rains and malnutrition occurs; during the rains the hard work of planting causes farmers to lose weight, while malaria and gastrointestinal disease increase. Very dry weather, be it hot, cold, at altitude or due to airconditioning, damages the upper respiratory mucosa, permitting infection. In sub-Saharan Africa this leads to annual epidemics of menigococcal meningitis in March and April. Figure 4.2 illustrates the effect of seasonal climate on disease.

Drought poses special problems (Fig. 4.3) which predispose to famine and intercurrent illness. Relief camps, like all refugee camps, encourage epidemics of respiratory, diarrhoeal, louse borne and skin diseases, through crowding and lack of sanitation.

FACTORS OTHER THAN CLIMATE

Climate is not the only determination of the geo-graphical distribution of disease. Many other factors are involved, for example: evolution of insects producing reduvid bugs and permitting Chagas disease in South America (p. 163), evolution of haemoglobin S in West Africa permitting sickle cell disease (p. 719), human behaviour determining the distribution of hepato-cellular carcinoma (p. 535) and hydatid disease (p. 172), 'technical development' determining the pattern of nutritional disease.

DISEASES RELATED TO POLLUTION

The environment, external, at home or at work, may contribute to risks of diseases in which the environ-

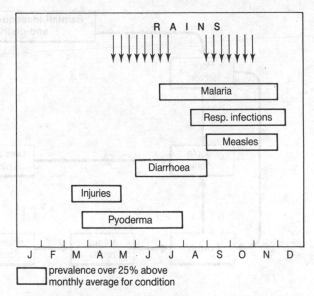

Fig. 4.2 **Seasonal variation of disease in a community in Southern Ghana.** (Parry, 1984.)

mental contribution is not easily recognised in the in-dividual patient, for instance chronic bronchitis or cancer of various organs. Occasionally environmental factors cause a distinctive clinical illness which may suggest the cause. This section describes some of these relatively distinctive illnesses, but does not attempt to address the much broader problem of the influence of the environment on health. The diseases included can result from factors in the general or home environment because an adequate description of occupational diseases is not possible here; instead, some suggestions are made to assist the general physician when seeking information on the health effects of agents encountered at work.

ACUTE TRACHEOBRONCHITIS AND PULMONARY OEDEMA

Air pollution from urban or industrial sources has occasionally reached disaster levels causing obvious acute disease and increased mortality. When this happens, the air contains a mixture of pollutants from local sources, and local climatic conditions cause polluted air to be retained close to the ground. For example in the London smogs of 1952 and 1956, burning of coal in domestic fires generated soot and sulphur dioxide; the disasters in the Meuse Valley in Belgium in 1930 and Donora, Pennsylvania in 1948 were associated additionally with fluorides from local metal smelters; and in the smog disasters in Los Angeles

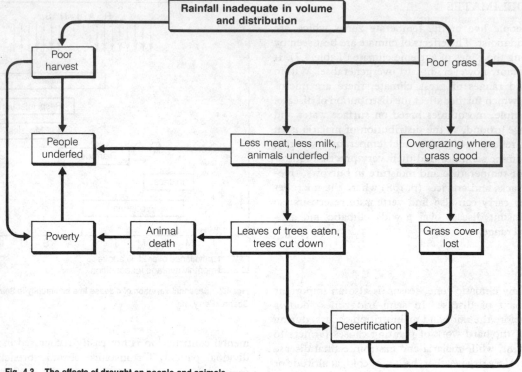

Fig. 4.3 The effects of drought on people and animals.

in 1942, 1954 and 1955, and in Piscatawar, New Jersey, the effect of sunshine on pollutants from vehicle exhausts and factories caused high levels of oxidants to be produced, particularly ozone. Sometimes local disasters have been the result of an accidental release of a gas from an industrial source, such as of chlorine or ammonia from a damaged road or rail tanker, or an explosion such as the release of isocyanates in the disaster at Bhopal, India. At work, exposure to leakages of chlorine, ammonia, oxides of nitrogen, sulphur dioxide, acids, alkalis and many other irritant or toxic substances may occur.

The elderly, and those already suffering from respiratory or cardiac disease, are particularly susceptible to the high levels of pollutants occurring in disasters, and in some instances, footballers, presumably by virtue of their outdoor activity and increased ventilation, have been notably, though temporarily, affected.

Clinical features

The symptoms are those of acute irritation, oedema and hypersecretion of respiratory mucosal surfaces; eye irritation, rhinitis, sore throat, chest pains, cough and wheeze. Symptoms may be worsened in asthmatic subjects, and in others, breathlessness and in extreme cases, frothy sputum, cyanosis, basal crackles and hypoxia indicate pulmonary oedema. Onset of symptoms may be delayed several hours after acute exposures. Deaths may occur, numbering from scores in several of the above mentioned disasters to several thousand in the London smogs. Deaths are commonly due to cardiac, as well as to respiratory, failure.

Management

This consists of withdrawal from the polluted atmosphere (even returning home and keeping the windows closed has been reported to relieve symptoms temporarily), and supportive measures including controlled oxygen, treatment of bronchospasm and cardiac failure, and ventilatory support when required.

CHRONIC BRONCHITIS AND AIRFLOW OBSTRUCTION

While the most important cause of chronic bronchitis (chronic mucous hypersecretion) and chronic airflow obstruction is smoking, urban and industrial air pollution also contribute. Either morbidity or mortality from these causes have been shown to be related to urbanisation, air pollution and fog. In Britain the improvement in air pollution brought about by the Clean Air Acts has been associated with a reduction of mortality from chronic bronchitis or emphysema (no doubt also influenced by changes in smoking habits), and day-to-day correlations between air pollution and rates of bronchitic morbidity can no longer be demonstrated.

The clinical features and management of chronic bronchitis, airflow obstruction and emphysema, are described in Chapter 9, p. 341.

EXTRINSIC ASTHMA, SEASONAL RHINITIS, CONJUNCTIVITIS

Extrinsic asthma, seasonal rhinitis (hay fever) and conjunctivitis in atopic individuals are strongly influenced by allergens in the air. Well-known examples are grass pollen in Europe and ragweed pollen in North America, though local variants are common. *Aspergillus fumigatus* is a universal soil mould whose airborne spores may colonise the bronchial mucus and cause an allergic pneumonia in asthmatics (allergic bronchopulmonary aspergillosis) or colonise lung cysts or cavities in the form of a fungus ball (mycetoma). These diseases are described in Chapter 9, p. 373. Many agents at work can cause asthma (for example, isocyanates, or colophony in solder fumes).

LEAD POISONING

In the general population the major contribution of lead to the total daily intake is usually from food and drink, though, in industry, inhalation of contaminated air may be more important. The major sources of lead in the environment are fuel additives released in automobile emissions, and various industrial sources. Lead is deposited near roads and in the vicinity of lead smelters, or where discarded battery cases are being burned. It may deposit on fruit and vegetables. Other sources include lead water pipes and tanks, and storage of food, wine or beverages in lead-soldered cans or pottery in which lead in the glaze and pigments has not been adequately stabilised; or illicit whisky made in stills improvised from discarded automobile radiators. Children are particularly at risk if they chew and eat lead-based paint from old houses or the soil around these houses.

The earliest effects of lead are interference with the enzymes responsible for manufacturing haemoglobin, notably aminolaevulinic acid dehydratase (ALAD) and haem synthetase, with accumulation of the substrates ALA and protoporphyrin IX in red cells, and ALA and coproporphyrins in the urine. Disturbances of ALA metabolism may occur at lower blood lead levels than any obvious clinical illness, the earliest feature of which is anaemia. The anaemia, of the microcytic variety with siderocytes, may be accompanied by basophilic stippling of red cells.

Clinical features

Symptoms may include fatigue and lassitude, generalised aches and pains in muscles and joints, abdominal discomfort, diarrhoea or a bad taste in the mouth. Severely affected patients may have abdominal pains, colic, constipation and a motor peripheral neuropathy. In extreme cases renal tubular damage occurs and encephalopathy, particularly in children. Blue lines on the gum margins and radiographic lead lines on long bones (except in children) are rare.

Investigations

Laboratory investigations show an elevated blood lead (whole blood, the lead is almost all bound to red cells) and increased urinary concentrations of ALA and coproporphyrin. Red cell concentrations of ALAD are decreased. Normal blood lead levels increase with age in children, for example an average value of about $3\,\mu g/100\,ml$ is to be found in the first year of life to about $13\,\mu g/100$ on average for ages between 4 and 13 years. Adult levels are between 10 and $25\,\mu g/100\,ml$, irrespective of age. On average, extrapolating from exposure-response studies, the no-detected effect blood level for ALAD activity in red cells is about $10\,\mu g/100\,ml$. The no-effect level for anaemia is between 50 and $100\,\mu g/100\,ml$, $(40\,\mu g/100$ in iron-deficient children). For noticeable brain dysfunction the level is about $50\,\mu g/100\,ml$ in children, $60–70\,\mu g/m^3$ in adults. There is currently a debate on the influence of intermediate blood lead levels on intellectual ability in children.

Management

Treatment consists of prompt removal from exposure, and supportive measures which in severe cases may include treatment of seizures with diazepam (0.5% solution, 10–20 mg, at rate of 0.5 ml (2.5 mg) per 30 s), maintenance of fluid and electrolyte balance, and treatment of cerebral oedema with dexamethasone (10 mg i.v. followed by 4 mg i.m. every 6 h for 2–10 days) and mannitol (50–200 g i.v. over 24 h). Chelation therapy should be instituted in symptomatic patients or those with blood levels greater than $100\,\mu g/100\,ml$. Edetate calcium sodium (up to 40 mg/kg twice daily i.v. in 0.9% NaCl infusion), and dimercaprol (2.5–3 mg/kg i.m. every 4 h for 2 days and then reduce dose) are used parenterally, and d-penicillamine orally.

As with other occupational or environmental diseases, when lead poisoning is diagnosed, the Employment Medical Advisor, or Environmental Health Officer (whichever is appropriate to the source of the poisoning) should be informed so that others may be protected against the hazard.

MERCURY POISONING

The major environmental source of mercury is the natural degassing of the earth's crust. Sources of additional production by man include burning of fossil fuels, production of steel, cement and phosphate, and the smelting of metals from their sulphide ores. Food is the main route of entry in non-occupational exposures, since methyl mercury compounds accumulate in fish, to high levels in contaminated waters. Outbreaks of chronic mercury poisoning in the general population occurred in the villages round Minimata Bay, and also the Niigata river, in Japan. In both circumstances mercury compounds from local industry had contaminated the water and fish. Over a thousand cases of chronic mercury poisoning were identified. Other epidemics have occurred due to ethyl or methyl mercury fungicides on wheat intended for planting but actually used for making bread. The largest of these was in Iraq, when over 6000 people were admitted to hospital.

Clinical features

The most common signs and symptoms of chronic mercury poisoning are paraesthesia, constriction of the visual fields, impairment of hearing and ataxia. Classical symptoms of severe poisoning include erethism (irritability, excitability, loss of memory, insomnia, excessive sweating and flushing), intention tremor and gingivitis. Renal damage may occur. The clinical affects may not reverse much even after exposure ceases. Acute mercury poisoning due to the ingestion of large amounts of any mercurial compound leads to bleeding from, and necrosis of, the gut; vomiting, circulatory collapse and renal failure. Acute pulmonary oedema may result from the inhalation of mercury vapour.

Management

Chronic inorganic mercury poisoning

This is treated with dimercaprol for high exposures or symptomatic patients, or penicillamine for lower exposures or asymptomatic patients. Haemodialysis may be required for renal failure in occasional cases.

Acute poisoning

This may require respiratory support, attention to fluid and electrolyte balance, gastric lavage, oral charcoal (5–10 g in 100–200 ml water repeated every 15–20 min) and a magnesium cathartic. Treatment of organic mercury poisoning is less effective. Penicillamine (1–2 g daily orally in divided doses before food) and an oral non-absorbable thiol resin can reduce blood concentrations of mercury, though this may not be associated with much clinical benefit. Dimercaprol is contraindicated, since it increases the mercury concentrations in the brain.

FLUOROSIS

Skeletal fluorosis occurs endemically in some tropical and sub-tropical areas with high fluoride concentrations in soil and water. In non-endemic areas it may occur as a result of occupational exposure in aluminium production, magnesium foundries, fluorspar processing and superphosphate manufacture. The bones become sclerotic, and calcification occurs in other organs.

Clinical features

In children the more severe effects include genu valgus and varum, lateral bowing of the femora, sabre shins, deformities of ribs, thorax, vertebral bodies, pelvis and joints. Milder forms include mottling of the teeth. In adults, occupational exposure may lead to increased bone density and thickening of long bones, the development of exostoses and osteophytes (e.g. calcaneal spur); calcification in ligaments, tendons and muscle insertions, polyarthralgia and arthroses. The spine may become rigid and contractures of hips and knees may occur. Occupational exposure to leaks of fluorides or hydrofluoric acid may cause severe acute illness, with skin and eye burns, acute tracheobronchitis and pulmonary oedema, and hypocalcaemia due to consumption of calcium converted to calcium fluoride.

Management

No treatment is effective for fluorosis. The effects of leaks of fluoride should be treated with calcium gluconate (gel locally, and by injection).

POLYCHLORINATED BIPHENYLS

Polychlorinated biphenyls (PCBs) are liquids, first manufactured in the 1930s, which have become widely distributed in the environment; particularly in water, fish and fish-eating birds; and in soils near sources of contamination. PCBs have been used for their electrical insulating properties in transformers, capacitors (even in some domestic equipment), heat transfer and cooling systems, hydraulic systems and vacuum pumps, and a variety of other uses. Use of PCBs has now been restricted or stopped in numerous countries, but certain occupational groups are still exposed, notably in the handling of chemical wastes, dealing with fires or accidents, working in or cleaning contaminated areas or servicing and dismantling old electrical apparatus; and the public in the vicinity of incinerators if the temperature is not high enough. Low levels of PCBs can be detected in many members of most industrial populations, and are concentrated in human milk. Poisoning by PCBs has been recognised as a result of occupational exposure, and in outbreaks in the general population, such as occurred in Japan (Yusho disease), and in Taiwan, due to contamination of rice oil.

Clinical features

The most striking effects are hypersecretion of tears, pigmentation and acneform eruptions of the skin (chloracne, also caused by dioxins), and persistent productive cough. Headaches and other non-specific central nervous system disturbances occur, and paraesthesiae; also liver damage and immunosuppression. Some deaths have occurred, mostly from liver disease, including hepatomas. Babies of exposed mothers are small and pigmented, and fetal deaths and abnormalities were common in the Yusho outbreak. Acute exposure irritates the eyes, skin and respiratory tract.

Management

Treatment consists of withdrawal from exposure, and general supportive measures. No specific treatment is available.

BUILDING SICKNESS SYNDROME

This benign syndrome occurs in workers in modern air-conditioned offices. The causes are unknown, but relevant factors may include fluctuating temperatures, possibly variations in humidity, the cyclical flashing of fluorescent lights, low levels of volatile organic chemicals such as formaldehyde or solvents, and psychological factors.

Clinical features

There are various combinations of itching, burning and discomfort of the eyes, nasal stuffiness, discomfort in the throat, headache, dryness of the skin and lethargy.

Symptoms are worse in the second half of the working shift, and towards the end of the week, and are more common in females. They resolve rapidly on leaving the building

Management

No specific treatment is required, though alterations in the office environment may be helpful.

Contamination of air-conditioning systems have also occasionally been associated with asthma, humidifier fever, extrinsic allergic alveolitis, and some infections, notably legionnaires disease. These are not generally classified as building sickness syndrome.

SOURCES OF INFORMATION ON HAZARDS OF SUBSTANCES USED AT WORK

Information about the potential hazards of substances used at work are listed in the information box below.

The label
Information carried on labels complying with the regulations provides a useful guide to compositions if chemical names are given.

Data hazard sheets
These are provided by the manufacturer or supplier to the employer. The information is not always adequate, however, and it may be necessary to contact the manufacturer for further information, which he is obliged to supply under Section 6 of the Health and Safety at Work Act.

Textbooks
Textbooks of occupational medicine.

An Encyclopaedia of Occupational Health and Safety

Health and Safety Executive Guidance Notes
These are notes on substances and processes, which may be obtained from HMSO bookshops or specialist libraries.

The American Conference of Governmental Industrial Hygienists
They publish an exhaustive and authoritative series of guidance notes on substances and processes, available from specialist libraries or ACGIH head office in Cincinnatti.

The Employment Medical Advisors of the Health and Safety Executive in Britain
They can give advice, and themselves have access to sources of information. The HSE library in Sheffield will give information over the telephone during office hours.

Some other organisations
For example the Institute of Occupational Medicine in Edinburgh, provide information services for subscribers.

FURTHER READING

Bardwell A R et al 1986 Effect of acetazolamide on exercise performance and muscle mass at high altitude. Lancet 1: 1001–1005

Dickinson J C 1982 Terminology and classification of acute mountain sickness. British Medical Journal 285: 720

Ellis F G 1976 Heat illness. Transactions of the Royal Society of Tropical Medicine and Hygiene 70: 402–411

Heath D, Williams D R 1981 Man at high altitudes, 2nd Edn. Churchill Livingstone, Edinburgh

Environmental health criteria: Lead (no. 3) 1976; Mercury (no. 1) 1976; Fluorides (no. 36) 1984; Polychlorinated Biphenyls and Terphenyls (no. 2) 2976. World Health Organisation, Geneva

Environmental Health 23: PCBs, PCDDs and PCDFs:

Prevention and Control of Accidental and Environmental Exposures 1987. World Health Organisation, Geneva

McElroy C, Auerbach P S 1983 Heat illness: current perspectives. Management of wilderness and environment emergencies. Macmillan, New York, pp 64–81

Margulies A D C 1987 A short course in diving medicine. Annals of Emergency Medicine 16: 689–701

Pickering C A C Building Sickness Syndrome. Respiratory Medicine 1989 83: 91–92

Raffle P A B, Lee W R, McCallum R I, Murray R eds 1987 Hunter's Diseases of Occupations. Hodder & Stoughton, London

Waldbot G L 1973 Health Effects of Environmental Pollutants. The C.V. Mosby Company, Saint Lewis

Diseases due to Infection

Infection can involve any organ or system of the body and thus embraces all medical disciplines. It is discussed in every chapter of this book. In this chapter an introductory account is given of general aspects, spread, diagnosis and prevention of infection as well as descriptions of individual infectious diseases. The term infectious disease has commonly been used to denote infections that are contagious or communicable, i.e. transmissible from man to man. The present trend is to refer to all diseases caused by microorganisms as infectious diseases.

Infection differs from other diseases in a number of aspects; most important is that it is caused by a living microorganism, which can frequently be identified, thus establishing the aetiology early in the illness. Many of these organisms, including all bacteria, are sensitive to antibiotics and most infections are potentially curable, unlike non-infectious diseases many of which are degenerative and frequently become chronic. The communicability of infection is another factor which differentiates infectious from non-infectious diseases; this leads to the transmission of pathogenic organisms to other people and if large numbers are involved an epidemic may result. Finally, many infections are preventable by hygienic measures or by vaccines. In certain circumstances, infection may be prevented by the judicious use of drugs (chemoprophylaxis).

PATTERN OF INFECTION IN DEVELOPED COUNTRIES

During the past 50 years there has been a dramatic fall in the incidence of communicable diseases in developed countries. This is due to several factors such as immunisation, antimicrobial chemotherapy, improved nutrition, and better sanitation and housing. Infections which have decreased, and in some instances almost disappeared in these countries include diphtheria, poliomyelitis, tuberculosis, leprosy, brucellosis, bacillary dysentery and malaria.

Despite economic development certain infections continue to pose problems and some are even increasing. These infections are listed in Table 5.1. Within the past ten years a number of 'new' infections have been recognised. Some represent changing patterns of human behaviour such as Ebola fever from penetration into the forests of Zaire and HIV infection from homosexual activity. Others represent the results of improved laboratory diagnostic techniques and better epidemiological methods including the establishment of national centres for the surveillance of communicable disease. These centres monitor incidents and outbreaks of infection and exchange information with similar organisations in other countries. The information box (p. 97) illustrates the present patterns of infection in Britain.

PATTERNS OF INFECTION IN UNDERDEVELOPED COUNTRIES

In less advanced countries, however, especially in the tropics, infection continues to be one of the commonest causes of disease and death, particularly in children, and determines the strength of the working man, the health of the mother and the pattern of systemic disease in the community, including neoplasia. The battle against acute infection is often a single episode in a long

Table 5.1   Infections which are increasing or causing concern in developed countries

Infection	Reasons
Sexually transmitted diseases (incl. AIDS)	Promiscuity, sexual 'liberation'
Food poisoning (esp. salmonella and campylobacter)	Fast food; battery-rearing of poultry
Hospital-acquired infection	Modern medical practices, use of antibiotics, inadequate hygiene, resistant bacteria (e.g. MRSA)
Travel-acquired infections (inc. malaria)	Package holidays, air travel
Recently recognised infections (e.g. legionellosis; rotavirus, cryptosporidium and isospora intestinal infections; Lyme disease, parvovirus infection)	Immunosuppression, contaminated water supplies, improved diagnostic techniques leading to recognition of new organisms
Common childhood infections (esp. measles and whooping cough)	Inadequate uptake of immunisation

PATTERNS OF INFECTION IN BRITAIN TODAY

Extinct infection
Smallpox

Decreasing or uncommon infections
Diphtheria
Poliomyelitis
Tetanus
Brucellosis
Tuberculosis

Increasing endemic infections
Salmonella infections
Campylobacter infections
Measles
Whooping cough
Meningococcal infections
Viral hepatitis
Listeria infection

Imported infections
Malaria
Giardiasis
Bacillary and amoebic dysentery
Typhoid and paratyphoid fever
Leishmaniasis
Schistosomiasis
Filariasis
Leprosy

Recently recognised (and increasing) infections
Human immunodeficiency virus infection (AIDS)
Pneumocystis carinii infection (in AIDS)
Legionella infection
Rotavirus infection
Chlamydia pneumoniae (TWAR) infection
Methicillin-resistant *Staph. aureus* infection
Cryptosporidium infection
Isospora belli infection (in AIDS)
Lyme disease
Parvovirus B19 infection
Verocytotoxin-producing *E. coli* infections
Herpes virus type 6 infections

campaign against chronic infection and malnutrition. Multiple disease entities are the rule and the clinical patterns of illness differ in many ways from those in temperate zones. The complex interaction between chronic parasitism, acute respiratory and diarrhoeal diseases, malnutrition and its immunosuppressive effects, pose special problems for the health of children. Up to 40% of children may die before they reach 5 years of age.

Chronic infections do serious damage to important organs, such as liver and kidneys in schistosomiasis, the heart in trypanosomiasis cruzi, the lungs, bones and lymph nodes in tuberculosis, the bone marrow reserves in malaria and hookworm infections, the gut in tropical

sprue and the nerves in leprosy. These organs may then fail if the demand upon them is increased through work, pregnancy or additional disease. Such diseases impose chronic ill health on millions of children and adults in the tropics.

Many of the decimating diseases of the past are controllable by vaccination (yellow fever), vector control (malaria and sleeping sickness) and general improvement in living standards (plague and relapsing fever), but control is imperfect and the diseases reappear. Other epidemic diseases such as cholera in Asia and meningococcal meningitis in Africa remain largely uncontrolled, and kill hundreds of thousands of people annually. Efficient vaccines exist for many diseases such as poliomyelitis, measles, rubella and tetanus, but in many countries they have made little impact because of the cost and practical difficulty in delivering them.

Development, especially in the form of dams and irrigation has often encouraged the spread of vector borne disease such as malaria and schistosomiasis, while the exploitation of the Amazonian forests has caused mutilating outbreaks of mucocutaneous leishmaniasis. Migration to urban slums increases the risk of gastrointestinal disease and tuberculosis and of 'Western' diseases such as hypertension, and in some countries has contributed materially to the AIDS epidemic.

EFFECTS OF INFECTION ON THE BODY

Infection has far-reaching effects on the body. These are summarised in Table 5.2. They may be acute, chronic or allergic. Chronic effects are seen especially in children in tropical countries.

PATHOLOGY OF INFECTION

Disease due to infection is the result of interaction between a microorganism and the natural defence mechanisms of the body. The outcome of this interaction can range from no demonstrable effect to death, and will depend on the number and virulence of the organism, the physiological and anatomical effects that they induce and the effectiveness of the natural defences (Table 5.3).

The several mechanisms by which microorganisms cause disease are summarised in Table 5.4 and discussed in other sections of this book. Organisms act directly and through their toxins. Many of these effects are general, but some act at certain anatomical sites, for example poliomyelitis virus in anterior horn cells, hepatitis virus in hepatocytes, pneumococcus in the

Table 5.2   Clinical effects of infection on the body

Acute	Fever	Anorexia, protein catabolism, nitrogen balance, acute phase proteins, albumin, serum iron, sequestration of iron, anaemia, neutrophilia
	Inflammation	Pain, dysfunction, tissue damage
	Convulsions	Especially in children
	Shock	Sustained fall in circulating blood volume associated with lowered systemic vascular resistance
	Haemorrhage	
	Organ failure	Kidneys, liver, lung, heart, brain
Chronic	Weight loss and muscle wasting	
	Malnutrition; especially associated with diarrhoea	
	Retardation of growth and intellect in children	
	Anaemia; iron sequestration, maturation arrest in marrow, folate deficiency	
	Tissue destruction; lung in pneumonia or tuberculosis, nerves in leprosy, liver in hepatitis B	
	Post-infective syndromes; lactose intolerance, malabsorption, irritable colon, depression, post-viral fatigue syndrome	
Allergic	Rash	Erythema with streptococci, urticaria with helminths, maculopapular in typhoid and endocarditis, erythema nodosum in tuberculosis
	Arthritis	In rheumatic fever, Reiter's syndrome
	Pericarditis	In meningococcal infection
	Encephalitis	In measles or following vaccines
	Peripheral neuropathy	In post-infective polyneuritis
	Haemolytic anaemia	In infectious mononucleosis
	Nephritis	In streptococcal infection

alveoli, tetanus and diphtheria toxins at different nerve terminals. Numbers of infecting organisms also affect the severity and outcome of the infection.

Shock is an especial problem in severe infections. It may be due to myocardial infarction or haemorrhage, but usually its aetiology is more complex and results from the reduced systemic vascular resistance brought about by dilated small vessels and leaky capillaries

under the influence of several mediators, which include kinins, complement components, histamine, monokines and endogenous opiates. The commonest cause of shock in infection is endotoxin from Gram-negative bacteria (Fig. 5.1). The cycle of shock, tissue anoxia and organ failure is difficult to break and may kill the patient quickly.

REDUCED RESISTANCE TO INFECTION

Resistance to infection may be decreased as a result of extremes of age, disease, medical or surgical treatment, or a combination of these factors. A person whose

Table 5.3   Natural defences against infection

Non-specific
Anatomical
  Skin and its secretions, sebum
  Mucous membranes and their secretions:
    Lysozymes
    Gastric acid
    Intestinal enzymes
    Bronchial secretions
    Vaginal secretions

Chemical
  Interferons
  Acute phase proteins
  Complement

Cellular
  Neutrophils (bacterial infection)
  Monocytes
  Macrophages
  Eosinophils (parasitic infection)

Specific
Humoral:	B lymphocytes and antibodies
Cellular:	T lymphocytes, macrophages, cytokines

Table 5.4   Pathology of infection

Microbe mediated	Host mediated
Direct	
Cell destruction poliomyelitis, rabies hepatitis	Neutrophils and macrophages
Exotoxin	
Tetanus, cholera, botulism, diphtheria	Complement activation Activation of clotting cascade
Endotoxin	
Typhoid, meningococcal infection	Immune mechanism Secondary autoimmune mechanisms

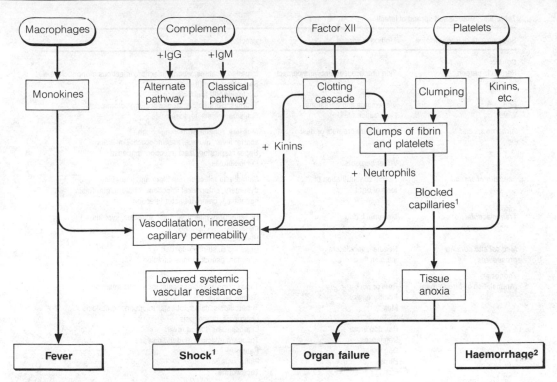

Fig. 5.1 Synopsis of the effects of bacterial endotoxinaemia. [1]Shock (low systemic arterial pressure) leads to poor perfusion and further tissue anoxia.
[2]Haemorrhage is the product of defibrination, consumption of clotting factors and platelets, and damaged capillaries (disseminated intravascular coagulation).

resistance to infection is decreased as a result of a congenital or acquired abnormality in the immune response is referred to as being *immunocompromised.*

SOURCE AND SPREAD OF INFECTION

Infection may originate from the patient (autogenous) usually from the skin, nasopharynx or bowel, or from outside sources (exogenous), commonly from another person who may either be suffering from an infection or carrying a pathogenic microorganism. Carriers are usually healthy and may harbour the organism in the throat (diphtheria) or bowel (salmonella).

Microorganisms may be transmitted by several routes. Autogenous infection may develop as a result of local spread, e.g. from bowel to peritoneum, or by the blood stream. An example of the latter is infective endocarditis caused by *Streptococcus sanguis* originating in the patient's mouth and entering the blood during dental procedures. Exogenous infection may be acquired directly or indirectly by one of the routes shown in Table 5.5.

Incubation period is the period of time which elapses between the invasion of the tissues by pathogens and the appearance of clinical symptoms and signs of infection (Table 5.6).
Period of infectivity is the time that the patient is infectious to others (Table 5.7).

DIAGNOSIS OF INFECTION

A knowledge of infections prevailing in the locality is an essential guide to diagnosis especially with imported infections. It is wise to enquire about contacts among the family, friends and workmates. Persons following certain occupations may be exposed to infection, e.g. leptospirosis occurs in abattoir and farm workers and anthrax in handlers of hides and bone meal.

A recent history of laparotomy or of obscure abdominal pain should suggest subphrenic or intrahepatic abscess as a cause of unexplained fever. Residence or travel abroad raises the possibility of malaria, amoebic abscess of the liver or other exotic disease.

In many infections a diagnosis beyond all reasonable

Table 5.5   Source and spread of infection

Source/route of transmission	Method of spread	Infection
Contact		
Person to person	Skin or mucous membrane contact	Impetigo, scabies, wound infection, infectious mononucleosis Sexually transmitted diseases (including HIV and hepatitis B)
Soil	Via wounds and abrasions	Tetanus, Buruli ulcer, hookworm, mycetoma
Water	Penetration of skin	Schistosomiasis, leptospirosis
Airborne spread	Respiratory droplets or dust	Measles, rubella, whooping cough, scarlet fever, mumps, meningococcal infection Upper respiratory tract infection, influenza
	Water aerosols	Legionellosis
Faecal/oral spread	Faecal contamination of food or drink	Salmonella infection, bacillary and amoebic dysentery, enteroviral infections, cholera, giardiasis hepatitis A, campylobacter infection
Transplacental	Maternal blood	Rubella, CMV infection, toxoplasmosis, syphilis, malaria HIV infection
Medical and nursing procedures	Needles, ventilators infusion fluid	Hepatitis B, staphylococcal infection, pseudomonas infection
Zoonoses (Animal, fish or bird to man)	Beef or pork	Tapeworms, toxoplasmosis, trichinella infection
	Poultry/eggs	Salmonellosis
	Milk	Tuberculosis, campylobacter infection, brucellosis
	Cheese	Listeriosis, brucellosis
	Rat, dog urine	Leptospirosis, Lassa fever
	Dog faeces	Toxocara infection, hydatid disease
	Dog bite	Rabies
	Birds	Psittacosis
	Fish	Tapeworms
Arthropods (see Table 5.39)		

doubt may be made on clinical grounds, e.g. measles or chickenpox. In others a diagnosis may require confirmation by microbiological, immunological, haematological or histopathological examination, radiography or scanning (Table 5.8).

PYREXIA OF UNKNOWN ORIGIN

Occasionally the cause of a febrile illness remains uncertain in spite of investigation and such a case is categorised as PUO (pyrexia of unknown origin). In order to establish the diagnosis certain measures should be undertaken which are listed in the information box (right).

It should be remembered that most causes of PUO are due to a common disorder with an unusual presentation. In Britain the most frequent causes of prolonged PUO are tumours (especially lymphomas), chronic infections (among which tuberculosis is important), connective tissue disorders and drug hypersensitivity reactions. In the tropics and elsewhere a wider variety of infections must be considered.

Mysterious fevers, particularly in patients who have some knowledge of medicine or nursing, may be due to deceit (factitious fever). Doubt should be raised if the skin of a supposedly febrile patient does not feel hot or if the general health does not deteriorate in spite of persistent fever. The occurrence of some bizarre symptom or sign may arouse suspicion that the temperature is being falsified. There are both subtle

---

INVESTIGATION OF PYREXIA OF UNKNOWN ORIGIN

Retake the history
Contact with infection
Contact with animals
Travel abroad
Drug therapy
Occupation

Repeat the examination
Heart murmur
Splenomegaly
Lymph glands
Fundal changes

Review results of investigations
(and repeat if indicated)
Re-examine chest x-ray
Biochemical results abnormal
Haematology results abnormal
Microbiology results abnormal

Consider further investigations
Serological investigations
Immunological investigations
Isotope scanning
CT scanning
Tissue Biopsy

Consider therapeutic trial
Antimicrobial therapy (esp.
tuberculous)
Corticosteroid therapy
Cytotoxic therapy

Table 5.6   Incubation periods of important infections

Infection	Incubation period Maximum range	Normal range
Short incubation periods (<7 days)		
Anthrax	2–5 days	
Bacillary dysentery	1–7 days	
Cholera	Hours–5 days	2–3 hours
Diphtheria	2–5 days	
Gonorrhoea	2–5 days	
Meningococcaemia	2–10 days	3–4 days
Scarlet fever	1–3 days	
Intermediate incubation periods (7–21 days)		
Amoebiasis	14 days–months	21 days
Chickenpox	14–21 days	
Lassa fever	7–14 days	
Malaria	8 days–months	
Measles	7–14 days	10 days
Mumps	12–21 days	18 days
Poliomyelitis	3–21 days	7–10 days
Psittacosis	4–14 days	10 days
Rubella	14–21 days	18 days
Trypanosoma rhodesiense infection	14–21 days	
Typhoid fever	7–21 days	
Typhus fever	7–14 days	12 days
Whooping cough	7–10 days	7 days
Long incubation periods (>21 days)		
Brucellosis	Days–months	
Filariasis	3 months–years	
Hepatitis A	2–6 weeks	4 weeks
Hepatitis B	6 weeks–6 months	12 weeks
Leishmaniasis		
Cutaneous	1 week–months	
Visceral	2 weeks–2 years	2–4 months
Leprosy	Years	2–5 years
Rabies	Variable	2–8 weeks
Schistosomiasis	Weeks–years	
Tuberculosis	Months–years	
Trypanosoma gambiense infection	Weeks–years	

and simple techniques for doing this. The latter include holding the thermometer close to a hot water bottle or other source of heat, dipping it into a hot drink,

Table 5.7   Periods of infectivity in childhood infectious diseases

Chickenpox
5 days before rash to 6 days after last crop of vesicles

Diphtheria
2–3 weeks (shorter with antibiotic therapy)

Measles
From onset of prodromal symptoms to 4 days after onset of rash

Mumps
3 days before salivary swelling to 7 days after

Rubella
7 days before onset of rash to 4 days after

Scarlet fever
10–21 days after onset of rash (shortened to 1 day by penicillin)

Whooping cough
7 days after exposure to 3 weeks after onset of symptoms (shortened to 7 days by antibiotics)

Table 5.8   Methods used to diagnose infection, and some examples

Microbiological

Recognition of causative agent
● In stained or fresh preparation, usually a smear:[1] malaria in blood slide, vibrio cholera in stool, diphtheria in throat swab, bacilli in urine, staphylococci in pus smear, entamoeba in rectal scrape, plague bacilli in buboe aspirate, schistosome ova in rectal snip, rickettsia in rash aspirate,[2] fungi in skin scrapings, pneumococci in purulent sputum, spirochaetes in condylomata,[3] leprosy bacilli and leishmania in slit skin smear.
● By electron microscopy: rotavirus in stool, pox virus in vesicle fluid.
● By histology of biopsy specimen: acid-fast bacilli in leprosy and tuberculosis, pneumocystis in pneumonia, hepatitis B in liver, rabies virus in brain.[2]
Culture of causative organism
● From blood: typhoid, brucellosis, Gram-negative septicaemia, pneumococcal pneumonia.
● From bone marrow: tuberculosis, brucellosis, leishmaniasis, histoplasmosis.
● From other body fluids, faeces or tissues: urinary tract infection, bacillary dysentery, sputum in pneumonia, liver in tuberculosis.

Immunological

Detection of microbial antigen
● Meningococcal and pneumococcal disease (blood, cerebrospinal fluid, sputum) sputum)
Detection of antibody of IgM class
● Toxoplasmosis, hepatitis A
Demonstration of antibody
● Rising titre: typhoid, brucellosis
● Closely linked to active disease: amoebic abscess, visceral leishmaniasis
● Screening for latent disease: syphilis, schistosomiasis, trypanosomiasis cruzi
Delayed hypersensitivity skin testing
● Tuberculosis, histoplasmosis, leishmaniasis. These tests may be difficult to interpret epidemiologically

Non-specific

Tissue biopsy
● Characteristic histology: chronic active hepatitis, leprosy
● Suggestive histology: tuberculosis
Radiology
● Association of site and pattern with infection: lobar pneumonia, renal tuberculosis, muscular cysticercosis
Scans
● Isotope: detection of abscess, osteomyelitis
● Ultrasound: abscess, hydatid cyst
● Computed tomography: intracranial infection, deep abscess, mediastinal lymph node enlargement

[1]Most of these are simple side room techniques which clinicians should be able to perform.
[2]Usually performed using immunofluorescent staining.
[3]Dark ground microscopy.

applying friction to the bulb, or shaking it in a retrograde manner.

When a diagnosis still cannot be established and the patient's condition is deteriorating, various remedies, e.g. antibiotics, may be tried empirically in the hope of influencing the course of the disease. A therapeutic trial should not be regarded as a satisfactory diagnostic test as it can further obscure the diagnosis by suppressing but not curing the infection. It is most useful in suspected tuberculosis.

THE PREVENTION OF INFECTION

The prevention of infection depends on three concepts

which may be interrelated. These concepts are listed in the information box below.

PREVENTION OF INFECTION

Elimination of the source
Examples: Screen donated blood for hepatitis B and HIV
             Eradication of tuberculosis and brucellosis from
             cattle
             Pasteurise milk
             Elimination of animal reservoir eg dogs and
             rabies
             Chemotherapy for tuberculosis, schistosomiasis,
             leprosy

Prevention of transmission
Examples: Hand washing
             Antisepsis in operating theatres
             Sterilisation of instruments
             Isolation of infected patients (source isolation)
             Control of insect vectors and animal reservoirs
             Quarantine of people and animals

Protection of susceptible persons
Examples: Active and passive immunisation
             Prophylactic antibiotics (e.g. endocarditis
             prevention)
             Isolation of immunosuppressed (protective
             isolation)
             Malarial chemoprophylaxis
             Use of mosquito nets

Table 5.10   Vaccines and toxoids

	Live attenuated vaccines	Inactivated vaccines	Toxoid (inactivated toxin)
For childhood immunisation	Measles Mumps Rubella Poliomyelitis* BCG (tuberculosis)	Pertussis	Diphtheria Tetanus
For travel	Yellow fever	Typhoid Cholera Rabies Japanese encephalitis	
Other vaccines	Influenza*	Pneumococcal Hepatitis B Influenza* Meningococcal (A & C only) Plague Poliomyelitis*	

* Both live and attenuated vaccines available.

IMMUNISATION AGAINST INFECTIOUS DISEASES

This involves active or passive immunisation.

Active immunisation

Vaccines may be live attenuated, inactivated or toxoids (Table 5.10). In Britain parents should be advised to have their children immunised against whooping cough, diphtheria, tetanus, measles, mumps, rubella, poliomyelitis and tuberculosis (Table 5.9). The World Health Organisation (WHO) has provided guidelines

---

Table 5.9   Immunisation schedule recommended in Britain

Age	Visits	Vaccine	Intervals
2–4 months	3	Three administrations of DTP+OPV	4 weeks
12–24 months	1	MMR vaccination	
First year at school	1	Booster DT+OPV	
10–13 years	1	BCG for the tuberculin negative	
Girls: 11–13 years	1	Rubella vaccination	
15–19 years or on leaving school	1	TT+OPV	

Immunisation schedule recommended by WHO for developing countries

Age	Vaccine
Birth or first contact:	BCG and OPV
6, 10, 14 weeks:	DPT and OPV
9 months:	Measles

DTP Diphtheria, tetanus, pertussis ('triple') vaccine
OPV Oral poliomyelitis vaccine
DT Diphtheria, tetanus vaccine
TT Tetanus toxoid
MMR Measles, mumps and rubella vaccine

for immunisation of children in developing countries (Table 5.10). The indications for immunisation against influenza, hepatitis B, typhoid fever, cholera, plague, typhus, yellow fever, Japanese encephalitis and rabies depend upon the likelihood of exposure or upon international health regulations (Table 5.11).

Acute demyelinating encephalomyelitis and poly-neuropathy are rare complications of immunisation. General guidelines for immunisation are given in the information box (right).

HIV infected persons should be immunised in the same way as normal individuals but should not be given BCG, live poliomyelitis or yellow fever vaccines.

GUIDELINES FOR IMMUNISATION AGAINST INFECTIOUS DISEASE

- The principle contra-indication to inactivated vaccines is a significant reaction to a previous dose
- Live vaccines should not be given to pregnant women or to immunosuppressed patients
- If two live vaccines are required either give them simultaneously in opposite arms or three weeks apart
- Live vaccines should not be given for three months after an injection of human normal immunoglobin (HNI)
- No HNI to be given for two weeks after a live vaccine
- Hay fever, asthma, eczema, topical steroid therapy, antibiotic therapy, prematurity and chronic heart and lung diseases are *not* contraindications to immunisation

---

Table 5.11   Medically recommended immunisations for travellers

Inoculation	Where advised	Course programme	Validity	Minimum age advised	Other comments
Yellow fever	Central Africa South and Central America	1 subcutaneous injection	After 10 days for 10 years	9 months	The only immunisation currently required by International Health Regulations
Cholera	Entering or transiting a cholera zone	2 subcutaneous injections, 4–6 weeks apart	After 6 days for 6 months	1 year	Poor protection. Very few countries require it
Typhoid	Wherever sanitation is poor	2 subcutaneous injections, 4–6 weeks apart	Booster injection every 3 years	2 years	0.1 ml intradermal adequate for second and booster, less toxic
Tetanus	Everywhere	3 subcutaneous injections, 4–6 weeks apart	Booster injection every 10 years	None	See also p. 885
Poliomyelitis	Everywhere	3 oral doses of attenuated virus at monthly intervals	Booster every 5 years, 3 doses better than 1	None	See also p. 878
Rabies	Endemic countries	3 intramuscular or intradermal injections 4 weeks and 4–12 months apart	Over 5 years	1 year	Groups at risk, using human diploid cell vaccine. Use deltoid muscle. Avoid chloroquine
Plague	Parts of S.E. Asia, E. Africa, USA	2 injections, 10–20 day intervals, 3rd 6 months later	6 months	1 year	Only special groups at risk
Hepatitis B	Endemic countries	3 intramuscular injections 4 weeks and 6 months apart	Over 5 weeks	1 year	Special groups at risk, resident expatriates
Gammaglobulin (type A hepatitis)	Countries where sanitation is poor	Intramuscular injection 250 mg or 500 mg. Age under 10 years, half dose	4–6 months	16 years	Also protects against measles, rubella
Japanese encephalitis	Areas of S.E. Asia India/China	3 doses subcutaneously 2 and 4 weeks apart	1–4 years	1 year	Rural travellers only
European tick encephalitis	Central Europe USSR, Mediterranean	3 intramuscular injections 4 weeks and 9/12 months apart	3 years	1 year	Campers and hikers at greatest risk
Meningococcal meningitis	Africa, South of the Sahara, S. America Middle and Near East, Asia (esp. India + Nepal)	1 subcutaneous injection	3 years	18 months except in epidemic situations (then 2 doses)	Risk is often seasonal Protects against Types A & C only

---

INDICATIONS FOR PROPHYLACTIC IMMUNOGLOBULINS

Human normal immunoglobulin (pooled immunoglobulin)
Virus A hepatitis (travellers and debilitated children)
Measles (child with heart or lung disease)

Human specific inmmunoglobulin
Virus B hepatitis (needlestick injuries, sexual partner)
Tetanus (susceptible injured patients)
Rabies (post-exposure protection)
Chickenpox (immunosuppressed children)

Passive immunisation

An injection of immunoglobulin will give temporary protection usually for 2–6 months against certain infectious diseases by providing pre-formed antibodies to protect against that infection. The indication for use are listed in the information box above.

Notification of infectious diseases. Clinicians in Britain have a statutory obligation to notify certain infectious diseases (Table 5.12) to the appropriate Public Health Authority.

Table 5.12 Notifiable infectious diseases in Britain

Under the Public Health (Control of Diseases) Act 1984
Cholera
Food poisoning
Plague
Relapsing fever
Smallpox
Typhus

Under the Public Health (Infectious Diseases) Regulations 1988
Acute encephalitis
Acute poliomyelitis
Anthrax
Diphtheria
Dysentery (amoebic or bacillary)
Leprosy
Leptospirosis
Malaria
Measles
Meningitis
Meningococcal septicaemia (without meningitis)
Mumps
Ophthalmia neonatorum
Paratyphoid fever
Rabies
Rubella
Scarlet fever
Tetanus
Tuberculosis
Typhoid fever
Viral haemorrhagic fever
Viral hepatitis
Whooping cough
Yellow fever

The individual infections in the chapter will be described according to the infecting agent as follows:

● Viruses
● Chlamydiae
● Rickettsiae
● Bacteria
● Spirochaetes
● Fungi
● Protozoa
● Helminths
● Arthropods

DISEASES DUE TO VIRUSES

No single classification of viral diseases is entirely satisfactory for the clinician, whether by viral structure and nomenclature, by method of transmission or by type of disease. Viruses are divided into two groups according to whether they contain DNA or RNA in their genome, and are sub-divided further into families according to their structure.

HUMAN IMMUNODEFICIENCY VIRAL INFECTION (INCLUDING AIDS)

Aetiology

The occurrence in 1981 of severe and often fatal pneumonia caused by the opportunist pathogen *Pneumocystis carinii* in apparently healthy male homosexuals in the United States led to the recognition of the acquired immune deficiency syndrome (AIDS). Two years later the infectious agent causing this apparently new disease was identified as a previously unknown retrovirus which was first called the human T cell lymphotrophic virus (HTLV 3). It was also known as the lymphadenopathy associated virus (LAV). The agreed name is now human immunodeficiency virus (HIV). Almost all infections in Europe and North America are caused by HIV 1. In Africa HIV 1 is still the commonest cause but a second virus HIV 2 is an increasing cause of AIDS. These viruses have a tropism particularly for helper T lymphocytes which play a crucial role in regulating the immune system. Damages to, or destruction of, helper lymphocytes leads to the development of a cellular immunodeficiency disease rendering the patient susceptible to a wide variety of infections but particularly to those caused by viruses, protozoa, fungi and intracellular bacteria.

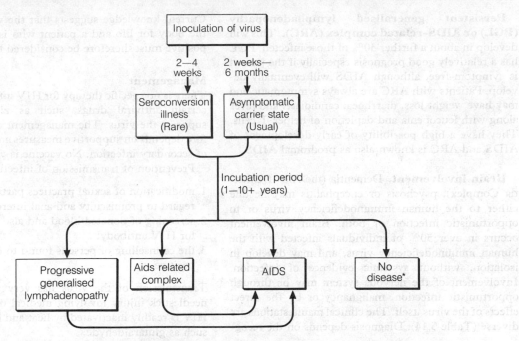

Fig. 5.2   HIV infection: progression of disease. *It is not known whether all HIV infected patients will eventually develop symptomatic disease.

Patients suffering from AIDS also develop various malignancies, most notably Kaposi's sarcoma and lymphomas. The HIV virus attacks cells of the nervous system including the brain.

In Europe and North America HIV infection is most commonly a sexually transmitted disease amongst homosexual males but it can also be transmitted heterosexually and by blood and blood products such as factor VIII. The routes of transmission are therefore similar to those of virus B hepatitis and infected persons include drug addicts and haemophiliacs. Infection can also be transmitted transplacentally.

HIV infection has been classified into four groups by the Communicable Disease Centre in the United States and by the World Health Organisation (Table 5.13).

Clinical features (see Fig. 5.2)

The initial infection with HIV is usually subclinical although a very small number of patients can develop an infectious mononucleosis-like illness with fever, lymphadenopathy and rash within 2–3 weeks of infection. The large majority, however, remain symptom-free. After an incubation period of between 1 and 10 years about 80% of these will develop one of the following syndromes:

AIDS. This syndrome is associated with depletion of T4 lymphocytes, profound cellular immunodeficiency, serious opportunistic infections, especially *Pn. carinii* pneumonia and Kaposi's sarcoma. It has been estimated that about 50% of HIV infected persons will develop the full AIDS syndrome within 10 years of infection.

Table 5.13   Classification of HIV infection

Group I		Acute HIV infection (a mononucleosis-like syndrome)
Group II		Asymptomatic HIV infection: no signs or symptoms
Group III		Patients with persistent generalised lymphadenopathy (PGL)
Group IV		Other HIV disease (the subgroups are not mutually exclusive)
A		Constitutional disease (aids-related complex—ARC)
B		With neurological disease (ARC)
C		With a symptomatic or invasive secondary infectious disease
	C1	(AIDS): one or more of 12 specified diseases, e.g. pneumocystis carinii pneumonia, toxoplasmosis, histoplasmosis, cytomegalovirus infection
	C2	(ARC): one of 6 other specified diseases, e.g. hairy leukoplakia, oral candidiasis, tuberculosis
D		With secondary cancers, e.g. Kaposi sarcoma, non-Hodgkin lymphoma (AIDS)
E		With other clinical findings not classified above, attributable to HIV infection, e.g. thrombocytopenia

Persistent generalised lymphadenopathy (PGL) or AIDS-related complex (ARC). This will develop in about a further 30% of those infected. PGL has a relatively good prognosis especially if the patient is symptom-free, although AIDS will eventually develop. Patients with ARC are always symptomatic and may have weight loss, diarrhoea, candidiasis and fever along with leucopenia and depletion of helper T cells. They have a high possibility of early development of AIDS and ARC is known also as prodromal AIDS.

Brain involvement. Dementia (the Aids Dementia Complex), psychosis or encephalitis may be due either to the human immunodeficiency virus or to opportunistic infection or both. Brain involvement occurs in over 50% of individuals infected with the human immunodeficiency virus, and may develop in isolation, without systemic evidence of infection. Involvement of the nervous system may be through opportunistic infection, malignancy or by the direct effects of the virus itself. The clinical manifestations are diverse (Table 5.14). Diagnosis depends on the recog-

Table 5.14 Neurological complications of HIV infection

Opportunistic infection	Direct viral effects	Neoplasia/other
Cerebral toxoplasmosis	Dementia encephalopathy	Cerebral lymphoma Primary Secondary
CMV encephalitis	Myelopathy	Kaposi's sarcoma
Herpes encephalitis	Neuropathy	Stroke
Fungal infections	Myopathy	
Mycobacterial infection		

nition of the possibility of HIV infection in a patient presenting with an atypical neurological syndrome (multiple cerebral abscess, dementia in a young patient) or the development of neurological signs in an individual from a high risk group. The demography of the epidemic, the difficulty in distinguishing between complications of HIV infection and other neurological disorders, and the increasingly diverse nature of these complications underlines the importance of considering HIV infection in any neurological patient. Serological tests are positive in the great majority of affected patients.

Thrombocytopenic purpura. This may be an isolated manifestation of HIV infection.

Diagnosis

The diagnosis of HIV infection is confirmed by the demonstration of serum antibodies to the virus.

Current knowledge suggests that the virus persists in the body for life and a patient who is HIV antibody positive must therefore be considered to be infectious.

Management

There is no specific therapy for HIV infection although certain antiviral drugs, such as zidovudine, will suppress the virus. The management of AIDS therefore depends on supportive measures and the treatment of secondary infection. No vaccine is yet available.

Prevention of transmission of infection depends on:

1. modification of sexual practices particularly with regard to promiscuity and anal intercourse;
2. screening of donated blood and also blood products for HIV antibody;
3. the counselling of persons found to be antibody positive.

Transmission of the virus has very rarely followed needlestick injury involving medical or nursing staff, HIV is readily inactivated by heat and by disinfectants such as glutaraldehyde.

At the end of 1989 over 75 000 cases of AIDS had been diagnosed in the United States, and 2500 in Britain. Eighty percent of patients with AIDS have died within 2 years of diagnosis.

AIDS in Africa

AIDS is epidemic in Central and East Africa and is rapidly becoming commoner in West Africa. The infection is spread principally by heterosexual contact and the male to female ratio is 1:1 as compared with almost 20:1 in Europe and North America. As a consequence large numbers of children are infected. Severe weight loss is a common presenting feature of African AIDS hence the name 'Slim disease'. Multiple parasite infection is common in African patients suffering from HIV infection and diarrhoea is therefore almost invariable.

HTLV1 INFECTION

This retrovirus, which does not cause AIDS, is endemic in Japan, the Caribbean and some areas of Africa. It can be transmitted by blood transfusion, by drug abusers sharing needles and from mother to child, principally through breast-feeding. Sexual transmission is thought to be uncommon.

Clinical features

HTLV1 is associated with adult T cell leukaemia/lymphoma and with a degenerative neurological disease known as tropical spastic paraplegia in the Caribbean and HTLV1-associated myelopathy in Japan. These diseases have been seen in Britain and America in immigrants from parts of the world where HTLV1 infection is endemic.

MEASLES

Measles is caused by a paramyxovirus which spreads by droplet infection. One attack confers a high degree of immunity. Most people suffer from measles in childhood, and a mother who has had the disease confers passive immunity on her infant for the first 6 months of life. Measles is very severe with a high mortality in many tropical countries. The incubation period is about 10 days to the commencement of the catarrhal stage.

Clinical features

Catarrhal stage. Measles commences in much the same way as a common cold. There is a febrile onset, with nasal catarrh, sneezing, redness of the conjuctivae and watering of the eyes. In addition cough, hoarseness of the voice due to laryngitis, and photophobia usually appear by the second day. At this stage, a diagnosis of measles may be made from the presence of Koplik's spots on the mucous membrane of the mouth. These are small white spots surrounded by a narrow zone of inflammation. The disease is highly infectious during the catarrhal stage and the child is miserable and irritable.

Exanthematous stage. After 3 or 4 days the diagnostic Koplik's spots disappear while the dark red macular or maculopapular rash develops first at the back of the ears and at the junction of the forehead and the hair. Within a few hours there is invasion of the whole skin and as the spots rapidly become more numerous they fuse to form the characteristic blotchy appearance of measles. When the rash is fully erupted, usually in 2 or 3 days, it tends to deepen in colour and then fade into a faint brown staining followed by a fine desquamation. The malaise and the fever subside as the rash fades.

Complications

These are listed in the information box (right).

Management

The patient should be isolated if possible and excluded from school for 10 days from the appearance of the rash. Most patients, in spite of the high temperature,

---

COMPLICATIONS OF MEASLES

Effects of measles virus
Stomatitis
Enteritis
Pneumonia
Keratitis

Secondary bacterial infection
Otitis media
Bronchopneumonia
Conjunctivitis

Neurological complications
Post-viral encephalitis
Sub-acute sclerosing panencephalitis

Nutritional
Severe weight loss
Kwashiorkor (tropics)
Corneal ulceration (tropics — vit. A deficiency)

---

remain uncomplicated and antibiotics should be prescribed only for unequivocal bacterial complications.

Prevention

Active immunisation. One injection of live attenuated measles virus (in association with mumps and rubella vaccines) should be given subcutaneously in children over 1 year old who have not had the disease. In the United States an aggressive immunisation programme has led to the virtual eradication of measles.

Passive immunisation. Human normal immunoglobulin, given intramuscularly, is recommended for the prevention or attenuation of measles, for contacts under 18 months of age and for debilitated children, especially those with malignant disease. The dose is 250 mg for children under 1 year old and 500 mg for those over this age.

RUBELLA (GERMAN MEASLES)

Rubella is caused by a togavirus which spreads by droplet infection. One attack confers a high degree of immunity. It tends to affect older children, adolescents and young adults and spreads less readily than measles. The incubation period is usually about 18 days. The disease in children is trivial. In adults the illness may be more severe, but of short duration and of little importance except when it develops in a woman during the first 4 months of pregnancy. In such cases the child

RUBELLA AND THE FETUS

Causes congenital abnormalities of:
Heart (septal defect)
Eye (cataract)
Brain (mental retardation)

Risk of congenital abnormality:
1st four weeks of pregnancy — 80%
16th week of pregnancy — less than 5%

may be born with a congenital malformation. Congenital abnormalities are listed in the information box above.

Clinical features

In children the constitutional symptoms are so slight that the illness is rarely suspected until the rash is seen. The spots are pink macules which appear first behind the ears and on the forehead. The rash spreads rapidly, first to the trunk and then to the limbs. Tender enlargement of the suboccipital lymph nodes is usual. In adolescents and adults the onset may be acute with fever and generalised aches, but even then the illness lasts for only 2 or 3 days. Polyarthritis is the commonest complication. Encephalomyelitis and thrombocytopenic purpura are very rare. Complete recovery from all of them is the rule.

Diagnosis

The rash of rubella is very similar to that due to certain drugs, enteroviruses and also parvovirus B19 which causes *erythema infectiosum* (Fifth disease). The latter infection may be differentiated clinically by redness of the patient's cheeks ('slapped cheek' appearance). Parvovirus B19 can also cause aplastic crises in sickle cell disease.

Serological tests are necessary for a definitive diagnosis of rubella.

Management

No treatment is available. If infection is known to have occurred during the first 16 weeks of pregnancy there is such a high chance of fetal abnormality that termination should be recommended.

Prevention

Rubella vaccine should be given to all children at the age of 15 months along with measles and mumps vaccine (MMR vaccine). A second dose of rubella vaccine alone is given to girls aged 11–13 years. Women of child-bearing age who are found to be serologically negative should also be offered vaccine provided that they are not pregnant and are willing to avoid pregnancy for 12 weeks after vaccination.

MUMPS

Mumps is caused by a paramyxovirus which spreads by droplet infection and affects mainly children of school age and young adults. The infectivity rate is not high and there is serological evidence that 30–40% of infections are clinically unapparent. The incubation period is about 18 days.

Clinical features

Malaise, fever, trismus and pain near the angle of the jaw is soon followed by tender swelling of one or both parotid glands. Parotid swelling alone is often the first feature. The submandibular salivary glands may also be involved. The swollen glands subside in a few days, and may be succeeded by swelling of a previously unaffected gland. Orchitis occurs in about one in four males who develop mumps after puberty; it is usually on one side only, but if it is bilateral, sterility may be a sequel. Obscure abdominal pain may be due to pancreatitis or oophoritis. Acute lymphocytic meningitis is another mode of presentation. Encephalomyelitis is rare.

Diagnosis

Most cases of mumps can be diagnosed on clinical grounds alone, but if in doubt the diagnosis can be confirmed by the demonstration of specific antibodies; or the virus may be cultured from the saliva, or from the cerebrospinal fluid in meningitis.

Management

Oral hygiene is important when the mouth is very dry from lack of saliva. Apart from the relief of symptoms as they appear, no other treatment is necessary. Orchitis can be relieved by prednisolone (40 mg orally daily for 4 days).

Prevention

Mumps vaccine is given at the age of 15 months along with measles and rubella vaccines.

ENTEROVIRUS INFECTION

Enteroviruses, so-called because they enter the body via the intestinal tract, cause a spectrum of disease. They are listed in the information box (p. 109). They are excreted in the stool and also, if there is respiratory infection, from the nasopharynx.

Most of the infections caused by enteroviruses are

INFECTIONS CAUSED BY ENTEROVIRUSES

Echoviruses
(approximately 40 strains)
Meningitis
Encephalitis
Conjunctivitis
Gastroenteritis
Pharyngitis
Fever and rash
Neonatal infection

Coxsackieviruses
(24 type A strains, 6 type B strains)
Myocarditis
Pericarditis
Meningitis
Herpangina
Bornholm disease
Hand, foot and mouth
disease
Gastroenteritis
Pharyngitis
Neonatal infection

Polioviruses (3 strains)
Poliomyelitis

Table 5.15   Herpes virus infections

Virus		Infection
Herpes virus hominis (Herpes simplex)	*Type 1*	Herpes labialis ('cold sores') Keratoconjunctivitis Finger infections ('whitlows') Encephalitis Primary stomatitis Genital infections (40%)
	Type 2	Genital infections (60%) Neonatal infection (acquired during vaginal delivery)
Cytomegalovirus (CMV)		Congenital infection Infection in immunocompromised patients Pneumonitis Retinitis Generalised infection
Epstein-Barr virus (EBV)		Infectious mononucleosis Burkitt's lymphoma Nasopharyngeal carcinoma Hairy leukoplakia (AIDS patients)
Varicella/zoster virus (VSV)		Chickenpox Shingles (Herpes zoster)
Human herpes virus 6 (HHV6)		Exanthem subitum ?Cervical lymphadenopathy

described elsewhere in the book with the exception of *herpangina* which produces a vesicular rash on the soft palate, and *hand, foot and mouth disease*, a highly infectious disease of childhood characterised by vesicles on the hands and feet and in the mouth.

HERPES VIRUS INFECTIONS

There are six herpes viruses which cause infection in man (Table 5.15). Herpes simplex virus (HSV) type 1, the cytomegalovirus (CMV) and the Epstein-Barr virus (EBV) are ubiquitous agents which commonly cause asymptomatic infection in early life — hence many adults have serological evidence of past infection with these agents. Chickenpox usually causes clinical infection in childhood and 80% of adults will have antibodies to the virus in their blood. Once a herpes virus has entered a person's body it is there for life. The varicella/zoster virus (VSV) may reappear as shingles in later life and HSV as recurrent lesions on lip or external genitalia. CMV and EBV, however, will only cause disease in later life if the patient has become immunosuppressed.

Human herpes virus 6 is a recently discovered virus which is the cause of *exanthem subitum*, a febrile illness with rash of childhood. It has also been associated with lymphadenopathy and may cause infection in the immunosuppressed.

INFECTIOUS MONONUCLEOSIS (GLANDULAR FEVER)

Infectious mononucleosis is an acute infectious disease caused by the Epstein-Barr virus which principally occurs in teenagers and young adults although occasionally other age groups may be affected. The virus infects, and replicates in B lymphocytes and is shed in the throat following the acute disease. Transmission is, therefore, usually by oral contact, possibly with the exchange of saliva. The incubation period is probably between 7–10 days.

Clinical features

The infection usually presents with malaise, tiredness, headache, abdominal discomfort, anorexia and fever. The clinical features can be variable. They are listed in the information box (p. 110).

The rash is especially common if ampicillin or amoxycillin has been given for the sore throat occurring in around 90% of patients.

Diagnosis

The diagnosis is suspected by the finding of a predominance of atypical lymphocytes in the peripheral blood and confirmed by a positive Monospot or Paul-Bunnell test. Specific virus serological tests are also available for diagnosis but are usually not required in most cases.

Conditions to be excluded in the differential diagno-

CLINICAL FEATURES OF INFECTIOUS MONONUCLEOSIS

Acute illness
Exudative tonsillitis
Petechial rash on palate
Lymph gland enlargement
Splenomegaly
Maculo-papular rash

Abnormal laboratory tests
Atypical lymphocytosis
Positive Monospot test
Elevation of liver enzymes

Complications
Chronic fatigue syndrome (common)
Hepatitis (rare)
Haemolytic anaemia (rare)
Thrombocytopenia (rare)
Rupture of spleen (rare)
Meningo-encephalitis (rare)

CLINICAL FEATURES OF CYTOMEGALOVIRUS INFECTION

Congenital infection
Hepatosplenomegaly
Purpura
Encephalitis

Acquired infection
In immunocompetent
    Asymptomatic infection
    Mononucleosis-like illness
    Retinitis (rare)
    Hepatitis (rare)
In immunosuppressed
    Retinitis
    Pneumonitis
    Enteritis
    Generalised infection

---

sis include cytomegalovirus infection, toxoplasmosis and acute HIV infection which can all present with lymphadenopathy, splenomegaly and fever with an atypical lymphocytosis (but not usually sore throat).

Complications
These are listed in the information box above. The chronic fatigue syndrome with debility, inability to concentrate, depression, tiredness and low-grade fever is the most important complication and may be associated with abnormalities of lymphocyte numbers and function. It can follow other virus infections.

Management
This is entirely symptomatic. Rest is important during the acute illness. A 48-hour course of corticosteroids is indicated for severe tonsillar enlargement causing dysphagia or difficulty in breathing.

CYTOMEGALOVIRUS INFECTION

Clinical features
The various features of CMV infection are listed in the information box (right).

Asymptomatic disease is the commonest manifestation in the immunocompetent. The cytomegalovirus is one of the most important pathogens in the immunosuppressed (including those with AIDS) causing much morbidity and mortality in these patients. The cytomegalovirus (along with rubella, toxoplasmosis and syphilis) is an important, although rare, cause of congenital infection which is acquired during a pregnancy in which the mother develops symptomatic or asymptomatic CMV infection. The child may be stillborn.

Diagnosis
CMV may be cultured from urine of infected patients. Diagnosis may also be confirmed by biopsy of infected tissue (e.g. lung or bowel) or by serology.

Management
The only drug which is active against CMV is ganciclovir which is toxic and expensive and is only indicated for serious infections in the immunosuppressed.

HERPES SIMPLEX INFECTIONS

Herpes simplex is a common DNA virus which frequently causes non-specific illness; hence many people have serum antibodies to the organism. It has assumed greater importance as a cause of serious, and sometimes fatal, infections in immunocompromised patients. There are two strains of *Herpes simplex virus* type 1 and type 2, the latter being principally responsible for sexually transmitted anogenital infections. Infections caused by these viruses can be categorised as primary or recurrent.

Clinical features
Primary infections. These include ulcerative stomatitis (commonest in infants), keratitis (dendritic ulcer), finger infections, vulvo-vaginitis, balanitis and encephalitis. In neonates and in the immunosuppressed the infection may be disseminated, involving many organs and tissues, and can be fatal. The newborn may contract the infection from the mother's genital tract

during birth and active genital *H. simplex* infection is therefore an indication for Caesarean section.

Recurrent infections. These are commonest on the lips and adjoining skin (herpes labialis or 'cold sore'). The lesions start as macules, become vesicular and then pustular. Attacks of herpes labialis may be precipitated by various stimuli including sunlight, menstruation and viral and bacterial infections. Genital lesions also commonly recur.

Diagnosis
The virus can readily be cultured from lesions and infection is confirmed by rising serum antibody titres.

Management
The *H. simplex* virus is susceptible to idoxuridine and acyclovir although most infections resolve spontaneously. Drops containing idoxuridine or acyclovir are effective in eye infections. Intravenous acyclovir is indicated for disseminated infections in immunocompromised patients and is also indicated for *H. simplex* encephalitis, which has a mortality of up to 80%. An oral preparation of acyclovir is available for the treatment of infections of the skin and mucous membranes. Acyclovir will not eradicate the *H. simplex* virus from posterior root ganglia and recurrent attacks cannot therefore be prevented.

CHICKENPOX (VARICELLA)

Chickenpox (varicella) is caused by the varicella-zoster virus which spreads by droplets from the upper respiratory tract or from the discharge from ruptured lesions on the skin or through contact with herpes zoster. Herpes zoster is due to reactivation of the varicella-zoster virus and may be accompanied by a varicelliform rash.

Chickenpox is highly infectious and chiefly affects children under 10 years of age. Most children tolerate this disease well but, as often happens with viral infections, adults may develop a more severe illness. In patients with leukaemia or who are otherwise immunocompromised, the disease may be severe or even fatal. The incubation period is 14–21 days.

Clinical features
Constitutional symptoms are usually brief and mild, and the first sign of the disease is often the rash. Lesions are sometimes present on the palate before the characteristic rash appears on the trunk on the second day of the illness. Then the face and finally the limbs are involved. The spots reach their maximum density upon the trunk, and are more sparse on the periphery of the limbs. Macules appear first and within a few hours the lesions become papular and then vesicular and, within 24 hours, pustular. Damage from scratching is frequent, since itching may be troublesome. Whether or not the pustules rupture, they dry up in a few days to form scabs. The spots appear in crops, so that lesions at all stages of development are seen in any area at the same time.

Complications
The course of the disease is usually uneventful but complications occasionally occur. These are listed in the information box below.

COMPLICATIONS OF CHICKENPOX

Direct viral effects
Pneumonia (usually adults or immunosuppressed)
Myocarditis (usually adults or immunosuppressed)

Post-viral effects
Encephalitis (cerebellar)
Glomerulonephritis

Secondary bacterial infection
Skin
Septicaemia
Osteomyelitis/septic arthritis

Intra-uterine infection
Congenital limb defects (rare)

Management
No treatment is required in the majority of patients but acyclovir can be used in the immunocompromised patient. If there is secondary infection a local antiseptic should be applied to the skin, e.g. chlorhexidine. If bacterial infection progresses, an antibiotic such as *flucloxacillin* should be prescribed. Immunocompromised children who have been in contact with chickenpox or shingles should have an injection of *human anti-varicella gammaglobulin* (zoster immune globulin).

VIRUS INFECTIONS OF THE NERVOUS SYSTEM

Herpes zoster, viral meningitis, viral encephalitis, poliomyelitis, postviral syndromes, slow virus infections, rabies (see pp. 880–881).

LASSA FEVER

Since the first report, in 1969, the disease has so far been limited to sub-Saharan West Africa where

Table 5.16   Common viral haemorrhagic fevers

Disease	Viral agent	Reservoir	Transmission	Geography	Case mortality
Lassa fever	Arenavirus	Multimammate rat (*Mastomys natalensis*) Patient	Urine Body fluids	West Africa	Up to 50% (responds to ribavirin)
Marburg/Ebola virus disease	Unclassified	? Patient	via monkeys, Body fluids	Central Africa	25–90%
Yellow fever	Togavirus	Monkeys	Mosquitoes	Tropical Africa S. and C. America	10–60%
Dengue	Togavirus (dengue types 1–4)	Man	*Aedes aegypti* et al	Tropical and sub-tropical coasts	Nil–10%*
Omsk	Togavirus	Musk rat	Ticks	Siberia	2%
Crimean-Congo	Bunyanwera	Ixodes tick	Ixodes tick	Africa, Asia, E. Europe	15–70%
Bolivian and Argentinian	Arenavirus (Machupa and Junin)	Rodents (*Calomys spp.*)	Urine	S. America	?
Haemorrhagic fever with renal syndrome	Hantaan virus	Rodents	Faeces	North Asia North Europe	30%

*Mortality of uncomplicated and haemorrhagic dengue fever, respectively.

serological studies have shown that the infection is widespread. Isolated cases and small rural outbreaks are commonest, but outbreaks in hospital have also occurred (Table 5.16).

Clinical features

The disease has the general features of a viral infection, high fever, intercostal myalgia, bradycardia, low blood pressure and leucopenia. Adherent yellow exudates on the pharynx are particularly characteristic. The fever lasts between 7 and 17 days. In severe cases liver and renal failure, electrolyte imbalance, haemorrhage and acute circulatory failure develop. Case mortality is high, but mild and subclinical infections also occur.

The virus may be isolated, or antigen detected, in maximum security laboratories from serum, pharynx, pleural exudate and urine but diagnosis will usually be established from 'paired sera', the later specimen being taken 6–8 weeks after the onset of infection. The diagnosis should be considered in Britain in patients presenting with fever within 21 days of leaving West Africa.

Management

Strict isolation and general supportive measures, preferably in a special unit, are required. Ribavirin is given intravenously (100 mg/kg, then 25 mg/kg/d for 3 days and 12.5 mg/kg/d for 4 days).

Prevention

The administration of convalescent immune plasma has been followed by recovery and is therefore recommended for prophylaxis after accidental exposure to infection.

MARBURG AND EBOLA VIRAL DISEASE

In 1967 a severe infectious illness broke out among laboratory workers in Marburg, West Germany, who had handled tissues from a batch of vervet monkeys imported from Uganda. In 1976 outbreaks of the disease occurred in Sudan and Zaire from a focus on the Ebola River. The viruses causing these two outbreaks have a unique identical structure but are antigenically distinct. Sporadic cases have occurred elsewhere in Africa (Table 5.16). In man-to-man outbreaks the mortality is high, but successive human passage seems to reduce virulence. The incubation period is 5–9 days.

Clinical features

The illness presents suddenly with fever, severe myalgia and diarrhoea. By the fourth or fifth day the fauces become inflamed and a bright red follicular rash appears on the extensor surfaces of the limbs; it spreads to the trunk and face, becomes maculopapular and finally confluent and livid. There may be lymphadeno-pathy. About the sixth day, in severe cases, bleeding associated with thrombocytopenia starts usually in the gastrointestinal tract. The virus also attacks the brain, kidneys and lungs. Fatal complications, often occurring between the sixth and tenth days of the illness, include haemorrhage, secondary infection, encephalitis, renal failure and pneumonia.

Management
Treatment consists of supportive measures, replacement of blood and the management of complications. Immune plasma may be beneficial if given at an early stage. No vaccine is available.

OTHER HAEMORRHAGIC FEVERS

The term haemorrhagic fevers is increasing in popularity but covers too wide a field of medicine to be of much value. Infections due to many different organisms may cause bleeding, and through several different mechanisms. The causes are listed in the information box (right).

Bolivian and Argentinian haemorrhagic fever
These cause epidemics in rural workers, characterised by fever, with severe haemorrhage developing about the fifth day. Treatment with convalescent plasma greatly reduces the mortality.

Haemorrhagic fever with renal syndrome
This has occurred in outbreaks in Korea, Manchuria and Eastern Europe. The infection causes severe capillary congestion, leakage and haemorrhage, especially in the renal medulla, so that oedema and acute renal failure develop, with oliguria and the passage of cells and protein in the urine. Untreated the mortality is high, but with proper treatment for acute renal failure (p. 588) and blood transfusion if necessary, patients should recover. A less severe form of the disease, nephropathia epidemica, is found in Scandinavia.

ARBOVIRAL INFECTIONS

Classification
So called because they are *arthropod-borne*, the hundred or so arboviruses are divided into groups according to their antigenic characters.

Group A are togaviruses all of which are transmitted by mosquitoes. The group includes three important causes of encephalitis in the New World, Eastern, Western and Venezuelan equine encephalitis, and several important fevers of Africa (Chikungunya, O'nyong-nyong, Sindbis and Semilki Forest fevers), South America and Australia (Ross River fever).

Group B are also togaviruses, many of which cause encephalitis or haemorrhagic fevers. Yellow fever, dengue, Japanese B encephalitis, and West Nile, St Louis and Murray Valley fevers are transmitted by mosquitoes. Russian and European Spring-Summer encephalitis, Omsk haemorrhagic fever, Kyasanur

---

CAUSES OF HAEMORRHAGIC FEVERS
Viruses (See Table 5.17)
Rickettsia Rocky Mountain spotted fever
Bacteria Meningococcaemia, plague, Gram-negative septicaemia
Spirochaetes Relapsing fever
Protozoa African trypanosomiasis

forest disease of India and louping ill of Britain are transmitted by ticks.

Bunyamwera group of bunyaviruses, all of which are mosquito borne, are responsible for a large number of fevers, especially in the New World, including California encephalitis.

The remaining arboviruses, many of which are bunyaviruses, are placed in small groups or are ungrouped. Included here are the sandfly fevers, Rift Valley fever, and the haemorrhagic fevers of Crimea, Congo and Korea.

Arboviruses often cause epidemics. Clinically many infections are mild; even with the potentially serious ones, subclinical cases outnumber the severe one hundred or one thousand times. The immunity that follows is often life-long and is an important determinant of the pattern of disease in the exposed community. Normally immunity protects and prevents further epidemics, but in the case of dengue, it may also sensitise and predispose to more severe disease if the person is infected with a different, but cross-reacting type. The incubation period is usually less than a week.

Clinical features
The presentation is with fever which may disappear after a few days, either permanently or to return accompanied by the clinical features and complications characteristic of the particular infection. In many arbovirus infections there is a maculopapular rash, conjunctival suffusion, photophobia and orbital pain. Arthralgia and myalgia are common; pain may be severe and immobilising. Lymphadenopathy is found in a few infections.

Complications
The most serious complications of arboviral infections are encephalitis and haemorrhage. When inoculated

into mice most arboviruses cause encephalitis, but relatively few do so in man. The important ones are listed above, but their distribution is wider than their names suggest. The clinical features of encephalitis are described on page 877.

The causes of haemorrhage in arboviral infections are not fully understood. In some, such as dengue, disseminated intravascular coagulation is important; in others, notably yellow fever, haemorrhage follows severe hepatitis when deficiency of prothrombin and other coagulation factors develop. Thrombocytopenia occurs in many arboviral infections, and may contribute. Acute circulatory failure may follow haemorrhage, or occur on its own, possibly due to increased capillary permeability, as in dengue.

Diagnosis

This may be possible on clinical grounds during the course of an epidemic. For virological confirmation blood is transported on ice for inoculation into mice or tissue culture. It may be possible to isolate virus from CSF if there are signs of encephalitis. Serological diagnosis depends on demonstrating rising titres of antibodies, usually by complement fixation or haemagglutination-inhibition. Such antibodies are, however, usually only group specific. Neutralising antibodies may be genus specific, but are more time consuming and expensive to assay.

Management

Treatment is supportive with attention to fluid and electrolyte balance and the circulatory state.

Prevention

This rests mainly on vector or reservoir control, but vaccines are available for some, including yellow fever, Kyasanur forest disease, European Spring-Summer encephalitis and Japanese B encephalitis.

YELLOW FEVER

Yellow fever is normally a zoonosis of monkeys that inhabit tropical rain forests in West and Central Africa and South and Central America, among whom it may cause devastating epidemics (Fig. 5.3). It is transmitted by mosquitoes living in tree tops (Fig. 5.4). *Aedes africanus* is the vector in Africa and the Haemagogus species in America. The infection is brought down to man either by infected mosquitoes when trees are felled, or by monkeys raiding human plantations. In the latter case *Aedes simpsoni*, which breeds in the axils of banana plants, may transmit the disease to man. In

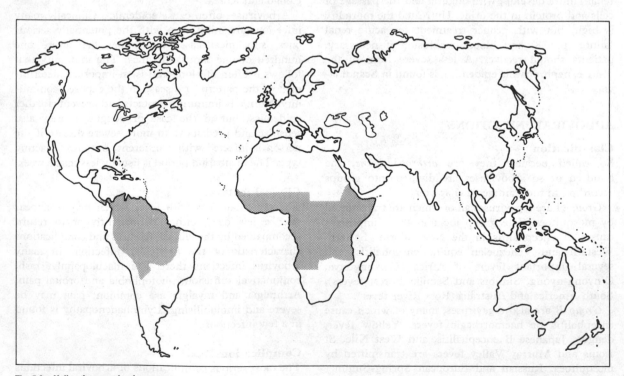

Fig. 5.3 Yellow fever endemic zones.

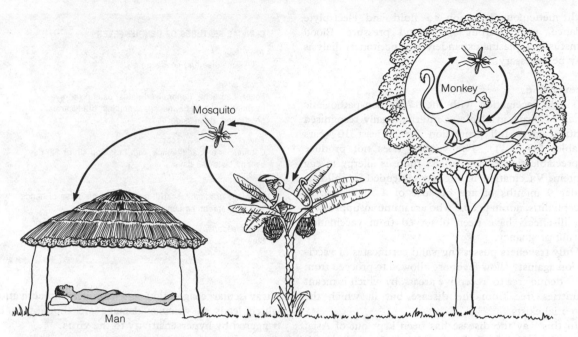

Fig. 5.4 Transmission of yellow fever. From tree top cycle, via paridomestic cycle, to man.

towns yellow fever may be transmitted between humans by *Aedes aegypti* which breeds efficiently in small collections of water. The distribution of this mosquito is far wider than that of yellow fever and poses a continual risk of spread.

Man is infectious during the viraemic phase which starts 3 to 6 days after the bite of the infected mosquito and lasts for 4 to 5 days. Mosquitoes become infectious 8–12 days after biting a patient and remain so for the rest of their 6–8 weeks' life span. They may pass on the virus transovarially. The incubation period is 3–6 days.

Pathology

In the liver, acute mid-zonal necrosis leads to deposits of hyalin called Councilman bodies (p. 506), and intranuclear eosinophilic inclusions called Torres bodies; another characteristic feature is the absence of inflammatory infiltrate. The kidneys show tubular degeneration, which may partly be due to reduced blood flow. Widespread petechial haemorrhages are most marked in the stomach and duodenum. Haemorrhage is due to liver damage and disseminated intravascular coagulation.

Clinical features

Yellow fever is often solely a mild febrile illness lasting less than a week. The classical disease starts suddenly with rigors and high fever. Backache, headache and bone pains are severe. Nausea and vomiting start. The face is flushed and the conjunctivae infected. Bradycardia and leucopenia are also characteristic of this phase of the illness, which lasts 3 days and is followed by a remission lasting a few hours or days.

The third stage is characterised by return of fever, and the onset of jaundice, petechial haemorrhages in the mucosae, ecchymoses, haematemesis and oliguria. Patients commonly die in the third stage, often after a period of coma.

Diagnosis

Diagnostic procedures are listed in the information box below.

DIAGNOSIS OF YELLOW FEVER

- Clinical features in endemic area
- Virus isolation from blood in first 4 days (p. 114)
- Fourfold rise in antibody titre
- Postmortem liver biopsy
- Differentiate from viral hepatitis, haemorrhagic fevers, malaria, typhoid, leptospirosis, afla toxin poisoning

Management

Patients should be nursed under a mosquito net until the viraemic stage has passed. Treatment is supportive, with meticulous attention to fluid and electrolyte balance, urine output and blood pressure. Blood transfusions, plasma expanders and peritoneal dialysis may be necessary.

Prevention

A single vaccination with the 17 D non-pathogenic strain of virus, available at internationally recognised centres, gives full protection for at least 10 years (Tables 5.9, 5.11). The vaccine does not produce appreciable side-effects, unless there is allergy to egg protein. Vaccination is not recommended in children under 9 months of age because of a slight risk of encephalitis, nor in people who are immunosuppressed. No ill-effects have been observed from vaccination during pregnancy.

Only travellers possessing valid certificates of vaccination against yellow fever are allowed to proceed from an endemic area to 'receptive areas', by which is meant countries free from the disease but in which the potential exists.

In this way the disease has been kept out of Asia. Mosquito control of airports should be maintained. The urban disease can be eradicated by the abolition of the breeding places of *Aedes aegypti* by the use of residual insecticides in houses and by mass vaccination in endemic areas. Vaccination is the only means to prevent humans being infected from forest reservoirs.

DENGUE

The disease is a risk in many tropical and subtropical countries, especially in coastal areas (Table 5.16) during the hot season when mosquitoes are numerous. Many large epidemics have occurred. One attack usually gives immunity for about 9 months and after several attacks a degree of permanent immunity is attained. Some cross-immunity exists between dengue and other members of the B group of arboviruses, including the virus of yellow fever. The incubation period is usually 5–6 days.

Clinical features

The disease varies in severity. The clinical features are listed in the information box (right). Subclinical infections are common.

Dengue haemorrhagic fever

This occurs in S.E. Asia, rarely elsewhere. After 3 to 4 days of fever bleeding starts with petechiae, ecchymoses, epistaxis and melaena, and proceeds to acute circulatory failure. Even with treatment of these complications, 10% of patients die. Disseminated

---

CLINICAL FEATURES OF DENGUE FEVER

Prodrome
2 days malaise and headache

Acute onset
Fever, backache, generalised pains, painful red eyes, lacrimation, anorexia, nausea, vomiting, bradycardia, prostration, depression

Fever
Continuous or 'saddle-back' with break on 4th or 5th day; usually lasts 7–8 days

Rash
Develops gradually, scarlet morbilliform on dorsa of hands and feet, spreading centripetally

Convalescence
Slow

---

intravascular coagulation and complement activation which leads to vascular damage are thought to be triggered by hypersensitivity to the virus.

Diagnosis

This is usually easy in an endemic area when a patient has the characteristic symptoms and signs. However, the mild cases may resemble other viral diseases and a severe attack may be mistaken for anicteric yellow fever, but the absence of urinary changes will help to differentiate it. The virus can be recovered from the blood and antibody titres rise. Leucopenia is usual.

Management

There is no specific treatment. The severe pains can be relieved by paracetamol, but occasionally opiates are required. Fluid replacement, blood transfusions and corticosteroids are indicated in the haemorrhagic varieties.

Prevention

Patients are nursed under a mosquito net. Breeding places of Aedes mosquitoes should be abolished and the adults destroyed by insecticides.

RIFT VALLEY FEVER

This disease is caused by an arbovirus which normally infects sheep and goats in East and South Africa. It is usually conveyed by a culicine mosquito, especially *Culex pipiens*. Cattle and other domestic animals may act as amplifying hosts. Sporadic infections have followed direct contact with infected meat and from inhalation.

Clinical features

There have been large outbreaks, with four clinical types characterised by:

1. uncomplicated fever resembling dengue
2. retinal changes
3. haemorrhages and jaundice
4. meningoencephalitis.

Deaths occurred in the last two groups.

Management

There is no specific treatment.

JAPANESE ENCEPHALITIS (see p. 881)

SMALLPOX AND MONKEYPOX

As a result of the WHO programme of case detection and vaccination, it is confidently believed that smallpox has been eradicated world-wide. Apart from two laboratory-acquired infections in 1978, the last known case occurred in Somalia in 1977.

Clinical features

Major smallpox produces a severe constitutional illness associated with a peripherally distributed rash with lesions which, in any one area, progress in unison from macules through papules, and vesicles, to pustules. The mortality rate may be as high as 40%.

A similar virus causes monkeypox in primates in jungle areas of Central Africa, with lesions resembling those of smallpox. Some human cases have occurred in those in contact with infected primates but inter-human spread is exceptional.

The virus of smallpox is maintained in two designated laboratories, in order to be able to differentiate such diseases as monkeypox from smallpox. Only staff employed in these designated laboratories, of which there are none in Britain, now require to be vaccinated against smallpox. Limited stocks of smallpox vaccine are available for this purpose, and in case the disease should reappear.

DISEASES DUE TO CHLAMYDIAE

Chlamydia causes psittacosis and ornithosis (p. 361), urethritis (p. 190), lymphogranuloma venereum (p. 191) and trachoma.

TRACHOMA

Trachoma is a specific communicable keratoconjunc-tivitis caused by *Chlamydia trachomatis*. Transmission is usually by contact or from fomites in unhygienic surroundings. Some infections occur during birth from infected genital passages.

Vast numbers of people suffer from trachoma in the hot dry dusty areas of the subtropics and tropics but it is also present in Southern Europe, and among immigrants in Britain. The disease varies markedly in incidence and in severity in different geographical areas. In endemic areas the disease is commonest in children.

Pathology

The infection lasts for years, may be latent over long periods and may recrudesce. The conjunctiva of the upper lid is first affected with vascularisation and cellular infiltration; pannus, spreading to the cornea causes opacity and impairment of vision.

Clinical features

The onset is usually insidious and infection may not be apparent to the patient. Early symptoms include conjunctival irritation and blepharospasm, but the problem may not be detected until vision begins to fail. Trachoma may also present as an acute ophthalmia neonatorum.

The early follicles of trachoma are characteristic, but clinical differentiation from conjunctivitis due to other viruses may be difficult at this stage. Scarring of the lids causes entropion.

Diagnosis

Intracellular inclusions may be demonstrated in conjunctival scrapings by staining with iodine or immunofluorescence. Chlamydia may be isolated in chick embryo or cell culture.

Management

Ophthalmic ointment or oily drops of 1–3% tetracycline should be applied twice daily for 3 months. In mass therapy in endemic areas topical application twice daily for 3–6 consecutive days each month for 6 months has given good results. Oral tetracycline (15 mg/kg/d), doxycycline (15 mg/kg/d) or sulphonamide (30 mg/kg/d) given for 3 weeks is just as effective. Deformity and scarring of the lids, corneal opacities, ulceration and scarring require surgical treatment, after control of local infection.

Prevention

Personal and family cleanliness should be improved. Proper care of the eyes of newborn and young children is essential. Family contacts should be examined.

Population surveys lead to discovery and treatment of asymptomatic infections. Trachoma clinics are required in areas of high endemicity.

DISEASES DUE TO RICKETTSIAE

Rickettsiae are natural parasites of the cells of the intestinal canal of arthropods. Some species may parasitise higher mammals including man. Infection is usually conveyed to man through the skin from excreta of arthropods but the saliva of some biting vectors is infected. Essential features of rickettsial infections are compared in Table 5.17. Transovarian infection to the next generation occurs in ticks and mites, which serve as reservoirs as well as vectors of infection.

Pathology
In man rickettsiae multiply in vascular endothelial cells especially of capillaries, producing lesions in the skin, central nervous system, heart, lungs, kidneys and skeletal muscles. Endothelial proliferation, associated with a perivascular reaction (nodules of Fraenkel) may cause thromboses and small haemorrhages. In epidemic typhus the brain and in scrub typhus the cardiovascular system and lungs are particularly attacked.

The common clinical findings are fever, severe prostration, mental disturbance and often a rash.

An eschar is often found in tick and mite borne typhus. An eschar is a necrotic sore, often scabbed, at the site of the bite and is due to vasculitis following immunological recognition of the inoculated organism. Regional lymph nodes often enlarge. There are epidemic, endemic, tick and scrub typhus fevers.

EPIDEMIC TYPHUS FEVER

Louse-borne or epidemic typhus is caused by *R. prowazeki* and is transmitted by infected faeces of the human body louse, *Pediculus humanus*, usually through scratching the skin, or sometimes by inhalation. Patients suffering from epidemic typhus infect the lice which leave when the patient is febrile. In conditions of overcrowding the disease spreads rapidly. During interepidemic periods the disease may be maintained by inapparent or latent cases or perhaps by infected fleas and rats. The disease is prevalent in parts of Africa especially Ethiopia and Rwanda, the South American Andes and Afghanistan. Large epidemics have occurred in Europe, usually as a sequel to war. The incubation period is usually 12–14 days.

Clinical features
There may be a few days of malaise but the onset is more often sudden with rigors, fever, frontal headaches, pains in the back and limbs, constipation and bronchitis. The face is flushed and cyanotic, eyes congested, and the patient soon becomes dull and confused.

The rash appears on the fourth to the sixth day and

Table 5.17 Essential features of rickettsial infections

Disease	Reservoir	Vector	Primary Complex[1]	Rash	Gangrene	Target organs	Mortality
Epidemic typhus	Man	Louse		Morbilliform Haemorrhagic	Often	Brain, skin, bronchitis, myocarditis	Up to 40%
Endemic typhus	Rat	Flea		Slight			Rare[2]
Rocky Mountain Spotted fever	Rodents, dogs, ticks	*Ixodid* ticks	Often	Morbilliform Haemorrhagic	Often	Bronchitis, myocarditis, brain, skin	2–12%[3]
Other tick-borne typhus	Rodents, dogs, ticks	*Ixodid* ticks	Usual	Maculopapular	—	Skin, meninges	Rare[2]
Scrub typhus	Rodents, mites	*Trombiculid* mites	Often	Maculopapular	Unusual	Bronchitis, myocarditis, brain, skin	Rare[2]
Rickettsial pox	Domestic mouse	Mite	Usual	Maculopapular	—	—	Rare[2]
Trench fever	Man	Louse	—	Maculopapular	—	—	Rare[2]

[1]Eschar at bite site and local lymphadenopathy.
[2]Except in infants, elderly and debilitated.
[3]Highest in adult males.

often resembles measles. In its early stages it disappears on pressure but soon becomes petechial with subcutaneous mottling. It appears first on the anterior folds of the axillae, sides of the abdomen or back of hands, then on the trunk and forearms. The neck and face are seldom affected.

During the second week symptoms increase in severity. Sores collect on the lips. The tongue becomes dry, brown, shrunken and tremulous. The spleen is palpable, the pulse feeble and the patient stuporous and delirious. The temperature falls rapidly at the end of the second week and the patient recovers gradually. In fatal cases the patient usually dies in the second week from toxaemia, cardiac or renal failure or pneumonia.

Complications

Common complications are listed in the information box below.

COMPLICATIONS OF LOUSE-BORNE TYPHUS

Vascular
Venous thrombosis, gangrene of fingers, toes, nose and genitalia

Infective
Parotitis, bronchopneumonia

Brill's disease
A mild relapse many years later

Diagnosis

The clinical features are diagnostic when there is an epidemic of the disease but in mild cases may be less distinctive. Laboratory aids to diagnosis are discovered on page 120.

Management

See page 120.

ENDEMIC TYPHUS FEVER

Flea-borne or 'endemic' typhus caused by *R. mooseri* is endemic world-wide. Man is infected when, by scratching, he introduces the faeces or contents of a crushed flea which has fed on an infected rat. The incubation period is 8–14 days. The symptoms resemble those of a mild louse-borne typhus. The rash may be scanty and transient. Laboratory aids to diagnosis are discussed on page 120 and treatment on page 120.

TICK-BORNE TYPHUS FEVERS

ROCKY MOUNTAIN SPOTTED FEVER

The casual organism, *R. rickettsii* is transmitted by the bite of hard (*Ixodid*) ticks which carry the infection to rodents and dogs and on occasion to man. It is widely distributed and increasing in western and south-eastern states of the USA and also in South America. The pathological changes are similar to those in epidemic typhus. The incubation period is about 7 days.

Clinical features

There may be eschar at the site of the bite, with enlargement of the regional lymph nodes. Symptoms closely resemble those of louse-borne typhus. The rash appears about the third or fourth day, at first like measles, but in a few hours the typical maculopapular eruption develops. Each day it becomes more distinct and papular and finally petechial. The rash first appears on the wrists, forearms and ankles, spreads in 24–48 hours to the back, limbs and chest and lastly to the abdomen where it is least pronounced. The fully developed rash often affects also the palms, soles and face. Petechiae may appear in crops. Larger cutaneous and subcutaneous haemorrhages may appear in severe cases. The liver and spleen become palpable. Complications are as in louse-borne typhus, but gangrene is more common. Untreated, the course of the disease may be mild or rapidly fatal.

Diagnosis

There may be a history of a bite by a tick. The character of the rash, appearing first at the periphery, is helpful. Laboratory aids to diagnosis are discussed on page 120. Detection of organisms by immunofluorescence in frozen sections of skin biopsies is quick and efficient.

OTHER FORMS OF TICK-BORNE TYPHUS FEVER

The causal agents of African tick-borne typhus in South and East Africa are *R. conori* and a substrain *R. conori pijperi*, the reservoir hosts being dogs and rodents. 'Fievre boutonneuse' of the Mediterranean is similar, as is also the infection in Queensland where *R. australis* is the causal organism. Infected hard ticks may be picked up by walking on grasslands, or dogs may bring the ticks into the house. Tourists often acquire tick typhus and import it into Britain. A careful search is needed to find the tell-tale eschar, and maculopapular rash on the trunk, limbs, palms and soles. There may be delirium and meningeal signs in severe infections but recovery is the rule.

SCRUB TYPHUS FEVER

Mite-borne or 'scrub' typhus is caused by *R. tsutsuga-mushi* transmitted by the bite of infective larval trombiculid mites. It occurs in the Far East, Assam, Burma, Pakistan, Bangladesh, India, Indonesia, S. Pacific Islands and Queensland.

Pathology
The pathology is similar to that of louse-borne typhus, but lesions in the lungs are more prominent. In many patients one or more eschars develop, surrounded by an area of cellulitis and enlargement of regional lymph nodes. The incubation period is about 9 days.

Clinical features
Mild or subclinical cases are common. The onset of symptoms is usually sudden with headache, often retro-orbital, fever, malaise, weakness and cough. In severe illness the general symptoms increase with apathy and prostration. An erythematous maculopapular rash often appears on about the fifth to the seventh day and spreads to the trunk, face and limbs including the palms and soles with generalised painless lymphadenopathy. The rash fades by the fourteenth day. The temperature rises rapidly and continues as a remittent fever with sweating until it falls by lysis about the twelfth to the eighteenth day. In severe infection the patient is prostrate with cough, pneumonia, confusion and deafness. Cardiac failure, renal failure and haemorrhage may develop. Convalescence is often slow and tachycardia may persist for some weeks.

Diagnosis
In endemic areas diagnosis is often possible on the clinical findings. Laboratory aids to diagnosis are discussed below.

Management
This is discussed below.

OTHER RICKETTSIAL DISEASES

RICKETTSIALPOX

This is due to *R. akari*, transmitted from the domestic mouse by a mite. It appears to be restricted to New York and Philadelphia where mice are now adapted to live in communal rubbish chutes of apartment houses.

Clinical features
The illness starts with a papule, which develops into an eschar, and is followed a week later by the sudden onset of fever, sweating, backache and a rash, maculopapular at first but which soon vesiculates and crusts, healing without scarring.

TRENCH FEVER

This is caused by *R. quintana* and is spread to man by louse faeces. It was prevalent in the First World War in Europe among troops in the trenches and again in the Second World War in the USSR. The disease is otherwise rare. The incubation period is 10–20 days.

Clinical features
The onset is sudden with headache, severe pains in trunk and limbs. The temperature rises sharply and remains raised for 5–7 days. The initial illness is like a mild case of typhus fever but febrile relapses are common, usually at intervals of 5–6 days and may be debilitating.

Diagnosis of rickettsial infections
The Weil-Felix reaction, which is the non-specific agglutination by the patient's serum of the strains of organisms Proteus OX 19 or OXK, helps in the differentiation of human infections (Table 5.17). A four-fold rise in titre is diagnostic.

Species-specific antibodies may be detected by complement fixation, microagglutination and fluorescence in specialised laboratories. Rickettsiae may be isolated from the blood in the first week of illness by intraperitoneal inoculation into male guinea-pigs or mice.

Management of the rickettsial diseases
The various fevers due to rickettsiae vary greatly in severity but all respond to tetracycline or chloramphenicol. Tetracycline is administered in a dose of 500 mg 4 times daily. The fever usually settles within 2 or 3 days. Tetracycline should be continued for 2–3 days after the patient is afebrile as there is a tendency to relapse. In endemic areas good results have been obtained in louse-borne typhus and scrub typhus by a single dose of 100 mg doxycycline.

Nursing care is important, especially in epidemic typhus. Sedation may be required for delirium and blood transfusion for haemorrhage. Relapsing fever and typhoid are common intercurrent infections in epidemic typhus, and pneumonia in scrub typhus. They must be sought and treated. Convalescence is usually protracted especially in older people.

Prevention

For louse and flea-borne typhus and in trench fever steps should be taken to get rid of all lice and fleas and their faeces. An insecticide powder can be insufflated in to the undergarments of those at risk without their undressing; 5% carboryl or 0.5% malathion are replacing 2% gamma-benzene hexachloride and DDT to which lice are often resistant. Residual insecticide powder on floors and bedding kills hatching fleas. To prevent flea-borne typhus, food stores and granaries should be protected from rats. Rats and their fleas must be destroyed.

Attendants on patients with louse-borne typhus should wear protective clothing smeared with an insect repellent such as dimethylphtalate (DMP). The patient should be washed, and an insecticide applied all over. They are a danger to others unless their clothes have been disinfected with insecticide in plastic bags, or sterilised in a domestic tumble drier or autoclaved.

Dogs should be regularly disinfected of ticks with forceps to guard against tick-borne typhus and should not be allowed to sleep in bedrooms. Protection of the legs when walking through grasslands may reduce the risk of picking up infected ticks. The early removal of ticks and cleansing the site of the bite are also important. Floors of log cabins in the USA should be creosoted annually.

Mite-borne typhus is acquired when man enters scrub country in endemic areas. Protection against the larval mite can be secured by wearing suitable clothing, the inside of which has been smeared once a week with insect repellent. Mites can be destroyed by aerial spraying of infected areas with Aldrin or Dieldrin, repeated every 3 months.

Active immunisation. Vaccines can be prepared from killed *R. prowazeki*, *R. mooseri* or *R. rickettsi* cultured in eggs, but they are not generally available.

Chemoprophylaxis. It is likely that doxycycline (100 mg/weekly) will protect those at risk.

Q FEVER

Q (Query) fever is caused by *Coxiella burnettii*, a rickettsia-like organism, which is widespread in nature and is highly resistant to drying. It is carried by ticks among animals, including cattle and sheep. Transmission to humans is air-borne through aerosols from birth products and contaminated dust. Unpasteurised milk is another source of infection. The incubation period of Q fever is from 7 to 14 days.

Clinical features

The clinical features of the illness are protean ranging from subclinical infection to fatal encephalitis or endocarditis (p. 301). Acute Q fever usually starts like influenza with pyrexia followed by myalgia, headache and sweating. Many cases resolve without specific therapy. Some patients have a cough and radiological examination may reveal a pneumonitis. Less common features of Q fever include hepatitis, myocarditis, epididymo-orchitis, iritis and osteomyelitis.

Diagnosis

The diagnosis of Q fever should be considered in patients living in rural areas, especially if there is occupational contact work with livestock. *C. burnettii* does not grow in the media used for routine blood cultures and it is therefore important to consider Q fever as a possible cause in patients with clinical evidence of endocarditis who have sterile blood cultures. The diagnosis of Q fever is confirmed by the detection of serum antibodies to the two polysaccharide antigens of *C. burnettii*; acute infection is confirmed by a four-fold rise in phase II antibody titre in paired specimens of blood taken at intervals of between 10 and 14 days. Phase 1 antibody titres rise more slowly than phase II and the persistence of both suggest chronic infection.

Management

C. burnettii is sensitive to the tetracyclines, clindamycin, chloramphenicol and rifampicin. Acute infections respond within a few days to tetracycline in a dose of 500 mg 4 times daily for 2–3 weeks, or doxycycline 200 mg daily. Treatment is continued for 2 weeks. The treatment of chronic infections, especially if there is endocarditis, requires prolonged therapy with tetracycline plus clindamycin or rifampicin.

DISEASES DUE TO BACTERIA

DIPHTHERIA

In many parts of the world diphtheria is still an important cause of illness. It is very rare in Britain.

Pathology

Infection with *Corynebacterium diphtheriae* occurs most commonly in the upper respiratory tract and sore throat is frequently the presenting feature. The disease is usually spread by droplet infection from cases or carriers. The organisms remain localised at the site of infection and the serious consequences result from the absorption of a soluble exotoxin which damages the heart muscle and the nervous system. The infection may occur rarely on the conjunctiva or the genital tract, or it may complicate wounds, abrasions or diseases of the skin.

The average incubation period is 2–4 days. Cases are isolated until cultures from 6 daily nose and throat swabs are negative.

Clinical features

These are listed in the information box below. The disease begins insidiously. The temperature is seldom much raised although tachycardia is usually marked. The diagnostic feature is the 'wash-leather' elevated greyish-green membrane of variable extent on the tonsils with a well-defined edge and surrounded by a zone of inflammation. The membrane is firm and adherent. There may be swelling of the neck ('bull-neck') and tender enlargement of the lymph nodes. In the mildest infections, especially in the presence of a high degree of immunity, a membrane may never appear and the throat is merely slightly injected.

With anterior nasal infection there is also nasal discharge often tinged with blood. In laryngeal diphtheria there is a husky voice, a high-pitched cough, and a danger of respiratory obstruction which can be fatal if tracheostomy is not carried out. When the infection spreads towards the uvula, to the fauces and then to the nasopharynx, the patient is often gravely ill. The pulse is rapid and of poor volume and the blood pressure low. Death from acute circulatory failure may occur within the first 10 days. Those who survive the earlier toxaemia may later develop arrhythmias or cardiac failure. Electrocardiographic changes are common and are due to myocarditis. These are reversible and there is no permanent damage to the heart in those who survive.

CLINICAL FEATURES OF DIPHTHERIA

Acute infection
Membranous tonsillitis
or Nasal infection
or Laryngeal infection
or Skin/wound/conjunctival infection (rare)

Complications
Laryngeal obstruction or paralysis
Myocarditis
Peripheral neuropathy

Involvement of the nervous system sometimes occurs, and after tonsillar or pharyngeal diphtheria it usually commences with palatal palsy on about the tenth day of the illness. Paralysis of accommodation often follows and may be inferred from the patient's complaint of difficulty in reading small print. A week or two later, though somewhat rarely, weakness and paraesthesia in the limbs due to polyneuritis may develop. Recovery from such neuritis is always ultimately complete.

Management

Procedures for managing diphtheria are listed in the information box below.

MANAGEMENT OF DIPHTHERIA

- Admit to isolation facility
- Administer antitoxin (4000–32 000 units i.m. — test dose first)
- Give benzylpenicillin 600 mg 6-hourly i.v. for 7 days
- Notify public health authorities
- Treat complications
  Tracheostomy for respiratory obstruction
  Monitor heart if myocarditis
- Protect close contacts
  Erythromycin prophylaxis
  Immunisation

Upon making a clinical diagnosis of diphtheria, the case should be notified to the public health authorities and sent urgently to a hospital for infectious diseases. Antitoxin should be injected intramuscularly without awaiting the report on a throat swab if the clinician considers that diphtheria is likely to be the cause of the illness. Delay increases the danger to the patient, because toxin, once fixed to the tissues, can no longer be neutralised by antitoxin. However, horse serum, in which antitoxin is contained is liable to cause undesirable reactions being a foreign protein. There may be an immediate anaphylactic reaction with dyspnoea, pallor and collapse or even death. Serum sickness, with fever, urticaria and joint pains may occur 7–12 days later. If there is a previous history of inoculation of horse serum, the symptoms commonly appear in 3–4 days. As anaphylaxis is potentially lethal, all patients must be asked whether they have ever had antiserum before and whether they suffer from any allergic disorder. A small test injection of antitoxin should be given half an hour before the full dose in every patient.

Rapid desensitisation must be undertaken with extreme caution when a reaction does occur after the test dose in an allergic subject. An ampoule of 1/1000 adrenaline solution must be close at hand to deal with any immediate type of reaction (0.5–1.0 ml i.m.). An antihistamine is also given.

In a very severely ill patient the risk of anaphylactic shock is outweighed by the mortal danger of diphtheritic toxaemia and up to 100 000 units of antitoxin is injected intravenously if the test dose has not given rise to symptoms. For disease of moderate severity 16 000–32 000 units i.m. will suffice, and for mild cases 4000–8000 units.

Penicillin should be administered for 1 week to eliminate *C. diphtheriae*. Patients allergic to penicillin can be given erythromycin.

Prevention

Active immunisation should be given to all children.

If diphtheria occurs in a closed community, all close contacts should be given erythromycin which is more effective than penicillin in eradicating the organism in carriers. All contacts should be advised to have active immunisation or a booster dose of toxoid.

ANTHRAX

Anthrax is a disease of domestic animals which become infected by inhaling or ingesting spores of *Bacillus anthracis* passed in faeces. Grazing lands remain infective for years. In man anthrax is an occupational disease of farmers, butchers and dealers in hides, hair, wool and bone meal from endemic areas. Anthrax is endemic in communities where skins are used as sleeping mats, for clothing or for carrying water, and where diseased cattle are eaten. Inoculation of spores subcutaneously is more common than their spread by inhalation or ingestion. The incubation period is usually 1–3 days.

Clinical features

A cutaneous lesion begins as an itching papule which enlarges and forms a vesicle filled with serosanguineous fluid surrounded by gross oedema — the 'malignant pustule'. The lesion is relatively painless and accompanied by slight enlargement of regional lymph nodes. The vesicle dries to form a thick black 'eschar' surrounded by blebs. Occasionally there are multiple lesions. In endemic areas patients may exhibit only slight constitutional symptoms and little oedema but in non-immune persons high fever, toxaemia and fatal septicaemia may develop.

An ulcer with much surrounding oedema may be seen in the pharynx or more commonly the infection causes a severe, fatal gastroenteritis when infected meat is eaten. Older people may escape unscathed presumably because of previously acquired immunity.

Those who acquire the infection by inhalation may develop an acute laryngitis or a virulent haemorrhagic bronchopneumonia 'wool sorters' disease. Anthrax may also present as meningitis.

Diagnosis

The appearance of a cutaneous lesion and the environmental and occupational history should suggest the diagnosis. A stained smear of fluid taken from the edge of a malignant pustule demonstrates the organism, which may be confirmed in an atypical case by culture and pathogenicity tests in mice, rabbits or guinea-pigs. *B. anthracis* is also recoverable from laryngeal and pulmonary anthrax and from the CSF in meningitis. Anthrax should be suspected if a group of people who have feasted on an animal which has sickened and died are taken abruptly ill with fulminating gastroenteritis. *B. anthracis* may be cultured from the faeces.

Management

Treatment is with penicillin. The organism is also sensitive to sulphonamides, erythromycin, tetracycline, chloramphenicol and streptomycin.

Prevention

The disease is controlled in cattle by slaughter and deep burial of the diseased animal and by vaccination of healthy animals at risk. Imports from endemic areas should be subject to strict control and sterilisation. Persons at risk through their occupation should be vaccinated.

WHOOPING COUGH

Whooping cough (pertussis) is a highly infectious disease caused by *Bordetella pertussis*. It is spread by droplet infection. Clinical diagnosis in the early and most infectious stage is virtually impossible so that epidemics occur. Whooping cough occurs at all ages but approximately 90% of cases are children under 5 years of age. The incubation period is 7–14 days.

Clinical features

The first stage of whooping cough consists of a highly infectious upper respiratory catarrh lasting about 1 week during which conjunctivitis, rhinitis and an unproductive cough are present. The distinctive paroxysmal stage follows and is characterised by severe bouts of coughing. The number of such paroxysms in 24 hours varies from an occasional attack to 40 to 50 and they are more severe at night. Each paroxysm consists of a succession of short sharp coughs, gathering in speed and duration and ending in a deep inspiration during which the characteristic whoop may be heard. It may be absent in older children and in adults because the air passages are so much wider. The last paroxysm of a series frequently ends with vomiting. The paroxysmal stage lasts from one to several weeks and is followed by the stage of convalescence during which the cough becomes less frequent and the sputum less tenacious.

Complications

The complications of whooping cough are listed in the information box below.

COMPLICATIONS OF WHOOPING COUGH

Respiratory
Bronchopneumonia
Atelectasis
Bronchiectasis

Other
Convulsions
Conjunctival haemorrhage
Ulceration of frenum
Prolapse of rectum

Diagnosis

The diagnosis of whooping cough is very difficult in the catarrhal stage when the disease is most infectious. It can be confirmed in the laboratory by the isolation of *Bordetella pertussis* taken from the posterior wall of the nasopharynx on small swabs passed along the floor of the nose. Examination of the blood shows a lymphocytosis which, however, may not develop until the disease is well established. The diagnosis is easy in the paroxysmal stage when the whoop has developed, but by this time the danger of transmission of infection has largely disappeared.

Management

Erythromycin may reduce the severity of the infection if given during the catarrhal stage. A cough suppressant such as methadone may be helpful in controlling the severity of paroxysms. When the illness is of long duration and vomiting is frequent, skilled nursing will be required to maintain nutrition, especially in infants and young children. Feeds are usually accepted and retained if they are given immediately after the vomiting which frequently follows a paroxysm of coughing.

Prevention

Active immunisation (Table 5.10) can very rarely (one in over 300 000 doses) cause fits or neurological damage and adverse publicity regarding this has led to a decrease in the number of children who are immunised against the disease. However, the adverse effects of the vaccine have to be balanced against the risk of contracting a potentially serious disease, especially in young children. Many of the deaths from whooping cough occur in the first 3 months of life and hence very special care must be taken to avoid exposure of infants to the risk of contracting the disease. Those who are exposed should be given prophylactic erythromycin.

STREPTOCOCCAL INFECTIONS

Streptococci produce a wide variety of infections. They are listed in the information box below. All species can cause septicaemia.

STREPTOCOCCAL INFECTIONS

Streptococcus pyogenes
Skin and soft tissue infection (including erysipelas and impetigo)
Bone and joint infection
Tonsillitis
Scarlet fever
Glomerulonephritis
Rheumatic fever

Streptococcus (entercoccus) faecalis
Endocarditis
Urinary tract infection

Viridans streptococci (Strep. mitior, sanguis, mutans, salivarius)
Endocarditis

Group B streptococci
Neonatal infections

Anaerobic streptococci
Peritonitis
Dental infections
Liver abscess

Streptococcus pyogenes infections result in features which vary with the invasiveness of the organism, its capacity to produce toxins, the site involved and the reaction of the host. If the resistance is low and the invasive properties of the streptococcus are high, a rapidly spreading erysipelas, cellulitis, lymphangitis or bacteraemia, may result. The organism may produce a specific exotoxin causing a widespread punctate erythema. When the infection is associated with such a rash the syndrome is known as scarlet fever. The same type of streptococcus may produce in one person acute tonsillitis, in another scarlet fever and in a third erysipelas.

SCARLET FEVER

Although scarlet fever is at present a mild disease, it may not necessarily remain so, as fluctuations in its severity have been recorded for the past 300 years. The primary site of infection in scarlet fever is usually the pharynx or the tonsils but the disease may follow streptococcal infection in other sites, e.g. in the genital tract after childbirth or in wounds. It is transmitted by air-borne infection, or more rarely by milk or ice-cream contaminated by streptococci. The incubation period is 2–4 days.

Clinical features

Scarlet fever occurs most commonly in children. It has a sudden onset and the more severe cases present with a sore throat, shivering, pyrexia, headache and vomiting. There is inflammation of the fauces; the tonsils are enlarged and may be covered with a follicular exudate. The exudate may be distinguished from the membrane seen in diphtheria by its yellow appearance and by being more easily wiped off. There is tender enlargement of the tonsillar lymph nodes. The rash, which usually appears first behind the ears on the second day, rapidly becomes a generalised punctate erythema. It is most intense in the flexures of the arms and legs. The face is not affected by the rash, though it is usually flushed due to fever, and the region round the mouth is pale. The tongue is initially furred but later shows prominent red papillae. The rash fades in about 1 week and is succeeded by desquamation. A profuse growth of S. pyogenes can usually be obtained from a throat swab.

Complications

The complications are less common than formerly because of the mild form of the disease and the introduction of effective chemotherapy. Acute otitis media, cervical adenitis and sinusitis may occur. Rheumatic fever and glomerulonephritis are rare sequelae which develop 2 or 3 weeks after the onset of any haemolytic streptococcal infection.

Management

The treatment of scarlet fever is the same as for streptococcal sore throat. Most patients respond rapidly to phenoxymethypenicillin (250 mg for children and 500 mg for adults t.i.d. for 7 days).

ERYSIPELAS

Erysipelas is an acute streptococcal infection of the skin, commoner in the elderly.

Clinical features

The onset is abrupt with heat and pain in the infected skin together with a systemic upset. There is a rapidly spreading red patch of inflamed skin with underlying oedema of the subcutaneous tissues. The edge of the patch is palpably raised and clearly defined and the lymph nodes draining the area become enlarged and tender. As the oedema subsides vesicles and bullae appear in the central part of the affected area. The face is involved in at least 80% of all cases of erysipelas from the spread of streptococci from the nose.

Management

Erysipelas is usually brought under control within 48 hours with penicillin; hence the prognosis is excellent for a disease which used to be very serious.

STAPHYLOCOCCAL INFECTIONS

Staphylococcus aureus is responsible for a wide variety of infections which are listed in the information box below.

INFECTION CAUSED BY STAPHYLOCOCCUS AUREUS

Skin infections	*CNS infections*
Wound infections	Meningitis
Boils, styes, carbuncles,	Brain abscess
abscesses	
	Blood-stream infections
Bone and joint infections	Septicaemia
Osteomyelitis	pyaemic abscesses
Septic arthritis	
Respiratory tract infections	
Pneumonia	
Lung abscess	
Empyema	
Intestinal infections	
Enterocolitis	
Cardiac infections	
Endocarditis	
Pericarditis	

Many infections, particularly boils, carbuncles and abscesses, are due to autogenous infection as the organisms can be grown from nasopharynx and skin of up to 30% of persons.

The staphylococcus is readily spread from these sites and from clothing to contaminate the dust in which it survives in the dry state for weeks or months. In hospital this organism is an important cause of wound infection, pneumonia and neonatal sepsis. Under suitable conditions it multiplies freely in food and milk to produce a heat-stable toxin which is an important cause of food poisoning.

Staphylococcal endocarditis

This occurs in drug addicts, in whom it usually causes right-sided heart valve lesions, and as a complication of septic thrombophlebitis associated with intravenous cannulae and lines.

The toxic shock syndrome

This is a condition caused by the toxins of certain *S. aureus* strains and occurs in women using some types of tampon, the infection originating in the vagina and presenting with fever, rash and shock. The syndrome has also been described in men and women as a complication of staphylococcal infections of the skin, lungs and breasts.

Management

90% of *S. aureus* strains are now resistant to penicillin which should be used only if the organism is known to be sensitive. If the illness is severe, treatment should be commenced with flucloxacillin, unless the patient is known to be allergic to the penicillins when erythromycin, fusidic acid or clindamycin should be given. Nasal carriage of staphylococci can be eradicated by topical application of neomycin plus chlorhexidine or mupirocin.

S. aureus strains resistant to all antibiotics except vancomycin (and sometimes also rifampicin) are causing outbreaks of hospital infection in many countries. Known as methicillin (or multiply) resistant *S. aureus* (MRSA), these organisms can cause serious and often fatal infections. Patients colonised by MRSA must be placed in isolation.

Staphylococcus epidermidis

This is a skin commensal organism which can cause serious infections in the immunosuppressed and in those with prosthetic heart valves and joint implants. Endocarditis due to this organism is particularly difficult to cure.

Methicillin-resistant *S. epidermidis* strains (MRSE) have now emerged as pathogens.

SALMONELLA INFECTIONS

There are approaching 2000 Salmonella serotypes most of which originate in animals, especially poultry, and are transmitted to man either directly or in food. The exception is *Salmonella typhi* which invariably has a

---

> **SALMONELLA INFECTIONS**
>
> - Typhoid and paratyphoid fever (enteric fever)
> - Gastroenteritis (food poisoning)
> - Enterocolitis
> - Septicaemia
> - Metastatic lesions (complicating septicaemia)
>   Osteomyelitis/septic arthritis
>   Liver abscess
>   Brain abscess
> - Asymptomatic carrier state

---

human source. There are 6 clinical syndromes caused by salmonellae and these are listed in the information box above.

TYPHOID AND PARATYPHOID (ENTERIC) FEVERS

In many countries where sanitation is primitive, typhoid and paratyphoid fevers, which are transmitted by the faecal-oral route, are an important cause of illness. Elsewhere they are relatively rare. Nevertheless, outbreaks occur from time to time and the infection may be contracted by persons travelling abroad.

Aetiology

The enteric fevers are caused by infection with *S. typhi* and *S. paratyphi A* and *B*. In Britain spread is usually by carriers, often food handlers, through the contamination of food, milk or water; infected shell fish are occasionally responsible for an outbreak. The bacilli may live in the gall bladder of carriers for months or years after clinical recovery and pass intermittently in the stool and less commonly in the urine. The incubation period of typhoid fever is about 10–14 days; that of paratyphoid is somewhat shorter.

Pathology

After a few days of bacteraemia, the bacilli localise mainly in the lymphoid tissue of the small intestine. The typical lesion is in the Peyer's patches and follicles. These swell at first, then ulcerate and ultimately heal, but during this sequence they may perforate or bleed.

Clinical features

Typhoid fever

The onset may be insidious. The temperature rises in a step-ladder fashion for 4 or 5 days. There is malaise, with increasing headache, drowsiness and aching in the limbs. Cough and epistaxis occur. Constipation may be present although in children diarrhoea and vomiting may be prominent early in the illness. The pulse is often slower than would be expected from the height of the temperature.

At the end of the first week the typical rash may appear on the upper abdomen and on the back as sparse slightly raised, rose-red spots which fade on pressure. It is usually visible only on white skin. About the seventh to tenth day the spleen becomes palpable. Often about this time constipation is succeeded by diarrhoea and abdominal distension with tenderness in the right iliac fossa. Bronchitis and delirium may develop. By the end of the second week the patient may be profoundly ill unless the disease is modified by antibiotic treatment. In the third week toxaemia increases and the patient may pass into coma and die.

Paratyphoid fever

The most common variety in Britain is due to *S. paratyphi B*. The course tends to be shorter and milder than that of typhoid fever but the onset is often more abrupt with acute enteritis. The rash may be more abundant and the intestinal complications less frequent.

Complications

Haemorrhage from, or a perforation of, the ulcerated Peyer's patches may occur at the end of the second week or during the third week of the illness. Additional complications may involve almost any viscus or system because of the septicaemia present during the first week. These include cholecystitis, pneumonia, myocarditis, arthritis, osteomyelitis and meningitis. Bone and joint infection is seen especially in children with sickle cell disease.

Diagnosis

In the first week the diagnosis may be difficult because in this invasive stage with bacteraemia the symptoms are those of a generalised infection without localising features. A white blood count may be helpful as there is typically a leucopenia. Blood culture is the most important diagnostic method in a suspected case. The faeces will contain the organism more frequently during the second and third weeks. The Widal reaction detects antibodies to the causative organisms and tests on paired sera may be useful in supporting a clinical diagnosis particularly when cultures are negative.

Management

The patient is treated in bed and preferably in isolation. Special attention must be paid to the maintenance of nutrition and fluid intake, care of the mouth and the prevention of pressure sores. Several antibiotics are effective in enteric fever. These include co-trimoxazole (2 tablets or i.v. equivalent 12-hourly), trimethoprim (300 mg 12-hourly), amoxycillin (750 mg 6-hourly), ciprofloxacin (500 mg 12-hourly) and chloramphenicol (500 mg 6-hourly). Chloramphenicol is the cheapest but can occasionally cause aplastic anaemia. Treatment should be continued for 14 days. Pyrexia may persist for up to 5 days after the start of specific therapy. Even with effective chemotherapy there is still a danger of complications, of recrudescence of the disease and of the development of a carrier state. The chronic carrier should be treated for 4 weeks with ciprofloxacin; cholecystectomy may be necessary in some patients.

The patient should be considered infective until six consecutive stools and urines are found to be negative on culture following treatment.

Prevention

Those who propose to travel to or live in countries where enteric infections are endemic should be inoculated with the monovalent typhoid vaccine.

FOOD POISONING

Food poisoning (gastroenteritis) can be due to many causes which are listed in the information box below.

It presents with vomiting, diarrhoea, or both, usually

CAUSES OF FOOD POISONING

Infective
Non-toxin mediated
   Salmonella species
   Campylobacter jejuni
   Bacillus cereus
   Viruses (e.g. Norwalk viruses)
   Listeria monocytogens (causing meningitis)
   Bacillus anthracis (anthrax)
   Protozoa (Giardia; Cryptosporidium)

Toxin mediated
   Staphylococcus aureus
   Clostridium perfringens
   Clostridium botulinum (botulism)
   E. coli 0157 (verocytotoxin-producing)

Non-infective
Allergic
   Shellfish, strawberries
Non-allergic
   Scrombotoxin (fish)
   Ciguatoxin (tropical fish)
   Fungi (e.g. Amanita phalloides)

within 48 hours of consumption of the contaminated food or drink. Outbreaks are common, especially in institutions and restaurants. Non-infective causes and bacterial toxins, which are pre-formed in the infected food produce symptoms within minutes or hours of a meal, whereas the other infections may not produce illness for up to 48 hours. Infective gastroenteritis can be classified as *non-toxin type* and *toxin type*.

Non-toxin type
Salmonella species (other than *S. typhi*) are very common causes of food poisoning. *S. typhimurium* and *S. enteritidis* are the most frequently isolated in Britain at present. The domestic fowl is the commonest source of infection which may be contracted from inadequately defrosted and undercooked chicken or from undercooked or raw eggs. Intensive rearing, infected poultry food and deep freezing of carcases all contribute to the high level of human salmonella infection. Symptomless faecal carriers of salmonella who are food-handlers are also a source of infection. The size of the infecting dose of bacteria bears a close relationship to the speed of onset of symptoms and to the severity of the illness. This indicates the dangers of bacterial multiplication which may take place when food is contaminated and thereafter remains warm for many hours or days.

Campylobacter jejuni. This is now the commonest bacterial cause of food poisoning in Britain. Sources of infection include poultry, dogs, water and unpasteurised milk.

Bacillus cereus infection. This is a hazard of eating rice which has been cooked and then consumed at a later date.

Listeria monocytogenes. This is an environmental bacterium which can contaminate food including poultry and cheese. It does not usually cause intestinal symptoms but is a cause of septicaemia and meningitis especially in pregnancy, the neonate, the immunosuppressed, diabetics and alcoholics.

Viruses. Viruses such as Norwalk viruses which can be identified by electron microscopy of stool but are not yet culturable and which often contaminate shell fish, can cause food poisoning.

Protozoal organisms. *Giardia lamblia* and cryptosporidium species can also cause food poisoning or waterborne outbreaks of diarrhoeal disease.

Toxin type
Such poisoning is most commonly caused by the enterotoxin of *S. aureus*. This frequently originates from a food handler with a septic lesion on the hand. Incubation at a suitable temperature leads to growth of the organism and production of toxin which is relatively heat resistant and may not be destroyed by cooking.

Strains of clostridia, many of them relatively resistant to heat, can also contaminate certain foods, particularly meat. Pre-cooking of stews and pies may not destroy all the spores and the keeping of such food will lead to the formation of heat-stable toxins which can give rise to gastroenteritis, sometimes severe.

A verocytotoxin-producing *Escherichia coli* strain (enterohaemorrhagic *E. coli* type 0157) has recently been found to cause food poisoning, possibly originating in meat, which may present as a haemorrhagic colitis. It is also a cause of the haemolytic/uraemic syndrome.

Clinical features
The simultaneous occurrence of symptoms in more than one member of a household or institution often simplifies diagnosis. The incubation period is a useful pointer to the aetiology. If vomiting starts within 30 minutes of the ingestion of suspected food, it is likely to be due to a chemical poison; if it arises 12–48 hours later, it is probably due to a salmonella or campylobacter infection. The incubation periods of staphylococcal and clostridial food poisoning are intermediate between these. The clinical features of food poisoning are shown in Table 5.18.

Table 5.18 Initial clinical features of food poisoning

Chemical poison	30 minutes	Vomiting
Staphylococcal or Clostridial toxin	2–6 hours	Vomiting initially – may be diarrhoea and abdominal pain later
Salmonella or Campylobacter infection	12–48 hours	Diarrhoea (bloody with campylobacter), abdominal pain, vomiting. Septicaemia can occur with salmonella infections.
Haemorrhagic colitis (*E. coli* 0157)	12–48 hours	Bloody diarrhoea predominates. May be abdominal pain

Botulism. This is a rare form of bacterial food poisoning due to the ingestion of the toxin produced by *C. botulinum* in imperfectly treated tinned food or preserved fish contaminated with the organism. The clinical features differ from all other types of bacterial food poisoning and consist chiefly of vomiting and pareses of skeletal, ocular, pharyngeal and respiratory muscles. The mortality rate can be high.

Diagnosis
A specimen of the patient's stool or vomit together with the suspected food, if available, should be sent for culture. Campylobacter and organisms of the salmonella group can usually be readily isolated. In more severe cases blood should be sent for culture. Notification of salmonella infection and other types of food poisoning is compulsory in Britain.

Management
Most cases are mild and symptoms subside in a few days. Solid food should be withheld and the patient instructed to take fluids only. Fluid and electrolytes can usually be replaced orally, but special care is needed with young children. Patients who are ill or dehydrated require intravenous fluid therapy. When acute symptoms cease, a semi-fluid low-roughage diet may be taken. Codeine phosphate or loperamide is useful in controlling diarrhoea in adults.

Antibiotics should not be given routinely for acute diarrhoea and vomiting as they are usually ineffective and frequently exacerbate symptoms. If salmonella bacteraemia is suspected or confirmed or if diarrhoea is severe or prolonged, ciprofloxacin or trimethoprim (p. 198) should be given. Campylobacter enteritis is treated with erythromycin or ciprofloxacin (p. 198). *Listeria monocytogenes* is susceptible to ampicillin. Gentamicin is given in combination with ampicillin in the immunosuppressed and for the treatment of meningitis.

If the poisoning is thought to be due to a chemical or a poisonous food, the patient's stomach should be washed out with tepid water, using the technique described on p. 974 and the stomach contents kept for analysis.

Prevention
A reduction in the high incidence of food poisoning can best be achieved by improving the standards of personal hygiene, especially in those handling food, and by stressing the importance of *hand-washing* after using the lavatory. Low-temperature storage is required for food which has to be kept for some hours or days before being consumed. It is essential to keep frozen poultry at room temperature for a least 12 hours before cooking or pathogens at the centre may survive unharmed. Improvements in poultry-rearing methods are urgently required.

DYSENTERY

Dysentery is an acute inflammation of the large intestine characterised by diarrhoea with blood and mucus in the stools. Its causes are bacillary or amoebic infection. The latter is described on p. 155.

BACILLARY DYSENTERY

The bacilli belong to the genus *Shigella* of which there are three main pathogenic groups, *dysenteriae*, *flexneri* and *sonnei* the first two having numerous serotypes. In Britain the majority of cases of bacillary dysentery are caused by *Shigella sonnei* although in recent years there has been a significant increase in imported infections caused by *S. flexneri* whereas sonnei dysentery has increased. Shigella strains, especially in tropical countries, are now commonly resistant to many antibiotics. These multi-resistant organisms have been responsible for epidemics of bacillary dysentery in Bangladesh and other tropical countries.

Epidemiology
Bacillary dysentery is endemic all over the world. It occurs in epidemic form wherever there is a crowded population with poor sanitation, and thus has been a constant accompaniment of wars and natural catastrophes. Spread may occur by contaminated food or flies but contact through unwashed hands after defecation is by far the most important factor. Hence the modern provision of handbasins, disposable towels and hot-air driers goes a long way towards the prevention of the faecal-oral spread of the disease. Outbreaks occur in mental hospitals, residential schools and other closed institutions. The disease is notifiable in Britain.

Pathology
There is inflammation of the large bowel which may involve the lower part of the small intestine. Sigmoidoscopy shows that the mucosa is red and swollen, the submucous veins are obscured and mucopus is seen on the surface. Bleeding points appear readily at the touch of the endoscope. Ulcers may form.

Clinical features
There is great variation in severity. Sonne infections may be so mild as to escape detection and the patient remains ambulant with a few loose stools and perhaps a

little colic. *S. flexneri* infections are usually more severe while those due to *dysenteriae* may be fulminating and cause death within 48 hours.

In a moderately severe illness, the patient complains of diarrhoea, colicky abdominal pain and tenesmus. The stools are usually small, and after the first few evacuations, contain blood and purulent exudate with little faecal material. There is frequently fever, with dehydration and weakness if the diarrhoea persists. There is tenderness over the colon more easily elicited in the left iliac fossa. In *S. sonnei* infection the patient may develop a febrile illness and diarrhoea may be mild or absent; there is usually some headache and muscular aching. Arthritis or ititis may occasionally complicate bacillary dysentery as in Reiter syndrome.

Diagnosis

Diagnosis depends on culture of faeces.

Management

Diarrhoea may be controlled by codeine (30 mg t.d.s.) or loperamide (1–2 tab. 3–4 times daily). A fluid or semifluid low roughage diet should be given depending on the severity of the diarrhoea but if this is severe, formal replacement of water and electrolyte loss will be necessary.

Sonne dysentery is usually a self-limiting disease and antibiotics are not indicated in most cases. In infections caused by dysenteriae or flexner strains trimethoprim 200 mg b.d. or ciprofloxacin 500 mg b.d. should be given.

Prevention

The prevention of faecal contamination of food and milk, the isolation of patients, and the identification of carriers, are methods which are theoretically important but may be difficult to apply except in limited outbreaks. Hand washing is very important.

INFECTIONS OF THE BRAIN, MENINGES AND SPINAL CORD

Infections of the nervous system may be caused by bacteria, viruses, protozoa, helminths or fungi. (see Chapter 16, pp. 876–888).

BACTERIAL INFECTIONS OF THE NERVOUS SYSTEM

(Bacterial meningitis, neisseria meningitidies, listeria monocytogenes, tuberculous meningitis, tetanus see pp. 883–886).

OTHER BACTERIAL INFECTIONS

BRUCELLOSIS (UNDULANT FEVER, MALTA FEVER, ABORTUS FEVER)

Brucellosis is caused in Northern Europe by infection with *Brucella abortus* which is usually spread to man by the ingestion of raw milk from infected cattle. It is also an occupational hazard of veterinary surgeons, laboratory personnel and slaughterhouse workers. The infection has now been virtually eradicated from cattle in Britain. In Malta and many Middle East countries the disease is frequently due to *B. melitensis* and is transmitted by infected goats or sheep. In the USA and the Far East *B. suis* acquired from pigs may be the causative organism. The incubation period is about 3 weeks. Subclinical infections are common in farmers and veterinarians.

Clinical features

The disease has features both of a bloodstream infection, and an intracellular infection. These are listed in the information box below. Untreated, the disease may last for a few days or for many months, and in the latter event the patient often becomes extremely depressed. Neutropenia and lymphocytosis occur in the more severely affected.

CLINICAL FEATURES OF BRUCELLOSIS

Onset
Acute with high continuous fever *or* insidious with fever undulating over 7–10 day periods

Symptoms
Fever, sweating, weakness, headache, anorexia, pain in limbs and back, rigors, joint pains

Signs
Fever and splenomegaly

Complications
- Relapse within 2 years of recovery
- Localised disease causing suppurative or granulomatous lesions including arthritis, spondylitis, bursitis, osteomyelitis, meningoencephalitis, endocarditis, epididymo-orchitis, pneumonia, hepatitis
- Chronic brucellosis: low-grade fever and neuropsychiatric symptoms

---

Diagnosis

Blood, and especially bone marrow, cultured under special conditions usually yields the organism in acutely ill patients. Brucella serology is unreliable: a four-fold rise in titre of agglutinating antibody, which detects IgM antibody, may be diagnostic but cross reactions are common. Complement fixation and anti-human globulin tests are more useful in chronic infections.

Management

Tetracycline 500 mg 6-hourly, plus rifampicin 600 mg daily for 4 weeks is curative and relapses are unusual. Streptomycin 1 g daily may be used instead of rifampicin. Tetracycline alone or cotrimoxazole 2 tablets twice daily are usually effective, but the disease may relapse.

Prevention

Infected herds of cattle can be identified and destroyed. The spread of brucellosis by milk is prevented by pasteurisation or boiling. Veterinary surgeons and others handling infected animals need to exercise scrupulous hygiene.

PLAGUE

Epidemics of plague, such as the 'Black Death', have attacked man since ancient times. Now, the disease is limited to rodents in the wild with occasional sporadic human cases or local outbreaks. The causative organisms, *Yersinia pestis*, is a small Gram-negative bacillus. It is spread between rodents by their fleas and if domestic rats become infected then infected fleas may bite man. In the late stages of human plague *Y. pestis* may be expectorated and inter-human spread by droplets, 'pneumonic plague', may follow. This can also be caused by the accidental inhalation of a laboratory culture or by hunters inhaling dust containing viable organisms from infected wild rodents or fleas. Recent outbreaks have predominantly been in Vietnam and East Africa with sporadic cases in the USA and elsewhere.

Pathology

Organisms inoculated through the skin are phagocytosed and taken rapidly to the draining lymph nodes where they elicit a severe inflammatory response that may be haemorrhagic. If the infection is not contained, septicaemia ensues and necrotic, purulent or haemorrhagic lesions develop in many organs. Vascular damage and fluid loss may lead to oliguria and shock, and disseminated intravascular coagulation may result in widespread haemorrhage. Inhalation of *Y. pestis* causes alveolar damage and copious exudation. The incubation period is short, 3–6 days, but less in pneumonic plague.

Bubonic plague

In this, the commonest form of the disease, the onset is usually sudden with a rigor, high fever, dry skin and severe headache. Soon aching and swelling at the site of the affected lymph nodes begin. The most common site of the bubo, made up of the swollen lymph nodes and surrounding tissue, is one groin. Some infections are relatively mild but in the majority of patients toxaemia rapidly increases with a rapid pulse, hypotension and mental confusion. The spleen is usually palpable.

Septicaemic plague

Those not exhibiting a bubo usually deteriorate rapidly. Meningitis and pneumonia and expectoration of blood-stained sputum containing *Y. pestis* may complicate bubonic or septicaemic plague.

Pneumonic plague

The onset is very sudden with cough and dyspnoea. The patient soon expectorates copious blood-stained frothy, highly infective sputum, becomes cyanosed and dies. Radiographs of the lung show a lobar opacity.

Diagnosis

A report of deaths among rats should alert suspicion of an outbreak. Early diagnosis is urgent. An aspirate from a bubo, sputum, or the buffy coat is used to show the characteristic organism by staining with methylene blue, or by immunofluorescence. Blood, sputum and aspirate should be cultured. Plague is notifiable under the International Health Regulations.

Management

If the diagnosis is suspected on clinical and epidemiological grounds, treatment must be started as soon as, or even before, samples have been collected for laboratory diagnosis. Streptomycin is given by intra-muscular or intravenous injection every 6 or 12 hours, at a daily dose of 30 mg/kg for 10 days, or tetracycline, 10 mg/kg every 6 hours orally or intravenously, for 10 days. Treatment may also be needed for acute circulatory failure, disseminated intravascular coagulation or hypoxia.

Prevention

This largely depends on preventing biting by fleas carrying plague. Rats should be controlled. Powders containing 1.5% Dieldrin or 2% Aldrin applied to floor and blown into rat holes kill all the fleas and remain active for 9–12 weeks. In endemic areas people should avoid handling and skinning wild animals.

A formalin-killed vaccine is available for those at occupational risk. Patients are isolated and attendants must wear gowns, masks and gloves. Contacts should be protected by tetracyline 2 g daily, or a sulphonamide 3–6 g daily for a week. Postmortem examination is dangerous.

TULARAEMIA

Tularaemia is an infection due to *Francisella tularensis* transmitted to mammals and birds by the bites of infected blood-sucking flies and ticks. It is often seasonal. Man may be infected by ticks or accidentally in a laboratory or while skinning infected wild rabbits or hares. In Norway lemmings are another source. The microorganisms enter through dermal abrasions, the conjunctiva or mouth. Contaminated water and infected meat are less common sources of human infection. The disease is found in the Americas, Japan, the USSR, and most European countries excluding Britain.

Pathology
Focal areas of necrosis occur especially in lymph nodes, spleen, liver, kidneys and lungs. There may be cutaneous, oral or ophthalmic lesions when infection is by these routes.

Clinical features
The commonest presentation is of a papule at the site of inoculation which becomes swollen and painful and suppurates, causing an ulcer up to 2 cm in diameter. Regional lymph nodes become tender, enlarged and may suppurate. There may be a systemic illness with fever, often prolonged. Sometimes the conjunctiva is the site of entry, and is inflamed. Occasionally the presentation is only with lymphadenopathy

Septicaemia is the rarest, but most severe form of the disease. There is a sudden onset of high fever, prostration, aching limbs, vomiting, diarrhoea and mental confusion. Pneumonia, pleurisy and pericarditis are serious complications.

Diagnosis
The organism may be isolated with difficulty and danger by culture on special medial or guinea-pig inoculation. Agglutination and complement-fixation tests become positive after 10–12 days.

Management
Streptomycin, as for plague (p. 131), or gentamicin is the treatment of choice, though tetracycline (500 mg 6-hourly for 2 weeks) is also likely to be effective.

Prevention
Masks should be worn in the laboratory and gloves are used when skinning rabbits and hares in endemic areas. Adequate cooking renders infected meat safe for eating.

MELIOIDOSIS

Melioidosis is caused by *Pseudomonas pseudomallei*, a microorganism closely related to *P. mallei*, the cause of glanders, which is a rare disease of horses and rarely their grooms. *P. pseudomallei* is a saphrophyte found in puddles following recent rain. Infection is through abrasions of the skin. Diabetics and patients with severe burns are particularly susceptible. The disease is commonest in the Far East and S.E. Asia and occurs rarely in India, Africa, Australia and America.

Pathology
A bacteraemia is followed by the formation of abscesses in the lungs, liver and spleen.

Clinical features
There is high fever, prostration and sometimes diarrhoea with signs of pneumonia and enlargement of the liver and spleen. A chest radiograph resembles that of acute caseous tuberculosis. In more chronic forms multiple abscesses recur in subcutaneous tissue and bone.

Diagnosis
Culture of blood, sputum or pus may yield *P. pseudomallei*. Except in fulminating infections, antibodies may be detected by indirect haemoagglutination, direct agglutination, and complement-fixation tests.

Management
In acute illness prompt treatment, without waiting for cultural confirmation may be life-saving. Tetracycline 3 g daily is given with chloramphenicol 3 g daily, in divided doses. Treatment is maintained for weeks or months until pulmonary cavities have healed.

CHOLERA

Cholera is a severe acute gastrointestinal infection, caused by *Vibrio cholerae*. Its home is in the valleys of the Ganges and other great rivers of the Far East where high humidity and population density have maintained the disease. In these valleys devastating epidemics have occurred often following large religious festivals, and pandemics have spread throughout Asia and Europe even to North America. The present, seventh, pandemic began in 1961. Good hygiene has prevented its spread to Europe, but cholera is present in the Near East and Africa, where it has for the first time become endemic. The biotype of *V. cholerae*, El Tor, that is responsible for the pandemic, is more resistant than the classical vibrio, and amenable to more prolonged carriage following infection. In 1982 the classical vibrio began to re-establish itself in Bangladesh.

The organism is passed in stools, or vomit, or patients with cholera and the very much larger number of subclinical cases, who excrete it for a few days. Chronic carriage is rare. The organism survives up to 2 weeks in fresh water and 8 weeks in salt water. Transmission is normally through infected drinking water, through shellfish and contamination of food by flies and hands also occurs.

Pathology

Cholera vibrios multiply in the lumen of the small bowel and are noninvasive. They secrete a powerful exotoxin (enterotoxin) which stimulates the adenyl cyclase-adenosine monophosphate pathway of the mucosa, resulting in an outpouring of normal alkaline, small bowel fluid. Severe dehydration follows rapidly even though absorption of fluid by the bowel is hardly impaired.

There may be acidosis and depletion of sodium and potassium with attendant complications, of which renal failure is the most important. The incubation period is a few hours to 5 days.

Clinical features

Severe diarrhoea without pain or colic, followed by vomiting, begins suddenly. After the faecal contents of the gut have been evacuated the typical 'rice-water' material is passed which consists of clear fluid with flecks of mucus. The enormous loss of fluid and electrolytes leads to intense dehydration with muscular cramps. The skin becomes cold, clammy and wrinkled and the eyes sunken. The blood pressure falls, the pulse becomes imperceptible, and the urine output diminishes. The patient usually remains mentally clear. Death from acute circulatory failure may occur within a few hours unless fluid and electrolytes are replaced.

COMPLICATIONS OF CHOLERA IN CHILDREN

- Electrolyte imbalance with hypocalcaemia, tetany, hypoglycaemia, hypernatraemia, acidosis
- Febrile convulsions
- Risk of over-treatment causing pulmonary oedema
- High mortality, 15% cf 5% in adults

Improvement is rapid, however, with proper treatment. Rarely, anuria persists and may lead to death.

Although this is the classical picture of cholera the majority of infections cause only mild illness with slight diarrhoea. Occasionally a very intense illness, 'cholera sicca', occurs in which the loss of fluid into the dilated bowel kills the patient before typical gastrointestinal symptoms appear. The disease is more dangerous in children. The complications are listed in the information box (left).

Diagnosis

Clinical diagnosis is usually easy during an epidemic but in other situations it is important to confirm the diagnosis bacteriologically so that an outbreak may be brought rapidly under control. *V. cholerae* has a characteristic movement that can be seen under the microscope. Culture of the stool or a rectal swab is used to isolate and identify the organism. Other diseases such as acute bacillary dysentery, viral enteritis, *P. falciparum* malaria, food poisoning, including *Vibria parahaemolyticus* infections from eating infected shellfish and certain chemical poisons may produce symptoms like those of cholera. Cholera is notifiable under the International Health Regulations.

Management

The chief aim is to maintain the circulation by replacement of water and electrolytes; the earlier this is started the better the prognosis. A quick clinical assessment of the state of dehydration is made from the appearance of the patient, the pulse, blood pressure and skin turgor. Fluids are given intravenously in severe cases or when there is vomiting. A large needle is inserted into a large vein (the femoral for example) and fluid is run in as fast as possible until pulse and blood pressure return. The rest of the estimated deficit is replaced more slowly. If intravenous fluids or i.v. drip apparatus are unavailable, fluid is administered via a nasogastric tube.

Vomiting usually stops once the patient is rehydrated and fluid should then be given orally every hour. Patients are made to drink up to 500 ml hourly. The quantity of fluid required is calculated every 8 hours from the output of urine, stool, vomit, and estimated insensible loss which may be as much as 5 litres in 24 hours in a hot humid climate.

Total fluid requirements can be in excess of 50 litres over a period of 2–5 days. Accurate records are essential and are greatly facilitated by the use of a 'cholera cot' which has a reinforced hole under the patient's buttocks beneath which a graded bucket is placed.

Table 5.19   Recommended solutions for treatment of cholera

Intravenous	g/l	mmol/l		Oral	g/i
Sodium chloride	5	Na	133	Commercial salt (NaCl)	3.5
		Cl	98		
Potassium chloride	1	K	13	Potassium chloride	1.5
				or citrate	2.7
Sodium bicarbonate	4	HCO₃	48	Sodium bicarbonate	2.5
or acetate	6.5			Glucose	20

The ideal solutions are shown in Table 5.19. Other satisfactory fluids include Ringer lactate (BP) or Hartman's solution or Darrow's solution, in which event supplements of potassium are given as 10 mmol/l of intravenous fluid or 2–4 g potassium chloride or citrate 3 times daily by mouth. Isotonic saline is better than nothing but every 2 litres should be alternated with 1 litre of isotonic sodium lactate (18.7 g/l) or bicarbonate (14 g/l) and added potassium. Acetate is a satisfactory substitute for bicarbonate, and more stable. The presence of glucose in the oral fluid has been shown to promote electrolyte absorption. Chlorpromazine, 50 mg 6-hourly, reduces intestinal secretion and fluid loss.

The use of correct fluids for replacement has eliminated the need for the estimation of plasma electrolytes. In children, the elderly, the anaemic and those with underlying heart disease overvigorous intravenous rehydration readily causes pulmonary oedema. Children require most careful attention to fluid balance. Ringer lactate is the fluid of choice. They are prone to hypoglycaemia. Any deterioration despite adequate rehydration is an indication for a bolus infusion of 25% glucose, 4 ml/kg and maintenance with 10 mg/kg/h. The management of renal failure is given on p. 585.

Three days' treatment with tetracycline 250 mg 6-hourly or co-trimoxazole one tablet daily reduces the duration of excretion of vibrios and the total volume of fluid needed for replacement.

Prevention

Personal prophylaxis means strict personal hygiene. Water for drinking should come from a clean piped supply or be boiled. Flies must not be allowed access to food. Vaccination with a killed suspension of *V. cholera* may provide limited protection (Table 5.11).

Control of water sources and of population movement and public education are most important in an epidemic. Mass vaccination with a single dose of vaccine and mass treatment with tetracycline are valuable. Disinfection of infective discharges and soiled clothing and scrupulous hand washing by medical attendants reduces the danger of spread from treatment centres.

BARTONELLOSIS (CARRION'S DISEASE, OROYA FEVER, VERRUGA PERUANA)

This disease is caused by *Bartonella baciliformis* transmitted by sandflies. It is prevalent in narrow hot valleys on the western slopes of the Andes at heights between 600–3000 m, in Peru, Ecuador, Bolivia, Colombia and Chile. The incubation period is 21 days.

Clinical features

Fever and haemolysis develop suddenly, accompanied by pains in muscles and joints, nausea, vomiting and diarrhoea, delirium or coma. The spleen and liver are enlarged and tender. Bartonellae are present in large numbers in the erythrocytes and also in the endothelial cells lining small blood vessels. Untreated the mortality is 90%. Secondary infection by salmonella is a frequent cause of death.

Verruga peruana

The cutaneous form, usually follows 30–40 days later with crops of cherry-red haemangioma-like cutaneous nodules 2–10 mm in diameter. They are distributed peripherally on the head and limbs and occasionally on the mucosa of the mouth and pharynx and heal in 2–3 months.

Diagnosis

The disease is confirmed by the demonstration of bartonellae in the erythrocytes, blood cultures or skin lesions.

Management

In the early febrile stage, chloramphenicol 500 mg every 6 hours is preferred because of the risk of concurrent salmonella infection, but the disease also responds to penicillin and tetracycline. Blood transfusions, fluids and electrolytes may be required.

Prevention

The use of insecticides, insect repellents and sleeping under fine mesh nets are advisable for personal protection.

LEPROSY

Leprosy is the commonest cause of peripheral neuritis in the world. It is a chronic granulomatous disease caused by *Mycobacterium leprae*, an acid and alcohol fast bacillus that has a very slow multiplication time of 12–14 days. Leprosy is one of the most seriously disabling and economically important diseases of the world and it is estimated that 20 million people are affected. *M. leprae* will grow in mice and the armadillo, but not in artificial media. Local multiplication of the organism in the foot-pads of mice is a useful technique for demonstrating the identity and viability of *M. leprae*, and the existence of drug-resistant strains for the screening of drugs, and for studying vaccines. The most important mode of spread of *M. leprae* is by droplets from the sneezes of lepromatous patients whose nasal mucosa is heavily infected. The organism may enter the body through the nasal mucosa or by inoculation through the skin.

The disease is common in tropical Asia, the Far East, tropical Africa, Central and South America, and in some Pacific Islands. It is still endemic in Southern Europe, North Africa and the Middle East.

Pathology

The organisms show a predilection for peripheral nerves, skin and mucosa of the upper respiratory tract. The response of the host to their presence varies widely. The early infection, usually transient and self-healing, is called 'indeterminate'. The histological appearances are non-specific. If the infection does not heal it develops into one of the determinate types, tuberculoid, lepromatous and borderline or dimorphous leprosy, whose features reflect the balance between the host cell-mediated immune response and bacillary multiplication (Fig. 5.5).

Tuberculoid leprosy

In tuberculoid leprosy there is a marked response of epithelial cells, lymphocytes and giant cells, around nerves, sweat glands and hair follicles. Caseation does not occur except occasionally in a nerve. Organisms are scanty, and difficult to find.

Lepromatous leprosy

In the infective form of this disease, there is no cell-mediated immune response to *M. leprae*. Organisms are present in great abundance in the dermis, in histocytes, Schwann cells, erectores pilorum muscles and endothelial cells of blood vessels. They may form globi, or large clumps of organisms, in showing foamy degeneration. Organisms are carried in the bloodstream to the peripheral nerves, eye and mucosa of the nose and upper respiratory tract, the testes and small muscles and bones of the hands, feet and face, in which they multiply. Nephritis and amyloidosis are common late complications.

Borderline or dimorphous leprosy

Between these two 'polar' types of leprosy, there is a

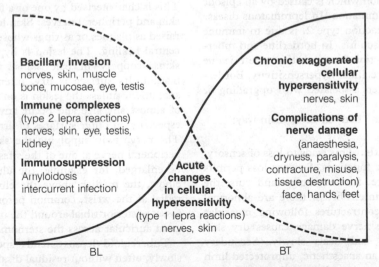

Fig. 5.5 Leprosy: mechanisms of damage and tissue affected. Mechanisms under the broken line are characteristic of disease near the lepromatous end of the spectrum and those under the solid line of the tuberculoid end. They overlap in the centre where, in addition, instability predisposes to type 1 lepra reactions. At the peak in the centre neither bacillary growth nor cell-mediated immunity has the upper hand BL = borderline lepromatous; BT = borderline tuberculoid. (From Bryceson A, Pfaltzgraff R E 1989 Leprosy, 3rd Edn. Churchill Livingstone, Edinburgh.)

spectrum of manifestations grouped under the terms 'borderline' or 'dimorphous'. The host reaction varies from the near-lepromatous to the near-tuberculoid. *M. leprae* are demonstrable in varying numbers. In the centre of the spectrum the disease is unstable. Immunity may diminish (downgrading) in untreated patients, especially in pregnancy or other times of stress and the disease becomes more lepromatous. Alternatively immunity may increase (upgrading or reversal), especially in response to successful chemotherapy, and the disease becomes more tuberculoid.

The lepromin test

Lepromin is a suspension of dead *M. leprae*. The test is performed like the tuberculin test, but is read after 4 weeks. The result indicates the degree of cellular immunity that an individual can mount against the organism. Positive reactions are obtained in tuberculoid leprosy, negative responses in lepromatous leprosy and negative or weak positive responses in borderline leprosy. This test is of no value in establishing the diagnosis of leprosy because positive results are also found in many normal people, but it is useful in helping to classify the disease, and so determine treatment and prognosis.

Lepra reactions

Any determinate form of leprosy may undergo an acute exacerbation or reaction which is caused by an episode of acute allergic inflammation. In lepromatous disease the reaction, lepra reaction type 2, is due to immune complex mediated vasculitis. In borderline and tuberculoid disease the reaction, lepra reaction type 1, is due to sudden increase in cellular hypersensitivity. Borderline reactions are often associated with upgrading or downgrading.

Leprosy damages the body in three main way:

Peripheral neuritis. This leads to loss of sensory, motor and autonomic functions. Sensory loss permits trauma from pressure, friction, burns and cuts, the effects of which are intensified if there are abnormal pressures from the contractures following muscular paralysis. Autonomic nerve damage causes dry skin which cracks easily and heals slowly. Secondary bacterial infection in an anaesthetic, unprotected limb leads to cellulitis, osteomyelitis and gross tissue destruction which produces the deformities with which the disease is still, so unnecessarily, associated. Paralyses result in claw hand and dropped foot from damage respectively to the ulnar and peroneal nerves. A combination of fifth and seventh cranial nerve damage exposes an anaesthetic cornea to trauma and sepsis, so the eye is easily blinded.

Lepromatous leprosy. In this bacillary growth insidiously damages the infiltrated organs and renders then liable to type 2 lepra reactions. Bones of hands and feet are easily fractured.

Acute lepra reactions. These may destroy nerves overnight, or cause severe eye damage.

In children, the incubation period is 2–5 years, but post primary disease is common in young adults, as in tuberculosis (p. 370). The disease may also appear in old people, as immunity declines.

Clinical features

The onset is usually gradual. The most common first symptom is a small but persistent area of impaired sensation or numbness. In other patients the first noticeable feature maybe macules, which are usually hypopigmented and erythematous. The disease may also present acutely, in a lepra reaction, with neuritis, iritis or erythema nodosum leprosum.

The macule of indeterminate leprosy is an inconspicuous lesion 2–3 cm in diameter, situated anywhere on the body, exhibiting slight pigmentary and sensory changes. This lesion usually heals spontaneously.

Tuberculoid leprosy

This is characterised by one or a few solitary lesions in skin and peripheral nerves. Skin lesions are macular or raised as plaques or as rings whose flat centres indicate central healing. The lesion is hypopigmented in dark skins, coppery in pale skins, with a well-defined margin. Its surface is dry, often scaly, and usually anaesthetic unless the lesion is on the face. Lesions are of almost any size and occur anywhere on the body, especially on outer surfaces of arms, legs or buttocks. The nerve twig supplying the skin lesion or a large peripheral nerve at one of the sites of predilection may be enlarged, for example, the ulnar nerve above the elbow, the median above the elbow or at the wrist, radial at the wrist, common peroneal in the popliteal fossa, posterior tibial around the medial malleolus, and great auricular across the sternomastoid muscle.

Tuberculoid leprosy tends spontaneously to heal slowly, often without residual disability. Sometimes its course is punctuated by a reaction and occasionally it downgrades into the borderline part of the spectrum.

Lepromatous lesions of the skin

These are initially macules (Table 5.20). They are numerous, hypopigmented and erythematous. They

Table 5.20   Clinical characteristics of the polar forms of leprosy

	Lepromatous	Tuberculoid
Skin and nerves		
Number and distribution	Widely disseminated	One or a few sites, asymmetrical
Skin lesions		
Definition		
Clarity of margin	Poor	Good
Elevation of margin	Never	Common
Colour		
Dark skin	Slight hypopigmentation	Marked hypopigmentation
Light skin	Slight erythema	Coppery or red
Surface	Smooth, shiny	Dry, scaly
Central healing	None	Common
Sweat and hair growth	Impaired late	Impaired early
Loss of sensation	Late	Early and marked
Nerve enlargement and damage	Late	Early and marked
Bacilli (Bacterial Index)	Many (5 or 6 +)	Absent (0)
Natural outcome	Progression	Healing
Other tissues	Upper respiratory mucosa, eye, testes, bones, muscle	None
Reactions	Immune complexes	Cell mediated

differ from tuberculoid macules in that they are small, inconspicuous, widely scattered on the body, usually symmetrically, and with margins that merge imperceptibily with normal skin. Overlying sensation is not impaired. As the disease advances, the macular lesions become infiltrated and succulent; in advanced lepromatous leprosy nodular lesions appear, especially on the ears and face, and eyebrows are lost. Diffuse symmetrical thickening of the skin causes thickened brow and lobes of the ear, producing the 'leonine facies'.

Clinical evidence of nerve damage appears relatively late in lepromatous leprosy. Anaesthesia and anhidrosis are first detected in the distal aspects of the forearms and lower legs, later in a 'glove and stocking' distribution and eventually over the trunk and face, although the palms, soles, axillae and groins may be spared. The effects on other organs are summarised in the information box (left). Untreated lepromatous leprosy gradually gets worse.

Borderline or dimorphous leprosy
This may present with lesions intermediate in character between lepromatous and tuberculoid or as a mixture of them. Skin lesions are often bizarre. The eyes and nose are spared. Nerve lesions are more numerous than in tuberculoid disease. In Asia, the majority of patients have borderline lepromatous leprosy. In Africa the majority have borderline tuberculoid leprosy. If the disease upgrades, nerve damage may increase with severe residual disability. If it downgrades the complications of extensive bacillary multiplication are added to those of widespread nerve damage. In either event the patient is liable to undergo reactions.

Lepra reactions
These may be defined as episodes of acute inflammation in pre-existing lesions of leprosy (Table 5.21). Sometimes a reaction is the first clinical manifestation of the disease. One half of patients with lepromatous leprosy and one quarter with borderline lepromatous disease will suffer *type 2 lepra reactions* at some time during the course of their disease, most commonly in

THE EFFECTS OF BACILLARY INFILTRATION IN LEPROMATOUS LEPROSY

Skin and nerves
(See text)

Muscles of hands, feet and face
Weakness and wasting

Testes
Atrophy, impotence, gynaecomastia

Mucosa of nose, mouth, pharynx and larynx
Rhinitis, hoarseness, perforation of nasal septum and palate, laryngeal obstruction

Bones of hands, feet and face
Cystic lesions of phalanges permitting fractures, loss of upper incisor teeth and nasal spine leading to nasal collapse

Eye
Keratitis, iridocyclitis, corneal anaesthesia leading to blindness

Table 5.21 Reactions in leprosy

Lepra reaction	Type 1	Type 2
Mechanism	Cell mediated hypersensitivity	Immune complexes Arthus phenomenon
Clinical features	Painful tender nerves, loss of function. Swollen skin lesions New skin lesions Rarely fever	Tender roseolar papules, may ulcerate Painful tender nerves, loss of function Iritis, orchitis, myositis, lymphadenitis Fever, oedema
Management	Mild: aspirin 600 mg every 6 hours Severe[1]: prednisone 40–80 mg, reducing over 3–9 months	Mild: aspirin 600 mg every 6 hours Severe[1]: Thalidomide[2] or prednisone 20–40 mg reducing over 1–3 months Local if eye involved[3]

[1]Includes any threat to nerve or eye function.
[2]See text for details.
[3]1% hydrocortisone drops or ointment and 1% atropine drops.

their second year of treatment. These reactions are characterised by fever and the appearance of crops of painful red papules or nodules, called *erythema nodosum leprosum*, which may necrose and discharge sterile pus, before subsiding.

Type 1 lepra reactions are especially common in borderline tuberculoid patients. They occur spontaneously or may be precipitated by treatment. Nerve function is rapidly lost, irretrievably so unless the reaction is promptly treated.

Diagnosis

Lepromatous and borderline lepromatous disease ('multibacillary leprosy') is diagnosed by demonstration of *M. leprae* in material obtained by a slit skin smear. The skin is pinched between finger and thumb to expel blood, incised with the point of a scalpel and the exposed dermis scraped with the flat of the blade. The tissue juice obtained is smeared on a microscope slide and stained by a modified Ziehl Neelsen's method. Smears are made from skin lesions, earlobes and dorsum of the ring of middle finger — sites in which bacilli multiply readily and persist. Nasal mucus may also contain the organisms in lepromatous leprosy and this is a good indication of infectivity. *M. leprae* are less readily demonstrable in skin smears in borderline disease and are undetectable in tuberculoid disease.

In borderline, and especially tuberculoid disease ('paucibacillary leprosy'), the cardinal signs of leprosy are enlarged nerves and anaesthesia. Nerves are usually enlarged at sites of predilection asymmetrically and irregularly; they may be tender.

Loss or diminution of sensation, or misreference (the inability to locate accurately the site stimulated) may be detected in a skin lesion or in the distribution of a large peripheral nerve. Biopsy of skin or nerve is seldom necessary except for accurate classification.

Management

Treatment of leprosy is long and often complicated. The patient must understand the disease and its complications, comply and persevere in the treatment and learn to look after anaesthetic limbs, control fear and cope with any stigma that exists in the community. Admission to hospital for a few days is useful to establish rapport and start education.

Specific chemotherapy

The essential features of the available drugs are given in Table 5.22.

Table 5.22 Main features of drugs available to treat leprosy

Drugs	Dose (mg)	Peak serum level/MIC*	Duration of MIC: days	Bactericidal activity
Dapsone	100	100–500	4–12	+
Rifampicin	600	30	1	+ + +
Clofazimine	100	(Stored in M.P. cells, possible depot)		?
Ethionamide	500	60	1	+ +
Thiacetazone	150	8	1	−

*MIC minimum inhibitory concentration.

Patients with multi-bacillary disease (lepromatous and borderline lepromatous). These are preferably isolated until they are rendered non-infectious, which takes only a few days with rifampicin. Ideally treatment should be with three drugs, rifampicin, clofazimine and dapsone to prevent the emergence of drug resistance. Rifampicin, the most expensive but most efficient bactericidal drug, need only be given monthly, because of the long generation time of *M. leprae*. It is most effective if given for two consecutive days in a daily dose of 600 mg, or 450 mg for patients under 35 kg in weight. Clofazimine is given in a dose of 50 mg daily, or 100 mg 3 times in the week (totalling

6 mg/kg/week for children). Dapsone is given in a dose of 2 mg/kg daily, not exceeding 100 mg. For mass treatment campaigns when compliance is often poor, WHO recommends that rifampicin be given in a single supervised monthly dose of 600 mg, and that a supervised monthly dose of clofazimine 300 mg be given in addition to the self-administered daily dose of clofazimine and dapsone. Treatment is continued for 2 years.

Patients with paucibacillary disease (intermediate, tuberculoid and borderline tuberculoid). These are treated with rifampicin once monthly and dapsone daily for 1 year. Patients should be followed up for 5 years.

Side-effects of dapsone are rare. They include psychosis, dermatitis and haemolytic anaemia. Should they occur the drug is temporarily withheld, and resumed at half the dose.

Secondary dapsone resistant. This occurs in up to 15% of lepromatous patients who have been treated for 10–20 years with dapsone alone. It presents as the re-emergence of solitary nodules or as a more generalised relapse. In the last 10 years primary dapsone resistance has been emerging as a new and increasing problem in several countries. Resistance is confirmed by mouse footpad inoculation, or by supervised full dose dapsone treatment. It is treated either by clofazimine alone, to which no resistance has yet appeared, or by combined treatment with ethionamide 500 mg daily and rifampicin given on the first two days of each month.

Clofazimine is a red-brown dye that gradually colours the skin and all bodily secretions and is therefore not always acceptable to paled-skinned patients. It does, however, reduce the incidence of lepra reaction type 2. Doses in excess of those recommended may cause severe abdominal pain. *Ethionamide* causes jaundice, especially in Asians. *Thiacetazone* is a cheap reserve drug; it is weak, and cross resistance may develop with the more useful ethionamide.

Treatment of reactions
Chemotherapy for leprosy is maintained and appropriate anti-inflammatory drugs used (Table 5.22). Reactional neuritis is a medical emergency as irreversible paralysis may occur overnight.

Type 2 reactions in lepromatous patients respond rapidly to thalidomide in a dose of 100 mg 4 times daily. The dose is reduced slowly over weeks or months. This drug must never be given to premeno-pausal women because of its disastrous teratogenic effects. If thalidomide is contraindicated or unavailable prednisolone is used. Increasing the dose of clofazimine to 200 mg or 300 mg daily for a few weeks will help control the reaction and permit prednisolone to be reduced or withdrawn. Iritis is a dangerous complication but can usually be managed by local measures.

Management of nerve damage
In the event of acute paralysis complicating reactional neuritis, the affected limb is splinted and exercised passively each day until function begins to return when active exercises can be added. A patient with an anaesthetic limb must be taught to accept the limitations it imposes, to adjust life accordingly, to inspect the limb daily for trauma or infection and to learn how not to damage it.

Tarsorrhaphy helps protect an exposed anaesthetic cornea. Secondary sepsis is treated with appropriate antibiotics and osteomyelitis and its sequelae are managed in the most conservative manner possible. Patients with plantar ulcers are confined to bed, or given crutches or a walking plaster until healing is complete. Shoes must fit and protect anaesthetic feet against trauma and must be made specially if there is added deformity.

Prevention
In endemic areas the disease is commonest among intimate contacts of patients, and children and young adults are especially susceptible. *M. leprae* is easily spread and two-thirds of contacts undergo sub-clinical immunising infections within 2 years of regular exposure. Of the small proportion of contacts (about 1%) that develop clinical disease only about 2% will be lepromatous. It is at present impossible to identify this small group at risk and logical prophylaxis is impossible. No specific vaccine is available. Bacille Calmette-Guérin (BCG) is of some value, especially in Africa, and should be given to all child contacts of lepromatous patients. Dapsone and rifampicin may be given as for paucibacillary disease (above) for 6 months to child contacts of lepromatous patients. Neither measure is a substitute for 6-monthly examination of contacts.

Mass prophylaxis is impossible, but treatment and follow-up of all cases identified during a population survey reduces deformity and lowers the incidence of leprosy. With improvement of socio-economic conditions the disease tends to disappear. The rapid spread of dapsone resistance poses a great problem to existing control schemes.

MYCOBACTERIAL ULCER

This condition, first accurately described in Australia and New Guinea, later named Buruli ulcer from its frequency in the Nile valley of Uganda, is caused by *Mycobacterium ulcerans*. The epidemiology is unknown.

Clinical features

It begins as a single small subcutaneous nodule situated commonly on the leg or forearm. The skin over the centre of the nodule ulcerates. Untreated, the ulcer extends to involve a progressively larger area. Histologically there is much necrosis of subcutaneous fat and mycobacteria are abundant in the necrotic tissue in the base of the ulcer.

Management

The nodule should be excised if the disease is suspected before ulceration. Ulcers require to be excised and skin grafted. Antimycobacterial chemotherapy is disappointing.

DISEASES DUE TO SPIROCHAETES

LEPTOSPIROSIS

Although over 100 serotypes of leptospiras have been identified only *Leptospira icterohaemorrhagiae*, *L. hardjo* and *L. canicola* have been shown to cause human disease in Britain (Table 5.23).

Table 5.23   Leptospiral infections in UK

Organism	Source
Leptospira icterohaemorrhagiae Hepatitis Renal tubular necrosis Myocarditis Purpura Haemorrhagic conjunctivitis	Water contamined by rats' urine
Leptospira canicola Non-specific febrile illness Aseptic meningitis	Dogs
Leptospira hardjo Non-specific febrile illness Chronic ill health Aseptic meningitis	Cattle

The natural host of Weil's disease, caused by *L. icterohaemorrhagiae*, is the rat and other rodents. Infected urine contains spirochaetes which can penetrate the skin or mucosa of man. Abattoir and farm workers, veterinarians, and vagrants are most at risk. It

has become uncommon in sewer workers, fish cleaners and miners because of better working conditions. Immersion in canals and stagnant water may result in sporadic infection. In patients dying from Weil's disease, there is a combination of hepatic, renal and cardiac failure.

Infection by *L. canicola*, which is contracted from dogs and pigs, usually presents as aseptic meningitis. It is not often associated with jaundice and is less severe than Weil's disease.

L. hardjo is increasing in farm workers, in contact with cattle, in whom it can cause ill health resembling chronic brucellosis. It can also cause aseptic meningitis.

The average incubation period of leptospirosis is 10 days, the range being 4–21 days.

Clinical features

A high proportion of infections are subclinical or cause mild undiagnosed fever. In the more severe infections the illness begins abruptly with headache, severe myalgia, pyrexia, conjunctival suffusion, anorexia and vomiting. Infrequently, there are rashes or petechiae and enlargement of the liver and spleen.

After about a week leptospiral antibodies appear in the blood. The temperature falls by lysis and is usually normal for 2 or 3 days. In the majority of patients, there is further pyrexia for a few days and transient meningism followed by prompt recovery. In illness caused by *L. icterohaemorrhagiae* hepatitis, renal tubular necrosis, myocarditis and meningitis may occur during this phase. The condition may progress to acute liver necrosis. Renal tubular necrosis may lead to acute renal failure. Myocarditis is suggested by tachycardia, fall in blood pressure and cardiac enlargement. The development of profound hypotension, arrhythmias and cardiac failure are ominous signs.

The majority of patients enter the convalescent phase by the third and fourth week of the illness. When there has been serious involvement of the liver, kidneys and heart, mortality in Weil's disease is in the region of 15–20%. Those who recover do so completely.

Diagnosis

A rising titre of specific leptospiral antibodies is found from the second week onwards. When there is liver involvement, liver function tests indicate a hepatocellular jaundice with an intrahepatic obstructive element; bilirubin and urobilinogen are present in the urine. The urine contains protein, red blood cells and cellular and granular casts in patients with renal failure; in severe cases the rise in blood urea is progressive.

Table 5.24 Comparison of the major treponemal diseases

| | | | | | Lesions | | |
Disease	Organism	Source	Transmission	At risk	Primary	Early*	Late*
Yaws	T. perternue	Skin	Contact	Children	Ulcero nodule	Skin Bones	Skin, bones, palms and soles
Endemic syphilis	T. pallidum T. carateum	Skin Mouth	Contact Utensils	Children Parents	Papule or none	Skin Mucosae Bones	Skin, bones, palms and soles
Venereal syphilis	T. pallidum	Genital sores Mouth	Sexual Placenta	Sexual partners Foetus	Genital ulcer Lymphaden-opathy	Skin Mucosae Bones Meninges	Cardiovascular Central nervous Bones, etc.

*Early and late correspond with secondary and tertiary lesions.

Management

Leptospiras are sensitive to penicillin in vitro. Benzyl-penicillin, 600–1200 mg 6-hourly for 7 days is effective provided it is given early enough; it shortens the average illness and reduces the incidence of complications. Penicillin is of doubtful value if treatment is initiated late in the infection. In severely affected patients supportive treatment for liver necrosis, renal failure, arrhythmias and cardiac failure may be required.

YAWS

Yaws is a granulomatous disease mainly involving the skin and bones and caused by *Treponema pertenue*, morphologically indistinguishable from the causative organisms of syphilis and pinta (Table 5.24). The three infections induce similar serological changes and possibly some degree of cross immunity. Organisms are transmitted by bodily contact from a patient with infectious yaws through minor abrasions of the skin of another patient, usually a child. Infection is most likely to take place in huts at night when the temperature and humidity are high and families use communal sleeping mats. The mass campaigns by WHO between 1950 and 1960 treated over 60 million people and eradicated yaws from many areas, but the disease has persisted patchily throughout the tropics and there has been a resurgence in the 1980s in West and Central Africa and the South Pacific.

Pathology

A proliferative granuloma containing numerous trepo-nemes develops at the site of the inoculation. This primary lesion is followed by eruptions, with a histology similar to the primary lesion. In addition there may be hypertrophic periosteal lesions of many bones with underlying cortical rarefaction. Lesions of late yaws are characterised by destructive changes which closely resemble the osteitis and gummas of tertiary syphilis and which heal with much scarring and deformity. The incubation period is 3–4 weeks.

Clinical features

Early yaws. The primary lesion or 'mother yaw' is usually on the leg or buttocks. The secondary eruption usually follows a few weeks or months later, sometimes before the primary lesion has healed. Most typical are numerous crops of papillomas covered with a whitish-yellow exudate, especially in the flexures and around the mouth. Sometimes a lesion erupts through the palm or sole, when walking becomes painful, 'wet crab yaws'. Bones of the fingers may rarefy and be surrounded by periosteal deposits. There may be a swelling of the nasal bones (gondou). The distorted tibia may remain as the 'sabre tibia' but most of the lesions of early yaws will eventually subside, even if untreated.

Latent yaws. Following the spontaneous resolution of 'early yaws' serological changes may persist to be followed by further manifestations of 'early yaws', or, after an interval of as much as 5–10 years, by the tertiary lesions or 'late yaws'.

Late yaws. Solitary or multiple lesions appear as nodules or ulcers in the skin, hyperkeratotic lesions of palms or soles 'dry crab yaws' and gummatous lesions of bone that may ulcerate through the skin. They heal with scarring. Lesions of the facial and palatal bones cause terrible disfigurement (gangosa).

Management

Lesions of early and late yaws respond rapidly to the intramuscular administration of 750 mg of procaine penicillin on two occasions at an interval of 1 week, or to tetracycline 1–2 g daily for 5 days. Early yaws heals complete but late yaws may leave deformity.

Prevention

The disease disappears with improved housing and cleanliness. In few fields of medicine have chemotherapy and improved hygiene achieved such dramatic success as in the control of yaws.

ENDEMIC (NON-VENEREAL) SYPHILIS

In certain tropical countries, where hygiene is poor, this treponematosis occurs as a family disease. The causative organisms are regarded as modified strains of *Treponema pallidum*, with which they are morphologically identical but biologically distinct (Table 5.24).

Congenital infections are rare and sexual transmission unusual. The common mode of infection is through an abrasion, the disease being transmitted from child to parent. Sometimes it spreads in a closed community by the use of common drinking vessels, and possibly mechanically by flies.

The poor social conditions in which the disease prevails are similar to those where yaws is found but the clinical lesions resemble those of juvenile syphilis.

Clinical features

In contrast to venereal syphilis the primary lesion is rarely seen. The secondary and tertiary lesions include all the common types of skin, mucosal and bone manifestation of syphilis.

Diagnosis

This is given in the information box below.

DIAGNOSIS OF NON-VENEREAL TREPONEMATOSIS

Early stages
Detection of spirochaetes in exudate of lesions by dark background microscopy

Latent and late stages
Positive serological tests as for syphilis (p. 188)

Management

The disease responds to treatment by penicillin in the same way as venereal syphilis (Table 5.42, p. 189).

Prevention

Prevention depends on the development of improved social and economic conditions and the mass treatment of affected communities.

PINTA

Pinta is a classical and geographic variant of endemic

syphilis caused by the related organism *Treponema carateum*. It is endemic in localised areas in Central and South America and in some West Indian and South Pacific Islands. The incubation period is 14–20 days.

Clinical features

There is a primary scaly papular lesion on the exposed part, usually the leg, which enlarges slowly, up to 10 cm in diameter and is surrounded by smaller papules. Regional lymph nodes enlarge and like the primary lesion contain treponemes. The secondary stage is manifest 5–12 months later and consists of a generalised eruption of macules and miliary papules, 'pintids', pinkish and slightly scaly. Most of these heal but others coalesce and form hyperpigmented patches, commonly on the face and exposed parts. The secondary lesions may persist for years and may be accompanied by hyperkeratosis of palms and soles. In the tertiary stage the affected patches become atrophic and depigmented.

Diagnosis

(See information box (left).)

Management

Treatment is by a long-acting penicillin (p. 189).

THE RELAPSING FEVERS

The relapsing fevers are a group of diseases due to infections by spirochaetes of the genus *Borrelia* transmitted by body lice or soft (Argasid) ticks. Sodoku, due to *Spirillum minus*, also relapses (Table 5.25). The louse-borne *Borrelia recurrentis* infects only man and is not transmitted from a louse to its progeny. This disease appears in epidemics particularly during wars or famine when refugees are crowded together in conditions under which infestation with the human body louse *Pediculus humanus* is frequent. It may accompany louse-borne typhus. The disease is endemic in Ethiopia from where recently recorded epidemics have probably arisen.

Species of Borrelia that cause tick-borne relapsing fever, are transmitted by various species of the genus *Ornithodoros*. Ticks live for years and once infected remain so for life and may convey the infection to the offspring. Tick-borne relapsing fever is thus an endemic disease.

LOUSE-BORNE RELAPSING FEVER

Lice cause itching. Borreliae are liberated from the infected louse when it is crushed during scratching which also inoculates the borreliae into the skin.

Table 5.25   Comparative features of the 'relapsing fevers' due to Borrelia and Spirillum

	LBRF[1]	TBRF[2]	Sodoku	Haverhill	Lyme disease
Incubation	2–12 days	2–12 days	5–21 days	1–5 days	4d–months
Fever	4–10 days	3–5 days	7 days	3 days	Weeks
Remission	7 days	3–5 days	3–5 days	—	No consistent pattern
Relapses	0–3 days	Up to 10	Numerous	None	
JHR[3]	Severe	Mild	Mild/none	None	None
Mortality	Up to 40%	Under 10%	None	None	? None
Major complications	Hepatitis Carditis Meningitis Shock Bleeding	Similar to LBRF but less severe Neurological in relapses	Adenitis Rash	Arthritis	Rash Arthritis Carditis Meningitis

[1]Louse-borne relapsing fever.
[2]Tick-borne relapsing fever.
[3]Jarisch–Herxheimer reaction.

Pathology

The borreliae multiply in the blood, where they are abundant in the febrile phases, and invade most tissues, especially the liver, spleen and meninges. Hepatitis causing jaundice is frequent in severe infections and there may be petechial haemorrhages in the skin, mucous membranes and serous surfaces of internal organs. Thrombocytopenia is marked. The urine frequently contains protein and sometimes there is frank haematuria.

Clinical features

Onset is sudden with fever. The temperature rises to 39.5–40.5°C and is accompanied by a rapid pulse, headache, generalised aching, injected conjunctivae and frequently a petechial rash, epistaxis and herpes labialis. As the disease progresses, the liver and spleen frequently become tender and palpable and jaundice is common. There may be severe serosal and intestinal haemorrhage. Mental confusion and meningism may occur. The fever ends by crisis between the fourth and tenth day, often associated with profuse sweating, hypotension, circulatory and cardiac failure (Table 5.25, above). There may be no further fever but, in a proportion of patients, after an afebrile period of about 7 days there may be one or more relapses which are usually milder and less prolonged. In the absence of specific treatment the mortality rate may be as high as 40%, especially among the elderly and malnourished.

Diagnosis

The organisms are demonstrated in the blood during fever either by dark ground illumination of a wet film or by staining thick and thin films.

Management

The problems of treatment are to eradicate the infection and to minimise the severe Jarisch-Herxheimer reaction (p. 163) which inevitably follows successful chemotherapy and to prevent relapses. The safest treatment is procaine penicillin 300 mg intramuscularly followed the next day by 0.5 g tetracycline. Tetracycline alone is effective and prevents relapse, but gives rise to a worse reaction. Doxycycline, 200 mg once by mouth, as an alternative to tetracycline has the advantage of being curative also for typhus, which often accompanies epidemics of relapsing fever.

Treatment is followed within a half to 3 hours by a chill or rigor, a brisk rise of temperature to 40–42°C, tachypnoea, tachycardia and often cough, confusion, distress, delirium and, occasionally, convulsions and coma. This phase is rapidly followed by profound hypotension and vasodilatation which may last from 8–12 hours and may be complicated by cardiac failure. The patient must be confined strictly to bed for 48 hours after treatment, carefully observed and managed as complications demand. Tepid sponging for fever over 41°C, careful attention to hydration, preferably by oral fluids, and prompt treatment of cardiac failure are required.

Prevention

The patient, clothing and all contacts must be freed from lice as in epidemic typhus (p. 121).

TICK-BORNE RELAPSING FEVER

This disease is conveyed by a variety of soft ticks and its endemicity is governed by the presence of the vector. In the Mediterranean area *Ornithodoros tholozani* is responsible; in the Middle East, Iran, Afghanistan and India and in the New World there are other vectors. These ticks can become infected from rodents or bats as well as by congenital transmission and man is only an incidental host. In Central and East Africa, however, where *O. moubata* is the vector of *Borrelia duttoni*, man is probably the only important mammalian host. The disease in these areas is thus confined to old camp sites, old houses and their surroundings where *O. moubata* lives in dried mud floors and walls.

The pathological changes resemble those of louse-borne relapsing fever but with late neurological lesions.

Clinical features
These are similar to those of louse-borne relapsing fever (Table 5.25, p. 143). The febrile bouts, although severe, last usually only for 3–5 days, and the apyrexial periods may also be shorter. Relapses are, however, more frequent. Iritis and neurological complications, including cranial nerve palsies, optic atrophy, localised palsies and spastic paraplegia, may develop during these later relapses.

Diagnosis
The methods used in diagnosis are similar to those for louse-borne relapsing fever. *B. duttoni* are, however, scantier in the peripheral blood but young mice are readily infected.

Management
Because many strains are resistant to penicillin, tetracycline 1 g daily for 7 days is given and the course repeated after an interval of a week. Good results may follow a single dose of 200 mg doxycycline.

Prevention
Ticks can be killed by lindane applied to the inside of the walls, floors and across the entrance to houses.

OTHER SPIROCHAETAL INFECTIONS

RAT-BITE FEVERS

There are two rat-bite fevers, one caused by *Spirillum minus*, the other by *Streptobacillus moniliformis*. The latter, in addition to being transmitted by a rat-bite, has also occurred as an epidemic due to infected milk (Haverhill fever); in other cases there has been no known contact with rats or mice. Both infections are world-wide. The incubation period of Streptobacillus fever is 1–5 days, and if *S. minus* 1–4 weeks.

Clinical features
The manifestations of both fevers are very similar (Table 5.25, p. 143). In *S. minus* infection (Sodoku) the bite wound usually heals. After 5 to 21 days it suddenly becomes inflamed, indurated, purplish and painful; it may ulcerate and is accompanied by lymphangitis, regional lymphadenitis, leucocytosis, splenomegaly and fever. After a week the local and general reactions subside but recur after a further few days. Without treatment, periods of fever lasting 24–48 hours may recur for weeks and the patient becomes anaemic. A macular or maculopapular dusky red rash, sparse over the trunk and extremities, appears during the febrile phases.

In *Streptobacillus* fever the rat-bite usually heals well but occasionally an abscess forms. Regional lymphadenopathy is not marked. The general symptoms resemble those of *S. minus* infections but there is frequently painful arthritis and it is unusual to have recurrences of fever after the initial bout which lasts only 48–72 hours.

Diagnosis
S. minus can be demonstrated in the exudate from the inflamed bite or in fluid aspirated from a lymph node, by darkground illumination, or be isolated by injection of exudate or blood into an uninfected mouse. There are serological cross-reactions with syphilis. In *Strep. moniliformis* infections agglutinating antibodies are demonstrable after 10 days. Serological tests for syphilis are negative. The organism can be recovered from the blood or, more easily, from an effusion into an inflamed joint.

Management
Both infections are readily cured by penicillin, streptomycin or tetracycline (pp. 193, 195).

TROPICAL ULCER

Tropical ulcer is a specific infection with *Borrelia vincenti* and anaerobic bacteria. Minor injury in the presence of undernourishment, poor hygiene and debilitating disease are predisposing factors. It is most common in adolescent males, on the lower third of the leg.

Clinical features
The initial lesion is a bleb filled with sanguineous fluid. The bleb ruptures and a green-grey slough is exposed which spreads, rapidly and painfully, in the skin and subcutaneous tissue up to a diameter of 5 cm or more. In a few days these tissues slough and liquefy releasing

an offensive discharge. After about a week there is usually no further spread and the necrotic tissue separates, exposing an ulcer.

In a chronic ulcer the edges are raised and slope sharply. The damage may be limited to the skin and superficial fascia, but in severe cases deep structures, including tendons and periosteum may be invaded. The ulcer is usually solitary and heals slowly with a tissue-paper-like scar which breaks down easily. Big ulcers fail to heal and may develop malignant changes after many years.

Management
Local treatment consists in thorough cleaning of the ulcer with hypertonic saline or magnesium sulphate. Acute ulcers heal in response to procaine penicillin 300 mg i.m., metronidazole 400 mg t.i.d., or tetracycline 2 g daily for 7 days. Ulcers over 5 cm diameter need grafting. Chronic ulcers are excised and grafted.

Prevention
Where tropical ulcers are a risk, abrasions should be cleaned and covered. The provision of a good diet, washing facilities and a first-aid service have abolished tropical ulcers from labour forces on well-run estates.

CANCRUM ORIS

Cancrum oris is rare except in poorly nourished children in the tropics. It is characteristically preceded by an infective illness, especially measles.

Clinical features
The manifestation is that of a rapidly developing gangrene, beginning inside of the mouth and penetrating through the lips and cheek. Gangrene becomes demarcated and ulceration follows resulting in severe disfigurement. Untreated it frequently causes death.

Diagnosis
Bor. vincenti and an anaerobic bacterium are frequently found in the ulcer.

Management
Penicillin (p. 193) arrests the infection but does not prevent gangrene of already diseased tissue. Coexistent malnutrition, anaemia or dehydration should be corrected. Subsequently skilled plastic surgery may do much to overcome the hideous defects.

Prevention
This depends on improved nutrition and hygiene in the community and on control of acute infectious diseases.

BACTERAEMIA, SEPTICAEMIA AND BACTERAEMIC (SEPTIC) SHOCK

Spread of infection to the blood stream is known as *bacteraemia* and, if the organisms multiply there, as *septicaemia*. Further dissemination may result in 'metastatic' foci of infection especially in bone, liver, brain or heart valves. The site of the primary infection varies but can be in diverticular disease, the skin or the urinary tract. Figure 5.6 provides a schematic description of septicaemia and its complications.

Bacteraemic shock occurs in up to one-third of episodes of Gram-negative septicaemia: it is due to potent bacterial endotoxins which affect cell walls, promote the release of vasoactive substances such as histamine and bradykinin and cause endothelial damage.

Initially there is a hyperdynamic reaction with high cardiac output, vasodilation and low peripheral resis-

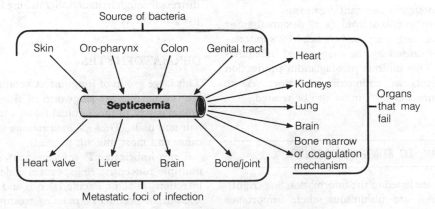

Fig. 5.6 Septicaemia: source of infection, metastatic lesions and complications.

tance followed by fluid loss from the vascular compartment as a result of extensive capillary leakage; this leads to hypovolaemia, peripheral vasoconstriction and acute circulatory failure. The endotoxin may initiate disseminated intravascular coagulation (DIC) by endothelial injury activating the clotting mechanisms and leading to tissue damage and organ failure (p. 757).

Clinical features

The pyrexia of the infection may be overtaken by the hypothermia of acute circulatory failure. Leucopenia, thrombocytopenia and a prolonged bleeding time point to DIC. Progressive impairment of blood flow may then lead to organ failure particularly of the brain, kidneys, liver and lungs. Mortality can be over 60% in Gram-negative sepsis causing severe hypotension and a low cardiac output.

Management

Antimicrobial therapy must be commenced immediately with a combination such as gentamicin and an agent active against Gram-positive cocci (e.g. penicillin or flucloxacillin) plus, if indicated clinically, an antibiotic active against anaerobes (e.g. metronidazole). This is adjusted when the nature of the infection has been determined. Alternatively, a broad-spectrum agent such as a cephalosporin or imipenem may be given (pp. 194, 195).

When Gram-positive cocci are the cause of the infection, benzylpenicillin should be given if the organism is known to be sensitive to penicillin. Flucloxacillin is indicated if penicillinase-producing staphylococci are responsible for the infection. If the patient is allergic to penicillin or the organism is resistant to cloxacillin, the next choice is clindamycin. Metronidazole is indicated for anaerobic infections. Gentamicin alone will suffice for other Gram-negative infections but not for pseudomonas. Amikacin is reserved for gentamicin-resistant organisms.

Two doses of corticosteroid (e.g. dexamethasone 1.5 mg/kg) given early may be beneficial by suppressing the damage caused by the exaggerated inflammatory response. This inhibits prostaglandin production and possibly acts as endotoxin mediators. Acute circulatory failure and DIC must also be treated.

DISEASES DUE TO FUNGI (MYCOSES)

These diseases are listed in the information box (right). Pathogenic fungi are ubiquitous; their importance varies between different parts of the world. Some fungi

---

FUNGAL DISEASE IN MAN

Cutaneous infections
Dermatophytes
Candidiasis
Pityriasis versicolor

Subcutaneous infections
Mycetoma (numerous species) (Table 5.26)
Other soft tissue infections (Table 5.27)

Systemic infections
Histoplasmosis
Aspergillosis
Coccidioidomycosis
Paracoccidioidomycosis
Blastomycosis
Cryptococcosis

---

are opportunistic and will not normally invade unless the defence mechanisms are impaired, as in the immunocompromised host. Fungal infections are transmitted by spores or hyphae, and normally enter the body through the lungs or skin, where they may cause disease, or from where they may disseminate to other parts of the body. Fungal infections tend to be chronic, and often require prolonged chemotherapy. For some infections there is still no effective treatment. Fungi also cause disease through allergy (p. 36) and from toxins such as ergot, muscarine and aflatoxin.

Fungal infections commonly present as skin disease, as subcutaneous swellings or as systemic infections.

CUTANEOUS FUNGAL INFECTIONS

An intact healthy skin is especially important in the tropics, where fungal infections are common. Extensive infections may impair sweating and heat loss, and cause distress through irritation. Scratching leads to secondary pyogenic infection.

DERMATOPHYTES

This large group of fungi infect keratinised tissues and are responsible for ringworm of the body and scalp, 'dhobi's itch' in the inguinal folds, and infection of the hair and nails. *Trichophytum rubrum* is the commonest cause and most difficult to treat.

Tinea imbricata (*T. concentricum*), characterised by multiple concentric rings, causes widespread disabling infections in some Pacific Islands and in S.E. Asia. *T. schoenleinii* produces a mass of creamy white material, with an offensive odour, on the scalp, known as favus.

Many dermatophytes are primarily parasites of domestic and farm animals.

Management

Dermatophytes are treated with topical antifungal ointments if mild, or if severe with griseofulvin 500 mg twice daily or ketoconazole 200–400 mg daily, by mouth. (p. 198)

CANDIDOSIS (MONILIASIS)

A yeast, *Candida albicans*, is the commonest fungus of medical importance.

Clinical features

Infections of skin or nails may resemble those caused by dermatophytes. Infections of skin folds and on the buttocks of babies are common. Mucosal infection (thrush) is also frequent, especially in the mouth (p. 423), on the vulvae of a diabetic woman and of the nails in hypocalcaemia (p. 642). Chronic mucocutaneous or disseminated candidosis occurs in immunocompromised individuals.

Management

Superficial infections may respond to topical treatment with gentian violet or nystatin, but otherwise ketoconazole (p. 199) is administered orally in a dose of 200–600 mg daily according to severity. Amphotericin (p. 149) may be required for systemic infections.

PITYRIASIS VERSICOLOR

This is due to a yeast that causes a widespread very superficial infection, especially of the chest, back and upper arms.

SUBCUTANEOUS FUNGAL INFECTIONS

MYCETOMA (MADURA FOOT)

Mycetoma, in this restricted sense, is a chronic fungal infection of the deep soft tissues and bones, most commonly of the limbs, but also of the abdominal or chest wall or head. It is produced by members of two groups of organisms classified as *Eumycetes* and aerobic *Actinomycetes*. A feature common to both groups is the formation of grains which are colonies of matted organisms with characteristic colours, ranging from 60 microns to 3 mm in diameter. The incidence appears to be related to climate, being especially high when an arid hot season ends in rains. The more common

Table 5.26 Fungi causing mycetoma

Species	Type of grains
Eumycetoma	
Madurella mycetomatis	Brown or black (big)
Madurella grisea	Black or brown (big)
Exophiala jeanselmei	Black
Pseudallescheria boydil	White or yellow (big)
Acremonium spp.	White or yellow
Actinomycetoma	
Actinomadura madurae	White, yellow, red (big)
Actinomadura pelletieri	Red (small)
Streptomyces somaliensis	White or yellow (big)
Nocardia brasilensis	White, yellow (microscopic)

species of fungi causing mycetoma are shown in Table 5.26.

Pathology

The histology is that of a chronic granuloma with a fibrous stroma and cyst-like spaces in which lie the characteristic grains. Nodules develop under the epidermis and these rupture revealing sinuses through which mucopus containing coloured grains is discharged. Some sinuses may heal with scarring while fresh sinuses appear elsewhere.

Clinical features

The lesions may occur in any part of the body but as the fungus is usually introduced by a thorn they are more common in the foot and leg in those who walk bare-footed. The mycetoma begins as a painless swelling at the site of implantation which grows and spreads steadily within the soft tissues causing swelling, and eventually penetrates bones.

There is little pain and usually no fever, but progressive disability. Secondary pyogenic infection does not usually penetrate far down the sinuses, possibly because of antibiotic activity of the fungi. It is unusual of the fungus to reach the lymph nodes unless there has been surgical interference. When the lesion is in the scalp, the skull may be affected but the dura mater appears to be an effective barrier. Apart from involvement of bones by a spreading mycetoma, intraosseous lesions may be found in the metaphysis of a long bone, especially at the upper end of the tibia and sometimes there may be an encapsulated periosteal mass. *Norcardia brasiliensis* often affects the skin of the back. It is seldom localised and may spread widely.

Diagnosis

Diagnosis is confirmed by demonstration of fungal grains in pus or tissue biopsy. Culture is usually necessary for species identification. Specific antibodies can usually be detected by precipitation.

Table 5.27   Subcutaneous fungal infections, other than mycetoma

	Zygomycosis	Chromoblasto-mycosis	Rhinospodidiosis	Sporothrichosis
Agent	Several	Several	*Rhinosporidium seeberi*	*Sporothrix schnekii*
Geography	Tropics	Tropics	S. America, India, etc. E. Africa	C. and S. Africa
Site	Face, limbs, systemic in immunocompromised or diabetic	Feet, others	Nose, cheeks	Limbs, rarely systemic
Presentation	Subcutaneous swellings	Mossy foot	Nasal polyps, subcutaneous nodules	Subcutaneous-swellings, ulcer, lymphatic spread
Treatment	Potassium iodide 1.5–3.5 g daily or amphotericin B	Flucytosine and/or itraconazole	Surgery	Potassium iodide 10 g daily, itraconazole

Management

The difference between *Eumycetes* and *Actinomycetes* is crucial because there is no drug of proven efficacy for the former. Sporadic successes against *Eumycetes* have been reported with griseofulvin and ketoconazole in the case of *M. mycetomatis*, but the results have been mostly disappointing and eumycetoma requires to be excised. It has a strong tendency to recur.

The treatment of actinomycetoma is more helpful. It consists of rifampicin (4 mg/kg/d by mouth) or streptomycin (14 mg/kg/d i.m.) for 3 months plus oral dapsone (1.5 mg/kg b.d.) or oral cotrimoxazole for 4–24 months. *Nocardia* infection may respond to dapsone alone. Precipitating antibodies disappear if treatment is successful.

OTHER SUBCUTANEOUS MYCOSES

These are summarised in Table 5.27.

SYSTEMIC FUNGAL INFECTIONS

HISTOPLASMOSIS

Histoplasmosis is caused by *Histoplasma capsulatum* (Darling) which is a yeast in its parasitic phase but is a filamentous fungus of soil at other times. A variant, *Histoplasma duboisii*, is found in parts of tropical Africa.

Histoplasma capsulatum

Histoplasma capsulatum multiplies in soil enriched by the droppings of birds and bats and the spores remain viable for years. Natural infections are found in several species of small mammals, including bats. Infection is by inhalation of infected dust. The infection is an especial hazard for explorers of caves, and people who clear out bird, including chicken, roosts.

Histoplasma capsulatum is found in all parts of the United States of America, especially in the east central states, and less commonly in Latin America from Mexico to Argentina, in Europe, North, South and East Africa, Nigeria, Malaysia, Indonesia and Australia.

Pathology

The parasite in its yeast phase multiplies mainly in monocytes and macrophages and produces areas of necrosis in which the parasites may abound. From these foci the blood stream may be invaded producing metastatic lesions in the liver, spleen and lymph nodes. Pulmonary histoplasmosis may cause pathological changes similar to those of tuberculosis, including the production of a primary complex with enlarged regional lymph nodes, multiple small discrete lesions and occasionally cavitation. Healed lesions may calcify.

Clinical features

These are listed in the information box (p. 149).

Diagnosis

In an area where the disease occurs histoplasmosis should be suspected in every obscure infection in which there are pulmonary signs or where there are enlarged lymph nodes or hepatosplenomegaly. Tissue is obtained by biopsy for an impression smear, histology, and culture. Radiological examination in long-standing cases may show calcified lesions in the lungs, spleen or other organs. In the more acute phases of the disease single or multiple soft pulmonary shadows with enlarged tracheo-bronchial nodes are seen.

CLINICAL SYNDROMES ASSOCIATED WITH INFECTIONS WITH HISTOPLASMA CAPSULATUM

Infection by inhalation
Subclinical disease: the majority of infections
Self limiting
Fever, chills, cough, chest pain, fatigue
Added dyspnoea, occasionally fatal pulmonary insufficiency due to heavy infection causing severe alveolitis

Inoculation
Solitary lesion of skin or mucosa

Disseminated histoplasmosis
Pattern depends on age and immunity
   Acute in children: severe, with fever, hepatosplenomegaly, cough, pancytopenia
   Subacute in the majority: fever, lymphadenopathy, hepatosplenomegaly, focal lesions of oropharynx, gut, adrenals, endocardium, meninges, brain
   Chronic in adults: low grade fever with fatigue. Various focal lesions possible

Chronic localised infection
Notably pulmonary bullae resembling cavitating tuberculosis

Delayed hypersensitivity to the intradermal injection of histoplasmin develops in patients with either active or healed infections but is usually negative in acute disseminated disease. Complement-fixing antibodies are detected within 3 weeks of the onset of an acute primary infection and increase in titre as the disease progresses. Precipitating antibodies may also be detected.

Management
Specific treatment with amphotericin is indicated only in severe infections, the dosage 0.5 mg/kg, in 500 ml of 5% glucose is given intravenously over a 6-hour period, gradually increasing to a maximum of 1.0 mg/kg. Treatment is given on alternate days. If badly tolerated, the dose may have to be reduced. Side-effects are anorexia, nausea, fever, headache and venous thrombosis which may be controlled by the addition of 10 mg prednisolone to the intravenous solution. Plasma urea rises and haemoglobin falls during treatment but later return to normal. Amphotericin may have to be continued for up to 3 months or longer, depending on the clinical response. Severe dyspnoea in histoplasmosis should be treated with prednisolone 20–40 mg daily for a few days.

Histoplasma duboisii
Histoplasma duboisii, the fungus of African histoplasmosis, is larger than the classical *H. capsulatum*. It is found throughout East, Central and West Africa.

Clinical features
This disease differs in several ways from *H. capsulatum* infection. The bones, skin, lymph nodes and liver develop granulomatous lesions or cold abscesses resembling tuberculosis, but the lungs are seldom involved. The visceral form with liver and splenic invasion is often fatal, while ulcerative skin lesions and bone abscesses follow a more benign course.

Radiological examination may show rounded foci of bone destruction sometimes associated with abscess formation. Multiple lesions of the ribs are common and the bones of the limbs may be involved.

Diagnosis
This is by isolation of the fungus. Immunodiagnostic tests are helpful.

Management
Systemic disease is treated in the same way as *H. capsulatum* infections. A solitary lesion in bone may require only local surgical treatment.

OTHER SYSTEMIC MYCOSES

ASPERGILLOSIS

This is the most common respiratory mycosis in Britain and is discussed on page 373.

COCCIDIOIDOMYCOSIS

This is caused by *Coccidioides immitis* and found in Southern United States, and Central and South America. The disease is acquired by inhalation.

Clinical features
In 40% of cases it affects the lungs, lymph nodes and skin. Rarely it may be carried by the blood stream to the bones, adrenals, meninges and other organs. In 60% of patients the infection is asymptomatic. Infections, including subclinical attacks, are followed by immunity.

Diagnosis
The fungi grow readily on culture media but as they are highly infective, diagnostic investigations are usually limited to intradermal, complement fixation and precipitin tests. Some localised pulmonary lesions can be treated by surgery.

Management
Amphotericin (above) or ketoconazole (200–400 mg daily for 1 year) may be helpful, but relapse is common.

PARACOCCIDIODOMYCOSIS

This is caused by *Paracoccicidiodes brasiliensis* and occurs in South America. Mucocutaneous lesions occur early. Involvement of lymphatic nodes and the lungs is prominent and the gastrointestinal tract may also be attacked. Most patients respond to ketoconazole, 200 mg/day for at least 6 months; liver function must be monitored; but for those who do not sulphonamides (60–100 mg/day in divided doses) or amphotericin (p. 149) may be used.

BLASTOMYCOSIS

North American blastomycosis is caused by *Blastomyces dermatitidis*. It also occurs in Africa. Systemic infection begins in the lungs and mediastinal lymph nodes and resembles pulmonary tuberculosis. Bones, skin and the genito-urinary tract may also be affected. Treatment is with amphotericin (p. 149).

CRYPTOCOCCOSIS

This is caused by *Cryptococcus neoformans*. Its distribution is world-wide.

Clinical features
It causes local gummatous-like tumours and granulomatous lesions of the lung, bones, brain and meninges. The CSF often contains the fungus when the nervous system is affected.

Diagnosis
The diagnosis is made by culture or recognition of spores in the CSF biopsy and serological detection of antigen.

Management
Amphotericin should be given intravenously (p. 149)

and flucytosine orally (p. 199). Surgical removal of local pulmonary lesions may be necessary. Recovery may be monitored by fall in antigen titre.

DISEASES DUE TO PROTOZOA

These diseases are listed in the information box below.

PROTOZOAL DISEASES OF MAN

In the blood
Malaria, trypanosomiasis

In the gut
Giardiasis, amoebiasis, balantidiasis

In the tissues
Toxoplasmosis, leishmaniasis

MALARIA

Human malaria is caused by *Plasmodium falciparum*, *P. vivax*, *P. ovale*, and *P. malariae*. It is transmitted by the bite of anopheline mosquitoes, in which the parasite undergoes a cycle of development which is temperature-dependent. Malaria is therefore predominantly a disease of hot wet climates, but it used to occur in Europe as far north as England and Denmark. Malaria may also be transmitted by blood transfusion or inoculation. Transplacental infection may occur in the child of a non-immune mother.

Malaria is endemic or sporadic throughout most of the tropics and subtropics below an altitude of 1500 m, excluding the Mediterranean littoral, the USA and Australia. One hundred million people are attacked

Table 5.28   Chemoprophylaxis of malaria

Area	Antimalarial tablets		Adult prophylactic dose
Chloroquine resistance present[2]	Chloroquine Proguanil	150 mg base *and* 100 mg or	Two tablets weekly Two tablets daily
	Chloroquine Pyrimethamine Dapsone	150 mg base *and* 12.5 mg plus 100 mg (maloprim)[1]	Two tablets weekly One tablet weekly
Chloroquine resistance absent	Chloroquine[3] Proguanil	150 mg base or 100 mg	Two tablets weekly One or two tablets daily

[1]Preferred in South East Asia (may not be needed in major cities – take advice before travelling).
[2]South America S.E. Asia including Southern China, Indonesia, Malaysia, Phillipines, Papua New Guinea, Bangladesh, India, Nepal, East, Central and West Africa.
[3]British preparations of chloroquine usually contain 150 mg base, French preparations 100 mg base and American preparations 300 mg base.

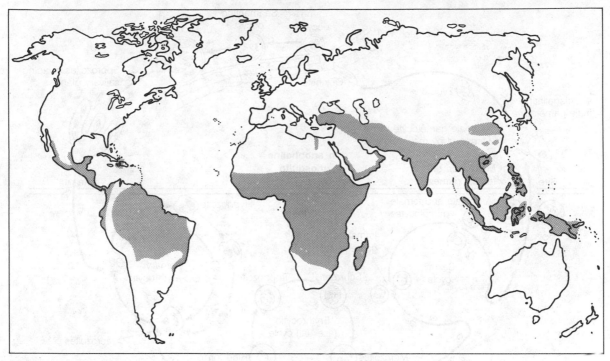

Fig. 5.7 Distribution of malaria.

annually of whom 1% die, mainly children. Following WHO sponsored campaigns of prevention and more effective treatment, the incidence of malaria was greatly reduced in 1950–60 but since 1970 there has been a resurgence. In the 1980s *P. falciparum* became resistant to chloroquine over a steadily increasing area (Table 5.28). Most serious is the emergence of resistance in East Africa, which has spread through Central Africa and in 1989 reached most parts of West Africa. Malaria due to this parasite is more severe than that due to the sensitive parasites.

Because of increased travel and neglect of chemoprophylaxis over 2000 cases are imported annually into Britain. Most are due to *P. vivax* from Asia. One in five, usually from Africa, is due to *P. falciparum* and of these 1% die because of late diagnosis. A few people living near airports in Europe have acquired malaria from accidentally imported mosquitoes.

Pathogenesis

Life cycle of parasite (Fig. 5.8)
The female anopheline mosquito becomes infected when it feeds on human blood containing gametocytes, the sexual forms of the malarial parasite. The development in the mosquito takes from 7–20 days. Sporozo-

ites inoculated by an infected mosquito disappear from human blood within half an hour and enter the liver. After some days (Table 5.29) merozoites leave the liver and invade red blood cells where further asexual cycles of multiplication take place, producing schizonts. Rupture of the schizont releases more merozoites into the blood and causes fever, whose periodicity depends on the species of parasite.

P. vivax and *P. ovale* may persist in liver cells as dormant forms, hypnozoites, that are capable of developing into merozoites months or years later. Thus the first attack of clinical malaria may occur long after the patient has left the endemic area, and the disease may relapse after treatment with drugs that kill only the erythrocytic stage of the parasite.

P. falciparum and *P. malariae* have no persistent exo-erythrocytic phase but recrudescences of fever may result from multiplication in the red cells of parasites which have not been eliminated by treatment and immune processes.

Effects on red blood cells and capillaries
Malaria is always accompanied by haemolysis and in a severe or prolonged attack anaemia may be profound. The causes of anaemia are listed in the information box (p. 152).

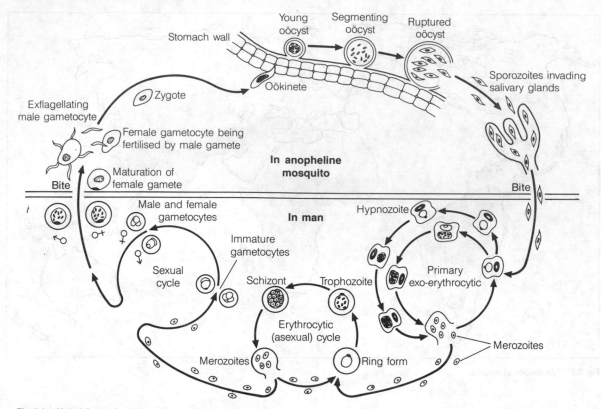

Fig. 5.8 Malarial parasites. Life cycle.

CAUSES OF ANAEMIA IN MALARIA

● Haemolysis of infected erythrocytes
● Haemolysis of uninfected erythrocytes
● Dyserythropoiesis
● Splenomegaly causing erythrocyte sequestration and haemodilution
● Depletion of folate stores

Haemolysis is most severe with *P. falciparum* which invades red cells of all ages, but especially young cells. *P. vivax* and *P. ovale* invade reticulocytes, and *P. malariae*, normoblasts, so that infections remain lighter.

In *P. falciparum* malaria, red cells containing schizonts adhere to the lining of capillaries in brain, kidney, liver, lungs and gut. The vessels become congested and the organs anoxic. Rupture of schizonts

Table 5.29 Relationships between life cycle of parasite and clinical features of malaria

Cycle/feature	P. vivax, P. ovale	P. malariae	P. falciparum
Pre patient period (minimum incubation)	8–25 days	15–30 days	8–25 days
Asexual cycle	48 hrs synchronous	72 hrs synchronous	<48 hrs asynchronous
Periodicity of fever	'tertian'	'quartan'	Aperiodic
Exoerythrocytic cycle	Persistent as hypnozoites	Pre-erythrocytic only	Pre-erythrocytic only
Delayed onset	Common	Rare	Rare
Relapses	Common up to 2 years	Recrudescence many years	Recrudescence up to 1 year

liberates toxic and antigenic substances which may cause further damage. Thus the main effects of malaria are haemolytic anaemia and, with *P. falciparum*, widespread organ damage.

P. falciparum does not grow well in red cells that contain haemoglobin F, C or especially S. Haemoglobin S heterozygotes (AS) are protected against the lethal complications of malaria. *P. vivax* cannot enter red cells that lack the Duffy blood group. West African negros and black Americans are protected.

Clinical features

Malaria in the non-immune
This is the pattern in children in an endemic area once they have lost the protection conferred by maternal antibodies, or in visitors of any age from a non-endemic area. The incubation period is often longer than the pre-erythrocytic cycle and may be up to several weeks for *P. falciparum* or months for *P. vivax*.

P. vivax and P. ovale malaria. In many cases the illness starts with a period of several days of continued fever before the development of classical bouts of fever on alternate days. Fever starts with a rigor. The patient feels cold and the temperature rises to about 40°C. After half to 1 hour the hot or flush phase begins. It lasts several hours and gives way to profuse perspiration and gradual fall in temperature. The cycle is repeated 48 hours later. Gradually the spleen and liver enlarge and may become tender. Anaemia develops slowly. Herpes simplex is common.

P. malariae infection. This is usually associated with mild symptoms and bouts of fever every third day. Parasitaemia may persist for many years without producing any symptoms. *P. malariae* causes glomerulonephritis and the nephrotic syndrome, in children.

Relapses. These are characteristic of vivax, ovale and malariae infections. They seldom occur more than 2 years after the patient has left the malarious area although much later recrudescence has been recorded with *P. malariae*.

P. falciparum infections. These are more dangerous than other forms of malaria. The onset, especially of primary attacks, is often insidious with malaise, headache and vomiting. Cough and mild diarrhoea are common suggesting influenza. The fever has no particular pattern and does not usually rise quite so high as in the other forms. The cold, hot and sweating stages are seldom found. Jaundice is common due to

hepatitis and haemolysis. The liver and spleen enlarge and become tender. Anaemia develops rapidly.

A patient with falciparum malaria, apparently not seriously ill, may develop serious complications. Children die rapidly without any special symptoms other than fever. Immunity is impaired in pregnancy and abortion from parasitisation of the maternal side of the placenta is frequent. Splenectomy increases the risk of severe malaria.

Mixed infections. Mixed infections with more than one species of malaria parasite may occur.

Complications of falciparum malaria
These are listed in the information box below.

COMPLICATIONS OF MALARIA DUE TO PLASMODIUM FALCIPARUM

Severe anaemia

Organ damage due to anoxia
Brain:
  confusion
  coma
Kidneys:
  oliguria
  uraemia (acute tubular necrosis)
Lungs:
  cough
  pulmonary oedoma
Intestine:
  diarrhoea
  congestion, possibly leaky to bacteria
Liver:
  jaundice
  encephalopathy (rare)

Intravascular haemolysis
Blackwater fever

Hypoglycaemia, especially with quinine treatment

Septicaemia secondary to shock

Hypotensive shock

Metabolic acidosis

Splenic rupture

In pregnancy
Maternal death, abortion, still birth, low birth weight

Cerebral malaria. This is the most urgent complication and is manifested either by confusion or coma, usually without localising signs.

Blackwater fever. This is associated with chronic falciparum malaria, most commonly in those who have taken antimalarial treatment irregularly, or are deficient in glucose-6-phosphate dehydrogenase. Haemolysis is unpredictable and severe destroying uninfected as well as parasitised red cells. The urine is dark or black.

Endemic malaria

The manifestations of malaria in people who grow up in an endemic area vary with the degree of endemicity, the age of the patient and the development of immunity.

In hypoendemic areas little immunity is acquired, epidemics of malaria are liable to occur and the disease does not differ materially from that in non-immunes.

In mesoendemic areas malaria is frequent but only seasonal. Repeated infections lead to anaemia, considerable enlargement of the spleen which is in danger of rupture, and chronic ill-health with bouts of fever. The growth and development of children may be retarded.

In hyperendemic areas malaria transmission takes place throughout the year but with seasonal increases; adults develop considerable immunity. Although affected individuals may have palpable spleens and parasitaemia, malaria causes only occasional short bouts of fever.

In holoendemic areas malarial transmission is intense throughout the year and adults do not suffer from the infection although they support a low parasitaemia and the spleen becomes impalpable. Pregnancy lowers resistance to malaria. The risks are greatest in the first pregnancy (see information box p. 153).

In hyperendemic and in holoendemic areas malaria may kill up to 15–20% of children below the age of 5 years. The regular taking of anti-malarial drugs prevents the manifestations of chronic malaria but may impair the development of immunity.

Tropical splenomegaly syndrome

In some hyperendemic areas gross splenomegaly is associated with an exaggerated immune response to malaria and is seen, unexpectedly, in adults who have high antibody titres to malaria and low parasitaemias. The condition, which is commoner in females and in certain racial and family groups is characterised by enormous overproduction of IgM, levels reaching 3–20 times the local mean value. Much of the IgM is aggregated with other immunoglobulin or complement and precipitates in the cold, in vitro. IgM aggregates are phagocytosed by reticuloendothelial cells in the spleen and liver, and the demonstration of this by immunofluorescence in a liver biopsy section is diagnostic. Light microscopy of the liver usually shows sinusoidal lymphocytosis. Anaemia and lymphocytosis

can be confused with leukaemia. Portal hypertension may develop.

Diagnosis

Malaria should be considered if a febrile patient is in or has recently left a malarious locality. Besides malaria there are many causes for acute febrile splenomegaly in the tropics. Gross enlargement of the spleen may also result from tuberculosis, visceral leishmaniasis, schistosomiasis and chronic brucellosis as well as leukaemia and lymphoma. Well-stained blood films, thick and thin, should be repeated if necessary. P. falciparum parasites may be very scanty, especially in patients who have been partially treated. With P. falciparum only ring forms are normally seen in the early stages. With the other species all stages of the erythrocytic cycle may be found. Gametocytes appear after about 2 weeks. Malaria may coexist with other diseases and not be the cause of the illness in semi-immune persons in endemic areas.

Management

Chemotherapy of the acute attack

The drug of choice is chloroquine. The usual course of treatment is 600 mg of the effective base (4 tablets) followed by 300 mg base in 6 hours then 150 mg base twice daily for 3–7 more days. The initial dose for children is 5–15 mg/kg. For semi-immune individuals a single dose, 600 mg for an adult, is usually adequate. Infections with P. falciparum from a chloroquine-resistant area (Table 5.28) should be treated with quinine dihydrochloride or sulphate 600 mg salt (10 mg/kg) 3 times daily for 5 days by mouth, followed by a single dose of sulfadoxine 1.5 g combined with pyrimethamine 75 mg, i.e. 3 tablets of Fansidar. The dose is reduced to twice daily if quinine toxicity develops. Amodiaquine may be used in the same dosage as chloroquine if quinine is not tolerated, or quinidine in the same dosage as quinine. If sulphonamide sensitivity is suspected, quinine may be followed by tetracycline 250 mg, 6-hourly for 7 days, or mefloquine 20 mg/kg in two or three divided doses 8 hours apart. Mefloquine is also useful on its own if quinine is not available.

Management of complicated P. falciparum malaria

Patients with 'cerebral malaria' or other severe manifestations, or non-immune with more than 1% of red cells infected are medical emergencies. The immediate administration of chloroquine or quinine is indicated, the drug being given as an intravenous infusion over 2–4 hours to avoid acute circulatory failure or acute encephalopathy. Quinine is indicated if a chloroquine-resistant infection is at all likely (Table 5.28). The dose of chloroquine is 5 mg/kg and of quinine 10 mg/kg. The dose should be repeated at intervals of 12 hours until the patient can take drugs orally. The drugs may instead be given intramuscularly but chloroquine may cause convulsions (especially in undernourished children) and quinine may cause necrosis of muscle; the hydrochloride is less irritant than the dihydrochloride. In a comatose patient lumbar puncture may be indicated to exclude coexisting bacterial meningitis.

Severe anaemia requires transfusion with packed red cells. If oliguria develops, frusemide or an infusion of mannitol may forestall renal failure. Intravenous fluid, if necessary, should be monitored by the central venous pressure because pulmonary oedema develops easily and total fluid should be restricted to less than 2 litres daily. Exchange blood transfusion is life-saving in complicated very heavy infections (over 10% of red cells infected). Hypoglycaemia, especially in children or in those treated with intravenous quinine, septicaemia may be the cause of failure to respond to treatment.

Management of tropical splenomegaly syndrome
Splenomegaly and anaemia usually resolve over a period of months of continuous treatment with proguanil 100 mg daily, which should be continued for life to prevent relapse. Complicating folate deficiency is treated wih folic acid 5 mg daily.

Radical cure of malaria due to P. vivax *and* P. ovale
Relapses can be prevented by taking one of the antimalarial drugs in suppressive doses. Radical cure is achieved in most patients by a course of primaquine (15 mg/d for 14 days) which destroys the hyponozoite phase in the liver. Haemolysis may develop in those who are glucose-6-phosphate dehydrogenase (G6PD) deficient. Cyanosis due to the formation of methaemoglobin in the red cells is more common but not dangerous.

Chemoprophylaxis
Clinical attacks of malaria can be prevented by drugs such as proguanil which attack the pre-erythrocytic form ('causal prophylaxis'), or by drugs after it has entered the erythrocyte ('suppression'). Maloprim (pyrimethamine 12.5 mg and dapsone 100 mg) and Fansidar (pyrimethamine 25 mg and sulfadoxine 500 mg) contain two compounds which block two successive enzymes in the parasite's folate pathway. Tables 5.28 and 5.30 give the recommended doses for protection of the non-immune. Chemoprophylaxis is begun 1 week before entering the malarious area and is

Table 5.30 Doses of antimalarials for children

Dose in relation to adult dose	Weight range	Age range
One-quarter	Under 5 kg	Under 1 year
One-half	5–20 kg	1–4 years
Three-quarters	20–40 kg	6–12 years
Adult dose	Over 40 kg	Over 12 years

Note: Doses according to weight are preferable to age.

continued until 4 weeks after leaving it. Resistance to the cheap and well-tolerated drugs proguanil and pyrimethamine is increasing and frequently coincides with the much more serious spread of chloroquine resistance. Resistance to maloprim and fansidar is also reported. Chloroquine should not be taken continuously as prophylactic for over 5 years, without regular ophthalmic examination as it may cause irreversible retinopathy. Infants under 8 weeks of age should not be given maloprim or fansidar. Pregnant and lactating women may take proguanil or chloroquine safely. Fansidar should be avoided for chemoprophylaxis if possible; allergic rashes are common and deaths have occurred, e.g. from agranulocytosis or Stevens-Johnson syndrome. Amodiaquine should not be used for prophylaxis for fear of agranulocytosis.

Prevention
Control of anopheline mosquitoes, especially by the spraying of houses with residual insecticides has greatly reduced or abolished the risk of malaria in many areas. However, unless eradication is complete, all visitors should take regular prophylactic drugs. Chemoprophylaxis alone may not be sufficient to prevent malaria. It is also important to avoid anopheline mosquitoes, which bite at night. Long sleeves and trousers should be worn outside the house. Repellent creams and sprays can be used. Screened windows and the use of a mosquito net and burning coils also reduce the risk.

AMOEBIASIS

Amoebiasis is usually caused by *Entamoeba histolytica*, a potentially pathogenic intestinal amoeba that is spread between humans by its cysts. *E. histolytica* must be distinguished from other species which are non-pathogenic, notably *E. hartmanii* and *E. coli*. In addition two amoebae of genera *Naegleria* and *Acanthamoeba* which inhabit polluted surface water and swimming pools all over the world are causes respec-

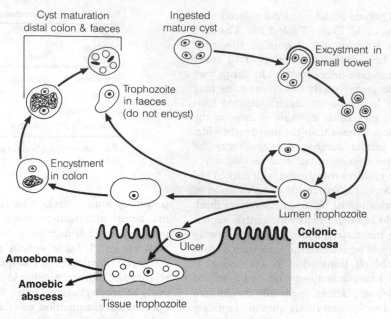

Fig. 5.9   Amoebiasis. Life cycle of *Entamoeba histolytica*. (Adapted from Knight R 1982 Parasitic disease in man. Churchill Livingstone, Edinburgh.)

tively of fulminating meningitis and granulomatous encephalitis.

Pathology

Cysts of *E. histolytica* survive well outside the body and are ingested in water or uncooked food which has been contaminated by human faeces. Lettuce is a common vehicle of infection. The disease is occasionally acquired in Britain.

In the colon the vegetative trophozoite forms emerge from the cysts (Fig. 5.9). While these remain free in the colon the condition is symptomless but some genetic strains, that can be distinguished enzymatically, may invade the mucous membrane of the large bowel. The lesions, which are usually maximal in the caecum but may be found as far down as the anal canal, are flask-shaped ulcers varying greatly in size and surrounded by healthy mucosa. A localised granuloma (amoeboma), presenting as a palpable mass in the rectum or causing a filling defect in the colon on radiography, is a rare complication. Because an amoeboma responds well to antiamoebic treatment it is important that it is not mistaken for a colonic carcinoma.

Amoebae may enter a portal venous radicle and be carried to the liver where they multiply rapidly and destroy the parenchyma causing an amoebic abscess. The liquid contents at first have a characteristic pinkish colour which later may change to chocolate brown. Amoebic ulcers may cause severe haemorrhage but rarely perforate the bowel wall. Cutaneous amoebiasis presents as progressive genital or perianal ulceration, usually in homosexuals, or around abdominal surgical wounds. The incubation period of amoebiasis varies from 2 weeks to many years.

Clinical features

Intestinal amoebiasis, or amoebic dysentery

This usually runs a chronic course with grumbling abdominal pains and two or more rather loose stools a day. Periods of diarrhoea alternating with constipation are common. Mucus is usually passed, sometimes with streaks of blood, and the stools often have an offensive odour. There may be tenderness along the line of the colon, usually more marked over the caecum and pelvic colon. The right iliac pain may simulate acute appendicitis. There may be more acute bowel symptoms, with very frequent motions and the passage of much blood and mucus, simulating bacillary dysentery or ulcerative colitis. This occurs particularly in the aged, in the puerperium and with superadded pyogenic infection of the ulcers.

Hepatic amoebiasis

This often occurs without a history of recent diarrhoea.

It is common in the tropics and an important cause of imported fever in Britain. The abscess is usually found in the right hepatic lobe. Early symptoms may be local discomfort only and malaise; later a swinging temperature, sweating and an enlarged, tender liver, cough and pain in the right shoulder are characteristic, but symptoms may remain vague and signs minimal. In particular, the less common abscess in the left lobe is difficult to diagnose. There is usually neutrophil leucocytosis and a raised diaphragm with diminished movement on the right side. A large abscess may penetrate the diaphragm and rupture into the lung from where its contents may be coughed up. Rupture into the pleural cavity, the peritoneal cavity or pericardial sac is less common but more serious.

Diagnosis

A careful naked-eye inspection of a freshly passed stool should be made. Any exudate is examined at once under the microscope for motile trophozoites which are about 30 microns in diameter, with a clear ectoplasm and a granular endoplasm, and usually contain red blood cells. Movements cease rapidly as the stool preparation cools. Sigmoidoscopy may reveal typical flask-shaped ulcers and a scraping should be examined for *E. histolytica*. Several stools may need to be examined in chronic amoebiasis before cysts are found. The presence of cysts in the faeces does not equate with invasive amoebiasis: in endemic areas one-third of the population are symptomless passers of amoebic cysts.

An amoebic abscess of the liver is suspected from the clinical and radiographic appearances and confirmed by radionuclide or ultrasonic scanning. Aspirated pus from an amoebic abscess has the characteristic appearance described above but only rarely contains free amoebae.

Antibodies are detectable by immunofluorescence in over 95% of patients with hepatic amoebiasis and intestinal amoeboma but in only about 60% of dysenteric amoebiasis. Tests for precipitating antibodies are less sensitive but become negative in a few months after cure.

Management

Invasive intestinal amoebiasis responds quickly to oral metronidazone (800 mg t.i.d. for 5 days), or tinidazole (single doses of 2 g daily for 3 days). Furamide 500 mg should be given orally t.i.d. for 10 days after treatment to eliminate luminal cysts. Stools are re-examined 4 weeks later.

Early hepatic amoebiasis responds promptly to treatment with metronidazole or tinidazole as above, or to chloroquine 300 mg base b.d. for 2 days, followed by 150 mg b.d. for 14 days. Furamide is given to eliminate the intestinal infection. Aspiration is also required and repeated if necessary if the abscess is large or threatens to burst, or if the response to chemotherapy is not prompt. If culture of the 'pus' indicates that there is secondary bacterial infection, treatment will be required with an appropriate antibiotic. Rupture of an abscess into the pleural cavity, pericardial sac or peritoneal cavity necessitates immediate aspiration or surgical drainage. Small serous effusions resolve without drainage.

Prevention

Personal precautions against contracting amoebiasis in the tropics and subtropics consist of not eating fresh uncooked vegetables nor drinking unboiled water.

GIARDIASIS

Infection with the flagellate *Gardia intestinalis* known also as *G. lamblia*, is world-wide but commoner in the tropics. It particularly affects children in endemic areas, tourists, and patients in mental hospitals and is the parasite most commonly imported into Britain. The flagellates attach to the mucosa of the duodenum and jejunum and cause inflammation and partial villous atrophy.

Clinical features

Recurrent attacks of urgent diarrhoea with abdominal discomfort and explosive loose pale stools are characteristic. There may be severe malabsorption. Lethargy, flatulence, abdominal distension, epigastric pain and nausea are common.

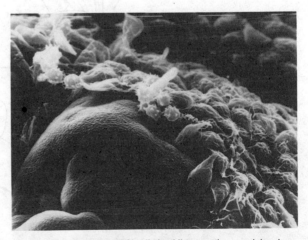

Fig. 5.10 **Trophozooites of *Giardia lamblia*** swarming over jejunal mucosa. Electron micrograph x925. (Professor K. Vickerman.)

Diagnosis

Giardiasis is diagnosed by recognising the cysts in stools or the flagellate form in jejunal juice or mucus, which can be obtained via a biopsy capsule or a string test (Enterotest capsule). Repeated examination may be necessary.

Management

Treatment is with a single dose of tinidazole 40 mg/kg in the range 0.5 g to 2 g, repeated after 1 week. Metronidazole 200–400 mg t.i.d. for 14 days is less efficient.

BALANTIDIASIS

Balantidium coli is a ciliate that causes dysentery in pigs and occasionally infects man in whom the disease resembles amoebic dysentery. Treatment is with tetracycline 10 mg/kg 4 times daily for 10 days or metronidazole 200–400 mg according to age 3 times daily for 7 days.

LEISHMANIASIS

This group of diseases is caused by protozoa of the genus *Leishmania*, conveyed to man by female phlebotomine sandflies in which the flagellate (promastigote) forms of leishmania develop. In man the leishmaniae are found in cells of the monocyte-macrophage system as oval forms known as amastigotes or Leishman-Donovan bodies (Fig. 5.11). Leishmaniasis may take the form of a generalised visceral infection, kala-azar, or of a purely cutaneous infection, known in the Old World as oriental sore. In South America cutaneous leishmaniasis may remain confined to the skin or metastasise to the nose and mouth.

Visceral leishmaniasis (kala-azar)

Visceral leishmaniasis is caused by *Leishmania donovani* and is prevalent in the Mediterranean and Red Sea littorals, Sudan, parts of East Africa, Asia Minor, mountainous regions of Southern Arabia, eastern parts of India, China and South America. In India, where the disease is epidemic, man appears to be the chief host. In most other areas, including the Mediterranean, dogs and foxes are the main reservoirs of infection. Here the disease is endemic and occurs chiefly in young children or tourists. In Africa various wild rodents provide the reservoir, and the disease is rural occurring in older children and visiting hunters and soldiers. Transmission has also been reported to follow blood transfusion in Northern Europe. The disease has presented unexpectedly in immunosuppressed patients, for example after renal transplantation and in AIDS.

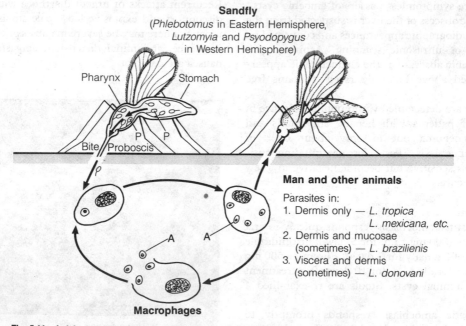

Sandfly
(*Phlebotomus* in Eastern Hemisphere,
Lutzomyia and *Psyodopygus*
in Western Hemisphere)

Pharynx   Stomach

Bite Proboscis

Man and other animals

Parasites in:
1. Dermis only — *L. tropica*
                  L. mexicana, etc.
2. Dermis and mucosae
   (sometimes) — *L. brazilienis*
3. Viscera and dermis
   (sometimes) — *L. donovani*

Macrophages

Fig. 5.11   Leishmaniasis. Life cycle of Leishmania: A = amastigole (L-D body); P = promastigote. (Adopted from Knight R 1982 Parasitic disease in man.)

Pathology

Multiplication, by simple fission, of leishmaniae takes place in monocytes and macrophages in various organs, especially in the liver and spleen which becomes greatly enlarged, the bone marrow, lymphoid tissue and the small intestinal submucosa. The disease is accompanied by malnutrition and immunosuppression which is both specific to leishmania and non-specific. Acute intercurrent infection or tuberculosis are common complications. Granulocytopenia and thrombocytopenia occur. Anaemia is due to haemolysis, hypersplenism and ineffective erythropoiesis. Serum albumin is low and globulin, mainly IgG, high. Hepatocellular damage and bleeding are late complications.

Clinical features

The incubation period is usually about 1 or 2 months but maybe up to 10 years. The onset is usually insidious with a low-grade fever, the patient remaining ambulant, or it may be abrupt with sweating and high intermittent fever, sometimes showing a double rise of temperature in 24 hours. The spleen soon becomes enlarged, often massively, hepatomegaly is less marked. If not treated, the patient will become anaemic and wasted, frequently with increased pigmentation especially on the face. Lymphadenopathy is common and rarely is the only clinical finding.

After recovery post kala-azar dermal leishmaniasis sometimes develops. It may present first as hypopigmented or erythematous macules on any part of the body or as a nodular eruption especially on the face. Amastigotes are scanty.

Diagnosis

This is established by demonstrating the parasite in stained smears of aspirates of bone marrow, lymph node, spleen or liver, or by culture of these aspirates. Antibody is detected by immunofluorescence or enzyme-linked immunosorbent assay early in the disease. The *leishmanin skin test* is negative; it is performed and read in the same way as the tuberculin test using a suspension of killed promastigotes as antigen.

Management

The response to treatment varies with the geographic area in which the disease has been acquired. In Europe and Asia the disease is readily cured, but in the Sudan and East Africa it is more resistant. Pentavalent antimonials are the drugs of choice. Sodium stibgluconate contains 100 mg Sb/ml, meglumine antimoniate contains 85 mg Sb/ml. Children are given 20 mg Sb/kg i.v. or i.m. daily for 20–30 days. The adult dose is 10–20 mg Sb/kg to a maximum of 850 mg.

Intercurrent infection is sought and treated. Rarely blood transfusion is needed for anaemia or bleeding. Measurement of spleen size, haemoglobin and serum albumin are useful in assessing progress. A small proportion of patients relapse, and should be re-treated for 2 months with a full 20 mg Sb/kg daily. Second-line drugs for patients who fail to respond to antimonials include pentamidine 3–4 mg/kg 1 or 2 times per week and amphotericin (p. 149).

Prevention

Infected or stray dogs should be destoyed in an endemic area where they are the reservoir. Sandflies should be combated. They are extremely sensitive to insecticides. Mosquito nets treated with permethrin will keep out the tiny sandfly. Insect-repellent creams may be helpful.

Early diagnosis and treatment of human infections reduces the reservoir and controls epidemic kala-azar in India. Serology is useful for case detection in the field. There is no vaccine.

CUTANEOUS LEISHMANIASIS OF THE OLD WORLD (ORIENTAL SORE)

Cutaneous leishmaniasis is found in the Old World around the Mediterranean littoral, throughout the Middle East and Central Asia as far as Pakistan, and in sub-Saharan West Africa and Sudan. It is caused either by zoonotic *L. major*, a parasite of gerbils and other desert rodents, or by the arthroponotic *L. tropica*, in towns. In the highlands of Ethiopia and Kenya a third parasite, of hyraxes, *L. aethiopica* is the cause. The disease is commonly imported into Britain. On inoculation the parasites are taken up by dermal histiocytes in which they multiply and around which lymphocytes and plasma cells accumulate. With time, the histological appearance becomes more tuberculoid and the overlying epidermis crusts and may ulcerate centrally. Healing is accompanied by subepidermal fibrosis. The incubation period is from 2 weeks to 5 years or more but usually is from 2 to 3 months.

Clinical features

Lesions, single or multiple on exposed parts of the body, start as small red papules which increase gradually in size, reaching 2–10 cm in diameter. A crust forms, overlying an ulcer with a granular base. Tiny satellite papules are characteristic. Untreated, the lesion heals in 3 months to 3 years, rarely longer. Healing produces a depressed mottled scar which may be disfiguring or disabling.

Two forms of cutaneous leishmaniasis occur that do

not heal spontaneously. Diffuse cutaneous leishmaniasis (*L. aethiopica*) in which an immune defect permits the disease to spread all over the skin, and recidivans (lupoid) leishmaniasis (*L. tropica*) in which apparently healed sores relapse persistently.

Diagnosis

The appearance of a typical lesion in a patient from an endemic area suggests the diagnosis. Amastigotes can be demonstrated by inserting a dry needle into the margin of the ulcer, or making a slit skin smear (p. 138) and staining the material obtained with Giemsa's stain or culturing it. Cultured parasites may be speciated by isoenzyme or DNA studies. The leishmanin skin is positive except in diffuse cutaneous leishmaniasis. Serology is unhelpful.

Management

The local application of heat by infra-red, hot water or a thermostatically controlled pad at 40°C may accelerate healing. When the lesions are multiple or in a disfiguring site it is better to treat the patient by parenteral injections of pentavalent antimonials (p. 159), but *L. aethiopica* is not sensitive to antimonials. Diffuse cutaneous leishmaniasis is treated with pentamidine once weekly.

Prevention

In addition to those prophylactic measures described under visceral leishmaniasis against animals and sandflies, a lasting immunity can be achieved by deliberate inoculation of a living culture of *L. major* on the upper arm, which produces a typical sore but protects against a subsequent, possibly disfiguring, lesion with the same species of parasite.

CUTANEOUS AND MUCOCUTANEOUS LEISHMANIASIS OF THE NEW WORLD

In South and Central America, cutaneous leishmaniasis is endemic and mostly caused by parasites of the *L. mexicana* and *L. braziliensis* groups, which occur in hot, moist, forest regions and are conveyed to man from a variety of rodents by several species of sandflies (Fig. 5.11). *L. mexicana* is responsible for chiclero's ulcer, the self-healing sores of Mexico, Guatemala and Honduras, and for some of the sores in the north of South America, including diffuse cutaneous leishmaniasis (*L. m. amazonensis*). *L. braziliensis* extends widely from the Amazon basin as far as Paraguay and Costa Rica and is responsible for self-healing sores and for mucocutaneous leishmaniasis. A third variety of the disease occurring in the Peruvian Andes is known as

'uta' and is caused by *L. peruviana*, dogs providing the reservoir.

Pathology

The microscopic appearances of the skin lesions may be similar to oriental sore. Mucocutaneous lesions begin as a perivascular infiltration; later endarteritis may cause destruction of the surrounding tissues.

Clinical features

Clinically, lesions of *L. mexicana* and *L. peruviana* closely resemble those seen in the Old World but lesions on the pinna of the ear are common and are chronic and destructive. The primary lesions of *L. braziliensis* are similar but in some areas up to 80% of infected persons develop 'espundia', metastatic lesions in the mucosa of the nose or mouth. Mucosal lesions usually occur 1–2 years after the skin lesions but may appear many years later. The nasal mucosa becomes congested and ulcerates; later all soft tissues of the nose may be destroyed. The lips, soft palate and fauces may also be invaded and destroyed leading to considerable suffering and deformity. Secondary bacterial infection is common. Two sub-species *L. b. guyanesis* and *L. b. panamensis* rarely cause espundia.

Diagnosis

Diagnosis depends on the history and clinical appearance, confirmed by demonstration of the parasites in smears, culture or histological section. As parasites are not easily found the leishmanin test is of value and serology may be useful.

Management

Purely cutaneous disease may be successfully treated by sodium stibogluconate given as recommended for visceral leishmaniasis (p. 159) but in established espundia amphotericin (p. 149) is sometimes necessary.

AFRICAN TRYPANOSOMIASIS (SLEEPING SICKNESS)

African sleeping sickness is caused by trypanosomes conveyed to man by the bites of infected tsetse flies of either sex. The disease is naturally acquired only in Africa between 12°N and 25°S. Two trypanosomes affect man, *Trypanosoma brucei gambiense* conveyed by *Glossina palpalis* and *G. tachinoides* and *T. b. rhodesiense* transmitted by *G. morsitans*, *G. pallidipes*, *G. swynnertoni* and *G. palpalis*.

Gambiense trypanosomiasis has a wide distribution in West and Central Africa reaching to Uganda and Kenya; rhodesiense trypanosomiasis is found in parts

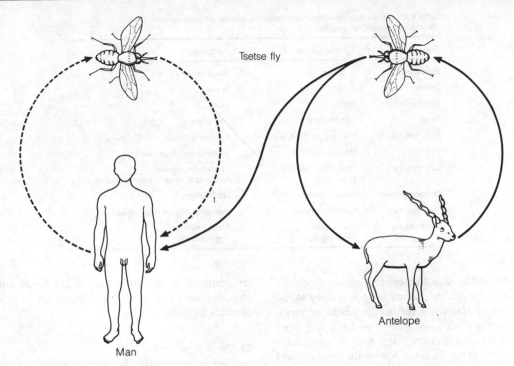

Tsetse fly

Man

Antelope

Fig. 5.12 Transmission of *trypanosomiasis gambiense* (left) and *trypanosomiasis rhodesiensie* (right).

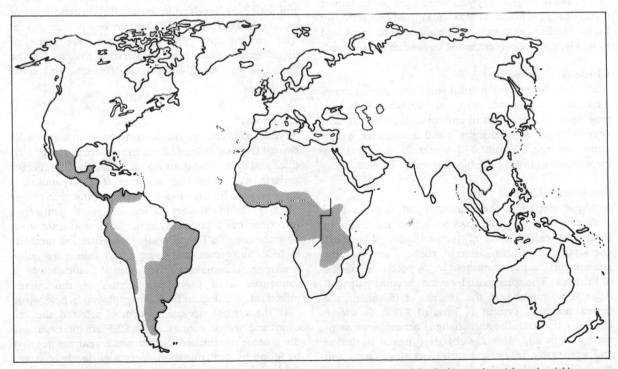

Fig. 5.13 Endemic zones of American and African trypanosomiasis. Within these zones, the actual distribution may be patchy and variable, especially in Africa.

Table 5.31   Comparison of the clinical and laboratory features of trypanosomiasis due to *T.b. rhodesiense* and *T.b. gambiense*

Feature	*T.b. rhodesiense*	*T.b. gambiense*
Incubation	7–14 days	Weeks–months
Onset	Abrupt	Insidious
Primary complex	Usual	Rare
Fever	High swinging	Low grade
Early features	Effusions, hepatitis, myocarditis	Lymphadenopathy
Rash	Macular, petechial	Erythematous, circinate
Late features	Drowsiness, tremors coma, death	Headache, insomnia, behavioural, tremors, paresis, wasting, coma
Duration of illness	Weeks or months	Months or years
Trypanosomes	Numerous in blood	Numerous in lymph node aspirate
Cerebrospinal fluid	Protein, cells Trypanosomes	Protein, cells Trypanosomes

of East and Central Africa where it is currently on the increase. In West Africa transmission is mainly at the riverside, where the fly rests in the shade of trees. Animal reservoirs of *T. b. gambiense* have not been identified although pigs may carry it. *T. b. rhodesiense* has a large reservoir in numerous wild animals and transmission takes place in the shade of woods bordering grasslands. Devastating epidemics of both types have occurred. Trypanosomiasis of cattle, caused mainly by *T. b. brucei*, is also widespread and seriously limits grazing land and the production of meat and milk. Only a low percentage of tsetse flies are infected.

Clinical features

A bite by a tsetse fly is painful and commonly becomes inflamed, but if trypanosomes are introduced, the site may again become painful and swollen about 10 days later ('trypanosomal chancre'), and the regional lymph nodes enlarge. Within 2–3 weeks of infection the trypanosomes invade the blood stream (Table 5.31).

Gambiense infections

In these infections the disease usually runs a slow course over months or years with irregular bouts of fever and enlargement of lymph nodes. These are characteristically firm, discrete, rubbery and painless and are particularly prominent in the posterior triangle of the neck. The spleen and liver may become palpable. After some months, in the absence of treatment, the central nervous system is invaded. This is shown clinically by headache and changed behaviour, insomnia by night and sleepiness by day, mental confusion and eventually tremors, pareses, wasting, coma and death. The histological changes in the brain are similar to those found in viral encephalitis but trypanosomes

are scattered in the substance of the brain and large mononuclear (morula) cells are found whose cytoplasm contains globules of IgM.

Rhodesiense infections

In these infections the disease is altogether more acute and severe than in gambiense infections, so that within days or a few weeks the patient is usually severely ill and may have developed pleural effusions and signs of myocarditis or hepatitis. There may be a petechial rash. The patient may die before there are signs of involvement of the central nervous system. If the illness is less acute, drowsiness, tremors, and coma develop.

Diagnosis

Trypanosomiasis should be considered in any febrile patient from an endemic area. In rhodesiense infections thick and thin blood films stained as for the detection of malaria, will reveal trypanosomes. The trypanosomes may be seen in the blood or from puncture of the primary lesion in the earliest stages of gambiense infections but it is usually easier to demonstrate them by puncture of a lymph node. Concentration methods include buffy coat microscopy and miniature anion exchange chromatography. Animal inoculation is sometimes used for the detection of rhodesiense infections. Serological tests are employed in field work.

If the central nervous system is affected the cell count and protein content of the CSF are increased and the glucose diminished. Sometimes trypanosomes may be found by centrifugation. Very high levels of serum IgM or the presence of IgM in the CSF are suggestive of trypanosomiasis.

Table 5.32   Chemotherapy of trypanosomiasis

Drug/route of administration	Dosage	Toxicity	Indications
Suramin, intravenous	Test dose 200 mg then 1 g in 10 ml water every 5 days, to total dose 5–6 g	Mild: protenuria, arthralgia Severe: dermatitis, diarrhoea, nephritis (red cells and casts)	Rhodesiense and gambiense infection before CNS involvement
Pentamidine as base intramuscular	4 mg/kg max 250 mg/dose, alternate days for 10 doses	Collapse if injected intravenously, hypoglycaemia, nephritis, diabetes mellitus, injection abscess.	As for suramin
Melarsoprol (Mel B) 3.6 percent in propylene glycol, intravenous	Three consecutive weeks for 4 weeks wk 1: 0.5 ml, 1 ml, 1 ml wk 2: 2.5 ml × 3 wk 3: 3.5 ml × 3 wk 4: 5 ml × 3	Jarisch–Herxheimer reaction, arsenical encephalopathy, mortality up to 10%*	Rhodesiense and gambiense disease after CNS involvement
Difluoromethyl ornithine, orally	200–400 mg/kg daily × 6 wk	Diarrhoea, abdominal pain	Cerebral gambiense infections
Nitrofurazone orally	10 mg/kg eight-hourly × 10 days	Haemolysis, neuropathy	Resistance to arsenicals

*Toxicity is greatly reduced if the blood has been cleared of trypanosomes with suramin (test dose plus 1 g) a few days previously.

Management

The prognosis is good if treatment is begun early before the brain has been invaded. At this stage either suramin or pentamidine may be used, the latter being employed only for gambiense infections. After the nervous system is affected an arsenical or difluoromethyl ornithine will be required. Details are given in Table 5.32.

Prevention

A single intramuscular injection of 250 mg pentamidine gives protection against *T. b. gambiense* for 6 months because of the slow excretion of the drug. As the protection against *T. b. rhodesiense* is less sure and shorter in duration, chemoprophylaxis is not advised in rhodesiense areas. In endemic gambiense areas various measures may be taken against tsetse flies and field teams detect and treat early human infection. In rhodesiense areas control is difficult.

AMERICAN TRYPANOSOMIASIS (CHAGAS' DISEASE)

Chagas' disease occurs widely in South and Central America. The cause is *Trypanosoma cruzi* transmitted to man from the faeces of a reduviid bug in which the trypanosomes have a cycle of development before becoming infective to man. Bugs live in the mud and wattle walls and thatch roofs of simple rural houses, and emerge at night to feed on the sleeping occupants. While feeding they defecate. Infected faeces are rubbed in through the conjunctiva, mucosa of mouth or nose or abrasions of the skin. Over 100 species of mammals,

domestic, peridomestic and wild may serve as reservoirs of infection. In some areas blood transfusion accounts for about 5% of cases. Congenital transmission occurs occasionally.

Pathology

The trypanosomes migrate via the blood stream and develop into amastigote forms in the tissues. These multiply in many sites, especially in the myocardium causing pseudocysts, in smooth muscle fibres, and also in the ganglion cells of the autonomic nervous system.

Clinical features

The entrance of *T. cruzi* through an abrasion produces a dusky red firm swelling and enlargement of regional lymph nodes. A conjunctival lesion, though less common, is more characteristic; the unilateral firm reddish swelling of the lids may close the eye and constitutes 'Romaña's sign'. Young children are most commonly affected. In a few patients an acute generalised infection soon appears, with fever, lymphadenopathy and enlargement of the spleen and liver. Neurological features include personality changes and signs of meningoencephalitis. The acute infection may be fatal to infants. In most patients the early infection is silent.

After a latent period of many years features of the chronic infection appear, notably damage to Auerbach's plexus with resulting dilatation of various parts of the alimentary canal, especially the colon and oesophagus, 'mega' disease. Dilatation of the bile ducts and bronchi are also recognised sequelae. Chronic low-grade myocarditis and damage to conducting fibres cause a cardiomyopathy characterised by cardiac dilatation, arrhythmias, partial or complete heart block and sudden death. Autoimmune processes may be responsible for much of the damage. There are geographical variations of the basic pattern of disease.

Diagnosis

T. cruzi may be seen in a blood film in the acute illness. In chronic disease it may be recovered by xenodiagnosis in which infection free, laboratory-bred, reduviid bugs are fed on the patient; subsequently the hind gut or faeces of the bug is examined for parasites. Complement fixation, direct agglutination and fluorescent antibody tests are positive in 95% of cases.

Management

Nifurtimox is given orally. The dose, which has to be carefully supervised to minimise toxicity while preserving parasiticidal activity, is for those under 10 years, 15–20 mg/kg; 10–17 years, 12.5–15 mg/kg; over 17 years 8–10 mg/kg for 90 days. Cure rates of 80% in acute disease and 90% of chronic disease are obtained, but established tissue damage is not reversed. Side-effects include anorexia, vomiting and epigastric pain; insomnia, headache, vertigo and excitability; myalgia and arthralgia; peripheral neuropathy. Surgery may be needed for 'mega' disease.

Prevention

Preventive measures include improving housing and destruction of reduviid bugs by spraying of houses with chlorinated hydrocarbon insecticides. Blood taken for transfusion in endemic areas is treated with gentian violet. Long-term resolution requires better housing.

TOXOPLASMOSIS

Toxoplasmosis is a world-wide infection caused by *Toxoplasma gondii*. Transmission from a mother infected during pregnancy to the fetus causes congenital toxoplasmosis. Infection after birth occurs from the ingestion of cysts excreted in the faeces of infected cats or from eating undercooked beef or lamb. Immuno-compromised patients are particularly at risk.

Pathology

In the congenital form of the disease the organism is widespread in the central nervous system, eyes, heart, lungs and adrenals. If the infant survives, the parasite soon disappears from most organs except the central nervous system and retina. The brain shows areas of necrosis with cyst formation and patchy calcification; the spinal cord may be similarly affected. The organism commonly invades lymph nodes and spleen in the acquired disease and less commonly liver and myocardium.

Clinical features

The manifestations in congenital infections are mainly cerebral. There may be hydrocephalus or microcephaly associated with convulsions, tremors or paralysis. Radiological examination may show patches of calcification in the brain. Microphthalmos, nystagmus and choriodoretinitis are common. The CSF is often xanthochromic with increased protein and mononuclear cells. An enlarged liver, jaundice, thrombocytopoenia and purpura may also occur. Congenital infections are usually fatal, and if the child survives it is frequently disabled and blind.

Many acquired infections are symptomless. In the acute form there may be pneumonia with fever, cough, generalised aches and pains, profound malaise, a maculopapular rash and rarely jaundice and myocarditis. More chronic infections are often afebrile and there may be only enlargement of the lymph nodes with a lymphocytosis showing atypical mononuclear cells similar to those present in infectious mononucleosis. Toxoplasmosis is a cause of choroidoretinitis and uveitis in adults.

Latent toxoplasmosis may reactivate and cause encephalitis and necrosis of brain in immunocompromised patients. Seronegative recipients of organ grafts may acquire the disease from seropositive donors.

Diagnosis

Serological tests are of value. Antibodies detectable by fluorescence or the dye test appear early in the disease and persist for years. Complement-fixing antibodies appear and decline more quickly. A rise in titre or IgM antibodies indicates acute infection. Antibodies may not be detectable in adult ocular toxoplasmosis. Antibodies persisting in an infant beyond 6 months of age imply congenital toxoplasmosis. Biopsy material from a lymph node may be inoculated into mice, or show characteristic histological changes. Toxoplasma may be found in CSF of immunocompromised patients.

Management

Most patients with acquired toxoplasmosis do not require specific therapy as the infection usually resolves spontaneously. Patients for whom treatment is essential include infants, the immunosuppressed and those with eye involvement. A combination of sulphadimidine 1 g 6-hourly and pyrimethamine in a single loading dose of 75 mg followed by 25 mg daily, both for 4 weeks, is given together with folic acid 10 mg daily. Blood count is monitored weekly.

Toxoplasmosis and pregnancy
A sero-negative woman who acquires toxoplasmosis during pregnancy, or who sero-converts, is at risk of producing a damaged fetus, especially if infection takes place in the first trimester; termination should be considered. Those who are sero-positive before becoming pregnant do not risk fetal damage.

DISEASES DUE TO HELMINTHS

Infections caused by the commoner helminths, or worms, are described in this section (see the information box below).

ZOOLOGICAL CLASSES WHICH PARASITISE MAN

- Trematodes or flukes
- Cestodes or tapeworms
- Nematodes or roundworms

Much morbidity is caused in the tropics by helminths and they are an important cause of imported disease in temperate countries.

The only prevalent parasitic helminth of humans in Britain is the nematode *Enterobius (Oxyuris) vermicularis* or threadworm. Other worms which may be acquired in Britain include the roundworms *Ascaris lumbricoides, Toxocara canis, Trichuris trichiura* (whipworm) *Trichinella spiralis, Taenia saginata* (beef tapeworm), *Echinococcus granulosus* causing hydatid disease, and *Fasciola hepatica*, the endemic fluke of sheep.

Many helminths have a complicated life cycle, often involving one or more intermediate host. Only *Strongyloides stercoralis* can complete its life cycle within man. Disease may be caused by invasive larval stages (e.g. tropical pulmonary eosinophilia), adult worms (e.g. hookworms) or their progeny, either eggs (e.g. schistosomiasis) or microfilariae (e.g. onchocerciasis). Adult worms may be present in the body before, or without, producing disease. Sometimes larval stages that normally develop in intermediate hosts cause disease in man (e.g. cysticercosis). Man may also suffer from invasion by larval stages of worms that normally only infect other animals (e.g. hydatid disease).

DISEASES DUE TO TREMATODES (FLUKES)

SCHISTOSOMIASIS (BILHARZIASIS)

Schistosomiasis is one of the most important causes of morbidity in the tropics and is being spread by irrigation schemes. Schistosome eggs have been found in Egyptian mummies dated 1250 BC.

There are three species of the genus *Schistosoma* which commonly cause disease in man *S. haematobium, S. mansoni* and *S. japonicum. S. haematobium* was discovered by Theodor Bilharz in Cairo in 1861 and the genus is sometimes called *Bilharzia* and the disease bilharziasis. The ovum is passed in the urine or faeces of infected individuals and gains access to fresh water where the ciliated miracidium inside it is liberated and enters its intermediate host, a species of fresh water snail, in which it multiplies. Large numbers of fork-tailed cercarie are then liberated into the water where they may survive for 2 to 3 day. Cercariae can penetrate the skin or the mucous membrane of the mouth of their definitive host, man. They transform into schistosomu-lae and moult as they pass through the lungs and are carried by the blood stream to the liver and so to the portal vein where they mature (Fig. 5.14). The male worm is up to 20 mm in length and the more slender cylindrical female, usually enfolded longitudinally by the male, is rather longer. Within 4–6 weeks of infection they migrate to the venules draining the pelvic viscera where the females deposit ova. The eggs of *S. haematobium* pass mainly through the walls of the bladder and rectum. The eggs of *S. mansoni* and *S. japonicum* pass mainly through the lower bowel wall or are carried to the liver.

Pathology

The pathological changes and symptoms depend on species and stage of infection (Table 5.33). Penetration of the skin by schistosomes not pathogenic in man in, for example, Scotland can produce a similar rash. Most of the disease is due to the passage of eggs through mucosa and to the granulomatous reaction to eggs deposited in tissues. Eggs of *S. haematobium* and of the other two species after the development of portal hypertension, may reach the lungs. The most serious consequence, though rare, of the ectopic deposition of eggs is transverse myelitis and paraplegia. Granulomas are composed of macrophages, eosinophils, epithelioid and giant cells around an ovum. Later there is fibrosis and eggs calcify, often in sufficient numbers to become radiologically visible.

S. haematobium infections also affect rectum, seminal

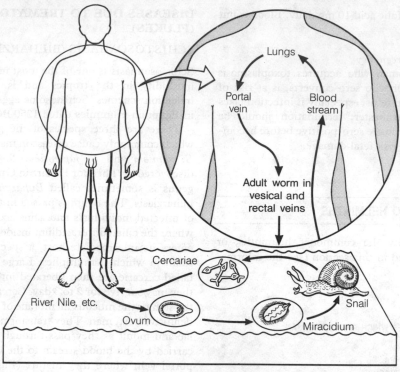

Fig. 5.14 Schistosoma. Life cycle.

vesicles, vagina, cervix and fallopian tubes. *S. japonicum* causes severe liver disease.

Clinical features

Early infection

Occasionally there may be itching at the site of cercarial penetration lasting 1–2 days. After a symptom-free period of 3–5 weeks allergic manifestations may develop such as urticaria, eosinophilia, fever, muscle aches, abdominal pain, splenomegaly, headaches, cough and sweating. Patches of pneumonia may be present. These allergic phenomena (Katayama syndrome) may be severe in infections with *S. mansoni* and *S. japonicum* but are rare with *S. haematobium*. The features subside after 1–2 weeks and for 2 or 3 months there may be no further symptoms. Further symptoms depend upon the deposition of eggs, the intensity of infection, and the species of infecting schistosome.

Table 5.33 Pathogenesis of schistosomiasis

Stage	Time	*S. haematobium*	*S. mansoni* and *S. japonicum*
Cercarial penetration	Days	Papular dermatitis at site of penetration	
Larval migration and maturation	Weeks	Pneumonitis, myositis, hepatitis, fever, 'serum sickness', eosinophilia, seroconversion	
Egg deposition:			
Early	Months	Cystitis haematuria	Colitis, granulomatous hepatitis, acute portal hypertension
		Ectopic granulomatous lesions; skin, CNS, etc.	
		Immune complex glomerulonephritis	
Late	Years	Fibrosis and calification of ureters, bladder, bacterial infection, calculi hydronephrosis, carcinoma	Colonic polyposis and strictures periportal fibrosis, portal hypertension
		Pulmonary granulomas and pulmonary hypertension	

Schistosomiasis haematobium

Man is the only natural host of *S. haematobium* which is highly endemic in Egypt, the east coast of Africa and the adjacent islands and occurs throughout most of Africa, in Iran, Iraq, Syria, Yemen, South Africa, Lebanon and Israel. It also occurs in Turkey, Cyprus and in solitary foci in Portugal and the Maharashtra State of India.

Clinical features

Painless terminal haematuria is usually the first and commonest symptom. Frequency of micturition follows, due to the contracted fibrosed or calcified bladder. Pain is often felt in the iliac fossa or in the loin and radiates to the groin. In advanced disease, pyelonephritis, hydronephrosis or pyonephrosis may lead to hypertension or uraemia. Disease of the seminal vesicles may lead to haemospermia. Females may be sterile and schistosomal lesions of the cervix may be mistaken for cancer. Intestinal symptoms may follow involvement of the bowel wall.

The severity of *S. haematobium* infection varies greatly, and many with a light infection suffer little. However, as adult worms can live for 20 years or more and lesions may progress, these patients should always be treated (p. 168).

Schistosomiasis mansoni

Man is the only natural host of importance although the infection is also found in baboons. *S. mansoni* is endemic in the Nile Delta and Libya, Southern Sudan, East Africa continuing as far south as the Transvaal and in West Africa from Senegal and Gambia to Cameroun, throughout Zaire and also in the Arabian peninsula. It is found in Venezuela, Brazil and in the West Indian Islands of the lesser Antilles, Puerto Rico and Dominica.

Clinical features

Characteristic symptoms begin 2 months or later after infection. They may be slight, no more than malaise, or consist of abdominal pain and frequent stools which contain blood-stained mucus. With severe advanced disease increased discomfort from rectal polypi may be experienced. The early hepatomegaly is reversible but portal hypertension may cause massive splenomegaly, fatal haematemesis from oesophageal varices, or progressive ascites. Jaundice and hepatic failure are uncommon. *S. mansoni* infections predispose to the carriage of Salmonella.

Schistosomiasis japonicum

The adult worm infects, in addition to man, the dog,

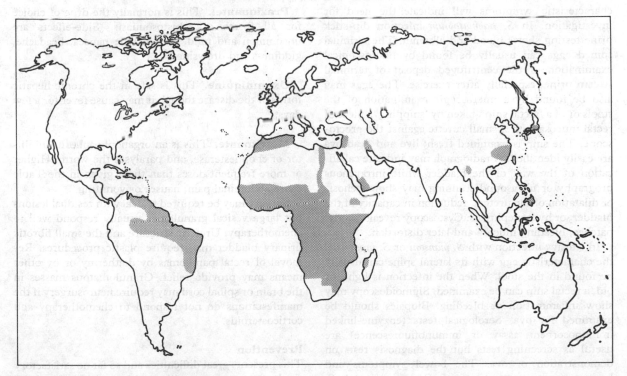

Fig. 5.15 Geographical distribution of schistosomiasis.

rat, field mouse, water buffalo, ox, cat, pig, horse and sheep. *S. japonicum* is prevalent in the Yellow River and Yangste-Kiang basins in China where the infection is a major public health problem. It also has a focal distribution in Japan, the Philippines, Celebes, and Vietnam. A related parasite *S. mekongi* occurs in Laos, Thailand and the Shan States of Burma.

Pathology

The pathology of *S. japonicum* is similar to that of *S. mansoni* but as this worm produces more eggs the lesions tend to be more extensive and widespread. The small bowel as well as the large may be affected, and hepatic fibrosis with splenic enlargement is usual. Deposition of eggs or worms in the central nervous system, especially in the brain, causes symptoms of cerebral irritation or compression in about 5% of infections. Evidence of cerebral involvement includes epilepsy, hemiplegia, blindness and paraplegia.

Clinical features

These resemble those of severe infection with *S. mansoni*.

Diagnosis

A history of residence in an endemic area with characteristic symptoms will indicate the need for investigation. In *S. haematobium* infection dip-stick urine testing shows blood and albumin. The terminal spined eggs can usually be found by microscopical examination of the centrifuged deposit of terminal stream urine, especially after exercise. The eggs may also be found by a microscopic examination of the stools or of a 'rectal snip', taken by 'snipping' a piece of rectal mucosa with a small curette against the proctoscope. The snip is examined fresh; live and dead ova are easily identified. A radiograph may indicate calcification of the wall of the bladder while intravenous urography or ultrasound scanning may show stenosis or dilatation of the ureters, reduction in capacity of the bladder, or hydronephrosis. Cystoscopy reveals 'sandy' patches, bleeding mucosa and later distortion.

In a heavy infection with *S. mansoni* or *S. japonicum* the characteristic egg with its lateral spine can usually be found in the stool. When the infection is light, or old, a rectal snip can be examined. Sigmoidoscopy may show inflammation or bleeding. Biopsies should be examined for ova. Serological tests (enzyme-linked immunosorbent assay or immunofluorescence) are useful as screening tests but the diagnosis rests on demonstration of ova. The bowel symptoms and barium enema appearances of *S. mansoni* and *S.*

japonicum infection may resemble those of amoebiasis or a neoplasm of the large bowel.

Management

The object of specific treatment is to kill the adult schistosomes and so stop egg laying. It may not be possible or desirable to kill all adult worms by mass treatment campaigns in communities where reinfection is likely, but a reduction in egg output of around 90% is often achieved which significantly reduces morbidity, and possibly transmission without impairing what little acquired immunity there may be. Details of the drugs used are given in Table 5.34.

Table 5.34 Drugs used in the treatment of schistosomiasis

Infection	Praziquantel*	Oxamniquine	Metrifonate
S. mansoni	30 mg/kg twice in one day	15 mg/kg b.d. for 2 days	Not useful
S. japonicum	40 mg/kg once		Not useful
S. haematobium	40 mg/kg once	Not useful	70.5 mg/kg every 2 wks × 3

*Doses quoted give cure rates of about 90% and reduce egg excretion by over 99%, and are used in mass campaigns and in primary health care centres. A dose of 10 mg/kg t.d.s. × 3 days gives a cure rate of virtually 100% for all three species.

Praziquantel. This is normally the drug of choice for all forms of schistosomiasis. Side-effects are uncommon and mild, and include nausea, headache, giddiness and drowsiness.

Oxamniquine. This is safe in the chronic hepatic forms of the disease though it may cause fever for a few days.

Metrifonate. This is an organophosphorus inhibitor of cholinesterase, and paralyses the worm. Higher or more frequent doses than those given in the Table cause abdominal pain, nausea or vomiting.

Surgery may be required to deal with residual lesions but large vesical granulomas usually respond well to chemotherapy. Ureteric stricture and the small fibrotic urinary bladder may require plastic procedures. Removal of rectal papillomas by diathermy or by other means may provide relief. Granulomatous masses in the brain or spinal cord may require neurosurgery if the manifestations do not respond to chemotherapy and corticosteroids.

Prevention

This presents great difficulties and so far no satisfactory single means of controlling schistosomiasis has been established. The life cycle is terminated if the ova in urine or faeces are not allowed to contaminate fresh water containing the snail host. The provision of latrines and of a safe water supply, however, remains a major problem in rural areas throughout the tropics. In the case of *S. japonicum*, moreover, there are so many hosts besides man that the proper use of latrines would be of little avail. Mass treatment of the population helps against *S. haematobium* and *S. mansoni* but this method has so far had little success with *S. japonicum*. Attack on the intermediate host, the snail, presents many difficulties and has not on its own proved successful on any scale.

Personal protection. Contact with infected water must be avoided. Accidental immersion or contact should be followed by a shower and vigorous towelling. Storage of water, free of snails, for three days will usually kill cercariae.

PARAGONIMIASIS (ENDEMIC HAEMOPTYSIS)

There are several species of the flukes of the genus *Paragonimus* which may affect man, the commonest being *P. westermani*. The adult flukes measuring 10×6 mm live in small 'nests' in the lung and elsewhere. The sputum contains ova, which may be expectorated or swallowed and passed in the faeces. Myracidia emerge in water from these eggs and seek the first intermediate host, a freshwater snail. Larvae emerging from the snail encyst as metacercariae in freshwater crabs or crayfish. Man or certain other mammals become infected if they eat these crustacea raw or inadequately cooked. Human infections are most frequent in the Far East but there are also endemic foci in South America, West Africa, Somalia and India.

Pathology
The adults lie in cysts up to 1 cm in diameter, situated chiefly in the lung and containing reddish-brown fluid. There are seldom more than 20 such cysts present. In heavy infections, cysts may also be present in the pleural or peritoneal cavities, in the brain, muscles, skin or elsewhere.

Clinical features
The first symptoms are slight fever, cough and the expectoration of brown or black sputum. Occasionally there are bouts of frank haemoptysis with severe pain in the chest. Increasing clinical signs in the chest may simulate pneumonia or pulmonary tuberculosis which

may coexist. When the parasites lodge in the abdomen there may be symptoms of enteritis or hepatitis. If they settle in the abdominal wall they may produce sinuses which discharge through the skin. Cysts in the central nervous system may cause signs of cerebral irritation, encephalitis or myelitis. The disease may be very chronic as the adult worms may survive for 20 years.

Diagnosis
Ova may be found on microscopic examination of the faeces, sputum or a discharge. The radiological appearances of affected lungs are variable but the lesions are usually situated close to the pleural surfaces. Extrapulmonary lesions are diagnosed by biopsy.

Management
Praziquantel is given in a dose of 25 mg/kg twice daily for 2 days orally. Lesions localised to or maximal in one lobe of a lung may be treated surgically.

Prevention
In an endemic area crab or crayfish should not be eaten unless adequately cooked. Immersion of crustaceans in wine, vinegar or brine does not kill the parasites.

LIVER FLUKES

Table 5.35 sets out the main features of the disease caused by flukes which infect the bile ducts of man. In the Far East and S.E. Asia, liver flukes are an important cause of ill-health. Severe acute infections cause anorexia, abdominal pain, diarrhoea, eosinophilia and increased serum levels of liver enzymes. Chronic infections cause recurrent febrile jaundice from cholangitis, and rarely cirrhosis and biliary carcinoma. Many people with light infections remain symptom free.

FASCIOLOPSIASIS

Fasciolopsis buski is the largest fluke to infect man. The adults 2–7.5 cm long, inhabit the small intestine of man, pigs and dogs. The infection is common in Central and S. China and among Chinese in S.E. Asia. It is spread from ova passed in the faeces into water. The intermediate hosts are snails. Man becomes infected by ingesting metacercariae encysted on water plants particularly when they are peeled with the teeth.

Clinical features
Light infections are symptomless. Heavy infections give rise to epigastric pain and loose motions. Very heavy infections may be fatal. The diagnosis is made by detecting ova or adult flukes in the faeces.

Table 5.35 Diseases caused by flukes in the bile ducts

Disease	Clonorchiasis	Opisthorciasis	Fascioliasis
Parasite	Clonorchis sinensis	Opisthorcis felineus	Fasciola hepatica
Other mammalian hosts	Dogs, cats, pigs	Dogs, cats, foxes, pigs	Sheep, cattle
Mode of spread	Ova in faeces into water	As for C. sinensis	Ova in faeces on to wet pasture
1st intermediate host	Snails	Snails	Snails
2nd intermediate host	Freshwater fish	Freshwater fish	Encysts on vegetation
Geographical distribution	Far East, esp. S. China	Far East, esp. N.E. Thailand	Cosmopolitan incl. Britain
Pathology	E. coli cholangitis, abscesses, biliary carcinoma	As for C. sinensis	Toxaemia, cholangitis, eosinophilia
Symptoms	Often symptom-free, recurrent jaundice	As for C. sinensis	Obscure fever, tender liver, may be ectopic subcut, fluke
Diagnosis	Ova in stool or duodenal aspirate	As for C. sinensis	As for C. sinensis also immunofluorescence
Prevention	Cook fish	Cook fish	Avoid contaminated watercress
Treatment	Praziquantel 25 mg/kg 8-hourly for 2 days	As for C. sinensis but 1 day only	Bithionol 30 mg/kg daily for 10–15 days*

*In UK available from the Hospital of Tropical Diseases, London. In USA from the Centres of Disease Control, Atlanta, Georgia.

Management
Praziquantel is given in a single dose of 25 mg/kg.

Prevention
This is by the proper disposal of faeces. Edible water plants can be made safe by immersing them in boiling water.

DISEASES DUE TO CESTODES (TAPEWORMS)

Cestodes are ribbon-shaped worms which inhabit the intestinal tract. They have no alimentary system and absorb nutrients through the segmental surface. The anterior end, or scolex, is provided with suckers for attachment to the host. From the scolex arises a series of progressively developing segments, the proglottides, which when shed may continue to show active movements. Cross-fertilisation takes place between segments. Ova, present in large numbers in mature proglottides, remain viable for weeks and during this period they may be consumed by the intermediate host. Larvae liberated from the ingested ova pass into the tissues.

Man acquires tapeworm by eating undercooked beef infected with Cysticercus bovis, the larval stage of Taenia saginata (beef tapeworm), undercooked pork containing Cysticercus cellulosae, the larval stage of T. solium (pork tapeworm), or undercooked fresh water fish containing larvae of Diphyllobothrium latum (fish tapeworm). Usually only one adult tapeworm is present in the gut but up to 10 have been reported. The lifecycles of Diphylloboth-

rium mansoni, Dipylidium caninum and Hymenolepsis nana are different (Table 5.36). Echinococcus granulosus is a tapeworm of dogs.

TAENIA SAGINATA
This worm may be several metres long. The scolex, the size of a pin head, has four suckers; mature segments 1.3 cm × 1 cm, contain a central stemmed uterus with lateral branches which are easily seen if the segments are left in water for 24 hours. The ova of both T. saginata and T. solium are indistinguishable microscopically.

Clinical features
Infection with T. saginata occurs in all parts of the world, including Britain. The adult worm produces little or no intestinal upset in human beings, but knowledge of its presence, by noting segments in the faeces or on underclothing, may distress the patient. Ova may be found in the stool.

Management
Praziquantel is the drug of choice. In a single dose of 10 mg/kg.

Prevention
This depends on efficient meat inspection and the thorough cooking of beef.

Table 5.36   Essential features of the less common tapeworm infections of man

Species	Geography	Definitive host	Intermediate host(s)	Stage and site in man	Clinical features
Multiceps multiceps	E + S Africa	Dog	Sheep	Larval cysts/brain	CNS
Diphyllobothrium latum	Scandinavia Asia	Fish eating mammals	Cyclops Fish Diaptomus	Adult worm/gut	Nil or megaloblastic anaemia
Diphyllobothrium mansoni	Africa Far East	Cats and dogs	Cyclops, frogs	Sparaganum	Subcutaneous swellings
Dipylidium caninum	World-wide	Dogs and cats	Flea	Adult worm/gut	Ova in faeces
Hymenolepis nana	World-wide	Man	None	Adult worm/gut	Ova in faeces

Treatment of intestinal worms is with praziquantel 20 mg/kg once, or niclosamide (1 g repeated after 2 h). Treatment of larval cysts and sparganosis is surgical.

TAENIA SOLIUM AND CYSTICERCOSIS

T. solium, the pork tapeworm, is common in Central Europe, South Africa, South America and in parts of Asia. It is not so large as *T. saginata*. The scolex has, in addition to suckers, two circular rows of hooklets anterior to the suckers. The adult worm is found only in man following the eating of undercooked pork containing cysticerci.

Human cysticercosis

This results from ova being swallowed or gaining access to the human stomach by regurgitation from the person's own adult worm (Fig. 5.16). The larvae are liberated from eggs in the stomach, penetrate the intestinal mucosa and are carried to many parts of the body where they develop and form cysticerci. Common locations are the subcutaneous tissue and skeletal muscles.

Clinical features

When superficially placed, cysts can be palpated under the skin or mucosa as pea-like ovoid bodies. Here they cause few or no symptoms, and will eventually die and become calcified.

Equally common is infection in the central nervous system. Heavy brain infections, especially in children, may cause features of encephalitis. More commonly, however, cerebral signs do not occur until the larvae die, 5–20 years later. Epilepsy, personality changes, staggering gait or signs of internal hydrocephalus are the most common features.

Diagnosis

Calcified cysts in muscles can be recognised radiologically. In the brain, however, less calcification takes place and larvae are only occasionally demonstrated

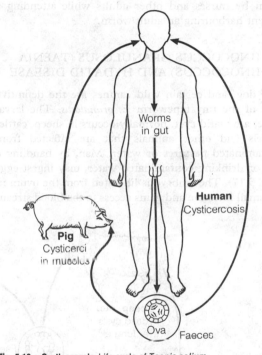

Fig. 5.16   **Cysticercosis.** Life cycle of *Taenia solium*.

radiologically but usually by computer tomography. Epileptic fits starting in adult life should suggest the possibility of cysticercosis if the patient has lived in an endemic area. The subcutaneous tissue should be palpated and any nodule excised for histology. Radiological examination of the skeletal muscles for calcified cysts must be made and repeated after intervals of 6 months, if at first negative.

Management

Adult *T. solium* can be destroyed by praziquantel or

niclosamide (Table 5.36). Praziquantel improves the prognosis of cerebral cysticercosis; the dose is 50 mg/kg in 3 divided doses daily for 10 days. Prednisone, 10 mg every 8 hours is also given for 14 days, starting one day before the praziquantel. In addition antiepileptic drugs should be given (p. 857) until the reaction in the brain has subsided. Operative intervention is indicated for hydrocephalus.

Prevention

Prevention of *T. solium* infection consists in cooking pork well before it is eaten. Cysticercosis is avoided if food is not contaminated by ova or segments. Patients with pork tapeworm probably acquire cysticercosis by ingesting ova from contaminated fingers, rather than from regurgitation of segments. Great care must be taken by nurses and other adults while attending a patient harbouring an adult worm.

ECHINOCOCCUS GRANULOSUS (TAENIA ECHINOCOCCUS) AND HYDATID DISEASE

The dog, and certain wild canines are the definitive host of the tiny tapeworm *E. granulosus*. The larval stage, a hydatid cyst, normally occurs in sheep, cattle, camels and other animals that are infected from contaminated pastures or water. Man, by handling a dog or drinking contaminated water, may ingest eggs (Fig. 5.17). The embryo is liberated from the ovum in the small intestine and gains access to the blood stream

and thus to the liver. The resultant cyst grows very slowly. It may calcify or may rupture giving rise to multiple cysts. The disease is common in the Middle East and North and East Africa, Australia and Argentina. Foci of infection persist in rural Wales and Scotland. A variant, *E. multilocularis* which has a cycle between foxes and voles, causes a similar but more severe infection, 'alveococcosis' which invades the liver like cancer.

Clinical features

A hydatid cyst is typically acquired in childhood and it may, after growing for some years, cause pressure symptoms. These vary, depending on the organ or tissue involved. In nearly 75% of patients with hydatid disease the right lobe of the liver is invaded and contains a single cyst. In others a cyst may be found in lung, bone, brain or elsewhere.

Diagnosis

The diagnosis depends on the clinical, radiological and ultrasound findings in a patient who has lived in close contact with dogs in an endemic area. Complement-fixation, immunofluorescent tests and enzyme-linked immunosorbent assay are positive in 70–90% of patients.

Management

Hydatid cysts should be excised wherever possible. Great care is taken to avoid spillage and cavities are

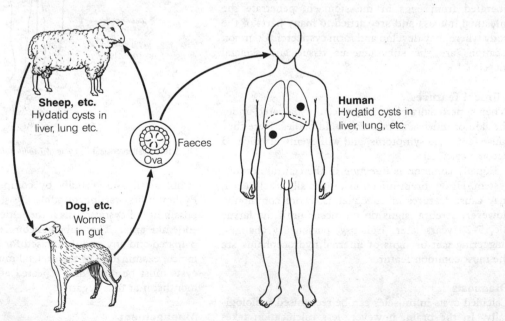

Fig. 5.17 Hydatid disease. Life cycle of *Echinococcus granulosus*.

Sheep, etc.
Hydatid cysts in liver, lung etc.

Ova Faeces

Dog, etc.
Worms in gut

Human
Hydatid cysts in liver, lung, etc.

sterilised with 0.5% silver nitrate or 2.7% sodium chloride. Albendazole (400 mg b.d. for 1–3 months) has been used for inoperable disease, and to reduce the infectivity of cysts preoperatively. Praziquantel 10 mg/kg t.d.s for 2 weeks kills protoscolices perioperatively.

Prevention
Prevention is difficult in situations where there is a close association with dogs and sheep. Personal hygiene, satisfactory disposal of carcases, meat inspection and deworming of dogs can greatly reduce the prevalence of disease.

OTHER TAPEWORMS
There are many other cestodes whose adult or larval stages may infect man, the commonest of which are summarised in Table 5.36.

DISEASES DUE TO NEMATODES (ROUNDWORMS)
Nematode infections of man may be divided into three groups:

Intestinal nematodes
The commonest that cause disease are *Enterobius vermicularis*, *Ascaris lumbricoides*, *Trichuris trichiura*, *Necator americanus*, *Ancylostoma duodenale*, *Strongyloides stercoralis* and *Capillaria philippinesis*. Others, notably *Trichostrongylus*, are not pathogenic.

Adult male and female worms live in the lumen of the gut and do not normally invade tissues. They often have complex life cycles and may cause a syndrome of fever, cough and eosinophila during the stage of larval invasion. Eggs or larvae are passed in the faeces and the worm does not normally complete its life cycle in man. Strongyloides, however, behaves differently and is potentially dangerous.

Tissue-dwelling human nematodes
These are the filarial worms (*Wuchereria bancrofti*, *Brugia malayi*, *Loa loa*, *Onchocerca volvulus*, and some others with a more restricted distribution), and the guinea worm *Drancunculus medinensis*.

These worms have complex life cycles, with an intermediate host that is also a vector. Disease may be due to the presence of the adult worms or to their progeny, the microfilariae, which migrate in the blood or tissues, provoking a massive eosinophilia; but often the infection is long lived and well tolerated.

Nematodes of other animals
These may cause ectopic infections in man. The most important are *Toxocara canis*, *Ancylostoma basiliensis*, *Oesophagostomum* species, *Angiostrongylus cantonensis*, *Trichinella spiralis*, *Gnasthostoma spinigerum* and *Anisakis marina*.

The infective larvae of these worms are unable to 'home' to their normal site for development into adults, in their abnormal host. They may wander or may become trapped in a particular organ. They tend to provoke severe inflammatory reactions characterised by eosinophilic granulomas.

ENTEROBIUS VERMICULARIS (THREADWORM)
This helminth is common throughout the world, including Britain. It affects children especially. The male worm is 2–5 mm long and the female 8–13 mm. After the ova are swallowed, development takes place in the small intestine, but the adult worms are found chiefly in the colon.

Clinical features
The gravid female worm lays ova around the anus, and causes intense itching, especially at night. The ova are often carried to the mouth on the fingers and so reinfection takes place (Fig. 5.18). In females the genitalia may be involved. The adult worms may be seen moving on the buttocks or in the stool.

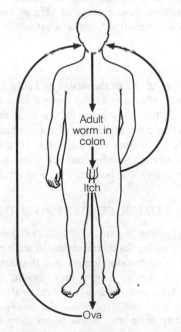

Adult worm in colon

Itch

Ova

Fig. 5.18 Threadworm. Life cycle of *Enterobius vermicularis*.

Table 5.37   Relative activity of drugs used for the common gut nematodes

	Ascaris	Hookworm	Enterobius	Trichuris	Strongyloides
Piperazine salts 100 mg/kg	+ + +	+	+ + +	−	−
Pyrantel pamoate 10 mg/kg	+ + +	+ +	+ + +	−	−
Oxantel pamoate 10 mg/kg	−	−	−	+ + +	−
Mebendazole 100 mg (any age)	+ +	+ +	+ + +	+ +	+
Albendazole 400 mg	+ +	+ +	+	+	+
Thiabendazole 25 mg/kg	(+ +)	(+ +)	(+ +)	(+)	+ + +
Levamisole 5 mg/kg	+ + +	+	+	−	−
Pyrvinium 5 mg/kg	+	−	+ + +	−	−

Size of a single dose is given. + = quite effective, + + = effective, + + + = very effective therapy; − = ineffective. Activities given in parenthesis indicate that the drug is not used for that species. Piperazine is cheap and safe, but with a limited range. Mebendazol given twice daily for 3 days is completely safe and eradicates most infections. Thiabendazole has a wide spectrum: it is absorbed and effective against many tissue-dwelling nematodes, but toxic, causing dizziness, headaches, anorexia, vomiting and drowsiness. A single dose antihelmintic is ideal for mass treatment and control schemes. Levamisole is the first choice for roundworms, and has a useful action against hookworms. A single dose of pyrantel pamoate and oxantel pamoate or of albendazole is used for multiple infections. (Adapted from Knight R 1982 Parasitic disease in man. Churchill Livingstone, Edinburgh.)

Diagnosis

Ova are detected by applying the adhesive surface of cellophane tape to the perianal skin in the morning. This is then examined on a glass slide under the microscope.

Management

A single dose of one of the drugs in Table 5.37 is given and repeated after 2 weeks to control auto-reinfection. Where infection constantly recurs in a family, each member should be treated with mebendazole 100 mg twice daily for 3 days repeated after 10 days. During this period all night clothes and bed linen are laundered and finger nails must be scrubbed before meals.

ASCARIS LUMBRICOIDES ('ROUNDWORM')

This pale-yellow worm is 20–35 cm long. Man is infected by eating food contaminated with mature ova. These hatch in the duodenum and the larvae migrate through the lungs, where they moult, ascend the bronchial tree and trachea and are swallowed. They mature in the small intestine. In heavy infections, larvae in the lung may cause pulmonary eosinophila (p. 383).

Clinical features

Adult worms commonly cause abdominal discomfort or colic. Sometimes a worm is vomited or passed per rectum. A tangled mass of worms may cause intestinal obstruction in children with severe infections. Heavy infestation will compete with the child for nourishment and contribute to malnutrition. Other complications include blockage of the bile or pancreatic duct and obstruction of the appendix by adult worms.

Diagnosis

The diagnosis is made microscopically by finding ova in the faeces or by observing an adult worm. A solely male infection is usually revealed only after the giving of an antihelminthic to a patient with an unexplained eosinophilia. Occasionally the worms are demonstrated radiographically by a barium examination.

Management

The appropriate drugs are listed in Table 5.37. Surgery is required if obstruction occurs and fails to respond to nasograstric suction and sedation; worms are 'milked' past the obstruction, or removed by enterostomy.

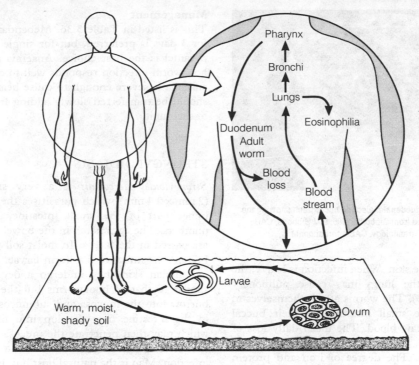

Fig. 5.19   Ancylostomiasis. Life cycle.

TRICHURIS TRICHIURA (WHIPWORM)

Infections with whipworm are common all over the world under unhygienic conditions. Infection takes place by the ingestion of earth or food contaminated with ova which have become infective after lying for 3 weeks or more in moist soil. The adult worm is 3–5 cm long and has a coiled anterior end resembling a whip. Whipworms inhabit the caecum, lower ileum, appendix, colon and anal canal.

Clinical features
There are usually no symptoms, but intense infections in children may cause persistent diarrhoea or rectal prolapse.

Diagnosis
The diagnosis is readily made by identifying ova in faeces.

Management
Treatment is with mebendazole in doses of 100 mg twice daily for 3–5 days or a single dose of oxantel (Table 5.37).

ANCYLOSTOMIASIS (HOOKWORM INFECTION)

Ancylostomiasis is caused by parasitisation of the small intestine with *Ancylostoma duodenale* or *Necator americanus*. It is one of the main causes of anaemia in the tropics. The adult hookworm is a greyish-white nematode about 1 cm long which lives, often in large numbers, in the duodenum and upper jejunum. Eggs are passed in the faeces. In warm, moist, shady soil the larvae develop and reach the filariform infective stage which penetrate human skin and are carried to the lungs (Fig. 5.19). After entering the alveoli they ascend the bronchi, are swallowed and develop in the small intestine, reaching maturity 4–7 weeks after infection.

Hookworm infection is widespread under insanitary conditions in the tropics and subtropics and used to be common in mines in Europe. *A. duodenale* is endemic in the Far East and Mediterranean coastal regions and is also present in Africa while *N. americanus* is endemic in West, East and Central Africa and Central and South America as well as in the Far East.

Pathology
The larvae may cause allergic inflammation at the site

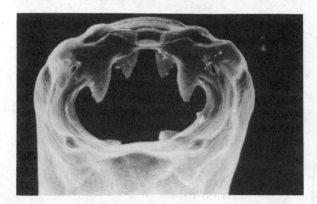

Fig. 5.20 Ancylostoma duodenale: electron micrograph showing the ventral teeth. (Reproduced from Gibbons, 1986, L M Gibbons, CAB International Institute of Parasitology, CAB International.)

of entry through the skin. When infection is heavy, the passage through the lungs may cause pulmonary eosinophilia (p. 383). The worms attach themselves to the mucosa of the small intestine by their buccal capsule and withdraw blood. The mean daily loss of blood from one *A. duodenale* is 0.15 ml and for *N. americanus* 0.03 ml. The degree of iron and protein deficiency which develops depends not only on the load of worms but also on the nutrition of the patient and especially on the iron stores. Thus, in a light infection there may be no anaemia. In the early stage of infection eosinophilia is common.

Clinical features
Dermatitis usually on the feet (ground itch) may be experienced at the time of infection. The passage of the larvae through the lungs in a heavy infection causes a paroxysmal cough with blood-stained sputum, associated with patchy pulmonary consolidation. When the worms have reached the small intestine, vomiting and epigastric pain resembling peptic ulcer disease, may ensue. Sometimes frequent loose stools are passed, the condition then resembling early sprue or giardiasis. Anaemia and hypoproteinaemia may develop in the undernourished. The mental and physical development of children may be retarded. There may be no symptoms in a well-nourished person with a light infection.

Diagnosis
The characteristic ovum can be recognised in the stool. If hookworms are present in numbers sufficient to cause anaemia, tests of the stool for occult blood will be positive and ova will be present in large numbers.

Management
This is listed in Table 5.36. Mebendazole twice daily for 3 days is preferred, but for single dose treatment pyrantel is the best choice. Anaemia associated with hookworm infection responds well to oral iron. When anaemia is severe enough to cause heart failure blood should be transferred slowly adding frusemide 20 mg to each unit.

STRONGYLOIDIASIS

Strongyloides stercoralis is a very small nematode (2 mm × 0.4 mm) which parasitises the mucosa of the upper part of the small intestine, often in large numbers. The eggs hatch in the bowel but only larvae are passed in the faeces. In moist soil they moult and become the infective filariform larvae. After penetrating human skin they undergo a development cycle similar to that of hookworms but the female worms burrow into the mucosa and submucosa. Some larvae in the intestine may develop into filariform larvae which may then penetrate the mucosa or the perianal skin and lead to auto-infection and a very persistent infection. Man is the natural host but dogs may also be infected. Strongyloidiasis occurs in the tropics and subtropics and is especially prevalent in the Far East.

Pathology
There may be a dermatitis at the time of entry of the larval worms. In the intestine female worms burrow into the mucosa and induce an inflammatory reaction; with heavy infections the mucosa may be severely damaged leading to malabsorption. Granulomatous changes, necrosis, and even perforation and peritonitis may occur. Eosinophilia commonly persists. Actively motile larvae are passed in the faeces. Immunosuppression may cause fatal systemic strongyloidiasis.

Clinical features
These are shown in the information box (p. 177).

Systemic strongyloidiasis occurs in association with immune suppression (intercurrent disease, HTLV1 infection, corticosteroids) and is rapidly fatal unless diagnosed and promptly treated.

Diagnosis
Motile larvae can be seen on microscopic examination of the faeces and occasionally in the sputum. Excretion is intermittent so repeated examinations or jejunal aspiration or a string test (p. 158) may be necessary. Filarial serology is positive in 15% of patients (p. 179).

CLINICAL FEATURES OF STRONGYLOIDIASIS

● Penetration of skin by infective larvae
    Itchy rash
● Presence of worms in gut
    Abdominal pain, diarrhoea, steatorrhoea, weight loss
● Allergic phenomena
    Urticarial plaques and papules, wheezing, arthralgia
● Auto-infection
    Transient itchy linear urticarial wheals across abdomen
    and buttocks (larva currens)
● Systemic (super-) infection
    Diarrhoea, pneumonia, meningo-encephalitis, death

Management

Thiabendazole is given orally in a dose of 25 mg/kg body weight twice daily for 2–4 days according to tolerance. A second course may be required. For systemic strongyloidiasis the drug is administered by nasogastric tube for a longer period.

CAPILLARIASIS

Infection with *Capillaria philippinensis* suddenly appeared as an epidemic in the Philippines in the 1960s and in Thailand. Freshwater fish are intermediate hosts.

Clinical features

Adult worms 2–4 mm long invade the jejunal mucosa, causing abdominal pain with severe diarrhoea and malabsorption.

Table 5.38 Pathology of filarial infections depends upon the site and stage of worms

Worm species	Adult worm	Microfilariae	
Wuchereria bancrofti and *Brugia malayi*	Lymphatic vessels +++	Blood,	Pulmonary capillaries ++
Loa Loa	Subcutaneous +	Blood +	
Onchocerca volvulus	Subcutaneous +	skin, +++	eye +++
Mansonella perstans	Retroperitoneal −	Blood −	
Mansonella streptocerca	Skin +	Skin ++	
Mansonella ozardi	Mesentery −	Blood −	

+++ = very severe
++ = severe
+   = quite severe
−   = not severe

Diagnosis

Eggs resembling those of *Trichuris* are passed in the faeces.

Management

Mortality is high in untreated subjects but mebendazole (200 mg b.d. for 2 weeks) is effective.

Prevention of intestinal nematode infections

Most of these worms are transmitted through contaminated soil or unwashed hands. Safe disposal of faeces, the provision of clean drinking water and strict personal hygiene form the basis of control. Mass treatment at yearly intervals is also useful (Table 5.37). Capillariasis is prevented by cooking fish.

FILARIASES

Several nematodes of the family *Filariidae* infect man. Larval stages are inoculated by biting flies, each specific to a particular filarial species. The larvae develop into adult worms (2–50 cm long) which, after mating, produce millions of microfilariae (170–320 microns long) that migrate in blood or skin. The life cycle is completed when the flies take up microfilaria while feeding on man. Man is normally the only host.

Disease is due to the host's immune response to the worms, particularly dying worms, and its pattern and severity vary with the site and stage of each species (Table 5.38). The worms are long lived; microfilariae survive 2–3 years and adult worms 10–15 years. The infections are chronic and worst in individuals constantly exposed to reinfection. Filarial infections cause the highest eosinophilia of all helminthic infections, and are normally diagnosed by the morphology of the microfilariae.

Bancroftian filariasis

Wuchereria bancrofti is conveyed to man by the bites of infected mosquitoes of a number of different species, the most common being *Culex fatigans*. The adult worms, 4–10 cm in length, live in the lymphatics, and the females produce microfilariae which at night circulate in large numbers in the peripheral blood. In the mosquito ingested microfilariae develop into infective larvae. As *Culex fatigans* bites at night the nocturnal periodicity of the microfilariae facilitates the spread of the infection. There is a non-periodic strain of *W. bancrofti* in some of the Pacific Islands maintained by mosquitoes which bite in the daytime. The microfilariae are chiefly in the capillaries in the lungs when not circulating in the peripheral blood and may cause pulmonary eosinophilia (p. 383). The infection is

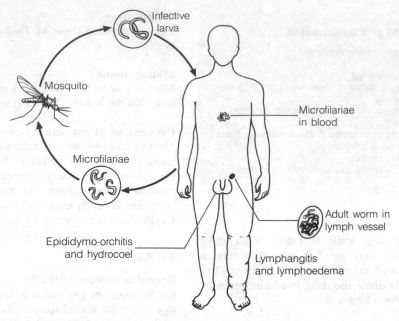

Fig. 5.21   Wuchereria bancrofti and Brugia malayi. Life cycle and pathogenesis of lymphatic filariasis.

widespread in tropical Africa, the North African coast, coastal areas of Asia, Indonesia and Northern Australia, South Pacific Islands, West Indies and also in North and South America.

Pathology
The presence of adult worms in the lymphatics causes allergic lymphangitis (Table 5.37). Recurrent episodes may lead to intermittent lymphatic obstruction and transient lymphoedema, which may later become permanent in the leg, arm, genitalia or breast; and hydrocoele. Obstructed lymphatics become dilated and tortuous and may rupture. Rupture into tissues leads to cellulitis, fibrosis and elephantiasis. Increased lymphatic pressure may cause retrograde flow or rupture, in turn causing chyluria, chylous ascites and chylous pleural effusions (Fig. 5.21). The incubation period is not less than 3 months.

Clinical features
There are bouts of fever accompanied by pain, tenderness and erythema along the course of inflamed lymphatic vessels. Inflammation of the spermatic cord, epididymitis and orchitis is common. The fever abates after a few days and the symptoms and signs subside.

Further attacks follow, temporary oedema becomes more persistant, and regional lymph nodes enlarge.

Progressive enlargement, coarsening, corrugation and fissuring of the skin and subcutaneous tissue with warty superficial excrescences develops gradually causing irreversible 'elephantiasis'. The scrotum may reach an enormous size. Chyluria and chylous effusions are milky and opalescent; on standing fat globules rise to the top. Eventually the adult worms may die but the lymphatics remain obstructed. The interval between infection and the onset of elephantiasis is usually not less than 10 years and elephantiasis develops only in association with repeated infections in highly endemic areas.

Diagnosis
In the earliest stages of lymphangitis the diagnosis is made on clinical grounds, supported by eosinophilia and sometimes by positive serology. Microfilariae appear in the blood at night after about a year from the time of infection and can be seen moving in a wet blood film or by microfiltration of a sample of lysed blood. They are usually present in hydrocoele fluid which may occasionally yield an adult filaria. By the time elephantiasis develops microfilariae become difficult to find. Calcified filariae may sometimes be demonstrable by radiography. An initial exaggeration of symptoms following the administration of diethylcarbamazine suggests a filarial infection.

Immunodiagnosis. Indirect fluorescence and enzyme-linked immunosorbent assay detect antibodies in over 95% of active cases and 70% of established elephantiasis. Cross-reactions occur in 15% of cases of strongyloides and 5% of other intestinal nematodes. The test becomes negative 1–2 years after cure. Intradermal tests of immediate hypersensitivity are positive and persist for life. None of these tests distinguishes between the different filarial infections.

Non-filarial elephantiasis. Usually affecting one or both legs; this occurs in certain geographical areas which are free from filariasis. It is attributable to damage to lymphatics by silicates absorbed from soil derived from volcanic rocks.

Management
Diethylcarbamazine kills microfilariae and adult worms. The dose is 9–12 mg/kg daily in 3 divided doses for 14 days orally. The full dose must be reached slowly, starting with 50 mg (one tablet) and doubling daily if no untoward allergic reactions ensue. This course may be repeated twice at intervals of 4–6 weeks. Antihistamines or corticosteroids may be required to control allergic phenomena. Plastic surgery may be indicated in established elephantiasis. Great relief can be obtained by removal of excess tissue but recurrences are probable unless new lymphatic drainage is established. Tight bandaging, or bed-rest with suspension or raising of the affected part or the nightly use of pneumatic stockings may control the swelling to some extent.

Prevention
Treatment of the whole population in endemic areas with diethylcarbamazine, 100 mg for adults (50 mg for children) 3 times daily for 7 days has reduced but not eliminated the infection. Children are given such a course on starting and before leaving school. This mass treatment should be combined with control of the vector by insecticides. Early chemotherapy prevents later elephantiasis. Individuals should avoid being bitten by mosquitoes (p. 155).

Brugia filariasis
Brugia malayi resembles *W. bancrofti* closely. The microfilariae usually exhibit nocturnal periodicity but a semiperiodic form, which may affect man, commonly infects animals. A similar filaria, *Brugia pahangi*, is found chiefly in animals but has been transmitted to man. It may be responsible for some cases of tropical pulmonary eosinophilia (p. 384). The vectors of *B. malayi* are mosquitoes mostly belonging to the genus *Mansonioides*. *B. malayi* is found in Indonesia, Borneo, Malaysia, Vietnam, South China, South India and Sri Lanka. A distinct, closely related, species, *B. timori* occurs in Timor.

The pathology, clinical manifestation treatment and personal prophylaxis are the same as for *W. bancrofti* except that elephantiasis is usually limited to the legs.

LOIASIS
Loiasis is caused by infection with the filaria *Loa loa*. The adults, 3–7 cm × 4 mm, parasitise chiefly the subcutaneous tissue of man. The larval microfilariae circulate harmlessly in the peripheral blood in the daytime. The vector is *Chrysops*, a day biting, forest dwelling, fly.

Pathology
The adult worms move harmlessly about in the subcutaneous tissues and other intestitial planes (Table 5.38). From time to time a short-lived, inflammatory, oedematous swelling (a *Calabar swelling*) is produced, presumably around an adult worm. Heavy infections, especially when treated, may cause encephalitis. The incubation period is commonly over a year but may be as short as 3 months.

Clinical features
The infection is often symptomless. The first sign is usually a Calabar swelling which is an irritating tense localised swelling that may be painful especially if it is near a joint. The swelling is generally on a limb; it measures a few centimetres in diameter but sometimes is more diffuse and extensive. It usually disappears after a few days but may persist for 2 or 3 weeks. A succession of such swellings may appear at irregular intervals, often in adjacent sites. Sometimes there is urticaria and pruritis elsewhere. Occasionally a worm may be seen wriggling under the skin, especially of an eyelid and may cross the eye under the conjunctiva, taking many minutes to do so. Severe unilateral headaches resembling migraine may be experienced when an adult worm moves in the retro-orbital tissues.

Diagnosis
This is made by demonstrating microfilariae in the blood, but they may not always be found in patients with Calabar swellings. Antifilarial antibodies are positive in 95% of patients and there is massive eosinophilia. Occasionally a calcified worm may be seen on a radiograph.

Management
Diethylcarbamazine (see above) is curative, gradually

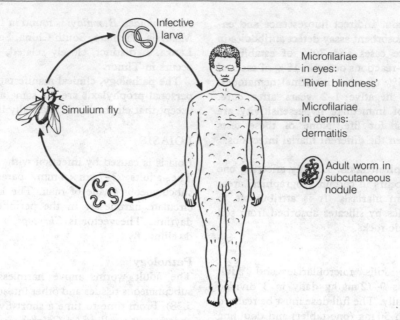

Fig. 5.22   Onchocerca volvulus. Life cycle and pathogenesis of onchocerciasis.

increased to a dose of 9–12 mg/kg daily which is continued for 21 days. Treatment may precipitate a severe reaction in patients with a heavy microfilaraemia characterised by fever, joint and muscle pain and encephalitis; these patients should be given steroid cover (p. 181).

Prevention
Protection is afforded by siting houses away from trees and by having dwellings wire-screened against the fly. Protective clothing and repellents are also useful. Treatment of the population with diethylcarbamazine will diminish the infective rate of the vector.

ONCHOCERCIASIS (RIVER BLINDNESS)

Onchocerciasis is the result of the infection by *Onchocerca volvulus*. Although only about 0.3 mm in diameter, the adult female may be as long as 50 cm; the male is 13 cm. The infection is conveyed by flies of the genus Simulium which inflict a painful bite. In West Africa the vector is *S. damnosum*, in Northern Nigeria also *S. bovis* and in East Africa and Zaire *S. neavei*. The flies breed in rapidly flowing well-aerated water, the larvae being attached to submerged vegetation, rocks or crabs. Adult flies bite during the daytime both inside and outside houses. Man is the only known definitive host.

Onchocerciasis is endemic in well-defined areas throughout tropical Africa, in Southern Arabia and Yemen and also in South Mexico, Guatemala, Colombia, Venezuela and Brazil. It is estimated that over 20 million people are infected. In parts of West and Central Africa it affects the whole adult population and blindness rates of 10% are common, reaching 35% in some parts of Ghana. Because of onchocerciasis huge tracts of fertile land lie virtually untilled, and individuals and communities are impoverished.

Pathology
Infective lavae of *O. volvulus* are introduced into the skin by the bite of an infected *Simulium*. The worms mature in 2–4 months and live for up to 17 years in small colonies in subcutaneous and connective tissues (Table 5.38). At sites of trauma, over bony prominences and around joints, fibrosis may form nodules around adult worms which otherwise cause no direct damage. Innumerable microfilariae, discharged by the female *O. volvulus*, move actively in these nodules, in the adjacent tissues and widely distributed in the skin and may invade the eye.

Live microfilariae elicit little tissue reaction, but dead microfilariae may cause severe allergic inflammation leading to hyaline necrosis and loss of collagen and elastin. Death of microfilariae in the eye causes conjunctivitis, sclerosing keratitis with pannus formation, iritis which may lead to glaucoma and cataract and, less commonly, choroidoretinitis and optic neuritis.

Clinical features

The infection may remain symptomless for months or years. The first symptom is usually itching, localised to one quadrant of the body and later becoming generalised and involving the eyes. Evanescent oedema of part or all of a limb in Europeans is an early sign, followed by papular urticaria spreading gradually from the site of infection. This is difficult to see on dark skins in which the commonest signs are papules excoriated by scratching, spotty hyperpigmentation from resolving inflammation and more chronic changes of a rough, thickened skin or inelastic wrinkled skin. Superficial lymph nodes enlarge and may hang down in folds of loose skin at the groins. Hydrocele, femoral hernias and scrotal elephantiasis occur. Firm subcutaneous nodules occur in chronic infection, (onchocercomas) which are palpable, 1 cm or more in diameter.

Eye disease is commonest in highly endemic areas and is associated with chronic heavy infections and nodules on the head. Early manifestations include itching, lacrimation, conjunctival injection and evidence of the features listed under pathology. Classically, 'snow flake' deposits are seen in the edges of the cornea.

Diagnosis

The finding of nodules or characteristic lesions of the skin or eyes, in a patient from an endemic area, associated with eosinophilia is suggestive. Aggravation of the dermatosis after a test dose of 50 mg of diethylcarbamazine supports the diagnosis. Skin snips or shavings, taken with a corneoscleral punch or scalpel blade from calf, buttock and shoulder are placed in saline under a cover slip on a microscope slide and examined after 4 hours. Microfilariae are seen wriggling free in all but the lightest infections. Slit lamp examination of the eye may reveal microfilariae moving in the anterior chamber of the eye, or trapped in the cornea. A nodule may be removed and incised, showing the coiled threadlike adult worm. Filarial antibodies may be detected in 95% of patients (p. 179).

Management

Ivermectin, in a single dose of 100–200 µg/kg, kills microfilariae and prevents their return for 9 months. It is non-toxic and does not trigger severe reactions. Diethylcarbamazine may be used if ivermectin is unavailable. It kills the microfilariae but is associated with a severe allergic reaction for the first few days of treatment. The itch increases, eye lesions are aggravated and there may be fever, painful joints, hypotension and respiratory distress. Only a small dose should be given initially, 25 mg on the first day, this being gradually increased as the drug is tolerated until, if possible, a dose of 9–12 mg/kg is reached. This dose is continued for 14 days. An antihistamine, such as chlorpheniramine maleate, may alleviate mild reactions but corticosteroids, locally as drops to the eyes and systemically, are needed in heavy infections or to control severe reactions. Prednisone 20–40 mg is given daily for a few days starting the day before treatment. Ideally the patient should be in bed for the first 24 hours of treatment.

Adult worms are killed by suramin (1 mg i.v. weekly for 5–6 doses). In endemic areas where reinfection is inevitable, and in patients with little or no eye involvement, repeated courses of diethylcarbamazine or long-term suppression with 50 mg daily may be preferred to the potential toxicity of suramin (Table 5.32). Palpable nodules should be excised.

Prevention

Mass treatment with ivermectin is under trial. Simulium can be destroyed in its larval stage by the application of insecticide to streams. Dimethylphthalate applied to skin or clothing will repel the fly for several hours. Long trousers, skirts and sleeves discourage the fly from biting.

OTHER FILARIASES

Mansonella perstans

This is transmitted by the midges *Culicoides austeni* and *C. grahami*. It is common throughout equatorial Africa as far south as Zambia, and also in Trinidad and parts of northern and eastern South America.

M. perstans has never been shown to cause disease but it may be responsible for a persistent eosinophilia and occasional allergic manifestations (Table 5.38). *M. perstans* is resistant to ivermectin and diethylcarbamazine and the infection may persist for many years.

Mansonella ozzardi

This is non-pathogenic and is found in the West Indies and South America.

Dracontiasis (Guinea worm infection)

The female *Dracunculus medinensis*, which measures over a metre in length and 0.9–1.7 mm in diameter, lives in the interstitial and subcutaneous tissues of man. The male worm, which is rarely seen, is only 2.5 cm long and dies earlier. Man is infected by ingesting a small crustacean, *Cyclops*, which inhabits the bottom of wells and ponds and which contains the infective larval stage of the worm.

Pathology

Ingested larvae mature and penetrate the intestinal wall and migrate through the connective tissues of the host. After 9–18 months the fully mature female surfaces under the skin, usually on the leg, where a vesicle is raised, ruptures and exposes the anterior end of the worm. The distended uterus ruptures and discharges its larvae externally. The worm is attracted to the surface by cooling, hence the larvae are likely to be expelled into water and complete the life cycle. Man is the most important host but *D. medinensis* has been found in dogs and cats.

The disease can be extremely disabling and is especially liable to affect women and children who collect water at water-holes or farmers at the beginning of the rains and thus seriously interfere with planting. It is found in sub-Saharan Africa, Egypt, the Arabian peninsula, Iran, Afghanistan and in parts of Pakistan and India.

Clinical features

The adult may sometimes be felt beneath the skin. Some hours before the head of the worm emerges from the skin there is painful, hot, local inflammation which vesiculates. It takes 3–4 weeks for the larvae to be discharged, during which time the ulcer persists and there is a variable degree of pain and local cellulitis, especially if it is close to an ankle or knee. There will be a marked allergic inflammation if the worm dies or is broken during extraction. The patient is immobilised by pain and swelling. Secondary infection is common and may cause cellulitis, arthritis or septicaemia. Tetanus is a well-recognised complication. Multiple infections may occur and reactions around aberrant worms may cause serious lesions, exceptionally spinal-cord compression.

Diagnosis

This is usually easy from the appearance of a vesicle, the protrusion of a worm and the recognition of the discharged larvae. A radiograph may show calcified worms.

Management

Traditionally the protruding worm has been extracted by winding it out gently over several days on a match stick. Niridazole in doses of 25 mg/kg daily in 2 divided doses for 10 days, or mebendazole 100 mg b.d. for 7 days, may reduce inflammation and aid the extraction of the worm. Antibiotics for secondary infection and prophylaxis of tetanus are also required.

Prevention

The provision of a satisfactory water supply will eradicate the infection. Where this is impracticable, wells and ponds may be protected or treated chemically to kill *Cyclops*.

TOXOCARA CANIS

This is a common intestinal worm of dogs. The ova are passed in the animal's faeces. Children who are in close contact with infected puppies are particularly liable to ingest ova of *Toxocara canis*.

Clinical features

Larvae, liberated in the stomach, migrate through the body and may cause allergic phenomena such as asthma, eosinophila and splenomegaly, ('visceral larva migrans'). The worms do not usually mature in the human host. Occasionally a granuloma develops around a dead larvae in the eye which resembles a neoplasm and may cause blindness.

Diagnosis

Serology may aid diagnosis.

Management

Larval worms are killed by diethylcarbamazine, 9–12 mg/kg daily for 3 weeks. Granulomas may require surgical treatment.

ANCYLOSTOMA BRASILIENSE AND ANCYLOSTOMA CANINUM

These are intestinal parasites of dogs with a similar life cycle to *A. duodenale*, but in man they cause a creeping eruption or cutaneous larva migrans. The larva burrows between the corium and stratum granulosum and progresses irregularly at about 1 cm in 24 hours.

Clinical features

The skin at the advancing end is erythematous and may vesiculate while that over the older part of the burrow is discoloured and scaly. Itching may be intense. The larva may remain active for months.

Management

Treatment is topical. One 0.5 g tablet of thiabendazole is ground into 5 g petroleum jelly and rubbed into the affected site twice daily for a few days.

OESOPHAGOSTOMIASIS

Species of the genus *Oesophagostomum*, a nematode related to hookworms, may cause a granuloma of the wall of the small intestine resembling a neoplasm. It has been reported chiefly from Uganda and is diagnosed at laparotomy.

ANGIOSTRONGYLUS

Angiostrongylus, a nematode affecting the lungs of rodents, has a larval stage in molluscs and freshwater shrimps. In the Far East and the Pacific, where infected crustacea are eaten or infected slugs on vegetables are inadvertently swallowed, the larvae may cause a serious eosinophilic meningitis and immature worms may be found in the CSF. Thiabendazole (p. 177) is effective but patients often recover spontaneously.

TRICHNELLA SPIRALIS

This parasite of rats and pigs is transmitted to man by eating partially cooked infected pork, usually as sausage or ham. Symptoms result from invasion of the body by larvae produced by the adult female worm in the small intestine and from their encystment in striated muscles. Outbreaks have occurred in Britain as well as in other countries where pork is eaten. Polar bear meat is another source.

Clinical features

The clinical features of trichinosis depends largely on the number of larvae. There may be no symptoms if there are only a few worms present, but many worms may cause nausea and diarrhoea 24–48 hours after the infected meal. Soon, however, these symptoms are overshadowed by those associated with the larval invasion, namely fever and oedema of the face, eyelids and conjunctivae. Invasion of the diaphragm may cause pain, cough and dyspnoea; involvement of the muscles of the limbs, chest and mouth causes stiffness, pain and tenderness in the affected muscle groups. Pyrexia may reach 40°C with daily remissions. Larval migration may cause acute myocarditis and encephalitis. An eosinophilia is usually found after the second week. An intense infection may prove fatal but those who survive recover completely.

Diagnosis

It is not uncommon for a group of persons who have eaten infected pork from a common source to develop symptoms about the same time. Biopsy from the deltoid or gastrocnemius after the third week of symptoms in suspected cases may reveal encysted larvae. Serological tests, if available, are also helpful.

Management

Thiabendazole, 25 mg/kg b.d. for 2 days may relieve muscle pain. Given early in the infection it may kill adult worms in the gut. Corticosteroids are given to control the serious effects of acute inflammation.

GNATHOSTOMIASIS

Gnasthostoma is a nematode of dogs and cats in Bangladesh, South East Asia and the Far East. Third-stage larva are ingested by people who eat inadequately cooked infected fish or by swallowing water containing infected *Cyclops*.

Clinical features

The immature worm usually migrates to the subcutaneous tissue where it causes recurrent swellings. The full grown adult worm, which may be as long as 3 cm, may be visible through the skin when it can be excised. In deeper tissues the worm may cause injury to the brain, kidney, lung, eye or other organs. Eosinophilia is usually pronounced.

Diagnosis

This is usually clinical, and is easy when the adult worm is visible. Serology, if available, is helpful.

Management

Treatment is not satisfactory but some success has been obtained with bithionol used as for fascioliasis (Table 5.35).

Anisakiasis (herring worm disease)

Anisarkis marina parasites herrings and other marine animals. Human infections occur in Holland and Japan from the consumption of raw herrings. An eosinophilic granuloma forms in the intestine and may give rise to colic, fever and intestinal obstruction. An indirect haemagglutination test has been used for diagnosis. Surgery may be required.

DISEASES DUE TO ARTHROPODS

Arthropods may be responsible for disease in four ways. They may act as vectors of infectious agents (Table 5.39); they may envenomate through stings or bites; they may infest or even infect the human body directly; and they may cause allergic dermatitis.

Table 5.39   Infections conveyed by arthropods

Name	Genus	Disease
House fly	*Musca*	Dysenteries, enteric fevers, salmonelloses; and possibly cholera, trachoma, tropical ulcer
House fly	*Tabanida*	Tularaemia, ?anthrax
Oscinid fly	*Hippelates*	Streptococcal dermatitis and nephritis, ?yaws
Tsetse fly	*Glossina*	African trypanosomiasis
Mosquito	*Anopheles*	Malaria, some arboviruses, Bancroftian and Brugia filarias in some areas
	Aedes	Yellow fever, dengue and other arboviruses
	Culex	Bancroftian and Brugia filariasis, Japanese encephalitis and other arboviruses
Black fly	*Simulium*	Onchocerciasis
Midges	*Culicoides*	*Mansonella perstans, M. streptocerca, M. ozzardi*
Soft ticks	*Ornithodoros*	Tick-borne relapsing fever, Lyme disease
Hard tick	(*Ixodidae*) *Rhipicephalus*, etc.	Some typhus fevers, Kyasanur Forest disease, tularaemia, ?Q fever
Sandflies	*Phlebotomus*, etc.	Leishmaniasis, sandfly fever, bartonellosis
Lice	*Pediculus*	Epidemic typhus fever, louse-borne relapsing fever, trench fever, *Dipylidium caninum*
Mites	*Leptotrombidium*	Scrub typhus fever
	Allodermanyssus	Rickettsial pox
Winged bug	*Triatoma*	Chagas' disease
Fleas	*Xenopsylla*	Plague, endemic typhus fever
	Ctenocephalides	*Dipylidium caninum*

LICE

As well as transmitting serious disease, the body louse *Pediculus humanus* causes dermatitis and sleeplessness through itching, especially in poor crowded communities in cold countries (for control see p. 121).

Clinical features

The head louse, *Pediculus capitis*, is cosmopolitan and increasing in prevalence in British schools. It makes the child itch and alarms parents and teachers. Tiny white oval eggs 'nits', are seen attached to the base of hairs on the scalp. The crab louse (p. 192) is transmitted while sharing beds.

Management

A single treatment with gammabenzene hexachloride (BHC) shampoo or lotion is usually curative. In countries, such as Britain, where resistance is developing to BHC, malathion or carbaryl is preferred.

SCABIES

This disease is due to the mite *Sarcoptes scabei*; it is common all over the world.

Clinical features

There is itching, initially between the fingers or on the buttocks or genitals where the mite burrows, and later all over the body. Secondary streptococcal infection is an important cause of glomerulonephritis in the tropics.

Diagnosis

The diagnosis of scabies is confirmed by finding the causative mite in a burrow.

Management

Scabies is treated by a single application of gammabenzene hexachloride 1% to the whole body below the neck or by 3 daily applications of benzyl benzoate 15%.

JIGGERS (TUNGIASIS)

This is due to infestation with *Tunga penetrans* (the chigoe or jigger flea). It is widespread in tropical America and Africa. Man and pigs are important hosts. The pregnant female flea burrows into the skin about the toes and soles and grows as large as a pea, packed with eggs which are subsequently discharged on to the surface.

Clinical features

The burrows irritate and become inflamed but the chief danger is from secondary pyogenic infection or tetanus.

Management

The chigoe or egg sac should be removed with a sterile

needle and a mild antiseptic ointment applied. Massive infestations, such as may be seen in neglected children and in senile persons, may be treated by immersing the feet in an aqueous solution containing benzene hexachloride 5% and centrimide 0.8%.

MYIASIS

This is an infestation of various tissues of man by the larvae of flies.

Cutaneous myiasis

A common cause of cutaneous myiasis is *Cordylobia anthropophaga* (Tumbu fly) which lays its eggs on laundry spread on grass. The larvae penetrate the skin and produce lesions like boils with central orifices through which they breathe. On reaching maturity they emerge. A drop of thick oil or petroleum jelly usually brings a larva out in search of air and facilitates its removal. Occasionally the common warble fly *Hypoderma bovis* may infest man.

Myiasis of wounds, sores and cavities

The larvae of many flies may infest necrotic tissues in open wounds or ulcers and occasionally invade living tissue. *Chrysomya bezziana* is found in Africa, India and South Vietnam. It may penetrate the nasal sinuses and cause great destruction. The application of 10% chloroform in a light vegetable oil is the treatment of choice for infested wounds.

Infested myiasis

In the tropics especially, vague digestive disturbances or abdominal cramps with diarrhoea and vomiting may be caused by fly larvae in the intestinal canal, the eggs having been ingested with food.

POROCEPHALOSIS

This disease is caused by invasion of the body by 'tongue worms', degenerative arthropods of which *Armillifer armillatus*, *A. moniliformis* and *Linguatula serrata* occur in man. Adult *Armillifer* parasitises the trachea and bronchi of snakes. Man is infected by ingesting ova on uncooked vegetables or by eating undercooked snakes. The condition is usually symptomless in man but calcified nymphs may be seen in the radiographs of the chest and abdomen.

Halzoun is the name given in the Middle East to a form of acute dysphagia and laryngeal obstruction from pharyngitis and oedema of the larynx. It is due to the ingestion of nymphs of *Linguatula serrata* in undercooked liver and lymph nodes of sheep and goats.

Foxes and dogs are the definitive hosts. Antihistamines and a local anaesthetic spray may be helpful.

SEXUALLY TRANSMITTED DISEASES (STD)

The number of conditions which are currently recognised as sexually transmitted has increased greatly in recent years. Only the more common will be considered. Two well-known diseases are gonorrhoea and syphilis; the incidence of gonorrhoea is falling and syphilis is at a low level in Britain. The other conditions are in general increasing. These include viral infections (herpes simplex, warts and human immunodeficiency virus (HIV) infection, chlamydial infections (e.g. non-gonococcal urethritis), protozoal infections such as trichomoniasis, and fungal conditions such as candidiasis.

APPROACH TO THE PATIENT WITH SUSPECTED OR CONFIRMED STD

Patients visiting their general practitioner, suspecting STD, or attending an STD clinic for the first time are frequently anxious and frightened. Staff should be friendly, sympathetic, patient and understanding. The doctor should put the patient at ease and stress that all information is completely confidential. Patients suspecting STD will usually expect questions related to the genital tract and their sexual habits, so it is often reasonably easy to discuss such details with these patients. The whole approach should be matter of fact and free from embarrassment.

It is usual to start with the present history of genital symptoms. In both sexes this will cover genital ulceration, rashes, itch, and urinary symptoms particularly burning on micturition. In men details of urethral discharge and in women vaginal discharge, and abdominal and pelvic pain must be noted. Information on general health is obtained together with any recent treatment especially with antibacterial or antiviral drugs. After this questioning should turn to sexual contacts, including dates, relationship to patient (casual or regular partner), duration of sexual relationship, and any symptoms mentioned by the contact. The different forms of genital contact such as genital to genital, anogenital and orogenital may need to be considered. Contraception should be recorded; whether a condom was worn by the male and if there was any contact at all without a condom is also recorded.

Details about previous STD should be requested, including dates and places of treatment where known.

Table 5.40 Investigations in sexually transmitted disease

Females	
Cervical os	Gram stain and culture for gonococci
	Culture for Chlamydiae
	Smear for cytological examination
Urethral meatus	Gram stain and culture for gonococci
Vagina	Gram stain and culture for candidal elements
	Saline mount (for microscopy) and culture for T. vaginalis
	Microscopy for bacteria causing anaerobic/bacterial vaginosis
	(Culture for Gardenerella vaginalis)
Males	
Urethra	Gram stain and culture for gonococci
	Saline mount and culture for T. vaginalis
	Culture for Chlamydiae
Males and Females	
(all patients)	
Blood for VDRL and TPHA serum antibody tests	
Urine for analysis for sugar and protein	
When indicated	
Genital ulcers	Scraping for herpes simplex virus culture
	Scraping for dark ground microscopy for T. pallidum
	Swab for bacterial culture if secondarily infected
Patients who	
are gonorrhoea contacts	Rectal Gram stain and culture for gonococci
	Throat culture for gonococci
Drug abusers and	Blood for serum markers for Hepatitis B
homosexual or bisexual men	Blood for HIV antibodies (after counselling)
plus others at risk	

Past general history and family history should be included. In all patients information about drug allergy must be recorded. In women details should be sought of the menstrual and obstetric history.

All patients must have a careful physical examination of the genitals and this will include passing a bivalve or similar speculum in the female. The best view of the female genitals is obtained in the lithotomy position. Ideally all patients should have a complete physical examination.

All patients should have the investigations outlined in Table 5.40 at their first visit. Relevant investigations must be repeated at follow up visits to ensure cure.

Contact tracing is part of the management of all sexually transmitted diseases. Many clinics in Britain have specialist staff, currently called health advisers in sexually transmitted diseases, who undertake this work for the more common and important STDs; they combine this with counselling including counselling for HIV infection.

SPREAD

The fundamental factor in spread is the acquisition of infection from one sexual partner and its transmission to another. This in turn depends on the availability of partners. A most important influence on the number of partners is population movement including the mi-

gration of people from rural to urban areas and world-wide travel. Other social factors which promote spread include affluence, alcohol consumption, increased leisure, personal freedom, prostitution, and ignorance. This last results in failure to recognise infection, and continuing to change partners. Additional factors are asymptomatic infection, antimicrobial resistance, and contraception. Antimicrobial resistance leads to treatment failure and spread of resistant infection. Unlike the condom and to a lesser extent the cap, oral contraceptives and the intrauterine device provide no barrier to infection.

All socio-economic groups can and do acquire STDs; people especially at risk are listed in the information box below.

INDIVIDUALS AT RISK FROM SEXUALLY TRANSMITTED DISEASES

- Men aged 18–34 years
- Women aged 16–24 years
- Frequent travellers
- Prostitutes
- Armed services personnel
- Merchant seamen
- Entertainers

CONTROL

Control of STD is based on effective treatment of established disease, contact tracing, education and screening. In Britain control is founded on good clinical medicine and most patients attend specialist clinics. The basis of clinical practice is listed in the information box below.

CLINICAL PRACTICE IN THE CONTROL OF STD

- Accurate diagnosis
- Effective treatment
- Careful follow up to ensure cure

Partner notification. This is the identification of potentially infected contacts and their attendance for examination and treatment.

Education on STD. This should be part of general health education.

Screening for STD outside specialist clinics. This is less important in Britain than in some countries with less developed clinical services; serological screening of groups such as blood donors and antenatal women remains important in all countries.

Problems in homosexual and bisexual men In the past homosexual and bisexual men changed partners frequently and had a high prevalence of HIV infection and AIDS. In Britain many homosexual males have modified their sexual behaviour and new infections with HIV and other sexually transmitted diseases such as syphilis and gonorrhoea are uncommon among homosexual and bisexual men.

BACTERIAL SEXUALLY TRANSMITTED DISEASES

SYPHILIS

Syphilis is due to *Treponema pallidum* and is:

1. a chronic infection
2. systemic from the beginning
3. characterised by florid features at some times
4. long periods of latency at other times
5. it responds well to penicillin and certain other antimicrobials such as tetracyclines. It is infectious during the first two years when it may be transferred to the fetus.

CLASSIFICATION OF SYPHILIS

Acquired
Early
  Primary
  Secondary
  Early latent
Late
  Tertiary (Benign gummatous)
  Quaternary
  Cardiovascular
  Neurosyphilis

Congenital
Early
Late
Stigmata (or scars)

The classification is shown in the information box above.

The division between early and late syphilis is 2 years. The course is variable and may be latent throughout. At any time clinical features may develop so all cases must be treated (Table 5.24).

Early stage

The incubation period is commonly 14–28 days but with extremes of 9–90 days.

Clinical features

The *primary* lesion or chancre develops at the site of infection usually on the genitals. A small pink macule appears which becomes papular and ulcerates. The regional lymph nodes are moderately enlarged, discrete, rubbery, painless and non-tender. The primary chancre heals without treatment.

Secondary syphilis develops 6–8 weeks after the appearance of the primary chancre starting with symptoms of generalised infection such as malaise, headache and low grade fever. Four cardinal signs may appear:

1. Rash
2. Condylomata lata
3. Lymphadenopathy
4. Mucosal ulceration.

Rash is present in 75% of patients. It starts as a faint macular eruption on the trunk and proximal limbs; it develops into a generalised papular rash which is characteristically dull red, polymorphic and symmetrical, does not itch and may become scaly. It characteristically affects the palms and soles.

Condylomata lata are flat papules that appear in warm moist areas such as around the anus.

Lymphadenopathy is found in 50% of patients and may be generalised. The nodes resemble those found in primary syphilis.

Mucosal ulcers are present in 30% of patients; they are superficial and appear on the mucous membranes of the genitals, mouth and throat. They may have a characteristic white base, narrow red margin and may coalesce to form 'snail track' ulcers. Sometimes they are so superficial as to be barely visible. In 30% of patients changes occur in the CSF indicating involvement of the nervous system; clinical features of low grade meningitis may rarely be present, sometimes with cranial nerve palsies. Rarely the eyes, bones, joints or abdominal viscera may be affected. After several months the secondary changes resolve to be followed by a latent period.

Late stage
Latency may persist for many years.

Tertiary stage
This takes 10 or more years to develop and affects skin, subcutaneous tissues, mucous membranes, submucosa, and bones (e.g. tibiae). Lesions run a prolonged benign course. The characteristic feature is a granulomatous lesion called a gumma.

Quaternary stage
Cardiovascular syphilis (p. 337) and neurosyphilis (p. 886) usually take longer to develop characteristic features and may lead to the patient's death.

Congenital syphilis
The fetus may contract syphilis from a mother with early acquired syphilis. There is no primary stage. The disease may be so severe that the child is born dead, or vesicles and bullae may be present on the skin at birth. The child may look normal at birth but fails to thrive, and within a few months develops a rash and signs of syphilitic disease of bones, joints, liver, kidneys and other organs. In a third group the disease remains latent for years until lesions of bones, joints, teeth, iritis, keratitis, nerve deafness, juvenile tabes or general paralysis appear. Alternatively the disease may remain latent.

Congenital syphilis is rare in countries where antenatal screening exists and treatment of a syphilitic woman during pregnancy usually ensures the birth of a normal baby.

Diagnosis
T. pallidum may be found in the chancre, papules or mucosal ulcers by dark ground microscopy in the primary and secondary stages (Table 5.40).

The serological tests for syphilis give positive results from about the fourth week and are always strongly positive in the secondary stage. Non-specific antigen is used in screening tests such as the Venereal Disease Research Laboratory (VDRL) test, but the specificity and sensitivity of such tests is variable. False positive results may be found in acute infections including infectious mononucleosis and chronic diseases, for example systemic lupus erythematosus, while negative findings may rarely be observed in older patients with late syphilis. Additional tests are required for diagnosis which use specific treponemal antigen such as the *T. pallidum* haemagglutination assay (TPHA) and the fluorescent treponemal antibody-absorbed (FTA-ABS) test. Any patient in whom latent syphilis is suspected should have all these tests repeated on two separate samples of blood. The CSF should be examined to exclude neurological disease, and chest radiographs taken to exclude calcification of the ascending aorta which indicates cardiovascular disease.

Course and prognosis
The primary stage may not be present or may not be noticed. The secondary stage may also be transient or absent. Many cases are found in the latent stage following serological tests. Modern antimicrobial therapy should give cure rates over 95%.

Primary syphilis must be considered in the differential diagnosis of all genital ulcers including herpes simplex, erosive balanitis and trauma. Less common causes of genital ulcers include secondary syphilis and scabies. The differential diagnosis of secondary syphilis is summarised in Table 5.41. Syphilis has to be distinguished clinically from yaws, endemic (non-venereal) syphilis and pinta. These diseases, caused by treponemes morphologically indistinguishable from *T. pallidum* are described on pages 141–142.

Management
Although *T. pallidum* remains very sensitive to penicillin, the infection needs prolonged treatment and longer

Table 5.41   Differential diagnosis of secondary syphilis

Macular rash	Papular rash	Condylomata lata
Drug eruption	Drug eruption	Viral warts
Rubella	Scabies	
Pityriasis rosea	Acne vulgaris	
Mouth ulcers	Genital ulcers	Lymphadenopathy
Herpes simplex	Herpes simplex	Infectious mononucleosis
Apthous ulcers	Erosive balanitis	Lymphoma
Ulcerative stomatitis		
Agranulocytosis		

Table 5.42 Management of syphilis

Stage	Medication	Regimen
Primary	Procaine penicillin	600 mg i.m. once daily for 12 days
	Oxytetracycline	500 mg orally 4 times daily for 15 days
	Doxycycline	100 mg orally 3 times daily for 15 days
Secondary	Procaine penicillin	600 mg i.m. once daily for 15 days
Tertiary	Oxytetracycline	500 mg orally 4 times daily for 15 days
Latent	Doxycycline	100 mg orally 3 times daily for 15 days
CVS	Procaine penicillin	900 mg i.m. once daily for 21 days
and	Oxytetracycline	500 mg orally 4 times daily for 28 days
CNS	Doxycycline	100 mg orally 3 times daily for 28 days

acting forms such as procaine penicillin are used. Details of regimens used for the various stages of syphilis are shown in Table 5.42. In heavier patients the daily dose should be increased from 600 mg–900 mg or 1.2 g especially in neurosyphilis. Tetracycline is given to patients allergic to penicillin. Pregnant women allergic to penicillin should be given erythromycin stearate in the same regimen as oxytetracycline; this antimicrobial crosses the placenta poorly so the new-born baby needs careful management. All patients must be followed up to ensure cure; contact tracing is an important part of management.

GONORRHOEA

Gonorrhoea is due to the Gram-negative diplococcus *Neisseria gonorrhoeae* which infects columnar epithelium in the lower genital tract, rectum, pharynx and eyes. The incubation period is usually 2–10 days.

Clinical features

The anterior urethra is the common site for infection in males. Anterior urethritis usually causes dysuria and a purulent discharge, but symptoms may be mild or absent.

In females the lower cervical canal is commonly infected but the urethra and rectum are also involved in 50% of patients. There may be vaginal discharge and dysuria but 50% of infected women have no symptoms.

The homosexual male may have rectal infection which is often asymptomatic. All groups occasionally have pharyngeal gonorrhoea.

Diagnosis

Gonorrhoea may be suspected clinically but diagnosis depends on laboratory investigations. Gram-negative intracellular diplococci may be seen in stained secretion from infected tracts and this allows rapid diagnosis. Confirmation by culture of exudate on selective media in the laboratory is important. (See Table 5.40 for specimens to be collected.)

COMPLICATIONS OF GONORRHOEA

- Epididymo-orchitis
- Salpingitis and pelvic infection
- Perihepatitis — characterised by right hypochondral pain and tenderness
- Bacteraemia is rare and causes fever, joint pains and sparse peripheral haemorrhagic pustules surrounded by erythema, though other skin lesions may occur
- Acute gonococcal arthritis (p. 786) and septicaemia are extremely rare in developed countries
- Acute purulent conjunctivitis in infants born to infected mothers (ophthalmia neonatorum) may progress to impairment of vision; this too is rare in the developed countries but remains an important cause of blindness in some tropical areas

Course and prognosis

Symptoms gradually resolve without treatment but it is not known how long patients remain infectious. The longer the delay in treatment the more likely are complications to develop. Most patients in developed countries seek treatment early and complications are rare.

Complications

Complications are listed in the information box above. The differential diagnosis is shown in Table 5.43.

Table 5.43 Differential diagnosis of uncomplicated gonorrhoea

Males	Females	Males and females
Nongonococcal urethritis	Urinary infection Trichomoniasis Candidiasis Anaerobic/ bacterial vaginosis	Proctitis Pharyngitis

Management

Uncomplicated gonorrhoea responds to a single adequate dose of a suitable antimicrobial. In Britain infections are usually sensitive to penicillin and some other antimicrobials.

The various regimens which can be used are listed in the information box (p. 190).

If one of these treatments fails it is important to establish whether the patient is infected with a gonococcus which is relatively resistant to penicillin or with one of the strains rare in Britain, totally resistant to penicillin. Totally penicillin resistant isolates are prevalent in several parts of the world including South East Asia and West Africa. Regimens for resistant

---

REGIMENS TO TREAT GONORRHOEA

- Procaine penicillin 2.4 g i.m. plus probenecid 1 g orally
- Ampicillin 2 g plus probenecid 1 g by mouth and in patients allergic to penicillin
- Co-trimoxazole 8 (480 mg) dispersible tablets in a single dose
- Co-trimoxazole 5 (480 mg) tablets 12-hourly for 3 doses

---

strains and for patients with complications are listed in the information box below.

It is essential to establish a cure of gonorrhoea, and any accompanying infection, by repeating culture of secretions from infected sites. Tracing contacts is also important in the management of gonorrhoea.

DRUG REGIMENS FOR MORE RESISTANT STRAINS OF GONORRHOEA

Relatively resistant
Procaine penicillin 4.8 g i.m. plus probenecid i g by mouth;
Ampicillin 3.5 g plus probenecid 1 g by mouth;
Spectinomycin 2 or 4 g i.m. for penicillin allergic patients.

Totally penicillin resistant isolates
Cefotaxime 0.5 to 1 g i.m.;
Ciprofloxacin 250 mg orally;
Spectinomycin 2 or 4 g i.m. for penicillin allergic patients.

Multiple dose therapy for patients with complications need
Ampicillin 2 g plus probenecid 1 g followed by
Ampicillin 500 mg plus probenecid 500 mg 4 times daily for 14 days.

NON-GONOCOCCAL INFECTION

Non-gonococcal urethritis (NGU) in men
In Britain, urethritis in males is more commonly non-gonococcal than gonococcal in origin. About half the non-gonococcal cases may be due to *Chlamydia trachomatis*, a member of the genus Chlamydia which also cause lymphogranuloma venereum (Table 5.44), and other diseases (p. 117). A few cases of NGU are due to ureaplasma urealyticum, herpes simplex virus, trauma and upper urinary infection, but many are of undetermined aetiology.

NGU also occurs in Reiter's disease (p. 781). The incubation period of NGU varies from a few days to a few weeks.

Clinical features
Clinical features resemble those of gonorrhoea but are milder.

Diagnosis
The usual investigations are undertaken to exclude gonorrhoea by Gram stain and culture of infected secretions. Where available, urethral exudate may be tested for chlamydiae by culture, or antigen detection.

Prognosis
Untreated non-gonococcal urethritis runs a prolonged low-grade course. Local complications resemble those due to gonorrhoea.

Management
Treatment is with oxytetracycline 250 mg 6-hourly or 500 mg twice daily for 14 days. Cure rates are lower than in syphilis or gonorrhoea; refractory patients may be given either erythromycin stearate 250 mg 6-hourly or 500 mg twice daily, both for 14 days.

Non-gonococcal genital infection in women
Chlamydiae may infect the cervical canal. It is therefore important to examine and treat partners of infected men.

Clinical features
Uncomplicated genital chlamydial infection in women causes no symptoms or signs. Chlamydiae may spread upwards and cause pelvic infection; this is a more common cause of pelvic infection than gonorrhoea.

Management
The treatment of uncomplicated infection is the same as for men. In the presence of complications treatment is with oxytetracycline or erythromycin 500 mg 6-hourly for at least 14 days. A woman with cervical chlamydial infection may infect her baby at birth causing eye infection and occasionally pharyngeal infection and pneumonia.

STD common in the tropics and sub-tropics
The salient features of these conditions are summarised in Table 5.44. They should be differentiated from each other, primary syphilis, secondary syphilis and genital herpes simplex.

SEXUALLY TRANSMITTED VIRAL DISEASES

ANOGENITAL HERPES SIMPLEX

This is due to *Herpes simplex* virus and resembles labial herpes or cold sores. The virus is spread by contact during sexual intercourse.

Table 5.44   Salient features of lymphogranuloma venereum (LGV) chancroid and granuloma inguinale (Donovanosis)

Distribution	Organism	Incubation period	Genital lesion	Lymph nodes	Diagnosis	Management
LGV Worldwide especially E. and W. Africa, India, S. E. Asia, S. America, Caribbean	Chlamydia trachomatis Types LI, II, III (intracellular inclusions)	1–5 weeks	Small transient often not recognised	Tender unilateral matted adherent suppurative multilocular	Culture or antigen identification. Circulating (micro IF) antibodies	Oxytetracycline 500 mg q.i.d. for 14 days. Increase and prolong if severe
Chancroid Africa, S.E. Asia	Haemophilus ducreyi (small Gram negative rod)	1–8 days	Multiple irregular tender ulcers	Tender unilateral matted adherent suppurative	Microscopy culture of scrapings	Erythromycin 500 mg q.i.d. for 7 days or cotrimoxazole 2 (80/400 mg) b.d. for 7 days
Granuloma inguinale S. India, S.E. Asia, Central and West Africa, Caribbean, S. America, Central Australian Aborgines	Donovania granulomatis (Bipolar rods)	Few days –3 months	Spreading granulomas pink and red velvety appearance	Only if secondary infected	Microscopy of scrapings	Streptomycin 1 g b.d. i.m. for 10–20 days or Oxytetracycline 500 mg q.i.d. for 14–21 days

Clinical features

Unlike labial herpes simplex infection, in anogenital infection there is a severe initial or primary attack with local discomfort followed by a crop of vesicles on the external genitals. The vesicles rupture and are followed by further crops. The lesions may be widespread on the genitals with painful regional lymph node enlargement, fever and malaise. There may be root pains in the second and third sacral dermatomes and occasionally retention of urine. In homosexual men, and rarely in heterosexuals and females, the anus may be affected. The initial illness lasts 2–4 weeks and afterwards most patients suffer recurrent attacks. These follow the same sequence of local discomfort and then a cluster of vesicles covering an area of about one square centimetre which become erosions and heal, the whole process lasting 5–10 days.

The virus may be identified in vesicular fluid or scrapings from fresh erosions. Syphilis must be excluded.

Management

Lesions always heal and local bathing with saline and treatment of secondary infection with co-trimoxazole 2 (480 mg) tablets twice daily for 7 days may suffice. Acyclovir will shorten the severe initial attack, but it does not yet have an established place in the treatment of recurrence.

ACQUIRED IMMUNE DEFICIENCY SYNDROME (AIDS)

(See p. 104.)

HEPATITIS (p. 518)

Hepatitis B is sexually transmitted between homosexual men but this mode of spread is rare in heterosexuals. The infection is usually transient and subclinical with only minor biochemical abnormalities. A few men develop chronic active hepatitis or cirrhosis. Vaccines have been introduced which give protection against hepatitis B.

Hepatitis A and hepatitis C may also be sexually transmitted.

WARTS, MOLLUSCUM CONTAGIOSUM AND CYTOMEGALOVIRUS DISEASE

Warts are common on the genitals and anus and spread by sexual contact. There is a link between genital warts and subsequent carcinoma, especially when the cervix is involved. Molluscum contagiosum is also found near the genitals and is sexually transmitted. Currently available antiviral drugs have no effect on these conditions which must be treated by destructive methods such as electrocautery or laser.

Cytomegalovirus disease of a subclinical type is widespread among homosexuals who occasionally develop mild clinical disease. Cytomegalovirus disease also spreads heterosexually.

MISCELLANEOUS CONDITIONS

Under this heading some conditions are included which are not sexually transmitted but have to be considered in the differential diagnosis of STD.

Balanitis

This is inflammation of the glans penis, but the undersurface of the prepuce is often also involved, when the correct term is balanoposthitis. It is more common in men with a long or tight prepuce who have difficulty with hygiene. Causal agents include; *Candida albicans*, *Trichomonas vaginalis*, *Streptococci* and some anaerobic bacteria; but no organism may be identified.

Clinical features

The affected areas are either generally or patchily erythematous with erosions in severe cases. There may be white or purulent exudate. Diagnosis is from the clinical appearance.

Management

If one of the causes can be identified, appropriate therapy should be given plus local saline bathing; if no cause can be identified then saline bathing alone will suffice. Immune deficiency conditions, diabetes mellitus, broad spectrum antimicrobials, corticosteroids and antimitotic drugs may predispose to candidiasis.

A characteristic form called circinate balanitis occurs in Reiter's disease (p. 781) with well-defined, round erosions which may coalesce. Balanitis xerotica obliterans is a local form of the skin condition lichen sclerosus et atrophicus; initially there is patchy erythema but later there is atrophy leading to meatal stenosis and phimosis.

Genital ulceration

Acute genital ulceration occurs in the Stevens-Johnson syndrome (p. 197), while recurrent genital ulceration occurs in Behçet's syndrome (p. 784). In the latter condition healing takes place leaving characteristic irregular scars. Trauma is a common cause of genital ulceration.

Vaginal discharge

This is a common complaint and may be due to a variety of causes.

Clinical features

These are summarised in Table 5.45. The organisms can be present without any clinical features. The different microorganisms can be identified by microscopy and culture (Table 5.40).

Management

Local antifungals are given for candidiasis and metronidazole for trichomoniasis and anaerobic/bacterial vaginosis.

Table 5.45   Causes and features of vaginal discharge

Causes	Features
Non-infective	
Chemicals, e.g. antiseptics	Soreness, redness variable discharge
Trauma	(as above)
Infective	
C. albicans	Itch, thick white discharge
T. vaginalis	Soreness, smell, redness, thin yellowish discharge
Bacteria Gardenerella vaginalis and anaerobes	Smell and off-white discharge

Infestations and other skin conditions

These can be sexually transmitted and contact tracing must be undertaken in its management. The lesions are modified on the genitals where the burrows are coiled to produce a dull red papule.

Pediculosis pubis (p. 184)

This is due to the crab louse, *phthirus pubis*, which is not confined to the pubic area but may be found in other body hair and the eyelashes. Characteristic crab-like adult lice and nits (eggs attached to hairs) are seen, better with a magnifying glass than by the naked eye. The adult causes an itch or the patient may notice the parasite. Diagnosis is made by recognising lice or nits and treatment, of pediculosis and scabies is by local application of gammabenzine hexachloride or benzyl benzoate lotion.

ANTIMICROBIAL THERAPY

The ability of one microorganism to interfere with the growth of another is called antibiosis and is due to specific diffusible metabolic products termed *antibiotics*. Since the introduction of penicillin in 1940, research has produced a wide range of antibiotics. A variety of chemotherapeutic agents such as metronidazole, trimethoprim, dapsone and isoniazid has also followed the demonstration of the therapeutic effects of sulphanilamide in 1935. A general term for all of these substances is *antimicrobial agent*.

Effective therapy is available against all known bacteria, rickettsiae, mycoplasmas and chlamydia. Specific antiprotozoal compounds are used in the treatment of diseases such as sleeping sickness, kala-azar, malaria and amoebic dysentery. Topical antifungal agents are widely prescribed, but fully effective, non-toxic, anti-fungal drugs have not yet been found for most systemic infections. Antimicrobial agents active against viruses have also been discovered but few have been successful therapeutically.

ANTIBACTERIAL DRUGS

THE BETA-LACTAM ANTIBIOTICS

These are the *penicillins* and *cephalosporins* and are so-called because of the 4-membered beta-lactam ring which forms part of their basic structure (Fig. 5.23). Resistance is commonly due to bacterial enzymes called beta-lactamases (penicillinases and cephalosporinases) which can cleave the ring and inactivate the antibiotic. The plasmids which code for these enzymes are transmissible between bacteria.

The penicillins

All penicillins are bactericidal and the range of activity of the group is wide as both Gram-positive and certain Gram-negative organisms are sensitive to individual penicillins. The outstanding adverse effect is the risk of inducing a hypersensitivity reaction. Even so the penicillins are the most useful antibiotics at present available (Table 5.46).

Benzylpenicillin. This is rapidly absorbed following intramuscular injection and is excreted by the kidneys within a few hours. The intramuscular injection of large doses is painful. Probenecid, 2 g daily by mouth, will raise the blood level of penicillin by delaying its excretion by the kidney and allow smaller doses to be used.

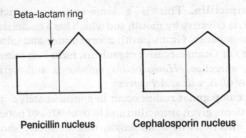

Fig. 5.23 Basic structure of penicillins and cephalosporins.

Penicillin is also used prophylactically to prevent endocarditis, tetanus and gas gangrene.

Procaine penicillin. This long-acting penicillin injection is used in the treatment of gonorrhoea and the treponemal diseases, syphilis and yaws.

Phenoxymethylpenicillin. This is incompletely absorbed from the stomach but frequent oral administration will usually produce reasonable blood levels although in some patients these are low. It is indicated for minor streptococcal infection such as tonsillitis. It is used prophylactically on a long-term basis following an attack of rheumatic fever to prevent recurrences.

Cloxacillin and flucloxacillin. These semi-synthetic penicillins are stable to staphylococcal beta-lactamases. The only indications for their use are infections caused by penicillin-resistant *S. aureus* and *S. epidermidis*. For oral therapy flucloxacillin is superior to cloxacillin as it is almost twice as well absorbed from the gut.

Table 5.46 The penicillins

	Beta-lactamase stable	Route of administration	Average adult dose (mg)	Indications
Benzylpenicillin	−	Parenteral	600–2400	Streptococcal and meningococcal infections, anthrax, diphtheria, gas gangrene, syphilis, yaws, gonorrhoea, actinomycosis, tetanus, endocarditis
Procaine penicillin	−	Parenteral	300 (daily)	As for benzylpenicillin
Pheoxymethylpenicillin	−	Oral	500	Mild streptococcal infections
Cloxacillin/flucloxacillin	+	Parenteral/oral	500–2000	Staphylococcal infections
Ampicillin/amoxycillin	−	Parenteral/oral	250–1000	Infections caused by aerobic Gram-negative bacilli, streptococci, salmonellae and shigellae
Amoxycillin + clavulanic acid ('Augmentin')	+	Parenteral/oral	250–1000 (Amox. dose)	As for amoxycillin + staphylococci and bacteroides species
Carbenicillin	−	Parenteral	1000–5000	Pseudomonas infections
Ticarcillin	−	Parenteral	1000–5000	Pseudomonas infections
Azlocillin	−	Parenteral	1000–5000	Pseudomonas infections
Mezlocillin	−	Parenteral	1000–5000	Infections caused by aerobic Gram-negative bacilli
Piperacillin	−	Parenteral	1000–5000	Infections caused by aerobic Gram-negative bacilli

Ampicillin. This is a semi-synthetic penicillin which is effective by mouth and which has a bactericidal action against Gram-positive organisms and also a variety of Gram-negative organisms, including salmonellae, shigellae, *Haemophilus influenzae* and certain strains of *E. coli* and *Proteus*.

Maculopapular rashes occur in approximately 5% of all patients given ampicillin and in over 90% of patients with infectious mononucleosis; this antibiotic should not therefore be prescribed for sore throats which may be due to infectious mononucleosis.

There are a number of ampicillin esters including talampicillin, bacampicillin and pivampicillin. These improve the absorption of ampicillin thus producing higher blood levels of the antibiotic.

Amoxycillin. This is an analogue of ampicillin which has a similar antibacterial range but is better absorbed from the gastrointestinal tract.

Clavulanic acid. This is a beta-lactam agent with only weak antibacterial activity. It is, however, a potent inhibitor of many beta-lactamases and can protect beta-lactamase-susceptible antibiotics, such as amoxycillin, from inactivation by these enzymes. A combination of amoxycillin plus sodium clavulanate is available (Augmentin).

Ticarcillin. Carbenicillin was initially the only penicillin with activity against *Ps. aeruginosa*. This organism, however, is only moderately sensitive to carbenicillin which has been replaced by its more active analogue ticarcillin. There is a preparation containing ticarcillin plus clavulanic acid (Timentin).

Mezlocillin, azlocillin and piperacillin. These acylureidopenicillins have a wider range of activity than ampicillin and are also more effective against many Gram-negative bacilli. They are used in combination with other antibiotics for the treatment of undiagnosed infections in immunocompromised patients.

Azlocillin is more active than ticarcillin against *Ps. aeruginosa*, an organism which is usually of relatively low virulence but is an important cause of disease in patients with impaired defence mechanisms. Treatment is with either ticarcillin or azlocillin but in *pseudomonas septicaemia* an aminoglycoside is also required; tobramycin plus azlocillin is probably the best choice.

Adverse effects of the penicillins
These are listed in the information box (right).

SIDE-EFFECTS OF THE PENICILLINS	
Hypersensitivity	*Related to high doses*
Skin rash	Encephalopathy
Urticaria	Neutropenia
Maculopapular	Haemolysis
Anaphylaxis	
Bronchospasm	
Drug fever	
Intestinal nephritis	

An increasing number of patients have acquired hypersensitivity to the systemic administration of the penicillins. This takes the form of urticaria and pyrexia or of an acute anaphylactic reaction which has occasionally proved fatal. Ampicillin commonly produces a maculopapular rash which differs from penicillin-induced urticaria and is specific for ampicillin. It is almost certainly unrelated to true penicillin allergy and is not a contraindication to future treatment with other penicillins. The patient should always be asked about previous allergy to any form of penicillin before treatment is commenced as a severe reaction may be provoked by the administration of only a few milligrams.

Skin sensitisation may result from topical applications of any antibiotic, but is so frequent with penicillin that it should never be applied locally.

Large doses of the penicillins can cause neutropenia or haemolytic anaemia.

Although penicillin is otherwise a safe antibiotic, its accumulation in patients with renal failure may lead to encephalopathy, so that dosage in these circumstances must be modified and guided by the blood levels.

Penicillin should never be given intrathecally.

The cephalosporins

The cephalosporins have a wide range of activity against many, but not all, important Gram-positive and Gram-negative bacteria and are therefore of value for the initial 'blind' therapy of undiagnosed infections. Cephalexin and cefaclor can only be given by mouth whereas cephradine and cefuroxime can be given by injection and by mouth. Cefoxitin, an injectable cephamycin antibiotic, has the additional advantage of activity against *Bacteroides fragilis*, an anaerobic bacillus which is a common cause of intra-abdominal sepsis. Cefuroxime and cefoxitin are resistant to degradation by many beta-lactamases.

Cefotaxime, latamoxef, ceftizoxime and ceftazidime. These are expensive injectable cephalosporins which are especially stable in the presence of beta-lactamases and have greater intrinsic activity against many Gram-negative bacilli than the earlier cephalosporins. They also have varying degrees of activity against *Ps. aeruginosa* and *B. fragilis* but are less active than cefuroxime against Gram-positive organisms, especially *Staph. aureus.*

Cefsulodin. This is a cephalosporin with only one indication, i.e. infection caused by *Ps. aeruginosa.*

The dose of the cephalosporins ranges from 250–1000 mg 6-hourly depending on the size of the patient, renal function, and severity of infection. For abdominal sepsis the dose of cefoxitin is 2 g. Cefuroxime is probably the best cephalosporin for general use and ceftazidime is the most active against Gram-negative bacilli.

Adverse reactions are similar to those of the penicillins. A small number of penicillin-sensitive patients may also be allergic to the cephalosporins which should be avoided if there is a history of significant hypersensitivity to the penicillins. Latamoxef can cause bleeding.

Other beta-lactum agents

Imipenem. This is a new beta-lactam antibiotic with a very broad spectrum which includes aerobic and anaerobic Gram-positive and Gram-negative organisms. It is partially inactivated by a renal enzyme and is therefore given along with an inhibitor of this enzyme called cilastatin. Side-effects are similar to other beta-lactam antibiotics.

Aztreonam. This is a new monocyclic beta-lactam antibiotic the efficacy of which is limited to Gram-negative aerobic bacteria including *Ps. aeruginosa, N. gonorrhoea* and *H. influenzae.* Side-effects are similar to those of other beta-lactam antibiotics.

THE TETRACYCLINES

Tetracycline, oxytetracycline and chlortetracycline are very closely related bacteriostatic agents which for practical purposes have an identical range of activity. The adult dose is 250–500 mg 6-hourly before meals because the absorption of most tetracyclines is reduced by chelation with calcium (e.g. in milk).

Doxycycline. This is an exception and also has the advantage that it is given only once daily, 200–300 mg on the first day and 100 mg thereafter.

The tetracyclines inhibit the growth of a wide range

of Gram-positive and Gram-negative bacteria and are particularly useful in the treatment of exacerbations of chronic bronchitis, but their value is limited by an increase in tetracycline-resistant pneumococci and *H. influenzae.* The tetracyclines are also active against rickettsiae (typhus fevers), *Coxiella burnetii* (Q fever), *Mycoplasma pneumoniae* and chlamydia (lymphogranuloma venereum, psittacosis and non-gonococcal urethritis) and are effective in brucellosis.

The tetracyclines are employed systemically in acne vulgaris and rosacea where their beneficial effect is almost certainly not due solely to their antibacterial action. Chlortetracycline is used for the local treatment of skin infections as it does not cause cutaneous sensitisation.

Adverse effects

The tetracyclines are safe with few side-effects. The commonest is diarrhoea which usually stops when the antibiotic is discontinued. Tetracyclines chelate with calcium and are deposited in developing bone and teeth causing a brown discoloration. They should not therefore be given to children or pregnant women. With the exception of doxycycline, the tetracyclines can exacerbate renal failure and should not be given to patients with kidney disease.

THE AMINOGLYCOSIDE ANTIBIOTICS

Streptomycin, kanamycin, gentamicin, tobramycin, netilmicin, amikacin and neomycin have similar chemical structures and adverse effects. They are not absorbed and for systemic treatment must be given by injection (except neomycin).

Streptomycin. The outstanding property of streptomycin is its bactericidal effect on the tubercle bacillus. It is given with two other antituberculous drugs and this triple therapy prevents the emergence of resistant strains. For long-term therapy the daily dose of streptomycin should not exceed 1 g.

Kanamycin. This is active against many Gram-negative bacilli but has been replaced by gentamicin for infections caused by Gram-negative bacilli.

Gentamicin. This has a range of activity similar to kanamycin but has the very important additional advantage of being effective against *Ps. aeruginosa.* It is also active against penicillin-resistant staphylococci but inactive against anaerobes and streptococci with the exception of *Strep. faecalis;* in serious infections caused by this organism gentamicin is combined with ampicillin. The dose of gentamicin depends on renal function and the age and weight of the patient. Five mg per kg body weight per 24 hours in divided doses (usually given 8-hourly) is indicated for most infections. Up to 7.5 mg per kg may be required for serious infections and in neonates. Two mg per kg is sufficient for uncomplicated urinary tract infections and for synergistic therapy with penicillin for the treatment of streptococcal endocarditis. Serum concentrations of gentamicin should be measured during therapy to ensure efficacy and also to prevent toxicity due to unduly high levels especially in renal failure and in the elderly. These are usually carried out on 2 specimens of blood, the first taken one hour after a dose and the second just before the next dose (trough concentration). One hour levels should be between 6 and 12 mg/l and trough levels less than 2 mg/l.

Tobramycin. This is more active than gentamicin against *Ps. aeruginosa* but has no other advantage.

Netilmicin. This is a gentamicin derivative. It is stable to three of nine aminoglycoside-inactivating enzymes, and like amikacin, should be reserved for infection caused by gentamicin-resistant organisms. Netilmicin is slightly less nephrotoxic than gentamicin to which it is preferred in the elderly and if renal function is impaired.

Amikacin. This is a derivative of kanamycin. It has less intrinsic antibacterial activity than gentamicin, but has the advantage of being stable to eight of the nine aminoglycoside-inactivating enzymes, in contrast to gentamicin which is susceptible to six of the nine. For this reason amikacin is active against many gentamicin-resistant Gram-negative bacilli and should be reserved for the treatment of infections caused by these organisms. The dose is 500 mg 12-hourly — this may have to be increased for serious infections.

Neomycin. This is too toxic to be given parenterally but local applications containing neomycin are used in infections of the skin and eye. Oral neomycin is used in hepatic encephalopathy to reduce the numbers of colonic bacteria.

Adverse effects
The aminoglycosides are all nephrotoxic and ototoxic. The commonest adverse effect of the aminoglycosides is on the eighth cranial nerve. With streptomycin and gentamicin the vestibular division is initially affected with resultant vertigo and inco-ordination; later deafness may also occur. Kanamycin tends to cause deafness first. Aminoglycosides, especially gentamicin, should not be administered together with the diuretic frusemide, as both can cause eighth nerve damage and additive ototoxicity may result from the combination.

The ototoxicity of the aminoglycosides is related to the age of the patient, the serum level of the antibiotic and the duration of administration. The aminoglycosides are principally excreted from the body by the kidneys and the risk of toxicity is increased when there is impairment of renal function. Serum levels of the aminoglycosides must be measured in all patients to prevent toxicity and also to ensure therapeutic blood levels.

OTHER ANTIBIOTICS AND CHEMOTHERAPEUTIC AGENTS

Chloramphenicol
Chloramphenicol has a range of activity similar to that of the tetracyclines with the important difference that it is effective in enteric fever. It is more active than the tetracyclines against *H. influenzae* and is the antibiotic of choice in meningitis due to this organism. The daily dose for an adult is 1–3 g. Preparations for parenteral administration are also available. Chloramphenicol eye drops and ointment are indicated for purulent conjunctivitis.

Adverse effects
Chloramphenicol has in its chemical structure a benzene ring of the type known to cause bone marrow aplasia. Although pancytopenia due to chloramphenicol is very uncommon, it is almost invariably fatal; this antibiotic should be used systemically for the treatment of typhoid fever and *H. influenzae* infections and only in other conditions if there is no alternative therapy.

Chloramphenicol should never be given to premature infants and very rarely to the newborn because of the risk of the development of the frequently fatal 'grey baby syndrome'. This is a state of acute circulatory failure caused by the very high blood levels of chloramphenicol due to its inadequate conjugation in the liver at this age.

Clindamycin
Clindamycin (7-chlorolincomycin) has a similar antibacterial spectrum to penicillin against most Gram-positive organisms including penicillin-resistant staphylococci. It penetrates well into bone and is therefore useful for osteomyelitis caused by *Staph. aureus*. The other principal indication is for the treatment of infections caused by *B. fragilis*. The dose is 300 mg 6-hourly, orally or by injection.

Clindamycin is the commonest cause of *antibiotic-associated colitis*. This adverse reaction, which can also complicate treatment with other antibiotics, especially ampicillin, is due to selective overgrowth of *Clostridium difficile* which produces a toxin detectable in the faeces and is the direct cause of the disease. Treatment is with vancomycin or metronidazole, the latter being less costly.

Erythromycin

Erythromycin has a similar although not identical spectrum to penicillin and is commonly used to treat infections caused by Gram-positive organisms in penicillin-allergic patients. It is also effective in whooping cough, campylobacter enteritis and Legionnaires' disease provided it is given early enough in the course of these illnesses. It is a safe and effective antibiotic for the treatment of respiratory infections in children in domiciliary practice. Erythromycin is prescribed in a dosage of 250–500 mg by mouth every 6 hours. There is a preparation for intravenous injection. Diarrhoea, vomiting and abdominal pain are the principal side-effects although cholestatic jaundice may rarely develop if the course of treatment exceeds 10 days.

Sodium fusidate

This sodium salt of fusidic acid is highly bactericidal against *Staph. aureus* and is useful in infections caused by penicillin-resistant staphylococci. Like clindamycin it is well concentrated in bone. Sodium fusidate is given orally in doses of 250–500 mg 3 times daily, is rapidly absorbed, attains high tissue levels and is reasonably well tolerated, although nausea and vomiting are not uncommon during therapy. An intravenous preparation is available. Jaundice has occasionally been associated with its use. This antibiotic is expensive and is indicated for serious infections due to staphylococci, especially osteomyelitis and endocarditis.

Spectinomycin

Spectinomycin is an aminocyclitol compound with certain structural similarity to streptomycin although it is not an aminoglycoside. Its only clinical use is for the treatment of gonorrhoea if penicillin is contra-indicated because of allergy or bacterial resistance.

Vancomycin

Vancomycin is a bactericidal antibiotic with a limited but important antibacterial spectrum. Indications for its use are shown in the information box (right).

Parenteral administration is by slow intravenous

INDICATIONS FOR VANCOMYCIN

Therapy
Treatment of serious streptococcal or staphylococcal infections, especially in the penicillin-allergic patient
Treatment of infections caused by multiply-resistant *S. aureus* or *S. epidermidis* (MRSE) organisms
Treatment of antibiotic-associated colitis caused by *Clostridium difficile*

Prophylaxis
Prevention of endocarditis in patients with heart valve lesions undergoing dental, urological or gynaecological surgery, especially if penicillin-allergic

---

infusion over 60 minutes. Side-effects include fever, rash and, rarely, nephrotoxicity and ototoxicity. The daily dose for injection is 1–2 g which must be reduced in renal failure when serum levels should be monitored. 125 mg 6-hourly is given by mouth for antibiotic-associated colitis.

The sulphonamides and trimethoprim

Although the sulphonamides have been superseded in many countries by antibiotics, their usefulness has been extended by co-trimoxazole, a combination of sulphonamide and trimethoprim. The sulphonamides most suitable for clinical use are the short-acting preparations, e.g. sulphadimidine, which is rapidly absorbed and quickly excreted in the urine in a soluble form.

The usual indication for sulphonamides is cystitis in a dose of 1 g 8-hourly orally. Sulphonamides have been used in the treatment of meningococcal infection, particularly meningitis but penicillin is now preferred. They are also used to treat toxoplasmosis.

Adverse effects
Sulphonamides have a wide range of potential hazards which are listed in the information box below.

ADVERSE EFFECTS OF THE SULPHONAMIDES

- Skin rash including Stevens-Johnson syndrome (erythema multiforme and mucous membrane ulceration)
- Drug fever
- Blood dyscrasias including haemolysis in glucose-6-phosphate deficiency
- Nephritis
- Photosensitivity (topical use)
- Interaction with warfarin and sulphonylurea drugs causing bleeding

Sulphonamides can detach protein-bound drugs such as warfarin and sulphonylurea antidiabetic agents and thereby cause overdosage.

Co-trimoxazole. The two components of this compound, trimethoprim and sulphamethoxazole, act by inhibiting enzymes at two successive stages in the synthesis of para-aminobenzoic acid to folic acid and DNA. Co-trimoxazole is used for exacerbations of chronic bronchitis and infections of the urinary tract. It is also effective in the treatment of invasive salmonella infections. The adult dose is 2 tablets twice daily and there is a preparation for injection. High-dose co-trimoxazole is used to treat pneumonia caused by *Pneumocystis carinii*.

The adverse effects are those of the sulphonamides but the clinician must also be on the alert for possible haematological reactions to trimethoprim and megaloblastic anaemia due to folate deficiency. Side-effects due to co-trimoxazole are commonest in the elderly.

Trimethoprim. This is available alone for the treatment of urinary tract infection for which it is given in a dose of 200 mg twice a day, or 100 mg each evening for long-term chemoprophylaxis. It is also used for the treatment of respiratory tract infections. Side-effects are less than with co-trimoxazole especially in the elderly.

Ciprofloxacin. This is a new 4-quinolone agent which, although broad-spectrum, has particularly high activity against aerobic Gram-negative bacilli including Salmonellae, Shigellae, Campylobacter and Pseudomonas species. It is active against chlamydia and some mycobacteria but not against most anaerobic bacteria. Ciprofloxacin diffuses readily into infected tissues and cells. The oral dose is 500 mg twice a day and for i.v. administration 200 mg twice a day. Recently introduced quinolone compounds include norfloxacin, enoxacin and ofloxacin.

Side-effects include rashes, gastrointestinal upset and headache. The drug is contraindicated in children and pregnant women as arthropathy has been demonstrated in studies on young animals.

Metronidazole

This imidazole compound has high activity against anaerobic bacteria and protozoa but none against aerobic organisms. It is the drug of choice for infections due to *Trichomonas vaginalis*, *Giardia lamblia* and *Entamoeba histolytica* and is widely used for the treatment and prophylaxis of infections caused by anaerobic bacteria, notably *B. fragilis*. It is active against *Clostridium tetani* and *Cl. difficile*.

Metronidazole is a non-toxic drug but should not be given to women during the first trimester of pregnancy as fetal abnormalities have been reported in animals given high doses for prolonged periods. Alcohol should be avoided during therapy with metronidazole which has a similar action to disulfiram. The oral dose varies from 200–400 mg given 3 or 4 times a day. Up to 800 mg 3 times a day is required for amoebic infections. There is a preparation for intravenous infusion.

Tinidazole. This is similar to metronidazole but has a longer serum half-life (12 hours as compared with 7 hours) allowing less frequent administration.

ANTITUBERCULOUS DRUGS

These are discussed on p. 367.

ANTIFUNGAL DRUGS (Table 5.47)

Fungal infections are classified as superficial (skin or mucous membranes) and systemic for therapeutic purposes. The former are commonly caused by *Candida albicans* and usually respond readily to topical applications of any anti-fungal agent. Systemic fungal infections often occur in a compromised host and can be extremely difficult to cure.

Nystatin. This is the most commonly prescribed agent for the treatment of Candida infections of skin and mucous membranes (thrush). It is not absorbed when given by mouth and cannot be administered

Table 5.47 Antifungal drugs

For topical application	
Nystatin	100 000 I.U. as suspension, cream, suppositories
Clotrimazole	1–2% skin cream; 10% vaginal cream
Miconazole	also vaginal suppositories, eardrops,
Econazole	oral gel
Amphotericin	3% skin cream
For oral administration	
Miconazole	250 mg 6-hourly (intestinal disease only)
Fluconazole	vaginal candidiasis – 150 mg single dose
	oropharyngeal candidiasis – 50 mg daily
Ketoconazole	200–400 mg daily
Flucytosine	30–50 mg/kg 6-hourly
Griseofulvin	500 mg once or twice daily
For intravenous administration	
Amphotericin	0.25 mg test dose – increasing to 1 mg/kg daily
Miconazole	600 mg 8-hourly
Flucytosine	50 mg/kg 6-hourly

parenterally because of its low solubility and toxicity. A suspension, tablets and pessaries are available for the treatment of oral, intestinal and vaginal thrush.

Imidazole antifungal agents. These include *clotrimazole*, *econazole*, *miconazole* and *ketoconazole*. They are effective against a wide range of fungi. The first two agents are used for the topical therapy of superficial fungal infections. Miconazole and ketoconazole are absorbed from the gut and have been successfully used for the treatment of systemic fungal infections as well as for superficial mycoses. There is also an intravenous formulation of miconazole. Hepatotoxicity has been reported during ketoconazole therapy. Liver function tests should, therefore, be performed during long-term therapy.

Fluconazole. This is a new triazole antifungal drug which is indicated for oral and vaginal candidiasis.

Amphotericin. This remains the most important antibiotic for the treatment of systemic fungal infections. It is a toxic drug and side-effects are relatively common. These include fever, vomiting, anaemia, thrombophlebitis and nephrotoxicity. The antibiotic is given by intravenous infusion in increasing daily doses usually commencing with 1 mg (p. 149).

Flucytosine. This is well absorbed from the gut and side-effects are relatively uncommon although bone-marrow depression can occur. It is active only against yeasts and has been used for the treatment of systemic candidiasis, sometimes in combination with amphotericin. *C. albicans* can develop resistance to flucytosine.

Griseofulvin. This is selectively concentrated in keratin and is the drug of choice for widespread or chronic dermatophyte infections such as ringworm. It is well absorbed from the gut and is given in a daily dose of 10 mg/kg (child) or 500 mg (adult). Skin lesions respond quickly but infection of the nails requires several months of therapy. Localised and minor ringworm lesions usually respond to a topical imidazole or Whitfield's ointment or miconazole.

ANTIVIRAL DRUGS

The main problem with antiviral chemotherapy is to find an agent which will arrest the replication of the virus without interfering with the metabolism of the host cell. Another difficulty is that by the time a viral infection has been diagnosed much of the damage has already been done to the host tissues. Table 5.48 provides information on currently available antiviral drugs.

SELECTION OF ANTIMICROBIAL AGENT

In addition to knowledge about the properties of available antimicrobial agents, important considerations

Table 5.48 Antiviral drugs

Drug	Route of administration	Indications	Side-effects
Acyclovir	Topical Oral Intravenous	Herpes zoster Chickenpox (immunosuppressed) Herpes simplex infection Encephalitis Genital tract Eye	Rash, headache Increase in urea and creatinine
Idoxuridine	Topical	Herpes zoster H. simplex keratitis	Local irritation
Amantadine	Oral	Prophylaxis of influenza A	CNS symptoms, nausea
Tribavirin	Oral	Lassa fever Respiratory syncitial virus infection in infants (inhalation)	Reticulocytosis Respiratory depression
Ganciclovir	Intraveous	Cytomegalovirus infection in immunosuppressed	Leukopenia Thrombocytopenia
Zidovudine	Oral	HIV infection (including AIDS)	CNS symptoms Anaemia Neutropenia Thrombocytopenia

in the choice of effective chemotherapy are the nature and site of the infection, the known or suspected causative organism, the infected patient and the available antibiotics.

The nature and site of the infection

In instances where the nature of the infection (and the likely causative organism) can usually be predicted from the clinical features of the illness, treatment can proceed without isolation of the causative organism as in the prescription of penicillin for acute follicular tonsillitis and lobar pneumonia. In exacerbations of chronic bronchitis the causative organisms are almost always pneumococci and *H. influenzae* and the use of ampicillin or co-trimoxazole is indicated without specific laboratory diagnosis.

If the patient is seriously ill, antibiotic therapy must be started on a 'best guess' (empirical) basis. The presentation of the illness may assist in the selection of the most appropriate agent. If there are no clues as to the nature of the infection, treatment should be started with a combination of antibiotics such as gentamicin plus a penicillin, or with a cephalosporin such as cefuroxime.

The known or suspected causative organism

Where there is uncertainty about the nature of the infection a bacteriological diagnosis should be made, if possible, so that the appropriate antibiotic can be given. If the organism is one such as *Streptococcus pyogenes*, which has a predictable susceptibility to the generally used antimicrobial agents, no further laboratory sensitivity tests are necessary.

Sensitivity tests will be required for bacteria known to vary in their susceptibility to antimicrobial agents. The acquisition of resistance occurs particularly with

staphylococci, Gram-negative bacilli and tubercle bacilli. Once the sensitivity of the organism has been determined, it is relatively rare for this to change in the course of treatment.

The infected patient

The age and sex of the patient, together with a knowledge of previous adverse reactions, immune function and renal and liver function must all be considered before a final selection of the antibiotic or antibiotics is made.

Pregnant women and children should not be given tetracyclines. Co-trimoxazole is also best avoided in pregnancy and this compound, together with other sulphonamides, must not be given to patients with glucose-6-phosphate dehydrogenase deficiency as haemolysis may be precipitated. Chloramphenicol should be prescribed only in the circumstances described on page 196 and is contraindicated in the neonate. Ampicillin must not be given to patients suffering from infectious mononucleosis and the aminoglycoside antibiotics should be used with caution in patients with renal disease and in the elderly. Clindamycin should not be used for trivial infection because of the risk of colitis.

The available antibiotics

Having considered the above factors the clinician selects an appropriate antibiotic with reference to its microbiological and pharmacological properties, adverse reactions and cost.

More than one (but rarely more than two) antibiotics may be required for the initial treatment of septicaemia or in the immunosuppressed. The use of two or more antibacterial drugs is only occasionally of proven value in other than the seriously ill. Thus in tuberculosis three agents are prescribed, at least initially, so as to

Table 5.49   Indications for chemoprophylaxis

Infection to be prevented	Indication for prophylaxis	Antimicrobial agent indicated
Diphtheria	Susceptible contacts	Erythromycin
Meningococcal infection	Susceptible contacts	Rifampicin
Whooping cough	Susceptible contacts	Erythromycin
Tuberculosis	Susceptible contacts	Isoniazid
Rheumatic fever	Following rheumatic fever	Penicillin
Endocarditis	Heart valve lesion	Amoxycillin or erythromycin
Tetanus	Wound or injury	Penicillin or metronidazole
Gas gangrene	Wound or injury	Penicillin or metronidazole
Abdominal/pelvic sepsis	Colonic or gynaecological surgery	Gentamicin or cefuroxime + metronidazole
Malaria	Travel to malarious country	e.g. Chloroquine
Leprosy	Childhood contacts	Rifampicin + dapsone

reduce the emergence of resistant strains. Drugs with differing ranges of activity may also be used when it has been shown that the effect of the combination is more potent than an equivalent amount of any one of the compounds acting alone. Co-trimoxazole is an example of such synergy.

The chemotherapy of infections can be very expensive, especially when newly introduced preparations are used. Unusual antibiotics should not be prescribed without good reason as the difference in cost can be over a hundred-fold.

Prophylactic use of antibiotics
The indications for this are limited (Table 5.49).

FURTHER READING

General
Christie A B 1987 Infectious Diseases: Epidemiology and Clinical Practice, 4th Edn. Churchill Livingstone, Edinburgh, London, Melbourne and New York
Dawood R (ed) 1987 Traveler's Health Guide. Oxford University Press, Oxford
Department of Health and Social Security 1990 Immunization Against Infectious Disease. HMSO, London
Grist N R, Ho-Yen D O, Walker E and Williams G R 1987 Diseases of Infection. An illustrated handbook. Oxford University Press, Oxford
Mandel, G L, Douglas R G and Bennett J E 1990 Principles and Practice of Infectious Diseases, 3rd Edn. John Wiley and Sons, New York
Manson-Bahr P E C and Bell D R (Eds) 1988 Manson's Tropical Diseases, 19th Edn. Bailliere Tindall, London
Mims C A 1982 The Pathogenesis of Infectious Diseases, 2nd Edn. Academic Press, London
Walker E and Williams G 1985 ABC of Healthy Travel, 2nd Edn. British Medical Association, London
WHO 1989 International Travel and Health; Vaccination Requirements and Health Advice. World Health Organisation, Geneva

Antimicrobial therapy
British National Formulary, British Medical Association and Royal Pharmaceutical Society of Great Britain

Krucers A, Bennett N McK 1987 The use of Antibiotics, 4th Edn. Heinemann, London

Parasitology
Beaver P C, Clifton Jung R, Wayne Cupp E 1985 Clinical Parasitology, 9th Edn. Lea and Febiger, Philadelphia
Knight R 1982 Parasitic Disease in Man. Churchill Livingstone, Edinburgh
Muller R 1975 Worms and Disease. Heinemann, London

Leprosy
Bryceson A D M and Pfaltzgraft R E 1990 Leprosy 3rd Edn. Churchill Livingstone, Edinburgh
Hastings E C (Ed) 1986 Leprosy. Churchill Livingstone, Edinburgh

Malaria
Bruce-Chwatt L J 1985 Essential malariology, 2nd Edn. Heinemann, London
Strickland G T (Ed) (1986) Clinics in Tropical Medicine and Communicable Diseases: Malaria. Saunders, London

Sexually transmitted disease
Holmes et al, Sexually Transmitted Diseases, 2nd Edn. Saunders, London (new edition to be published shortly — details will be notified as soon as available)
King A, Nicol C, Rodin P, 1982 Venereal diseases, 4th Edn. Bailliere Tindall, London

6

Disturbances in Water, Electrolyte and Acid Base Balance

The chemical events collectively called metabolism require the concentration of hydrogen ions, $[H^+]$, and electrolytes to remain within narrow limits in the cells and in the interstitial fluid which bathes them. Derangement of water and electrolyte balance and disturbance of $[H^+]$ occur in a wide variety of clinical conditions described in appropriate chapters of this book. It is convenient, however, to summarise here the relevant physiological facts and to describe briefly the more common abnormalities.

The kidney plays an important part in maintaining water, electrolyte and acid base balance; details of the movements of ions that occur in the nephron are given on pages 549 and 550.

NORMAL DISTRIBUTION OF WATER AND ELECTROLYTES

WATER

The body of a healthy 65-kg man contains approximately 40 litres of water distributed as shown in Figure 6.1. Water passes freely through almost all cell membranes and thus moves readily from one body compartment to another, its final distribution being determined by osmotic and hydrostatic forces. In health total body water remains remarkably constant despite wide variations of the intake of solute and water.

ELECTROLYTES

The inorganic ions dissolved in the body water and the manner in which they are distributed through the various body fluid compartments are shown in Figure 6.2.

The effective osmolality or tonicity of the plasma and interstitial fluid is determined by the concentration of sodium (Na^+) and chloride (Cl^-) in the extracellular fluid compartment (ECF), while that of the intracellular fluid (ICF) depends mainly on the concentrations of potassium (K^+), magnesium (Mg), sulphate and phosphate in cell water. The $[H^+]$ in ECF is only 40 nmol/l; the intracellular $[H^+]$ is higher and varies amongst different tissues.

The differences in ionic composition between cells and the fluid that bathes them are essential to life and are maintained by the activity of ionic pumps within the cell membrane. Despite ionic differences osmotic activity is believed to be virtually identical in intra- and extracellular fluids.

The concentration of electrolytes in plasma and interstitial fluid is very similar because of the permeability of the capillaries. Interchange of protein molecules between these extracellular compartments is limited, and the concentration of protein is much greater in plasma. The plasma volume is largely determined by the balance between capillary hydrostatic pressure which tends to force water and electrolytes outwards,

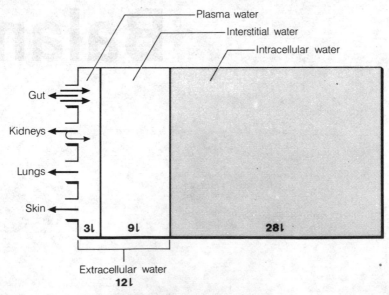

Fig. 6.1   Distribution of water in a 65-kg man. The vascular compartment is in contact with the environment at 4 portals. Nett gain or loss of water and electrolytes occurs by these routes.

and the colloid osmotic pressure of the plasma proteins which draws water and salts back into the vessels.

DISTURBANCES IN WATER AND ELECTROLYTE BALANCE

Changes in the volume and composition of body fluids occurs as a result of disease and as a consequence of treatment. Such disturbances contribute to the clinical picture of many disorders and can themselves hinder recovery or even endanger life. Thus it is important to maintain the volume and the chemical composition of body fluids. Specific disturbances must be identified

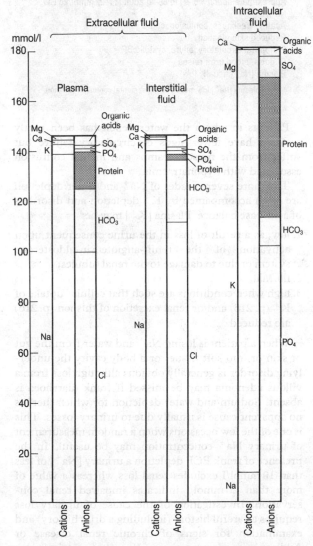

Fig. 6.2   Distribution of electrolytes in plasma, interstitial fluid and cell fluid.

and appropriately treated. In this chapter they are, therefore, described separately although in practice two or more often coexist.

SODIUM DEPLETION

Normal Na^+ balance depends upon equality between the amounts of Na^+ ingested and excreted. In health, in temperate climates negligible amounts of Na^+ are lost in stools and from the skin. Moreover, provided the kidneys are healthy, and the amount of solute excreted in the urine is not very large, renal conservation of Na^+ is extremely efficient and normal Na^+ balance can be maintained on a very small daily intake. Thus Na^+ depletion results from excessive salt loss rather than inadequate intake.

Because of the intimate relation between Na^+ balance and water balance, loss of Na^+ is almost always accompanied by a reduction in body water. Pure Na^+ depletion without a significant water deficit is uncommon and occurs only when abnormal losses of salt and water are replaced by salt-free fluids. In these circumstances the change in total body water may be negligible despite a considerable deficit of body salt. More commonly Na^+ and water depletion coexist in varying degrees.

Causes of mixed sodium and water depletion

The important causes of this are shown in Table 6.1. In temperate climates this condition is due to excessive loss of Na^+ from the gastrointestinal tract, in the urine or in exudates or transudates.

In tropical countries large losses of salt and water can result from sweating and this often aggravates Na^+ depletion caused by concomitant disease (p. 85).

Consequences of mixed sodium and water depletion

Sodium depletion reduces the volume of the ECF. When proportionately more Na^+ than water is lost, the ECF also becomes hypotonic and the plasma $[Na^+]$ falls. Two mechanisms mitigate these changes in tonicity:

1. extracellular water migrates into cells
2. provided the ECF deficit does not exceed 2–3 litres secretion of antidiuretic hormone (ADH) is inhibited and the proportion of water to solute excreted in urine increases.

These physiological responses to a low plasma $[Na^+]$ result in further diminution in the ECF volume, including plasma volume, while the water content of cells increases.

Table 6.1 Causes of mixed sodium and water depletion

Loss from alimentary tract	External loss Vomiting Aspiration of GI contents Fistulae Diarrhoea Villous adenoma of large bowel
	Sequestration of fluid in bowel Ileus Intestinal obstruction
Loss in urine	Extrarenal factors acting on kidney Osmotic diuresis 　Diabetes mellitus 　Mannitol Diuretics Metabolic acidosis Adrenocortical insufficiency
	Renal disease Diuretic phase acute tubular necrosis Post obstructive diuresis Chronic renal insufficiency Proximal renal tubular acidosis Medullary cystic disease Congenital polycystic disease Chronic interstitial nephritis
Loss in sweat	Fevers, hot environment
Loss in exudates and transudates, 'third' space losses'	Loss from body surfaces Burns Extensive dermatitis Loss into body cavities or soft tissues Ascites Peritonitis Acute pancreatitis Rhabdomyolysis Inferior vena caval thrombosis

Reduction in plasma volume results in underfilling of the vascular system and stimulation of intravascular receptors. These initiate mechanisms which:

1. activate the renin-angiotensin-aldosterone system and the sympathetic nervous system resulting in a fall in glomerular filtration rate (GFR), and therefore in the amount of filtered Na^+, and in enhanced tubular reabsorption of Na^+. Thus when the kidneys are healthy, urinary Na^+ falls gradually to less than 10 mmol/day;
2. induce release of ADH to which the healthy kidney responds by producing a highly concentrated urine thus conserving water.

Clinical features

Reduction of the ECF volume is responsible for the clinical features common to all cases of mixed Na^+ and water depletion. Reduction of plasma volume results in diminished venous return and, despite compensatory tachycardia and selective vasoconstriction, a progressive fall in cardiac output and blood pressure occurs, renal perfusion is reduced and the blood urea rises. The clinical features are shown in the information box (right).

CLINICAL FEATURES OF SODIUM AND WATER DEPLETION

Mild
Approximate deficit 1–2 l in 65-kg adult (2.5–5 mmol/kg BW Na^+)
Lassitude, light headedness, postural hypotension

Moderate
Approximate deficit 2–4.5 l in 65-kg adult (5–11 mmol/kg BW Na^+)
Lassitude, giddiness, nausea, headache
Reduced skin elasticity
Tachycardia, peripheral vasoconstriction, systolic BP reduced but rarely < 90, marked postural hypotension
In larger deficits: oliguria, blood urea raised

Severe
Approximate deficit 4.5–9 l in 65-kg adult (11–22 mmol/kg BW Na^+)
Apathy, weakness, confusion, coma
Reduced skin elasticity
Peripheral circulatory failure, systolic BP < 90
Oliguria, blood urea raised
Plasma [Na^+] usually low*

* When plasma [Na^+] low muscle cramps, mental confusion common

---

Patients in whom the water deficit has been partly restored have fewer signs of circulatory failure but suffer from the muscle cramps and mental confusion associated with hyponatraemia.

The more severe grades of Na^+ and water depletion are often accompanied by K^+ depletion and disorders of acid-base balance. Plasma [K^+] may be:

1. low, as a result of loss in the urine consequent upon activation of the renin-angiotensin-aldosterone system or due to damage to the renal tubules;
2. normal;
3. high when conditions are such that cellular uptake of K^+ (p. 216) and/or renal excretion of this ion (p. 216) are reduced.

When a patient is losing Na^+ and water from the gut or skin or into soft tissues or a body cavity the underlying disorder is generally obvious although loss from a villous adenoma may be missed if frank diarrhoea is absent. Sodium and water depletion for which there is no apparent cause is usually due to urinary losses. This is one of the few occasions when a random measurement of urinary Na^+ concentration may be useful. In the presence of frank ECF depletion a urinary [Na^+] of less than 10 mmol/l excludes renal loss whereas a value of more than 20 mmol/l indicates impaired renal conservation. Investigation of the cause of urinary loss requires a careful history (including a drug history) and examination for signs of chronic renal disease or Addisonian pigmentation. If adrenocortical insufficiency is suspected a synacthen test should be performed (p. 650). Patients suspected of having organic renal disease require investigation of the renal tract and kidney function (Chapter 12).

Management

Both Na$^+$ and water must be replaced. Administration of water or glucose in water alone is dangerous because hypotonicity may be aggravated. Moreover, much of the administered water enters cells and, in less severe cases, the kidneys respond by excreting dilute urine in an attempt to restore extracellular tonicity; thus the ECF volume remains low. Guidelines are listed in the information box below.

GUIDELINES FOR REPLACEMENT OF SODIUM AND WATER DEFICITS IN A 65-KG ADULT

The size of deficit is assessed from the history and clinical features

Mild depletion
Slow sodium 6–10 tabs/day
(60–100 mmol NaCl) in divided doses ⎫
Water 2–3 l/day   ⎬ 2–3 days
or   ⎭
0.9% NaCl solution i.v. 1–2 l   24 hours

Moderate depletion
0.9% NaCl solution i.v. 2–4 l   1–2 days

Severe depletion
0.9% NaCl solution i.v. 4–9 l. The first ⎫
2–3 l to be infused rapidly over   ⎬ 2 days
2–3 hours   ⎭

Indications of circulatory overload during fluid administration
Rapid increase JVP, CVP or pulmonary capillary wedge pressure
Crackles at lung bases

Indications of correction if deficit
Normal pulse, BP, urine output
Restoration skin elasticity
Plasma [Na$^+$] in reference range, blood urea falling

Coexisting metabolic acidosis
Treat if indicated (p. 224) by giving 1/3–1/2 of total Na$^+$ requirement as 1.26% NaHCO$_3$ solution

Coexisting K$^+$ or Mg deficit
Add KCl (p. 218) or MgCl$_2$ (p. 221) to i.v. fluid when circulation and urine output restored

Maintenance therapy
Measure or estimate daily losses Na$^+$ and water
Replace losses daily
Weigh daily, examine for evidence fluid depletion or overload, measure plasma electrolytes daily, adjust therapy accordingly

---

The cause of the disturbance must be treated appropriately (see relevant sections this book), e.g. glucocorticoid and mineralocorticoid therapy for primary adrenal insufficiency, surgery for relief of intestinal obstruction, long-term salt supplements for patients with chronic Na$^+$ losing renal disease.

PRIMARY WATER DEPLETION

Pure or predominant water depletion is one of the simplest chemical disorders. The water content of the body is reduced both absolutely and relative to the Na$^+$ content, and the osmolal concentration of all body fluids rises.

An adult in a temperate climate has an insensible loss of between 0.5–1 l/day in expired air and by evaporation from the skin and this loss continues irrespective of water intake. Water is, if course, excreted in urine but can be conserved up to a limit determined by renal concentrating ability and the amount of solute to be excreted (Fig. 6.3).

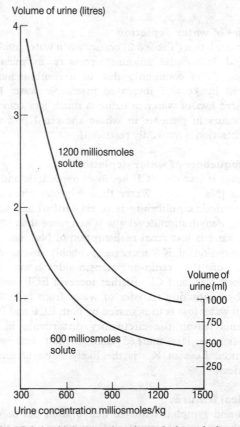

Fig. 6.3 Relationship between the volume of urine and urinary concentration at two levels of solute excretion. As concentrating ability falls the volume of urine required to excrete a given amount of solute rises. (Reproduced by permission from Lambie A T, Robson J S 1974 A companion to Medical Studies, vol 3. Blackwell Scientific Publications Ltd, Oxford.)

Table 6.2 Causes of pure or predominant water depletion

Reduced intake	Water unavailable Infants, aged, coma, apathy, depression Inability to swallow, nausea Primary hypodipsia
Increased loss from skin	Fever, hyperthyroidism Hot environment
Increased loss from respiratory tract	Hyperventilation, fever High altitudes
Increased loss in urine due to marked impairment of urinary concentrating mechanism	*ADH deficiency* Diabetes insipidus *Renal tubular lesions* Nephrogenic diabetes insipidus Hypercalcaemia, K^+ depletion Chronic interstitial nephritis Amyloidosis, obstructive uropathy Medullary cystic disease *Solute diuresis* Diabetes mellitus Tube ⎱ feeds with high solute Parenteral ⎰ concentration Infants feeds wrongly made up

---

CLINICAL FEATURES OF PURE OR PREDOMINANT WATER DEPLETION

Mild
Approximate deficit 1–2 l in 65-kg adult
Thirst[1], concentrated urine[2]

Moderate
Approximate deficit 2–4 l in 65-kg adult
Marked thirst[1], dry mouth, difficulty swallowing
Dizziness, slight personality changes
Slight muscle weakness
Oliguria, concentrated urine[2], slight rise blood urea
Plasma [Na^+] raised

Severe
Approximate deficit 4–10 l in 65-kg adult
Severe thirst[1], dry mouth, difficulty swallowing
Mental confusion, coma
Marked muscle weakness
'Doughy' skin and tissues
Tachycardia, vasoconstriction, systolic BP low
Oliguria, concentrated urine[2], blood urea raised
Plasma [Na^+] raised, Hb raised

[1]Unless senile or confused.
[2]Provided kidneys healthy, solute load not large and normal vasopressin production.

Causes of water depletion

Water depletion (Table 6.2) occurs when water intake is reduced below the amount necessary to maintain balance. It is commonly due to a combination of reduced intake and increased insensible water loss; excessive loss of water in urine is much less common and occurs in patients in whom the renal power of concentration is markedly restricted.

Consequences of water depletion

As water is lost the ECF becomes hypertonic and the plasma [Na^+] rises. Water then migrates from cells until osmotic equilibrium is re-established and intra-cellular dehydration develops. When more than 8% of body water is lost renal reabsorption of Na^+ and Cl^- and excretion of K^+ increase, probably due to activation of the renin-angiotensin-aldosterone axis. Retained Na^+ and Cl^- further increase ECF tonicity thereby facilitating transfer of water from cells. The overall water loss is thus shared by both ECF and ICF. For this reason the circulatory disturbance in dehydration is less marked than in salt and water depletion. Loss of K^+ is the likely cause of muscle weakness.

Clinical features

Signs and symptoms due to dehydration per se vary with the amount of water lost. Circulatory insufficiency is seen only in severe cases. The clinical features are shown in the information box (right).

The diagnosis is made on the basis of the history and clinical findings. The presence of hypernatraemia is of great diagnostic value provided that hypertonic solutions of Na^+ salts have not been infused recently. The underlying cause is usually obvious. It is, however, important to examine the urine even when there is an obvious extra-renal cause for dehydration, because inability to form a concentrated urine undoubtedly contributes to water depletion in patients with unsuspected renal impairment and this is not uncommon in the elderly. A small volume of urine of specific gravity (SG) 1020 or more excludes a significant renal component. In dehydrated patients in whom the urine is not concentrated urine should be tested for sugar to exclude diabetes mellitus and renal function assessed by measuring blood urea and plasma creatinine levels. Marked polyuria with a urine volume of more than 3 l/day and urine of less than 1010 SG (UOsm 290 mOsm/kg) suggests ADH deficient diabetes insipidus or nephrogenic diabetes insipidus or, rarely, one of the uncommon renal tubular lesions (Table 6.2). Administration of vasopressin results in a reduction in urine volume and increase in urine SG or osmolality only in those with ADH deficiency.

Management

Water depletion can be prevented by ensuring an adequate intake in patients unable to drink enough of their own accord. The daily requirements must be carefully assessed taking into consideration insensible loss and renal concentrating ability. For an adult 40 ml/kgBW/day usually suffices but more may be required when insensible or urinary losses are high. It is important to maintain this intake when tube feeds are given. Careful instructions must be given to the patient's attendants and whenever possible fluid balance charts should be kept and the patient weighed daily.

Guidelines for management of established dehydration are given in the information box below.

GUIDELINES FOR REPLACEMENT OF WATER DEFICITS IN A 65-KG ADULT

The size of deficit is assessed from the history and clinical features.

Mild depletion
Water 2 l by mouth	6–12 hours
or	
5% glucose solution i.v. 2 l	12 hours

Moderate depletion
5% glucose solution i.v. 2 4 l	24 hours

Severe depletion
0.9% NaCl solution i.v. 1 l	1 hour
5% dextrose solution i.v. 3 l	24 hours
5% dextrose solution i.v. 4 l or equivalent water by mouth	24–48 hours
5% dextrose solution i.v. or water by mouth to restore remaining deficit	48–96 hours

If plasma [K+] low give KCl by mouth or in i.v. fluids (p. 218) once urine output > 500 ml/day

Indications of correction of deficit
Restoration of circulation
Relief of thirst
Urine output > 1500 ml/24 hours in those previously oliguric
Plasma [Na+] in reference range

Maintenance therapy
Water 2.5 l/24 hours by mouth, more if polyuria or high fever present (some or all may be given as 5% glucose solution i.v.). Treat diabetes insipidus if present

---

It is essential that large water deficits are replaced gradually over several days to avoid sudden shift of water into cells which can cause severe disturbance of cerebral function.

The underlying cause should be corrected where possible, for example, synthetic analogues of ADH are given to patients with pituitary diabetes insipidus (p. 622). The polyuria of patients with nephrogenic diabetes insipidus can be mitigated by giving a diuretic, usually bendrofluazide, which induces mild Na+ depletion thereby increasing isotonic proximal tubular reabsorption of Na+ and water and reducing Na+

delivery to the diluting site where free water is generated (p. 214).

SODIUM AND WATER EXCESS

In health total body Na+ is kept within narrow limits despite considerable day to day variation in intake.

Aetiology
Accumulation of Na+ occurs when renal excretion fails to keep pace with the amount ingested. Since Na+ retention is accompanied by retention of an approximately isosmotic amount of water the volume of the ECF is increased but ECF [Na+] is not materially altered. Generalised oedema due to accumulation of fluid in the interstitial spaces is the clinical consequence of expansion of the ECF and becomes evident when the ECF volume is increased by about 15%.

Accumulation of generalised oedema requires:

1. a change in the forces acting upon the microcirculation which determine distribution of water and electrolytes between intravascular and interstitial fluid;
2. renal retention of Na+ and water in the face of increased body Na+ and expansion of the ECF.

The sequence of events differs depending upon the underlying disease and its stage of development. The simplest pattern (Fig. 6.4) is seen in patients with minimal lesion glomerulonephritis (p. 572) in whom heavy proteinuria coexists with a normal or raised GFR. Loss of water and electrolytes from plasma into the interstitial space results in underfilling of the vascular bed and stimulation of intravascular receptors. This leads to appropriate activation of mechanisms designed to maintain plasma volume all of which increase renal Na+ reabsorption. As a consequence, the disturbance of the physical forces acting across the capillary walls retains Na+ and water accumulates in the interstitium.

In patients with acute nephritic syndrome (p. 562) or nephrotics in whom GFR is low, the plasma volume appears to be normal or increased and the stimulus for increased Na+ reabsorption, as yet unknown, appears to arise in the kidney itself.

Sodium retention in congestive cardiac failure (Fig. 6.5) is probably initiated by stimulation of intra-arterial receptors by the reduced arterial blood flow which results from a fall in cardiac output. An increase in both pulmonary and systemic venous pressure leads to sequestration of retained Na+ and water in the interstitial spaces of both circuits; this further reduces effective arterial flow. The problem is compounded by loss of the

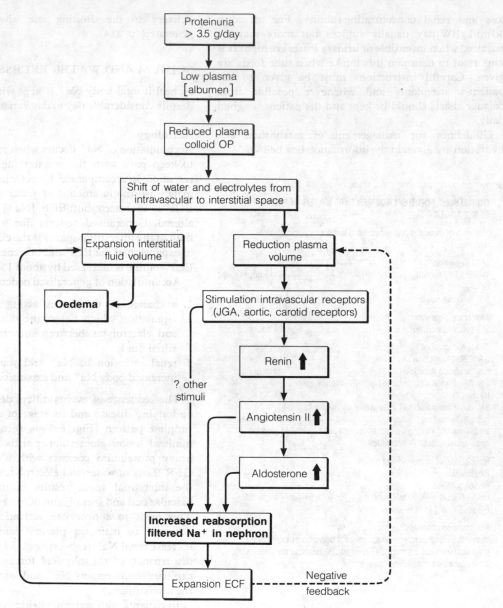

Fig. 6.4   Pathogenesis of oedema in nephrotic syndrome due to minimal lesion nephritis.

normal natriuretic response to atrial dilatation, atrial natriuretic peptide levels in plasma are raised but the kidney apparently fails to respond.

In hepatic cirrhosis gross distortion of intrahepatic architecture gives rise to obstruction to hepatic venous outflow, to portal hypertension and to the development of portal-systemic shunts (p. 520). The proposed sequence leading to the development of ascites and oedema is shown in Figure 6.6. Receptors within the

hepatic circulation are thought to respond to increased hepatic venous pressure and to initiate Na^+ retention before hypovolaemia develops. Subsequently there is underfilling of the vascular tree due both to loss of fluid from plasma and to an increase in vascular capacitance. Thus impulses from intravascular receptors further stimulate Na^+ retention.

Knowledge of this subject is incomplete and changing rapidly but clearly in all these disorders

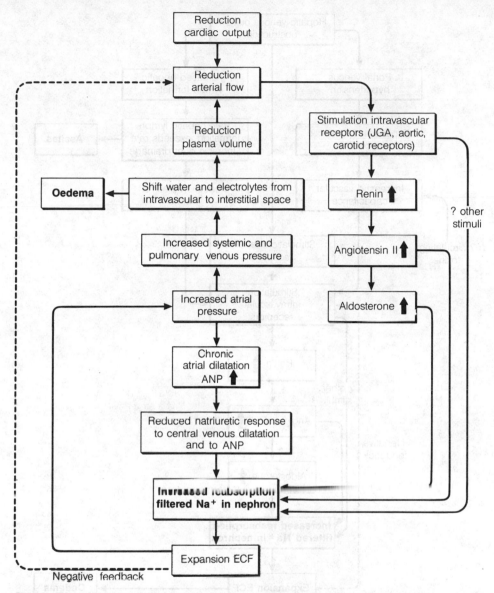

Fig. 6.5 Proposed mechanisms for pathogenesis of oedema in congestive heart failure. (Modified from Skorecki, KL and Brenner BM. American Journal of Medicine 72, 325, 1982.)

stimuli arising from an underperfused section of the vascular tree are important in initiating and maintaining renal Na^+ retention despite increased total body Na^+. Conditions associated with generalised oedema are shown in the information box (p. 213).

Clinical features

These depend to some extent on the distribution of retained fluid and are described under the various diseases.

Management

The principles of management are simple and are shown in the information box (p. 213).

Diuretic therapy

Drugs which block Na^+ reabsorption also increase urinary volume because reabsorption of water in the nephron is passive and depends on Na^+ reabsorption.

Table 6.3 provides information about commonly used diuretics. The choice of drugs depends upon the

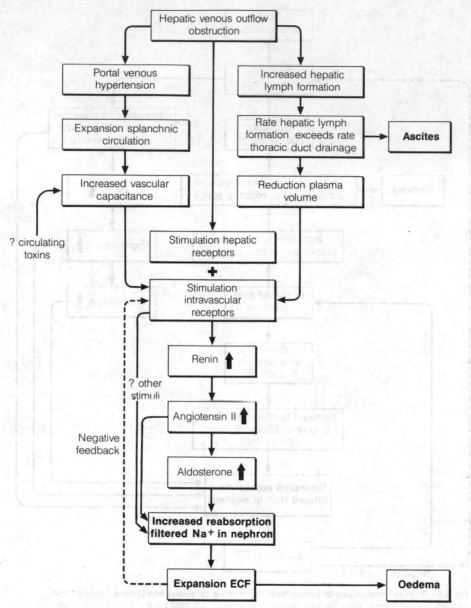

Fig. 6.6 Proposed mechanisms for pathogenesis of oedema in cirrhosis. At a later stage hypoalbuminaemia may contribute to oedema formation. (Modified from Skorecki KL and Brenner BM, American Journal of Medicine 72, 325, 1982.)

severity of the oedema and whether or not the patient is resistant to the effects of diuretics. Mild cases, e.g. ankle oedema in an elderly person with mild cardiac failure, usually respond to a combination of moderate salt restriction and benzothiadiazine diuretic. Hydrochlorothiazide 50–100 mg/day or bendrofluazide 5–10 mg/day may be given or, if a slower and more prolonged diuresis is desired, chlorthalidone 100–200 mg/day can be used. More severe cases should receive a high potency diuretic, oral frusemide 40–120 mg/day or an equivalent dose of bumetanide, 1–3 mg/day, along with a diet containing 100 mmol/day Na^+. Intravenous frusemide, 20–40 mg, is valuable in treating acute pulmonary oedema. Intravenous ethacrynic acid should be avoided because of ototoxicity. Causes of resistance to the effects of diuretics are given in the information box (p. 213).

Patients with chronic renal failure often respond to

CONDITIONS ASSOCIATED WITH GENERALISED OEDEMA

- Congestive cardiac failure
- Hepatic cirrhosis, acute liver failure, hepatic vein thrombosis
- Acute oliguric renal failure, advanced chronic renal failure (GFR < 15 ml/min), acute nephritic syndrome, nephrotic syndrome
- Protein-losing gastroenteropathy
- Starvation, thiamine deficiency
- Pregnancy, premenstrual
- Acute anaphylaxis
- Drugs which induce renal Na^+ retention: Antihypertensives (particularly vasodilators), corticosteroids, liquorice, carbenoxolone, oestrogens, NSAID

MANAGEMENT OF OEDEMA

- Measures designed to correct specific factors causing oedema, e.g. corticosteroids in steroid sensitive nephropathy; salt poor albumen in hypoproteinaemia; rest, vasodilators, digoxin in heart failure
- Restriction of dietary Na^+ to about 100 mmol/day ('no added salt diet') in mild and moderate cases or 50 mmol/day in severe resistant cases
- Diuretics to increase rate of urinary excretion of Na^+ and water

CAUSES OF RESISTANCE TO THE EFFECTS OF DIURETICS

- Reduced renal blood flow. GFR < 20 ml/min
- Severe hypoproteinaemia
- Severe secondary aldosteronism

large doses of frusemide (500–2000 mg by mouth) or bumetanide (5 mg by mouth) but if this fails a combination of one of these diuretics which act on the loop with metolazone (10 mg) or bendrofluazide (10 mg) may

Table 6.3   Commonly used diuretic drugs

Class	Drugs	Principle sites of action in nephron	Extrarenal actions	Principal side-effects of the group	Individual side-effects
High potency	Frusemide	1 Inhibition reabsorption NaCl thick ascending limb loop of Henle 2 Minor inhibition reabsorption NaCl proximal tubule 3 Increase renal blood flow	Increase venous capacitance	Postural hypotension K^+ depletion, Mg^{++} depletion, alkalosis, hyperuricaemia, hyperglycaemia, hypersensitivity (rash, myelosuppression, hepatic dysfunction, interstitial nephritis)	Ototoxic
	Bumetanide	As above		Bumetanide myalgia IV Frusemide } IV Ethacrynic acid }	Myalgia
	Ethacrynic acid	As above			Ototoxic
Medium potency	Benzothiadiazines (thiazides)	1 Inhibition reabsorption NaCl early distal tubule (diluting site) 2 Inhibition reabsorption NaCl proximal tubule 3 Some inhibit reabsorption $NaHCO_3$ in proximal and distal tubules (minor)	Antihypertensive	K^+ depletion, alkalosis, hyponatraemia, hyperuricaemia, hyperglycaemia, hyperlipidaemia hypersensitivity (rash, myelosuppression, acute pancreatitis, hepatic dysfunction, interstitial nephritis)	
	Metolazone	As above 1 and 2			
Low potency	Acetazolamide	Inhibits reabsorption $NaHCO_3$ in proximal and distal tubule	Decreased rate formation aqueous humour	K^+ depletion, acidosis, drowsiness, hypersensitivity, (rash, myelosuppression, interstitial nephritis, renal stone)
K^+ sparing low potency	Spironolactone	Aldosterone antagonist inhibits aldosterone sensitive Na^+/K^+ exchange in collecting tubule	Gynaecomastia	Hyperkalaemia, acidosis
	Triamterene	Inhibits reabsorption Na^+ in collecting tubule thus indirectly inhibits K^+ secretion at that site			Hyperkalaemia, acidosis formation renal stones containing triamterene, acute renal failure when given with indomethacin
	Amiloride	As triamterene			Hyperkalaemia, acidosis

succeed since the drugs, which have different sites of action, act synergistically. In patients with resistant oedema due to cirrhosis or severe cardiac failure whose renal function is not compromised a combination of spironolactone (100–200 mg), triamterene (200 mg) or amiloride (20 mg) with frusemide or bumetanide may induce diuresis. The low potency drugs are, per se, poor diuretics but are of value when combined with a loop diuretic as they inhibit Na^+ reabsorption in exchange for K^+ or H^+ in the lower nephron. Since they reduce K^+ excretion, they must not be given along with K^+ supplements nor used when renal function is impaired lest dangerous hyperkalaemia results. When severe hypoproteinaemia is present addition of salt poor albumen to the regime (p. 564) usually induces diuresis.

Adverse effects of diuretic therapy on water and electrolyte balance

Potassium depletion. High and medium potency diuretics, which deliver an increased amount of Na^+ to the distal nephron, induce K^+ depletion, (p. 216) especially when given repeatedly over long periods and when combined with a low Na^+ diet. Symptoms of K^+ deficiency may arise before satisfactory loss of oedema has been achieved and are then superimposed upon clinical features of Na^+ and water accumulation. This is prone to occur during the treatment of severe heart failure (p. 289) and may be responsible for development of digitalis toxicity before the heart failure has been controlled. In hepatic disease with ascites and oedema K^+ depletion may aggravate or precipitate hepatic encephalopathy.

Prophylactic administration of K^+ is essential when diuretics are given frequently, e.g. on alternate days. Potassium chloride 3–4 g/day in divided doses is given, usually as slow release or effervescent tablets (p. 218).

Metabolic alkalosis due to diuretics (see p. 225).

Sodium depletion and oligaemia. Overtreatment with diuretics results in Na^+ and water depletion. This may occur when high potency drugs are given over prolonged periods without adequate supervision. The clinical features of Na^+ and water depletion are described on page 206.

Patients with severe oedema resistant to therapy, sometimes develop clinical features of oligaemia while still oedematous. In these cases hypotension, tachycardia and a raised blood urea are often associated with a low plasma $[Na^+]$. Such patients usually suffer from advanced cardiac, hepatic or renal disease associated with hypoproteinaemia. Persistent attempts to reduce the oedema usually lead to further deterioration. Diuretics should be withheld temporarily and a more liberal salt intake permitted. Cautious infusion of 25–100 g plasma protein fraction or 20–40 g salt poor albumen over a period of 3 or 4 hours to increase the blood volume may help. Signs of circulatory overload are an indication to stop the infusion.

Hyponatraemia. Patients with severe oedema may develop hyponatraemia because they are unable to excrete water normally (Table 6.4, p. 215). This is exacerbated by the use of thiazides or metolazone which interfere with urinary dilution. The clinical features associated with hyponatraemia and its management are discussed on page 215.

WATER EXCESS

Healthy adults can safely drink up to 20 l/day of water and respond with a vigorous water diuresis. The requirements for excretion of solute-free water are given in the information box below.

REQUIREMENTS FOR EXCRETION OF SOLUTE-FREE WATER

- Delivery of sufficient solute and water to the diluting sites in the ascending limb of Henle's loop and early distal tubule
- Unimpaired reabsorption of Na^+ and Cl^- without water at diluting sites
- Adequate flow through collecting duct
- Absence of ADH or ADH-like substances – collecting duct therefore largely impermeable to water

---

Aetiology

In the disorders shown in Tables 6.4 and 6.5 excretion of water is restricted because of disturbance of one or more of these physiological processes while in some patients with primary polydipsia the huge intake of water exceeds normal excretory capacity.

Retention of water reduces the plasma $[Na^+]$ and osmolality and induces a shift of water into cells.

Clinical features

The resultant symptoms are primarily those of disordered cerebral function, partly due to cerebral oedema and include dizziness, headache, anorexia, nausea, vomiting and mental confusion. Severe water intoxication can cause convulsions, coma and death. Diagnosis depends upon awareness of the circumstances in which water intoxication is likely to occur and demonstration of a plasma $[Na^+]$ below 130 mmol/l.

Table 6.4   Conditions associated with impaired excretion of water

Renal	Acute renal failure Chronic renal failure Nephrotic syndrome
Endocrine	SIADH[1] (Table 6.5) Primary or secondary adrenocortical insufficiency Hypothyroidism
Hepatic	Liver failure Hepatic cirrhosis
Congestive cardiac failure	
Extracellular fluid volume depletion	
Drugs	Diuretics which impair urinary dilution (frusemide, bumetanide, metolazone, benzothiadiazines) Drugs thought to induce SIADH (Table 6.5)

[1]Secretion of ADH from the posterior pituitary in the absence of recognised osmotic or haemodynamic stimuli or secretion of ADH or ADH-like peptides by a malignant neoplasm.

Table 6.5   Conditions associated with the syndrome of inappropriate secretion of ADH (SIADH)

Neoplasm	Carcinoma-lung (small cell), pancreas, duodenum, ureter, bladder, prostate, lymphoma, thymoma, mesothelioma
Disorders of CNS	Meningitis, encephalitis, brain abscess, head injury, cerebral tumour, cerebral vascular accident, hydrocephalus, cerebral or cerebellar atrophy, delirium tremens, psychosis, Guillain-Barré syndrome
Non-malignant pulmonary lesions	Tuberculosis, pneumonia (bacterial, viral)
Drugs	Narcotics, phenothiazines, carbamazepine, tricyclic antidepressants, monoamine oxidase inhibitors, clofibrate, vincristine, vinblastine, cyclophosphamide*, chlorpropamide, non-steroldal anti-inflammatory agents*
Miscellaneous	Pain, postoperative period, nausea

* Potentiate effect ADH on collecting duct.

Urinary osmolality, which in these circumstances should be less than 100 mosm/kg, is inappropriately high except in the rare patient with primary polydipsia.

Management

Water intake should be restricted and, simultaneously, the underlying cause identified and treated. To maintain water balance 400 ml/day (the difference between insensible losses and water produced by metabolic processes) plus a volume equal to the urinary output should be given to afebrile patients. More rigorous restriction is required to achieve negative water balance in the overhydrated. In severely symptomatic cases 100 ml 5% NaCl solution should be given intravenously and repeated in a few hours if there is little or no clinical improvement and the plasma [Na$^+$] remains below 130 mmol/l. Patients who have irremediable tumours producing ADH or ADH-like peptide can be treated with demethylchlortetracycline, 300 mg 4 times daily to inhibit the action of the peptide on the collecting duct. The drug is nephrotoxic and its use is best confined to such patients. It also commonly induces a photosensitive dermatitis and patients should be warned to avoid direct sunlight. Alternatively, when the cause cannot be treated, plasma [Na$^+$] may be kept within the reference range by increasing the Na$^+$ intake to about 200 mmol/day and giving frusemide, 40 mg/day, by mouth.

HYPONATRAEMIA

It is convenient, here, to summarise the conditions which give rise to hyponatraemia which develops when for any reason the proportion of Na$^+$ to water in the ECF is reduced (Table 6.6). When marked hyper-

Table 6.6   Hyponatraemia

Pathogenesis		Clinical condition	Extracellular fluid volume
Increased total body water	1 impaired water excretion	SIADH, adrenocortical insufficiency, hypopituitarism, hypothyroidism, (see Table 6.4)	Slightly increased. No oedema
	2 Excess water intake	Psychogenic polydipsia	
Relative increase extracellular water	Transfer of water from cells	Uncontrolled diabetes mellitus administration of mannitol	Normal or slightly reduced
Reduction in total body Na$^+$ exceeds reduction in total body water	1 Severe untreated Na$^+$ and water depletion	Any cause of mixed Na$^+$ and water depletion (Table 6.1)	Reduced. May be evidence of oligaemia
	2 Na$^+$ and water depletion treated by replacement of water without Na$^+$		
Increase in total body water exceeds increase in body Na$^+$	Retention of Na$^+$ associated with impaired water excretion	Congestive cardiac failure, nephrotic syndrome, liver failure, cirrhosis, acute or chronic renal failure, diuretics	Increased Oedema

lipaemia is present a falsely low value for plasma [Na^+] is obtained as Na^+ is confined to the aqueous phase. In such cases plasma osmolality is normal.

Clinical features

Manifestations of cellular overhydration (p. 213) are usually present when plasma [Na^+] falls below 128 mmol/l and are accompanied by signs and symptoms of the underlying disorder. The latter can usually be determined from the history, physical examination and specific investigations, e.g. tests of thyroid, adrenal or pituitary function, liver function tests, blood urea, creatinine clearance. A good history and clinical assessment of the state of the ECF are helpful in determining into which of the groups shown in Table 6.6 the patient fits.

Management

The underlying cause should be identified and if possible, treated. Patients in whom there is a straightforward excess of body water are treated along the lines indicated on page 213. In those in whom inability to excrete water complicates Na^+ retention the outlook is poor unless the underlying condition can be improved. Restriction of water, ideally to 400 ml/day, should be attempted but may prove intolerable. Patients depleted of Na^+ and water are treated by infusion of 0.9% Nacl solution (or a mixture of this solution with 1.26% $NHCO_3$ solution) to restore the ECF volume. It is useful to monitor the CVP throughout to avoid overload. Expansion of the ECF volume results in improved renal perfusion, the ability to excrete water is restored and the plasma [Na^+] gradually rises to normal. During this procedure the intake of water should be cut to the absolute minimum. Hyponatraemia associated with poorly controlled diabetes mellitus resolves when the blood glucose is lowered, ECF osmolality falls and water shifts into cells.

POTASSIUM DEPLETION

The adult body contains approximately 45 mmol/kg body weight of K^+ the great majority being in cells at a concentration between 140 and 150 mmol/l. The ECF contains less than 2% at a concentration of 3.5–5 mmol/l (Fig. 6.2, p. 205). In health both total body K^+ and the distribution of the ion between cells and ECF are maintained within narrow limits. The large concentration gradient across cells membranes, which is the main determinant of the resting membrane potential, is sustained by active transport mechanisms including the Na^+/K^+ pump. Cellular uptake of K^+ is enhanced by insulin, beta-adrenergic stimulation and

aldosterone and influenced by blood [H^+] and ECF tonicity.

Over 85% of the daily intake of 60–80 mmol K^+ is excreted in urine, the remainder in stools. Maintenance of K^+ balance thus depends on regulation of urinary K^+ excretion. Most filtered K^+ is reabsorbed in the upper nephron. Potassium enters the tubular fluid in the distal nephron by passive diffusion down a lumen negative electrochemical gradient. The amount is determined by the magnitude of this gradient which increases when:

1. cell [K^+] rises;
2. the rate of flow through the distal nephron increases;
3. the rate of reabsorption of Na^+ in the distal nephron increases;
4. there is an excess of poorly reabsorbed anions in distal tubular fluid.

When the intake of K^+ is excessive adaptive mechanisms come into play which increase its rate of excretion in urine and uptake by hepatic and muscle cells. When intake is reduced to 10–15 mmol/day urinary excretion falls gradually to about 15 mmol/day but this small continuing loss, together with the daily faecal losses of 8–10 mmol/l, results in moderate K^+ depletion.

Causes of potassium depletion (Table 6.7)

The condition usually results from excessive loss of K^+ from the gastrointestinal tract or in urine (Table 6.7). Most of the gastrointestinal disorders listed are associated with loss of Na^+ and water as well as K^+ and the resulting increase in circulating aldosterone leads to additional loss of K^+ in urine. Renal K^+ wastage usually develops because one or more of the factors discussed earlier augment transfer of K^+ into distal tubular fluid. Thus in mineralocorticoid excess, uptake of K^+ from the peritubular fluid into tubular cells, intracellular [K^+] and permeability of the luminal membrane to the ion are all increased. In alkalosis K^+ uptake and thus tubular cell [K^+] are increased and in addition urinary loss is further augmented by the presence of poorly reabsorbed HCO_3^- in distal tubular fluid. Tubular cell [K^+] is reduced in acidosis but paradoxically in chronic metabolic acidosis the increased delivery of Na^+ and water to the distal nephron actually augments K^+ excretion. Many diuretics facilitate K^+ loss by the same means. In diabetic ketoacidosis increased distal delivery of Na^+, water and poorly reabsorbable anions of ketoacids augment K^+ excretion. Circulating aldosterone is increased in the last three disorders. Loss of K^+ during recovery from acute tubular necrosis or after relief of

Table 6.7   Causes of potassium depletion

Reduced intake	Diet containing adequate calories and insufficient potassium
	Potassium-free intravenous fluid
Loss from alimentary tract	*External loss*
	Vomiting
	Aspiration of GI contents
	Fistulae
	Diarrhoea
	Acute
	Chronic (laxative addicts[1], malabsorption syndrome[1])
	Villous adenoma large bowel
	Ureterosigmoidostomy
	Sequestration of fluid in bowel
	Ileus
	Intestinal obstruction
Loss in urine	*Extrarenal factors acting on kidney*
	Primary aldosteronism[2]
	Bartters' syndrome
	Secondary aldosteronism (e.g. renovascular disease, accelerated hypertension[2], cirrhosis, cardiac failure, nephrotic syndrome)
	Cushing's syndrome[2]
	Diabetic ketoacidosis
	Metabolic alkalosis
	Chronic metabolic acidosis
	Drugs, e.g. diuretics, amphotericin B, corticosteroids[2], liquorice[2], carbenoxolone[2]
	Renal disease
	Recovery phase acute tubular necrosis
	Following relief urinary tract obstruction
	Renal tubular acidosis

[1]Considerable amounts of potassium may be lost in diarrhoea with formed stools.
[2]Associated with hypertension.

urinary obstruction is due to failure to reabsorb the ion in the upper nephron and also to increased delivery of Na^+, water and HCO_3^- to the distal nephron. In renal tubular acidosis (p. 599) it is likely that permeability of the luminal membrane of tubular cells for K^+ is increased. Amphotericin B may cause a similar defect. Elderly people taking a diet inadequate in K^+ often become mildly depleted. The precise mechanism is unknown but inappropriate urinary loss probably contributes.

Relationship of plasma potassium to total body potassium
Plasma $[K^+]$, which in general reflects changes in body stores of this ion, is low in most cases of K^+ depletion. However in the presence of severe ECF depletion, metabolic acidosis or deficiency of insulin or aldosterone (p. 216) clinically significant K^+ depletion can develop without a change in plasma $[K^+]$, e.g. untreated diabetic ketoacidosis. Conversely patients suffering from metabolic alkalosis and those who have received insulin or beta-adrenergic agonists may have hypokalaemia despite a normal total body K^+. Plasma $[K^+]$ often falls when patients with severe megalo-

blastic anaemia start treatment with vitamin B_{12} because K^+ is taken up in newly formed erythrocytes. Many cases of K^+ depletion are accompanied by mild metabolic alkalosis (p. 225).

Consequences of potassium depletion
The most important clinical features are due to changes in electrical potential difference across cell membranes and to effects on intra-cellular enzymes.

Clinical features
Deficits of less than 10% body K^+ give rise to few if any clinical features. The clinical picture in patients with larger deficits depends on the rapidity with which the condition develops and the presence or absence of ECF depletion and disturbances of acid base balance. The clinical features of chronic and acute potassium depletion are listed in the information boxes below and page 218.

CLINICAL FEATURES OF ACUTE POTASSIUM DEPLETION (DEFICIT > 10% BODY K^+)

Causes
Loss of large volumes of intestinal secretions, massive diuresis following relief of urinary tract obstruction, severe ketoacidosis

Associated disturbances
Severe Na^+ and water depletion, commonly metabolic acidosis, possible Mg^{++} depletion

Presentation
Initially features of ECF depletion predominate (p. 206) and plasma $[K^+]$ may be normal
When ECF volume restored unless K^+ salts are given plasma $[K^+]$ falls and features of acute K^+ depletion develop viz:
   Generalised muscle weakness, depression of tendon reflexes
   ECG changes (Fig. 6.7), arrhythmias, sensitivity to digitalis, reduced cardiac output
   Paraesthesiae, apathy, confusion, coma
Death may occur due to respiratory paralysis or cardiac arrest.

Diagnosis
On basis history, clinical findings
Low plasma $[K^+]$ confirms diagnosis (plasma $[K^+]$ may be normal at presentation)

When depletion results from a gastrointestinal disorder a diagnosis of the cause is often easily made. However, patients addicted to laxatives and those who induce surreptitious vomiting will usually deny these practices and the uncommon villous adenoma may give rise to no symptoms. When the cause of depletion is not clear the urinary K^+ should be measured. A value of less than 20 mmol/day excludes renal K^+ wasting while one of more than 30 mmol/day in a patient whose plasma K^+ has been low for some days suggests impaired renal

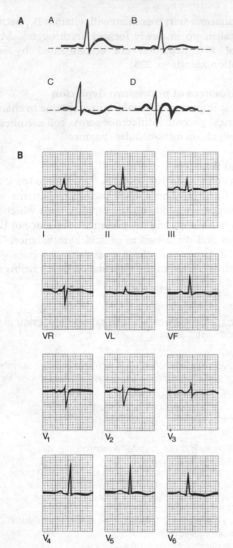

Fig. 6.7   Changes in the ECG associated with hypokalaemia.
A. Progressive ECG changes in hypokalaemia. A normal; B flattening of T wave and depression of S-T segment; C S-T segment depression resembling an inverted T wave; prolongation of Q-T interval; D inverted T wave; U wave appears. These patterns are not necessarily sequential; patterns C and D are most common. **B.** ECG showing effects of hypokalaemia. Sinus rhythm with normal QRS complexes. In all leads the T waves are flattened and it is difficult to measure the QT interval, but this is probably 0.44 seconds. U waves are present in most leads.

conservation. In patients losing K^+ in urine a careful history and examination will often suggest one of the disorders shown in Table 6.7 and appropriate investigations can be instigated. It is important to enquire about any drugs taken by the patient and to note whether or not hypertension or metabolic acidosis is present.

CLINICAL FEATURES OF CHRONIC POTASSIUM DEPLETION (DEFICIT > 10% BODY K^+)

Causes
Surreptitious vomiting, chronic diarrhoea, villous adenoma large bowel, chronic loss K^+ in urine

Associated disturbances
Mild metabolic alkalosis (sometimes a consequence of K^+ depletion)
Patients with renal tubular lesions often have metabolic acidosis
Mg^{++} depletion common
Na^+ and water balance depends on underlying cause

Presentation
A low plasma $[K^+]$ is usual
Muscle stiffness, weakness, depression tendon jerks, in severe cases attacks of muscle paralysis following carbohydrate meal or rest
ECG changes (Fig. 6.7), arrhythmias, digitalis sensitivity. In severe cases cardiac output, renal blood flow, GFR, reduced
Impaired urinary concentration, polyuria, nocturia, thirst
Drowsiness, apathy, impaired memory

Diagnosis
On basis history, clinical findings. Characteristic ECG suggestive
Low plasma $[K^+]$ confirms diagnosis

Management
Potassium depletion can be treated by giving a K^+ salt orally or intravenously. The former route is preferable as it carries much less risk of inducing hyperkalaemia and cardiac arrest and should be used whenever possible. Unless there is an associated metabolic acidosis KCl should be given. One gramme of KCl contains 13.4 mmol of K^+. This preparation sometimes causes gastrointestinal irritation especially when there is delay in intestinal transit. 'Slow release' tablets of KCl are less troublesome in this respect, each contains 600 mg (8 mmol) of KCl. Some patients tolerate the less nauseating effervescent K^+ tablets better.

Established deficiencies of moderate severity can be corrected by giving 8–15 g/day (107–201 mmol) of KCl, in divided doses, for several days and a diet rich in K^+, i.e. containing fruit juices, coffee, milk and meat. Treatment is stopped when the plasma $[K^+]$ is stable within the reference range.

In patients unable to take K^+ by mouth and those with frank muscle weakness or marked electrocardiogram (ECG) changes intravenous infusions of KCl are needed. This route should be used only when proven hypokalaemia is present. Associated salt and water depletion should be treated first; when significant sodium depletion or oliguria is present intravenous administration of potassium should be avoided unless

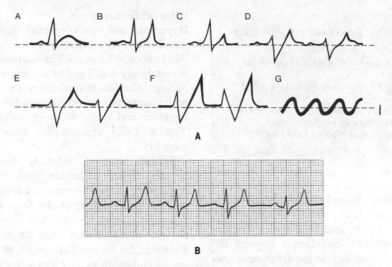

Fig. 6.8 Changes in the ECG associated with hyperkalaemia. A. Progressive ECG changes in hyperkalaemia. A Normal; B tall, peaked, symmetrical T waves, tentlike shape, narrow base; C T waves of normal amplitude, but with tentlike shape and narrow base; D P-R and QRS intervals lengthen; R wave and P wave decrease in height; S wave increases in depth; RS-T segment depressed. E, F P wave may disappear; QRS may lengthen further; ventricular rhythm may become grossly irregular at this point and may give appearance of bundle branch block; G QRS complexes lose angular shape and become smoother and wider; continuous sine wave; may give appearance of paroxysmal ventricular tachycardia. **B.** ECG showing hyperkalaemia. The T waves are tall, peaked, tentlike and the PR QRS complexes are lengthened.

dangerous hypokalaemia is present and facilities for repeated chemical analysis are available.

For intravenous administration, KCl 1.5 g can be added to 500 ml of isotonic NaCl or glucose solution. The solution then contains 20 mmol/l of K^+ and should be given over 2–3 hours. Repeated measurements of plasma $[K^+]$ are necessary to determine whether further KCl is required. It is rarely necessary to give more than 100 mmol of K^+ daily. As soon as possible oral KCl should be substituted for intravenous KCl. When K^+ depletion is due to persistent vomiting and is associated with alkalosis due to loss of gastric HCl, a solution containing KCl, NaCl and NH_4Cl is sometimes used (p. 227).

The cause of the K^+ depletion must be identified and treated. Wherever possible steps should be taken to prevent K^+ depletion. These steps are shown in the information box (right).

HYPERKALAEMIA

The plasma $[K^+]$ depends upon total body K^+ and the distribution of the ion between cells and ECF. Since the ECF contains less than 2% of body K^+ a small shift of

---

PREVENTION OF POTASSIUM DEPLETION

- Patients receiving benzothiadiazine diuretics, frusemide or bumetanide for treatment of oedema should receive KCl 20–60 mmol/day in whatever form is tolerated. Plasma $[K^+]$ should be monitored at intervals and the dose adjusted.
- Some patients receiving pharmacological doses of corticosteroids require KCl supplements.
- Patients receiving diuretics for treatment of hypertension may require KCl supplements.
- Patients unable to eat or drink, maintained on i.v. fluids, should receive sufficient KCl, distributed through the fluids, to maintain K^+ balance. 60–80 mmol/day is recommended for patients with no unusual K^+ loss. The plasma $[K^+]$ should be monitored at least daily and the dose adjusted.

---

this ion out of cells could, theoretically cause marked hyperkalaemia. In practice three factors are important in the genesis of significant hyperkalaemia and these are listed in the information box (p. 220).

Aetiology

It is common for several causal factors to be present in patients with hyperkalaemia. For example, in diabetic

CIRCUMSTANCES IN WHICH SIGNIFICANT HYPERKALAEMIA MAY OCCUR

- Tissue damage with release of K^+ from dead and injured cells
- Rapid administration of a large amount of K^+ by mouth or i.v.
- Impaired renal excretion of K^+ including administration of potassium-sparing diuretics such as spironolactone
- Combination of lesser degrees of points 1 and 2 with 3

ketoacidosis, in which hyperkalaemia is relatively common despite an overall K^+ deficit, lack of insulin, metabolic acidosis and increased ECF tonicity reduce cell uptake of K^+ while hypovolaemia impairs K^+ excretion. In chronic renal failure hyperkalaemia may be precipitated by any drug which further impairs K^+ excretion (Table 6.8) or by an excessive intake of the ion. In some chronic renal diseases, notably chronic interstitial nephritis and diabetic glomerulosclerosis, release of renin is impaired (hyporeninaemic hypo-aldosteronism) and hyperkalaemia develops at a time when overall renal function is still fairly good. The same pattern is seen in disorders such as lupus or amyloidosis which cause selective distal tubular damage.

Table 6.8   Causes of hyperkalaemia

Increased intake	i.v. fluid containing K^+, high K^+ foods
	Drugs containing K^+ (e.g. Sandocal)
Tissue breakdown	Bleeding into soft tissues, GI tract or body cavities
	Haemolysis, rhabdomyolysis
	Catabolic states
Shift of K^+ out of cells	Tissue damage (e.g. following ischaemia, shock)
	Acidosis
	Insulin deficiency
	Aldosterone deficiency
	Beta adrenergic blocking drugs
	ECF hypertonicity
Impaired excretion	*Renal disease*
	Acute renal failure
	Severe chronic renal failure (GFR < 15 ml/min)
	Impaired tubular secretion K^+ (SLE, transplanted kidney, amyloidosis, sickle cell disease)
	Acute circulatory failure
	Drugs which inhibit renal K^+ secretion
	Aldosterone antagonists, triamterene, amiloride
	Abnormalities of renin-angiotensin aldosterone axis
	Addison's disease, adrenal enzyme deficiencies
	Primary hypoaldosteronism
	Hyporeninaemic hypoaldosteronism
	Beta adrenergic blockers, NSAID, captopril
Pseudohyperkalaemia	Release K^+ in vitro from abnormal blood cells or incorrectly handled specimens

Clinical features

Hyperkalaemia causes partial depolarisation of cell membranes. As cardiac arrest can occur when plasma $[K^+]$ exceeds 7.5 mmol/l measurement of plasma $[K^+]$ is mandatory when any of the known causal factors are present. Cardiac disturbances are often the first and only manifestations of the disorder, the pulse becomes irregular and heart block of varying degree occurs. Typical ECG changes are shown in Figure 6.8, page 219.

Patients develop muscular weakness which may progress to loss of tendon jerks, flaccid paralysis and respiratory embarrassment. Abdominal distension due to ileus and tingling of the face, hands and feet are common. These features are indistinguishable from those of hypokalaemia – the diagnosis is suggested by knowing the circumstances in which hyperkalaemia occurs and confirmed by measuring plasma $[K^+]$.

Management

Hyperkalaemia must be prevented in conditions associated with oliguria and the recommendations about diet in acute renal failure have this end in view (p. 591). In dealing with established acute hyperkalaemia the measures shown in the information box below are advised.

MANAGEMENT OF ACUTE HYPERKALAEMIA

- Identify and if possible remove the cause
- When there are marked ECG changes inject 10 ml 10% calcium gluconate solution slowly, monitoring ECG throughout.
- Inject 50 ml 50% glucose +5 units soluble insulin i.v. to encourage shift of K^+ into cells. Monitor plasma $[K^+]$ at intervals and repeat procedure if hyperkalaemia recurs. Alternatively 500 ml of 20% glucose solution +5–10 units soluble insulin are infused over 6–12 hours.
- Infuse 1.26% $NaHCO_3$ solution until plasma $[HCO_3^-]$ is in the upper reference range to encourage shift of K^+ into cells and excretion of K^+ in urine. This must not be done if there is evidence of circulatory overload.
- Replace any Na^+ and water deficit to restore circulation, renal perfusion and K^+ excretion.
- Correct respiratory acidosis.
- If these measures fail haemodialysis or peritoneal dialysis is indicated.

Measures to prevent recurrence of hyperkalaemia include:

1. restriction of foods rich in K^+;
2. use of calcium resonium.

Resin adsorbs K^+ in the intestine and can be given orally as 15 g suspended in a small volume of water, or 30 g in

Table 6.9   Causes of magnesium depletion

Reduced intake	Protein calorie malnutrition
	Prolonged administration Mg^{++} free parenteral fluids
Loss from alimentary tract	Vomiting
	Aspiration of GI secretions, fistulae
	Chronic diarrhoea (malabsorption syndrome, laxative addicts)
Loss in urine	*Extrarenal factors acting on kidney*
	Ketoacidosis
	Hyperparathyroidism
	Primary aldosteronism, Bartters syndrome
	secondary aldosteronism
	Chronic alcoholism
	Drugs, e.g. loop diuretics, gentamicin, cisplatin
	Renal disease
	Renal tubular acidosis
	Post-obstructive diuresis
	Diuretic phase acute tubular necrosis
Miscellaneous	Excessive lactation
	Acute pancreatitis

water administered by retention enema as required, usually 3 or 4 times daily.

MAGNESIUM DEFICIENCY AND EXCESS

Disorders of magnesium metabolism are occasionally responsible for otherwise puzzling clinical features.

Aetiology of magnesium depletion

The important known causes of magnesium depletion are shown in Table 6.9.

Clinical features of magnesium depletion

These are predominantly neuromuscular, with tremor and choreiform movements. Depression, confusion, agitation, epileptic fits and hallucinations also occur. The diagnosis can be confirmed by finding the plasma magnesium less than 0.75 mmol/l. Since most magnesium is intracellular a body deficit of this ion can coexist with a normal plasma magnesium.

Management

The condition is best treated by giving 30–50 mmol $MgCl_2$ in a litre of isotonic saline or glucose over 12–24 hours. Thereafter 15–25 mmol $MgCl_2$ should be infused daily until plasma Mg^+ remains in the reference range. When renal function is impaired the amount of $MgCl_2$ should be halved.

Magnesium excess

This mainly occurs in acute and chronic renal disease and contributes to the central nervous features associated with uraemia. Its treatment is that of the primary disorder.

HYDROGEN ION CONCENTRATION

Life is possible only if the $[H^+]$ of body fluids is kept within a narrow range. In health a blood $[H^+]$ of 36–44 nmol/l (pH 7.37–7.45) is maintained by several closely integrated mechanisms. Some understanding of these is necessary to appreciate the clinical implications of acidosis and alkalosis.

Since $[H^+] = K[HA]/[A^-]$ where $[HA]$ is the concentration of the conjugate acid and $[A^-]$ the concentration of the conjugate base in any buffer system, K being the dissociation constant of the acid, the $[H^+]$ in any body fluid is determined by the ratio of the conjugate acids to the conjugate bases of the different buffer systems in that fluid. Thus in ECF the $[H^+]$ depends mainly upon the ratio of carbonic acid, (H_2CO_3) to HCO_3^-. The concentration of H_2CO_3 in plasma is determined by the partial pressure of carbon dioxide (P_{CO_2}) in the alveoli. The latter is normally about 5.3 kPa (Fig. 6.11) which gives rise to a little over 1 mmol/l of H_2CO_3 in physical solution in plasma. The alveolar P_{CO_2} is maintained steady because CO_2 is excreted by the lungs at the same rate as it is produced by tissues. The $[HCO_3^-]$ is regulated by the kidneys and, in health, is kept at about 22–27 mmol/l (p. 551).

Metabolic processes produce acids which must be eliminated from the body if the $[H^+]$ of body fluids is to remain within the normal range. The route of disposal of acids depends upon whether or not they can be oxidised completely to CO_2 and water. Carbon dioxide, which forms H_2CO_3 within the body, is eliminated by ventilation. Other acids such as phosphoric and sulphuric derived from the oxidation of phospholipids or sulphur-containing proteins respectively, are excreted by the kidneys. At the site of their production in tissues and during their carriage in blood all acids increase $[H^+]$ but this is minimised by the physiologically important buffers in both ECF and ICF.

Carbonic acid is produced in far greater amounts than any other acid. A small part of the CO_2 is transported reversibly bound to haemoglobin as a carbamino compound in erythrocytes but the greater part is converted to H_2CO_3 in these cells which are rich in carbonic anhydrase. Hydrogen ions from H_2CO_3 are taken up by haemoglobin in red cells after it has given up its oxygen to tissues while the HCO_3^- moves out from red cells to plasma in exchange for Cl^- (chloride shift, Fig. 6.9). Most of the carbonic acid added to the blood therefore appears not as acid but as HCO_3^-. When the blood passes through the lungs and haemoglobin is reoxygenated this process is reversed and the CO_2 formed is exhaled.

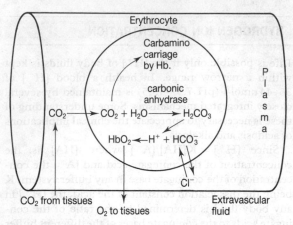

Fig. 6.9   Transport of CO_2.

Table 6.10   Changes in blood $[H^+]$, Pa_{CO_2} and plasma $[HCO_3^-]$ in acid base disturbances

Disorder	Compensation	Arterial blood gases	
		Uncompensated	Compensated
Metabolic acidosis	Ventilation ↑ Pa_{CO_2} ↓	$[H^+]$ ↑ $[HCO_3^-]$ ↓ Pa_{CO_2} normal	$[H^+]$ ↑ or normal $[HCO_3^-]$ ↓ Pa_{CO_2} ↓
Metabolic alkalosis	Ventilation ↓ Pa_{CO_2} ↑	$[H^+]$ ↓ $[HCO_3^-]$ ↑ Pa_{CO_2} normal	$[H^+]$ ↓ or normal $[HCO_3^-]$ ↑ Pa_{CO_2} ↑
Respiratory acidosis	Renal $[HCO_3^-]$ ↑	$[H^+]$ ↑ $[HCO_3^-]$ normal Pa_{CO_2} ↑	$[H^+]$ ↑ or normal $[HCO_3^-]$ ↑ Pa_{CO_2} ↑
Respiratory alkalosis	Renal $[HCO_3^-]$ ↓	$[H^+]$ ↓ $[HCO_3^-]$ normal Pa_{CO_2} ↓	$[H^+]$ ↓ or normal $[HCO_3^-]$ ↓ Pa_{CO_2} ↓

In health, on a normal diet, 40–80 mmol/day of non-volatile acids are excreted in the urine. In some disorders, notably diabetic ketoacidosis, large amounts of acid are formed. The tissues and blood are buffered against these acids by a different mechanism which involves in particular the $NaHCO_3$ and H_2CO_3 buffer system in the plasma.

The addition of acid to the plasma results in a movement of the reactions in the direction indicated by the broad arrow (Fig. 6.10). As a result of this and similar reactions on the part of the other buffer systems, many H^+ ions which would otherwise increase the acidity of plasma are removed to form increased amounts of poorly dissociated acids such as H_2CO_3. There is a corresponding diminution in the concentration of conjugate bases including HCO_3^-. By this means the $[H^+]$ of the plasma rises far less than it would if the buffers were not present.

The rise in $[H^+]$ stimulates ventilation and the excess H_2CO_3 is exhaled as CO_2. Removal of the anion of the acid (e.g. acetoacetate) and restoration of depleted body HCO_3^- occurs simultaneously within the kidney. The renal tubules form H_2CO_3 much of the H^+ of which is excreted in the form of NH_4^+ ions along with the acid anion. The HCO_3^- ion generated in this process is

returned to the blood and reconstitutes the depleted blood buffer (p. 551).

These buffering and excreting mechanisms are continually in operation in response to normal production of acids derived from metabolism. It is clear from this simplified description that the important

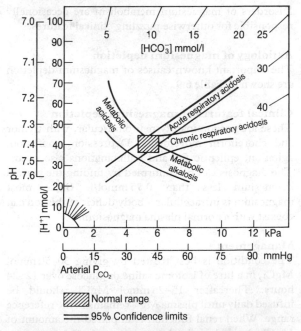

Fig. 6.11   Diagram showing changes in blood $[H^+]$, Pa_{CO_2} and plasma $[HCO_3^-]$ in stable compensated acid base disorders. The rectangle indicates limits of normal reference ranges for $[H^+]$ and Pa_{CO_2}. Diagram devised by Flenley using data from literature. The bands represent 95% confidence limits of single disturbances in human blood in vivo. When the point obtained by plotting $[H^+]$ against Pa_{CO_2} does not fall within one of labelled bands compensation is incomplete or a mixed disorder is present. (Dr D Flenley. The Lancet, 1971; 1: 1921)

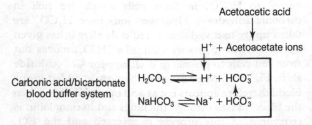

Fig. 6.10   Effect of acid on the blood buffer system.

limiting factor in the buffering power of blood is availability of haemoglobin and HCO_3^-. The excretory power of the kidneys is the limiting factor in the body's ability to rid itself of the H^+ and anions derived from acids other than H_2CO_3.

DISTURBANCES IN HYDROGEN ION CONCENTRATION

Abnormalities in the reaction of the body fluids are reflected in inter-related changes in blood $[H^+]$, $[H_2CO_3]$ (i.e. Pa_{CO_2}) and $[HCO_3^-]$. Determination of the quantity and quality of any change requires accurate measurement of at least two of these variables. pH and Pa_{CO_2} can be measured directly, $[HCO_3^-]$ is usually calculated from either Pa_{CO_2} or total CO_2 and pH using the Henderson-Hasselbach equation or a nomogram based on it. Since $[HCO_3^-]$ is itself influenced by Pa_{CO_2} it may be expressed as 'standard bicarbonate' namely the $[HCO_3^-]$ which would exist at a standard value of Pa_{CO_2}, 5.2 kPa.

METABOLIC ACIDOSIS

Metabolic acidosis is characterised by a reduction in plasma $[HCO_3^-]$ and a consequent rise in $[H^+]$. The

Pa_{CO_2} is reduced secondarily by hyperventilation induced by the acidaemia; this restores the $[H_2CO_3]/[HCO_3^-]$ ratio partially and mitigates the rise in $[H^+]$ (Table 6.10). The relationship between $[H^+]$ and Pa_{CO_2} in stable disorders of acid base balance is well defined and diagrams such as Figure 6.11 are sometimes helpful in defining the nature and extent of the disturbance present in a particular patient.

Aetiology
The physiological disturbances which give rise to metabolic acidosis are shown in the information box below while conditions in which these disturbances develop are listed in Table 6.11. The pathogenesis of the Na^+ and water depletion which usually accompanies metabolic acidosis is shown in Table 6.11.

DISTURBANCES WHICH GIVE RISE TO METABOLIC ACIDOSIS

- Overproduction of acids other than H_2CO_3. Ingestion of acids or potential acids
- Failure to excrete acids other than H_2CO_3 at a rate equal to that at which they are generated
- Loss of the base HCO_3^- in urine or from the GI tract

Table 6.11 Causes of metabolic acidosis

Mechanism	Clinical disorders	Accumulating acid	Anion gap[1]	Cause of associated Na^+ depletion
Addition of excessive acid				
1 Disorders of intermediary metabolism	Ketoacidosis	Acetoacetic β hydroxybutyric	Increased	Loss in urine with anion of abnormal acid
	Lactic acidosis	Lactic	Increased	Loss in urine with anion of abnormal acid
2 Induced by exogenous substances	Methanol poisoning	Formic	Increased	Loss in urine with anion of abnormal acid
	Ethylene glycol poisoning	Glycolic, oxalic	Increased	Loss in urine with anion of abnormal acid
	Salicylate poisoning[2]	Various organic	Increased	Loss in urine with anion of abnormal acid
	Overdose NH_4Cl or $CaCl_2$	Hydrochloric	Normal	Loss in urine with anion of abnormal acid
Failure to excrete acid at a normal rate				
1 Inadequate renal NH_4^+ production	Chronic renal failure	Sulphuric, phosphoric etc produced by metabolism	Increased	Impaired renal Na^+ conservation
2 Inability to maintain $[H^+]$ gradient between blood and urine	Distal renal tubular acidosis	Hydrochloric	Normal	Reduced Na^+/H^+ exchange in distal tubule
3 Oliguria	Acute renal failure	Sulphuric, phosphoric etc. produced by metabolism	Increased	Usually absent
Loss of bicarbonate				
1 In urine	Proximal renal tubular acidosis	Hydrochloric	Normal	Reduced Na^+/H^+ exchange in proximal tubule
	Carbonic anhydrase inhibitors	Hydrochloric	Normal	Reduced Na^+/H^+ exchange throughout nephron
2 From GI tract	Diarrhoea, fistulae	Hydrochloric	Normal	Loss of Na^+ in GI secretions
	Ureterosigmoidostomy	Hydrochloric	Normal	Loss of Na^+ in GI secretions

[1]Anion Gap = $[Na^+] - [Cl^-] - [HCO_3^-]$ normal 8–12 mmol/l
[2]Especially in children, in adults respiratory alkalosis usually predominates.

Lactic acid accumulates when its rate of production from pyruvate in muscle, skin, brain and erythrocytes exceeds its rate of removal by liver and kidney. As indicated by the equation

$$[lactate] = K\frac{[NADH]}{[NAD]} \times [pyruvate] \times [H^+]$$

Lactate production increases when oxidative metabolism is reduced, glycolysis increased and [pyruvate] and [NADH] rise. Causes of lactic acidosis are shown in the information box below.

CAUSES OF LACTIC ACIDOSIS

Group A
Shock due to any cause, respiratory failure, poisoning with cyanide or carbon monoxide, profound anaemia

Group B
Diabetes mellitus, hepatic failure, severe infection
Malignant neoplasm (lymphoma, leukaemia), fits
Drugs (biguanides, streptozotocin, salicylate, isoniazid, fructose, sorbitol)
Toxins (ethanol, methanol)
Congenital enzyme defects

Those in Group A produce hypotension or severe tissue hypoxia, disorders in Group B do not give rise to either but are nonetheless associated with impaired mitochondrial respiration and increased lactate production. Diabetic ketoacidosis is discussed on page 680. In chronic renal failure the most important factor limiting H^+ excretion is reduced production of the NH_4^+ ion by the diminished mass of tubules. Failure to conserve or to regenerate HCO_3^- characterises proximal and distal renal tubular acidosis respectively (p. 599).

Clinical features

The most obvious clinical consequence is stimulation of respiration by the raised blood $[H^+]$. In severe cases the respirations become deep and sighing (Kussmaul's respiration). When the blood $[H^+]$ exceeds 70 nmol/l myocardial function is compromised, cardiac output falls and this, in conjunction with peripheral vasodilation, results in a fall in blood pressure. These patients are frequently confused or stuporous.

In many cases the clinical picture is determined by the underlying disorder and the presence of concomitant Na^+, K^+ and water depletion.

The diagnosis is facilitated by awareness of those pathological conditions in which it is likely to arise. It should be confirmed by determining $[H^+]$ Pa_{CO_2} and $[HCO_3^-]$ in blood.

Information about the likely cause may be obtained by calculating delta (Δ), the anion gap, the concentration of unmeasured anions (albumin, sulphate, phosphate) in plasma using the equation:

$$\Delta = [Na^+] - ([Cl^-] + [HCO_3^-]),$$

In health Δ is less than 14. In metabolic acidosis due to diarrhoea, renal tubular acidosis or some forms of poisoning, hydrochloric acid (HCl) is added to body fluids, HCO_3^- is replaced by Cl^- and Δ is normal. In other forms of metabolic acidosis it is increased (Table 6.11).

Management

The cause of the acidosis should be identified and where possible corrected. Treatment of ketoacidosis and lactic acidosis results in metabolism of the accumulated acids to CO_2 and water, a process which regenerates HCO_3^-. Metabolic acidosis is commonly associated with Na^+ and water depletion (Table 6.11) and the size of the deficit should be assessed and it should be corrected using intravenous isotonic NaCl solution (p. 207). This neutral solution might be expected to have little influence on the reaction of body fluids; however, provided the kidneys are healthy, it is usuallly effective in correcting metabolic acidosis of moderate severity. Its success depends on the capacity of adequately perfused kidneys to generate HCO_3^- and to retain this with the infused Na^+, rejecting the Cl^- in urine.

When blood $[H^+]$ exceeds 70 nmol/l it is advisable to give sufficient 1.26% $NaHCO_3$ solution at the start of treatment to lower the $[H^+]$ below this value. Thereafter administration of saline usually suffices.

In the presence of renal disease or of markedly reduced renal function resulting from severe Na^+ and water depletion renal regeneration of bicarbonate is impaired and approximately 1/3 of the total requirements of Na^+ and water should be given in the form of isotonic $NaHCO_3$ rather than isotonic NaCl. Blood $[H^+]$ and plasma $[HCO_3^-]$ should be monitored and infusion of $NaHCO_3$ stopped when the $[H^+]$ is normal. If there is still evidence of Na^+ and water depletion infusion of NaCl solution should be continued.

In cardiogenic shock or cardiac arrest acidosis develops without salt depletion. However treatment with intravenous $NaHCO_3$ is seldom necessary.

The treatment of lactic acidosis in diabetes is given on page 682. When metabolic acidosis is due to chronic renal disease $NaHCO_3$ supplements must be continued on a long-term basis.

METABOLIC ALKALOSIS

Metabolic alkalosis, less common than metabolic acidosis, is characterised by an increased plasma $[HCO_3^-]$, a fall in blood $[H^+]$ and a small compensatory rise in Pa_{CO_2} (Fig. 6.12 and Table 6.10). In health when plasma $[HCO_3^-]$ rises above normal, filtered HCO_3^- exceeds the renal reabsorptive capacity for the ion and urinary excretion of HCO_3^- increases immediately. When renal function is normal it is, therefore, very difficult to induce metabolic alkalosis by giving $NaHCO_3$.

Metabolic alkalosis however induced, can be sustained only if certain conditions, shown in the information box below, are present.

CONDITIONS IN WHICH METABOLIC ALKALOSIS CAN BE SUSTAINED

Reduced filtered HCO_3^-
- Very low GFR
  Low plasma $[HCO_3^-]$

Increased proportion of filtered Na^+ reabsorbed with HCO_3^-
- Strong stimulus to reabsorb Na^+ (i.e. hypovolaemia) in presence low plasma (Cl^-) and thus reduced filtered Cl^-
- Increased secretion H^+ by renal tubular cells:
  Tubular cell K^+ depletion
  High P_{CO_2}
  Increased mineralocorticoid activity
  Increased delivery Na^+ to distal nephron

Commonly several factors contribute to the development of metabolic alkalosis and it is convenient to consider an initiation phase, in which plasma $[HCO_3^-]$ increases, and a maintenance phase during which the raised plasma $[HCO_3^-]$ is sustained because of altered renal function.

Aetiology

The important causes of this condition are shown in Table 6.12. Normally when H^+ ions are secreted into the gastric lumen HCO_3^- from parietal cells is added to the blood and this is neutralised by reabsorption of the secreted H^+ in the small bowel. Loss of H^+ in vomitus or by aspiration therefore initiates metabolic alkalosis. The disturbance is maintained because loss of Na^+, Cl^-, water and K^+ in vomitus gives rise to hypochloraemia, ECF depletion and a K^+ deficit all of which enhance renal reabsorption of Na^+ in exchange for protons (Fig. 6.12). The pattern is similar in congenital chloride diarrhoea. Prolonged use of potent diuretics in patients with resistant oedema results in selective loss of $NaCl$ and water from ECF and consequently induces hyper-

Table 6.12 Commonest causes of metabolic alkalosis

Underlying mechanism	Clinical condition
Loss Na^+, Cl^-, H^+ and water (ECF depletion)	Vomiting or aspiration gastric contents Congenital chloridorrhoea[1] Administration of diuretics (benzothiadiazines, frusemide, bumetanide)
Potassium depletion	See Table 6.7[2]
Excessive mineralocorticoid activity	Primary aldosteronism, Cushing's syndrome Bartter's syndrome, adrenal enzyme defects, secondary aldosteronism Administration of liquorice, carbenoxolone
Administration of exogenous alkali	Oral or i.v. HCO_3^-, citrate[3] Administration of gluconate, acetate, lactate

[1]A rare disorder associated with loss H^+ and Cl^- in diarrhoeal stools.
[2]Alkalosis is uncommon in K^+ depletion due to primary renal disease.
[3]Present in transfused blood.

bicarbonataemia. This is sustained because the drugs deliver increased amounts of Na^+ to the distal nephron where H^+ secretion is further enhanced by secondary aldosteronism and cell K^+ depletion (Fig. 6.13). In K^+ deficiency alkalosis may be initiated by transfer of H^+ into cells and maintained both by the increased secretion of protons by K^+ depleted tubular cells and by increased renal synthesis of NH_4^+. In the presence of increased mineralocorticoid alkalosis is initiated and maintained by steroid stimulated reabsorption of Na^+ in exchange for H^+ in the distal nephron. Potassium is also lost (p. 550) which further stimulates renal Na^+/H^+ exchange.

In the presence of a low GFR and/or any factor which enhances HCO_3^- reabsorption, administration of base causes alkalosis.

Consequences of metabolic alkalosis

The compensatory increase in Pa_{CO_2} which partially restores ECF $[H^+]$ actually stimulates H^+ secretion and thus HCO_3^- reabsorption by the kidney. Because of increased secretion of H^+ in the distal nephron the urine often remains acid.

Clinical features

Alkalosis is rarely attended by specific clinical disturbances. Acute alkalosis induces tetany which occurs spontaneously or may be produced by the Trousseau manoeuvre (p. 642) and which is associated with the reduction in the concentration of plasma ionised calcium. Enhanced release of acetylcholine is another cause of increased neuromuscular excitability. Apathy, personality changes, delirium and stupor may occur in

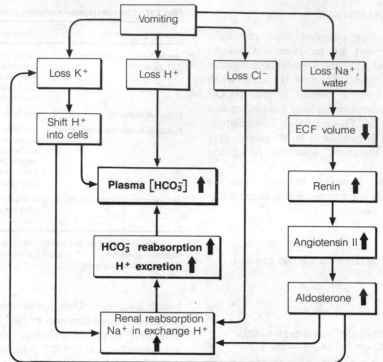

Fig. 6.12 Simplified scheme showing pathogenesis of metabolic alkalosis due to loss of gastric contents.

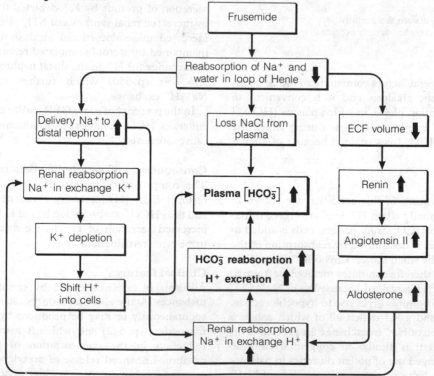

Fig. 6.13 Simplified scheme showing pathogenesis of diuretic induced metabolic alkalosis.

severe cases but since patients often suffer from associated Na^+, water, K^+ and Mg^{++} deficiency it is unwise to attribute such features solely to the effects of alkalosis. Severe longstanding alkalosis may be associated with depression of renal function and uraemia.

Management

Disturbances which initiate or maintain hyperbicarbonataemia should be corrected.

In patients with pyloric obstruction the volume of the ECF should be restored and hypochloraemia corrected using isotonic NaCl solution; usually 2–4 litres are required in 24 hours. Sufficient KCl should be added to repair the associated K^+ deficit, usually 40 mmol/l. Restoration of ECF volume, plasma $[Cl^-]$ and cell $[K^+]$ is associated with renal retention of Cl^- and excretion of excess of HCO_3^- in urine. Patients who require continuous gastric aspiration in preparation for surgery should have the volume of aspirate removed by aspiration replaced by intravenous infusion of an equal amount of isotonic saline containing KCl or by an equal volume of 'gastric solution'. The latter contains NaCl 63 mmol/l, KCl 17 mmol/l, NH_4Cl 90 mmol/l. One litre may be given in 4–6 hours. It is usually necessary to add more KCl to this solution.

Alkalosis associated with K^+ deficiency is corrected when sufficient KCl is given to restore body K^+ to normal (p. 218). Diuretic induced alkalosis is difficult to correct. If possible the diuretic should be stopped for a few days and the intake of NaCl increased. Failing this 500–1000 mg/day of the carbonic anhydrase inhibitor acetazolamide should be substituted for the diuretic for one or two days to induce excretion of $NaHCO_3$. Any K^+ deficit must be corrected. When alkalosis is due to mineralocorticoid excess the underlying disorder must be treated. Restriction of dietary salt and correction of K^+ deficiency with KCl mitigates the alkalosis. During treatment of metabolic alkalosis blood $[H^+]$, Pa_{CO_2} and plasma $[HCO_3]$ must be monitored regularly.

RESPIRATORY ACIDOSIS AND ALKALOSIS

Respiratory acidosis

This arises when the effective alveolar ventilation fails to keep pace with the rate of CO_2 production (p. 344). As a result Pa_{CO_2}, blood $[H_2CO_2]$ and $[H^+]$ rise. The kidney responds to raised Pa_{CO_2} with increased H^+ secretion so that the urine becomes acid, HCO_3^- is generated and added to blood and the blood $[H_2CO_3]$ is partly restored. The distinction between respiratory acidosis and metabolic alkalosis can usually be made from knowledge of the cause of the disturbance. Characteristically the blood $[H^+]$ is increased in res-

piratory acidosis and reduced in metabolic alkalosis while Pa_{CO_2} is raised in both disorders (Table 6.10, p. 222). Plotting these variables on a diagram such as that shown in Figure 6.12 is often helpful – particularly in stable cases in which compensation has occurred.

The aetiology and clinical features of respiratory acidosis are given on page 351.

Respiratory alkalosis

This occurs when there is excessive loss of CO_2 by over ventilation of the lungs. Pa_{CO_2} and blood $[H^+]$ fall; the low Pa_{CO_2} results in reduced renal Na^+/H^+ exchange, loss of HCO_3^- in the urine, a fall in plasma $[HCO_3^-]$ and consequent mitigation of the fall in blood $[H^+]$. Distinction between respiratory alkalosis and metabolic acidosis, in both of which Pa_{CO_2} is low is usually clear from the clinical circumstances and the changes in blood $[H^+]$ (Fig 6.11 and Table 6.10). The more common causes of respiratory alkalosis are shown in the information box below.

CAUSES OF RESPIRATORY ALKALOSIS

- Hysterical overbreathing
- Assisted ventilation – overventilation
- Lobar pneumonia, pulmonary embolism
- Meningitis, encephalitis
- Poisoning with salicylate
- Hepatic failure

Management

This should be directed at the underlying disorder, electrolyte solutions have no part in the treatment of these respiratory disturbances. The management of hypercapnia is described on page 393 and that of respiratory alkalosis due to hysterical overbreathing on page 642.

DIAGNOSIS OF DISTURBANCES IN WATER AND ELECTROLYTE BALANCE

Disturbances of water and electrolyte balance present considerable diagnostic difficulty and some are not characterised by pathognomonic signs or symptoms.

Accurate diagnosis depends upon a careful history and knowledge of the conditions which give rise to abnormalities in water and electrolyte balance. In patients with such disorders, the suspicion that these abnormalities may exist is strengthened by the presence of clinical features known to occur with them and possibly by the results of appropriate biochemical examinations.

FURTHER READING

Arieff A I, De Fronzo R A 1985 Fluid, electrolyte and acid-base disorders, vols 1 & 2. Churchill Livingstone, Edinburgh. A detailed account of the physiology and pathophysiology of water and electrolyte balance. Useful accounts of the electrolyte disturbances occurring in clinical situations.

Forrester J M 1986 Companion to medical studies, 4th Edn. vol. 1. Blackwell Scientific Publications, Oxford. For further information about acid-base metabolism and renal physiology.

Robinson J R 1975 Fundamentals of acid-base regulation, 5th Edn. Blackwell Scientific Publications, Oxford. A straightforward account of this difficult subject.

The New England Journal of Medicine frequently contains reviews of the physiological basis of medical progress. Recent reviews include:

Defense against hyperkalaemia, the roles of insulin and aldosterone (M Cox, R Sterns, I Singer)1978, 299, 525–532

Adrenergic control of serum potassium (F H Epstein, R N Rosa) 1983, 309, 1450–1451

Dehydration in the elderly (A Leaf) 1984, 311, 791–792

Treatment of hyponatraemia (R Schrier) 1984, 312, 1121–1123

Atrial natriuretic hormone, the renin-aldosterone axis and blood pressure-electrolyte homeostasis (J Laragh) 1985, 313, 1330–1340

Pathogenesis of sodium and water retention in high output and low output cardiac failure, nephrotic syndrome, cirrhosis and pregnancy (R Schrier) 1988, 319, 1065–1073, 1127–1134

7

Oncology

Oncology is the study of tumours. Neoplasia means abnormal new growth, which may be benign or malignant. Cancer is a term that is used to describe a wide variety of malignant diseases, the management of which requires several medical disciplines. Traditionally physicians have played a lesser role than surgeons or radiotherapists in the treatment of these diseases but the development of cytotoxic drugs and major advances in palliative care has resulted in the greater involvement of physicians in the overall management of malignancy. The use of cytotoxic drugs, and medicines to control the symptoms of advanced malignancy require specialised knowledge and experience but since cancer impinges on every medical discipline, it is necessary for all doctors to be aware of the basic principles of investigating and managing malignant diseases. This chapter reviews these basic principles and outlines some aspects of the aetiology and pathology of tumours, the assessment of tumour burden, the use of radiotherapy, chemotherapy and hormone therapy, and possible approaches to the prevention of these diseases, many of which may be associated with avoidable causes.

INCIDENCE

Cancer is second only to coronary artery disease as being the commonest cause of death in the Western world. In 1983 (the most recent year for which complete figures are available) 242 540 new cancer patients were registered in the UK. This gives an incidence of 4198 per million of population for males and 3875 for females. Based on current incidence rates it is estimated that 1 in 3 people will develop cancer at some time during their life.

Throughout the Western world the commonest sites of malignant disease are the lung, large bowel, breast and skin (Fig. 7.1). Over the past 25 years the incidence of lung cancer in men has increased by 125%, and even more significantly in women concomitant with their increased consumption of cigarettes. The incidence of colonic, prostatic and bladder cancer has also shown an increase but during the past decade there has been a decrease in the incidence of carcinomas arising in the stomach, uterus, rectum and oesophagus.

Progress in diagnosis and treatment has had a significant effect on survival for some cancers, but ironically the best results have been achieved in relatively rare cancers such as testicular and Hodgkins lymphoma. The commonest cancers such as lung and large bowel remain the most refractory. Figure 7.2 illustrates survival data for patients first diagnosed in 1979.

Age

Age has a bearing on the incidence of specific cancers, and more than 70% of all new cases occur in patients over 60 years old. In children, cancer is the leading cause of death between the ages of 3–13 years, about half of these being due to acute lymphoblastic leukaemia. For the age group in the third and fourth

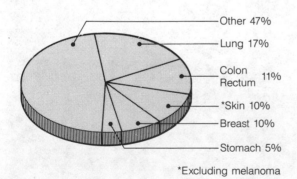

*Excluding melanoma

Fig. 7.1 Cancer incidence in the UK, 1984. (Statistical Factsheets: courtesy of Cancer Research Campaign, 2 Carlton Terrace, London.)

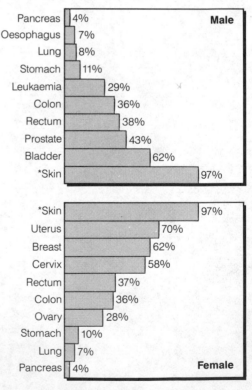

* Adjusted for non-cancer deaths

Fig. 7.2 Five-year survival rates in England and Wales, 1981. (Cancer Research Campaign.)

decades, cancer is three times as common in women as in men but men are at greater risk than women between the ages of 60–80.

AETIOLOGY

In a recent survey of the trend in mortality from cancer in the USA it has been estimated that up to 90% of all such deaths could be attributed to potentially avoidable factors, namely tobacco, alcohol, diet, reproductive and sexual behaviour, occupation, pollution and geographical features.

Cigarette smoking

The only cause whose effect is large, and has been reliably identified, is tobacco which is estimated to have been responsible for 50 000 deaths in the UK in 1987 – one third of all cancer deaths. The public health campaigns emphasising the indisputable association between cigarette tobacco and lung cancer are beginning to prove successful, and there are indications that cigarette consumption is at last starting to decline. There is, however, still a continuing need for such education – aimed particularly at the young to warn them of the dangers of cigarette smoking.

Diet

It appears easier to influence dietary habits but research is needed to identify the specific agents responsible for the development of tumours where diet appears to play a role such as gastrointestinal carcinomas.

Geographical distribution

Studies of the geographical distribution of the incidence of different cancers give some leads as to the possible influence of particular environmental or social factors in causation.

The incidence of carcinoma of the *oesophagus* varies greatly from country to country (over a 200-fold range) with a particularly high incidence in a geographical band covering eastern and southern Africa, Iran, Afghanistan, Soviet and central Asia, Mongolia and northern China. Suggestions that diet or cooking practices are involved are as yet unconfirmed.

The incidence of carcinoma of the *pancreas* is increasing in most of the developed countries but is relatively rare in Japan, whereas the reverse is true for stomach cancer which is particularly prevalent in Japan.

It has been known for a long time that the incidence of *breast* cancer varies appreciably in different parts of the world, being high in the USA and low in the Orient but increasing over two generations of orientals who emigrate to the USA. Population migration represents a

natural experiment where the assumption of incidence levels of the host country strongly suggests an environmental rather than a genetic aetiology. Breast cancer incidence rates increase with age, but the rate of increase is greater up to age 50 than afterwards. If the currently observed increases in incidence rates in younger women in previously low-risk parts of the world, such as Asia and South America, continue throughout their life-span, then it is estimated that by the year 2000 the annual world-wide incidence of breast cancer will be in excess of 1 million. Several aetiological factors are known to be associated with breast cancer, such as an increased risk for women having an early menarche and late menopause. The older the age at which a woman has her first full-time pregnancy the higher is the risk of developing breast cancer, but lactation has a protective influence.

The incidence of carcinoma of the *uterine cervix* has increased in recent years particularly amongst younger women. This has coincided with changing social patterns of greater sexual freedom and the use of oral contraception, suggesting that a sexually transmissable agent may be the aetiological factor responsible. The screening of women who have started sexual activity at an early age or have had multiple partners should be encouraged because early detection can be curative. As further aetiological factors are identified, it is reasonable to predict that other screening procedures will become useful for certain groups although at present there is no indication for screening the entire population.

There is evidence that both environmental and genetic factors are important in the pathogenesis of malignant *melanoma*. In the USA recent figures show an incidence of 4.2 cases per 100 000 population, but of great concern is the fact that the incidence is rising rapidly, doubling every 10–15 years. Between 1979–1983 the annual age-adjusted incidence rate for malignant melanoma in Scotland was 4.75 per 100 000 for females and 2.75 for males. The marked difference in incidence between the sexes is unusual and as yet unexplained, but during these years the incidence for both sexes rose by an annual average of 2.5%. Figure 7.3 shows the increasing incidence in England and Wales between 1974 and 1984. Melanoma is rare in black and oriental people suggesting that skin-pigment plays a genetic role in protecting against the development of melanoma. Although not proven, there is support for the fact that sunlight is environmentally involved in the aetiology of this disease. Although in most parts of the world the incidence between the sexes is equal, women tend to develop melanoma in the legs and exposed parts of the limbs more frequently than

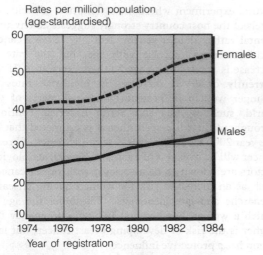

Rates per million population (age-standardised)

Fig. 7.3 Increasing incidence of malignant melanoma in England and Wales over a decade. (Cancer Research Campaign.)

men who have a higher incidence of lesions on the trunk (Fig. 7.4). Furthermore, studies from Norway, Canada, the USA and Australia show that the incidence of melanoma increases as one approaches the equator, consistent with greater exposure to ultraviolet light.

Viruses

It has been suspected that viruses may be involved in the pathogenesis of human neoplasms. Indirect evidence suggests that viruses may act as cofactors in the development of some malignant diseases; viral particles can be demonstrated in the cells of certain malignancies, the enzyme reverse transcriptase (or oncornavirus-type) has been demonstrated in human cancer cells, and the nuclei of some malignant cells have been shown to contain DNA base sequences complementary to the base sequences of known tumour viruses.

Oncogenes

The integration of viral information into the genome of the human cell that subsequently becomes malignant has led to the concept of 'oncogenes', whereby cancer results from the depression of these viral oncogenes to permit malignant transformation. De-repression may be caused by exposure to an external carcinogen, or by spontaneous mutation. The study of viral oncogenes has resulted in the first real evidence for the fact that the action of a few or even a single gene may result in the transformation of a cell from normal to the malignant state. In the accepted vocabulary of molecular biology any gene – viral or cellular – that transforms cells into tumours is called an oncogene. Cellular oncogenes are derived from normal cellular genes, the proto-oncogenes. Viral oncogenes carried by transforming retroviruses are derived from cellular proto-oncogenes, but those of the DNA tumour viruses have no obvious cellular progenitor. It is the conversion from proto-oncogene to oncogene (oncogene activation) which is thought to be the critical genetic event in malignant transformation.

It has been known for some time that direct genetic damage is found in the cells of some cancers, where there is no viral association. Such 'direct' damage includes translocation of parts of chromosomes to other chromosomes, deletions of a part of a chromosome, and abnormal amplification of large regions within a chromosome. It is now known that translocation and amplification affect the expression or function of proto-oncogenes, because the breakpoints where portions of two chromosomes are joined together by translocation may lie within or next to proto-oncogenes. Altered expression is illustrated by the translocation that joins the proto-oncogene known as c-myc to immunoglobulin genes in Burkitt's lymphoma. This results in uncontrolled transcription of c-myc into RNA allowing inappropriate expression of the gene.

Amplification of proto-oncogenes may occur as an occasional event in many types of tumour or consistently as an abnormality of a specific proto-oncogene in a particular tumour type. Some examples of the association of proto-oncogenes with specific cancers are

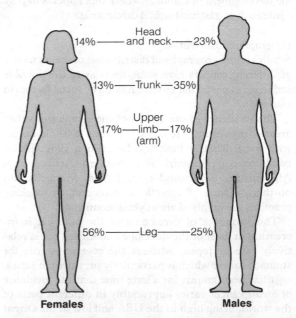

Fig. 7.4 Percentage distribution of malignant melanoma on parts of the body. (Cancer Research Campaign.)

Table 7.1   Association of proto-oncogenes with various cancers

Disease	Proto-oncogene	Mechanism
Small cell lung carcinoma	C-myc L-myc N-myc	Amplification
Breast carcinoma	C-myc C-erb-B2	Amplification
Cervical carcinoma	C-myc	Amplification
Burkitt's lymphoma	C-myc	Translocation
Chronic myelogenous leukaemia	C-myc	Translocation
Colon carcinoma	C-ras	Point mutation

illustrated in Table 7.1. The proteins encoded by the large number of oncogenes that have been identified are mostly unknown, and hence the effects of gene amplifications are unclear. In the case of C-erbB-2 the protein appears to be a transmembrane growth factor regulator. Recent evidence in patients with various cancers suggest that the greater the amplification of the oncogene the poorer the prognosis.

PATHOLOGY

A fundamental principle of oncology is to establish, usually by biopsy, the pathological nature of any lesion suspected of being neoplastic before making decisions about management.

The first distinction to be made is between benign and malignant lesions. Benign tumours represent the accumulation of cells which have been transformed to reproduce in abnormal numbers but under circumstances where they remain within the tissue of origin. Malignant tumours are comprised of cells which are capable of invading adjacent tissues and leaving the tissue of origin to disseminate and form metastases. The histological distinction between benign and malignant lesions will depend, amongst other factors, on the pleomorphism of the cells, the presence of aberrations in the nucleus, increased numbers of mitoses and whether or not there is evidence of invasion into surrounding tissues.

Table 7.2   Classification of cancers

Type	Tissue of origin	Examples
Carcinomas	Endoderm or ectoderm	Epithelial lining of gut (e.g. adenocarcinoma of colon) or bronchus (e.g. squamous cell or small cell carcinoma of bronchus)
Sarcomas	Mesoderm	Osteosarcoma Fibrosarcoma
Leukaemia	Haemopoetic (white blood cell)	Acute lymphoblastic leukaemia
Lymphoma	Monocyte macrophage	Hodgkin's disease

Cancers are classified into three major groups (Table 7.2). Within a given tissue there may be major differences in the cell type from which the tumour has arisen. Thus for example bronchogenic carcinomas are classified histologically into four major groups: squamous carcinomas, adenocarcinomas, small cell and large cell undifferentiated carcinomas.

Such distinctions are essential to clinical management since the choice between surgery, radiotherapy and chemotherapy will depend on whether or not the lesion is benign or malignant, and whether or not the particular histological subtype is sensitive to radiotherapy or chemotherapy. As regards the latter, there is a great variation in the sensitivity of different tumours to different cytotoxic drugs, and therefore appropriate therapy can be prescribed only when the tumour tissue has been accurately classified.

Although there is evidence to support the concept that many human tumours arise from the transformation of a single cell, i.e. are clonal in origin, it is not unusual to find a mixed histological picture; for example in the testis, teratomas and seminomatous tissue may occur together, and in the lung, squamous and small-cell undifferentiated tumours may present in the same biopsy specimen.

In addition to defining whether the tumour is benign or malignant and from which cell type it arises, it is useful to define the degree of differentiation or anaplasia of the cancer cell since for many tumour types this has been shown to correlate with prognosis and response to treatment.

Cytology

Whilst most histology is performed on tissue that is obtained by surgical biopsy, in certain circumstances it is possible to achieve excellent classification from cytology alone. Thus for example sputum may be examined for malignant bronchogenic cells, pleural or peritoneal effusions may provide suitable cells for diagnostic purposes and smears can be prepared from the uterine cervix. Increasing use is being made of needle aspiration for cytological diagnosis. A fine-gauge needle can be inserted into breast lumps, subcutaneous deposits, intrathoracic or hepatic lesions, and a smear for cytological evaluation can be made from the aspirated material. In experienced hands, this technique has many advantages over the more conventional surgical biopsy technique, mainly because of speed and simplicity.

Immunohistochemistry

The production of polyclonal and, more recently, monoclonal antibodies has made a very significant contribution to the further identification and classification of histological and cytological preparations of tumour tissues. Highly specific antibodies raised against tumour antigens can be labelled with fluorescine or used in immunohistochemical techniques to detect tumour cell products such as enzymes, hormones or receptors. This can be used for the more confident distinction between benign and malignant tissues, and to differentiate between histological subtypes of similar tumours; for example in a histologically undifferentiated bronchogenic tumour a monoclonal antibody that stains positively for mucin, used in conjunction with one that detects keratin may help distinguish an adenocarcinoma from a squamous carcinoma. Similarly immunophenotyping (as it is called) of lymphomas and leukaemias can greatly enhance the distinction between morphologically related subtypes. Such categorisation is important in predicting the natural history of an individual patient's illness and in selecting the most appropriate therapy.

TUMOUR MARKERS

Malignant cells appear different histologically and vary biochemically from their normal counterparts but attempts to identify biochemical abnormalities unique to the cancer cell have proved unrewarding. Nevertheless it is now appreciated that the presence of viable tumour tissue in the body may be detectable by the presence in the blood of biochemical products known as 'tumour markers'. These are normal metabolic constituents that are found either in abnormal amounts or at an inappropriate time of life, for example fetal proteins being re-expressed in adult life.

Tumour markers of this type can be useful in a number of different clinical situations. In theory tumour markers might be useful for screening whole populations for undetected cancers but in practice this has not proved useful for the following reasons. The predictive value of a screening test depends on the sensitivity of the test, its specificity and the prevalence of the particular disease. Sensitivity refers to the number of times a test is positive for patients known to have the disease, i.e. true positives, and specificity refers to the incidence of true negatives, i.e. that the test should prove negative in people known to be free of the disease. Unfortunately sensitivity is inversely related to specificity. For example it is known that some gastrointestinal tumours contain carcinoembryonic antigen (CEA), a substance that is present in the gut during fetal life but which is not found in normal adult gastrointestinal tissues. Radio-immunoassays of CEA in blood have shown an overall 67% positivity in patients

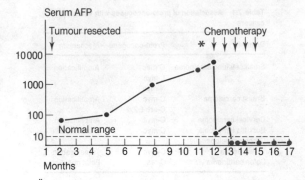

Fig. 7.5 Serum alpha-fetoprotein (AFP) levels in a young man with testicular teratoma. The levels of AFP fluctuate with disease state and can be used to monitor the effects of the treatment.

with colorectal carcinoma but the test is also positive in alcoholic cirrhosis (70%), emphysema (57%) and diabetes mellitus (38%) amongst many other diseases. Screening the population at large for subclinical carcinomas of the colon with this method would therefore fail because of lack of specificity.

However the presence of a tumour marker can be of clinical value in monitoring the progress of individual patients known to have a given malignancy. For example testicular teratomas not infrequently secrete another oncofetal protein – alpha-fetoprotein (AFP). Figure 7.5 illustrates a typical case where during the months following surgical resection of the primary tumour, a rising level of AFP was associated with (and preceded) the clinical appearance of metastases. The successful use of chemotherapy was associated with a disappearance of the abnormal tumour marker.

Human chorionic gonadotrophin (normally produced only by placental tissue) is another tumour marker seen in testicular teratoma while the production of placental alkaline phosphatase is associated with approximately 40% of testicular seminomas.

A variety of hormones can be produced ectopically by tumours (Table 7.3). The levels of these hormones, or the biochemical consequences of their production can be useful markers of the viability of residual tumour following treatment, therefore indicating whether or not further therapy is required.

CLINICAL FEATURES

Malignant diseases manifest themselves in a variety of ways. The presence of an abnormal accumulation of cells may, by virtue of its physical bulk alone, produce clinical symptoms and signs. Thus for example painless swellings in the breast or in muscle may indicate an

Table 7.3 Hormones produced by tumours

Ectopically-produced hormones	Clinical hormone syndromes	Associated neoplasms
ACTH	Cushing's syndrome	Small cell bronchogenic ca
HCG (human chorionic gonadotrophin)	Gynaecomastia, precocious puberty	Small cell bronchogenic ca, hepatoblastoma
AVP (arginine vasopressin)	Inappropriate ADH (AVP) syndrome	Small cell bronchogenic ca, ca pancreas (rare)
TGF (transforming growth factor)	Hypercalcaemia	Squamous cell bronchogenic ca, kidney ca, ovary ca
OAF (osteoclast activating factor)	Hypercalcaemia	Myeloma
Erythropoeitin	Erythrocytosis	Uterine fibromyoma, cerebellar haemangioblastoma
Chorionic somato-mammotropin or HPL (human placental lactogen)	None	Small cell bronchogenic ca
GH (growth hormone)	?Hypertrophic pulmonary osteoarthropathy	Small cell bronchogenic ca
GH releasing factor	Acromegaly	Bronchial carcinoid, pancreatic islet carcinoid
HCG (TSH-like)	Hyperthyroidism	Choriocarcinoma
Prolactin	Galactorrhoea	Hypernephroma
Enteroglucagon	Gastrointestinal abnormalities and symptoms	Renal tumour
CRF (corticotrophin-releasing factor)	Cushing's syndrome	Bronchial carcinoid, prostatic ca
Calcitonin	None	Small cell bronchogenic ca, medullary ca, thyroid and breast ca
VIP (vasoactive intestinal polypeptide)	Watery diarrhoea	Small cell bronchogenic ca

underlying carcinoma or sarcoma respectively. Lymphomas usually present as painless enlargements of lymph nodes or spleen. Intracranial space-occupying lesions may cause focal manifestations, fits, headaches, vomiting and papilloedema. Tumours in the distal colon may partially obstruct the lumen of the bowel with a resulting change in bowel habit. Bronchogenic tumours may cause cough or shortness of breath resulting from partial or complete occlusion of an airway.

Haemorrhage
Malignant tumours not infrequently present as haemorrhage from an eroded epithelial surface. For example bronchogenic carcinomas may present with haemoptysis, gastric carcinomas with iron deficiency anaemia or, occasionally, haematemesis, colonic carcinoma with bleeding per rectum, and renal and bladder carcinomas with haematuria.

Pain
This is often thought to be an inevitable accompaniment of malignant disease but in fact it is not a common symptom especially at presentation of most cancers. When pain does occur, it is due either to nerve compression or to distension of an organ. The most common peripheral nerve compressions are due to involvement of the brachial plexus (carcinomas of the lung or breast), the sacral plexus (carcinomas of the rectum or cervix) or the paraspinal nerves (carcinomas of the pancreas). Metastatic tumours in the liver may cause pain as a result of distension and stretching of its capsule. Bone pain resulting from primary, or more commonly, secondary deposits usually occurs in the weight-bearing bones, and results from compression

secondary to weakening of the structural component of the bone. Pathological fractures may arise as a consequence. Patients may present with referred pain, most frequently in the shoulder, hip or knee, as when a nerve root is involved directly or by metastases.

Cachexia
This is a profound state of general ill health – malnutrition, wasting, anaemia and muscle weakness. It is a clinical feature of many malignant diseases presenting at an advanced stage, especially carcinomas of the gastrointestinal tract, lung, ovary and testis. It is, however, not a universal phenomenon and is rare in breast cancer and in tumours of the central nervous system, and uncommon in leukaemia and lymphomas.

Cachexia may arise as a direct result of malnutrition from a tumour in the gastrointestinal tract. Malabsorption may arise rarely as a consequence of tumour replacing the absorptive epithelia but more commonly from reduced exocrine function (from carcinomas of the pancreas), or loss of bile from carcinomas of the upper gastrointestinal tract that obstruct biliary outflow. Loss of taste and the malaise that accompanies many malignant diseases may contribute to poor food intake but all of these factors in promoting malnutrition do not of themselves fully explain the cachexia of malignancy. Although many patients will have a negative nitrogen balance, others who are in positive balance may show a caloric deficit. It has been shown that in the cachexia accompanying malignant disease, caloric expenditure remains high with an elevated basal metabolic rate despite reduced dietary intake (the reverse of the situation that follows starvation) which indicates that this phenomenon results from a profound systemic derangement of host metabolism, the pathogenesis of which remains unclear.

Paraneoplastic features

In addition to generalised clinical features that are commonly associated with the presentation of a malignant disease, there are a variety of syndromes for which the term 'paraneoplastic' has been used. These syndromes include many that arise as a result of the secretion into the blood of tumour products (usually polypeptide hormones) which produce clinical signs as a consequence of their action on target organs remote from the primary tumour (see Table 7.3, p. 235).

A number of neurological paraneoplastic syndromes (p. 903) have been described for which the tumour product remains unknown. These include peripheral neuropathies, a myasthenia-like syndrome and subacute cerebellar degeneration. Whilst all of these syndromes may improve with successful treatment of the primary tumour, complete resolution is rare.

Dermatomyositis and polymyositis present as gradually progressive muscle weakness predominantly affecting the proximal musculature, coming on over a period of months. Whilst these disorders are not universally associated with malignancy, patients suffering from them have a greatly increased risk of an underlying neoplasm compared with the general public, and malignancies of the breast, lung, and gastrointestinal and genito-urinary tract should be considered.

Acanthosis nigricans is a rare condition characterised by the appearance of black velvety verrucose lesions in the flexures around the neck, axillae and groin. It is particularly seen in patients with carcinomas of the stomach.

PRINCIPLES OF TREATMENT

As a general rule, patients should be informed that they have a malignant disease prior to starting treatment but not necessarily of the exact prognosis.

The first interview with a patient suspected of having a malignant disease should be performed in a quiet and unhurried manner. In addition to a routine history of symptoms and previous illnesses, it is important to ascertain whether patients already know that they have a malignant disease and what this means to them. The patient will be helped very considerably by positive assurance that symptoms can almost always be improved even if the underlying disease cannot be eradicated.

Cure or palliation

In order to plan the optimal management for an individual patient, it is necessary to consider two questions:

1. Is the tumour still localised to its site of origin?
2. Is it a realistic aim to 'cure' the patient, or should treatment be focused on palliation of symptoms?

Tumours that have not metastasised are amenable to local forms of treatment (e.g. surgery or radiotherapy) whilst tumours that have already disseminated require systemic treatment with chemotherapy or hormonal therapy. It is frequently necessary to use a combination of these measures, particularly if aiming for complete eradication of the tumour. Surgery, radiotherapy and chemotherapy all cause some degree of host toxicity which may be enhanced by combining the treatments. It is important to decide whether or not cure is feasible and desirable in order to minimise any treatment-related toxicity in circumstances where an aggressive therapeutic approach would be inappropriate.

Staging

It is usually necessary to perform specialised investigations to determine the extent of dissemination of the tumour prior to selecting treatment – the process of 'staging' the tumour. Staging investigations take time and the delay causes anxiety for the patient.

The internationally recognised staging system is known as the TNM classification. This is shown in Table 7.4. An example for lung cancer is shown in Table 7.5.

The TNM system is a clinical staging system but if supplemented by the pathological examination of biopsied or resected speciments the suffix p is added. Having

Table 7.4 TNM classification

T*	Extent of primary tumour
N*	Extent of regional lymph node involvement
M	Presence or absence of metastases

Extent of disease

T0	Excised tumour
T1	
T2	Increases in primary tumour size
T3	

Increased involvement of nodes

N1	
N2	Increasing involvement
N3	

Presence of metastases

M0	Not present
M1	present

* Exact criteria of size and region of nodal involvement have been defined for each anatomical site.

Table 7.5 TNM for lung cancer

TX	Positive cytology	
T1	≤ 3 cm	
T2	> 3 cm/extends to hilar region/invades visceral pleura/partial atelectasis	Primary tumour
T3	Chest wall, diaphragm, pericardium, mediastinal pleura etc., total atelectasis	
T4	Mediastinum, heart, great vessels, trachea, oesophagus etc., malignant effusion	
N1	Peribronchial, ipsilateral hilar	
N2	Ipsilateral mediastinal	Lymph node
N3	Contralateral mediastinal, scalene or supraclavicular	

Table 7.6 Stage grouping for lung cancer

Stage	T	N	M
Occult carcinoma	TX	N0	M0
0	Tis	N0	M0
I	T1	N0	M0
	T2	N0	M0
II	T1	N1	M0
	T2	N1	M0
IIIA	T1	N2	M0
	T2	N2	M0
	T3	N0, N1, N2,	M0
IIIB	Any T	N3	M0
	T4	Any N	M0
IV	Any T	Any N	M1

INVESTIGATIONS TO DEFINE TNM STATUS

Tumour
Palpation
Inspection including endoscopy (e.g. bronchoscopy, cystoscopy)
Radiology
(conventional, CT, Nuclear magnetic resonance)
Cytology/aspiration/biopsy

Nodes
Palpation
Aspiration
Biopsy
Radiology
(Lymphangiogram/CT scanning)

Metastases
Biochemical screening (e.g. liver function tests)
Radionuclide scans (e.g. liver, brain, bone)
Ultrasound of liver
Radiology
(e.g. chest X-ray, CT scan of liver, brain, lung)
Peritoneoscopy
Laparotomy

Table 7.7 Eastern Cooperative Oncology Group performance status scale

0 Fully active, able to carry on all usual activities without restriction and without the aid of analgesics
1 Restricted in strenuous activity but ambulatory and able to carry out light work or pursue a sedentary occupation. This group also contains patients who are fully active, as in grade 0, but only with the aid of analgesics
2 Ambulatory and capable of all self-care but unable to work. Up and about more than 50% of waking hours
3 Capable of only limited self-care, confined to bed or chair more than 50% of waking hours
4 Completely disabled, unable to carry out any self-care and confined totally to bed or chair

---

defined the T, N and M status of the tumour, it is then possible to group patients into different stages. For example in lung cancers the stage groupings are as shown in Table 7.6.

The TNM system for the majority of malignant diseases is increasingly being used, particularly to facilitate comparisons of the results of treatments in different international centres. For certain diseases it has proved useful to define staging systems which differ from the TNM classification, as for example the Ann Arbor staging for Hodgkin's lymphoma (p. 740) and Duke's classification for carcinomas of the rectum.

The investigations required to define the T, N or M status of a tumour vary for different diseases. Examples are shown in the information box (right).

Performance status

In addition to the anatomical assessment of tumour extent evaluated by staging procedures, it is important to assess the overall degree of functional impairment that the disease is causing the patient at the time of diagnosis. A variety of 'performance status' scales have been devised such as the Eastern Cooperative Oncology Group (ECOG) scale shown in Table 7.7. These have been found useful in assessing prognosis and also the efficacy and toxicity of treatment.

Evaluation of response

With presently available therapies most methods of cancer treatment are associated with significant morbidity. It is thus essential to evaluate the response to therapy as accurately as possible and use properly defined criteria for evaluating response so as to make valid comparisons between different treatments. The concept of 'survival time', especially the traditional use of 'five year survival' places too much emphasis on cure. Since palliation is a much commoner objective in management planning, more subtle criteria are required than crude survival figures.

The terms universally accepted for evaluating treatment are defined as shown in the information box (p. 238).

The term 'complete response' may or may not indicate true eradication of the tumour and for any given disease these terms can only reflect the ability to detect viable tumour.

TERMS FOR EVALUATING TREATMENT

Objective response
Any response that fulfils the criteria of complete or partial response

Complete response
Complete disappearance of all known disease in the absence of any new lesions appearing

Partial response
A reduction in size by at least 50% of the tumour in the absence of any new lesions appearing

No response
No change, or an increase or decrease of 25% in the size of the tumour in the absence of new lesions

Progressive disease
Increase in the size of the tumour by 25% or the development of any new lesions

PRINCIPLES OF RADIOTHERAPY

It is important that physicians should be familiar with an outline of the procedures involved when their patients are referred for this form of treatment.

Radiotherapy involves the exposure of a defined area of the body to a source of ionising radiation under carefully controlled conditions. Treatment planning involves accurate localisation of the tumour and prescription of multiple daily fractions of irradiation for a specified period of time. The biological effect of radiation depends on the amount of energy absorbed per unit mass. The unit of absorbed dose is the gray and is equivalent to 1 joule per kilogram.

Ionising radiation damages cells by interaction with nuclear DNA thus preventing the normal reproduction of that cell. As with cytotoxic drugs there is only a relative selectivity in this process, and normal (non-malignant) cells are readily damaged by radiation. For this reason radiotherapy planning must take into account the exact anatomical distribution of the tumour in order to minimise the exposure of normal tissues whilst at the same time ensuring that all of the diseased tissues are included in the treated area. Great care is taken to ensure that the patient can be accurately and reproducibly repositioned whilst radiotherapy is being undertaken.

Patients are usually treated in the supine position although the prone position may be more suitable for some abdominal and pelvic tumours. In order to immobilise the area to be treated, moulds, casts and shells are constructed for the individual patient.

With the patient comfortably positioned and the treatment area immobilised, the tumour is localised by a variety of techniques such as the placement of radio-opaque seeds in the tumour or the use of contrast media as in conventional radiography. Increasingly computed tomography is being used to assist in planning radio-therapeutic treatment, especially since CT can provide information about tumour margins in the transverse plane in which most radiotherapy is administered.

Radiotherapy localisation is usually carried out on specialised equipment known as a simulator which is designed to allow isocentric rotation and thus to simulate the exact axis distance of the treatment machine. Computers are now used to integrate the information obtained from simulators in order to select the optimum configuration, energy and variable loading of different treatment beams. This ensures that the least possible dose of radiation will be given to critical normal tissues and that a homogeneous high level of dose will be given to the tumour.

To maximise the absorbed dose within the tumour area and minimise the dose to normal tissues, treatment is given through multiple portals, for example as a four-field box technique for the pelvis, or through fields at right angles to each other with compensating wedge filters to even the dose distribution where the beams overlap. Compensating filters are used to overcome variations in thickness of the areas to be treated through multiple ports. Since the human body is not a sym-metrical cube, the routine use of these filters compensates for the lack of consistent tissue thickness and ensures a more homogeneous dose distribution throughout the target.

Teletherapy

Most radiotherapy is performed with 'teletherapy' techniques, i.e. where a beam of photons is used to irradiate the tumour from outside the patient. Alternatively for specific sites, 'brachytherapy' is used whereby a source of radiation is implanted in a body cavity or within the tumour itself. Teletherapy techniques include the use of low energy ortho- or kilovoltage sources and the more widely used mega-voltage sources. Low energy radiation (50–100 kVp range) is useful for treating carcinomas of the skin and lip, and orthovoltage (250–300 kVp) machines are sometimes used for the palliative treatment of bone metastases and lesions of the chest wall. However, orthovoltage machines are unsuitable for the treatment of more deep-seated tumours.

^{60}Cobalt machines and linear accelerators are the most widely used teletherapy equipment. Both of these types can be used isocentrically, i.e. the radiation source can be mounted in a gantry which can be rotated around the axis of the patient thus allowing direction of multiple beams to the centre of the target volume with great accuracy. ^{60}Cobalt machines provide a less well-defined beam of radiation than a linear accelerator. In general, ^{60}cobalt or 4 MV linear accelerators are used for treating carcinomas of the head and neck and breast, 6 MV linear accelerators for lymphomas and lung cancers, and higher energy accelerators for some deep-seated abdominal and pelvic tumours. In addition to producing X-rays, the higher energy linear accelerators can be used to produce accelerated electrons. The latter are charged particles which are absorbed within a finite range of tissue and can be useful in the treatment of superficial lesions where it is desirable to spare under-lying tissues. Thus, for example, electrons may be employed (with advantage) for the treatment of some lesions of the head and neck, lymph nodes near the spinal cord, and lesions of the chest wall such as occur in breast carcinoma.

Brachytherapy

Brachytherapy is performed with sealed sources of radioactivity introduced for a few days into a body cavity or tumour, for example the insertion of ^{137}caesium into the uterus for treating carcinoma of the cervix. The advantages of brachytherapy are that a relatively high dose of radiation can be administered to a very limited volume of tissue thereby sparing any adverse effects on normal adjacent tissues. Such treat-ments are often supplemented by teletherapy to treat the larger volume where microscopic disease may be present.

Fractionation of dose

Radiotherapy is most frequently prescribed in daily fractions of 200 centigray (cGy) for 5 days a week where, depending on the tumour type and management plan, treatment may continue for 3–6 weeks. Many patients, particularly those treated with target volumes greater than 500 cm^3, will experience some malaise and fatigue. Nausea and anorexia are common and vomiting is a frequent problem if it is necessary to irradiate very large volumes, particularly in the upper abdomen. Acute skin reaction usually consists of mild erythema best treated by keeping the skin dry. Oral and pharyngeal mucosal reactions are common if the area receives high radiation doses. Particular attention to oral hygiene is required and close inspection for candidiasis essential.

Radiation effects on the bone marrow may occur. Minor decreases in lymphocyte count are common and a frequent check on the peripheral blood must be made throughout treatment. Maintenance of haemoglobin is important since hypoxia may render the tumour less sensitive to radiation damage. Irradiation of the gastro-intestinal tract may result in temporary dysphagia, diarrhoea, tenesmus or production of mucus per rectum.

PRINCIPLES OF CHEMOTHERAPY

During the 1940s research into the action of mustard gas showed that sulphur and nitrogen mustard could destroy dividing cells in lymph nodes and the bone marrow. The potential therapeutic benefit was explored in treating some lymphomas with nitrogen mustard which was then developed as the first clinically useful cytotoxic drug. Study of the effects of folic acid metabolism in leukaemic cells resulted in the second cytotoxic drug of therapeutic value – the antifolate, methotrexate. Thereafter many naturally occurring substances were tested resulting in some 30 effective antineoplastic drugs.

Classification

Anticancer drugs are divided into 6 main groups (Table 7.8). The site of action of each group is shown in Figure 7.6.

Table 7.8 Classification of anticancer drugs

Group	Examples
Antimetabolites (metabolism of substance in parenthesis is interrupted)	Methotrexate (folic acid)
	6-Mercaptopurine (hypoxanthine)
	6-Thioguanine (guanine)
	5-Fluorouracil (uracil)
	Cytosine arabinoside (cytidine)
Alkylating agents	Nitrogen mustard
	Cyclophosphamide
	Chlorambucil
	Busulphan
	Melphalan
	Iphosphamide
Plant alkaloids	Vinblastine
	Vincristine
	Vindesine
	VP-16-213
	VM 26
Antibiotics	Doxorubicin
	Daunorubicin
	Actinomycin D
	Bleomycin
	Mitomycin C
Nitrosoureas	BCNU
	CCNU
	TCNU
	Streptozotocin
Miscellaneous synthetic compounds	DTIC
	Cisplatin
	Procarbazine
	Hexamethylmelamine
	Hydroxyurea
	Mitozantrone

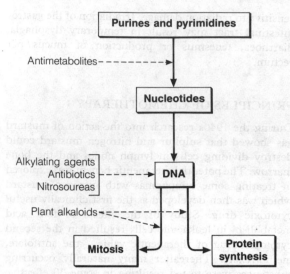

Fig. 7.6 **Anticancer drugs:** site of action of major groups.

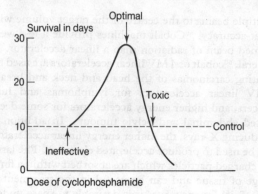

Fig. 7.7 **Dose-response curve for cyclophosphamide** in mice bearing the L1210 leukaemia. Too low a dose is ineffective but beyond a narrow therapeutic range too high a dose kills the animals from haematological toxicity.

Antimetabolites. Methotrexate acts to inhibit folate metabolism by preventing the cell from re-plenishing its source of reduced folates necessary for purine and pyrimidine synthesis (p. 711). The term 'anti-metabolite' is used for this group of drugs which includes mercaptopurine, thioguanine, fluorouracil and cytosine arabinoside.

Alkylating agents. Nitrogen mustard is thought to destroy cells by the process of alkylation – the addition of an alkyl group to constituents of DNA, thus inter-fering with replication and transcription of further nucleic acid. Busulphan, chlorambucil, cyclophos-phamide and melphalan are other clinically useful alky-lating agents.

Plant alkaloids. These inhibit cell division by binding to tubulin and disrupting the mitotic spindle.

Antibiotics. The compounds grouped together as antibiotics include doxorubicin and actinomycin which act by intercalating between base pairs in DNA and bleomycin which causes breaks in both single and double-stranded DNA.

Nitrosoureas. The mechanism of action of this group probably involves alkylation.

Miscellaneous synthetic compounds. Alkylation and other metabolic lesions may be involved.

Therapeutic index
Unfortunately none of these biochemical events is confined to the metabolism of malignant cells. Systemic exposure to these cellular poisons therefore must inevitably result in some damage to normal host tissues, particularly to those which rely on rapid cell division such as the bone marrow and gastrointestinal tract. In addition to their relative lack of selectivity, anticancer drugs are very potent because they act at low concentra-tions. Together with a tendency towards steep dose-response curves, these factors all account for the narrow 'therapeutic index' of cytotoxic drugs (see Fig. 7.7).

The narrow therapeutic index of antineoplastic drugs means that the greatest care is required in their ad-ministration. Whenever anticancer drugs are used, it is necessary to monitor the peripheral blood count and be aware of any functional disturbances such as dysphagia or diarrhoea. Since the maximum dose of any cytotoxic drug that can be prescribed on any one occasion is governed by its toxicity to normal cells, only partial tumour shrinkage results from any single treatment. It is therefore necessary to administer these drugs repeatedly, the total duration of treatment varying from a few months to several years. To prevent damage to host tissues, intermittent administration is necessary to allow host tissue to recover between treatments. Damage to bone marrow results in depression of the blood counts 10–14 days later. Thus many cytotoxic drug regimens are given on 21-day cycles to preserve bone marrow integrity.

Choice of drug
To select the most appropriate drug it is necessary to know the range of activity against disease for the various drugs, and to use one which has the minimum toxicities in relation to the particular patient. This information is obtained through a sequence of three phases of clinical trials which are shown in Table 7.9.

Table 7.9 Choice of drug – three phases of clinical trials

Phase	Aims	Type of malignant disease
I	Determine acute toxicology Discover pharmacokinetics and pharmacodynamics	Advanced disease refractory to therapy
II	Determine range of activity	Wide variety of malignant diseases
III	Determine efficacy in particular tumour types by large-scale randomised trials	Specific malignant diseases

Combination chemotherapy

The theory behind combination chemotherapy is that simultaneous disruption of the metabolism of a tumour cell at more than one site may have far more profound effects on the cell than a single metabolic lesion. Thus for example in Hodgkin's disease a treatment with the four-drug combination of nitrogen mustard, vincristine, procarbazine and prednisolone yields complete remissions in more than 80% of patients whereas when these same drugs were used singly they produce remissions in only 15–20% of cases. Similarly combination chemotherapy for acute leukaemia has increased the remission rate from 20% to 90%. Combination chemotherapy is valuable in many other malignant diseases including carcinomas of the breast, ovary, lung, testis and several of the childhood tumours. The five general principles governing the use of combination chemotherapy are listed in the information box below.

GENERAL PRINCIPLES OF COMBINATION CHEMOTHERAPY

- Each drug in the combination should have been demonstrated to have some activity on its own against the tumour type for which the combination is being used.
- Drugs with a similar mechanism of action should not be combined.
- As far as is possible the major dose-limiting toxicity of each drug should differ from that of the other components of the combination.
- Since it is rarely possible to avoid some overlap in toxicity to host tissues, it is usually necessary to reduce the dose of each of the component drugs compared with the optimal dose which would be used if the drugs were prescribed individually.
- There should be no known adverse interaction between the drugs.

Multimodality treatment

Since in many situations cytotoxic drugs are capable of shrinking only a proportion of the tumour, increasing attention has been paid to the use of chemotherapy in conjunction with surgery or radiotherapy. Thus chemotherapy can be used to reduce tumour bulk prior to local therapy with surgery or radiotherapy, as for example in treating head and neck tumours, or drug treatment can be introduced after primary resection or irradiation to prevent the growth of subclinical micrometastases. The latter use of chemotherapy is frequently referred to as 'adjuvant' chemotherapy, and is now widely used for treating breast carcinomas, lymphomas, and several tumours in children.

Caution must be exercised to prevent additive damage to host tissues, particularly the bone marrow if radiotherapy and chemotherapy are used together, but the principle of combining local and systemic therapy has many potential advantages since as a general principle small tumours are much more susceptible to chemotherapy than large ones. This is explained in part by the fact that drugs penetrate small tumours more effectively but also by the fact that the emergence of drug resistance may be related to the frequency of mutations in the tumour, and the potential number of such events increases with the growth of a tumour.

One major difficulty with adjuvant chemotherapy is to decide for how long it should be continued. In obvious advanced tumours, it is possible to measure tumour shrinkage and continue treatment for as long as benefit lasts. Conversely drug resistance is detectable and thus further inappropriate chemotherapy can be avoided. However, in the 'adjuvant' setting where there is no measurable tumour, it is not possible to be certain in the short term whether or not treatment is proving effective. Clinical trials have demonstrated that, for curable tumours in children, it is necessary to continue chemotherapy for 1–2 years. For lymphomas and carcinomas in adults, the optimum duration of adjuvant chemotherapy is less certain.

It is possible to rank many malignant diseases into groups comprising those for which chemotherapy contributes to cure, those for which effective control prolongs useful life and those for which benefit is less certain or unproven. These are listed in the information box (p. 242).

The side-effects of chemotherapy

Due to the relatively poor selectivity of presently available anticancer drugs, it is impossible to avoid some damage to normal host tissues, resulting in a variety of side-effects. Table 7.10 illustrates one representative study of side-effects. Nevertheless, when properly administered and monitored, many cytotoxic drugs can be given without producing symptomatic side-effects. For example, the effect on the bone marrow should not cause significant symptoms provided adequate time is allowed between cycles of treatment and the blood count is monitored prior to subsequent treatment.

Mouth ulceration and diarrhoea result from necrosis

CONTRIBUTION OF CHEMOTHERAPY TO VARIOUS MALIGNANT DISEASES

Tumours for which chemotherapy can be curative
Acute lymphoblastic leukaemia in children
Burkitt's lymphoma
Hodgkin's lymphoma
Wilms' tumour
Rhabdomyosarcoma
Testicular teratoma
Choriocarcinoma
Diffuse histiocytic lymphoma
Ewing's sarcoma

Tumours highly sensitive to chemotherapy – remissions prolong life
Breast carcinoma
Ovarian carcinoma
Small cell anaplastic lung carcinoma
Non-Hodgkin's lymphoma
Chronic lymphocytic leukaemia
Acute myeloid leukaemia
Medulloblastoma

Tumours sensitive to chemotherapy – life sometimes prolonged
Gastric carcinoma
Pancreatic carcinoma
Myeloma
Soft tissue sarcoma
Bladder carcinoma
Anaplastic thyroid carcinoma

Tumours refractory to available chemotherapy
Squamous cell lung carcinoma
Colorectal carcinoma
Carcinoma of oesophagus
Melanoma

Table 7.10   Rank order of the distressing side-effects of chemotherapy (From Coates et al., 1983)

Symptom	Rank
Being sick (vomiting)	1
Feeling sick (nausea)	2
Loss of hair	3
Thought of coming for treatment	4
Length of time treatment takes at clinic	5
Having to have a needle	6
Shortness of breath	7
Constantly tired	8
Difficulty sleeping	9
Affects family or partner	10
Affects work/home duties	11
Trouble finding somewhere to park	12
Feeling anxious or tense	13
Feeling low, miserable (depression)	14
Loss of weight	14

treatment must be continued for this period. For most patients given platinum the combination of metoclopramide and dexamethasone affords the best antiemetic treatment. It is important to prescribe both in adequate dosage and continuous infusions of metoclopramide – at least during the first 24 hours – are superior to intermittent administration. Unfortunately metoclopramide at the required dose of 3–4 mg/kg may produce unpleasant extrapyramidal side-effects (usually presenting as facial twitching and discoordination of tongue movements) especially in patients less than 30 years. The recently introduced 5-hydroxytryptamine antagonists do not produce such neurological side-effects and may offer an appropriate alternative for younger people requiring platinum treatment.

Cytotoxic drugs such as the alkylating agents cyclophosphamide, iphosphamide and nitrogen mustard

of the rapidly dividing epithelial cells lining the gut. Appropriate timing of chemotherapy can prevent this but sometimes it is necessary to adjust the dose of the drug if an individual is particularly sensitive. The events leading to nausea and vomiting almost certainly include a direct central nervous system response to many cytotoxic drugs, but the nature of such chemoreceptors is uncertain. For the cytotoxic drugs which are known to cause nausea and vomiting, it is necessary to prescribe antiemetics, prior to and following administration of the cytotoxic drug.

Nausea and vomiting

Not all cytotoxic drugs cause emesis, and individuals vary considerably in the degree to which they experience the problem. As illustrated in Table 7.11 cisplatinum and other platinum containing compounds are the most emetogenic of all cytotoxic drugs and hence prophylaxis is necessary. Nausea may persist for 5–7 days after starting therapy, and therefore antiemetic

Table 7.11   Common cytotoxic drugs in rank order of emetic potential

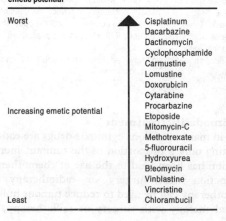

Worst	Cisplatinum
	Dacarbazine
	Dactinomycin
	Cyclophosphamide
	Carmustine
	Lomustine
	Doxorubicin
	Cytarabine
	Procarbazine
Increasing emetic potential	Etoposide
	Mitomycin-C
	Methotrexate
	5-fluorouracil
	Hydroxyurea
	Bleomycin
	Vinblastine
	Vincristine
Least	Chlorambucil

Table 7.12 Commonly used antiemetic regimes

Cytotoxic drug	Antiemetic	Dose-regime
Cisplatinum	Metoclopramide	3 mg/kg i.v. loading dose, then 4 mg/kg continuous infusion in normal saline. Start 30 min prior to cisplatinum and continue for 8 hours
	Dexamethasone	16 mg in 20 ml normal saline given i.v. over 10–15 minutes at time of cisplatinum administration
Cyclophosphamide Iphosphamide	Dexamethasone	As above
Nitrogen Mustard DTIC	Lorazepam	2–4 mg i.v. every four hours
Doxorubicin	Domperidone	10–20 mg orally or by suppository every 4–8 hours.

cause emesis of less severity and shorter duration. Antiemetic therapy should however be administered, and as with platinum therapy it is important to administer the antiemetic prior to the cytotoxic treatment, since prevention is very much more successful than trying to stop nausea and/or vomiting once they have started. For these alkylating agents and for the widely used anthracycline doxorubicin, dexamethasone, metoclopramide, lorazepam, prochlorperazine or domperidone are usually successful in abolishing emesis. Recommended doses of these antiemetics are given in Table 7.12. There is increasing use of antiemetics in combinations of two or more drugs.

Alopecia

Alopecia is associated with the administration of some cytotoxic drugs, particularly doxorubicin and cyclophosphamide. If such drugs are prescribed, it is important to warn the patient in advance and, if appropriate, to arrange for a wig to be fitted. Alopecia is almost always reversible on cessation of therapy.

Psychological effects

The psychological effect of chemotherapy over a period of many months is one which the physician must be aware of. If properly counselled, many patients tolerate being informed of their diagnosis and also their early treatment remarkably well, only to become anxious and depressed as treatment continues even though their tumour may be obviously responding. Awareness of this is essential and constant reassurance and support are necessary.

Growth

The chronic toxicity of cancer chemotherapy is important now that increasing numbers of patients are surviving for longer periods. Data from the follow-up of children cured of malignant disease have shown that physical growth can be stunted by the use of combinations of cytotoxic drugs with radiation but there is conflicting evidence as to whether or not these agents cause significant intellectual impairment.

Fertility

This is preserved for the majority of prepubertal children treated with cytotoxic drugs but for adults fertility may be lost. This is particularly the case for men. For women the problem is more variable depending on their premorbid menstrual pattern and the length of time prior to the expected menopause. Many patients suffering from malignant diseases may be subfertile at the time of diagnosis and amenorrhoea is common for the months during which women are receiving treatment. Nevertheless, this is not a universal finding and since cytotoxic drugs are potentially teratogenic, patients of both sexes should be advised to use contraceptive measures whilst they are receiving chemotherapy.

It is now established that children who receive curative treatment for cancer may successfully produce children of their own in adult life. The number of successful pregnancies in this situation is only approximately half that of the normal population, but the frequency of congenital malformations amongst second generation children is no greater than that expected.

Second malignancy

Cytotoxic drugs may be associated with the eventual development of a second malignancy in a small proportion of patients. The cases have usually been of acute myelomonocytic leukaemia developing 5–10 years following the use of alkylating agents. In a study of over 5000 cases of ovarian cancer treated with alkylating agents, it was shown that the risk of developing acute leukaemia was 36 times that of the normal population. However, only certain classes of anticancer drug are associated with this rare phenomenon which has arisen only as a result of developing therapies which may cure the primary tumour.

PRINCIPLES OF ENDOCRINE THERAPY

Tumours which develop in organs that are known to be under hormonal control sometimes retain hormonal dependency. This can be used therapeutically either by withdrawing the source of the hormone, by prescribing an anti-hormone or by the administration of another hormone. Carcinomas of the breast, prostate, endometrium and thyroid are the diseases currently amenable to endocrine therapy. The therapeutic use of adrenal corticosteroids is exceptional in that these compounds influence non-endocrine-related tumours, for example the lymphomas and leukaemias.

The biological effect of hormones such as oestrogen and progesterone is dependent on the hormone binding to a cytoplasmic receptor protein that transports the hormone to the nucleus where it interacts with DNA to modulate gene expression. An oestrogen receptor can be assayed in biopsies of breast tumours or lymph nodes containing metastases. It has been found that for about 65% of patients whose tumours possess a significant amount of this receptor protein, removal of the source of oestrogen drive will be therapeutically useful whilst for those in whom this protein is absent, hormonal therapy is usually of no benefit. The presence of progesterone-receptor further increases the likelihood of hormone sensitivity. The development of techniques to predict hormone sensitivity has had a major influence on the management of patients with breast carcinomas. If oestrogen receptor activity is present then premenopausal patients may benefit from oophorectomy and both pre- and postmenopausal patients may respond to the administration of tamoxifen, a compound that blocks oestrogen binding.

The use of ablative procedures such as adrenalectomy has now been superseded by the availability of aminoglutethimide which achieves the same result by 'medical' rather than surgical means. Aminoglutethimide inhibits the desmolase that catalyses the conversion of cholesterol to delta-5-pregnenolone, thus preventing the synthesis of corticosteroids, oestrogens and androgens. It also inhibits the aromatase that converts androgens to oestrogens in peripheral tissues. In order to prevent excess secretion of ACTH (as a result of the failure to produce the 11-hydroxycorticosteroids), it is necessary to prescribe hydrocortisone together with aminoglutethimide. Tumour response to tamoxifen and aminoglutethamide may not be manifest for 6–12 weeks from the start of therapy and it is therefore necessary to wait for this period before making decisions about further management. Androgen may produce responses in about 20% of patients with breast cancer, particularly in postmenopausal women with bone metastases.

Oestrogens are useful in the palliation of prostate cancer, but have very significant risks and have a similar response rate (c. 80%) to that of orchidectomy which removes the major source of testosterone.

A new class of endocrine compounds has recently been introduced into clinical practice which are long-acting agonists of luteinising hormone releasing hormone (LHRH). By down-regulating receptors on pituitary gonadotrophs these substances have the potential to suppress gonadal activity on a temporary basis and by a potentially reversible mechanism. This is not associated with the side-effects of direct suppression achieved with the use of oestrogens or androgens. The two malignant conditions in which LHRH agonists have been evaluated most thoroughly are the treatment of breast and prostatic cancer. For premenopausal women with hormonally sensitive breast cancer (oestrogen receptor positive) LHRH antagonists offer a medical alternative to the surgical removal of the ovaries or a permanent menopause induced by radiation. Clinical trials of the agonist leuprolide given as a subcutaneous injection of 1 mg show that it provides sustained suppression of plasma oestradiol. An alternative is administration of nasal spray preparations such as buserelin which has to be given 6 times daily. Although medical oophorectomy is achieved by this means the relative low morbidity and cost of ovariectomy considered together with the fact that breast cancer, even in pre-menopausal women, frequently occurs beyond the time at which women will wish to have further children suggests that surgery may for some be preferable.

For the management of prostate cancer it has been shown that daily subcutaneous injections of leuprolide produce marked suppression of testosterone. This provides a potential medical alternative to surgical castration, a procedure which even at the age span of typical patients with prostate cancer, is an unacceptable operation for many patients. More acceptable and equally effective is a subcapsular orchidectomy.

Progestogens are compounds related to the progesterone produced by the corpus luteum and placenta. Some women with metastatic endometrial carcinoma benefit from these drugs, particularly patients with well differentiated tumours.

Papillary carcinomas of the thyroid remain under the influence of thyroid-stimulating hormone (TSH) and the administration of thyroid hormone may be useful as a result of its inhibiting pituitary secretion of TSH. Initial treatment of these tumours is surgical with total thyroidectomy followed by ablation dose of radioactive iodine to remove any residual normal thyroid. The patient is then established on thyroid hormone replacement therapy and serum thyroglobulin levels used to monitor progress. If the levels rise then further assessment of thyroid replacement is necessary to determine whether a therapy dose of radioactive iodine is indicated.

The major advantage of hormonal therapy over chemotherapy is that the side-effects of endocrine treatment are usually less severe than those associated with cytotoxic drugs. Tamoxifen rarely causes toxicity but aminoglutethimide can cause drowsiness, depression and transient rashes in some patients. The use of oestrogen in elderly men with prostate cancer warrants special caution in view of its known propensity to exacerbate the fluid retention that may be associated with cardiovascular disease.

THE MANAGEMENT OF PAIN

Pain is relatively rare as a presenting symptom of early or localised malignant disease, but patients often associate the diagnosis of cancer as leading inevitably to severe and intractable pain, and many need reassurance that such a situation is both rare and preventable. However, advanced cancer is frequently associated with some degree of pain and its management forms an essential part of palliative medicine.

Classification

Accurate definition of the site and cause of pain
This is essential before deciding on therapy, for example, bone pain as caused by myeloma or metastases from tumours such as breast cancer often has two components – a background of diffuse aching pain unrelated to activity, and localised intensive pain triggered by touch or weight bearing. Abdominal colic is typically of sudden, intermittent type, whereas headache arising from raised intracranial pressure tends to be more constant. Musculo-skeletal and joint pains are usually localised, as are the consequences of nerve entrapment such as can result from tumour infiltration (for example of the brachial plexus), or collapsed vertebrae secondary to bone metastases.

Assessment of severity of pain
This should be recorded in the patients' notes so that the results of analgesic therapy can be *regularly reviewed*. Several grading systems are used such as the one shown in the information box below.

SCALE FOR GRADING PAIN

- Grade 1: Pain relieved by occasional mild analgesics
- Grade 2: Pain requiring regular mild analgesics
- Grade 3: Pain requiring regular medium strength analgesics
- Grade 4: Pain requiring regular strong analgesics
- Grade 5: Pain not controlled by regular strong analgesics

Only 10–15% of patients with cancer fall into the category of grade 4 or 5. It cannot be over-emphasised that successful pain control requires not only the selection of the analgesic most appropriate to the par-

ticular cause of painful stimulus, but the *regular* administration of therapy to constantly suppress pain and prevent its re-emergence. As indicated in the above grading of pain, analgesics can be classified as mild, medium or strong in terms of their effect.

Relief of pain

Mild analgesics
Widely used mild analgesics include paracetamol, aspirin, dextropropoxyphene, and flurbiprofen.

Table 7.13   Mild and medium strength analgesics

Mild	Dose	Side-effects
Paracetamol	1 g 4-hourly	Occasionally hepatotoxic
Aspirin (with codeine)	300–600 mg (with 8–16 mg codeine phosphate 4-hourly)	Gastritis
Dextropropoxyphene	65–150 mg 6-hourly	Constipation, sedation
Flurbiprofen	50–100 mg 4-hourly	Gastritis

Medium	Dose	Side-effects
Dihydrocodeine	30–60 mg 4-hourly	Constipation, sedation
Dipipanone with cyclizine	10 mg 30 mg } 6-hourly	Sedation

Medium strength analgesics
Dihydrocodeine, and dipipanone are useful as medium strength analgesics. Dihydrocodeine is the most commonly used of these and is well tolerated apart from causing constipation. Dipipanone is stronger than dihydrocodeine and provides useful analgesia for grade 3 symptoms. Examples of doses of mild and medium strength analgesics are given in Table 7.13.

Strong analgesics
Dextromoramide, morphine and diamorphine are the most widely used potent analgesics. Dextromoramide is limited by short duration of action (approximately 2 hours) but for the same reason is valuable for 'breakthrough' pain that may occur occasionally when a patient is on long-term opiates. Morphine and diamorphine play an essential role in the management of severe chronic pain, but these substances are all too often prescribed in sub-optimal ways. Two common mistakes are the overcautious prescription for fear of inducing addiction, and prescribing 'cocktails' containing substances such as cocaine and chlorpromazine (e.g. Brompton's mixture). Addiction is irrelevant in the management of severe pain in advanced malignancy, and the stimulant or sedative effects of cocaine or chlorpromazine can induce confusion, anxiety and emotional distress. There is little to choose between

morphine and diamorphine, but the availability of slow release oral morphine is useful for ambulant patients, and the greater solubility of diamorphine can be useful in reducing the volume of parenteral injection. MST Continus tablets contain morphine in different strengths; (10, 30, 60 and 100 mg) and are formulated to provide slow release for up to 12 hours. For these and standard formulations of morphine and diamorphine the dose must be titrated to the needs of the individual patient. For oral administration of standard preparations the dose must be repeated every 4 hours and dosage will vary from 20–100 mg or more. Intravenous administration of high dose may be appropriate for hospitalised patients, but the introduction of highly accurate slow-release pumps has enabled opiates to be given by continuous subcutaneous administration. The two major advantages of this are that these portable devices allow patients to remain ambulant, and that even very large doses can be given without causing significant central nervous system depression resulting in lethargy and confusion. Constipation is an inevitable consequence of prolonged administration of opiates and patients requiring these should always be given regular laxatives at the same time. Stool softeners such as dioctyl sodium sulphosuccinate and compounds that stimulate peristalsis such as bisacodyl are appropriate to ease constipation.

TERMINAL CARE

An essential component of oncological medicine is the management of patients in the terminal phase of their illness. Psychological support is the most important aspect but this can be provided only if positive measures are taken to relieve pain, to ensure adequate and appropriate nutrition and treat specific symptoms such as cough, pruritus and nausea. Successful symptomatic treatment allows patients to prepare themselves mentally for death, and the relief of physical distress will also help the patient's family to cope with impending bereavement.

An individual patient's reaction to the inevitability of death from a malignant disease depends on a host of interrelated variables including his or her cultural and religious background, age, education, the duration of the illness and the reactions of dependants. Nevertheless certain common patterns of behaviour are recognisable. A period of initial disbelief and denial is often replaced by resentment and anger. This in turn is followed by a period of depression which is almost universal but many patients, with or without medical intervention, enter a final phase of peacefully accepting the inevitability of death.

When to tell patients that they have a terminal illness is a matter of experience. Death does not necessarily represent a failure of treatment and it is essential that those caring for the terminally ill do not avoid discussion of the processes of terminal illness. Such avoidance can only enhance the patient's sense of loneliness and isolation.

It is not always appropriate to present all of the facts to a patient, most especially on a single occasion, and time must be spent to determine patients' awareness of their situation, and their expectations. Non-committal, even ambiguous statements about the future may be appropriate but the patient should never be told what is known to be untrue.

Preparation for death is not the sole responsibility of the medical profession and, especially for patients dying in hospitals, it is important to make provision for the adequate access of relatives, friends and other professionals such as the clergy when patients request their support. Religious belief does not necessarily make death any easier and even for patients who hold such beliefs it should not be forgotten that fear of the unknown is something shared by patients and all those who are caring for them.

The most important principle of managing terminal illness is to provide adequate time for talking with the patient. In a busy world this is difficult and it is sometimes easier to use the lack of time as an excuse for avoiding demanding consultations that drain the doctor's emotional resources. Nevertheless to develop the ability to listen to patients and to learn from them how best to provide psychological support during terminal illness can be one of the most rewarding experiences in medicine.

FURTHER READING

Bishop J M 1986 From Proto-Oncogene to Oncogene: The Molecular Genetics of Cancer. Advances in Oncology, Vol. 2, No 4

Chabner B 1982 Pharmacologic principles of cancer treatment. Saunders, Philadelphia. A detailed account both preclinical and clinical.

DeVita V T, Hellman S, Rosenburg S A 1982 Cancer, principles and practice of oncology. Lippincott, Philadelphia. This is a comprehensive textbook.

Doll R, Peto R 1981 The causes of cancer. Oxford Medical Publications, Oxford. This is a short resumé of the known epidemiological factors.

Doyle, D, 1984 Palliative Care: The Management of Far Advanced Illness. The Charles Press, Philadelphia

Glover D M, Hames B D 1989 Oncogenes. Oxford University Press, Oxford

Saunders Dame Cecily 1978 The management of terminal disease. The management of malignant disease, vol. 1. Arnold, London. A summary of the theory and practice of terminal care by the Medical Director of St Christopher's Hospice, London

8

Diseases of the Cardiovascular System

Heart disease is common. Minor congenital abnormalities affect one in one hundred live births and more serious abnormalities approximately one in five hundred. Acquired heart disease becomes increasingly common with age and in 'western' societies heart disease is the commonest cause of death from the fourth decade onwards. Over the last decade mortality from heart disease has begun to decline in the United States of America, in Australia, and very recently this decline has also been noted in the United Kingdom. It is not yet clear whether this reflects changing lifestyles, improved diagnosis and management, or other factors as yet unrecognised. Heart disease has two peculiarities when compared with diseases of other organs. First, it is very commonly latent, that is a disease process of, for example, the coronary arteries can proceed to an advanced stage before the patient notices any symptoms. Second, the number of symptoms attributable to heart disease is limited and it is common for many different pathologies to present through a final common symptomatic pathway. For this reason this chapter will start with a brief description of cardiac symptoms and of cardiac investigation before going on to discuss individual cardic diseases.

CLINICAL FEATURES

THE SYMPTOMS OF HEART DISEASE

Cardiac death

Cessation of the heart's activities is a traditional definition of death. There are three forms of cardiac death. *Asystole* is a lack of electrical activation of the ventricle. *Ventricular fibrillation* is due to inco-ordinate activation of ventricular muscle with consequent lack of ventricular contraction. *Electromechanical dissociation* occurs when the ventricle is activated but is unable to contract or to expel blood. Causes are summarised in the information box (right).

Breathlessness (Dyspnoea)

Breathlessness or dyspnoea is a common symptom of cardiac disease. It is commonly defined as a subjective awareness of increasing work in breathing, but the mechanisms responsible for this sensation are incompletely understood and may differ according to the circumstances.

Exertional dyspnoea. This is breathlessness which comes on during exertion and subsides on resting. It is commonly due either to heart failure or to

---

CAUSES OF CARDIAC DEATH

Asystole
Heart block
Myocardial infarction
Hypoxia

Ventricular fibrillation
Myocardial infarction
Myocardial ischaemia
Myocarditis
Cardiomyopathy
Electrolyte disturbances:
low or high K^+
low Ca^{++} or Mg^{++}
Electric shock
WPW (see p. 269), Long QT syndromes

Electromechanical dissociation
Cardiac rupture
Cardiac tamponade
low Ca^{++}
Cardiac depressant drugs

---

lung disease. Some patients with angina describe breathlessness rather than chest pain on exertion.

Pulmonary oedema. This is persistent breathlessness resulting from fluid accumulation in the lung as a manifestation of acute left heart failure. The patients looks and feels unwell, and there is peripheral vasoconstriction and tachycardia. Breathing is rapid and shallow, and there is a persistent cough. Sputum is white and frothy, sometimes tinged with pink. Crepitations are heard on auscultation of the chest, initially at the lung bases, later throughout the lungs. Orthopnoea and paroxysmal nocturnal dyspnoea are transient forms of pulmonary oedema.

Orthopnea. This is breathlessness brought on by lying flat. It is usually due to failure of the left side of the heart, and is attributed to redistribution of fluid from the lower extremities to the lungs.

Paroxysmal nocturnal dyspnoea. This is a variant of orthopnea in which the patient awakes from sleep extremely breathless, has a persistant cough, and may produce white frothy sputum. It is usually relieved at least initially by sitting upright. It is a manifestation of acute left heart failure. Paroxysmal nocturnal dyspnoea has to be distinguished from intermittent respiratory obstruction in the *sleep apnoea syndrome* (p. 352) This is usually associated with restlessness and snoring. Occasional deep sighing respirations either at rest or provoked by exertion may be a feature of cardiac neurosis but do not indicate heart disease.

Cheyne Stokes breathing. This is periodic breathing in which both the rate and depth of breathing increase to a maximum over a period of a few minutes, then decrease until breathing virtually ceases, when the cycle is repeated. It is a feature of severe heart failure, but may also be observed during sleep in normal subjects at high altitude, or in the elderly.

Other abnormal breathing patterns. Patients with heart failure tend to have rapid shallow respirations with similar inspiratory and expiratory times. This is distinct from the prolonged expiratory phase of obstructive airways disease. In some patients reversible airways obstruction does develop as a manifestation of left heart failure ('cardiac asthma'). In others, heart disease and chronic obstructive lung disease may co-exist. The differential diagnosis of dyspnoea is given in the information box below.

DIFFERENTIAL DIAGNOSIS OF DYSPNOEA

Cardiac failure
Exertional dyspnoea
Pulmonary oedema
Paroxysmal nocturnal dyspnoea
Orthopnoea

Respiratory disease
Asthma
Chronic obstructive lung disease
Pneumonia
Pulmonary neoplasm
Laryngeal/tracheal obstruction

Other
Anaphylaxis
Severe anaemia
Toxic gas inhalation
Psychogenic dyspnoea

Chest pain

Angina. This is a choking or constricting chest pain which comes on with exertion, is relieved by rest, and is due to myocardial ischaemia. It is commonly felt retrosternally and may radiate to the left or more rarely the right arm to the throat, jaws and teeth, or through to the back. The pain may be squeezing, crushing, burning or aching, but seldom stabbing. The pain may be brought on or exacerbated by emotion, and is frequently made worse by large meals or a cold wind. It is relieved by nitrates.

Myocardial infarction. The pain is similar in nature and distribution to angina but is more severe, persists at rest, and does not respond to nitrates. There are usually features of sympathetic nervous system activation, and vomiting is common. There may be anxiety and a feeling of impending death.

Dissecting aortic aneurysm. The pain is severe sharp and tearing often felt in or penetrating through to the back. It may be accompanied by vomiting. The pulse may be disproportionately slow for the severity of the pain, owing to stimulation of aortic baroreceptors.

Pericarditic pain. This is felt retrosternally, to the left of the sternum, or in the left or right shoulder. It characteristically varies in intensity with the phase of respiration.

Musculo-skeletal chest pain. This is very variable in site and intensity but does not usually fall into the patterns described above. It may or may not vary with posture or movement, it may be brought on by exertion but often does not cease instantly on rest and it is very commonly accompanied by local tenderness over a rib or costal cartilage.

Oesophageal spasm. The pain can mimic that of angina very closely, is sometimes precipitated by exercise and may be relieved by nitrates. It is usually possible to elicit some history of relation of chest pain to food or drink intake.

Types and differential diagnoses of chest pain are summarised in the information box below.

DIFFERENTIAL DIAGNOSIS OF CHEST PAIN

Cardiac
Angina (pain on exertion, remits at rest)
Myocardial infarction (severe, persists at rest)
Pericarditis (varies with breathing, audible rub)

Aortic
Dissecting aneurysm ('tearing' pain in back, asymmetric pulses, bradycardia)

Lung/Pleura
Pneumothorax (asymmetric air entry, percussion note)
Pleurisy (varies with breathing, pleural rub)

Musculoskeletal
Local tenderness common

Oesophageal
May be food related (but not invariably)

Oedema

Peripheral oedema. This is a feature of chronic heart failure and is due to excessive salt and water retention. In ambulant or sedentary patients it usually affects the ankles, legs, thighs and lower abdomen in that order. In a patient who is lying down it is most apparent over the sacrum. The oedema of heart failure is usually accompanied by at least some other symptoms of heart failure, and by a raised jugular venous pressure. Unless it is long-standing and the skin is very tense the oedema pits easily on pressure. A differential diagnosis is given in the information box below.

DIFFERENTIAL DIAGNOSIS OF PERIPHERAL OEDEMA

- Cardiac failure
- Chronic venous insufficiency
- *Hypoalbuminaemia* (nephrotic syndrome, liver disease, protein-losing enteropathy)
- Drugs
  Retaining sodium (fludrocortisone, non-steroidal anti-inflammatory agents); increasing capillary permeability (nifedipine)
- Idiopathic (women > men)

Oedema of chronic venous insufficiency. This together with immobility is very common in the elderly. It usually affects the ankles and lower legs only. The oedema pits readily and redistributes after a night's sleep. However there are no other features of cardiac failure. Oedema is a relatively late and unreliable feature of deep venous thrombosis. However ilio-femoral vein thrombosis can cause severe venous congestion and oedema.

Oedema of nephrotic syndrome. This tends to be more severe and more widely distributed than the oedema of heart failure, and often affects the face and arms. This is because patients with a nephrotic syndrome have normal cardiac output and normal or reduced circulating blood volume. A heart failure patient with the same degree of oedema would be profoundly ill. The presence of proteinuria confirms the diagnosis. Hypoproteinaemic oedema may also occur in liver disease and in protein losing enteropathy.

Palpitation

Palpitation is an abnormal subjective awareness of the heart beat. Patients can usually distinguish between sporadic and continuous palpitation (for example extrasystoles or a sustained tachycardia) and between an irregular and a regular pulse. It may be helpful to ask the patient to tap out the heart rhythm on the table. Palpitation with a regular rhythm and a normal heart rate may be due to sudden vasodilatation (e.g. during perimenopausal flushing).

Syncope

Syncope is loss of conciousness resulting from an inadequate blood supply to the brain. This may be due to sudden vasodilatation, to a sudden fall in cardiac output or to both simultaneously. Postural syncope when due to vasodilator or antihypertensive drugs is an example of the former, and diminished cardiac output from complete heart block or a very rapid tachycardia of the latter.

Vasovagal fainting. This involves both a reflex cardiac slowing mediated by the vagus and a sudden withdrawal of peripheral sympathetic tone. It is a complex centrally mediated reflex which tends to be initiated when pain or a powerful emotional stimulus is inflicted against a background of intense sympathetic stimulation. A very similar reflex can also be triggered by mechano-receptors from the endocardium of the left ventricle. This accounts for the fainting reflex which occurs in patients with pulmonary embolism or aortic stenosis (p. 297).

The causes are listed in the information box below.

CAUSES OF SYNCOPE

Cardiac dysrhythmia	*Excessive vasodilatation*
Heart block	Antihypertensive drugs
Paroxysmal tachycardia	Nitrates
	Anaphylaxis
Impaired venous return	
Hypovolaemia	*Vasovagal fainting*
Haemorrhage	
Diabetic pre-coma	*Acute heart failure*
Raised intrathoracic	Pulmonary embolus
pressure	Atrial myxoma
Cough syncope	Aortic stenosis
Micturiction syncope	

Other symptoms

Tiredness is a common complaint with severe heart failure and with ischaemic heart disease. Sometimes it is the consequence of treatment rather than the disease itself, e.g. beta-blockade or hypokalaemia from diuretics. In those with valvular disease without heart failure it should lead to a suspicion of infective endocarditis.

Nocturia, or a reversal of the usual diurnal rhythm of diuresis, sometimes occurs in ambulant patients with cardiac failure. It probably reflects improved renal perfusion during bed-rest rather than a simple mobilisation of oedema fluid from the ankles. Cough is a feature of pulmonary oedema. Anorexia, nausea and vomiting are all common in severe protracted heart failure; they may also be manifestations of digitalis intoxication (p. 276).

PHYSICAL EXAMINATION

GENERAL EXAMINATION

Certain features such as breathlessness or anxiety may have been obvious during the history taking.

Pallor. This may indicate anaemia, which may contribute to breathlessness or, in a patient with ischaemic heart disease, to angina. Conversely, anaemia may be due to infective endocarditis or to bleeding associated with anticoagulant therapy.

Cyanosis of the mucous membranes (central cyanosis). This is due to arterial hypoxaemia – either from poor gaseous exchange in the lungs resulting from respiratory disease or pulmonary oedema, or when there is a right-to-left shunt as in congenital heart disease.

Obesity. This is commonly associated with acquired hyperlipidaemia or maturity onset diabetes, both of which are causes of ischaemic heart disease. In a hypertensive patient it may be a manifestation of Cushing's syndrome.

Features of hyperlipidaemia. These are summarised in Fig. 8.1. A corneal arcus and xanthelasma are the most common, but do not reliably indicate hyperlipidaemia in patients over 50 years old.

Facial abnormalities. These are sometimes pointers to cardiac disease – for example the ptosis and frontal baldness of dystonia myotonica (cardiomyopathy and conduction abnormalities), the high-arched palate and ocular lens abnormalities of Marfan's Syndrome (aortic aneurysm) and the 'elfin' faces of congenital supravalvar aortic stenosis. Many children with congenital heart disease have unusual facial features.

Other observations. Skin temperature is a measure of skin blood flow – cold skin indicates

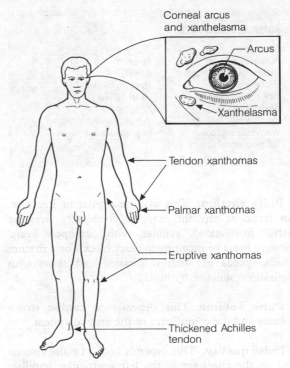

Fig. 8.1 Diagram to show sites of the cutaneous stigmata of hyperlipidaemia. The commonest features are a corneal arcus and xanthelasmata, but these are not necessarily indicative of severe hyperlipidaemia in the elderly. Tendon xanthomas are always indicative of severe hyperlipidaemia. Palmar and eruptive xanthomas are rare.

cutaneous vasoconstriction or a low cardiac output, a warm skin cutaneous vasodilatation. Unduly moist palms suggest anxiety if they are cold, or thyrotoxicosis if they are warm. Clubbing of the fingers occurs in cyanotic congenital heart disease and in advanced infective endocarditis, as well as in a variety of respiratory and other diseases (p. 346). Sublingual or 'splinter' haemorrhages may result from trauma and occur in normal individuals, but are also a feature of infective endocarditis.

EXAMINATION OF THE CARDIOVASCULAR SYSTEM

Arterial pulse

Although the *rate* and *rhythm* of the arterial pulse can be assessed from the radial pulse, the *volume* and *quality* are better assessed from the brachial, carotid or femoral pulses. Bradycardia is a resting pulse <60 beats per minute, tachycardia a resting pulse >100 beats per minute. Causes are shown in the information box (p. 254).

ARTERIAL PULSE: RATE

Bradycardia	Tachycardia
Athletes	Fever
Beta-blocking drugs	Anxiety
Hypothyroidism	Hyperthyroidism
Sick sinus syndrome	Heart failure
Heart block	Arrhythmias
Hypothermia	Sympathomimetic drugs
Vasovagal syncope	(e.g. salbutamol)
Coupled ectopic beats	

Pulse rhythm. This may be regular or irregular. An irregular rhythm may be completely irregular (atrial fibrillation), regular with 'dropped beats' (ectopic beats or incomplete heart block), or a rhythm which speeds up with inspiration and slows with expiration (sinus arrhythmia).

Pulse volume. This depends on cardiac stroke volume and the compliance of the arterial system.

Pulse quality. This depends both on pulse volume and on the character of the left ventricular impulse. The most striking abnormalities are the *slow rising* pulse of aortic stenosis, the *collapsing* pulse of aortic incompetence, and the *jerky* pulse of hypertrophic obstructive cardiomyopathy (Fig. 8.2)

Pulsus paradoxus. This is a pulse which gets smaller in volume with inspiration and large with expiration. 'True' or type 1 paradox is seen in pericardial tamponade. Type 2 paradox, in which there is no change in pulse volume, but systolic and diastolic pressures both rise and fall in phase with expiration and inspiration, this occurs in severe airways obstruction.

Pulsus alternans. This is an alternation of large and small volume beats. True pulsus alternans is a feature of severe cardiac failure, and is much less common than apparent pulsus alternans due to coupled ectopic beats. Pulsus alternans is best detected with a stethoscope and sphygmomanometer. There may be a difference of 10–40 mmHg in systolic pressure between beats.

Bisferiens pulse. This is a pulse with a double peak, usually best felt in the brachial artery, and indicative of combined aortic stenosis and regurgitation.

In old age, arteries become more rigid, and this may affect the way they transmit the pulse wave. They also elongate and become more tortuous. In elderly patients, particularly hypertensive women, an arterial pulsation may be seen above the right clavicle because of 'kinking' of a tortuous carotid artery.

Arterial pulsation in the neck is increased in aortic regurgitation and sometimes in coarctation of the aorta. A bruit heard over a carotid artery with the stethoscope bell is an important sign of partial obstruction, but needs to be distinguished from a murmur conducted from a stenosed aortic valve.

In hypertensive patients, and in children suspected of having congenital heart disease, the radial and femoral pulses should be palpated simultaneously in order to detect coarctation of the aorta. In this condition the femoral pulse is seldom absent, but it is of small volume, delayed after the radial pulse, and measurement of the arterial pressure in the legs with a suitably large cuff shows it to be lower than in the arms.

Jugular venous pulse
With the patient reclining against pillows at about 45°, and with the neck muscles relaxed, the jugular venous

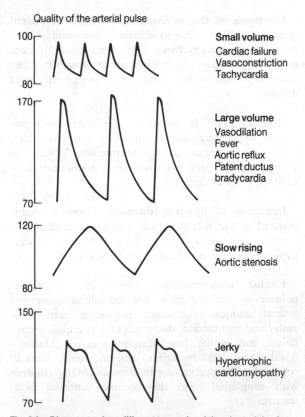

Quality of the arterial pulse

Small volume
Cardiac failure
Vasoconstriction
Tachycardia

Large volume
Vasodilation
Fever
Aortic reflux
Patent ductus
bradycardia

Slow rising
Aortic stenosis

Jerky
Hypertrophic
cardiomyopathy

Fig. 8.2 Diagram to show different types of peripheral arterial pulse wave. It is more reliable to assess the pulse waveform from a large artery such as carotid or femoral than from the radial pulse.

pulse may be examined from movement of the skin overlying the internal jugular vein, although the vein itself is not visible. Unlike arterial pulsation, jugular venous pulsation represents the zone of transition between distended and collapsed segments of vein, and the height of this above the level of the right atrium is a measure of the right atrial, or central venous, pressure. In normal subjects, or in those with a low central venous pressure, jugular pulsation is often hidden behind the clavicle in this position, and rarely extends for more than 2 or 3 cm above the sternal angle. When venous pressure is transiently increased by pressure on the abdomen, the level of pulsation moves upwards in the neck: this is called *hepato-jugular reflux* and is one of the ways in which the jugular pulse can be distinguished from arterial pulsation.

The venous pulse varies with the patient's position and the phase of respiration; it frequently exhibits two peaks to every one of the arterial pulse (Fig. 8.3), and the most prominent movement is often an inward one.

It is usual to express *jugular venous pressure* (which is equivalent to central venous pressure) as the vertical distance in centimetres between the zone of jugular pulsation and the sternal angle. Sometimes the jugular pressure is so high that pulsation is apparent only when the patient sits or stands upright. The commonest and most important cause of a raised jugular venous pressure is cardiac failure. Sometimes it is possible to find out more about the cause of the failure by analysing the wave form of the pulse. Causes are listed in the information box below.

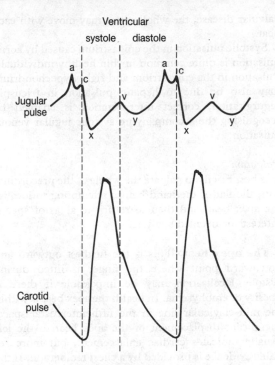

Fig. 8.3   Carotid and jugular pulses. Simultaneous central arterial and venous pulses to demonstrate carotid and jugular pulse wave form. a Atrial contraction, c Onset of ventricular contraction, v Pressure peak immediately prior to opening of tricuspid valve, c–x x descent, v–y y descent.

CAUSES OF RAISED JUGULAR VENOUS PRESSURE

Common
Heart failure (right heart failure or combined right and left heart failure)
Tricuspid reflux

Less common
Pulmonary embolism
Pericardial tamponade
Superior vena cava obstruction

Rare
Constrictive pericarditis
Tricuspid stenosis

The *wave form of the jugular venous pulse* in a patient in sinus rhythm is shown in Fig. 8.3. The *a* wave is due to atrial systole. It is absent in atrial fibrillation, and may be abnormally large when there is obstruction to right atrial discharge, as in tricuspid stenosis, or when the right ventricle is hypertrophied and stiff, as in pulmonary stenosis or pulmonary hypertension. With tricuspid regurgitation there are prominant waves in the venous pulse in time with ventricular systole; these are often called *v* waves but the mechanism and timing are different from the physiological *v* waves shown in Fig. 8.3.

In patients with atrioventricular dissociation (p. 277) intermittent large volume systolic waves may be seen in the venous pulse; these are called *cannon waves*, and occur when the atrium contracts against a closed tricuspid valve.

Inspection
In children, enlargement of the right ventricle during the growing period may show as a prominence to the left of the sternum. The apical impulse (see below) may be visible, and its position may give a clue to cardiac enlargement. The sustained apical impulse of left ventricular hypertrophy, and the diffuse pulsation over a left ventricular aneurysm can often be seen as well as felt. Occasionally an aneurysm of the aortic arch can be seen to move the upper sternum with each systole; when the heart is very much enlarged, as with advanced

valvular disease, the whole chest may move with each beat.

Systolic pulsation in the epigastrium caused by aortic pulsation is quite common in thin healthy individuals. Pulsation in the epigastrium and right hypochondrium may also be due to hepatic pulsation in tricuspid regurgitation; correct interpretation is enabled by recognising the accompanying systolic jugular venous pulsation.

Palpation
It is best briefly to palpate the whole of the precordium with the flat of the hand before attempting to localise the apex beat, and then to return to areas of special interest for detailed analysis.

The apex beat. This is the furthest outward and downward point where the finger is lifted during systole; localisation may be impossible if there is obesity or emphysema. In health the apex beat is within the mid-clavicular line in the fifth intercostal space. Significant displacement of the apex beat to the left usually indicates cardiac enlargement, but more reliable evidence is provided by a chest radiograph. If the mediastinum is displaced by fibrosis, collapse or removal of the lung on the left side or by a large pleural effusion on the right, the apex beat may lie to the left in the absence of cardiac enlargement. Abnormalities are listed in the information box below.

ABNORMALITIES OF THE APEX BEAT

- Displaced Apex
  Cardiac enlargement
  Pleural effusion or pneumothorax
  Dextrocardia
- Sustained ('heaving') impulse
  Left ventricular hypertrophy
- Double apical impulse
  Hypertrophic cardiomyopathy
- Diffuse apical impulse
  Dilated cardiomyopathy or ischaemic damage
- Tapping apical impulse ('palpable first sound')
  Mitral stenosis

The quality of the cardiac impulse should be noted. In left ventricular hypertrophy it is forceful and sustained, while abrupt closure of the mitral valve, either with anxiety or when associated with mitral stenosis, may give it a tapping quality. When the heart is dilated, as for exmple in dilated cardiomyopathy or advanced ischaemic heart disease, the apex is displaced

to the left but the impulse is diffuse rather than forceful.

With right ventricular hypertrophy a pulsation may be imparted to the hand on the chest to the left of the sternum. This may also result when the heart is displaced forward by a dilated left atrium. A dilated pulmonary artery under abnormally high pressure may cause a pulsation in the second left intercostal space beside the sternum. Closure of the semilunar valves under abnormal pressure may give a diastolic shock, or palpable second heart sound.

Thrills. Turbulent flow may impart a vibration to the hand; this thrill is the palpable equivalent of a murmur. Usually only loud murmurs are associated with thrills, but a low-pitched vibration is sometimes felt as readily as it is heard. A systolic thrill at the apex usually indicates mitral regurgitation, and a diastolic thrill mitral stenosis. A systolic thrill can often be felt at the lower left sternal edge with a ventricular septal defect, and at the upper sternal edge in aortic or pulmonary stenosis. An aortic diastolic thrill is very rare and usually indicates rupture of an aortic valve cusp.

Percussion
This is seldom used except when seeking abnormal dullness to the right of the sternum in a patient with a suspected pericardial effusion. One of the physical signs of emphysema is a loss of the normal area of cardiac dullness.

Heart sounds
Use a good stethoscope with both diaphragm and bell. The diaphragm, firmly pressed against the chest, preferentially conveys high pitched sounds and murmurs, whereas the bell, lightly applied to the skin, favours the transmission of lower pitched sounds.

First and *second* heart sounds can be heard in almost every patient, *third* and *fourth* sounds are associated with specific circumstances. The relation of the heart sounds to the cardiac cycle is show in Fig. 8.4.

The first heart sound. This results from closure of the mitral and to a lesser extent tricuspid valve, and is best heard at the cardiac apex. Its features are listed in the information box (p. 257).

The second heart sound. This is due to closure of aortic and pulmonary valves. Normally closure is synchronous in expiration, but in inspiration the pulmonary component is delayed because of increased right ventricular filling and the aortic component

FIRST HEART SOUND

Loud in:
    Patients with a large Cardiac output:
        Vasodilatation
        Exercise
        Fever
        Thyrotoxicosis
    Mitral stenosis (because of rigid valve)
Quiet in:
    Obesity
    Emphysema
    Impaired left ventricular function

advanced because of decreased left ventricular filling, so the second sound becomes split. This *physiological inspiratory splitting* is most prominent in children and young adults. Abnormally delayed closure of one of the semilunar valves may result from delayed conduction

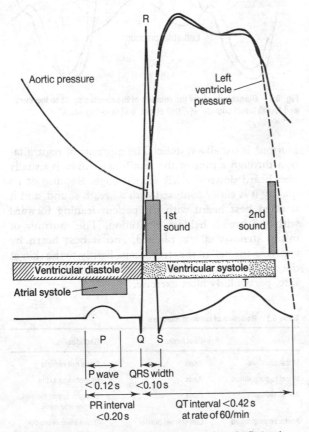

Fig. 8.4 Diagram to show relation of cardiac cycle to the first and second heart sounds, ventricular and atrial systole and diastole, and the ECG.

or mechanical factors, for example when aortic closure is delayed by left bundle branch block – this leads to *reversed splitting* of the second sound. Increased right ventricular stroke volume from a left-to-right shunt, together with equalisation of left and right atrial pressures, leads to wide *fixed* splitting of the second heart sound in atrial septal defect. The different features are listed in the information box below.

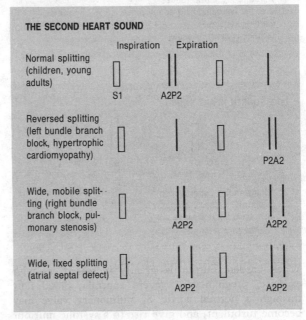

A third heart sound. This is a low pitched sound at the end of the rapid phase of diastolic left ventricular filling, best heard at the apex. It can be 'physiological' in children, pregnant women and athletes, but may also be associated with increased left ventricular stroke volume or diminished left vetricular compliance in heart failure. The features are listed in the information box (p. 258).

A fourth heart sound. This occurs as a result of forceful atrial contraction, and just precedes the first heart sound. It is shown in the information box (p. 258).

Other added sounds. These include the opening snap, ejection click, midsystolic click and prosthetic valve sounds. Their timing and relation to the cardiac cycle are shown in Fig. 8.5.

Cardiac Murmurs
Murmurs are associated with turbulent blood flow.

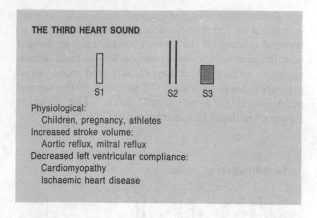

THE THIRD HEART SOUND

S1   S2   S3

Physiological:
    Children, pregnancy, athletes
Increased stroke volume:
    Aortic reflux, mitral reflux
Decreased left ventricular compliance:
    Cardiomyopathy
    Ischaemic heart disease

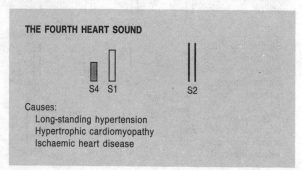

THE FOURTH HEART SOUND

S4 S1   S2

Causes:
    Long-standing hypertension
    Hypertrophic cardiomyopathy
    Ischaemic heart disease

When cardiac output is greatly increased, as with exercise, pregnancy or severe anaemia, blood flow through a normal aortic or pulmonary valve may become turbulent, and give rise to a systolic murmur usually best heard at the sternal border in the second left intercostal space. Murmurs also arise when blood is projected through, or leaks back through, abnormal valves, or through an abnormal channel such as a ventricular septal defect. The features are listed in the information box below.

FEATURES OF MURMURS

- Systolic or diastolic
- Pitch
- Quality
- Intensity
- Where is it heard best?
- Where does it radiate to?

Whether a murmur is systolic or diastolic is best assessed by timing it against the apex beat or carotid pulse. Changes in a murmur's intensity during the cardiac cycle are an important clue to its origin; they are usually depicted by a kind of shorthand based on how the murmur would look if depicted on a phonocardiogram (Fig. 8.6). As a general rule a harsh

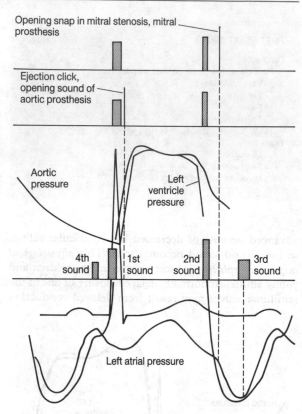

Fig. 8.5 Diagram to show the relation of the cardiac cycle to the third and fourth heart sounds, ejection clicks, and opening snap.

murmur is usually systolic. The murmur of regurgitation through either of the semilunar valves is usually best heard down the left sternal edge. Because of its quality it is easily confused with a breath sound, and it is often best heard with the patient leaning forward with the breath held in expiration. The murmur of mitral stenosis is low pitched, and is best heard by applying the bell of the stethoscope lightly to the skin at the cardiac apex, with the patient half turned to the left side, particularly after exercise.

Table 8.1 Radiation of common murmurs

	Best heard	Radiates
Mitral stenosis	Apex	Does not radiate
Mitral regurgitation	Apex	Radiates to axilla
Aortic stenosis	Apex	To right upper sternal border and neck
Aortic regurgitation	Left sternal border	Down sternal border
Tricuspid regurgitation	Lower left sternal border	Does not radiate
Pulmonary stenosis	Upper left sternal border	To left chest and back

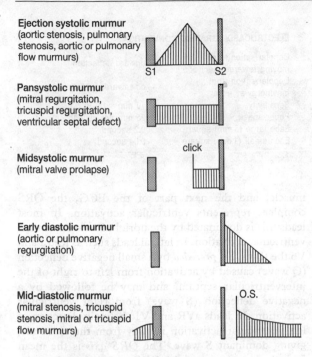

Ejection systolic murmur
(aortic stenosis, pulmonary stenosis, aortic or pulmonary flow murmurs)

S1   S2

Pansystolic murmur
(mitral regurgitation, tricuspid regurgitation, ventricular septal defect)

Midsystolic murmur
(mitral valve prolapse)

click

Early diastolic murmur
(aortic or pulmonary regurgitation)

Mid-diastolic murmur
(mitral stenosis, tricuspid stenosis, mitral or tricuspid flow murmurs)

O.S.

Fig. 8.6   Diagram to show the conventional 'shorthand' notation (based on phonocardiography) for recording different cardiac murmurs.

Murmurs tend to *radiate* in the direction of the blood flow which causes the murmur (Table 8.1).
The characteristics of the main murmurs are discussed with the lesions which cause them. More than one murmur may be present – learn to isolate different murmurs and diagnose them separately. Make full use of other clues, for example the slow rising pulse of aortic stenosis (p. 297).

Blood pressure
The inflatable cuff of a sphygmomanometer is wrapped carefully round the upper arm with the bag over the brachial artery and is connected with a mercury or aneroid manometer. The stethoscope is placed over the brachial artery and the cuff is inflated to a level well above that which abolishes the Korotkov sounds. The pressure in the cuff is then allowed to fall slowly and the point of return of the sounds is taken as the systolic pressure. As the pressure falls further the sounds become louder and then usually quite suddenly they become muffled (phase 4) and later disappear (phase 5). Although, in the past, some authorities have used phase 4 it is now universal practice to use phase 5 to define diastolic pressure. In some people there is a large gap between phase 4 and phase 5 and occasionally the sounds do not disappear; in such case it is good practice

to record both phase 4 and phase 5 (e.g. 140/80–45).

When the blood pressure is to be recorded in the leg the patient lies prone, a special large cuff is applied to the thigh, and the stethoscope is placed over the popliteal fossa.

The *pulse pressure* is the difference between the systolic and diastolic pressures; it tends to be increased in the elderly who have rigid arteries and in patients with conditions that give rise to an increased stroke volume.

Unfortunately conventional sphygmomanometry can produce misleading or inaccurate results for reasons that may be related to the apparatus, the observer or the patient. If the inflatable bladder is too small it will not occlude the brachial artery efficiently and both systolic and diastolic pressure may be overestimated by as much as 20–30 mmHg. Blood pressure is a dynamic variable and will reflect the patient's physical and emotional state at the time it is measured. Allowances must be made for beat to beat variation due to arrhythmias such as atrial fibrillation or ectopic beats. Respiration and posture may also affect the blood pressure. In some patients the very act of measuring blood pressure can itself induce a rise in the blood pressure (in exceptional cases this may be as much as 70 mmHg). Repeated blood pressure measurements are valuable because this phenomenon tends to diminish as the patient's confidence grows (habituation). Home blood pressure and ambulatory pressure recordings may also help to overcome the problem of unrepresentative blood pressure recordings.

It would be helpful if normal blood pressure could be clearly defined but this is not feasible because, like body weight, blood pressure has a unimodal distribution throughout the population. Hence, there is no clearcut dividing line between 'normotensive' and 'hypertensive' subjects. Furthermore allowances must be made for the fact the blood pressure is constantly changing and tends to rise with increasing age.

INVESTIGATION

Electrocardiography (ECG)
This helps to elucidate cardiac arrhythmias and conduction deficits, and to diagnose and localise myocardial hypertrophy, ischaemia or infarction. It also gives information about electrolyte inbalance and the toxicity of certain drugs.

The basis for electrocardiography is that the electrical activation of a heart muscle cell causes a depolarisation of its membrane. The depolarisation is propagated along the length of a cell or fibre, and transmitted to adjoining cells. The result is a moving wavefront of

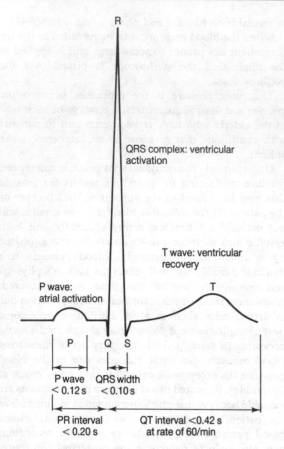

R

QRS complex: ventricular activation

T wave: ventricular recovery

P wave: atrial activation

T

P   Q   S

P wave   QRS width
<0.12 s   <0.10 s

PR interval
<0.20 s

QT interval <0.42 s
at rate of 60/min

Fig. 8.7   Diagram to show the components of a 'typical' ECG complex.

ELECTROCARDIOGRAPHIC CONVENTIONS

Depolarisation front moving towards electrode:	upward deflection
Depolarisation front moving away from:	downward deflection
Sensitivity:	10 mm = 1mV
Paper speed:	25 mm per second
Each large (5 mm) square =	0.2 second
Each small (1 mm) square =	0.04 second

muscle, and the next part of the ECG, the QRS complex, represents ventricular activation. In most leads this is dominated by the upright R wave from left ventricular activation. In lateral leads such as lead I and V6 the R wave is *preceded* by a small negative deflection (Q wave) caused by activation from left to right of the interventricular septum, and may be followed by a negative deflection (S wave) from right ventricular activation. In leads aVR and V1 the main direction of left ventricular activation is away from the electrode, giving dominant S wave. The *QRS axis* is the mean frontal plane vector of the QRS complex, and can be estimated roughly by seeing which limb lead has the biggest R wave (Fig. 8.10). Normally it lies between O° (largest R, smallest S in lead I) and 90° (largest R, smallest S in aVF).

There is a short period of inactivity of the QRS complex during which the whole of the ventricular mass is depolarised (the ST segment). Repolarisation then takes place, producing the T wave. Normally, repolarisation takes place in the *reverse direction* from depolarisation, so the T wave is normally in the same direction as the largest part of the QRS complex. Atrial depolarisation is usually hidden in the QRS complex. A normal ECG is shown in Fig. 8.11. Examples of abnormal, ECGs are given in the following pages. The information box below shows how rates can be worked out.

depolarisation which passes through the heart and sets up electrical currents which are detected by distant electrodes, amplified and displayed as the electrocardiograms. The ECG pattern recorded in a simple lead during one heart beat is called an ECG complex. Its components are explained in Fig. 8.7. Sets of electrodes are arranged as electrocardiographic *leads* and each of the twelve leads conventionally recorded 'looks at' the heart from a particular direction. Leads I, II, III aVR, aVL and aVF are called frontal plane or limb leads, (Fig. 8.8) and leads V1 to V6 chest leads (Fig. 8.9). These are shown in the information box (right, top).

Normally cardiac activation starts in the sino atrial (SA) node, but this cannot be detected on the ECG. The depolarisation then spreads through the atria, producing the P wave (normally upright in all leads except aVR). The only point at which the impulse can be transmitted to the ventricles is at the atrioventricular (AV) node, through which conduction is relatively slow (the PR interval). It then goes rapidly through the left and right branches of the bundle of His to ventricular

WORKING OUT THE RATE FROM THE ECG

Measure the distance between R waves in successive complexes:
Distance RR interval rate
1 large square 0.2 second 300/min
2 large squares 0.4 second 150/min
3 large squares 0.6 second 100/min
4 large squares 0.8 second 75/min
5 large squares 1 second 60/min
6 large squares 1.2 second 50/min

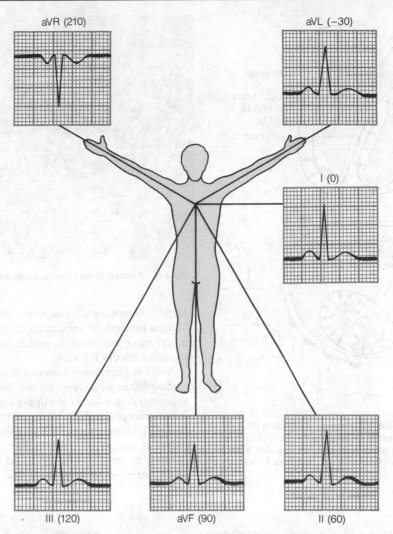

Fig. 8.8 Diagram to show the way in which the frontal plane or limb leads 'look at' the heart from different directions. Note that while the complexes in leads I,II,III, aVL and aVF look similar, the complex in lead aVR is almost a vertical 'mirror image' of lead II, because lead aVR 'looks at' depolarisation from the opposite direction.

Ambulatory ECG (Holter monitoring). Continuous recordings of one or two ECG leads may be obtained by attaching them to a small portable tape recorder. This technique is useful in detecting transient episodes of arrhythmia or ischaemia, which seldom occur at the time of routine 12-lead ECG recordings.

Radiological examination
This is important for determining the size and shape of the heart, and the state of the pulmonary blood vessels. Most information is given by a postero-anterior (PA) projection taken in full inspiration. Antero-posterior

(AP) projections are less useful because the heart outline is distorted owing to its distance from the film.

A rough estimate of overall heart size can be made by comparing the maximum width of the cardiac outline with the transverse diameter of the thoracic cavity at the same level. The cardiothoracic ratio so determined should be less than 0.5. Dilatation of individual cardiac chambers can be recognised by the characteristic alterations they cause to the cardiac silhouette (Figs. 8.12 and 8.13 and also the sections on valvular heart disease). A barium swallow to outline the oesophagus coupled with a lateral or oblique projection sometimes

A

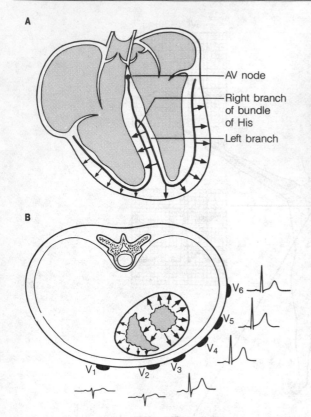

B

Fig. 8.9 **Activation of septum and ventricles. A.** Activation of the septum is from left to right by the left branch of the bundle of His and is followed by spread of the impulse throughout both ventricles. **B.** This also shows the placement of the chest leads and how each 'looks at' the heart.

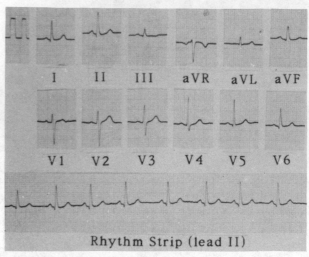

Rhythm Strip (lead II)

Fig. 8.11 **A normal 12-lead electrocardiogram.**

helps to determine the side of the left atrium. Lateral or oblique projections are also useful in detecting aortic or mitral valve calcification, which may be obscured by the spine on the PA view.

A rise in pulmonary venous pressure from left-sided cardiac failure first shows on the chest radiograph as an abnormal distension of the upper lobe pulmonary veins in the erect position. Subsequently, interstitial oedema causes thickened septa and dilated lymphatics which shows as horizontal lines in the costophrenic angles (Kerley 'B' lines). More advanced changes are a hazy opacification spreading from the hilar region, and

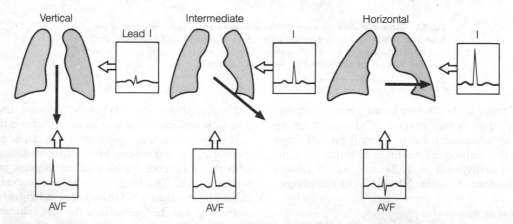

Fig. 8.10 **Diagram to show how alterations in the position of the cardiac axis can alter the relative size and shapes of the QRS complex in lead I and lead aVF.** The cardiac axis can simply reflect differences in cardiac position with different types of body habitus, as shown here, but it can also reflect differences in the relative size of left and right ventricles or in the pattern of intracardiac conduction.

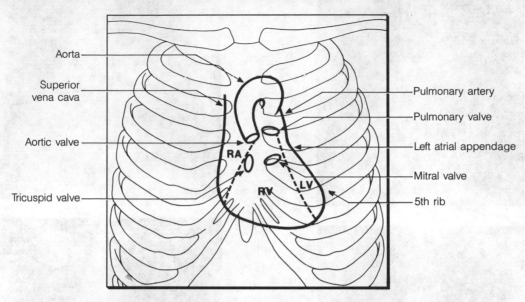

Fig. 8.12 The radiological outline of the heart and the surface projection of its valves.

pleural effusion. An increased pulmonary blood flow, as in congenital heart disease with a left-to-right shunt, causes enlargement of the pulmonary artery and a generalised increase in pulmonary vascular markings. Pulmonary arterial hypertension also causes an enlargement of the main pulmonary artery and of the proximal pulmonary arteries, but the peripheral lung vascular markings tend to be diminished.

Radioscopy

Screening of the heart, using an image intensifier, may help in the detection of abnormal cardiac pulsations and of valvular calcification. Its main use, however, is during cardiac catheterisation and pacemaker implantation.

Echocardiography

This uses ultrasound to study the disposition and movement of valves and other structures within the heart. It depends on the reflection of ultrasound waves at interfaces between blood and more solid tissues.

M-mode echocardiography. The ultrasound is focused into a narrow beam, and the output is a graph against time of the movement relative to the chest wall of those structures through which the beam passes (Fig. 8.14). Characteristic patterns of movement are produced in, for example, mitral stenosis, and pericardial effusions are easily recognised. Accurate measurements can be made of cardiac dimensions.

Two-dimensional (or cross-sectional) real-time echocardiography. The ultrasound beam is swung rapidly back and forth over an arc or sector and the resulting information synthesised into a two-dimensional map or picture of the position of the reflecting structures on a television screen (Fig. 8.15). The picture is the equivalent of a 'slice' through the heart, and the structures shown will depend on the position and orientation of the ultrasound crystal. Because the beam oscillates very rapidly, the ultrasound image accurately reproduces the movement of structures in the living heart (hence 'real time'). This type of echocardiography is particularly good at detecting intracardiac masses, such as thrombi or tumours, or endocarditic vegetations. It is also very useful in sorting out complex structural abnormalities in congenital heart disease.

Doppler cardiography. This depends on the fact that sound waves reflected from moving objects, such as intracardiac red blood cells, undergo a frequency shift. This can be used to detect the speed and direction of movement of the red cells, and thus of blood, in the heart chambers and great vessels. The greater the frequency shift, the faster the blood is moving. The information can be presented either as a plot of blood velocity against time for a particular point in the heart (Fig. 8.16) or as a colour overlay on a two-dimensional real-time echo picture (colour flow doppler). Doppler cardiography can be used to detect abnormal directions

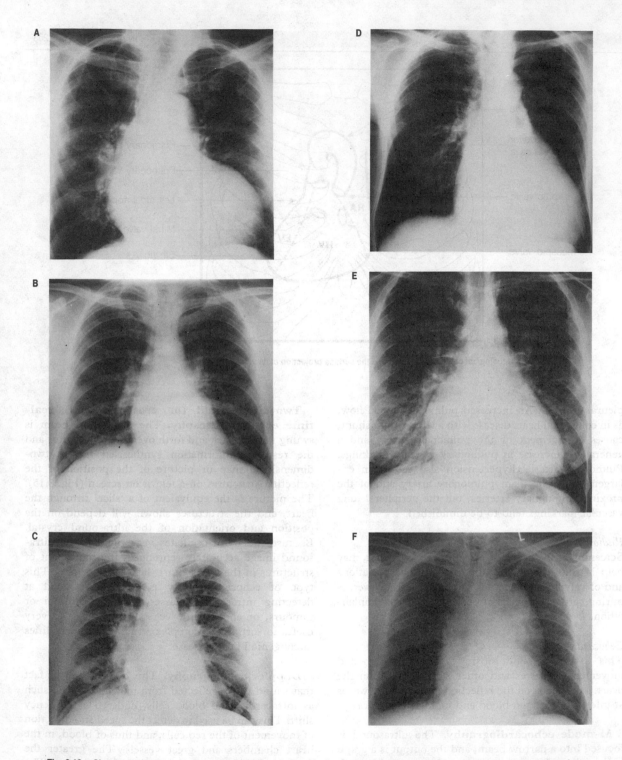

Fig. 8.13   Chest radiographs in cardiovascular disease. A. Chest radiograph from a patient with long-standing aortic stenosis and regurgitation. The heart shadow is enlarged, with a 'roman nose' contour to the left ventricle and dilatation of the ascending aorta. **B.** Mitral stenosis – there is enlargement of the left atrial appendage. **C.** The same patient as (**B**), but with the addition of pulmonary oedema. **D.** Chest radiograph from a patient with chronic mitral regurgitation. In addition to left atrial enlargement there is also left ventricular dilatation. **E.** Chest radiograph from a 40-year-old woman with a congenital ventricular septal defect (pulmonary to systemic flow ratio 2.5:1). There is cardiac enlargement and an increase in the pulmonary vascular markings. **F.** Chest radiograph from a patient with dissecting aneurysm of the aorta showing widening of the upper mediastinum.

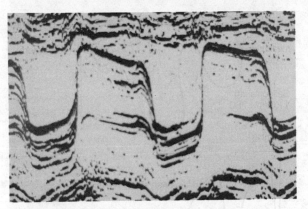

Fig. 8.14 M-mode echocardiogram of young patient with severe mitral stenosis. The movement of the fused mitral valve cusps is characteristic of this condition.

of blood flow, e.g. aortic or mitral reflux and in estimating pressure gradients, for example, the gradient across a stenosed aortic valve.

Phonocardiography
This records heart sounds and murmurs and may help to elucidate difficult problems of auscultation.

Cardiac catheterisation and angiocardiography
In contrast to the preceding investigations, these are invasive techniques. A catheter inserted into a vein can be advanced into the right atrium, and then manipulated into the right ventricle and pulmonary artery. In the presence of an artrial septal defect or patent foramen ovale, venous catheters can also enter the left atrium and left ventricle. If the atrial septum is intact, access to the left ventricle is usually by retrograde passage of a catheter across the aortic valve. Left atrial pressure can be measured directly by puncturing the interatrial septum with a special long, curved needle via a catheter passed up the femoral vein to the right atrium. For many purposes, however, a satisfactory approximation to left atrial pressure can be recorded by 'wedging' an end-hole venous catheter in a branch of the pulmonary artery.

Cardiac catheters are usually manipulated under radiographic control using an image-intensifier, but if a venous catheter is provided at its distal end with a small balloon which can be inflated when the catheter is in the right atrium then the blood stream itself will guide the catheter through the right ventricle and into the pulmonary artery. The balloon also makes it easy to 'wedge' the catheters so as to estimate left atrial pressure. These Swan-Ganz catheters (Fig. 8.17) are used in intensive and coronary care units, where they can be inserted without the need to transfer the patient to a radiology department.

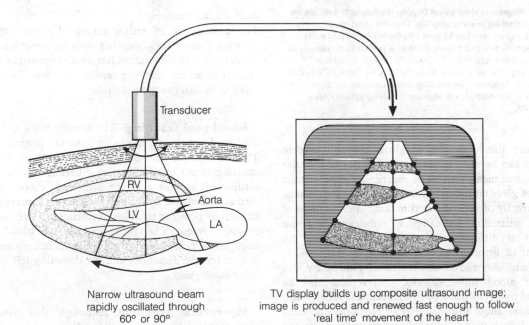

Fig. 8.15 Principles of two-dimensional (2D) real time echocardiography. A moving, two-dimensional image of the echoes detected from a 'slice' of heart can be built up by swinging the ultrasound beam rapidly back and forth.

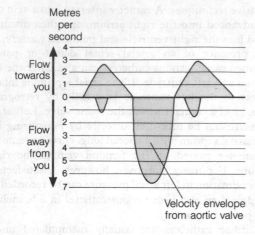

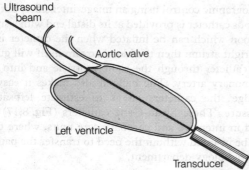

Fig. 8.16 Diagram to show use of Doppler ultrasound to estimate the aortic valve gradient in aortic stenosis. The ultrasound transducer is applied to the chest wall and aligned with the left ventricular outflow tract. The spectrum of blood flow velocities is presented graphically so that it is possible to determine the maximum systolic blood-flow velocity through the aortic valve. By simplifying the Bernouilli equation for the relation between pressure drop and velocity, an equation can be derived which will estimate the peak aortic valve gradient: Peak gradient $= 4V_{max^2}$.

Pressure measurements obtained through cardiac catheters can be used to assess the severity of valvular stenoses, and measurement of ventricular end-diastolic pressures gives an indication of ventricular compliance and indirectly of ventricular function. Measurement of oxygen saturation in samples withdrawn via the catheters at different sites in the heart allows the detection of intracardiac left-to-right or right-to-left shunts, and also allows calculation of pulmonary and systemic blood flow. Cardiac output can also be measured by dyedilution or thermodilution techniques.

Catheters allow the injection of radio-opaque contrast medium into individual chambers of the heart, the aorta or pulmonary artery, or, using specially shaped catheters, into either coronary artery (Fig. 8.18).

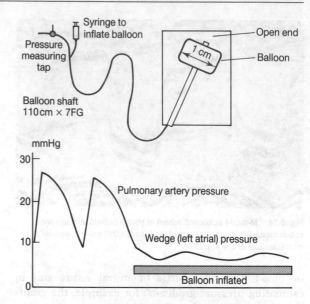

Fig. 8.17 Diagram to show principal of the Swan-Ganz catheter. The small balloon at the end of the catheter can be inflated to allow bood flow to pull the catheter into the pulmonary artery. If the balloon is then deflated pulmonary artery pressure will be recorded. By advancing the catheter and reinflating the balloon it is possible to record a 'wedged' pulmonary artery pressure, which is usually a good estimate of left atrial pressure.

Radionuclide scanning

The availability of radionuclides of short half life emitting gamma rays, together with the gamma camera for detecting this radiation has made it possible to use radionuclides for studying cardiac function. Two basic types of technique are available:

Blood pool scanning. The isotope is injected into the blood stream and mixes with the circulating blood. The gamma camera detects the amount of isotope-emitting blood in the heart at different phases of the cardiac cycle, and also the size and 'shape' of the cardiac chambers. By linking the gamma camera to the ECG it is possible to collect information over several cardiac cycles. The principal use of blood pool scanning is as an accurate and repoducible measure of left ventricular function, and for detecting left ventricular aneurysms.

Myocardial scanning. Although this uses the same gamma camera, both the radionuclides used and the concepts involved differ from blood pool scanning. The object is usually to distinguish between ischaemic

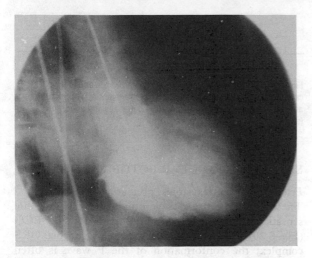

Fig. 8.18 Angiocardiography. A frame from a cineradiograph taken while radio-opaque contrast is being injected into the left ventricle though a catheter introduced via a femoral artery and passed retrogradely through the aortic valve. This technique allows measurements to be made of left ventricular size in systole and diastole, abnormal movements of the left ventricular wall to be seen, and leakage through the mitral valve to be assessed.

and non-ischaemic myocardium (using radioactive thallium) or between normal and damaged myocardium (using radioactive pyrophosphate).

Radionuclide scanning is also of great value in detecting pulmonary embolism, particularly if the injection of an isotope into the blood stream is combined with a study of the distribution of an inhaled radioactive gas (ventilation-perfusion scanning).

DISORDERS OF RATE AND RHYTHM

Ectopic rhythms
Supraventricular
  Ectopic beats
  Supraventricular tachycardia
  Atrial flutter
  Atrial fibrillation
Ventricular
  Ectopic beats
  Ventricular tachycardia
  Ventricular fibrillation

Heart Block
Sinoatrial block
Atrioventricular block
  First degree heart block
  Second degree heart block (Mobitz type I and II)
  Third degree (complete) heart block

DISORDERS OF CARDIAC RATE, RHYTHM AND CONDUCTION

These are listed in the information box (left).

The control of cardiac rate
Some cardiac cells have the faculty of self excitation. The pacemaking of the heart is due to this activity, and is normally controlled by the sinoatrial node. The SA node has its own intrinsic rate but is also under nervous control; vagal activity slows it and sympathetic activity accelerates it. If the sinus rate becomes unduly slow, lower centres may take over, e.g. either the AV node (junctional rhythm), or an ectopic ventricular focus. At other times the natural rate of lower centres may be increased as a result of disturbances of cellular metabolism due to electrolyte disorders, drug toxicity or cellular damage from myocardial disease.

Sometimes, as a consequence of congenital abnormality or acquired disease, there are alternative pathways for the conduction of the impulse. As shown in Fig. 8.19, this can lead to an abnormal re-entry movement of electrical activity and is the most common cause of paroxysmal tachycardia.

SINUS RHYTHMS

Sinus arrhythmia. This is a phasic alteration in heart rate in time with breathing; the rate increases in inspiration. It is a manifestation of normal autonomic nervous activity, and is often particularly pronounced in children. A complete absence of variation in heart

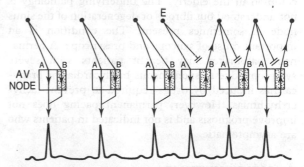

Fig. 8.19 Mechanism of re-entry tachycardia. In this example there are two alternative pathways, A and B, through the AV node. B has a longer refractory period than A. The atrial ectopic beat E finds pathway B refractory, but travels through A. On reaching the end of A, the impulse finds that B has now completed its refractory period, so the impulse can now travel retrogradely to give a further premature atrial beat, which repeats the process. The result is a re-entry or reciprocating tachycardia.

rate with breathing or with changes in posture may be a feature of autonomic neuropathy.

Sinus bradycardia. This is arbitrarily defined as a sinus rate of less than 60 per minute. This may occur in normal people during sleep, and is a common finding in athletes. It can be caused by several drugs, e.g. beta-adrenoceptor antagonists. It may also be a feature of myxoedema, jaundice or raised intracranial pressure, and occurs in some patients after myocardial infarction.

Sinus tachycardia. This is defined as a resting sinus rate of more than 100 per minute. It is a feature of anxiety, fever, hyperthyroidism and acute circulatory or cardiac failure. Except in infants, the rate seldom exceeds 160 per minute.

SINOATRIAL DISEASE (THE SICK SINUS SYNDROME)

The features are listed in the information box below.

COMMON FEATURES OF SINOATRIAL DISEASE

- Sinus bradycardia
- Sinoatrial block (sinus arrest) with pauses or escape rhythms
- Paroxysmal supraventricular tachycardia
- Paroxysmal atrial fibrillation
- Atrioventricular block

Sinoatrial disease may occur at any age, but is most common in the elderly. The underlying pathology is not understood but fibrosis or degeneration of the sinus node is sometimes present. The condition is an important cause of syncope and presyncope. A permanent pacemaker may benefit patients with severe symptoms due to spontaneous bradycardias or bradycardias induced by drugs required to prevent tachyarrhythmias. However, permanent pacing does not improve prognosis and is not indicated in patients who are asymptomatic.

ECTOPIC RHYTHMS

When impulses arise somewhere other than the SA node the rhythm is called ectopic; such rhythms may be due to increased automaticity or a re-entry circuit (Fig. 8.19). They can broadly be classified into supraventricular (arising in the atria, AV node or other AV junctional tissue) and ventricular.

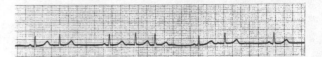

Fig. 8.20 Atrial ectopic beats. The first, third, sixth and eighth QRS complexes are normal sinus beats. They are followed by premature atrial ectopic beats with identical QRS complexes and abnormal (sometimes barely visible) p waves.

SUPRAVENTRICULAR ECTOPIC RHYTHMS

Ectopic beats (extrasystoles, premature beats)
These usually cause no symptoms but can give the sensation of an extra or thumping beat. The ECG (Fig. 8.20) shows a premature beat with a normal QRS complex; the conformation of the P wave is often different because the impulse starts at an abnormal site.

Supraventricular tachycardia (Fig. 8.21)
Paroxysmal tachycardia may occur with a rate of between 140 and 220 as a result of re-entry or a rapidly firing ectopic focus in the atria or AV node. This usually occurs in hearts which are otherwise normal and may last from a few seconds to many hours if left untreated. The patient is usually aware that the heart has suddenly started to beat fast, and may feel faint or breathless. Polyuria is sometimes a feature; cardiac pain and left ventricular failure may occur if there is co-existing structural heart disease. Coffee, alcohol, tobacco, anxiety or hyperthyroidism may be precipitating factors.

The ECG usually shows a tachycardia with normal QRS complexes but occasinally there may be rate-dependent bundle branch block.

Management

Treatment is not always necessary. However, if an attack is causing troublesome symptoms it may be terminated by carotid sinus massage or other measures that increase vagal tone (e.g. self-induced vomiting). Intravenous verapamil, beta-blockers or disopyramide

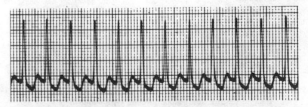

Fig. 8.21 Supraventricular tachycardia. The rate is 190 per minute. The QRS complexes are normal.

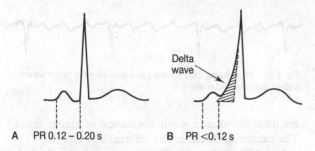

A PR 0.12 – 0.20 s   **B** PR <0.12 s

Delta wave

Fig. 8.22 Wolff-Parkinson-White syndrome. A. A normal ECG complex compared with one from a patient **B** with the Wolff-Parkinson-White syndrome. In this syndrome, premature excitation of part of the ventricles through an accessary atrioventricular conduction pathway produces the delta wave, which gives the appearance of a short PR interval and a broad QRS complex. These patients are prone to re-entry tachycardias.

may restore sinus rhythm but should not be given together (see p. 274 for dosages). Digoxin (see p. 276) is also effective but takes longer to act and can accelerate the tachycardia in patients with accessory conducting tissue (see below). In an emergency the tachycardia should be terminated by DC cardioversion (p. 279). If attacks are frequent or otherwise disabling, prophylactic oral therapy with any of the above drugs may be indicated. Further information on anti-arrhythmic drugs is given on pages 273–276. In resistant cases amiodarone (p. 275), surgery or an anti-tachycardia pacemaker may be helpful. Anti-tachycardia pacemakers are able to detect the onset of an abnormal rhythm and respond by emitting appropriately timed impulses which block the re-entry circuit (Fig. 8.19).

The Wolff-Parkinson-White (WPW) syndrome

This results from the presence of an abnormal band of atrial tissue which connects the atria and ventricles and can bypass the AV node. In normal sinus rhythm conduction takes place partly through the AV node and partly through the more rapidly conducting bypass tract. The ECG shows shortening of the PR interval and a slurring of the QRS complex called a delta wave (Fig. 8.22). Because the AV node and the bypass pathway have different conduction speeds and refractory periods, a re-entry circuit can develop causing paroxysms of tachycardia (Fig. 8.23). Because the bypass pathway lacks the rate-limiting properties of the normal AV node, patients are at risk from very rapid ventricular rates, and sometimes ventricular fibrillation and death. Atrial fibrillation is a particularly dangerous event.

Treatment is aimed at reducing conduction rate and increasing the refractory period of the bypass tract, using disopyramide, quinidine or amiodarone (pp. 273–276).

Atrial tachycardia with atrioventricular block

In this condition there is an atrial tachycardia of 140–220 per minute accompanied by atrioventricular block, usually either 2:1 or variable (p. 277). Carotid sinus massage may slow the pulse by increasing the degree of block (Fig. 8.24), but seldom terminates the attack. Atrial tachycardia with block seldom occurs in otherwise normal hearts, and is sometimes a manifestation of digitalis toxicity. If this arrhythmia develops in a patient not already taking a digitalis preparation, then digoxin is, paradoxically, the drug of choice for

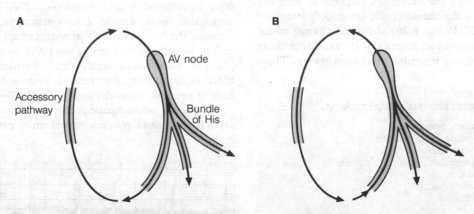

A   **B**

AV node

Accessory pathway   Bundle of His

Fig. 8.23 Wolff-Parkinson-White syndrome – re-entry tachycardias. A. Usually ventricular activation takes place through the AV node with retrograde conduction to the atria through the accessory pathway. This is known as an *orthodromic* tachycardia and produces an ECG with normal QRS complexes. **B.** More rarely ventricular activation takes place through the accessory pathway with retrograde conduction through the AV node. This is known as an *antidromic* tachycardia and produces an ECG with broad complex QRS complexes, depending on the exact site of the accessory pathway.

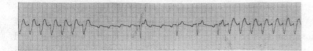

CSP ──────────►

Fig. 8.24   Atrial tachycardia with atrioventricular block induced by carotid sinus pressure (CSP).

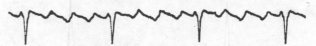

Fig. 8.25   Atrial flutter. ECG showing saw-toothed atrial flutter waves and 4:1 atrioventricular block.

controlling the ventricular rate. (See p. 274 for dosage schedule.)

Atrial flutter
This is a condition in which a rapid atrial rate of around 300/min is associated with 2:1, 3:1, or 4:1 atrioventricular block. The ECG shows characteristic saw-toothed flutter waves (Fig. 8.25). With a regular 2:1 AV block it may be difficult to distinguish atrial flutter from supraventricular or even sinus tachycardia, but carotid sinus pressure may help by temporarily increasing the degree of block.

Management
Digoxin, beta-blockers or verapamil can be used to control the ventricular rate (for details see p. 274). However, in many cases it may be preferable to try and restore sinus rhythm by means of atrial overdrive pacing, DC cardioversion or drug therapy. Amiodarone, disopyramide, flecainide or quinidine may be effective and can also be used to prevent recurrent episodes of atrial flutter (see pp. 273–276).

Atrial fibrillation
In this arrhythmia the atria beat rapidly, chaotically and ineffectively; the ventricles respond at irregular intervals giving the characteristic 'irregularly irregular' pulse. The ECG (Fig. 8.26) shows no change in the QRS complexes and an absence of P waves; sometimes the baseline shows irregular fibrillation waves. These

are most obvious in atrial fibrillation of recent onset. The causes are listed in the information box (left).

Atrial fibrillation may be asymptomatic, particularly in the elderly. Patients with paroxysmal atrial fibrillation are usually more aware of the arrhythmia than those in whom it is established. Atrial fibrillation frequently precipitates or aggravates cardiac failure in those with an abnormal heart, particularly those with mitral stenosis or poor left ventricular function.

Ineffective atrial contraction coupled with left atrial dilatation predisposes to stasis, thrombosis, and a risk of systemic thromboembolism. The risk is greatest when atrial fibrillation coexists with mitral valve disease, in patients with paroxysmal atrial fibrillation, and in the weeks immediately following the onset of fibrillation; however there is some risk of systemic embolism in all patients with atrial fibrillation.

Management
Digoxin (p. 276) is used to reduce the ventricular rate by increasing the degree of AV block, and this alone may result in a striking improvement particularly in patients with mitral stenosis. In atrial fibrillation due to thyrotoxicosis, beta-blockade (p. 275) may be better than digoxin. When atrial fibrillation persists after correction of the underlying cause sinus rhythm can often be restored by cardioversion (p. 279). In chronic rheumatic heart disease cardioversion is pointless, because the arrhythmia is almost certain to return unless the valve lesions can be improved by surgery. In patients with paroxysmal atrial fibrillation beta-blockers, quinidine, disopyramide or amiodarone may help to preserve sinus rhythm (see pp. 273–276).

Long-term anticoagulant therapy with warfarin reduces the risk of systemic embolism in patients with

---

COMMON CAUSES OF ATRIAL FIBRILLATION

- Coronary artery disease
  (especially acute myocardial infarction)
- Valvular heart disease
  (especially rheumatic mitral valve disease)
- Hypertension
- Thyrotoxicosis
- Sino-atrial disease
- Alcohol
- Cardiomyopathy
- Congenital heart disease
- Pulmonary embolism
- Pericardial disease

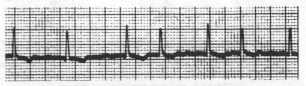

Fig. 8.26   Atrial fibrillation. The ventricular complexes are irregular, there are no P waves and irregular oscillations (f waves) disturb the baseline.

mitral valve disease, and is probably also indicated in patients with paroxysmal atrial fibrillation and to cover elective cardioversion. The potential benefits have to be weighed against the risks of anticoagulant therapy in each case. Although patients with lone atrial fibrillation or sinoatrial disease have an increased risk of stroke, there is no evidence that this is reduced by anticoagulation.

In exceptional cases refractory supraventricular or junctional tachyarrhythmias may be abolished by implanting an anti-tachycardia pacemaker or by deliberately inducing complete heart block. The latter can be achieved by surgery or by delivering a high energy shock to the bundle of His through a transvenous catheter; a permanent pacemaker must be implanted at the same time.

VENTRICULAR ECTOPIC RHYTHMS

Ectopic beats

The symptoms and signs are the same as those of atrial ectopic beats, from which they can be distinguished by the abnormally widened QRS complex on the ECG (Fig. 8.27). They are fairly frequent in normal people, and their prevalence increases with age. They are sometimes precipitated by excessive tea, coffee or alcohol consumption. Ectopic beats in patients with otherwise normal hearts are often more prominent at rest, and tend to disappear with exercise.

Ventricular ectopic beats are sometimes a manifestation of underlying heart disease, particularly disease of ventricular muscle which enhances ventricular excitability and increases the scope for ventricular re-entry circuits. Examples include acute myocardial infarction and myocarditis. Under these conditions an unusually premature ectopic beat falling on the T wave of a normal beat ('R on T') may initiate ventricular tachycardia or ventricular fibrillation.

Frequent ventricular ectopic beats, often against a background of bradycardia, are a feature of digitalis intoxication, and here too they may be a herald of more serious arrhythmias. Hypokalaemia may cause ventricular ectopic beats on its own, and will potentiate other

causes. Ventricular ectopic beats are sometimes a feature of mitral valve prolapse, and occasionally they occur as 'escape beats' in the presence of an underlying bradycardia.

Management

Treatment should be directed at the underlying causes. The use of lignocaine to suppress ventricular ectopic beats after myocardial infarction does not appear to improve survival. If frequent ectopic beats are causing annoyance in an otherwise healthy patient, betablockers, disopyramide or mexiletine may help to suppress them (pp. 273–276).

Ventricular tachycardia (Fig. 8.28)

This is a grave arrhythmia because it is nearly always associated with serious heart disease, because the ventricular rate may be very rapid, and because it may degenerate into ventricular fibrillation. Patients sometimes complain of palpitation, but more often the symptoms are those of a low cardiac output – dizziness and dyspnoea, or even loss of consciousness. The ventricular rate is usually between 140 and 220 per minute, and carotid sinus pressure is ineffective. The ECG shows broad, abnormal QRS complexes and may be difficult to distinguish from supraventricular tachycardia with bundle branch block. Extreme left axis deviation, very broad QRS complexes (>140 msec) or evidence of dissociated atrial activity favour a diagnosis of ventricular tachycardia. An intracardiac or oesophageal ECG may also help to establish the diagnosis. When there is doubt, it is safer to treat for ventricular tachycardia.

The commonest cause of ventricular tachycardia is acute myocardial infarction. It may also be due to myocarditis, cardiomyopathy, or chronic ischaemic heart disease, especially when the last is associated with a ventricular aneurysm. In a few individuals a predisposition to ventricular arrhythmia is associated with abnormal prolongation of the QT interval of the ECG, a trait which is sometimes hereditary and may also be

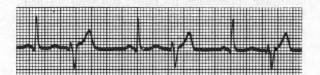

Fig. 8.27 Ventricular ectopic beats. Alternate beats have an abnormally wide QRS complex with no preceding P waves, i.e. coupling of the pulse results.

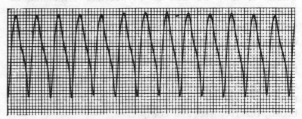

Fig. 8.28 Ventricular tachycardia. The rate is 220 per minute. The complexes are broad and abnormal.

due to hypokalaemia, hypomagnesaemia, and drugs such as quinidine or amiodarone.

Patients recovering from myocardial infarction sometimes have periods of idioventricular rhythm ('slow' ventricular tachycardia) at a rate only slightly above the preceding sinus rate. These episodes are usually self limiting, asymptomatic, and do not require treatment. Most other instances of ventricular tachycardia, if they last for more than a few beats, will require treatment, often as an emergency.

Management

Prompt action to restore sinus rhythm is required and in most cases should be followed by prophylactic therapy. Cardioversion is often the initial treatment of choice but if this is not available or the arrhythmia is well tolerated intravenous lignocaine may be given as a bolus (1.5 mg per kg) followed by an infusion of 4 mg per minute reducing to 2 mg per minute over a period of 2–4 hours. The dose may need to be reduced in the elderly, the frail and those with liver disease. Lignocaine toxicity causes confusion, paraesthesiae and twitching; if these are observed the dose should be reduced. Mexilitine, flecainide, disopyramide and amiodarone are suitable alternatives (see pp. 273–276). Hypokalaemia, hypomagnesaemia and acidosis must be corrected. Cardioversion should be avoided if digitalis toxicity is likely; if it is considered necessary in these circumstances the first attempts should be made at low energy settings.

Urgent treatment of ventricular tachycardia should be followed by oral prophylaxis with mexilitine, disopyramide, flecainide or amiodarone (pp. 273–276).

CARDIAC ARREST

Cardiac arrest is the sudden and complete loss of cardiac function. It may be due to ventricular fibrillation, asystole, or electromechanical dissociation.

Ventricular fibrillation. This is the commonest cause and the most easily treatable cause of sudden death. It may be due to myocardial ischaemia or inappropriate electrical stimulation such as electrocution. The presence of structural heart disease, electrolyte disturbance such as hypokalaemia, or inappropriate medication may increase susceptibility to ventricular fibrillation. The arrhythmia produces rapid ineffective unco-ordinated movement of the ventricles, which therefore produce no pulse. The ECG (Fig. 8.29) has broad, bizarre, irregular complexes.

Within seconds of the onset of ventricular fibrillation the patient loses consciousness. Respiration ceases and

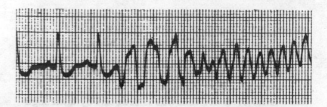

Fig. 8.29 Ventricular fibrillation. The change from sinus rhythm to ventricular fibrillation occurs when a ventricular ectopic beat falls on the T of the previous complex.

death is virtually inevitable unless treatment is started promptly. If a defibrillator is available the immediate application of a direct current shock may restore sinus rhythm within seconds. Under other circumstances the circulation must be maintained by the resuscitation procedures described below.

Ventricular asystole. This occurs when there is no electrical activity of the ventricles. It may be due to a localised failure of impulse conducting tissue with delay in the emergence of a ventricular escape rhythm, or massive ventricular damage complicating myocardial infarction. With the former, cardiac massage or a blow to the chest will often restore cardiac activity, although an artificial pacemaker may be needed to prevent recurrent attacks. When asystole occurs as a consequence of massive myocardial damage, it is nearly always resistant to treatment.

Electromechanical dissociation. This occurs when there is no effective cardiac output despite the presence of normal or near normal electrical activity. This may complicate cardiac rupture or massive pulmonary embolism and is seldom amenable to treatment.

The management of cardiac arrest

Cardiopulmonary resuscitation
Prompt treatment is essential because irreversible brain damage will occur unless some circulation of oxygenated blood can be achieved within two or three minutes. First, confirm the diagnosis (unconscious, death-like appearance, no pulse) and send for help. Next, deliver a sharp blow to the centre of the chest. If the heart does not start immediately, as indicated by the return of the carotid or femoral pulse, start basic life-support (Fig. 8.30). The patient should be placed on his back, on the floor or on some other firm surface, and his legs should be elevated. Mouth to mouth, mouth to nose, or mouth to airway ventilation should be used until a facemask and bag become available.

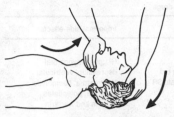

A   Airway
Clear the airway of vomitus
or debris, extend the neck and raise the chin

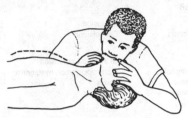

B   Breathing
1. Direct mouth-to-mouth breathing

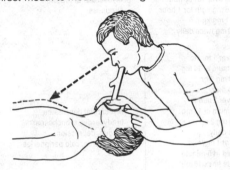

2. Indirect mouth-to-mouth breathing

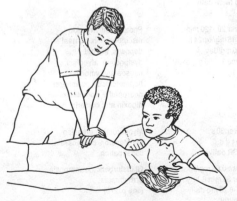

C   Circulation
Cardiac massage (see text)

Fig. 8.30   Emergency resuscitation. The ABC of basic life support.
A. Airway. Clear the airway of vomitus or debris, extend the neck and
raise the chin. **B.** Breathing. 1. Direct mouth-to-mouth breathing. 2.
Indirect mouth-to-mouth breathing. **C.** Circulation. Cardiac massage.

Cardiac massage should be given by placing both hands on the lower sternum (Fig. 8.30) and applying short sharp, forceful compressions at a rate of 60 to 100 per minute (practice with a dummy or manikin is very helpful).

Obtain an ECG as soon as possible (many defibrillators have a facility for reading the ECG through the paddles). When there is ventricular fibrillation give a 200 joule shock as soon as possible. If in doubt defibrillate. If this fails give a further 200 joule shock and if necessary repeat the shock using 360 joules.

If ventricular fibrillation remains, defibrillation should be repeated after giving 1 mg (10 ml of 1 in 10 000) adrenaline intravenously (using a central or large vein) and then after giving lignocaine 100 mg intravenously.

If the diagnosis is asystole give intravenous atropine (0.6–1.2 mg) and if this fails intravenous adrenaline (1 mg) and consider temporary pacing (see p. 279).

Resuscitation is most likely to succeed when cardiac arrest is due to ventricular fibrillation particularly if this occurs as a result of an accident or an otherwise uncomplicated myocardial infarct.

ANTIARRHYTHMIC DRUGS

Some of the drugs used to treat individual arrhythmias have already been mentioned. These agents may be classified according to their mode of action or their main site of action. These classifications are listed in the information boxes below and page 275. The main uses, dosages and side-effects of the most widely used drugs are summarised in Table 8.2.

Class 1 drugs
These act principally by suppressing excitability and slowing conduction in atrial or ventricular muscle.

Quinidine. This is excreted in the urine and accumulates in renal failure. Gastrointestinal side-effects (abdominal discomfort, nausea, and diarrhoea) are common; more serious side-effects include myocar-

> **CLASSIFICATION OF ANTIARRHYTHMIC DRUGS ACCORDING TO THEIR MAIN SITE OF ACTION**
>
> - AV node
>   (beta-blockers, verapamil, digoxin)
> - Ventricles
>   (lignocaine, mexilitine)
> - Atria, ventricles and accessory conducting tissue
>   (quinidine, disopyramide, flecainide, amiodarone)

Table 8.2 The main uses, dosages and side-effects of the most widely used arrhythmic drugs

Drug	Main uses		Dose (adult)	Important side-effects
Class I				
Quinidine	Prevention of VE's and AF	oral	test dose, 250 mg maintenance, 500 mg b.d. as Quinidine bisulphate SR	GI upset, myocardial depression, ventricular tachycardia, haemolytic anaemia, potentiates digoxin and warfarin
Disopyramide	Prevention and treatment of all tachyarrhythmias	i.v.	2 mg/kg slowly at <30 mg/min then 0.4 mg/kg/h (max 800 mg/d)	Myocardial depression Hypotension Dry mouth Urinary retention
		oral	100–150 mg q.d.s. or 250–375 mg b.d. SR	
Lignocaine	Treatment and short-term prevention of VT and VF	i.v.	bolus 1.5 mg/kg 4 mg/min for 2–4 hours then 2 mg/min	Confusion Convulsions
Mexilitine	Prevention and treatment of ventricular tachyarrhythmias	i.v.	*loading dose* 100–250 mg at 25 mg/min then 250 mg in 1 hour then 250 mg in 2 hours *maintenance therapy* 0.5 mg/min	GI irritation, confusion dizziness, tremor, nystagmus ataxia
		oral	250 mg 8-hourly	
Flecainide	Prevention and treatment of all tachyarrhythmias	i.v.	2 mg/kg over 10–30 min then 1.5 mg/kg/h for 1 hour then 0.1 mg/kg/h	Myocardial depression Dizziness
		oral	50–100 mg twice daily	
Class II				
Propranolol		i.v.	1 mg over 1 min to a maximum of 10 mg	
		oral	10–160 mg 3 or 4 times daily	
Metoprolol	Treatment and prevention of SVT and AF prevention of VEs and exercise induced VT	i.v.	5 mg over 2 min to a maximum of 15 mg	Myocardial depression, bradycardia, bronchospasm, fatigue, depression, nightmares, cold peripheries
		oral	50–100 mg 2 or 3 times daily	
Atenolol		i.v.	2.5 mg at 1 mg/min repeated at 5-minute intervals (max 10 mg)	
		oral	50–100 mg daily	
Sotalol		i.v.	10–20 mg slowly	
		oral	40–160 mg twice daily	
Class III				
Amiodarone	Serious atrial and ventricular tachyarrhythmias, particularly in the WPW syndrome	i.v.	5 mg/kg over 20–120 min then up to 15 mg/kg/24 h	Photosensitivity, skin discolouration, corneal deposits, thyroid dysfunction, alveolitis, nausea and vomiting, hepatotoxicity, peripheral neuropathy, potentiates digoxin and warfarin
		oral	initially 600 mg/day maintenance 1–200 mg daily	
Class IV				
Verapamil	Treatment of SVT control of AF	i.v.	5–10 mg over 30 s	Myocardial depression hypotension, bradycardia, constipation
		oral	40–120 mg t.d.s. or 240 mg SR daily	
Digoxin	Treatment and prevention of SVT control of AF		*loading dose 0.02 mg/kg*	GI disturbance, xanthopsia arrhythmias (see p. 276)
		i.v.	0.5 mg over 30 min 6-hrly then 0.125–0.25 mg daily	
		oral	0.5 mg 6-hourly then 0.125–0.25 mg daily	

SVT Supraventricular tachycardia
AF Atrial fibrillation
VE Ventricular ectopic
VT Ventricular tachycardia
VF Ventricular fibrillation
SR Sustained release formulation

CLASSIFICATION OF ANTI-ARRHYTHMIC DRUGS ACCORDING TO THEIR EFFECT ON THE INTRACELLULAR ACTION POTENTIAL (after Singh and Vaughan-Williams)

Class I – inhibit fast sodium current
- Also prolong action potential
  Quinidine, disopyramide
- Also shorten action potential
  Lignocaine, mexilitine
- No effect on action potential, slow conduction in
  His-purkinje tissue
  Flecainide

Class II – beta-blockers
Propranolol, metoprolol, atenolol, sotalol

Class III – prolong action potential
Amiodarone, sotalol

Class IV – inhibit slow calcium channel
Verapamil

dial depression, ventricular tachycardia (often heralded by prolongation of the QT interval) and idiosyncratic autoimmune thrombocytopenia or haemolytic anaemia. Quinidine potentiates digoxin, by increasing plasma digoxin concentrations, and is subject to many other important drug interactions. In view of these problems it is usually used as a second or third line agent.

Disopyramide. This has weak atropine-like effects and may cause urinary retention or precipitate glaucoma. It has a depressant effect on ventricular function and should be avoided in cardiac failure. The drug is cleared through the kidneys and liver. If it is used in patients with atrial flutter and AV block, there is a risk of a paradoxical increase in heart rate as the atria slow and 2:1 block changes to 1:1 conduction; this can be prevented by pretreatment with digoxin.

Lignocaine. This has to be given parenterally, and has a very short plasma half-life, so plasma concentration will depend on the rate of infusion. It is mainly used for the urgent treatment or prophylaxis of ventricular tachycardia or fibrillation.

Mexilitine. This can be given intravenously or orally and is used for the treatment or prophylaxis of ventricular arrhythmias. Side-effects include nausea, vomiting, confusion, dizziness, tremor, nystagmus and ataxia. Metabolism is mainly hepatic and the drug may accumulate in liver disease.

Flecainide. This can be given intravenously or orally for the treatment or prophylaxis of supraventri-

cular or ventricular arrhythmias. Unfortunately it is a potent myocardial depressant and cannot, therefore, be used safely in patients with poor left ventricular function. Like all anti-arrhythmic drugs it can in some circumstances be pro-arrhythmic. This may explain why long-term therapy appears to increase mortality in patients with impaired left ventricular function due to previous myocardial infarction.

Class II drugs
These comprise the beta-adrenoceptor antagonists (beta-blockers). The agents used most commonly are:

Propranolol. This is not cardioselective and is subject to extensive first pass metabolism in the liver. The effective oral dose is therefore unpredictable and must be titrated after starting treatment with a small dose. For the same reason intravenous propranolol is very potent. CNS side-effects are common because the drug readily crosses the blood-brain barrier.

Metoprolol. This is a cardioselective beta-blocker and may therefore have fewer side-effects than propranolol. However, it is also lipid soluble and therefore crosses the blood-brain barrier.

Atenolol. This is a cardioselective beta-blocker with a long duration of action. It is water soluble and is largely excreted unchanged through the kidneys.

Sotalol. This is not cardioselective, but has a long half-life and also has some class III anti-arrhythmic activity.

Class III drugs
These act by prolonging the plateau phase of the action potential, thus lengthening the refractory period.

Amiodarone. This is the principal drug in this class although both disopyramide and sotalolol have class III activity. Amiodarone has unusual pharmacokinetics and is effective against a wide variety of atrial and ventricular arrhythmias. It is probably the most effective drug currently available for controlling paroxysmal atrial fibrillation and the arrhythmias associated with the Wolff-Parkinson-White syndrome. Furthermore, it is very useful in preventing episodes of recurrent ventricular tachycardia, particularly in patients with poor left ventricular function. Amiodarone has an extraordinarily long tissue half.life (25–110 days). This means that the onset of action after oral and intravenous therapy is delayed; indeed it may take several months to reach steady state. For the same reason the drug's effects may last for weeks or months after treatment has been stopped. Side-effects are numerous and potentially serious (see Table 8.2). The common side-effects, notably photosensitisation, corneal deposits and gastrointestinal problems are usually reversible. Drug interactions are also common; for example, the effects of digoxin and warfarin are potentiated by amiodarone.

Class IV drugs

These block the 'slow calcium channel' (p. 308) which is particularly important for impulse generation and conduction in atrial and nodal tissue, although it is also present in ventricular muscle.

Verapamil. This is the most widely used antiarrhythmic drug in this class; nifedipine (p. 309) has no significant antiarrhythmic effect in man. Intravenous verapamil may cause profound bradycardia and/or hypotension and should not be used in conjunction with oral or intravenous beta-blockers.

Digoxin

This is an important anti-arrhythmic drug which does not feature in the Vaughan-Williams classification. Its principal value lies in its ability to slow conduction and prolong the refractory period in the AV node. This effect helps to control the ventricular rate in atrial fibrillation or paroxysmal atrial tachycardia, and will often interrupt re-entry tachycardias involving the AV node. On the other hand digoxin tends to shorten the refractory period and enhance excitability and conduction in other parts of the heart (including accessory conduction pathways); it may therefore increase atrial and ventricular ectopic activity and can lead to more complex atrial and ventricular tachyarrhythmias.

Digoxin is a purified glycoside from the European foxglove, *Digitalis lanata*. Digitalis is a less precise term sometimes used for the powdered leaves of *D. lanata*, sometimes as a generic term for the whole family of cardiac glycosides.

Digoxin is largely excreted by the kidneys, and the maintenance dose should be reduced in children, the elderly and those with renal impairment. It is widely distributed and has a long tissue half-life so that effects may persist 24–36 hours after the last dose. Measurements of plasma digoxin concentration are useful in demonstrating that the dose being used is inadequate and in confirming a clinical impression of toxicity. Its manifestations are listed in the information box (right, top).

Principles of anti-arrhythmic therapy are listed in the information box (right, bottom).

DIGOXIN TOXICITY

Extracardiac manifestations
Anorexia, nausea, vomiting
Diarrhoea
Altered colour vision (xanthopsia)

Cardiac manifestations
Bradycardia
Multiple ventricular ectopics
Ventricular bigeminy (alternate ventricular ectopics)
Paroxysmal atrial tachycardia
Ventricular tachycardia
Ventricular fibrillation

Management
Stop digoxin
Check urea, electrolytes and plasma digoxin concentration
Correct hypokalaemia and/or dehydration
Correct bradycardia using atropine (0.6 mg i.v.) and/or temporary pacing
Treat atrial tachycardia with beta-blockers (p. 275)
Treat ventricular tachycardia with lignocaine (p. 275)
N.B. cardioversion carries an increased risk of provoking ventricular fibrillation
In overdose specific anti-digoxin antibodies may be of value

PRINCIPLES OF ANTI-ARRHYTHMIC THERAPY

- Many arrhythmias are benign and do not require specific treatment.
- Precipitating or causal factors should be corrected if possible. These may include excess alcohol or caffeine consumption, myocardial ischaemia, hyperthyroidism, acidosis, hypokalaemia and hypomagnesaemia.
- If drug therapy is required it is best to use as few drugs as possible.
- In difficult cases programmed electrical stimulation (electrophysiological study) may help to identify the optimum therapy.
- When dealing with life-threatening arrhythmias it is essential to ensure that prophylactic treatment is effective. Ambulatory monitoring, exercise testing, and programmed electrical stimulation may be of value.
- Patients on long-term antiarrhythmic drugs should be reviewed regularly and attempts made to withdraw therapy if the factors which precipitated the arrhythmias are no longer operative.
- Patients who do not respond to drug therapy may benefit from other forms of therapy such as anti-tachycardia pacing, arrhythmia surgery or His bundle ablation.

HEART BLOCK

SINOATRIAL (SA) BLOCK

In this condition a complete cardiac cycle is missed so that a gap appears in the pulse. The electrocardiogram

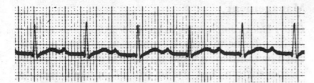

Fig. 8.31   First degree heart block. The PR interval is 0.26 seconds.

shows that both atrial and ventricular complexes are absent. Sinoatrial block is one of the features of the sick sinus syndrome.

Sinoatrial block does not require treatment if it is asymptomatic. Sinoatrial disorders causing symptoms may require the implantation of an artificial pacemaker.

ATRIOVENTRICULAR (AV) BLOCK

In this condition conduction between the atria and ventricles is impaired. AV block may coexist with a variety of atrial tachyarrhythmias, e.g. atrial flutter (Fig. 8.25, p. 270).

First degree heart block (delayed AV conduction). The PR interval is prolonged beyond the upper limit of normal (0.20 second) (Fig. 8.31).

Second degree heart block (partial heart block). Some impulses from the atria fail to get through to the ventricles, i.e. dropped beats occur. In *Mobitz type I* second degree AV block there is progressive lengthening of successive PR intervals followed by a dropped beat. This is known as *Wenckebach's phenomenon* (Fig. 8.32) and is due to progressive fatigue of the AV bundle with recovery following the rest period when the dropped beat occurs.

In *Mobitz type II* second degree AV block the PR interval of the conducted impulses remains constant but some p waves are not conducted. This is usually caused by disease below the bundle of His and is more serious than Mobitz type I. Both forms of second degree heart block can cause 2:1 block (Fig. 8.33).

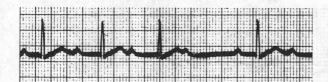

Fig. 8.32   Second degree heart block (Wenckebach's phenomenon). The first beat in the cycle has a PR of 0.28 seconds; it lengthens with the next two beats and the fourth P wave is not followed by a QRS – the dropped beat.

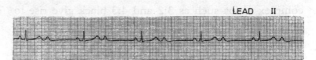

LEAD   II

Fig. 8.33   Second degree heart block with fixed two to one block. Alternate P waves are not conducted. This may be due to Mobitz type I or Mobitz type II block.

Complete heart block. No impulses from the atria reach the ventricles. Cardiac action is maintained by an escape rhythm arising in the bundle of His (narrow QRS complexes) or in the ventricles (broad QRS complexes). A ventricular escape rhythm is less reliable and carries a worse prognosis (Fig. 8.34).

Aetiology
The aetiology is shown in the information box below.

THE AETIOLOGY OF COMPLETE HEART BLOCK

- Congenital
- Acquired
  Idiopathic fibrosis
  Myocardial infarction/ischaemia
  Inflammation – acute e.g. aortic root abscess in infective
    endocarditis
  Inflammation – chronic e.g. sarcoidosis, Chaga's disease
    (p. 163)
  Trauma e.g. cardiac surgery
  Drugs, e.g. digoxin
  Excess vagal activity

Clinical features

First degree heart block. This can be diagnosed only by ECG (Fig. 8.31).

Second degree heart block. When the atrial and ventricular contractions bear a simple ratio to one another such as in 2:1 and 3:1 block, the pulse is slow and regular. Change in the degree of heart block may give rise to sudden changes in the pulse rate. More

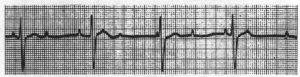

Fig. 8.34   Complete heart block. There is complete dissociation of atrial and ventricular complexes. The atrial rate is 90 and the ventricular rate 40 per minute.

complex ratios such as 3:2 and 4:3 block give rise to dropped beats. Mobitz type I second degree AV block may be physiological and is sometimes observed at rest or during sleep in athletic young adults with a high vagal tone.

Complete heart block. This may be chronic or intermittent. Chronic complete heart block should be suspected when the pulse is slow (30–40 per minute and regular), and except in the case of congenital complete heart block, does not vary with exercise. Venous cannon waves may occur (p. 255). The arterial pulse volume is large and the increased stroke volume may produce a systolic murmur. The intensity of the first heart sound varies with each beat due to the presence of AV dissociation.

Episodes of ventricular asystole may complicate complete heart block or Mobitz type II second degree block and can also occur in patients with sino-atrial disease and episodes of prolonged sinus arrest. Episodes of ventricular asystole may cause cardiac syncope which are sometimes called Adams-Stokes attacks. These attacks often occur without warning although some patients describe a prodrome. There is rapid loss of consciousness and the patient may fall. Convulsions may occur if the heart does not begin to beat again within about 10 seconds, and death will result if the arrest is prolonged. The skin blanches at the beginning of an attack but when the heart starts beating again there is a characteristic flush. In contrast to epilepsy recovery is rapid.

Management

Heart block complicating acute myocardial infarction

Acute inferior myocardial infarction is often complicated by transient AV block. There is usually a reliable escape rhythm and if the patient remains well no treatment is required. Clinical deterioration due to second degree or complete heart block may respond to atropine (0.6 mg i.v., repeated as necessary) or, if this fails, a temporary pacemaker. In the vast majority of cases the AV block will resolve within 7–10 days.

Second degree or complete heart block complicating acute anterior myocardial infarction is usually a sign of extensive myocardial damage and carries a poor prognosis. Asystole often occurs and a temporary pacemaker should be inserted as soon as possible. If the patient presents with asystole atropine (0.6 mg i.v., repeated if necessary) and isoprenaline (1–5 mg in 500 ml 5% dextrose, infused intravenously at the minimum rate needed to produce a satisfactory heart rhythm) may help to maintain the circulation until a temporary pacing electrode can be inserted.

Chronic atrio-ventricular block

Patients with symptomatic bradyarrhythmias with complicating AV block should receive a permanent pacemaker. Asymptomatic first degree or Mobitz type I second degree AV block does not require treatment but may be an indication of serious underlying heart disease or a contraindication to the use of drugs that impair AV conduction. Permanent pacing may be

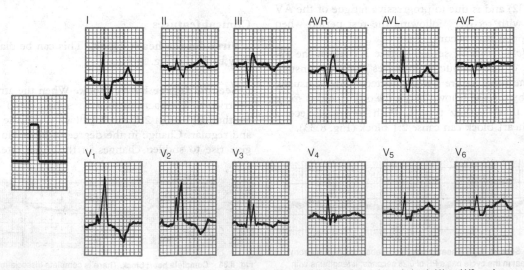

Fig. 8.35   Right bundle branch block. Note the wide QRS complexes with 'M'-shaped complexes in leads V1 and V2, and a wide S wave in lead V6.

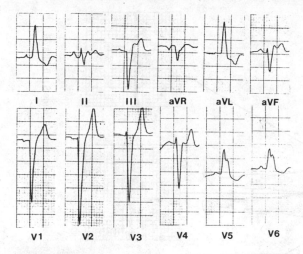

I   II   III   aVR   aVL   aVF

V1   V2   V3   V4   V5   V6

Fig. 8.36   Left bundle branch block from a patient with ischaemic heart disease. The QRS complexes are broad, with a large broad S wave in V2 and V3, and an 'M'-shaped QRS in V5 and V6. The normal septal Q wave is absent in V5 and V6. The T wave in bundle branch block usually goes in the opposite direction to the terminal part of the QRS complex, i.e. upright in V1, 2, 3, inverted in V5 and V6.

indicated in patients with asymptomatic Mobitz type II second degree or complete heart block because there is evidence that pacing may improve their prognosis. An exception may be made in young asymptomatic patients with congenital complete heart block who have a mean day-time heart rate of more than 50 per minute.

BUNDLE BRANCH BLOCK AND HEMIBLOCK

Interruption of the left or right branches of the bundle of His causes delay in the activation of the appropriate ventricle, broadening of the QRS complex on the ECG to 0.12 seconds or more, and characteristic alterations to QRS morphology shown in Figures 8.35 and 8.36.

Right and left bundle branch block may be due to conducting tissue disease but are also features of other types of heart disease (Table 8.3). The left branch of the bundle of His rapidly divides into a fan-like array of conducting tissue on the left side of the interventricular septum. Partial interruption of the bundle at this point (hemiblock) does not broaden the QRS complex, but alters the mean direction of ventricular depolarisation (cardiac axis) as shown in Figure 8.37, p. 280.

The treatment and prognosis of bundle branch block are in general those of the underlying disease. The development of left bundle branch block, or of right bundle branch block plus anterior or posterior hemiblock after myocardial infarction indicates extensive myocardial damage, and often a poor prognosis.

Table 8.3   The common causes of bundle branch block

LBBB	RBBB
Coronary artery disease	Normal variant
Hypertension	Right ventricular hypertrophy or strain
Aortic valve disease	e.g. pulmonary embolism
Cardiomyopathy	Congenital heart disease e.g. ASD
	Coronary artery disease

ELECTRICAL TREATMENT OF ARRHYTHMIAS

Defibrillation and cardioversion

The heart can be completely depolarised by passing a sufficiently large electrical current through it from an external source. When the current has stopped there is a period of asystole followed, usually, by the resumption of normal sinus rhythm. Modern defibrillators use direct current (d.c.) stored in a bank of electrical capacitors to deliver a shock of high energy but short duration. The current is transmitted to the chest wall by large-area electrodes which must be coated with electrically conducting jelly. One electrode is applied over the sternum and the other is pressed against the chest wall beneath the left scapula or in the left axilla.

The precise timing of the discharge is not important in ventricular fibrillation, but when the technique is used to treat supraventricular or ventricular tachycardia or atrial fibrillation discharge should be synchronised with the R wave of the ECG. This is because a current, not large enough to cause total depolarisation, applied during a critical period at the end of the T wave may provoke ventricular fibrillation.

In ventricular fibrillation neither preparation anaesthesia nor synchronisation are required. Discharge energy should be set at 200 Joules (Watt-seconds) and the sooner the shock is applied the more likely it is to succeed. For other arrhythmias there is less urgency, a synchronised discharge should be used, and the patient should be anaesthetised. *Atrial fibrillation* often requires energies of 150 to 200 J to restore sinus rhythm. In *atrial flutter* or *supraventricular tachycardia* lower energies of 50 J or less may suffice.

Digitalis intoxication increases the risk of untoward arrhythmias after cardioversion, and ideally digitalis therapy should be withdrawn 36 hours before elective cardioversion. Patients with long-standing atrial arrhythmias are at risk of systemic embolism after cardioversion, so it is wise to delay elective cardioversion until the patient has been adequately anticoagulated for at least 6 weeks.

Artificial pacemakers

Temporary procedures. In an emergency it is sometimes

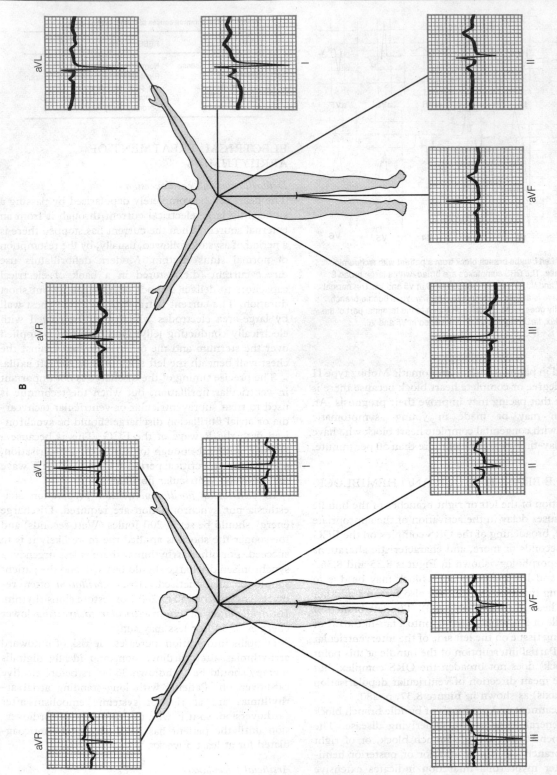

Fig. 8.37   Bundle branch hemiblock. A. Damage to the anterior part of the left bundle (left anterior hemiblock) shifts the axis to the left (large R in lead I and aVL, large S in II, III, aVF).
B. Damage to the posterior part of the left bundle shifts the axis to the right (large S in I, aVL, large R in III, aVF).

possible to stimulate the heart by passing an electric current through electrodes placed on the chest wall, passed down the oesophagus, or inserted directly through the chest wall into the myocardium. None of these methods is satisfactory for longer than a few minutes, if at all, and the most effective technique for temporary artificial pacemaking is to insert a bipolar pacing electrode via an antecubital, subclavian or femoral vein and position it under radioscopic control in the apex of the right ventricle. The electrode is connected to an external pulse generator. The threshold for reliable ventricular stimulation should be less than 1 volt, and the pulse generator should be set to deliver at least three times this figure – usually 3 to 4 volts.

The ECG of a patient whose rhythm is controlled by an artificial ventricular pacemaker shows regular broad QRS complexes with a left bundle branch block pattern and left axis deviation. Each complex is immediately preceded by a 'pacing spike' (Fig. 8.38). Nearly all pulse generators are used in a 'demand' or 'ventricular-inhibited' mode whereby a spontaneously generated QRS complex can inhibit the artificial impulse. In other words, if the patient's spontaneous rhythm recovers and its rate exceeds that at which the artificial pacemaker is set, the latter is inhibited, but if the patient's spontaneous rate drops below that set on the pulse generator then artificial pacing will be resumed.

It is also possible to pace the atria, using a J-shaped electrode inserted percutaneously and positioned in the right atrial appendage. Sequential pacing of atria and ventricles, using a special pulse generator, reproduces the physiological sequence of atrial and ventricular contraction, and gives a better cardiac output than ventricular pacing alone. This may be important when there is impaired left ventricular function, e.g. after myocardial infarction.

Temporary pacemakers are invaluable where heart block is transient, as is usually the case after myocardial infarction, but their long-term use is inconvenient and the insertion site is prone to infection. Only in very exceptional circumstances should one be used for longer than 2 weeks.

Permanent artificial pacemakers utilise the same principles, but the pulse generator is smaller, completely enclosed, and can be implanted under the skin. Many pacemakers are programmable, i.e. the rate, output, etc. can be altered by external radio frequency or magnetic stimuli. This facility allows the cardiologist to prolong the life of the pacemaker by choosing optimum settings and may provide the means to overcome a wide range of pacing problems. For example, programming can be used to increase output in the face of an unexpected increase in threshold, or to alter sensitivity if the pacemaker is inappropriately inhibited by electrical potentials generated in the pectoral muscles.

Atrial electrodes can also be used with permanent pacemakers. They can detect the atrial P wave and use it to initiate the impulse delivered to the ventricle. This has the dual advantage that atrioventricular synchrony is preserved and that the ventricular rate can increase together with the atrial rate during exercise. Atrial-triggered permanent pacemakers are the treatment of choice in physically active patients with complete heart block but normal atrial rhythm. Conversion to an atrial triggered pacing system may cure 'pacemaker syndrome' – a fall in blood pressure and dizziness precipitated by the start of ventricular pacing. Pacing the atrium probably reduces the prevalence of atrial tachyarrhythmias in patients with sino-atrial disease. There are also 'rate-responsive' pacemakers which react (by changing the pacing rate) to parameters such as the QT interval (an index of sympathetic activity), respiration, or physical movement. This type of pacemaker helps to maintain an optimum heart rate and can be used in patients who are not suitable for atrial triggered pacing, e.g. patients with atrial fibrillation.

ACUTE CIRCULATORY FAILURE

Acute circulatory failure, shock and *low output state* are terms used to describe a clinical syndrome of hypotension, peripheral vasoconstriction, oliguria, and often impairment of consciousness. The basic cause is an inadequate cardiac output with compensatory vasoconstriction and renal and cerebral hypoperfusion. The features of acute circulatory failure are listed in the information box (p. 282).

Onset may be sudden or gradual. The skin is cold, pale and sweaty and in advanced cases there may be peripheral cyanosis or gangrene. The systolic blood

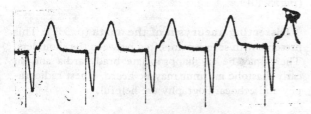

Fig. 8.38   ECG of a patient with a ventricular pacemaker. The QRS complexes are broad and each is immediately preceded by a narrow pacemaker 'spike'.

FEATURES OF ACUTE CIRCULATORY FAILURE

- Blood pressure < 100 mm Hg systolic
- Pulse: weak, usually > 100/minute
- Skin: cold, clammy
- Respiration: rapid, may be Cheyne-Stokes pattern
- Urine < 30 ml/hour

---

pressure is usually low, often under 100 mmHg. With peripheral constriction the blood pressure, measured by cuff, is often an underestimate of central pressure. Consciousness may be preserved, but frequently there is confusion and irritability.

If treatment is not prompt and effective, systemic consequences may ensue (Fig. 8.39). Oliguria may progress to acute tubular necrosis (p. 589). A rising plasma potassium concentration and progressive acidosis both from renal failure and ischaemic necrosis of skeletal muscle cause cardiac arrhythmias which may eventually be intractable. Even if recovery occurs permanent cerebral damage or loss of peripheral tissues may be inevitable.

Successful treatment of acute circulatory failure is absolutely dependent on identification of the cause; this requires meticulous assessment of the history and physical signs, and efficient use of investigation. While this is being done the patient should be protected from fuss, unnecessary disturbance and hypothermia;

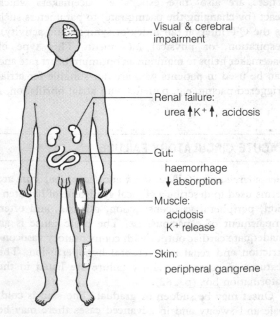

Fig. 8.39 Systemic consequences of acute circulatory failure.

Visual & cerebral impairment

Renal failure:
urea ↑ K+ ↑, acidosis

Gut:
haemorrhage
↓ absorption

Muscle:
acidosis
K+ release

Skin:
peripheral gangrene

anxiety and pain should be relieved using small intravenous doses of morphine if necessary. Oxygen should be administered by facemask or nasal prongs. A catheter should be inserted to monitor urine output, and great care taken to protect ischaemic skin from damage.

Aetiology

The causes of acute circulatory failure can be divided into those associated with a low central venous pressure (hypovolaemic shock) and those characterised by a raised venous pressure (cardiogenic shock). Central venous pressure can be difficult to assess with the patient lying flat, and if there is doubt a central venous catheter should be inserted and the pressure measured with a saline manometer.

Hypovolaemic shock

The commonest cause of hypovolaemia is haemorrhage – external, into the bowel, or into a body cavity. Gastrointestinal haemorrhage can often be diagnosed on the basis of history and rectal examination; its further assessment is considered on page 436. Intra-abdominal haemorrhage, from a leaking aortic aneurysm in the elderly or a ruptured spleen or ectopic pregnancy in a younger patient, is often insidious in its presentation, and atypical in its physical signs.

Less common causes of hypovolaemia include plasma loss in severe burns, or into the abdominal cavity in acute pancreatitis, inappropriate vasodilation in bacteraemic shock (p. 145) and anaphylactic shock (p. 37), and excess urinary fluid loss as in diabetic ketoacidosis.

Cardiogenic shock

Acute circulatory failure with a raised central venous pressure is caused by problems affecting the left or right side of the heart or the pulmonary circulation. The two most common causes are acute myocardial infarction and acute massive pulmonary embolism. When the diagnosis is not immediately apparent, it is useful to consider possible causes in a methodical order (Fig. 8.40).

Dissecting aneurysm of the aorta (p. 337). This presents with severe pain, often between the shoulders. There may be an inappropriate bradycardia and an early diastolic murmur may be heard. Chest radiography and echocardiography are helpful.

Pericardial tamponade (p. 327). This is an important cause of acute circulatory failure because it carries a high mortality if neglected and because it

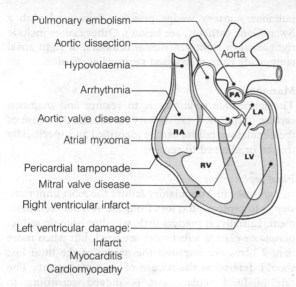

Pulmonary embolism

Aortic dissection

Hypovolaemia

Arrhythmia

Aortic valve disease

Atrial myxoma

Pericardial tamponade

Mitral valve disease

Right ventricular infarct

Left ventricular damage:
Infarct
Myocarditis
Cardiomyopathy

Aorta
PA
LA
RA
LV
RV

Fig. 8.40   Some possible cardiac causes of acute circulatory failure.

usually responds dramatically to treatment. The features are listed in the information box below. Echocardiography, which may be done at the bedside, is the best way of confirming the diagnosis, and helps to indicate the best site for paracentesis.

FEATURES OF PERICARDIAL TAMPONADE

- Hypotension
- Grossly elevated venous pressure
- Pulsus paradoxus
- CXR: enlarged heart shadow
- ECG: small voltages, electrical alternans
- Echocardiography: pericardial effusion
- Management: pericardiocentesis

Aortic valve disease. This may precipitate acute circulatory failure by causing left ventricular failure and pulmonary oedema. The signs of *aortic stenosis* (p. 297) may be masked by a low cardiac output, the characteristic murmur becoming quiet. Acute severe *aortic regurgitation*, from cusp rupture or endocarditis, may also be atypical, with an unimpressive murmur and little cardiac enlargement on the chest radiograph. Echocardiography is helpful.

Myocardial infarction. When this is extensive enough to cause acute circulatory failure it is usually obvious from the ECG, but occasionally ECG changes of ischaemia are a secondary result of circulatory failure

from some other catastrophe such as pulmonary embolism. Usually, circulatory failure from myocardial infarction is associated with pulmonary oedema, but if the infarct predominantly affects the right ventricle (see below) this is not always the case.

Drugs. These may sometimes precipitate severe cardiac failure, either directly or when they interact with other drugs (e.g. intravenous verapamil in a patient taking beta-blockers) or underlying disease (e.g. beta-blockers in a patient with unsuspected cardiomyopathy). The drugs are listed in the information box below.

DRUGS CAUSING CARDIAC FAILURE

- Directly toxic
Daunorubicin
Adriamycin
Ethanol
- Cardiac Failure complicating Overdose
Tricyclic antidepressants
Salicylates
Calcium antagonists
Beta blockers
Class I antiarrhythmic drugs
(Flecainide, disopyramide)
Organic solvents

Progressive myocarditis. Including that of rheumatic fever, sometimes presents as acute circulatory failure; the chest radiograph usually shows an enlarged heart and echocardiography reveals severely impaired left ventricular function.

Tachyarrhythmias. These are usually obvious clinically and from the ECG. The onset of atrial fibrillation may precipitate acute circulatory failure, often with severe pulmonary oedema, in patients with impaired left ventricular function or *mitral stenosis*. The murmur of mitral stenosis (p. 257) is difficult to hear in the presence of tachycardia, but the history, chest radiograph and echocardiogram will confirm the diagnosis.

Acute massive pulmonary embolism (p. 324). This is a sequel to leg or pelvic vein thrombosis. Collapse is sudden, often with extreme breathlessness. The features are listed in the information box (p. 284). Pulmonary angiography is the definitive diagnostic procedure, but is not without risks – including those of moving a severely ill patient and of delay in instituting treatment.

FEATURES OF ACUTE MASSIVE PULMONARY EMBOLISM

- Usually
    Breathlessness
    Raised JVP
    Tachycardia
- Sometimes:
    Parasternal lift
    Wide splitting S_2
    Right ventricular S_3
- ECG
    RV strain (Fig. 8.41) or normal
- CXR
    Usually normal
- Echo
    Large RV, small LV
- Blood gases
    Low Po_2, normal Pco_2
- Pulmonary Angiography
    Diagnostic

Pure 'right-sided' causes of acute circulatory failure. These are rare apart from pulmonary embolism. Probably the most common is the combination of a right ventricular infarct with excessive diuretic therapy; this can be suspected if cardiac output and urine production decline after an inferior infarct in the absence of pulmonary congestion, and confirmed by demonstrating a high central venous pressure but a low pulmonary artery wedge pressure (measured with a Swan-Ganz catheter, see below). Other causes include right atrial or right ventricular tumours, or right atrial tamponade from a localised pericardial effusion.

Management

The immediate objective is to restore and maintain cardiac output at a satisfactory level until the cause of the circulatory failure can be identified and specifically treated or allowed to resolve.

Fluid replacement

In hypovolaemic circulatory failure the most important step is to replace fluid lost from the vascular compartment. Initially, it matters little whether isotonic saline, plasma or plasma substitutes are used, but when more than 2 litres are required the nature of the fluid lost should determine the nature of its replacement. The rate of fluid replacement is judged according to estimates of the fluid lost, the clinical state of the patient, observation of the jugular venous pressure, and in severely ill patients by manometer measurement of the central venous pressure. Where large transfusions are needed rapidly it is important to warm the fluid used to body temperature.

Hypovolaemic shock sometimes occurs in patients with pre-existing cardiac disease. Under these conditions central venous or right atrial pressure may be an

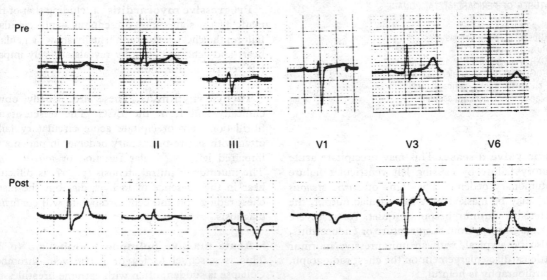

Fig. 8.41 ECGs from a patient before and immediately after a massive pulmonary embolism (the embolus was successfully removed surgically shortly after this record was taken). Right ventricular dilatation and strain are manifested by the development of an S wave in lead I and a Q wave plus T inversion in lead III (the 'S$_1$Q$_3$T$_3$' pattern). There is also acute T wave inversion in V1 and a shift from a left ventricular to a right ventricular pattern in V3. Note that many of these features can be seen in ECGs from normal subjects, and it is only by taking the pattern as a whole, and particularly by comparison with a previous ECG, that the full significance is appreciated.

unreliable guide to fluid replacement, and it is better to obtain an estimate of pulmonary venous or left atrial pressure by *bedside haemodynamic monitoring*. This can be done using a Swan-Ganz catheter (Fig. 8.17). The mean left atrial pressure is normally between 5 and 10 mmHg; in left-sided cardiac failure it may rise as high as 30 mmHg. In managing patients with acute circulatory failure a left atrial pressure of about 15 mmHg is usually aimed at; this is high enough to give good left ventricular filling but carries a low risk of pulmonary oedema.

Acute pulmonary oedema
This is usually a feature of circulatory failure caused by left-sided cardiac problems. The three initial steps in its management are the administration of:

1. morphine, to alleviate breathlessness and reverse reflex peripheral vasoconstriction
2. a powerful diuretic such as frusemide (40–80 mg i.v.) both for its diuretic effect and also as a vasodilator
3. a high concentration of oxygen.

If these immediate measures are inadequate, one may try to stimulate the heart using inotropic agents, or to reduce left ventricular load by using more powerful vasodilators.

Controlled vasodilatation
This is an important concept in the management of pulmonary oedema and of left-sided cardiac failure in general. *Venodilatation* reduces central venous pressure and right ventricular output, and slows the accumulation of pulmonary oedema, while *arteriolar dilatation* improves left ventricular function by reducing the afterload against which it has to work.

Glyceryl trinitrate. This as a spray (400–800 µg) or buccal tablet (slow release GTN 5mg) is a useful 'first aid' vasodilator, but controlled intravenous administration of nitrates is preferable, e.g. isosorbide dinitrate 2–10 mg/hour via infusion pump. In severe heart failure nitrates tend to act both as venous and arteriolar dilators. Ideally, vasodilator therapy should be controlled by measuring the pulmonary wedge pressure using a Swan-Ganz catheter aiming at a mean wedge pressure of 14–15 mm/Hg. The main complication of vasodilator therapy is hypotension, the systolic pressure should not be allowed to fall below 90 mmHg. Intravenous nitrate therapy can be followed up with oral angiotensin converting enzyme inhibitors – starting with low dose and gradually increasing (p. 290).

Dopamine. At low doses this has a selective renal vasodilator effect (2–5 µg/kg/min) and is a useful adjunct to diuretic therapy. At higher doses it has a systemic vasodilator effect plus some inotropic effect, and at higher doses still it is a vasoconstrictor. It needs to be given via a central venous catheter as local extravasation causes tissue necrosis.

Inotropic agents. These increase ventricular output for a given filling pressure, but at the cost of increased oxygen consumption. They are most useful in reversing the effects of cardiac depressant drugs (including anaesthetics), or for tiding over a patient until a metabolic disturbance can be corrected or a mechanical defect repaired. Dobutamine (2–10 µg/kg/minute) by infusion is the most effective inotrope for severe heart failure due to medical causes. Overdosage is indicated by hypertension or tachycardia. Adrenaline is sometimes preferred by anaesthetists for postoperative myocardial depression, perhaps because of its peripheral vasoconstrictor and dilator effects.

Circulatory assist devices
A variety of devices are now available to provide mechanical assistance to the circulation. The most widely used is the intra-aortic balloon pump. Their principal use is to support a patient with a cardiac problem amenable to surgical correction while surgery can be arranged, or to support post-surgical patients in the immediate postoperative period while the myocardium is recovering from the effects of surgery. These devices are listed in the information box below.

CIRCULATORY ASSIST DEVICES

- Intra-aortic balloon pump
- Partial cardiac bypass
  Right ventricular assist (RVAD)
  Left ventricular assist (LVAD)
  Biventricular assist (BVAD)
- Extracorporeal membrane oxygenator (ECMO)

In pure right-sided cardiac failure it is important to maintain an adequate filling pressure for the right side of the heart, and the left atrial pressure may be a better guide to this than the central venous pressure. Inotropic agents may be helpful, but diuretics should be used with care and venodilators are contraindicated.

Care of other systems
Renal failure (p. 589) is a common complication of

acute circulatory failure. The kidney responds to a severe fall in blood pressure by vasoconstriction and by redistribution of blood flow between medulla and cortex. If this vasoconstriction persists, tubular necrosis may ensue. Inducing a diuresis with frusemide or the osmotic diuretic mannitol may help protect the kidney from vasoconstriction, but the most effective antidote to renal vasoconstriction is low-dose dopamine (2– 4 µg/kg/minute. Once tubular necrosis has occurred it is important to restrict fluid intake, or pulmonary oedema will follow. Correction of the acidosis which often accompanies circulatory failure presents a dilemma in the presence of tubular necrosis, because of the sodium and fluid load involved. Peritoneal or haemodialysis are sometimes needed.

Hypoxaemia is common in acute circulatory failure, particularly when there is pulmonary oedema. If it does not respond rapidly to oxygen and diuretic therapy, early consideration should be given to endotracheal intubation and positive-pressure ventilation. Sometimes oxygenation can be further improved by using positive end-expiratory pressure (PEEP) or continuous positive airway pressure (CPAP).

Prognosis
In acute circulatory failure this is determined by the underlying cause. No amount of medication can compensate for massive and irretrievable myocardial damage, and the prognosis for circulatory failure complicating extensive myocardial infarction is poor. In contrast the prognosis after drainage of a pericardial effusion, replacement of a diseased valve, or dissolution of a pulmonary embolus may be excellent.

CARDIAC FAILURE

Heart failure is an imprecise term used to describe the state that develops when the heart cannot maintain an adequate cardiac output or can do so only at the expense of an elevated filling pressure. In the mildest forms of heart failure cardiac output is adequate at rest and becomes inadequate only when the metabolic demand increases during exccrcise or some other form of stress. Almost all forms of heart disease may lead to heart failure and it is important to appreciate that, like anaemia, the term refers to a clinical syndrome rather than a specific diagnosis. Good management depends on an accurate aetiological diagnosis, partly because in some situations a specific remedy may be available, but mainly because a clear understanding of the pathophysiology is essential to logical drug therapy.

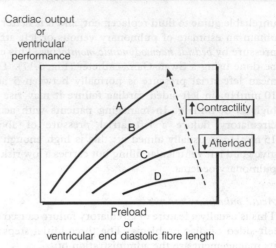

Fig. 8.42 Starling's law. A. Normal, **B.** Mild, **C.** Moderate, **D.** Severe heart failure. Ventricular performance is related to the degree of myocardial stretching. An increase in end diastolic volume (preload) will enhance function, although overstretching causes marked deterioration. An increase in myocardial contractility or a reduction in afterload (arterial resistance/blood pressure) will shift the curve upwards. Whereas, in heart failure the curve moves to the right and becomes flatter.

PATHOPHYSIOLOGY AND AETIOLOGY

The cardiac output is a function of the preload (the volume and pressure of blood in the ventricle at the end of diastole), the afterload (the arterial resistance) and myocardial contractility. The interaction of these variables is shown in Figure 8.42, which is based on Starling's law of the heart. In heart failure the curve relating cardiac output to preload moves to the right and becomes flatter (Fig. 8.42). This is associated with important pathophysiological changes in the peripheral circulation which are largely due to neuro-hormonal activation as a result of impaired renal perfusion due to a low cardiac output and treatment with diuretics. These changes may help to optimise cardiac function by increasing myocardial contractility or by altering the afterload or preload (Fig. 8.43). However, they can also be counterproductive; for example, activation of the sympathetic nervous system and the renin-angiotensin system may lead to an inappropriate and excessive increase in peripheral vascular resistance; similarly, impaired renal perfusion and secondary aldosteronism often lead to salt and water retention and oedema.

TYPES OF HEART FAILURE

Heart failure may be classified in several ways:

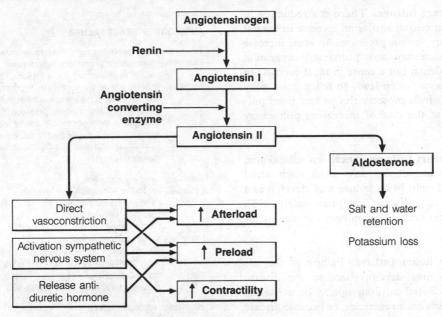

Fig. 8.43   The renin-angiotensin-aldosterone system in heart failure. Impaired renal perfusion and diuretic therapy lead to the release of renin; the activation of the renin-angiotensin system then causes changes in the afterload, preload and myocardial contractility as shown.

Acute and chronic heart failure
Heart failure may develop suddenly, as in myocardial infarction, or gradually, as in progressive valvular heart disease. When there is gradual impairment of cardiac function a variety of compensatory changes may take place. Although initially these changes may improve overall cardiac function, as the disease progresses they often become counterproductive and a vicious circle develops. The changes are listed in the information box below.

COMPENSATORY CHANGES IN HEART FAILURE

Local changes
Chamber enlargement
Myocardial hypertrophy
Increased heart rate

Systemic changes
Activation of the sympathetic nervous system
Activation of the Renin-angiotensin-aldosterone system
(Fig. 8.43)
Release of antidiuretic hormone
Release of atrial natriuretic peptide

The term *compensated heart failure* is sometimes used to describe a patient with impaired cardiac function in whom adaptive changes have prevented the development of overt heart failure. A minor event, such as an intercurrent infection, may precipitate severe heart failure in this type of patient. Some factors that may precipitate or aggravate heart failure are listed in the information box below.

FACTORS THAT MAY PRECIPITATE OR AGGRAVATE HEART FAILURE

● Inappropriate reduction of therapy
● Administration of a drug with negative inotropic or fluid retaining properties (e.g. corticosteroids)
● Physical or emotional stress
● Arrhythmia
● Intercurrent illness (e.g. infection)
● Pulmonary embolism
● Conditions associated with increased metabolic demand (e.g. pregnancy, thyrotoxicosis, anaemia)
● Second form of heart disease

Left, right and biventricular heart failure
The left side of the heart is a term for the functional unit of the left atrium and left ventricle together with the mitral and aortic valves, and the right side stands for the right atrium, right ventricle, tricuspid and pulmonary valves.

Left-sided heart failure. There is a reduction in the left ventricular output and/or an increase in the left atrial or pulmonary venous pressure. An acute increase in left atrial pressure may cause pulmonary congestion or pulmonary oedema; but a more gradual increase in the left atrial pressure often leads to reflex pulmonary vasoconstriction which protects the patient from pulmonary oedema at the cost of increasing pulmonary hypertension.

Right-sided heart failure. There is a reduction in right ventricular output for any given right atrial pressure. Isolated right heart failure may develop as a result of chronic lung disease (cor pulmonale p. 395), multiple pulmonary emboli, pulmonary valvular stenosis, etc.

Biventricular heart failure. Failure of the left and right heart, may develop because the disease process, such as dilated cardiomyopathy or ischaemic heart disease, affects both ventricles, or because disease of the left heart leads to chronic elevation of the left atrial pressure, pulmonary hypertension and subsequent right heart failure.

Forward and backward heart failure
In some patients with heart failure the predominant problem is an inadequate cardiac output (forward failure) whilst other patients may have a normal or near normal cardiac output with marked salt and water retention, and pulmonary and systemic venous congestion (backward failure).

Diastolic and systolic dysfunction
Heart failure may develop as a result of impaired myocardial contraction (systolic dysfunction) but can also be due to poor ventricular filling and high filling pressures caused by abnormal ventricular relaxation (diastolic dysfunction). The latter is commonly found in patients with left ventricular hypertrophy and/or fibrosis and occurs in many forms of heart disease. Systolic and diastolic dysfunction often coexist, particularly in patients with coronary artery disease.

High output failure. Conditions that can lead to a very high cardiac output, e.g. a large AV shunt, severe anaemia or thyrotoxicosis, can occasionally cause heart failure. In many cases additional causes of heart failure are present.

The causes of heart failure
These can be divided into four groups and are listed in the information box (right).

AETIOLOGY OF HEART FAILURE

Ventricular outflow obstruction (pressure overload)
Examples – systemic or pulmonary hypertension
aortic or pulmonary valve stenosis
Features – initially concentric ventricular hypertrophy allows the ventricle to maintain a normal output by generating a high systolic pressure. Secondary changes in the myocardium and/or increasing obstruction eventually lead to failure with ventricular dilatation and rapid clinical deterioration.

Ventricular inflow obstruction
Examples – mitral or tricuspid valve stenosis
endomyocardial fibrosis and other disorders that cause a stiff myocardium e.g. left ventricular hypertrophy, constrictive pericarditis
Features – small vigorous ventricle
dilated hypertrophied atrium
atrial fibrillation is common and often causes marked deterioration because ventricular filling depends heavily on atrial contraction.

Ventricular volume overload
Examples – increased metabolic demand
intracardiac shunting e.g. ASD (right ventricular volume overload)
valvular incompetence e.g. mitral or aortic incompetence (left ventricular volume overload)
Features – dilatation and hypertrophy allows the ventricle to generate a high stroke volume and therefore helps to maintain a normal cardiac output. However, secondary changes in the myocardium eventually lead to impaired contractility and worsening heart failure.

Impaired ventricular function
a) diffuse myocardial disease
Examples – myocarditis, cardiomyopathy
this is also a feature of chronic ventricular pressure or volume overload
Features – impaired myocardial contractility, progressive ventricular dilatation
b) Segmental myocardial disease
Example – myocardial infarction
Features – 'akinetic' or 'dyskinetic' segments contract poorly and may impede the function of the normal segments by distorting their contraction and relaxation patterns.

Clinical features
The clinical picture depends on the nature of the underlying heart disease, the type of heart failure that it has evoked and the neural and endocrine changes that have developed.

Symptoms, signs and investigations
Left heart failure may cause breathlessness, orthopnoea, and paroxysmal nocturnal dyspnoea with inspira-

tory crepitations over the lung bases. These features may be absent if there is marked pulmonary vasoconstriction (p. 322). The chest X-ray shows characteristic abnormalities (p. 262) and is usually a more sensitive indicator of pulmonary venous congestion than the physical signs.

A low cardiac output causes fatigue, listlessness and a poor effort tolerance. The peripheries are cold and the blood pressure is low. Poor renal perfusion may lead to oliguria and uraemia.

Right heart failure produces a high jugular venous pressure, with hepatic congestion and dependent peripheral oedema. In ambulant patients the oedema affects the ankles whereas in bedbound patients it collects around the thighs and sacrum. Massive accumulation of fluid may cause ascites or pleural effusion.

In many cases a specific diagnosis can be made on the basis of the clinical findings, the ECG, and chest X-ray. Echocardiography is also extremely valuable and may demonstrate the cause and the severity of the underlying problem.

Complications

In advanced heart failure a number of non-specific complications may occur – and these are listed in the information box (right).

Management of heart failure

General measures

Physical rest is helpful. Bed-rest increases renal blood flow and will often initiate a diuresis without any

---

COMPLICATIONS OF HEART FAILURE

Uraemia due to:
Diuretic therapy
Low cardiac output
Treatment with vasodilators or dopamine may improve renal perfusion

Hypokalaemia due to:
Diuretic therapy
Hyperaldosteronism (activation of the renin-angiotensin system and impaired aldosterone metabolism due to hepatic congestion)
N.B. most of the body's potassium is intracellular, and there may be substantial depletion of potassium stores even when the plasma potassium concentration is in the normal range.

Hyponatraemia, due to:
Diuretic therapy
Inappropriate water retention (may respond to fluid restriction – p. 215)
Failure of cell membrane ion pump

Impaired liver function due to:
Hepatic congestion and poor hepatic perfusion;
Abnormal liver function tests, mild jaundice;
Anticoagulants potentiated

Thromboembolism due to:
Deep vein thrombosis and pulmonary embolism (low cardiac output, immobility – information box p. 338)
Systemic emboli (intracardiac thrombus e.g. mitral stenosis, LV aneurysm and arrhythmias e.g. atrial fibrillation)

Arrhythmias due to:
Underlying heart disease
Electrolyte changes (e.g. hypokalaemia)
Increased circulating catecholamines
Drug effects (e.g. digoxin toxicity – information box p. 276)

---

adjustment in diuretic therapy. Conversely, patients often need a larger dose of diuretic when they become more active. Patients should be advised to avoid a high dietary salt intake, excess alcohol, and salt or fluid retaining drugs (e.g. non-steroidal anti-inflammatory drugs).

Drug therapy

Cardiac function can be improved by increasing contractility, optimising preload or decreasing afterload. The effects of these measures are illustrated in Fig. 8.44. Drugs that reduce preload are most appropriate in patients with high end-diastolic filling pressures and evidence of pulmonary or systemic venous congestion (backward failure). Whereas, drugs that reduce afterload or increase myocardial contractility are particularly valuable in patients with signs and symptoms of a low cardiac output (forward failure).

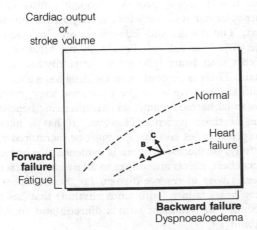

Fig. 8.44   The effect of treatment on ventricular performance curves in heart failure. A. Diuretics and venodilators. **B.** Angiotensin converting enzyme inhibitors, mixed vasodilators. **C.** Positive inotropic agents.

Diuretics. These are usually the first line of treatment. The main types, mode of action, dosage, and side-effects of these drugs are described on page 213. In heart failure they will produce an increase in urinary sodium excretion, leading to a reduction in blood and plasma volume, and may also cause a small but significant degree of arterial and venous dilatation. They will, therefore, reduce preload with a reduction in ventricular filling pressures and an improvement in pulmonary and systemic venous congestion. There may also be a small reduction in afterload and a reduction in ventricular volume leading to a fall in wall tension and increased cardiac efficiency.

Although a fall in ventricular filling pressure tends to reduce cardiac output the 'Starling curve' in heart failure is flat so there may be a substantial and beneficial fall in filling pressure with little change in cardiac output (Fig. 8.44). Nevertheless, excessive diuretic therapy may cause an undesirable fall in cardiac output with a rising blood urea, hypotension and increasing lethargy.

In severe heart failure treatment with combinations of diuretics from different classes (loop, thiazide, and potassium-sparing – p. 213) may increase the diuretic effect and may help to prevent hypokalaemia.

Vasodilators. The use of vasodilators in acute circulatory failure is described on page 285. These drugs are also valuable in chronic heart failure; venodilators (e.g. organic nitrates) reduce preload and arterial dilators (e.g. hydralazine) reduce afterload (Fig. 8.44). However, their use is limited by pharmacological tolerance and hypotension, and treatment with angiotensin converting enzyme inhibitors is usually preferable.

Angiotensin converting enzyme inhibitors. The advent of these drugs has been a major advance in the treatment of heart failure. They act to prevent the conversion of angiotensin I to angiotensin II, thereby counteracting salt and water retention, peripheral arterial and venous vasoconstriction, and activation of the sympathetic nervous system (Fig. 8.43). This will interrupt the vicious circle of neurohumoral activation that is characteristic of moderate and severe heart failure and will also prevent the undesirable activation of the renin-angiotensin system caused by diuretic therapy. Treatment will, therefore, improve cardiac function by reducing the preload and afterload (Fig. 8.43); there may also be a diuresis with an increase in plasma potassium concentration. Clearly a combination of a diuretic and an ACE inhibitor has many potential advantages.

Clinical trials have shown that in moderate and severe heart failure ACE inhibitors can produce a substantial improvement in effort tolerance and in mortality. Unfortunately they may cause profound hypotension with postural symptoms and a deterioration in renal function (especially in patients with bilateral renal artery stenosis or pre-existing renal disease). There may be a potentially catastrophic fall in blood pressure following the first dose of an ACE inhibitor, particularly if the drug is given when there is evidence of hypovolaemia or hyponatraemia due to prior diuretic therapy. Accordingly, it is wise to withold diuretics for 24 hours before starting treatment with a low dose of a short acting agent such as captopril 6.25 mg, while the patient is supine and under close observation. If hypotension occurs this can be counteracted by elevating the foot of the bed, intravenous saline or, in extreme circumstances intravenous angiotensin II.

Captopril (average dose 25 mg t.i.d.) is a short-acting agent with an elimination half life of 6–8 hours. Unwanted effects include hypotension, hyperkalaemia, deterioration in renal function, cough, skin rash, altered taste and neutropenia.

Enalapril (average dose 20 mg daily) is a long-acting agent that is only active after conversion, in the liver, to the active metabolite *enalaprilat*. Unwanted effects are similar to those caused by captopril.

Lisinopril (average dose 10 mg daily) is a new agent that has a long half life and a similar range of side-effects.

Digoxin. This should be used as first-line therapy in patients with heart failure and atrial fibrillation when it will usually provide adequate control of the ventricular rate together with a small positive inotropic effect. The dosage and side-effects are discussed on page 276. The role of digoxin in the treatment of patients with heart failure and sinus rhythm is less certain. There is no doubt that the drug has a small but significant positive inotropic effect and may produce substantial haemodynamic and symptomatic benefit in some of these patients. However, it has a narrow therapeutic index and therapy must be monitored very carefully; furthermore, there is evidence that some of its beneficial effects are subject to tolerance. In practice it seems wise to reserve digoxin for the treatment of severe heart failure (with sinus rhythm) that has not responded to treatment with a diuretic and an ACE inhibitor.

Other drugs. A number of alternative oral positive inotropic agents have been developed but have largely proved disappointing. Anticoagulants may be used to treat or prevent thrombo-embolism. Although not firmly established, there is growing interest in the use of antiarrhythmic drugs to prevent potentially fatal arrhythmias.

Prognosis

Heart failure carries a poor prognosis. Although the outlook depends, to some extent, on the underlying cause of the problem approximately 50% of patients with severe heart failure will die within two years. Many patients die suddenly, often due to maligant ventricular arrhythmias or myocardial infarction.

RHEUMATIC DISEASE

ACUTE RHEUMATIC FEVER

Aetiology

Acute rheumatic fever is an autoallergic disease triggered by infection with specific strains of *streptococcus pyogenes* which express antigens cross-reactive with those on human connective tissue. It usually affects children or young adults, and there is a definite family variation in susceptibility. Its prevalence in Western Europe and North America has progressively declined, for poorly understood reasons, over the last 40 years, but may now be rising again.

Clinical features

Rheumatic fever is a systemic illness nearly always accompanied by arthritis, and sometimes by skin rashes, carditis and neurological features (Sydenham's chorea). The arthritis of rheumatic fever (sometimes called acute rheumatism, but not to be confused with rheumatoid arthritis) is an acute painful inflammation of one or several joints. Characteristically the arthritis 'flits' from joint to joint (i.e. a migratory polyarthralgia). There is pain, tenderness and redness, and sometimes an effusion. The joints affected include those of the limbs, spine, and sometimes temporomandibular and costoclavicular joints. There is commonly, but not invariably, a history of sore throat 2–4 weeks before the onset of joint symptoms. In adults, joint symptoms tend to be more prominent than carditis, in children under six years old the converse may be true.

Skin lesions

Skin lesions which may accompany rheumatic fever include non-specific rashes, erythema marginatum, erythema nodosum and subcutaneous nodules.

Erythema marginatum. This occurs in 10–20% of children with rheumatic fever. It starts as red macules (blotches) which fade in the centre but remain red at the edges. The resulting red rings or 'margins' may coalesce or overlap.

Erythema nodosum. These dusky red raised papules or nodules, usually on the front of the shins are less common, and less specific. Subcutaneous nodules are firm painless nodules best felt over bone or tendons. They are usually much smaller than the nodules of rheumatoid arthritis. They are uncommon, but associated with more severe carditis.

Carditis. This is the most important manifestation of rheumatic fever. It presents as palpitation, chest pain (usually due to pericarditis) or breathlessness. There is usually a tachycardia and often cardiac enlargement. A soft systolic murmur is common but non-specific. A soft mid-diastolic murmur (Carey-Coombs murmur) is much more specific – it is thought to be due to nodules forming on the mitral valve leaflets. There may be a pericardial friction rub – often intermittent. Cardiac failure may result either from impaired function of ventricular muscle or from mitral or aortic incompetence caused by valve damage. Severe mitral or aortic incompetence tend to be features of a 'fulminant' form of rheumatic fever more common in developing countries. Conduction defects sometimes occur and may cause syncope.

Sydenham's chorea. This rarely occurs at the same time as acute arthritis or acute carditis. It is often delayed for up to six months after an initial streptococcal infection. It is characterised by jerky, involuntary movements. Spontaneous recovery is usual, though it may be followed by chronic cardiac disease.

Other systemic manifestations of rheumatic fever include pleurisy, pleural effusion and pneumonia, but are rare.

Investigations

These are listed in the information box (p. 292, top).

The Duckett-Jones criteria

Because of the therapeutic and other implications of a diagnosis of acute rheumatic fever, and because the diagnosis is essentially clinical, it is useful to have a scheme for 'weighting' the various clinical findings. These criteria were originally proposed by Duckett-Jones, and subsequently modified by the American Heart Association. A diagnosis of rheumatic fever is *likely* in the presence of two major manifestations, or one major and two minor manifestations, *plus* evidence

---

INVESTIGATIONS IN ACUTE RHEUMATIC FEVER

Evidence of a systemic illness
A fever, leukocytosis and raised ESR are usual, non-specific but useful for following the progress of the disease once diagnosed.

Evidence of preceding streptococcal infection
Culture of group A beta haemolytic streptococci from a throat swab is positive in only a minority by the time rheumatic fever is clinically manifest. Positive cultures can sometimes be obtained from family members and contacts.
Antistreptolysin O antibodies (ASO titre) are useful evidence of recent streptococcal infection, especially if a rising titre can be shown. In the absence of a rising titre, a level of >200 units or >300 units in children is also usually evidence of recent infection. ASO titres are normal in about a fifth of adult cases of rheumatic fever and most cases of chorea.

Evidence of carditis
The chest radiograph may show cardiac enlargement or pulmonary congestion. ECG changes include first and second degree heart block, features of pericarditis, T wave inversion and reduction in QRS voltages. Echocardiography is useful for showing cardiac dilatation and valve abnormalities.

MANIFESTATIONS OF RHEUMATIC FEVER

Major manifestations
Carditis, polyarthritis, chorea, erythema marginatum, subcutaneous nodules
Minor manifestations
Fever, arthralgia, previous rheumatic fever, raised ESR, first degree or second degree AV block

Plus supporting evidence of preceding streptococcal infection
Recent scarlet fever, raised ASO or other streptococcal antibody titre, positive throat culture
N.B. Evidence of recent streptococcal infection is particularly important if there is only one major manifestation

---

of previous streptococcal infection. The manifestations are listed in the information box above.

Management

Bed-rest. During the acute phase of rheumatic fever the patient feels unwell and welcomes bed-rest. Later, the patient may feel well although temperature and erythrocyte sedimentation rate (ESR) remain elevated. Bed-rest must be continued until these indices of continuing disease activity have settled, as otherwise there is a risk of recurrence of symptoms. In patients who have had carditis, it is traditional to continue to bed-rest for 2–6 weeks after ESR and temperature have returned to normal.

Aspirin. In large regular doses this is effective in providing symptomatic relief of arthritis. 60 mg/kg bodyweight per day is a reasonable starting dose, divided into 6 doses. In adults up to 120 mg/kg/day may be needed, up to a maximum of 8g per day. Mild toxic effects include nausea, tinnitus and deafness, more serious ones are vomiting, tachypnoea and acidosis. Aspirin should be continued until the ESR has fallen, and then gradually tailed off.

Corticosteroids. These produce more rapid symptomatic relief than aspirin, and are preferable in cases with severe arthritis or carditis. There is no evidence that the long-term effects are superior. Prednisolone or prednisone 0.25 mg/kg/day in divided doses should be continued until ESR is normal, then gradually tailed off.

Antistreptococcal therapy. Clearance of streptococcal infections and prevention of recurrence is important. Benzathine penicillin 1 200 000 units (916 mg) should be given on diagnosis, once a week for 3 weeks, and then monthly for the first year. Subsequent prophylaxis may be with oral phenoxymethylpenicillin 500 mg daily, continued until the patient reaches the age of 20.

Supportive therapy. Cardiac failure should be treated as necessary (see p. 290). Valve replacement may be necessary for severe acute mitral or aortic incompetence. Heart block is seldom progressive, and pacemaker therapy is rarely needed. Prolonged bed-rest, particularly in children or adolescents, produces problems of boredom and depression that need to be anticipated and dealt with.

Follow up. If carditis is going to occur, it usually does so within a week or two of the onset of arthritis. Chronic rheumatic heart disease is much commoner in patients who have had carditis during the initial attack or a recurrence. It is important to prevent recurrence by continuing antistreptococcal prophylaxis, and to recognise and follow up chronic valve lesions, but at the same time it is important not to induce a cardiac neurosis. Echocardiography is useful in detecting valve problems; if it is normal initial yearly follow-ups can be extended to two yearly, and discontinued ten years after the initial attack.

CHRONIC RHEUMATIC HEART DISEASE

Aetiology
In 'Western' countries rheumatic mitral stenosis usually presents between the ages of 20 and 50, but it may

present much earlier in tropical countries. The individual valve lesions which may result from chronic rheumatic heart disease are described in detail below.

Clinical features

The main pathological process in chronic rheumatic heart disease is a progressive fibrosis particularly affecting the heart valves. This is in contrast to the destructive lytic process in acute rheumatic fever. In the mitral valve the result is often fusion of the cusps with a reduction in size of the valve orifice and consequent mitral stenosis. Distortion and rigidity of the cusps can also cause incompetence. Aortic stenosis and incompetence can similarly result from damage to the aortic valve. Once valve damage has proceeded beyond a certain point, the altered haemodynamic stresses on the valve help to perpetuate the damage even in the absence of a continuing rheumatic process.

DISEASES OF THE HEART VALVES

GENERAL PRINCIPLES

A diseased valve may be narrowed (stenosed) or it may fail to close adequately, and thus permit regurgitation of blood. The term 'incompetence' may be used synonymously with regurgitation or reflux, but the latter are preferable. The principal causes of valve disease are summarised in the information box below.

PRINCIPAL CAUSES OF VALVE DISEASE

Valve stenosis	*Valve regurgitation*
Congenital	Congenital
Acute rheumatic carditis	Acute rheumatic carditis
Chronic rheumatic carditis	Chronic rheumatic carditis
Senile degeneration	Infective endocarditis
	Syphilitic aortitis
	Valve ring dilatation
	Traumatic valve rupture
	Senile degeneration

The aetiology of individual valve lesions is considered separately below.

MITRAL STENOSIS

Aetiology

In about half the patients there is a history of rheumatic fever or chorea. The gradual scarring process in the heart takes many years to develop fully. The commis-

sures of the mitral valve become adherent and the chordae tendineae are short and deformed. The mitral valve orifice is about 5 cm^2 in diastole in health, and is reducted to about 1 cm^2 in severe mitral stenosis. With the reduction in size of the valve orifice, cardiac output can be maintained only by a rise in left atrial, pulmonary venous and pulmonary capillary pressures, with resulting loss of lung compliance. A sudden increase in pulmonary venous pressure, caused perhaps by the onset of atrial fibrillation, may precipitate pulmonary oedema. With a more gradual rise in pressure, there tends to be an increase in pulmonary vascular resistance which protects against pulmonary oedema.

In about 80% of cases left atrial dilatation is prominent, and may be accompanied by atrial fibrillation. In a minority, the left atrium remains small but becomes hypertrophied and sinus rhythm tends to persist in spite of severe stenosis. All cases may develop pulmonary hypertension and right ventricular hypertrophy, but this is often more severe in those who remain in sinus rhythm. All patients with mitral stenosis are at risk from left atrial thrombosis and systemic thromboembolism, particularly those with atrial fibrillation. Mitral stenosis is frequently associated with mitral regurgitation or disease of the aortic or tricuspid valves.

Clinical features

The main features of mitral stenosis are tabulated in the information box below.

CLINICAL FEATURES OF MITRAL STENOSIS

- Cause
  - Usually rheumatic
- Clinical presentation
  - Exertional dyspnoea
  - Acute pulmonary oedema (esp. with pregnancy or AF)
  - Chronic right heart failure
- Clinical diagnosis
  - Loud first heart sound
  - Opening snap
  - Mid-diastolic murmur
- ECG
  - Left atrial hypertrophy or AF
  - Right ventricular hypertrophy
- CXR
  - Prominent left atrial appendage
- Echo
  - Characteristic M-mode, 2D and Doppler features
- Treatment
  - Medical – diuretics, digoxin, anticoagulants
  - Surgical – mitral valvulotomy, valvuloplasty or valve replacement

---

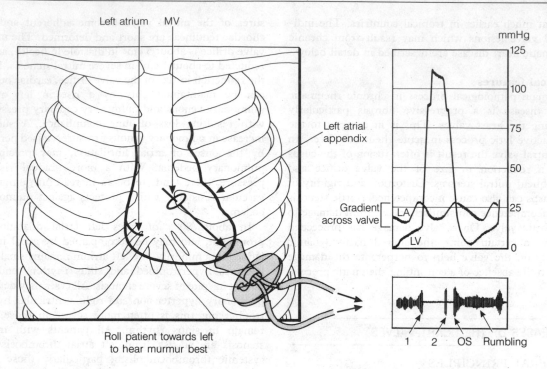

Fig. 8.45 Features of mitral stenosis. The opening snap is often best heard at the left sternal edge, the rumbling mid-diastolic murmur is characteristically loudest at the apex. A phonocardiogram is shown at the bottom right. Above it are left ventricular and left atrial pressure traces to show the relation of the murmur to the left atrial – left ventricular pressure gradient in diastole.

The gradual reduction in the mitral valve orifice usually produces breathlessness in about the third decade. The extra demands of pregnancy, or the impairment of function brought about by tachycardia or atrial fibrillation may precipitate a deterioration, and may bring on breathlessness even at rest. Pulmonary congestion may cause a cough, and pulmonary hypertension lead to haemoptysis. Systemic embolism is sometimes presenting feature.

Diastolic murmur
In some patients with mitral stenosis the face may have a malar flush but this is not specific. The major signs are those which are due to the abnormal valve (p. 258). It closes with an unusually loud sound which may be palpable – the tapping apex beat. The turbulent flow, which is heralded by the opening snap, causes the characteristic diastolic murmur, and often a thrill (Fig. 8.45). The murmur may be accentuated during atrial systole, and in early or asymptomatic patients this presystolic murmur may be the only auscultatory abnormality. In patients with symptoms the murmur usually extends from the opening snap to the first heart sound. The opening snap may be inaudible if the valve

is heavily calcified. Accompanying mitral regurgitation may cause a pansystolic murmur.

Signs of pulmonary hypertension
An *abnormal pulsation* is often felt to the left of the sternum; this may be due either to right ventricular hypertrophy or to forward displacement of the heart by a dilated left atrium. Pulmonary hypertension may cause a loud pulmonary component of the second heart sound, and right atrial hypertrophy may produce a prominent *a* wave in the jugular venous pulse. Tricuspid regurgitation secondary to right ventricular dilatation causes a systolic murmur and systolic waves in the venous pulse.

Asymptomatic mitral stenosis
The physical signs of mitral stenosis are often found before symptoms develop, and their recognition is of particular importance in the obstetric department, since the identification of mitral disease allows appropriate decisions to be made about its management.

Investigation
The ECG may show either the bifid P waves associated

with left atrial hypertrophy or atrial fibrillation. There may be evidence of right ventricular hypertrophy; one of the earliest signs is a reduction in the size of the usual QS complex in lead V1. Enlargement of the left atrium and its appendage and of the main pulmonary artery may be seen on the chest radiograph (Fig. 8.45). There may be enlargement of the upper pulmonary veins and horizontal linear shadows in the costophrenic angles as indications of a high left atrial and pulmonary venous pressure. In the lateral and right anterior oblique position an enlarged left atrium causes a backward displacement of the barium-filled oesophagus.

Echocardiography is very useful in the evaluation of mitral stenosis; apart from confirming the diagnosis it allows an estimate to be made of its severity and it also provides information on the rigidity and state of calcification of the valve cusps, the size of the left atrium, and the state of left ventricular function (Fig. 8.14, p. 265). Cardiac catheterisation has been extensively used to confirm the severity of mitral stenosis by measurement of the gradient across the mitral valve from recording pressures simultaneously in the left ventricle and left atrium (or pulmonary arterial wedge position). Increasing confidence in echocardiography has considerably reduced the need for this, although catheterisation may still have a role in assessing mitral regurgitation and associated coronary disease.

The main features of mitral reflux are listed in the information box below.

CLINICAL FEATURES OF MITRAL REFLUX

- Cause
   Rheumatic
   Valve degeneration
   Ruptured chorda or papillary muscle
- Clinical presentation
   Exertional dyspnoea
   Pulmonary oedema
   Chronic cardiac failure
- Clinical diagnosis
   Active, dilated left ventricle
   apical pansystolic murmur
- ECG
   Non-specific, AF common
- CXR
   Heart usually enlarged, left atrial enlargement
- Echo
   Dilated left ventricle with vigorous contraction
   Reflux detectable on Doppler
- Treatment
   Medical – Diuretics, afterload reduction, digoxin and anticoagulants for AF
   Surgical – Valve repair or replacement

Management
Patients with minor symptoms should be treated medically, but the definitive treatment of mitral stenosis is surgical – by mitral valvotomy, balloon valvuloplasty or mitral valve replacement. Management in relation to pregnancy is discussed on page 334.

Medical management
This consists of anticoagulants (p. 759) to reduce the risk of systemic embolism, digoxin (0.125–0.25 mg/d) to control the ventricular rate in atrial fibrillation (or to prevent a rapid ventricular rate if atrial fibrillation should develop), diuretics to control pulmonary congestion (p. 290) and antibiotic prophylaxis against infective endocarditis p. 303.

Mitral balloon valvuloplasty. This is the treatment of choice if the appropriate criteria are fulfilled. Closed or open mitral valvotomy has similar criteria, and may be used if the facilities or expertise for valvuloplasty are not available. The criteria are listed in the information box below.

CRITERIA FOR MITRAL VALVULOPLASTY

- Significant symptoms
- Pure mitral stenosis
- No mitral regurgitation
- Mobile, non calcified valve on echo
- Left atrium free of thrombus

Mitral valve replacement. This is indicated if there is substantial mitral reflux, or if the valve is rigid and calcified.

Monitoring and after care. Clinical symptoms are a good guide to the severity of mitral stenosis. The ECG gives evidence of increasing pulmonary hypertension, and the heart size on chest radiography is a useful but not infallible guide to severity. Patients who have had a mitral valvuloplasty or valvotomy should be followed up at 1–2 yearly intervals because restenosis may eventually occur.

MITRAL REGURGITATION

Aetiology

Mitral prolapse
This is also known as 'floppy' mitral valve. It is one of the more common causes of mild mitral regurgitation, and is caused by a congenital abnormality or degenerative myxomatous changes. Mitral prolapse is some-

times a feature of connective tissue disorders such as Marfan's syndrome.

In the mildest forms of mitral prolapse the valve bulges back into the atrium during systole, causing a mid-systolic click, but remains competent and so produces no murmur. Frequently however the click is followed by a late systolic murmur, and the combination of mid-systolic click and late systolic murmur is the clinical hallmark of mitral prolapse. Sometimes multiple clicks are heard, while in other cases prolapse occurs at the start of systole, the click is obscured by the first heart sound, and the pansystolic murmur is indistinguishable from other causes of mitral regurgitation. The physical signs may vary with posture or respiration.

Progressive elongation of the chordae tendineae may lead to increasing mitral regurgitation, while if chordal rupture occurs, regurgitation may suddenly become severe. These complications are rare before the fifth or sixth decade.

Mitral prolapse is associated with an increased incidence of arrhythmias; these are usually benign but a small minority of patients have frequent and bizarre arrhythmias and perhaps an increased risk of sudden death. Many patients found to have mitral prolapse present with atypical chest pain but the specificity of this association is uncertain. Telling a patient there is an abnormal valve sometimes exacerbates or perpetuates a cardiac neurosis. Mitral prolapse is more common than would be expected in young people with embolic stroke or transient cerebral ischaemic attacks, but the overall risk of the complication is very small and prophylactic treatment unwarranted in the absence of previous embolic symptoms. Mitral prolapse can predispose to infective endocarditis but overall, the long-term prognosis is good.

Other causes of mitral regurgitation
This can also result from dilatation of the mitral valve ring in association with diseases involving the myocardium, such as rheumatic fever, diphtheria, myocarditis or cardiomyopathy. Papillary muscle dysfunction or rupture may follow myocardial infarction. The valve cusps may be damaged gradually from chronic rheumatic heart disease, in which case there is often coexisting mitral stenosis and/or aortic valve disease. Mitral regurgitation may develop quickly with infective endocarditis.

Clinical features
These are summarised in the information box (p. 295).

The symptoms depend on how suddenly the regurgitation develops. When the valve damage is a slow process the symptoms are similar to those in mitral stenosis. In myocardial disease, the mitral regurgitation exacerbates an already serious situation.

The physical signs arise from the regurgitant jet which causes an apical systolic murmur. This often radiates into the axilla, and may be accompanied by a thrill. The apex beat is usually displaced to the left as a result of dilatation of the left ventricle. The abnormal valve closure is often associated with a quiet first heart sound, and the increased forward flow through the mitral valve may give rise to a loud third heart sound or a short mid-diastolic murmur.

Investigation
The radiograph and ECG often give evidence of left atrial or left ventricular hypertrophy. Atrial fibrillation is common as a consequence of atrial dilatation. Echocardiography provides information about the state of the mitral valve, but Doppler cardiography gives a better estimate of the extent of regurgitation. At cardiac catheterisation the severity of mitral regurgitation may be indicated by the size of the v waves in the left atrial or pulmonary artery wedge trace, or by left ventricular angiography. In practice, the usual problem lies in deciding the extent to which cardiac failure is due to mitral regurgitation and the extent to which it reflects impaired left ventricular function.

Management
If mitral regurgitation is due to myocardial disease, treatment when available is directed to the latter. When the valve disease is predominant and symptoms severe, mitral valve replacement is indicated. Infective endocarditis should be treated if possible before surgery. Mitral regurgitation of moderate severity can be treated medically as shown in the information box (below).

MEDICAL MANAGEMENT OF MITRAL REGURGITATION

- Diuretics (see p. 212 for dose)
- Vasodilators e.g. captopril (p. 290)
- Digoxin if atrial fibrillation is present (p. 276)
- Anticoagulants if atrial fibrillation is present.

Patients who are being managed medically should be reviewed at regular intervals; worsening symptoms or progressive radiological cardiac enlargement are indications for surgical intervention.

AORTIC STENOSIS

Aetiology
The likely aetiology of aortic stenosis varies with the

age of the patient, and possible causes are summarised in the information box below.

CAUSES OF AORTIC STENOSIS

- Infants, children, adolescents
  Congenital aortic stenosis
  Congenital subvalvar aortic stenosis
  Congenital supravalvar aortic stenosis
- Young adults to middle age
  Calcification and fibrosis of congenitally bicuspid aortic valve, rheumatic aortic stenosis
- Middle age to elderly
  Rheumatic aortic stenosis
  Calcification of bicuspid valve
  Senile degenerative aortic stenosis

Except in the congenital forms, aortic stenosis develops slowly; the cardiac output is maintained at the cost of a steadily increasing gradient across the aortic valve. The left ventricle becomes increasingly hypertrophied, and coronary blood flow may become inadequate. In elderly patients aortic stenosis and coronary atheroma may coexist.

Clinical features

These are summarised in the information box below.

CLINICAL FEATURES OF AORTIC STENOSIS

- Clinical presentation
  Exertional dyspnoea
  Angina
  Exertional syncope
  Pulmonary oedema
  Secondary right heart failure
- Clinical diagnosis
  Ejection systolic murmur
  Slow rising carotid pulse
  Left ventricular hypertrophy
- ECG
  Left ventricular hypertrophy (usually)
- CXR
  May be normal. Sometimes enlarged left ventricle and dilated ascending aorta on PA view, calcified valve on lateral view
- Echo
  Calcified valve, thick walled LV, Doppler estimate of gradient
- Management
  Medical – for short-term palliation and inoperable patients
  Valvuloplasty – palliative only
  Surgical – aortic valve replacement

Investigation

The ECG may show left atrial and ventricular hypertrophy, and in advanced cases changes of the latter are gross (Fig. 8.47). In elderly patients the ECG may be normal despite severe stenosis. The postero-anterior chest radiograph is frequently normal, but may show left ventricular enlargement and post stenotic dilatation of the ascending aorta (shown diagrammatically in Fig. 8.46). A lateral radiograph, or radiographic screening, may show valve calcification. Fluttering of the mitral leaflet produces a soft mid-diastolic murmur called an Austin Flint murmur.

Echocardiography will show an abnormal aortic valve, usually heavily calcified and disorganised in the elderly, and a hypertrophied left ventricle. Doppler cardiography can calculate the systolic gradient across the aortic valve from the velocity of the ejected jet of blood. Cardiac catheterisation is indicated if the ultrasound studies are unsatisfactory or if it is wished to assess the state of the coronary arteries.

Management

Patients with severe aortic stenosis (gradient > 70 mm mercury with a normal cardiac output at rest) should have aortic valve replacement irrespective of the severity of symptoms. To wait too long exposes the patient to the risk of sudden death, or irreversible deterioration in ventricular function. In severe congenital aortic stenosis aortic valvotomy may be required as an intermediate measure until an adult-size valve can be inserted. Old age is not a contraindication to valve replacement, and results remain very good even into the ninth decade.

Aortic balloon valvuloplasty is a palliative measure in patients with severe heart failure or intercurrent illness, but long-term results are bad.

Patients with mild aortic stenosis should be followed up with regular cardiac ultrasound examination to detect progression of stenosis.

Anticoagulants are only required in patients who have had a valve replacement with a mechanical prosthesis.

AORTIC REGURGITATION

Aetiology

This results from abnormal aortic cusps as in congenital bicuspid valves, or when valves have been damaged by rheumatic heart disease or infective endocarditis. Aortic regurgitation may also be due to dilatation of the first part of the aorta in cystic medial necrosis, Marfan's syndrome, ankylosing spondylitis, late syphilis or atheroma. When the leak is large the stroke output of

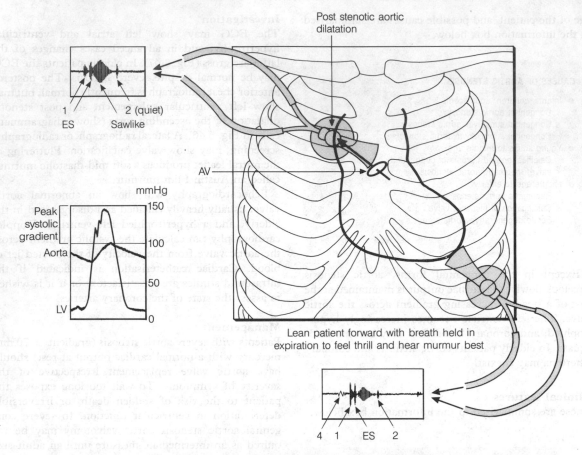

Fig. 8.46 Diagrammatic representation of features of aortic stenosis. The drawing (bottom left) represents pressure tracings from left ventricle and aorta during a cardiac cycle. The phonocardiogram above it shows an ejection sound (ES) as the IV pressure rises above aortic pressure and the valve opens. The ejection systolic murmur corresponds to the period blood is being ejected through the narrow valve. The second heart sound is quiet because the valve is rigid. Note the 'slow rising' aortic pulse contour.

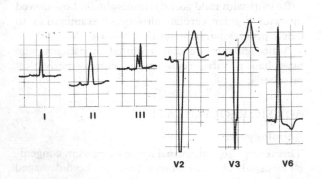

Fig. 8.47 Left ventricular hypertrophy from a 75-year-old woman with aortic stenosis. The QRS complexes in the limb leads I, II and III are slightly widened to 0.10 seconds, but of normal amplitude in this case. However there is a very large S wave in V2 and a large R wave in V6, with T wave inversion in V6.

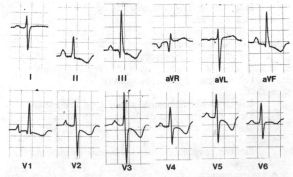

Fig. 8.48 Right ventricular hypertrophy and right atrial hypertrophy. ECG from a 38-year-old woman with primary pulmonary hypertension. There is a tall (3 mm) peaked P wave in leads II and aVF; there is a tall R wave with T wave inversion in the right-sided chest leads V1–V3 and a deep S wave in the left-sided chest leads V4–V6 (see p. 322).

the left ventricle may be doubled or trebled. The major arteries are then conspicuously pulsatile; the left ventricle dilates and hypertrophies and initially compensates for the fault in the valve. The left ventricular diastolic pressure rises, at first only with exercise; the pulmonary vascular pressures then also increase and breathlessness develops.

Clinical features

These are listed in the information box (right). Until the onset of breathlessness the only symptom may be an awareness of the heartbeat, particularly when lying on the left side. Paroxysmal nocturnal dyspnoea may be the first symptom. Peripheral oedema may follow. Angina may occur particularly when there is coexisting coronary atheroma or when the coronary ostia are involved in syphilitic aortitis.

The characteristic murmur is illustrated in Fig. 8.49; although it is usually best heard to the left of the sternum it is sometimes louder to the right, particularly with syphilitic aortitis. A thrill is uncommon. When the leak is small the murmur will be heard only if the steps shown in Fig. 8.49 are followed: this is of crucial importance in the early detection of infective endocarditis affecting the aortic valve. A systolic murmur due to the increased stroke volume is common and should not be regarded as due to accompanying stenosis

CLINICAL FEATURES OF AORTIC REFLUX

- Clinical presentation
  Often asymptomatic
  Left Heart Failure
- Clinical diagnosis
  Collapsing pulse
  Early diastolic murmur
  Austin Flint murmur
  Enlarged left ventricle

- ECG
  Initially normal, later LV hypertrophy and T wave inversion
- CXR
  Cardiac dilatation, may be aortic dilatation
- Echo
  Dilated left ventricle, fluttering anterior mitral leaflet, Doppler detects reflux
- Management
  Medical – diuretics if symptoms mild or patient inoperable. Avoid vasodilators
  Surgical – aortic valve replacement

without other evidence of the latter. When the leak is large the diagnosis is usually easy, with gross pulsation in the large arteries, a collapsing pulse, a low diastolic and an increased pulse pressure. There is usually a thrusting apical impulse and often a presystolic impulse

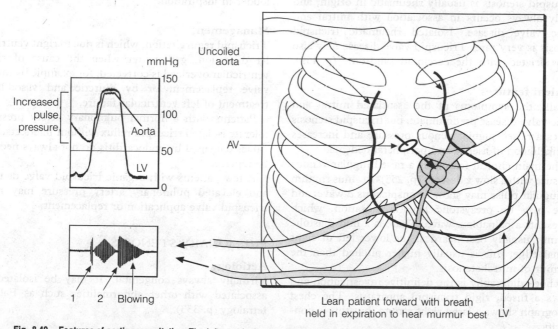

Fig. 8.49 Features of aortic regurgitation. The left ventricular and aortic pressure traces (top left) show the absence of an aortic valve gradient in systole. Aortic pressure falls rapidly in diastole, as blood leaks back through the aortic valve. This is accompanied by an early diastolic murmur best heard at the lower left sternal edge with the patient leaning forward and breathing out.

and a fourth heart sound as evidence of left atrial hypertrophy.

Investigation

The change in the radiographic outline is illustrated in Figure 8.13, page 264. The ECG usually shows left ventricular hypertrophy (Fig. 8.47). Echocardiography in aortic regurgitation often shows fluttering of the anterior mitral leaflet in the regurgitant jet and the jet is usually readily detected by Doppler cardiography. In severe aortic regurgitation the mitral valve may close completely before the onset of ventricular systole. The echocardiogram may reveal vegetations in infective endocarditis, and gives information about left ventricular function. Cardiac catheterisation and aortography are also helpful in assessing severity.

Management

Aortic valve replacement under cardiopulmonary bypass is indicated when aortic regurgitation is beginning to cause symptoms or when an enlarging heart or progressive ECG changes give evidence of increasing left ventricular overload.

TRICUSPID STENOSIS

Aetiology

Tricuspid stenosis is usually rheumatic in origin, and nearly always occurs in association with mitral and aortic valve disease. Isolated rheumatic tricuspid stenosis is very rare. Tricuspid valve disease may also be associated with the carcinoid syndrome (p. 459).

Clinical features

Usually the symptoms of the associated mitral and aortic valve disease predominate, but tricuspid stenosis causes a raised jugular venous pressure and increases the likelihood of ascites and peripheral oedema.

The main clinical feature is a raised jugular venous pressure with a slow x descent (p. 255). In sinus rhythm the jugular pulse may show a conspicuous *a* wave, and there may be presystolic hepatic pulsation, which represents a palpable *a* wave. There is a mid-diastolic murmur usually best heard at the lower left or right sternal edge; this is usually higher pitched than the murmur of mitral stenosis.

Echocardiography is the definitive investigation and shows a fused, rigid tricuspid apparatus. The chest radiograph shows a large right atrium, but this is non-specific.

Management

In patients who require surgery to other valves, the tricuspid valve is either replaced or subjected to valvotomy at the same time. Balloon valvuloplasty is a promising technique for the rare instances of isolated tricuspid stenosis.

TRICUSPID REGURGITATION

Aetiology

Tricuspid regurgitation is common. The most frequent causes are shown in the information box below.

CAUSES OF TRICUSPID REGURGITATION

- Right ventricular dilatation secondary to pulmonary hypertension
- Rheumatic heart disease
- Endocarditis, particularly in intravenous drug abusers
- Right ventricular infarction

Clinical features

Symptoms are usually non-specific. The most prominent clinical feature is a large systolic wave in the jugular venous pulse. Systolic hepatic pulsation may also be present. There is a pansystolic murmur, similar to that of mitral regurgitation but best heard at the lower left or right sternal edge. The murmur gets louder in inspiration.

Management

Tricuspid regurgitation, which is due to right ventricular dilatation, gets better when the cause of right ventricular overload is corrected, for example by mitral valve replacement or by diuretic and vasodilator treatment of left ventricular failure.

Patients with a normal pulmonary artery pressure tolerate isolated tricuspid reflux without ill effects, and valves damaged by endocarditis do not always need to be replaced.

A few patients with organic tricuspid valve damage and elevated pulmonary artery pressure may need tricuspid valve application or replacement.

PULMONARY STENOSIS

Aetiology

Virtually always congenital. It may be isolated or associated with other abnormalities such as Fallot's tetralogy (p. 333).

Clinical features

Mild or moderate pulmonary stenosis is asymptomatic, severe pulmonary stenosis causes right heart failure.

The principal finding on examination is an ejection systolic murmur loudest to the left of the upper sternum, radiating towards the left shoulder. There may be a thrill, best felt when the patient leans forward and breathes out. The murmur is often preceded by an ejection sound. Delay in right ventricular ejection may cause wide splitting of the second heart sound (p. 257).

Severe pulmonary stenosis is characterised clinically by a loud harsh murmur, an increased right ventricular thrust, prominent *a* waves in the jugular pulse, ECG evidence of right ventricular hypertrophy, and post-stenotic dilatation on the chest radiograph. The severity of stenosis can be further assessed by Doppler ultrasound or cardiac catheterisation.

Management

Mild to moderate isolated pulmonary stenosis (resting gradient < 50 mmHg with a normal cardiac output) is common, does not usually progress, and does not require treatment. It is a low-risk lesion for infective endocarditis.

Severe pulmonary stenosis is treated by percutaneous pulmonary balloon valvuloplasty or, if the valve is very rigid, by surgical balloon valvotomy. Long-term results are very good. Postoperative pulmonary regurgitation is common but harmless.

PULMONARY REGURGITATION

Aetiology

Pulmonary regurgitation is rare as an isolated lesion. Most commonly it is associated with pulmonary artery dilatation which is due to pulmonary hypertension (Graham Steell murmur). The pulmonary hypertension may be secondary to disease of the left side of the heart, to primary pulmonary vascular disease, or to Eisenmenger's syndrome.

INFECTIVE ENDOCARDITIS

Aetiology

Infective endocarditis is due to microbial infection of a heart valve or the lining of a cardiac chamber. The causative organism is usually a bacterium, but may be *Coxiella burnettii* (Q fever endocarditis) or a fungus. Clinically and pathologically endocarditis can be divided into *subacute*, *acute* and *postoperative*.

Subacute endocarditis

This is usually due to an organism of relatively low virulence but which is able, under the particular conditions of endocardial infection, to resist the usual defence mechanisms of the host. It occurs at sites where the endothelium is damaged by a high pressure jet of blood (ventricular septal defect, persistent ductus arteriosus, or regurgitant mitral or aortic valves) or on the damaged valves themselves. Endothelial damage leads to the deposition of platelets and fibrin, which are colonised by blood-borne organisms. The avascular valve tissue and presence of fibrin aggregates help to protect the proliferating organisms. Affected valves develop vegetations composed of organisms, fibrin and platelets, which may become large enough to cause obstruction or break away as emboli. Regurgitation may develop or increase owing to the perforation of a cusp. *Mycotic aneurysm* may develop in arteries at the site of infected emboli. At postmortem it is common to find infarction of the spleen and kidneys, and sometimes an immune glomerulonephritis.

The commonest organism is *Streptococcus sanguis* (alpha-haemolytic streptococcus) which is a common cause of peridontal infection and may enter the blood stream at the time of dental treatment. Other streptococci including *Streptococcus faecalis*, *S. milleri* and *S. bovis*, may enter the blood from the bowel or urinary tract. *S. milleri* and *S. bovis* are sometimes associated with large bowel neoplasms. *Coxiella burnettii* is more common in, but not confined to, those who work with sheep or carcases.

Acute endocarditis

This is usually due to a highly virulent and invasive organism, usually *Staphylococcus aureus*, less often *Streptococcus pneumoniae* or *Neisseria gonorrhoea*. It can affect damaged valves, but can also occur in hearts with no previous defect. The tricuspid valve is particularly likely to be affected in main-line drug addicts. Vegetations are more florid and valve destruction greater than in subacute endocarditis, and abscess formation is common.

Postoperative endocarditis

This is endocarditis following cardiac surgery in which prosthetic heart valves or other prosthetic materials are used. The commonest organism is a coagulase – negative staphylococcus (*Staphylococcus albus*). There is frequently a history of postoperative wound infection with the same organism. These patients are also susceptible to the organism causing subacute and acute endocarditis.

Clinical features

Subacute endocarditis. It should be suspected when a patient known to have congenital or valvular heart disease develops a persistent fever or complains of unusual tiredness or depression. Less often, it presents as an embolic stroke or peripheral arterial embolism. Other features include purpura and petechial haemorrhages in the skin and mucous membranes, and splinter haemorrhages under the fingernails. Osler's nodes are painful tender swellings at the finger tips, probably the result of vasculitis. They are rare. Finger clubbing is a late sign. The spleen is frequently palpable; in coxiella infections both it and the liver may be considerably enlarged. Microscopic haematuria is common. The finding of any of these features in a patient with persistent fever or malaise is an indication for re-examination for hitherto unrecognised heart disease.

Acute endocarditis. This usually presents as a severe febrile illness with prominent and changing heart murmurs. Embolic events are common, and cardiac or renal failure may develop rapidly. Partially treated acute endocarditis behaves like subacute endocarditis.

Postoperative endocarditis. This may resemble subacute or acute endocarditis depending on the virulence of the organism. Any unexplained fever in a patient who has had heart valve surgery should be regarded as endocarditis until this can be excluded.

Investigation

Blood culture is the crucial investigation. It should identify the infection and give guidance about management. Three specimens taken at intervals of 2–3 hours should be sufficient.

Echocardiography is valuable for detecting and following the progress of vegetations, for investigating valve damage, and for detecting abscess formation. Vegetations are sometimes too small for echocardiographic detection, especially against the background of a chronically-diseased valve.

Elevation of the ESR, a normocytic, normochromic anaemia and leukocytosis are common but not invariable. Measurement of plasma C-reactive protein is sometimes more reliable than the ESR in assessing progress.

Management

The basic objective is to give a suitable antibiotic for a long enough period (Table 8.4). Any source of infection should be removed if possible, for example a tooth with an apical abscess should be extracted. Cardiac surgery is indicated if valve damage causes progressive cardiac failure, if the endocarditis involves a prosthetic valve, if there are large vegetations on a left-sided valve (risk of embolism) or if active infection persists in spite of adequate treatment. Persisting

Table 8.4 Antibiotic treatment of infective endocarditis

Organism	Antibiotic	Dose		Period	Notes
Streptococci highly sensitive to penicillin	Benzylpenicillin plus gentamycin followed by: ampicillin (oral)	1.2g i.v. 80 mg 500 mg	6-hourly 8-hourly 6-hourly	2 weeks 2 weeks 2 weeks	1, 2
Streptococci less sensitive to penicillin	as above but continue gentamycin for 4 weeks				
Staphylococci	Flucloxacillin Fusidic acid	2g i.v. 580 mg i.v.	6-hourly 8-hourly	6 weeks	3
Staphylococci in patients allergic to penicillin	Vancomycin Fusidic acid	500 mg i.v. 580 mg i.v.	6-hourly 8-hourly	6 weeks	4
Anaerobic streptococci	Benzylpenicillin Metronidazole	as above 500 mg oral or i.v. 8-hourly		4–6 weeks	
Coxiella Burnetii	Tetracycline	500 mg-1g i.v.	12-hourly		5

Notes:
1. Gentamycin: reduce dose to 60 mg if patient <60 kg. Reduce frequency if renal function impaired. Monitor plasma concentration to be <10 μg/ml (peak) and <2 μg/ml (trough).
2. Netilmycin may be used instead of gentamycin in the elderly or if renal function is impaired.
3. It may be possible to change to oral medication after 4 weeks depending on response.
4. Adjust dose of vancomycin if renal function impaired.
5. May change to oral therapy after 2 weeks (500 mg 6-hourly).
Doses and intervals shown are based on manufacturer's data sheets, which must be consulted for details. Choice of antibiotic should be based on the known sensitivities of the actual organism, and doses should be adjusted to give an appropriate bactericidal concentration in the patient's serum. Duration of treatment should be guided by clinical response, ESR and protein C measurements.

infection is indicated by continuing fever, changing murmurs, and a persistently elevated ESR or CRP concentration. Antibiotic therapy must be started before surgery.

Prevention

Every patient with heart disease susceptible to infective endocarditis – for practical purposes, every patient with a murmur – should be aware of the risk of endocarditis and of the need to avoid bacteraemia. Measures to be taken are summarised in the information box (right).

PREVENTION OF INFECTIVE ENDOCARDITIS

- Ensure and maintain good dental health
- Antibiotic cover for events likely to lead to bacteraemia
- Dental procedures which go below the gum margin, or scaling
    Amoxycillin 3 g orally 1 hour before
    Erythromycin 1.5 g orally 1 hour before plus 500 mg 6 hours after (for penicillin sensitive patients)
- Operations on G.I. or urinary tract
    Ampicillin 1 g i.m. 1 hour before, 500 mg 8-hourly for 48 hours after
  Avoid prolonged antibiotic prophylaxis
  'Blind' antibiotics for undiagnosed fever

ISCHAEMIC (CORONARY) HEART DISEASE

The coronary circulation
The right coronary artery arises from the right sinus of Valsalva and passes in the right atrioventricular groove to supply the right ventricle, part of the interventricular septum and the inferior part of the left ventricle; a branch supplies the AV node. The left coronary artery arises from the left sinus and divides into:

1. an anterior descending branch, which supplies part of the septum and the anterior and apical parts of the heart;
2. the circumflex branch, which passes in the left atrioventricular groove and supplies the lateral and posterior surfaces of the heart (Fig. 8.50)

In health there are small anastomoses between the coronary arteries; these enlarge under the influence of ischaemia if the flow through a neighbouring coronary artery is compromised. With advancing years an extensive network of anastomotic vessels may develop.

Aetiology

Apart from rare congenital anomalies, most coronary disease is due to atheroma and its complications. The basic atheromatous lesion is the plaque – this is a fibrous thickening of the intima of the vessel with destruction of the internal elastic lamina and invasion of the intima by medial smooth muscle cells. In some plaques cholesterol-rich material accumulates and lies

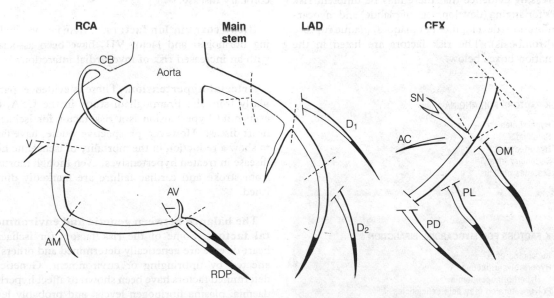

Fig. 8.50   Diagram of the human coronary arterial system. RCA Right coronary artery, LAD Left anterior descending coronary artery, CFX Circumflex coronary artery. D1 Diagonal branches, OM Obtuse marginal branch of circumflex.

between the fibrous 'cap' of the plaque and the rest of the vessel wall. These lesions tend to bulge into the lumen of the coronary artery and narrow it. Sometimes haemorrhage occurs into a plaque, or its fibrous cap becomes cracked or partially detached. The unsupported 'flap' of intima may further narrow the lumen, and the exposed thrombogenic material with the plaque may precipitate thrombosis, thus completely blocking the vessel. In Western countries, evidence of coronary atheroma is often apparent in young adulthood. The number and state of evolution of plaques both increase with age, but the rate of progression of individual plaques, even in the same patient, is very variable.

The causes of coronary disease can be studied either in animal models or by looking for associations between clinical coronary disease and variables such as smoking and plasma cholesterol. Animal models do not accurately reproduce human pathology, and epidemiological studies are often unable to distinguish between risk *factors*, which bear a causative relation to the disease, and risk *marker*, where the variable measured is not the cause, but is linked to something which is. It is also important to distinguish between *relative risk* and *absolute risk*. Thus a man of 35 with a plasma cholesterol of 10 mMol/litre who smokes 40 cigarettes a day is many times more likely to die from coronary disease within the next decade than a non-smoking woman of the same age with a normal cholesterol, but his actual likelihood of dying during this time is still very small (high relative risk, low absolute risk). There is increasing evidence that there may be different risk factors for angina (development of plaque) and myocardial infarction (development of plaques, plaque rupture and thrombosis). The risk factors are listed in the information boxes below.

RISK FACTORS FOR ANGINA

- Hypercholesterolaemia
- Smoking
- Hypertension
- Sedentary lifestyle
- Diabetes mellitus

RISK FACTORS FOR MYOCARDIAL INFARCTION

As for angina plus
- Hypertriglyceridaemia
  Hyperfibrinogenaemia
- Polyunsaturated fatty acid deficiencies
- Raised plasma factor VII levels

Smoking. There is evidence of a strong, consistent and dose-linked relationship between cigarette smoking and ischaemic heart disease. The relative risk of death from ischaemic heart disease for smokers compared to non-smokers is highest in younger patients and declines in older age groups.

Cholesterol. Patients with hereditary hypercholesterolaemia have a high incidence of precocious coronary disease. In population studies, there is a positive correlation between mean population plasma cholesterol concentration and morbidity and death from coronary disease. Clinical trials have been shown that lowering high cholesterol concentrations by diet or drugs reduce the risk of cardiac events (though sometimes at the cost of other morbidity).

Other dietary factors. Diets deficient in polyunsaturated fatty acids are associated with an increased risk of coronary disease. This may be independent of the tendency of diets with a high polyunsaturated/saturated ratio to lower cholesterol. Low vitamin C and vitamin E are risk factors for coronary disease, but part of this may be explained by a smoker's dislike for foods rich in vitamin C.

Diabetes mellitus. This is associated with an increased incidence of ischaemic heart disease and with a tendency to diffuse coronary atheroma. In some part of the world, diabetes is one of the major risk factors for coronary disease.

Blood coagulation factors. These factors, including fibrinogen and factor VII, have been associated with an increased risk of myocardial infarction.

Arterial hypertension. There is evidence, particularly from the Framingham study in the USA, that even mild hypertension is a risk factor for ischaemic heart disease. However, prospective studies have failed to show a reduction in the mortality of ischaemic heart disease in treated hypertensives, even though mortality from stroke and cardiac failure are markedly diminished.

The balance between genetic and environmental factors. Some of the risk factors for ischaemic heart disease are genetically determined and others are affected by upbringing or environment. Genetically determined factors have been shown to affect hyperlipidaemia, plasma fibrinogen levels, and probably levels of other blood coagulation factors. At present it is estimated that about 40% of the risk of developing ischaemic heart disease is controlled by genetic, and 60% by environmental factors.

ANGINA PECTORIS

Angina pectoris is the name for a clinical syndrome rather than a disease. The term is used to describe a discomfort due to transient myocardial ischaemia. Coronary atheroma is the commonest cause. The obstruction produced by atheroma may be exacerbated by spasm; occasionally coronary spasm occurs in the absence of atheroma. Angina is made worse by factors which increase myocardial oxygen requirements. These factors are listed in the information box below.

FACTORS WHICH INCREASE MYOCARDIAL OXYGEN REQUIREMENT OR REDUCE SUPPLY

- Increase preload
    Exercise
    Anaemia
    Hyperthyroidism
- Increase afterload
    Hypertension
    Aortic stenosis
- Reduced diastolic
    coronary flow
    Tachycardia
    Aortic regurgitation

Clinical features

The history is by far the most important factor in making the diagnosis. Angina pectoris is usually experienced as a sense of oppression or tightness in the middle of the chest – 'like a band round the chest'; when describing it the patient commonly places the hand or clenched fist on the sternum, or both hands on the lower chest with the fingers touching at the sternum. It is usually induced by exertion and relieved by rest, lasting only a few minutes. Angina is likely to be worse when walking against a wind, uphill, on a cold day, and particularly after meals. Some patients find that the pain comes when they start walking and that later it does not return despite greater effort. Others can 'walk it off'. Some experience the pain when lying flat (*angina decubitus*), and some are awakened by it (*nocturnal angina*) particularly with 'energetic' or alarming dreams. Rarely, pain may come capriciously as a result of coronary arterial spasm, and be accompanied by transient ST elevation in the ECG (*Prinzmetal's or variant angina*). The situations precipitating angina are listed in the information box (right, top).

The pain is often accompanied by discomfort in the arms, more commonly the left, the wrists and sometimes the hands; the patient may describe a feeling of uselessness in the limbs. Angina may more rarely be

---

CLINICAL SITUATIONS PRECIPITATING ANGINA

- Physical exertion e.g. walking
- Cold exposure
- Heavy meals
- Intense emotion
- Lying flat (decubitus angina)
- Violent dreams (nocturnal angina)

---

epigastric or interscapular or may radiate to the neck and jaw, or occur at any of these places of reference without chest discomfort. The precipitation by effort or anxiety, and the relief by rest or with the use of glyceryl trinitrate, should allow the pain to be recognised. There may be accompanying breathlessness. Pain may sometimes be induced by a cardiac arrhythmia.

Physical examination is frequently negative, but evidence of contributory or concomitant disease should be sought. The presence of tendon xanthomas, thickening of the achilles tendons and an arcus lipidis in a young patient may indicate a hereditary hyperlipidaemia. Aortic valve disease, particularly aortic stenosis, may cause angina. The patient should be examined for anaemia, obesity, diabetes, thyroid and peripheral vascular disease. Other diseases are listed in the information box below.

ANGINA: CONTRIBUTORY OR CONCOMITANT DISEASE

- Hypertension
- Hyperlipidaemia
    Tendon xanthomas, corneal arcus, xanthelasma
- Anaemia
- Obesity
- Diabetes mellitus
- Myxoedema
- Peripheral vascular disease

Investigation

Electrocardiography. The ECG is normal in most patients at rest between attacks. Occasionally T wave flattening or inversion may be seen in some leads; this is non-specific evidence of myocardial ischaemia or damage. A few patients may show ECG signs of established infarction (p. 312). The most convincing ECG evidence is the demonstration of reversible ST segment depression or elevation, with or without T wave inversion, at the time the patient is experiencing symptoms – whether spontaneous or induced by exer-

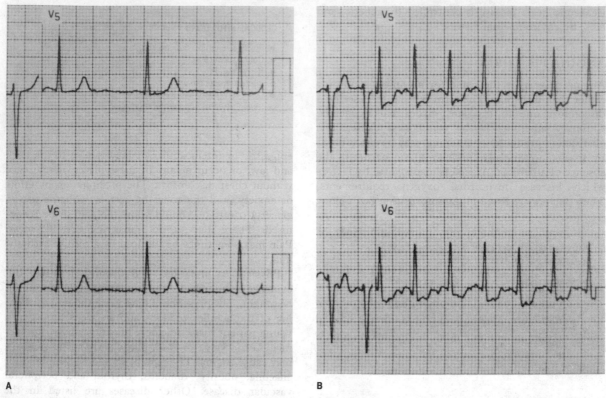

A   **B**

Fig. 8.51   Electrocardiogram showing ST segment depression during exercise on a treadmill. A. V_5 and V_6 from resting ECG in patient with angina. **B.** V_5 and V_6 from same patient during exercise test showing ST segment depression.

cise testing (Fig. 8.51). Formal exercise testing is usually done using a treadmill or bicycle ergometer and a standard procedure which ensures a progressive and reproducible increase in work load. Exercise testing should be done only where resuscitation facilities are available and the test should be stopped if the patient develops significant chest pain or discomfort or suffers arrhythmias or a fall in blood pressure. The amount of exercise which can be tolerated under these conditions is a useful guide to the extent of coronary disease.

Scanning. Myocardial perfusion scanning using radioactive thallium may be helpful, in conjunction with exercise testing, in evaluating the minority of patients with an atypical history, or the small group who have severe symptoms but no significant ECG abnormality on exercise testing. Echocardiography or radionuclide bloodpool scanning provide information about ventricular function, which may be relevant in making a decision about coronary arteriography.

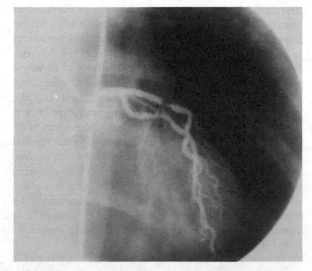

Fig. 8.52   Coronary arteriogram from a patient with angina. There is a severe stenosis (narrowing) of the left anterior descending coronary artery.

Coronary arteriography. This provides detailed information about the extent and site of coronary artery stenosis. It is usually performed with a view to subsequent coronary bypass grafting or angioplasty (p. 309). In a small minority it may be indicated when a full range of non-invasive tests have failed to elucidate the cause of atypical chest pain.

Differential diagnosis

This includes musculoskeletal, pericardial and oesophageal pain. Musculoskeletal pains are provoked by specific movement rather than by walking, and background pain often persists at rest. There may be marked tenderness over the coastal cartilages and manubriosternal angle. The pain of pericarditis is occasionally provoked by exercise, but its other characteristics (p. 327) should help to make the distinction. Angina occurring at rest may be confused with oesophagitis, with or without a hiatus hernia, but pain due to oesophagitis usually has a burning quality and is relieved by alkalis. Oesophageal spasm however causes a different type of pain which may be difficult to distinguish from variant angina.

Management

Management of angina pectoris involves three phases: a proper assessment of the severity of the symptoms and the likely extent of the disease; the use of measures to control symptoms; and treatment which will improve life expectancy. The first phase has been discussed under diagnosis, and a suggested sequence of investigation is shown as a flow chart in Fig. 8.53.

Control of symptoms should start with an explanation of how they are caused. Patients usually respond to a careful presentation of the problem as what it is – a mismatch between coronary supply and cardiac needs. The natural process of repair by development of anastomoses should be stressed. Patients can then learn how to help themselves, e.g. by avoiding walking after meals, particularly in the cold or against a wind, and by avoiding severe unaccustomed exertion. They may need encouragement and support in their endeavours to stop smoking and to lose weight. In a few patients

---

ADVICE TO PATIENTS WITH ANGINA

- Do not smoke
- Aim at ideal body weight
- Take regular exercise – exercise up to, but not beyond, point of chest pain is beneficial
- Avoid severe unaccustomed exertion, vigorous exercise after a heavy meal, or in very cold weather

---

hyperlipidaemia requires treatment by diet and other measures (p. 697). The information box (left) lists advice for patients.

Drug treatment

There are three principal groups of drugs which help to relieve or prevent the symptoms of angina: nitrates, beta-adrenoceptor antagonists (beta-blockers) and calcium antagonists.

Nitrates. Fresh glyceryl trinitrate (GTN 500 micrograms), allowed to dissolve under the tongue or crunched for more rapid effect and retained in the mouth, usually relieves the pain in 2–3 minutes, and about the same time it often produces a slight headache. The headache may become severe in some patients if the tablet is left in the mouth, so the patient should be instructed to spit it out or swallow it once the angina is relieved.

The best use of GTN is prophylactically before exercise known as liable to produce pain. The beneficial effect comes from venous and arteriolar dilatation, which lowers the blood pressure and also dilates the coronary vessels provided their disease does not prevent this. Patients can be reassured that GTN is not dangerous or habit forming. The tablets themselves have a limited shelf life, particularly if kept in a warm place. Not more than about 2 tablets per hour should be used; if the requirement for it increases significantly the patient should seek medical advice. The appropriate use of GTN (or other drugs) allows more exercise to be taken; this should be encouraged because physical activity promotes the formation of collateral vessels.

As sublingual GTN has a short duration of action, there has been much interest in ways of giving more prolonged nitrate therapy. GTN can be given percutaneously as a paste or plasters (5–10 mg 12-hourly), or as a slow-release buccal tablet (1–5 mg 6-hourly). Some patients find these helpful, but they are more expensive than sublingual tablets. GTN is virtually ineffective when swallowed, but other nitrates such as isosorbide dinitrate (10 mg or more, 3–6 per day) can be given by mouth. Headache is common when patients are started on oral nitrates, but tends to improve on persevering with the therapy. Tolerance frequently occurs, and the dose needs to be increased to maintain efficacy. A nitrate free period of 1–2 hours every 24 hours helps to prevent the development of tachyphylaxis, and long-acting oral nitrates should not be administered more frequently than every 12 hours.

Beta-blockade. This is an important and effective way of preventing angina. It helps to reduce myocardial

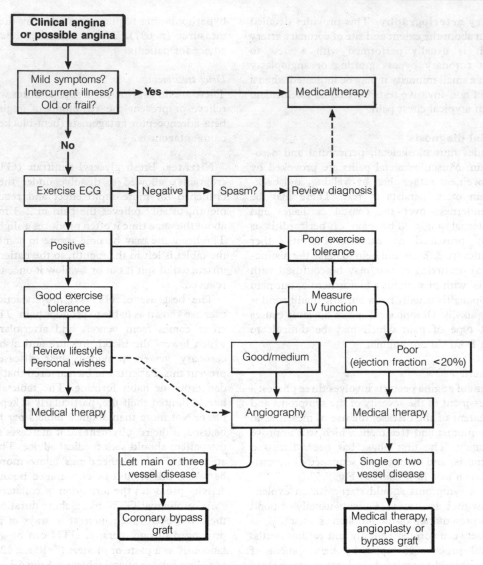

Fig. 8.53 Angina pectoris – sequence of investigation and treatment.

oxygen demand, largely by reducing the heart rate for a given level of exercise, and by reducing the heart rate response to anxiety. *Propranolol* can be prescribed initially in small doses (e.g. 20 mg 6-hourly) with progressive increments until benefit is obtained, which is often not until the resting heart rate has been significantly slowed. There is considerable individual variation and as much as 160 mg 6-hourly or even more may be required. Other beta-blockers are probably no more effective than propranolol but may have the advantages of less individual dose variation, once daily administration and possibly, in the case of cardioselec-

tive agents, fewer peripheral side-effects. These matters are discussed, together with other properties of beta-blocking drugs, on page 320. A beta-blocking drug should not be withdrawn abruptly because of the risks of dangerous arrhythmias and myocardial infarction.

Calcium antagonists. These are so-called because they inhibit the slow inward current caused by the entry of extracellular calcium through the cell membrane of excited cells, particularly arteriolar smooth muscle and cardiac atrial cells. In arterioles, the result is vasodilatation and hence a fall in blood pressure. In

Table 8.5   Calcium antagonists in angina

Name	Dose	Comment	Side-effects
Nifedipine	5–20 mg t.i.d.	Can cause tachycardia, best combined with beta-blocker	Oedema, rashes, myocardial depression
Nicardipine	20–40 mg t.i.d.	Less myocardial depression than nifedipine	
Verapamil	120–240 mg t.i.d.	May cause bradycardia	Constipation
Diltiazem	60–120 mg t.i.d.	Similar to verapamil but less bradycardia	

cardiac muscle, the principal effects are a reduction in excitability and conductivity, with large doses causing reduced contractility (Table 8.5).

Although each of these groups of drugs can be shown to be superior to placebo in treating symptoms of angina, there is little convincing evidence that one group is more effective than another. The author's present policy is to start with sublingual GTN, to progress to a beta-blocker unless there are contraindications and then to add nifedipine or a long-acting nitrate such as isosorbide dinitrate. The ultimate aim of achieving excellent control of angina with minimal side-effects and the simplest possible tablet regimen is unlikely to be reached without trial and error.

Surgical treatment

'Surgical' treatment of ischaemic heart disease may involve coronary angioplasty (sometimes called PTCA for percutaneous transluminal coronary angioplasty), saphenous vein bypass grafting or internal mammary artery grafting.

Coronary angioplasty. This is performed by passing a fine guidewire across a coronary stenosis under radiographic control and using it to position a balloon which is then inflated to dilate the stenosis (Fig. 8.54). It is mainly used in single or two-vessel disease. The main complication is occlusion of the vessel by thrombus or by a loose flap of intima. This occurs in about 2–5% of procedures and may necessitate urgent coronary bypass grafting. The stenosis reoccurs in 20–30% of cases, but can usually be redilated. Aspirin reduces the risk of early thrombosis, but not of restenosis. Coronary angioplasty is an effective symptomatic treatment for chronic stable angina. It has mainly been used in groups with a low mortality risk, and there is no evidence it improves survival. It is also used in unstable angina and post-infarct angina. There is no evidence that routine angioplasty is indicated following thrombolytic therapy for myocardial infarction.

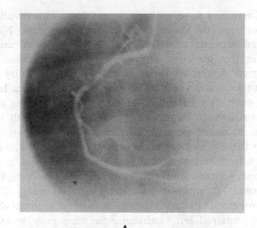

A

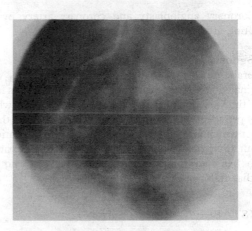

B

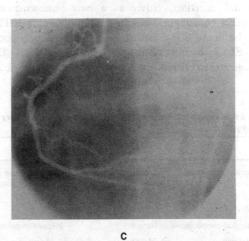

C

Fig. 8.54   Coronary angioplasty. Series of frames of a coronary arteriogram of the right coronary artery. **A.** shows a coronary stenosis. **B.** A balloon has been guided across the stenosis and inflated. **C.** The stenosis has been dilated.

Coronary artery bypass grafting. This involves major surgery under cardiopulmonary bypass. Narrowed segments of coronary artery are bypassed using either free grafts of saphenous vein or the patient's internal mammary arteries. Operative mortality is about 1%, and about 80% of patients are angina free one year after surgery. Coronary bypass grafting has been shown to improve survival in patients with left main coronary stenosis, and in symptomatic patients with three vessel coronary disease (i.e. disease involving left anterior descending, circumflex and right coronary arteries) or two vessel disease involving the proximal left anterior descending coronary artery. The improvement in survival is most marked in those who have impaired left ventricular function prior to surgery.

Coronary angioplasty and coronary artery bypass grafting are compared in Table 8.6 below.

Prognosis

Overall, more than half of a group of patients with angina will live for 5 years, and a third for 10 years from the time of diagnosis. Spontaneous recovery, which may prove temporary, may occur in as many as a third, a fact which is useful to remember in talking to patients about their disease. Prognosis is worse in the patient who has had multiple cardiac infarcts or who has cardiac failure.

UNSTABLE ANGINA

Unstable angina is anginal pain coming on at rest or minimal exertion, either as a new phenomenon or against a background of chronic stable angina. There may be acute ST segment elevation or depression on the ECG during symptoms, but permanent ECG changes or enzymatic evidence of infarction are absent.

Mechanism

Most cases of unstable angina are due to rupture of an atheromatous plaque in a coronary artery. Either the partially detached 'cap' of the plaque, or associated thrombus, cause severe narrowing of the vessel.

Management

Patients should be admitted to hospital because there is a 10–15% risk of progression to acute myocardial infarction. Initial treatment is with aspirin 300 mg daily to inhibit platelet activation, bed-rest, and a beta-blocker (e.g. metoprolol 100 mg b.d.) to minimise disturbance of the ruptured plaque. Nifedipine can be added to the beta-blocker but should not be used alone – verapamil or diltiagem are preferable if beta-blockers are contraindicated. If pain persists, intravenous nitrates should be started (e.g. isosorbide dinitrate 1–2 mg/h) and the patient referred for coronary angiography. This often shows an isolated severe coronary stenosis which can be treated with angioplasty. If pain settles, the patient can gradually be mobilised as for myocardial infarction, and exercise testing undertaken after 3–4 weeks when the plaque has stabilised.

MYOCARDIAL INFARCTION

This is myocardial necrosis occurring as a result of a critical imbalance between coronary blood supply and myocardial demand.

It is usually due to the formation of occlusive thrombus at the site of rupture of an atheromatous plaque in a coronary artery. The thrombus usually undergoes spontaneous lysis over the course of the next few days, but by this time the damage has been done.

In its mildest forms the infarct may be unrecognised ('silent') and be disclosed subsequently only by ECG evidence; at the other end of the range there is permanent severe disability or death. At the onset of the illness, sudden death, presumably from ventricular

Table 8.6 Comparison between coronary angioplasty and coronary artery bypass grafting

	PTCA	Surgery
Predominately used for	Single vessel disease Two vessel disease Unstable angina	Left main stenosis Three vessel disease
Mortality	<1%	<1%
Neurological complications	None	5%, seldom permanent
Hospital stay	24–36 h	7–10 days
Recurrence	30%, PTCA May be repeated	10% in 1 year then 5% per year
Complications	Vascular	Infection Wound pain

CLINICAL FEATURES OF MYOCARDIAL INFARCTION

- Symptoms
  Pain – like angina but persistent and more severe
  Anxiety – may be fear of impending death
  Vomiting
- Physical findings
  Pallor, sweating and other signs of autonomic activity
  Tachycardia (occasionally bradycardia)
  Low systolic pressure and reduced pulse pressure
  Frequent extrasystoles

fibrillation or asystole, may occur immediately, and many of the patients who die do so within the first hour. If the patient survives this most critical stage, the liability to dangerous arrhythmias remains, but diminishes as each hour goes by. The development of cardiac failure reflects the extent of myocardial damage; its severity may range from slight reduction in skin perfusion and basal lung crepitations at one end to acute circulatory failure at the other. Cardiac failure is the major cause of death in those who survive the first few hours of infarction.

Clinical features

The clinical features are listed in the information box (p. 310). The cardinal symptom is pain, but breathlessness, syncope, vomiting and extreme tiredness are common. The pain occurs in the same sites as for angina but is usually more severe and lasts longer. It is most often described as a tightness, heaviness or constriction in the chest. At its worst the pain is one of the most severe which can be explained and the patient's expression and pallor may vividly convey the seriousness of the situation.

Many patients are breathless and in some this is the only symptom; a few develop pulmonary oedema at the onset. Syncope may occur and the blood pressure falls particularly if the patient is upright, or from the development of a serious arrhythmia or heart block. Vomiting is common, particularly in the more severe cases. It may also result from morphine given for pain relief. In rare cases the infarct may go unnoticed until endocardial thrombosis resulting from it leads to systemic embolism.

At any time after the first 12 hours or so the patient may recognise that a different pain has developed, even though it is at the same site. It is worse, or only appears, on inspiration and may be altered by a change of position. It is due to pericarditis consequent on the infarct, and the diagnosis is confirmed if a pericardial rub is heard.

The principal *physical signs* are summarised in the information box (left). Sometimes infarction may occur in the absence of signs.

Complications

Arrhythmias

Nearly all patients with myocardial infarction have some form of arrhythmia, but in most cases this is mild and of no haemodynamic or prognostic significance. Various degrees of heart block (p. 277) are also frequent.

Ventricular fibrillation occurs in about 5–10% of patients in hospital. The risk is much higher in the first hour after infarction, and ventricular fibrillation is thought to be the major cause of death before reaching hospital. Its potential reversibility in those patients who do not have extensive myocardial damage is one of the main foundations on which the policy of acute coronary care is built. The different arrhythmias are listed in the information box below. Management of these arrythmias is discussed on page 272.

ARRHYTHMIAS IN MYOCARDIAL INFARCTION

- Ventricular fibrillation
- Ventricular tachycardia
- Accelerated idioventricular rhythm
- Ventricular ectopics
- Atrial fibrillation
- Atrial tachycardia
- Heart block

Acute circulatory failure

If there is a reversible arrhythmia as an important contributory factor its correction may bring about considerable improvement. In a few cases excessive diuretic therapy leading to hypovolaemia may be the cause. If neither of these is responsible, acute circulatory failure usually reflects extensive myocardial damage and indicates a bad prognosis. In its presence, all the other complications of myocardial infarction are more likely.

Other complications

Cardiac failure may occur, and pulmonary oedema is its

PHYSICAL SIGNS OF MYOCARDIAL INFARCTION

- Signs of sympathetic activation
  Pallor, sweating, tachycardia
- Signs of vagal activation
  Vomiting, sometimes bradycardia
- Signs of impaired myocardial function
  Raised JVP
  Narrow pulse pressure
  3rd heart sound
  Quiet 1st heart sound
  Diffuse apical impulse
  Lung crepitations
- Signs of tissue damage
  Fever
  Pericardial friction rub
- Complications
  Arrhythmias
  Murmur of ventricular septal defect, mitral regurgitation

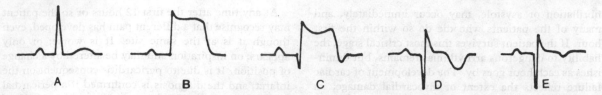

Fig. 8.55   The serial evolution of ECG changes in myocardial infarction. A. Pre-infarct; **B.** ST elevation owing to a myocardial 'injury current', also some reduction in R wave size; **C.** Developing Q wave and terminal T wave inversion; **D.** Established Q wave and T inversion; **E.** 'Old infarct' pattern – the Q wave tends to persist but T wave changes become less marked. The rate of evolution is very variable. In general stage C is usually reached in hours, stage D in days and stage E after some months. This diagrammatic representation should be compared with the actual ECGs in Figures 8.56 and 8.57.

commonest form. Regular examination for basal lung crepitations and chest radiography should lead to its early detection.

Rarer complications include *infarction of a mitral papillary muscle*, which leads to mitral regurgitation and may precipitate pulmonary oedema. *Rupture of the interventricular septum* is diagnosed by the development of the characteristic murmur of a ventricular septal defect (p. 331) and may cause severe hypotension and venous hypertension. Rupture of the ventricle into the pericardial space may lead to *cardiac tamponade* (p. 327).

Embolism, cerebral or peripheral, can occur when a thrombus forms on the endocardium of the left ventricle. *Venous thrombosis* is less common now than when patients were routinely kept in bed for 6 weeks; it often first announces its presence by pulmonary embolism.

The *post-myocardial infarction syndrome* (Dressler's syndrome), which is probably an autoimmune reaction to necrotic myocardium, is characterised by persistent fever, pericarditis and pleurisy. It occurs a few weeks or even months after the infarct and often subsides after a few days but may require aspirin, other anti-inflammatory drugs or corticosteroids for its control if symptoms are prolonged.

Ventricular aneurysm and dyskinetic or akinetic segments (information box, p. 288) can develop later.

Investigation

Electrocardiography

The ECG is usually a sensitive and specific way of confirming the diagnosis, but the typical changes may take some hours to develop. The ECG may also be difficult to interpret after previous infarction and occasionally it will not be significantly altered in spite of clinical and biochemical evidence of re-infarction. The earliest ECG change is usually ST elevation, which reflects acute myocardial injury. At the same time or slightly later there is diminution in the size of

the R wave, and a Q wave begins to develop. One explanation for the Q wave is that the myocardial infarct acts as an 'electrical window' transmitting the changes of potential from within the ventricular cavity, and allowing the ECG to 'see' the reciprocal R wave from the other wall of the ventricle. Subsequently the T wave becomes inverted because of a change in ventricular repolarisation, and this change persists after the ST segment has returned to normal. These features are shown diagrammatically in Fig. 8.55 and their sequence is sufficiently reliable for the approximate age of the infarct to be deduced. In contrast to transmural lesions, with subendocardial infarction there is usually no Q wave or ST elevation, but symmetrical T wave inversion develops.

The ECG changes are best seen in the leads which 'face' the infarcted areas (Fig. 8.8). When there has been anteroseptal infarction abnormalities are found in one or more leads from V1 to V4 (Fig. 8.56) while

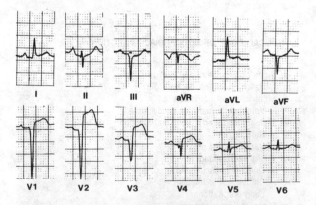

Fig. 8.56   Established anterior myocardial infarct, from a 43-year-old man with chest pain starting 6 hours previously. There are Q waves in leads V2, V3 and V4, ST elevation in the same leads, and loss of the normal R wave pattern in all the chest leads. Anterior infarcts with Q waves most prominent in leads V2, V3 and V4 are sometimes called 'anteroseptal' infarcts to distinguish them from 'anterolateral' infarcts with Q waves most prominent in leads V4, V5 and V6.

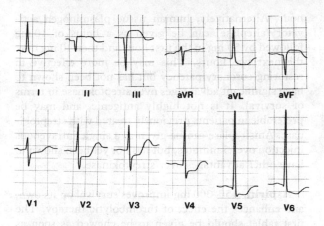

Fig. 8.57 Established inferior myocardial infarction with Q waves and ST elevation in leads II, III and aVF, from a 55-year-old man with a severe episode of chest pain 24 hours before. In this patient there is also 'reciprocal' ST depression in the chest leads V2 to V6.

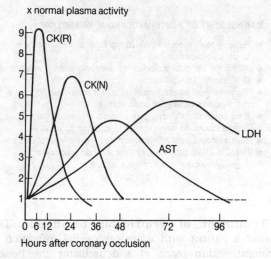

Fig. 8.58 Changes in plasma enzyme concentrations after myocardial infarction. Creatine kinase (CK) is the first to rise, followed by aspartate aminotransferase (AST) and then lactate (hydroxybutyrate) dehydrogenase (LDH). In patients treated with a thrombolytic agent reperfusion is usually accompanied by a rapid rise in plasma creatine kinase (curve CK(R)), whereas if reperfusion does not occur the rise is less rapid (curve CK (N)).

anterolateral infarction produces changes from V4 to V6, in aVL and hence also in lead I. In strict anterior infarction the changes may be confined to V3 and V4. Inferior infarction is best shown in leads II, III and aVF, while leads I, aVL and the lateral chest leads show 'reciprocal' changes of ST depression (Fig. 8.57). Infarction of the posterior wall of the left ventricle is not recorded in the standard leads by ST elevation or Q waves, but the reciprocal changes of ST depression and a tall R wave may be seen in leads V1–V4.

Plasma enzymes
Myocardial infarction leads to a detectable rise in the plasma concentration of enzymes normally confined within cardiac cells. The enzymes most widely used in the detection of myocardial infarction are creatine kinase (CK), asparate aminotransferase (AST) and lactate dehydrogenase (LD). CK starts to rise at 4–6 hours, peaks about 12 hours and falls to normal in 48–72 hours. CK is also present in skeletal muscle, and a rise in CK may be due to an intramuscular injection or vigorous physical exercise. Measurement of the myocardial isoenzyme of CK (CK-MB) is more specific for myocardial damage. AST starts to rise about 12 hours after infarction, and reaches a peak on the first or second day. LD is also liberated from haemolysed red cells and is therefore less specific. It starts to rise after 12 hours, reaches a peak after 2 or 3 days and may be elevated for about a week. LD estimation may be useful when the diagnosis is uncertain several days after a possible infarct. Serial estimations are necessary in doubtful cases, for it is the change in enzyme levels which is of diagnostic value (Fig. 8.58).

Other blood tests
A leucocytosis is usual, reaching a peak on the first day. The ESR becomes raised and may remain so for several days.

Chest radiography
This may demonstrate pulmonary oedema which has been undetected clinically. The heart size is usually normal. Enlargement of the cardiac shadow may indicate previous myocardial damage or a developing pericardial effusion.

Radionuclide scanning (p. 266)
A pyrophosphate scan may show the site of myocardial necrosis. A radionuclide ventriculogram indicates the extent of impairment of ventricular function and may give useful prognostic information.

Management
The essentials in the management of acute myocardial infarction are summarised in the information box (p. 314).

Pain relief. An intravenous cannula should be inserted and opiate analgesia given, e.g. morphine 10 mg plus cyclizine 50 mg ('cyclimorph'). Analgesia should be titrated against the response: patients with large infarcts may need more analgesia.

MANAGEMENT OF ACUTE MYOCARDIAL INFARCTION

- Relieve pain: morphine 10–20 mg i.v. plus cyclizine 50 mg or prochlorperazine 12.5–25 mg
- Watch for ventricular fibrillation and defibrillate if needed
- Oral aspirin 150–300 mg
- Thrombolysis: streptokinase 1 500 000 units over 60 minutes *or* alteplase *or* anistreplase
- If no cointraindications, give atenolol or metoprolol i.v., 5 mg aliquots, to maximum of 15 mg over 30 minutes
- Watch for and treat maemodynamic or rhythm complications
- Rehabilitation, long-term oral beta-blocker, consider angiotensin converting enzyme inhibitor

---

Treatment of ventricular fibrillation. The earlier a patient with acute myocardial infarction is brought within reach of a defibrillator the better. Ideally an ambulance or general practitioner responding to a call from a patient with chest pain should carry a defibrillator. Patients should then be admitted to hospital for further observation and monitoring. If the infarct has occurred more than 24 hours earlier, the patient is free from pain or complications, and there is adequate domestic support then the patient may be cared for at home.

Acute coronary thrombolysis. Coronary thrombolysis helps restore coronary patency, preserves left ventricular function, and improves survival. The best results are obtained in patients treated as soon as possible after the onset of symptoms. It is reasonable to give thrombolytic therapy to all patients presenting within 6 hours of the onset of major symptoms, and to selected patients with a longer history but evidence of persisting ischaemia (e.g. persistent pain and ST elevation on the ECG). The major contraindications to thrombolytic therapy are given in the information box below.

The most widely used (and cheapest) thrombolytic drug is streptokinase: a dose of 1 500 000 units is given as an intravenous infusion in 100 ml of saline over 1 hour. Alternatively, human tissue plasminogen activator (alteplase) can be given as a bolus of 10 mg followed by 50 mg in the first hour and then 40 mg over the next two hours. This may be more effective in restoring coronary patency but has not been shown to have significant advantages over streptokinase in terms of survival. It is not highly antigenic, and may be preferable in patients previously treated with streptokinase. Anistreplase can be given as a single intravenous injection over 5 minutes, but has not yet been shown to have other advantages over streptokinase.

Aspirin. 150–300 mg improves survival on its own, and enhances the effect of thrombolytic therapy. The first tablet should be given to be chewed as soon as possible, and this therapy should be continued (150 mg on alternate days) for at least a month if tolerated.

Nitrates. Coronary spasm may contribute to acute coronary occlusion, and may hinder development of a collateral circulation. Sublingual glyceryl trinitrate (500 µg, or two puffs of spray) is a useful first-aid measure in threatened infarction. Intravenous glyceryl trinitrate (2–10 mg per hour) is useful both for treating left ventricular failure and for recurrent or persistent ischaemic pain.

Beta-blockers. Acute beta-blockade with intravenous atenolol or metoprolol (15 mg in 5 mg aliquots at 10-minute intervals) reduces the risk of cardiac rupture. It should be avoided in patients with heart failure or severe bradycardia. Chronic beta-blockade (timolol 5 mg b.d. or equivalent) improves one-year survival, and should be given to all patients who can tolerate it.

Anticoagulants. Subcutaneous heparin (5000 units 8–12-hourly) is indicated in immobile patients at risk of venous thrombosis, and long-term warfarin therapy should be considered in patients with extensive anterior infarcts, who are at increased risk of systemic thromboembolism.

Angiotensin converting enzyme inhibitors. These have been shown to prevent, or at least reduce, left ventricular dilatation after anterior infarcts (captopril 12.5–50 mg t.i.d., enalapril 2–10 mg b.d.). The blood pressure needs to be carefully monitored, as they can cause severe hypotension, especially in patients with an activated renin-angiotensin system.

Post-infarct angina

Post-infarct angina occurs in up to 50% of patients.

CONTRAINDICATIONS TO THROMBOLYTIC THERAPY

- Active internal bleeding
- Previous subarachnoid or intracerebral haemorrhage
- Recent surgery (within 1 month)
- Recent trauma (including traumatic resuscitation)
- High probability of peptic ulcer &c
- Pregnancy or current menstruation
- Severe diabetic proliferative retinopathy

Most patients have a residual stenosis despite successful thrombolysis, and this may cause angina if there is still viable myocardium downstream. In other patients occlusion of a vessel may disturb a system of collateral flow compensating for stenosis elsewhere. Angina at rest or on minimal exertion after infarction should be managed as described for unstable angina, if possible with early coronary angiography and either angioplasty or coronary grafting. There is however no evidence that elective angioplasty improves outcome after thrombolysis. Patients who are able to do so should have a symptom limited exercise test about one month after infarction. Those with residual ischaemia in the form of chest pain or ECG changes at low exercise levels are at risk of further ischaemic events and should be considered for angiography.

Complications of infarction

Arrhythmias
Pain relief, rest, reassurance and the correction of hypokalaemia all play a major role in preventing arrhythmias. Lignocaine (p. 275) is given after resuscitation from ventricular fibrillation or to treat ventricular tachycardia with a rapid rate. In some units lignocaine is also given if multiple ectopic beats, or the potentially dangerous 'R on T' ectopics are observed during the acute phase of the illness. If lignocaine is ineffective, mexiletine (p. 275) may be used instead; sometimes an intravenous beta-blocker (e.g. atenolol 5–10 mg or sotalol 10 mg) may be helpful.

Ventricular fibrillation should be treated with an immediate d.c. shock (p. 279). Failing this, the cardiac resuscitation procedure (p. 272) should be used until the defibrillator is available. Atrial tachycardia, flutter or fibrillation are best treated with digoxin if the ventricular rate is rapid, and spontaneous reversion to sinus rhythm is common. If the arrhythmia causes severe hypotension, synchronised d.c. shock treatment should be considered.

Sinus bradycardia does not usually require treatment, but if there is hypotension or ventricular escape, atropine may be given (0.3 mg i.v. every 5 min to a maximum of 1.5 mg). Heart block complicating inferior infarction often responds to atropine and a temporary pacemaker is needed only if this drug is ineffective in preventing hypotension. Heart block complicating anterior infarction is an indication for the prophylactic insertion of a temporary pacemaker, as asystole may suddenly supervene. Asystole sometimes responds to cardiac massage, and following this a pacemaker electrode should be inserted.

Acute circulatory and cardiac failure
These are treated as described on pages 281 and 289.

Aftercare and rehabilitation
There is histological evidence that an infarct takes 4–6 weeks to become replaced with fibrous tissue. Accordingly it is generally thought reasonable to restrict physical activities during this period. When there are no complications the patient can sit in a chair within a few days, be ambulant within a week, return home in 7–10 days and gradually increase activity with the prospect of a return to work after 6 weeks. When there are complications the regimen has to be adjusted accordingly. Reassurance is essential at every stage because many patients are severely and even permanently incapacitated as a result of psychological rather than physical effects of myocardial infarction. The success of restoring a patient to normal life depends very much on the attitudes of the physician. The naturally vigorous person may require restraint in the early stages but more often the anxious will need encouragement. In general, patients can be reassured that exercise within the limits set by angina and tiredness will do no harm and much good. The same limits apply to sexual activity. The spouse has often to learn to stop reminding the patient of former disability. Formal rehabilitation programmes based on graded exercise and counselling may be of great psychological benefit, although it has not been possible to show convincing effects on eventual exercise ability or survival.

Much advice given to patients after myocardial infarction is based on common sense rather than on objective demonstration of benefit, but control of obesity, regular exercise and the adoption of a less frenetic way of life are unlikely to do harm. Stopping smoking improves survival, more so in younger than in older patients. There is no overall evidence that control of plasma lipids, by dietary or other means, affects survival in patients who have had an infarct, but lipid control may still be worthwhile in young patients with familial hyperlipidaemias.

Prognosis
In about a quarter of all cases of myocardial infarction death occurs within a few minutes without medical care. Half the deaths from myocardial infarction occur within 2 hours of the onset of symptoms and three-quarters within 24 hours. About 40% of all affected patients die within the first month. Unfavourable features are poor left ventricular function, heart block and persistent ventricular arrhythmias. The prognosis is worse for anterior than for inferior infarcts. Bundle

branch block and high enzyme levels both indicate extensive myocardial damage. Old age, stress and social isolation are also associated with a higher mortality. In the absence of unfavourable features, the outlook is as good for those who survive ventricular fibrillation as for the others. Of those who survive an acute attack, more than 80% live for a further year, about 75% for 5 years, 50% for 10 years and 25% for 20 years. It is therefore appropriate to be reassuring to patients about their prospects.

SUDDEN DEATH

This term can be applied when a person previously in apparent good health falls ill and dies within minutes or at most a few hours. Some of these patients have an identifiable non-cardiac cause of death such as cerebral haemorrhage or a ruptured aortic aneurysm. Many have extensive coronary atherosclerosis; the proportion of these who have thrombotic occlusion of a coronary vessel is small when death is virtually instantaneous but higher in those who survive for a few hours. The explanation for this is uncertain but possibly coronary spasm may occlude a vessel for long enough to produce fatal consequences without a thrombus developing. Alternatively, death might be due to an arrhythmia in the absence of coronary occlusion. Arrhythmias are probably the immediate cause of sudden death in patients with other cardiac abnormalities such as severe aortic or pulmonary stenosis or hypertrophic cardio-myopathy.

A small group of patients who die suddenly have no obvious pathological cause of death on postmortem examination; cardiac arrhythmia seems the most likely cause in this group also, and in some cases a previous ECG has been found to be abnormal. There is evidence both from patients who have died during ambulatory ECG monitoring and from acute resuscitation services that ventricular fibrillation is the commonest arrhyth-mia causing sudden death, and resuscitation, if promptly applied, may restore effective cardiac action.

Relatives of patients who have died suddenly often seek reassurance, and should be examined, if appropri-ate, for evidence of hypertrophic cardiomyopathy, Marfan's syndrome and hyperlipidaemia. A family history of sudden death in childhood or young adult life is sometimes associated with prolongation of the QT interval on the ECG, and beta-blockade may improve prognosis in this group.

Prevention of coronary disease

There is excellent evidence that morbidity and mor-tality from coronary artery disease can be reduced by stopping smoking in any patient at any age, and by reducing plasma cholesterol concentrations in male patients with a total plasma cholesterol of over 7 mmol per litre and a plasma total cholesterol/high density lipoprotein cholesterol ratio of 5 or greater. There is suggestive epidemiological evidence that lower plasma total cholesterol concentrations, of 6 mmol per litre or higher, are still associated with an increased incidence of coronary disease, and that this may apply to women as well as men, but intervention trials have not yet demonstrated benefit from treatment.

Patients with hypercholesterolaemia should stop smoking, take exercise and reduce their body weight to the 'ideal' weight for their height. Diet should be adjusted so that no more than 30% of total energy is supplied from fat, and the ratio of polyunsaturated to saturated fat should be 2:1 or greater. Patients who remain hypercholesterolaemic after 3 months despite dietary compliance may need further medication. The most useful drugs are gemfibrosil (600 mg b.d.) and cholestyramine 12–24 g daily. Gemfibrosil can cause gastrointestinal disturbances, blurred vision, headache, dizzyness and myalgia. It is contraindicated in patients with liver impairment, and should be used with caution if there is renal impairment. Cholestyramine is un-pleasant to take, may cause diarrhoea or constipation, and may cause deficiency of fat soluble vitamins. Patients with severe hyperlipidaemia are best managed in a specialist lipid clinic.

There is controversy over whether efforts to prevent coronary disease should concentrate on identifying and treating those at the highest risk, or should try to persuade whole populations to modify their habits. The two are not incompatible. Reasonable 'population' advice is summarised in the information box below.

POPULATION ADVICE TO PREVENT CORONARY DISEASE

- Do not smoke
- Take regular exercise
- Aim for 'ideal' bodyweight
- Eat a mixed diet with fruit and vegetables as well as meat and dairy products
- Aim to get no more than 30% of energy intake from fat
- Avoid more than 30 g alcohol per day

SYSTEMIC HYPERTENSION

In Western societies the average systolic and diastolic blood pressures gradually rise with age. Hypertension is defined arbitrarily at levels above generally accepted 'normals', for example 140/90 at the age of 20, 160/95 at the age of 50 and 170/105 at the age of 75. Exercise, anxiety, discomfort and unfamiliar surroundings can all lead to a transient rise in blood pressure, and measurements should be repeated when the patient is resting and relaxed until consistent readings are obtained. Patients who have a high blood pressure on first examination which subsequently settles with rest may not require treatment but should be kept under review because they are more likely to develop sustained hypertension. According to these criteria, some 15% of the population can be regarded as hypertensive, though only a proportion of these will be diagnosed or receive treatment.

Aetiology

In about 5–10% of cases, hypertension can be shown to be a consequence of a specific disease or abnormality. The causes are listed in the information box below.

CAUSES OF SECONDARY HYPERTENSION

- Coarctation of the aorta
- Renal disease
    Parenchymal renal disease, e.g. glomerulonephritis, chronic pyelonephritis, collagen vascular diseases
    Polycystic kidney disease
    Renal artery stenosis
- Endocrine disorders
    Phaeochromocytoma
    Cushing's syndrome
    Conn's syndrome (primary hyperaldosteronism)
    Hyperparathyroidism
    Acromegaly
    Primary hypothyroidism
    Congenital adrenal hyperplasia
    11 beta-hydroxylase, 17-hydroxylase deficiency
- Alcohol
- Drugs
    e.g. Oral contraceptives containing oestrogens, anabolic steroids, corticosteroids, non-steroidal anti-inflammatory drugs, carbenoxolone, sympathomimetic agents
- Pregnancy
    Pre-eclamptic toxaemia

These conditions give an insight into the possible mechanisms by which hypertension may be caused. In phaeochromocytoma, it results from an increased cardiac output and/or a raised peripheral resistance due to excessive catecholamines. Conn's syndrome is associated with sodium retention, and probably an alteration in the reactivity of vascular smooth muscle. Renal causes of hypertension are also often associated with sodium retention, and in many cases with high plasma concentrations of renin, which causes the production of the potent vasoconstrictor agent angiotensin II. The latter stimulates aldosterone secretion and thus also encourages sodium retention.

In the majority of patients with hypertension, although some of these mechanisms may be operating, it is not possible to define a specific underlying cause, and they are said to have *essential hypertension*. In 70% of such patients another member of the family is affected. Essential hypertension is especially frequent in some races, particularly American Blacks and Japanese and it is commoner in countries where there is a high salt intake.

The pathogenesis of essential hypertension is not clearly understood. However, it is known that the underlying defect is an increase in peripheral vascular resistance. Some authorities believe that this is due to an increase in sympathetic nervous activity while others believe that there is a fundamental defect in the vascular smooth muscle.

Long-standing hypertension causes important structural changes in the peripheral resistance vessels and kidneys. These changes may lead to an increase in peripheral vascular resistance and a further rise in blood pressure. Hence, the factors that cause a rise in blood pressure may differ from those that sustain high blood pressure once it is established.

Clinical features

Hypertension occasionally causes headache or polyuria but, provided there are no complications, most patients remain asymptomatic. Accordingly, the diagnosis is usually made at routine examination or when a complication arises.

Non-specific physical signs may include left ventricular hypertrophy, accentuation of the aortic component of the second heart sound, a fourth heart sound, and a short early diastolic murmur. The optic fundi are often abnormal (see below).

The three main objectives of clinical examination in a hypertensive patient are to identify any underlying causes (most commonly found in young patients with no family history of hypertension), to recognise risk factors for the development of complications and to detect any complications already present.

A careful history should identify those patients with drug or alcohol induced hypertension. Panic attacks, paroxysmal headache or palpitation should prompt a careful search for a phaeochromocytoma. Similarly, recurrent backache or urinary tract infection may be due to chronic pyelonephritis.

Physical examination should detect the delay between radial and femoral pulses characteristic of coarctation of the aorta, and the enlarged kidneys in polycystic disease. The characteristic facies and habitus of Cushing's syndrome may be recognised, and a bruit is sometimes audible over the abdomen in renal artery stenosis.

It is important to identify risk factors such as smoking, obesity and hyperlipidaemia which may interact with hypertension, particularly in the genesis of ischaemic heart disease.

Complications

The adverse effects of hypertension principally involve the central nervous system, the retina, the heart and the kidneys.

Central nervous system

Stroke. When this results from cerebral haemorrhage or from cerebral ischaemia it is a common complication of hypertension and a major cause of death in hypertensive patients. Carotid atheroma and transient cerebral ischaemic attacks are more common in hypertensive patients.

Hypertensive encephalopathy. This is a rare condition characterised by a very high blood pressure and neurological symptoms including transient disturbances of speech or vision, paraesthesiae, disorientation, fits and loss of consciousness. Papilloedema is common. The neurological deficit is usually reversible if the hypertension is properly controlled.

Subarachnoid haemorrhage. This is more common in hypertensive patients.

Retina

Hypertensive retinopathy. In long-standing hypertension there may be thickening of the walls of retinal arterioles, causing diffuse or segmental narrowing of the blood columns, varying width of the light reflex from the vessel wall and often some arterio-venous nipping. With more severe hypertension, retinal haemorrhages occur, and are usually flame shaped. Soft (cotton wool) exudates are associated with retinal ischaemia or infarction and fade in a few weeks. Hard exudates are small white dense deposits of lipid which may persist for years. Papilloedema indicates the most advanced stage of hypertension. In early retinopathy there is little effect on visual acuity, but extensive exudates or haemorrhages can cause visual field defects, or blindness if the macula is affected.

Heart

Hypertension places a pressure load on the heart and may lead to left ventricular hypertrophy (Fig. 8.59) and ultimately left ventricular failure (p. 288). However, the excess cardiac mortality and morbidity associated with hypertension is largely due to a higher incidence of coronary artery disease (pp. 303–316). Hypertension is also implicated in the pathogenesis of aortic aneurysm and aortic dissection.

Kidneys

In addition to being a cause, renal disease may also be a result of hypertensive damage to the renal vessels. Long-standing hypertension may cause proteinuria and progressive renal failure. Sometimes, renal damage resulting from hypertension produces an increased release of renin, and a vicious circle may be set up with worsening renal failure and very severe hypertension. This *accelerated phase* or *malignant hypertension* has a bad prognosis unless the cycle is interrupted. There is fibrinoid necrosis in the small arterioles of the kidney and also in those of the heart, brain and retina where the presence of soft exudates haemorrhages and later papilloedema are pathognomonic.

Investigation

Investigation of the hypertensive patient has the same basic objectives as the clinical examination, but because hypertension is so common it is prudent to be selective

---

INVESTIGATION OF HYPERTENSION

- Urine analysis for protein (may indicate renal disease) glucose (diabetes may coexist and is a risk factor for vascular disease)
- Plasma urea/creatinine to assess renal function
- Plasma electrolytes – hypokalaemic alkalosis may indicate primary or secondary hyperaldosteronism (NB diuretic therapy is the commonest cause)
- Plasma cholesterol – hypercholesterolaemia is an important risk factor for vascular disease
- Chest X-ray – look for cardiomegaly, heart failure, rib notching in coarctation (page 330)
- ECG – left ventricular hypertrophy (Fig. 8.59)

Special investigations
- 24-hour urine collection for metanephrine or vanillylmandelic acid (VMA) excretion – if history suggests phaeochromocytoma
- Intravenous urogram – if renal disease is suspected
- Radionuclide renography or renal arteriography – if there is evidence of renal artery stenosis
- Lying plasma renin activity and aldosterone – if Conn's syndrome (p. 647) suspected due to hypokalaemic alkalosis
- Urinary cortisol, dexamethasone suppression test (see p. 643–646) – if there are signs of Cushing's syndrome

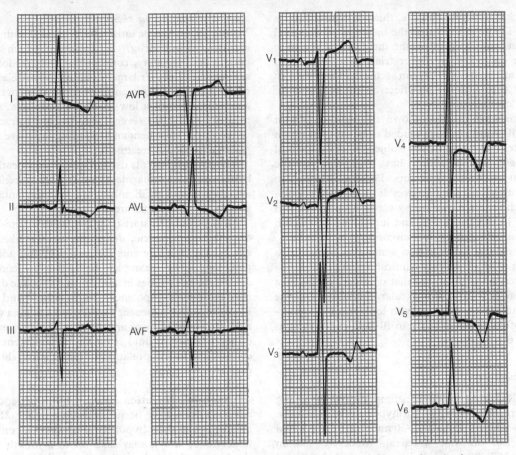

Fig. 8.59 An ECG showing gross left ventricular hypertrophy and strain from a patient with severe hypertension.

in the use of resources. Some investigations need to be done on all patients, while others can be reserved for those with specific features of a particular condition or who are refractory to the initial treatment. Investigations are listed in the information box (p. 318).

Renal artery stenosis often causes refractory hypertension and should be considered in patients with severe hypertension that is difficult to control or has developed rapidly. Renal arteriography provides the most detailed information about the renal vessels, and can sometimes be combined with percutaneous balloon dilatation of a renal artery stenosis.

Management

The object of treating systemic arterial hypertension is to reduce the risk of complications and to improve patient survival. The benefits of treatment have to be weighed against its inconvenience and the possibility that the agents used may themselves have potentially harmful effects. In most instances, the discovery of

hypertension commits the patient to a lifetime of supervision and treatment. It is important to treat the whole patient, and not just the blood pressure. Because of these considerations it is not particularly helpful to set up arbitrary levels of blood pressure at which treatment should be commenced. Decisions about treatment should also take into account the fact that the natural history of hypertension tends to be more benign in women than in men, and that Black people and diabetics are more prone to hypertensive complications.

There is general agreement that hypertension should be treated with antihypertensive drugs if it is severe (e.g. over 160/100 at age 20, 170/110 in men aged 50) or if it is associated with retinal, cardiac or renal damage. There is less certainty concerning the benefits of such treatment in mild or 'borderline' hypertensives, e.g. 140/90 at age 20, 160/95 at age 50. A large-scale trial conducted in Britain by the Medical Research Council tested the effects of treating mild hypertension with a beta-blocker (propranolol), a thiazide diuretic or a placebo. Treatment reduced the incidence of non-fatal stroke but had no effect on the incidence of coronary events or on mortality. Other trials have also shown that treating mild hypertension seems to reduce the risk of stroke with little or no effect on the incidence of coronary events.

The trials which have shown the most consistent benefits of treatment have tended to be those in which the 'treated' group has been subject to close medical supervision, and attention has been paid to the correction of other risk factors. Perhaps it is best to regard borderline hypertensives as an 'at risk' population which requires continuing supervision, redoubled efforts at health education, and judicious intervention as determined by individual circumstances.

In the elderly hypertension sometimes responds to treatment with gratifying clinical results; indeed, a large European trial showed that treatment produced a substantial fall in cardiovascular mortality. On the other hand elderly patients with long-standing hypertension often respond badly to ill-judged attempts at lowering the pressure.

General measures

Diet. Reducing alcohol consumption and correcting obesity are both effective antihypertensive measures. Very low sodium diets (10–20 mmol/d) lower blood pressure but are not practical. Moderate sodium restriction (70–80 mmol/d) is sometimes helpful and patients should, therefore, be advised to stop adding salt to food and to avoid foods with a very high sodium content (p. 528).

Smoking. The effects of cigarette smoking and hypertension on cardiovascular morbidity are additive, and smoking should be strongly discouraged.

Exercise. Regular exercise improves physical fitness and may lower blood pressure.

Relaxation. It is customary to advise patients to 'avoid stress' but this is usually a pious hope. Spouses should be dissuaded from perpetually reminding patients of their hypertension. Formal relaxation classes, meditation and biofeedback have all been shown to reduce blood pressure in small groups of patients; their efficacy is usually proportional to the enthusiasm of the teacher and the commitment of the participant; it is unusual, however, for such treatment to replace the need for antihypertensive drug therapy.

Antihypertensive drug therapy

Many patients can be satisfactorily treated with a single antihypertensive drug, the choice of which will be determined by safety, convenience and freedom from side-effects. Another large group will require a combination of two or three antihypertensive agents to give good control with a low level of side-effects. A small minority will have severe hypertension refractory to conventional treatment and requiring intensive investigation and special treatment.

The principal agents used in single drug treatment of hypertension are thiazide diuretics, beta-adrenoceptor antagonists and ACE inhibitors; calcium antagonists and some vasodilators are also effective.

Most physicians start treatment with a beta-blocker or a thiazide diuretic, depending on the likely side-effects and the presence of any relevant additional pathology. For example, beta-blockers commonly cause cold extremities in women, and thiazide diuretics may cause male impotence. On the other hand a beta-blocker is likely to benefit a patient with angina whereas a diuretic may be more appropriate if there is evidence of heart failure or fluid retention. If one agent fails to control the blood pressure a combination should be prescribed.

Thiazide diuretics. These diuretics and their adverse effects have been discussed on page 213. The mechanism of their hypotensive action is incompletely understood, and it may take up to a month for the maximum effect to be observed.

A daily dose of 5 mg bendrofluazide or 0.5 mg cyclopenthiazide is appropriate. More potent loop acting diuretics such as frusemide (40 mg daily) or bumetanide (1 mg daily) have few advantages over thiazides in the treatment of hypertension unless there is substantial renal impairment or if they are used in conjunction with an ACE inhibitor, when their greater ability to cause sodium excretion may be useful.

Beta-adrenoceptor antagonists. A large number of beta-blockers are available and these differ in several important respects. Those with a short half-life are mostly available in slow release, once daily, formulations. *Metoprolol* (100–200 mg daily) and *atenolol* (50–100 mg daily) are cardioselective and therefore preferentially block the cardiac β_1 receptors as opposed to the β_2 receptors which mediate vasodilatation and bronchodilatation. *Pindolol* (15–30 mg daily) and *oxprenolol* (160–320 mg daily) have partial agonist (intrinsic sympathomimetic) activity and therefore tend to cause less bradycardia. *Propranolol* is subject to extensive first pass metabolism which means that a large and variable proportion of the drug is destroyed in its first passage through the liver. The dose of propranolol must, therefore, be carefully titrated according to the patient's individual needs; in some patients a dose of 40 mg twice daily will suffice whilst others may need as much as 320 mg 6-hourly. Propranolol is lipid soluble and crosses the blood-brain barrier; this may explain why it commonly causes CNS side-effects such as nightmares, drowsiness and depression. In contrast atenolol is water soluble and is largely excreted unchanged through the kidneys; CNS side-effects are therefore unusual.

Metabolic side-effects of beta-blocking drugs include a tendency to increase plasma concentrations of cholesterol in low density lipoproteins, which could in theory have a deleterious effect on the progression of atheroma. Non specific beta-blockers may cause a small rise in plasma potassium concentration.

Labetalol. This is a combined alpha and beta adrenoceptor antagonist which is sometimes more effective than pure beta-blockers. The usual dose is 100–200 mg twice daily.

Angiotensin converting enzyme (ACE) inhibitors (p. 290). These have been a major advance in the treatment of moderate to severe hypertension. They have few side-effects and compliance tends to be good. They should be used with care in patients with impaired renal function or bilateral renal artery stenosis, as a sudden reduction in renal perfusion may precipitate renal failure. As in the treatment of cardiac failure it is best to start with a small dose (e.g. captopril 6.25 mg daily) and build up to an effective maintenance dose (e.g. captopril 25–75 mg twice daily, or enalapril 20 mg daily).

Calcium antagonists. Slow release as verapamil (240 mg daily) or nifedipine (20 mg twice daily) are effective and usually well tolerated antihypertensive drugs. They are particularly useful when hypertension coexists with angina.

Drug combinations. This may allow control of hypertension refractory to either drug alone at doses insufficient to cause serious side-effects. In some respects the drugs have complementary actions; thiazides increase renin production while beta-blockers depress it, and the hypokalaemic effect of thiazides may be countered by the hyperkalaemic effect of a nonselective beta-blocker. On the other hand the complexity of combination therapy may discourage compliance and

the risk of side-effects unrelated to the dose of drug is increased. A number of beta-blocker/thiazide combination tablets have been marketed, but the proportion of the two drugs is not necessarily optimal for every patient.

If satisfactory hypertensive control (usually defined as a phase 5 diastolic pressure of 90 or less) cannot be achieved with a beta-blocker and thiazide combination, a third drug may be added – usually a peripheral vasodilator such as *hydralazine*. This drug is rarely used alone as it tends to cause a tachycardia. The usual dose of hydralazine is 50–200 mg daily in divided doses. It is sometimes the cause of an allergic vasculitis or a syndrome resembling SLE (p. 791). In severe hypertension the more potent vasodilator minoxidil (10–50 mg daily) may be useful. However, this produces marked fluid retention and increased facial hair and is therefore unsuitable for female patients.

The emergency treatment of hypertension
It is virtually never necessary or desirable to cause an instantaneous fall in blood pressure. Even in the presence of cardiac failure or hypertensive encephalopathy a controlled reduction over a period of 30–60 minutes to a level of about 150/90 is adequate, and there is often less urgency. Too rapid a fall in pressure may cause permanent cerebral ischaemic damage, including blindness, and may sometimes precipitate coronary or renal insufficiency.

The most effective agent for blood pressure reduction in an emergency is a controlled intravenous infusion of sodium nitroprusside (0.3– 1.0 µg/kg body weight/minute), but this requires very careful supervision, preferably in an intensive care unit. Alternatives are intravenous or intramuscular labetalol (2 mg/min to a maximum of 200 mg) or intramuscular hydralazine (5 or 10 mg aliquots repeated at half-hourly intervals and titrated against the blood pressure response). In many patients, however, it is possible to avoid parenteral therapy; for example, chewing a nifedipine 10 mg capsule is often sufficient to produce a graded reduction in blood pressure. Bed-rest, sedation and a diuretic are also helpful. Urinary output and plasma electrolytes should be monitored, and urgent enquiry made into the cause of the hypertension.

Hypertensive emergencies in young patients may result from acute glomerulonephritis or from an acute exacerbation of chronic renal failure. The latter is also an important cause in older patients, but these are also likely to suffer from acute renal ischaemia caused by atheroma or embolism. The possibility of phaeochromocytoma should also be considered.

Refractory hypertension

The common causes of treatment failure in hypertension are non-compliance with drug therapy, inadequate therapy, and failure to recognise an underlying cause such as renal artery stenosis or phaeochromocytoma; of these the first is by far the most prevalent. There is no easy solution to compliance problems, but a simple treatment regimen, attempts to improve rapport with the patient, and careful supervision may all help.

DISEASES OF THE PULMONARY CIRCULATION

PULMONARY ARTERIAL HYPERTENSION

Aetiology

The principal cause of severe pulmonary hypertension in adults is an increase in pulmonary vascular resistance. In infancy another important cause is an increased pulmonary blood flow resulting from left-to-right shunting, as in atrial and ventricular septal defects and in persistent ductus arteriosus. While this is initially reversible when the shunt is corrected, prolonged exposure of a child's lungs to pulmonary hypertension causes irreversible vascular damage, and a rise in pulmonary vascular resistance perpetuates the hypertension.

Causes of pulmonary hypertension in adult life are summarised in the information box below.

Any cause of left-sided cardiac failure may produce pulmonary hypertension, but it is most prominent when there has been a very gradual rise in left atrial

---

CAUSES OF PULMONARY HYPERTENSION IN ADULTS

- Reflex vasoconstriction from a rise in pulmonary capillary pressure
    Left-sided heart failure
    Pulmonary veno-occlusive disease
- Alveolar hypoxia
    'Blue bloater' cor pulmonale
    Chronic altitude sickness
- Destructive lung disease
    Chronic emphysema
    'Pink puffer' cor pulmonale, antitrypsin deficiency
- Thromboembolism
- Diseases primarily affecting the pulmonary vessels
    Systemic sclerosis
    Schistosomiasis
- Drugs
    Fenfluramine
    Diethylpropion
- Unknown cause
    'Primary pulmonary hypertension'

---

pressure, as in some cases of mitral stenosis. The combined burden of a raised left atrial pressure and an increased pulmonary vascular resistance may produce secondary right heart failure. Provided the left-sided failure is relieved, e.g. by mitral valvotomy, the pulmonary hypertension will usually regress.

Pulmonary vasoconstriction in response to hypoxia is to some extent a protective reflex, which will divert blood flow away from poorly ventilated alveoli. It may be responsible however for the chronic pulmonary hypertension seen in some people who live at high altitude, and for the pulmonary hypertension and right heart failure associated with chronic alveolar hypoventilation. Another important cause of right heart failure in association with chronic lung disease (*cor pulmonale*) is a rise in pulmonary vascular resistance as the result of loss of pulmonary vessels in destructive lung diseases such as emphysema (p. 394). Pulmonary thromboembolism is particularly important and is considered in the next section. Pulmonary vessels can be affected by connective tissue diseases such as systemic sclerosis, by drugs such as fenfluramine and by schistosomiasis (p. 165).

In primary pulmonary hypertension the underlying cause is obscure. This is a rare disease most common in young women, and there is sometimes a family history.

Clinical features

There may be a left parasternal impulse either from right ventricular hypertrophy, or from an enlarged pulmonary artery, or both. If there is accompanying right atrial hypertrophy a large *a* wave is to be expected in the jugular venous pulse. There may be an ejection sound and a loud second heart sound over the pulmonary valve, and pulmonary regurgitation may produce a soft early diastolic murmur. Associated conditions such as left-sided cardiac failure or chronic lung disease may also produce their own clinical features.

Investigation

The ECG usually shows evidence of right atrial and right ventricular hypertrophy (Fig. 8.48, p. 298). The *chest radiograph* may show enlargement of the pulmonary artery and its main branches (Fig. 8.60). *Echocardiography* is important to exclude left-sided obstructive lesions such as 'silent' mitral stenosis, and radionuclide lung scanning may suggest pulmonary embolism. Pulmonary arteriography and lung biopsy have a role in a few selected cases.

Management

This is basically that of the underlying cause. Prognosis

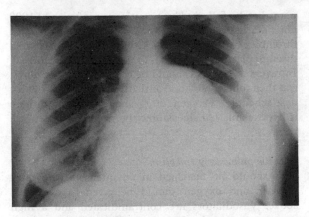

Fig. 8.60   Chest radiograph from a patient with severe pulmonary hypertension showing dilatation of the main pulmonary artery and absence of vascular markings in the peripheral lung fields.

is fairly good if the hypertension is due to correctable left-heart failure, treatable hypoxia or to drugs which can be withdrawn; the outlook is poor if the cause is advanced lung disease or thromboembolism. Primary pulmonary hypertension generally has a poor prognosis; vasodilators have been tried but with inconsistent results. Continuous intravenous infusion of prostacyclin has been successful in some patients. Very occasionally, spontaneous recovery has been reported. Patients with irreversible pulmonary hypertension may be candidates for heart-lung transplantation.

PULMONARY EMBOLISM AND INFARCTION

Pulmonary embolism occurs when a portion of thrombus in a systemic vein, or less commonly the right side of the heart, is discharged into the circulation. It may lodge in the main pulmonary artery and cause sudden death, or in a smaller pulmonary artery and result in pulmonary infarction. Recurrent 'silent' pulmonary embolism may come to light only when pulmonary hypertension and chronic right-heart failure develop.

Aetiology

Thrombosis in a pelvic vein or a deep vein of the legs (p. 338) is the most frequent source. As this is usually the result of stasis, pulmonary embolism most often affects people who have been confined to bed. It is paticularly liable to occur within 10 days after a surgical operation or after childbirth. A long journey in an aircraft or car can cause thrombosis in a leg vein. The presence of phlebothrombosis is frequently not recognised until after the embolism.

In less than 10% of cases thrombi responsible for pulmonary embolism form in the right atrium in patients with atrial fibrillation, especially if cardiac failure is present.

Clinical features

Massive pulmonary embolism has been described on page 283. In cases of lesser severity, symptoms and signs may be absent or there may be transient dyspnoea, tachycardia or syncope. In *pulmonary infarction*, which is usually due to a small peripheral embolus, the signs are pleural pain which may be severe, and haemoptysis which may be profuse and repetitive. There may be dyspnoea, tachycardia, central cyanosis, pyrexia and polymorphonuclear leucocytosis. Secondary infection may occur. Often, pulmonary infarction produces no symptoms.

Investigation

Radiological examination

In massive pulmonary embolism the lung fields often appear normal but sometimes there is a hilar opacity from the blocked vessel and ischaemia distal to the embolus causes a reduction in the usual vascular markings of a lung or lobe. Pulmonary angiography is the most reliable method of diagnosis, but should not be allowed to delay urgent treatment (Fig. 8.61). The radiological features are listed in the information box below.

Venous thrombosis can be demonstrated by bilateral ascending phlebography.

RADIOLOGICAL FEATURES OF PULMONARY EMBOLISM

- Small emboli
    Linear or wedge shaped opacities
    Pleural effusion
    Elevation of hemidiaphragm
    May be no changes
- Massive emboli
    May be no diagnostic changes
    Unilateral hyperlucency

Radionuclide scanning

The intravenous injection of radionuclide-labelled macroaggregated albumin can be used to delineate underperfused areas of lung not detected on a plain radiograph. This technique is of value in the diagnosis of pulmonary embolism, especially if combined with ventilation scanning following the inhalation of a radionuclide-labelled gas. Radionuclide lung scans may be difficult to interpret if the chest radiograph is abnormal.

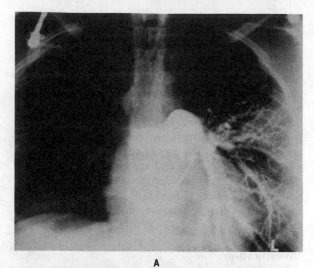

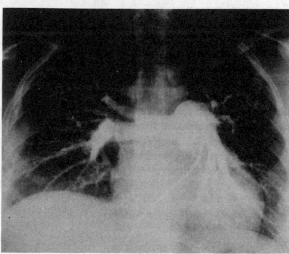

Fig. 8.61 Pulmonary angiograms from a patient with massive pulmonary embolism. A. Before. **B.** After thrombolytic therapy. In the first film there is complete obstruction to blood flow to the right lung, and smaller emboli in many of the other pulmonary vessels.

Electrocardiography
This may show evidence of right ventricular dilatation and strain in cases of massive pulmonary embolism (right axis deviation, T wave inversion in the right ventricular leads and displacement of the interventricular septum to the left), or the pattern of incomplete right bundle branch block (Fig. 8.27). In cases of lesser severity the ECG is usually normal, except for a sinus tachycardia.

Management
Intravenous heparin 5000–10 000 units should be given

immediately, followed by a continuous infusion of 1000 units per hour. The dose should be adjusted to give a thrombin clotting time (TCT) or activated partial thromboplastin time (APTT) of 1.5–2 times normal. Intravenous heparin should be continued for 5–7 days, and then followed by oral anticoagulants (see p. 759 for dose schedule). Oxygen (60%) should be given if there is hypoxaemia. Analgesia may be needed for pleuritic pain.

Massive pulmonary embolism
This should be managed in an intensive care unit. Heparin and oxygen should be given as described above. Vasodilators are contraindicated and a high venous pressure should be maintained, if necessary by infusing saline and/or noradrenaline (2 mg in 500 ml 0.9% NaCl, infused initially at 1 ml/min (4 µg/min), titrated against blood pressure response). If there is no detectable cardiac output cardiac massage may help by fragmenting pulmonary artery thrombus.

Pulmonary angiography helps confirm the diagnosis, and may improve cardiac output by displacing thrombus in the right ventricular outflow tract.

Patients with angiographically proven thrombus and circulatory failure (systolic blood pressure < 100 mmHg, tachycardia, PO_2 < 10 KPa and oliguria) should receive thrombolytic therapy.

Prevention
Prevention of pulmonary embolism and infarction is summarised in the information box below.

PREVENTION OF PULMONARY EMBOLISM

- Immobile medical patients (e.g. post myocardial infarction)
  Subcutaneous heparin 5000–10 000 units 12-hourly
- Postoperative surgical patients
  Early mobilisation *plus* heparin as above *and/or* pneumatic boots/calf muscle stimulation
- Patients with previous documented embolism
  Oral anticoagulation
  Mobin-Uddin vena cava filter
  Vena cava plication

Course and prognosis
Massive pulmonary embolism is frequently fatal. Minor and medium sized emboli are much less dangerous, but may herald subsequent massive embolism. Recurrent emboli may cause pulmonary hypertension and right ventricular failure. The vast majority of pulmonary infarcts resolve completely. Occasionally an infarct may become secondarily infected and result in a lung abscess.

DISEASES OF THE MYOCARDIUM

Although the myocardium is involved in most types of heart disease the terms myocarditis and cardiomyopathy are usually applied to conditions that primarily affect the heart muscle. An international commission has recommended using specific terminology, e.g. 'sarcoid heart disease', when the cause of heart muscle disease is known and using the term 'cardiomyopathy' only if a cause cannot be identified.

SPECIFIC DISEASES OF HEART MUSCLE

Specific diseases are shown in the information box below.

SPECIFIC DISEASES OF HEART MUSCLE

- Infections
  Viral – e.g. coxsackie A and B, influenza
  Bacterial – e.g. diphtheria, chickenpox
  Protozoal – e.g. trypanosomiasis (Chaga's disease p. 163)
- Endocrine and metabolic disorders
  e.g. diabetes, hypo- and hyperthyroidism, acromegaly, carcinoid syndrome, inherited storage diseases
- Connective tissue diseases
  e.g. scleroderma, SLE, polyarteritis nodosa
- Infiltrative disorders
  e.g. haemochromatosis, haemosiderosis, sarcoidosis, amyloidosis
- Endomyocardial fibrosis and eosinophilic heart disease
- Toxins
  e.g. drugs, alcohol, irradiation
- Neuromuscular disorders
  e.g. dystrophia myotonica, Freidreich's ataxia

Acute myocarditis

This is an acute inflammatory and potentially reversible condition that may complicate a wide variety of infections, due to direct invasion of the myocardium or the effects of a toxin. Viral infection is the commonest cause of myocarditis in the UK.

The clinical picture ranges from a symptomless disorder, sometimes recognised by the presence of an inappropriate tachycardia, to fulminant heart failure. Any ECG changes are non-specific; but, if necessary, the diagnosis can be confirmed by endomyocardial biopsy. Although death may occur, due to a ventricular arrhythmia or rapidly progressive heart failure, the immediate prognosis is excellent. However, there is strong evidence that some forms of myocarditis may lead to chronic low grade myocarditis or dilated cardiomyopathy; for example, in Chaga's disease (p. 163) the patient usually recovers from the acute infection but often develops a chronic and potentially fatal dilated cardiomyopathy 10 or 20 years later.

There is no specific therapy for acute myocarditis; corticosteroids have been tried but are of no proven value. Treatment for cardiac failure or arrhythmias may be required. Prolonged rest is sometimes necessary.

Chronic specific heart muscle disease

Many forms of specific heart muscle disease produce a clinical picture that is indistinguishable from dilated cardiomyopathy (e.g. connective tissue disorders, sarcoidosis, haemochromatosis, alcoholic heart muscle disease). In contrast, amyloidosis and eosinophilic heart disease produce symptoms and signs similar to those found in restrictive cardiomyopathy (see below), whereas Friedreich's ataxia (p. 901) often mimics hypertrophic cardiomyopathy (see below).

The treatment and prognosis is determined by the underlying disorder. Abstention from alcohol may lead to a dramatic improvement in patients with alcoholic heart disease.

CARDIOMYOPATHY

There are three types of cardiomyopathy (Fig. 8.62).

Dilated cardiomyopathy

In this condition there is impaired ventricular contraction (often affecting both ventricles) leading to progressive left-sided and, later, right-sided heart failure. Functional mitral and/or tricuspid regurgitation may occur; arrhythmias are also common. The ECG usually shows non-specific changes but echocardiography is useful in making the diagnosis. The differential diagnosis includes most forms of specific heart muscle disease (e.g. alcoholic heart disease) and ischaemic heart disease. Treatment is aimed at controlling the resulting heart failure. Although some patients remain well for many years the prognosis is generally poor and cardiac transplantation may be indicated.

Restrictive or obliterative cardiomyopathy

In this condition ventricular filling is impaired because the ventricles are 'stiff'. This leads to high atrial pressures with atrial hypertrophy, dilatation and later atrial fibrillation. The differential diagnosis includes endomyocardial fibrosis, eosinophilic heart disease and amyloidosis. Diagnosis can be very difficult and may require doppler echocardiography, CT or MRI scanning and endomyocardial biopsy. Treatment is usually

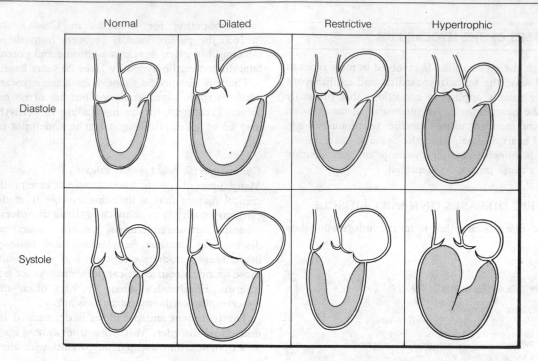

Fig. 8.62 The cardiomyopathies. In dilated cardiomyopathy the ventricle is enlarged and contracts poorly. In restrictive cardiomyopathy the ventricle is small and stiff with impaired diastolic filling and a large atrium. In hypertrophic cardiomyopathy there is reduced filling in diastole and in some forms there is also impaired ejection due to ventricular outflow tract obstruction.

symptomatic, but excision of fibrotic endocardium may benefit some patients.

Hypertrophic cardiomyopathy
This condition is often familial and is characterised by increased thickness of the ventricular wall. The hypertrophy may be generalised or may principally affect the interventricular septum. If asymmetrical septal hypertrophy is present it may cause left ventricular outflow tract obstruction, but this is not invariable. Mitral regurgitation is often present. In many cases the diagnosis is made only at autopsy following sudden death in a young person. In others, the condition may present with syncopal episodes or with angina.

On examination there is usually palpable left ventricular hypertrophy, and there may be a double impulse at the apex due to additional atrial hypertrophy. The pulse is characteristically 'jerky' and on auscultation there may be a mid-systolic murmur (due to left ventricular outflow tract obstruction) heard at the base and a pansystolic murmur (due to mitral regurgitation) heard at the apex. The ECG usually shows left ventricular hypertrophy, but may show a

wide variety of often bizarre abnormalities. Echocardiography is usually diagnostic.

The natural history is variable. The prognosis tends to be better in those who have the condition discovered incidentally in adult life than in those who present with symptoms in childhood or adolescence.

No treatment is definitely known to improve prognosis, but beta-blockers help to relieve angina and sometimes prevent syncopal attacks, particularly in those with ventricular outflow obstruction. Arrhythmias are common, and amiodarone is useful in their control. Digoxin and vasodilators may increase outflow tract obstruction and should be avoided.

DISEASES OF THE PERICARDIUM

ACUTE PERICARDITIS

Aetiology
Pericarditis may be fibrinous, serous, haemorrhagic or purulent. In the first there is a fibrinous exudate on the surface which may eventually lead to varying degrees of adhesion formation. In serous pericarditis there is in

addition an exudate of anything from a few millilitres to a litre or more. The effusion is straw-coloured and often slightly turbid with a high protein content. A haemorrhagic effusion suggests a malignant origin. Purulent pericarditis is due to a pyogenic infection. The aetiology is given in the information box below.

AETIOLOGY OF ACUTE PERICARDITIS

- Common
    Acute myocardial infarction
    Viral (e.g. Coxsackie B, but often not identified)
- Less common
    Secondary to bacterial infection
    Uraemia
    Malignant disease
    Trauma
    Connective tissue disease (e.g. SLE)
- Rare (in UK)
    Rheumatic fever
    Tuberculosis

Clinical features

The characteristic pain of pericarditis is retrosternal and often radiates to the shoulders and neck. It may be present on, or made worse by, a deep breath, movement, change of position, exercise or swallowing.

A friction rub is the diagnostic sign of pericarditis. It consists of a superficial scratching sound, best heard to the left of the lower sternum; it is usually systolic but may be audible also in diastole. It frequently has a 'to-and-fro' quality. Friction is often better heard when the stethoscope diaphragm is pressed firmly upon the chest, the patient's breath being held for a time in inspiration and then in expiration. If a pericardial effusion develops there is sometimes a sensation of retrosternal oppression. An effusion may be difficult to detect clinically – the heart sounds may become quieter, but pericardial friction is not always abolished.

Cardiac tamponade

This refers to compression of the heart by a large or rapidly developing effusion which interferes with diastolic filling. Atypical presentations may occur when the effusion is loculated as a result of previous pericarditis or cardiac surgery.

Investigation

The ECG shows ST elevation with upward concavity over the affected area, which may be widespread. Later, there may be T wave inversion. QRS voltage is often reduced in the presence of an effusion. Serial radio-graphs may show a rapid increase in the size of the cardiac shadow over days or even hours, and with a large effusion the heart may have a pear-shaped appearance. *Echocardiography* is particularly useful in detecting pericardial effusion.

Management

The pain can usually be relieved by aspirin (600 mg 4-hourly), but a more potent anti-inflammatory agent such as indomethacin (25 mg 8-hourly) may be required.

Paracentesis of a pericardial effusion may be indicated for diagnostic purposes or to relieve symptoms from cardiac tamponade. Either of two approaches may be used depending on the experience of the operator and the configuration of the patient:

1. the needle is inserted to the left of the xiphoid process, insinuated deep to the left costal margin, and then directed towards the left shoulder;
2. the needle is inserted medial to the cardiac apex at a point where echocardiography reveals the presence of a layer of fluid lying in front of the heart.

For diagnostic purposes it is usually enough to withdraw a few millilitres of fluid. If therapeutic drainage is needed it may be safer to use a plastic cannula inserted over a needle or guidewire than to attempt aspiration of the whole effusion through a rigid needle. A viscous or loculated effusion may require surgical drainage. The main dangers of pericardiocentesis are arrhythmia, damage to a coronary artery, and exacerbation of tamponade as a result of injury to the right ventricle. It is however life saving in the presence of severe tamponade.

VIRAL, TUBERCULOUS AND PURULENT PERICARDITIS

Viral pericarditis

This may follow an upper respiratory infection, and in about 10% of cases a Coxsackie infection can be established. Recovery usually occurs within a few days or weeks, but there may be recurrences. There is no specific treatment; corticosteroids may help suppress symptoms but there is little evidence they accelerate cure.

Tuberculous pericarditis

This may be secondary to manifest pulmonary tuberculosis, or the primary source may not be detectable. The disease is commonly insidious in onset and the subsequent course is chronic. An effusion usually develops and the pericardium may become thick and unyielding so that the heart is compressed. Pleural effusions are often associated.

The diagnosis may be confirmed by aspiration of the fluid and direct examination or culture for tubercle bacilli. Antituberculous chemotherapy is prescribed (p. 367). Corticosteroids may help to prevent the development of constrictive pericarditis. Pericardial aspiration may be carried out as required to relieve symptoms. In the inactive stage surgical relief may be necessary.

Purulent pericarditis

This is rare. It occurs as a complication of septicaemia, by direct spread from an intrathoracic infection, or from a penetrating injury. Treatment is by antimicrobial therapy, paracentesis if needed to relieve tamponade, and if necessary surgical drainage.

CHRONIC PERICARDIAL CONSTRICTION

Tuberculosis is a frequent cause. Some cases accompany rheumatoid arthritis and others follow a haemopericardium or, rarely, acute pericarditis. Often the cause is obscure. A slowly progressive fibrosis of the pericardium develops and constricts the movement of the heart, so that it cannot expand in diastole. The fibrous tissue is dense and inelastic and calcification is common. The inflow to the heart is impeded, so that cardiac output is diminished and systemic venous pressure raised.

Clinical features

Breathlessness is not a prominent symptom as the lungs are seldom congested. A raised jugular venous pressure is present, with a rapid and transitory *y* descent (Fig. 8.1). The arterial pulse tends to be rapid, of small volume, and pulsus paradoxus may be present. Hepatomegaly and ascites occur relatively early compared with peripheral oedema. The heart is usually not enlarged but chest radiography may show pericardial calcification. The main differential diagnosis is from restrictive cardiomyopathy. In countries where constrictive pericarditis is common the diagnosis can usually be made clinically. Where both constrictive pericarditis and restrictive cardiomyopathy are rare, and there is no pericardial calcification, cardiac catheterisation is indicated (Fig. 8.63).

Management

The problem is primarily a mechanical one, and rapid improvement is usual if surgical resection of the pericardium is performed.

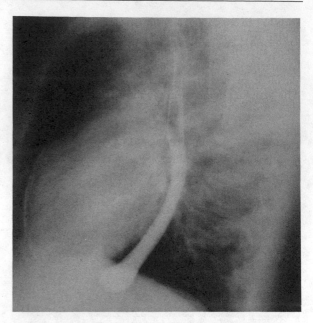

Fig. 8.63 Lateral chest radiograph from a patient with calcific pericarditis. The oesophagus has been outlined with barium, the calcified rim of pericardium is best seen on the anterior border of the heart.

CONGENITAL HEART DISEASE

Aetiology

The incidence of haemodynamically significant congenital cardiac abnormalities is about 1% of live births. In most cases the cause of the abnormality is unknown, but some fetal defects are due to maternal infections in the early weeks of pregnancy, e.g. rubella. All degrees of severity occur. Many defects are not compatible with extrauterine life, or only for a short time. Early diagnosis is important because most types are amenable to surgical treatment, but this opportunity may be lost if secondary changes, for example pulmonary vascular damage, occur.

Symptoms may be absent, or the child may be noticed to be breathless, or may fail to thrive and grow normally. Local signs vary with the anatomical lesion.

Central cyanosis

This occurs when desaturated blood enters the systemic circulation without passing through the lungs (i.e. there is a right-to-left shunt). In the neonate the commonest cause of this is transposition of the great arteries, in which the aorta derives from the right ventricular and the pulmonary artery from the left. In older children cyanosis is usually the consequence of a

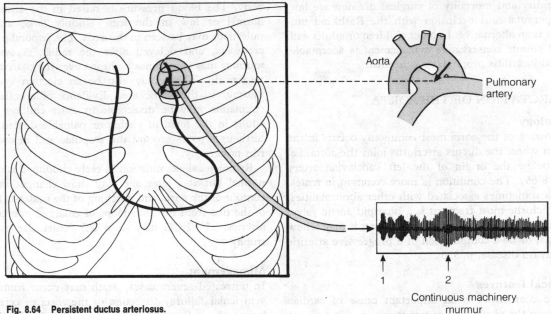

Fig. 8.64 Persistent ductus arteriosus.

ventricular septal defect combined with severe pulmonary stenosis (tetralogy of Fallot, p. 333) or with pulmonary vascular disease (Eisenmeger's syndrome, p. 332).

PERSISTENT DUCTUS ARTERIOSUS

Aetiology
During fetal life, before the lungs begin to function, most of the blood from the pulmonary artery passes through the ductus arteriosus into the aorta just below the origin of the left subclavian artery. Normally the ductus closes soon after birth but sometimes it fails to do so. Since the pressure in the aorta is higher than that in the pulmonary artery there will be a continuous arteriovenous shunt, the volume of which depends on the size of the ductus. As much as 50% of the left ventricular output may be recirculated through the lungs, with a consequent increase in the work of the heart. The condition, which may be associated with other abnormalities, is much commoner in females.

Clinical features
With small shunts there may be no symptoms for years but, if the ductus is large, growth and development are retarded. There is usually no disability, but cardiac failure may eventually ensue, dyspnoea being the first symptom. A continuous 'machinery' murmur is heard with late systolic accentuation, maximal at the second left rib near the sternum (Fig. 8.64). It is frequently accompanied by a thrill. Enlargement of the pulmonary artery may be detected radiologically. The ECG is usually normal.

A large left-to-right shunt in infancy may cause a considerable rise in pulmonary artery pressure, and sometimes this leads to progressive pulmonary vascular damage. With the resulting rise in pulmonary vascular resistance, pulmonary artery pressure rises further until it equals or exceeds aortic pressure. The shunt through the defect may then reverse, causing central cyanosis; with a persistent ductus arteriosus this cyanosis may be more apparent in the feet and toes than in the upper part of the body. The murmur becomes quieter, may be confined to systole, or may disappear. The ECG shows evidence of right ventricular hypertrophy.

Management
The treatment options in the management of persistent ductus arteriosus are listed below in Table 8.7. The

Table 8.7 Management of persistent ductus arteriosus

Age	Pulmonary resistance	Shunt flow	Treatment
Infant/neonate	Low	Large	Surgical division
Child/adult	Low	Large	Division or percutaneous occlusion
Child/adult	Low	Small	Conservative or percutaneous occlusion
Any	High	Reversed	None

morbidity and mortality of surgical division are low, but percutaneous occlusion with the Rashkind umbrella is an alternative. In older children or adults with small shunts conservative management is acceptable, but endocarditis prophylaxis is needed.

COARCTATION OF THE AORTA

Aetiology

Narrowing of the aorta most commonly occurs in the region where the ductus arteriosus joins the aorta, i.e. just below the origin of the left subclavian artery (Fig. 8.65). The condition is more common in males, and is sometimes associated with other abnormalities, of which the most frequent is a bicuspid aortic valve. Acquired coarctation of the aorta is rare; it may follow trauma, or be a complication of a progressive arteritis (Takayasu disease, p. 336).

Clinical features

Aortic coarctation is an important cause of cardiac failure in the newborn, but symptoms are often absent in older children or adults. Headaches may occur from hypertension in the upper part of the body, and occasionally weakness or cramps in the legs may result from decreased circulation in the lower part of the

body. The blood pressure is raised in the arms but normal or low in the legs. Unduly large arterial pulsations may be seen in the neck. The femoral pulses are weak, and delayed after the radial. A systolic murmur may sometimes be heard over the coarctation posteriorly. There may also be an ejection systolic murmur in the aortic area. Evidence of a collateral circulation may be detectable in older children and adults in the form of visible or palpable dilated and tortuous arteries around the scapulae and below the ribs posteriorly.

Radiological examination in early childhood is often normal but at a later age may show changes in the contour of the aorta and notching of the undersurfaces of the ribs from tortuous loops of enlarged intercostal arteries. The ECG may show left ventricular hypertrophy.

Management

In untreated severe cases, death may occur from left ventricular failure, dissection of the aorta or cerebral haemorrhage. Surgical correction is advisable in all but the mildest cases. If this is done early enough in childhood the risk of persistent hypertension may be avoided, but patients operated on in late childhood or adult life often remain hypertensive or become hypertensive again. Coexistent aortic valve disease is another reason for long-term follow-up.

ATRIAL SEPTAL DEFECT

Aetiology

Atrial septal defect is more common in females. Since the normal right ventricle is much more compliant than the left, a large volume of blood shunts through the defect from the left to right atrium and thence to the right ventricle and pulmonary arteries (Fig. 8.66). As a result there is gradual enlargement of the right side of the heart and of the pulmonary artery and its main branches. Pulmonary hypertension and shunt reversal sometimes complicate atrial septal defect, but are less common and tend to occur later in life than with other types of left-to-right shunt.

Clinical features

There may be no symptoms for many years and the condition is often detected after a routine chest radiograph. Dyspnoea, cardiac failure and arrhythmias such as atrial fibrillation are other possible modes of presentation. The characteristic physical signs are:

1. wide fixed splitting of the second heart sound –
   wide because of delay in right ventricular ejection,

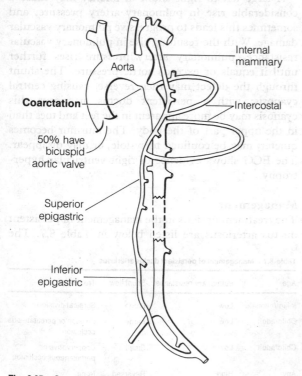

Fig. 8.65   Coarctation of the aorta.

(labels within figure: Internal mammary; Aorta; Coarctation; Intercostal; 50% have bicuspid aortic valve; Superior epigastric; Inferior epigastric)

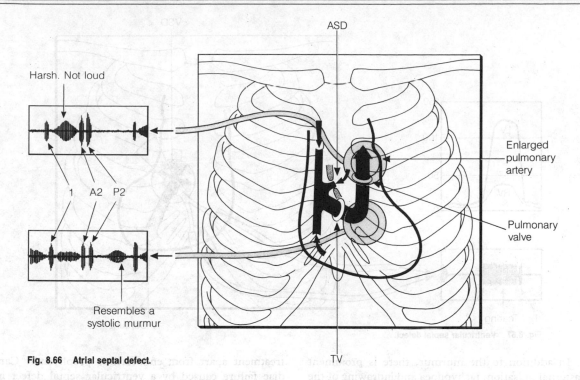

Fig. 8.66   Atrial septal defect.

fixed because the septal defect equalises left and right atrial pressures throughout the respiratory cycle;

2. a systolic flow murmur over the pulmonary valve.

In children with a large shunt there may be a diastolic flow murmur over the tricuspid valve; unlike a mitral flow murmur, this is usually high-pitched.

The chest radiograph shows enlargement of the heart and of the pulmonary artery; increased pulsation of these vessels can be seen on screening. The ECG usually shows incomplete right bundle branch block because right ventricular depolarisation is delayed as a result of ventricular dilatation. Echocardiography is very useful, and cross-sectional echocardiography may directly demonstrate the defect.

Management
Atrial septal defects large enough to be clinically recognisable should be closed surgically, and the long-term prognosis thereafter is excellent. Pulmonary hypertension and shunt reversal are contraindications to surgery.

VENTRICULAR SEPTAL DEFECT

Aetiology
Congenital ventricular septal defect occurs as a result of incomplete septation of the ventricles. Embryologically, the interventricular septum has a membranous and a muscular portion, and the latter is further divided into inflow, trabecular and outflow portions. Most congenital defects are 'perimembranous', i.e. at the junction of the membranous and muscular portions.

Acquired ventricular septal defect may result from stab wounds, or from rupture of an infarcted interventricular septum as a complication of acute myocardial infarction.

Clinical features
Flow from the high pressure left ventricle to the low pressure right ventricle during systole produces a *pansystolic* murmur usually heard best at the left sternal edge but radiating all over the praecardium (Fig. 8.67). The murmur will be absent if pressure in the right vetricle is elevated. This may be the case immediately after birth, while pulmonary vascular resistance remains high, or in Eisenmenger's syndrome (described below). Congenital ventricular septal defect may present as cardiac failure in infants, as a murmur with only minor haemodynamic disturbance in older children or adults, or rarely as Eisenmenger's syndrome.

Cardiac failure
This is usually absent in the immediate postnatal period but becomes apparent in the first 4–6 weeks of

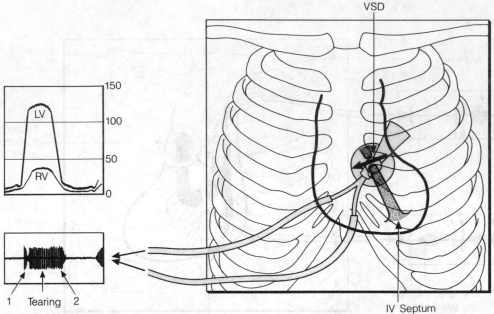

Fig. 8.67   Ventricular septal defect.

life. In addition to the murmur, there is prominent parasternal pulsation, tachypnoea and indrawing of the lower ribs on inspiration. The chest X-ray shows pulmonary plethora and the ECG shows right and left ventricular enlargement. In a proportion of infants, cardiac failure regresses and the murmur gets quieter or disappears. This may be due to *spontaneous closure* of the defect or to the development of Eisenmenger's syndrome. *Small ventricular septal defects* present in older children as a loud pansystolic murmur without other haemodynamic changes (Maladie de Roger). The ECG is normal, the chest radiograph may show a slightly enlarged heart and pulmonary plethora.

Eisenmenger's syndrome
This is pulmonary hypertension complicating an initial left-to-right shunt. Progressive changes take place in the pulmonary vessels, and once established the increased pulmonary resistance is irreversible. It is more common with large ventricular septal defects or persistent ductus arteriosus than with atrial septal defect. The murmur disappears, and the cardiac action is less forceful. Central cyanosis appears, and finger clubbing develops. The chest radiograph shows a small heart shadow, enlarged central pulmonary arteries and peripheral 'pruning' of the pulmonary vessels. The ECG shows right ventricular hypertrophy.

Management
Small ventricular septal defects require no specific treatment apart from endocarditis prophylaxis. Cardiac failure caused by a ventricular septal defect in infancy is initially treated medically with digoxin (10–20 µg/kg/d) and frusemide (1–3 mg/kg/d). Persisting failure is an indication for surgery: either repair of the defect or banding of the pulmonary artery to raise right ventricular pressure and reduce the shunt (banding is a prelude to definitive closure and debanding when the child is larger). Echocardiography helps to predict which septal defects are likely to close spontaneously. Eisenmenger's syndrome is prevented by monitoring (repeated ECG and echocardiography) for signs of rising pulmonary resistance and carrying out pulmonary artery banding or repair as appropriate. A fully developed Eisenmenger's syndrome is irreversible. Periodic venesection helps if there is extreme polycythaemia (as a reaction to arterial hypoxia), and heart-lung transplantation may be considered.

Post-myocardial infarct. Septal defects require urgent surgical closure, usually with resection of infarcted tissue, and sometimes coronary grafting.

Outcome and prognosis
Except in the case of Eisenmenger's syndrome, long-term prognosis is very good in congenital ventricular septal defect. Most patients with Eisenmenger's syndrome die in the second or third decades of life, but a few survive to the fifth decade. Post-myocardial infarct VSD carries a high mortality.

PULMONARY STENOSIS

Pulmonary stenosis with an intact interventricular septum has already been considered on page 300.

TETRALOGY OF FALLOT

This comprises pulmonary stenosis, a ventricular septal defect, 'overriding' of the ventricular septal defect by the aorta, and right ventricular hypertrophy (Fig. 8.68). It is distinct anatomically and embryologically from the coincidence of pulmonary stenosis and ventricular septal defect in the same patient.

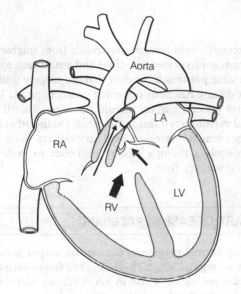

Fig. 8.68 Fallot's tetralogy. The stenosis is in the infundibulum of the right ventricle.

Aetiology

The embryological cause is abnormal development of the bulbar septum which separates the ascending aorta from the pulmonary artery, and which normally aligns and fuses with the outflow part of the interventricular septum. The defect occurs in about 1 in 2000 births.

Clinical features

Tetralogy of Fallot is the commonest congenital condition causing cyanosis in infancy, but cyanosis may not be present in the newborn child. It is only when right ventricular pressure rises to equal or exceed left ventricular pressure that a large right-to-left shunt develops. The right ventricular outflow obstruction is partly valvar and partly subvalvar. The subvalvar

obstruction is dynamic, and may increase suddenly under adrenergic stimulation. The affected child, often after feeding or a crying attack, suddenly becomes increasingly cyanosed, and may become pulseless and apnoeic. These attacks are called 'Fallot spells'. In other children Fallot spells are uncommon, but cyanosis becomes increasingly apparent, with stunting of growth, finger clubbing and polycythaemia. The natural history before the development of surgical correction was variable, with most patients dying in infancy or childhood, but some surviving to adulthood to die of cerebral thrombosis or right heart failure.

On examination the most characteristic feature is usually the combination of cyanosis with a loud ejection systolic murmur in the pulmonary area (as for pulmonary stenosis). Cyanosis may be absent in the newborn, or, in patients where right ventricular outflow obstruction is mild ('acyanotic tetralogy of Fallot'). The murmur becomes very quiet or disappears during a 'spell' (because blood flow through the pulmonary valve virtually ceases).

Investigations

ECG shows right ventricular hypertrophy, and the chest radiograph shows an abnormally small pulmonary artery. Echocardiography is diagnostic.

Management

The definitive management is total correction of the defect by surgical relief of the pulmonary stenosis and closure of the ventricular septal defect. If the child is too small or too frail for definitive correction, a Blalock-Taussig shunt can be performed by anastomosing one of the subclavian arteries to a pulmonary artery. This improves pulmonary blood flow and does not preclude definitive correction at a later stage.

Follow-up

Patients with uncorrected tetralogy of Fallot usually die in childhood or adolecence. The prognosis after total correction is good, especially if the operation is done in childhood. Follow-up is needed to look for residual pulmonary stenosis, recurrence of the septal defect, or rhythm disorders.

OTHER CAUSES OF CYNOTIC CONGENITAL HEART DISEASE

Other causes of cyanotic congenital heart disease are summarised in Table 8.8. Echocardiography is usually the definitive diagnostic procedure, supplemented if necessary by cardiac catheterisation.

Table 8.8   Other causes of cyanotic congenital heart disease

Name	Cause of cyanosis	Treatment	Comments
Tricuspid atresia	Blood diverted from RA to LA	Fontan operation (conduit from right atrium to pulmonary artery)	Surgery feasible in selected cases only
Pulmonary atresia	Venous blood diverted to LA	Shunt *may* be possible from aorta to vestigial pulmonary artery	
Transposition of the great arteries	Aorta arises from right, pulmonary artery from left ventricle	Balloon rupture of interatrial septum to allow mixing of arterial and venous blood followed by *either* Mustard's operation (intertatrial baffle) *or* Switch operation (reconnect aorta to LV, PA to RV)	

SURGERY AND HEART DISEASE

THE SURGICAL TREATMENT OF HEART DISEASE

Surgery is playing an increasingly important role in the management of heart disease; it is now possible, for example, to correct, to varying degrees, most types of congenital heart disease.

SURGERY IN PATIENTS WITH HEART DISEASE

Patients with heart disease undergoing surgery are at risk from the anaesthetic and from the surgery itself. Skilled anaesthesia is particularly important. Continuous monitoring of the ECG, systemic arterial pressure, central venous pressure or pulmonary artery and pulmonary artery wedge pressure may be advisable in appropriate cases, both during surgery and in the early postoperative period.

On the whole, patients with heart disease tolerate surgery remarkably well. Exceptions to this rule are patients with recent myocardial infarction and those who have cardiac or respiratory failure. Only in exceptional circumstances should patients be operated on within 3 months of myocardial infarction; cardiac and respiratory failure should be brought under control before operation if possible. If heart block is present, a pacemaker should be inserted prior to surgery. Surgical diathermy should be avoided if possible in patients with pacemakers; if it is essential, the diathermy electrodes should be kept as far from the pacemaker as possible.

Hypertension is not usually a contraindication to surgery, but it is necessary for the anaesthetist to be aware of what antihypertensive therapy is being used,

as excessive hypotension may result from interactions between antihypertensive drugs and anaesthetic agents.

In some patients it is better to defer surgery until the heart disease has been corrected or ameliorated. Thus, elective general surgery should be deferred until after mitral valvotomy, if this is indicated. On the other hand if the cardiac surgery will necessitate long-term anticoagulant therapy it may be better to undertake general surgery first.

HEART DISEASE IN PREGNANCY

During normal pregnancy the cardiac output increases by an average of 30%. This is due to a fall in peripheral vascular resistance, a rise in blood volume and a small increase in the heart rate. These changes produce characteristic physical signs which are listed in the information box below. The heart may be slightly enlarged and tends to be displaced upwards and outwards by the high diaphragm.

The increased load on the heart often provokes or worsens symptoms in patients with heart disease.

CARDIOVASCULAR SIGNS IN NORMAL PREGNANCY

- Warm peripheries
- Large volume pulse
- Increased venous pressure
- Increased heart rate
- Reduced diastolic BP
- Loud first heart sound
- Third heart sound
- Pulmonary and aortic systolic flow murmurs
- Modest ankle oedema

These do not usually occur before the 12th week, and tend to become maximal from the 24th week onwards. The main symptom of heart disease in pregnancy is breathlessness, but oedema may also occur. Symptoms are a poor guide to the severity of heart disease as some patients are totally asymptomatic until they develop acute pulmonary oedema in late pregnancy or shortly after delivery.

The commonest major form of heart disease encountered in pregnancy is mitral stenosis. Pregnancy should be deferred in patients with severe mitral stenosis, but is usually safe after valvotomy has been performed. If a patient with advanced mitral stenosis does become pregnant either valvotomy or termination should be carried out before the 16th week. With less serious degrees of mitral stenosis and with most other forms of heart disease, pregnancy can be allowed to continue and is usually uncomplicated. However, if objective evidence of deterioration is apparent, bed-rest must be enforced, combined if necessary with digoxin and diuretics. With careful management, even those with advanced heart disease can be carried successfully through pregnancy and delivery.

Patients with mechanical heart valves who require continuous anticoagulation pose a particular problem during pregnancy because warfarin commonly causes fetal abnormalities and may lead to haemorrhagic complications. In some cases the risks can be reduced by switching to heparin, which does not cross the placenta; nevertheless, it is wise to try and avoid mechanical valve replacement in patients who may become pregnant.

Patients with congenital heart disease are being seen with increasing frequency during pregnancy. Usually the lesion has been corrected beforehand and in most cases no problems arise. However, pregnancy is a formidable hazard in those who have severe pulmonary vascular disease.

Ischaemic heart disease in pregnancy is rare but is also associated with a high fetal and maternal mortality.

Women with cardiac lesions susceptible to infective endocarditis should receive prophylactic antibiotics if labour is complicated. Since it is impossible to predict some complications many authorities advise prophylactic antibiotics in every patient at risk.

VASCULAR DISEASES

PERIPHERAL ARTERIAL DISEASE

Aetiology
Disease of the peripheral arteries is most commonly due to atheroma. Less common causes are thromboembolism, vasculitis, Raynaud's disease and cold injury (frostbite).

A variant of atheromatous peripheral vascular disease occurs in diabetics: here the major arterial pulses may be preserved despite soft tissue ischaemia, infection and ulceration are common, and diabetic peripheral neuropathy may affect sensation.

ATHEROMATOUS PERIPHERAL VASCULAR DISEASE

Clinical features
Atheromatous peripheral vascular disease is more common in men than women, is strongly associated with smoking, and affects the legs more than the arms. Patients are usually over 50 years old. The commonest presenting symptom is intermittent claudication – a discomfort or ache in the calves or buttocks which comes on with walking and disappears with rest. Pulses in the leg and foot are absent or diminished.

Eventually the patient may develop rest pain in the affected limb. Characteristically this is worse at night, and the patient may get temporary relief by allowing the limb to hang over the side of the bed outside the bedclothes. It is common at this stage for the limb to feel cold to the examiner's touch, for the skin to be pale or discoloured, and for hair growth to be absent. Small patches of skin necrosis may appear, often related to pressure points or minor injury. Finally, frank gangrene may occur, usually starting with one or more toes. At this stage there may be much pain, and if infection occurs a foul smelling discharge.

Investigation
Doppler ultrasound allows a more accurate assessment of peripheral pulse pressure. Plain radiographs of the abdomen and legs may detect vascular calcification. Angiography allows an accurate assessment of the presence and extent of vascular stenoses. It is important to assess the whole patient for evidence of coronary or cerebrovascular disease and for smoking related lung disease.

Management
Management advice is summarised in the information box (p. 336).

Because the failure rate after angioplasty or surgical reconstruction is appreciable, these are usually reserved for patients with crippling symptoms or in whom the limb is in jeopardy. Sympathectomy may produce temporary improvement sufficient to heal an ischaemic ulcer. Amputation my be necessary for a painful,

---

MANAGEMENT OF PERIPHERAL ARTERIAL DISEASE

- Stop smoking, lose weight if obese
- Stop vasoconstrictor drugs, e.g. beta-blockers
- If diabetic, optimise blood glucose control
- Encourage exercise (increases collateral flow)
- Arrange chiropody
- Vasodilator drugs unhelpful
- Surgery only for severe disability, intractable pain, limb in jeopardy:

  Surgical options
  Angioplasty
  Vascular reconstruction
  Sympathectomy: phenol injection
                   surgical
  Amputation

---

infected and non-viable limb. Medication has little role in atheromatous peripheral vascular disease, but vasodilators may be useful where there is a substantial vasospastic component (nifedipine 5–10 mg t.i.d.). Severe pain, especially if there is a neuropathic component, may be helped by amitryptilene (25–50 mg nocte).

Follow-up

The major cause of death in patients with atheromatous peripheral vascular disease is myocardial infarction. It is important to reduce risk factors for this as far as possible. Patients should have specialised chiropody because of the increased risk of infection from minor injury to the feet.

VASCULITIS

Clinical features

Vasculitis is a generic term for inflammatory diseases affecting blood vessels. Vasculitides affecting medium-sized or large vessels may cause symptoms of peripheral artery disease. The most important are polyarteritis nodosa (p. 794), giant cell arteritis (p. 794) and Takayasu's disease (pulseless disease or aortic arch syndrome). The latter characteristically affects young women aged 20–30 and is common in Oriental races. There may be an association with HLA-B5. It is an inflammatory arteritis predominantly affecting the aorta and its branches, and also the pulmonary artery. It starts with a generalised systemic illness with fever, myalgia and arthralgia. The upper limbs are more affected than the lower, and in the late stages the major pulses are impalpable. The ESR is usually raised.

Management

Corticosteroid treatment (prednisolone 40 mg daily initially, tailing down to 10 mg a day at a rate determined by symptoms and the ESR) may be helpful in Takayasu's disease and in giant cell arteritis. Corticosteroids and other immunosuppressants may be useful in polyarteritis nodosa (p. 794).

RAYNAUD'S PHENOMENON

Clinical features

This is an intense vasospasm of peripheral arteries. On exposure to cold the fingers (and less commonly the toes) become initially very pale from vasoconstriction. This is followed by cyanosis secondary to the poor blood flow. Eventually when the blood flow returns there is redness and discomfort. When the phenomenon occurs without other associated illness or precipitating cause it is called Raynaud's disease. This occurs more frequently in women than in men, and is common, affecting about 5% of the population. Other associations are listed in the information box below.

CAUSES OF RAYNAUD'S PHENOMENON

- Idiopathic (Raynaud's disease)
- Drugs
  Beta-blockers
  Ergotamine and derivatives
- Occupational exposure to vibrating tools
- Occupational exposure to cold
- Scleroderma/systemic sclerosis
- Cryoglobulinaemia
- CRST syndrome (calcinosis, Raynaud's, sclerodactyly, telangiectasia)

Management

Patients should stop smoking, and vasoconstrictor drugs or beta blockers should be withdrawn. Cold exposure should be avoided. Nifedipine (5–10 mg t.i.d.) is sometimes helpful. Severe cold injury causes occlusion of peripheral arterioles while leaving large vessels patent. Initially the limb or digits are white and anaesthetic; as warming occurs they become dusky and painful. Vasodilators are unhelpful and analgesia with conservative treatment is best. Amputation is sometimes necessary, but should be delayed until there is clear demarcation of dead tissue.

AORTIC ANEURYSM

Aetiology

An aortic aneurysm is an abnormal dilatation of the

aortic wall. Aneurysms may be due to atheromatous disease, connective tissue disease, or syphilis. Dissecting aneurysm has a different pathology and is considered separately. *Atheromatous aortic aneurysm* is the commonest form. Atheroma may weaken the aortic wall and lead to local aneurysm formation. The commonest site is the abdominal aorta between renal and iliac arteries, but the thoracic aorta may also be affected.

Clinical features

Abdominal aneurysms usually occur in men over 60: they may be asymptomatic, may cause backache or be associated with claudication, or may present acutely with abdominal pain and hypotension as a consequence of rupture. Clinical diagnosis is by palpation – the 'expansile' pulsation of an aneurysm is different from 'transmitted' pulsation from a normal aorta. Confirmation is by *ultrasound* scanning, followed up by angiography. The natural history of an aneurysm is for it to expand and eventually rupture.

Management

Elective surgical repair has a much lower mortality than emergency surgery for rupture. Suggested management for abdominal aneurysms is shown in the information box below. The mortality for surgical repair of thoracic aneurysms is higher, and they are usually treated conservatively unless there are signs of progressive enlargement.

MANAGEMENT OF ABDOMINAL AORTIC ANEURYSMS

- Symptoms of rupture
  Emergency surgery
- Backache or abdominal pain
  Ultrasound, angiography
  Surgery
- Asymptomatic
  Ultrasound – if < 4 cm, follow with serial ultrasound
              if > 4 cm, angiography and consider surgery

Aneurysms associated with connective tissue disease
Connective tissue diseases such as Marfan's disease and Ehlers Danlos syndrome are associated with aneurysm, usually of the thoracic aorta. These may rupture directly or cause dissecting aneurysm. Patients are usually 20–50 years old: they may have the characteristic facial and skeletal features of the fully fledged syndrome, but formes frustes occur and a family history is helpful. Screening by chest radiography or CT scan may detect aortic dilatation at an early stage.

Elective replacement of the ascending aorta has been recommended, but carries a mortality of 5–10%. Beta-blockade may also reduce the risk of dilatation and rupture. Pregnancy is a particularly hazardous time, and rest in hospital may be indicated.

Syphilitic aortic aneurysm
This is now rare. It usually presents as a chance radiographic finding, as angina-like chest pain, or as heart failure via aortic reflux. Besides a dilated ascending aorta, the X-ray may show fine 'egg-shell' calcification. Serology is usually positive. Surgical treatment may be required for progressive enlargement, angina due to coronary ostial stenosis, or aortic reflux. Otherwise, treatment is that of the underlying syphilis.

Dissecting aneurysm of the aorta
A dissecting aneurysm is the result of a tear in the tunica intima of the aorta followed by entry of blood into the plane of the tunica media and separation of a 'flap' of intima from the rest of the aortic wall. It may go on to external rupture of the aorta, or the flap may cause ischaemia of vital organs by occluding the origins of their supplying arteries from the aorta.

Two predisposing factors are hypertension, and a connective tissue disorder causing weakness of the aortic tissues. A useful classification of dissecting aneurysms distinguishes Type 1 aneurysms which arise in the ascending aorta, Type 2 which arise distal to the origin of the brachiocephalic artery but may extend into ascending or descending aorta, and Type 3 aneurysms which arise distal to the left subclavian and do not extend into the aortic arch.

Clinical features

Clinical presentation is usually acute, with severe pain in the chest and back, often starting between the shoulder blades and described as 'tearing'. On examination there may be assymetry of the brachial, carotid or femoral pulses. In Type 1 dissection there may be a diastolic murmur of aortic reflux. There is sometimes an inappropriate bradycardia from stimulation of aortic baroreceptors. The chest radiograph characteristically shows broadening of the upper mediastinum and distortion of the aortic 'knuckle', but these appearances are not invariable. A pleural effusion is common in Type 3 dissection. The most useful investigations are transoesophageal echocardiography, CT scanning and angiography. Type 1 dissecting aneurysms require emergency surgical repair under cardiopulmonary bypass. Type 2 aneurysms usually also require surgery. Type 3 aneurysms can initially be treated medically, with bed-rest and careful control of blood pressure. Surgical intervention may be needed if there is evidence of leakage or extension, or for renal or bowel ischaemia from the intimal flap.

SUDDEN OCCLUSION OF A MAJOR ARTERY

This is usually due to embolism from the heart as a result of rheumatic heart disease, myocardial infarction or, rarely, an atrial myxoma. Emboli lodge commonly at the aortic, iliac or popliteal bifurcations. The limb becomes painful, cold, numb and pale, and pulses distal to the block are absent. Surgical embolectomy should be considered without delay. A Fogarty balloon catheter is used to extract the embolus through a small arteriotomy, and the procedure is often performed under local anaesthesia. While preparations for surgery are being made, pain should be relieved and the limb kept at rest and at room temperature.

VENOUS THROMBOSIS

Thrombo-occlusive disease of peripheral veins may present as superficial thrombophlebitis or deep vein thrombosis.

Superficial thrombophlebitis

This is characterised by a tender painful superficial vein. The condition usually occurs in patients with varicose veins and often affects the saphenous vein. Pulmonary embolism is extremely rare. The problem usually resolves spontaneously but analgesics and bed-rest may be necessary for a few days.

Deep vein thrombosis

This is most common in the lower limbs particularly in the venous sinuses of the soleus muscle in the calf and in the femoral and iliac veins. It is much less frequent in the upper limb but the axillary vein may be involved as a complication of trauma, neoplasm or radiotherapy.

Pathology

At first the thrombus consists mainly of dense layers of platelets and fibrin; later it is a loose, friable, jelly-like mass of fibrin and red cells which readily becomes detached to form an embolus. After a few days inflammatory changes occur in the wall of the vein. The thrombus may undergo lysis or organisation.

Aetiology

A number of factors may encourage venous thrombosis and these are listed in the information box right. Although deep vein thrombosis can occur in an

---

> **FACTORS THAT MAY PREDISPOSE TO VENOUS THROMBOSIS**
>
> - Venous stasis
>   Immobility (bed-rest, surgery, limb paralysis)
>   Low cardiac output
> - Venous injury
>   Trauma
>   Intravenous cannulation
> - Increased coagulability
>   Malignant disease, drugs (e.g. oestrogens or oestrogen containing oral contraceptives), dehydration, polycythaemia, nephrotic syndrome, ulcerative colitis, antithrombin III deficiency
> - Increasing age

---

otherwise normal individual a careful search will usually uncover one or more aetiological factors. The condition is extremely common in elderly women with fractured neck of femur and elderly hemiplegic patients; it is also a common complication of abdominal or gynaecological surgery and of myocardial infarction.

Clinical features

Deep vein thrombosis may be clinically silent in up to 50% of cases. Some patients may present with pulmonary embolism (p. 323) and, occasionally, hospitalised patients may present with a low-grade pyrexia. There may be pain, swelling, and cyanotic discolouration of the affected limb. If the lumen of the main vein is occluded there may be dilatation of the superficial veins with warm pink skin. In the most severe cases the limb may become deeply cyanosed with gross oedema and venous gangrene may supervene.

Post-phlebitic syndrome

This is due to long-standing deep venous obstruction with destruction of the deep venous valves. This leads to high pressure in the remaining leg veins and can cause chronic pain, oedema, venous staining, eczema and ulceration.

Diagnosis

Unfortunately the clinical features of deep vein thrombosis are very variable and clinical diagnosis is notoriously unreliable. Ascending venography is the definitive investigation and will also help to define the extent and site of thrombus. This may influence the choice of treatment because thrombus that extends into the ileo-femoral vessels is more likely to lead to the post-phlebitic syndrome or pulmonary embolism.

Ultrasound examination of the calf may help in the differential diagnosis; this includes simple muscle strain, haematoma and ruptured Baker's cyst (p. 767).

Other potentially useful investigations include Doppler flow meter studies, impedence plethysmography and 125 I fibrinogen scanning (this is particularly useful in detecting early, often asymptomatic thrombus).

Management

Treatment is aimed at preventing the propagation of thrombus, pulmonary embolism, and damage to the valves of the vein leading to chronic venous insufficiency. Unless there is a major contraindication, such as active peptic ulceration or bleeding, treatment is initiated with heparin (using the same dose as in pulmonary embolism, see p. 324) and continued with warfarin (p. 759). Thrombolysis with streptokinase (p. 314) has been shown to improve the outcome in selected cases and should be considered in patients with recent, extensive ileo-femoral thrombosis. Thrombectomy may occasionally be required.

Oral anticoagulants are normally continued for three months. However, indefinite therapy may be indicated in patients with persisting risk factors (see information box right) or recurrent episodes of deep vein thrombosis.

Most patients require a short period of bed-rest with the legs elevated to 15%. Mobilisation and physiotherapy can begin as soon as the patient can walk without undue discomfort. Graduated elastic stockings accelerate venous flow and may reduce oedema and encourage

recanalisation. However, care must be taken to avoid a constricting effect by the hose rolling up. Support of this kind may be necessary to control chronic venous insufficiency. Straining at stool often causes separation of venous thrombi and should be avoided.

Prevention

A variety of measures have been shown to reduce the incidence of deep vein thrombosis and pulmonary embolism in patients at risk. These are most applicable to patients confined to bed or undergoing surgery when the period of risk can be easily defined. (See information box below.)

PREVENTION OF VENOUS THROMBO-EMBOLISM

- Avoid venous stasis
  Graduated support stockings
  Active leg exercises in bed
  Early mobilisation
- Anticoagulants
  Intravenous dextrans (e.g. 30 gm dextran, mol wt 70 000, In 500 ml 5% dextrose infused over 6 hours immediately after surgery)
  subcutaneous heparin
  (e.g. 5000 units 8-hourly for the duration of the high-risk period)
  Full dose i.v. heparin or oral warfarin for patients at high risk

---

FURTHER READING

Bhattacharyya S and Tandon R 1986 The diagnosis of rheumatic fever – evolution of the Jones criteria. International Journal Cardiology 12: 285–294.

de Bono D P 1989 Examination of the cardiovascular system. In: Munro J, Edwards C R W (eds) Macleod's clinical examination. 8th Edn. Churchill Livingstone, Edinburgh.

Bradley R D 1977 Studies in acute heart failure. Arnold, London. An elegant discussion of the application of physiological principles to the management of acute heart failure.

Brandenburg R O, Fuster V, Giuliani E R, McGoon D C 1987 'Cardiology – fundamentals and practice'. Chicago, Year Book Medical Publishers. An alternative to Braunwald as a major cardiological text.

Braunwald E 1988 Heart disease: a text book of cardiovascular medicine. Saunders, Philadelophia. A detailed and comprehensive textbook.

ISIS-2 (Second International Study of Infarct Survival)

Collaborative Group 1988 Randomised trial of intravenous streptokinase, oral aspirin, both or neither among 17 187 cases of suspected myocardial infarction: ISIS-2. Lancet ii: 349–60.

Julian D G 1987 Cardiology, 5th edn., Balliere Tindall, London. An introduction to cardiology for the nonspecialist.

Orme S 1988 Aspirin all round? British Medical Journal 296: 207–308. This issue of the British Medical Journal also contains three major reports of aspirin in the prevention of vascular disease.

Report of a Working Party of the British Society for Antimicrobial Chemotherapy 1985 Antibiotic treatment of streptococcal and staphylococcal endocarditis. Lancet; 2: 815–7.

The CONSENSUS Trial Study Group 1987 Effects of enalapril on mortality in severe congestive cardiac failure. New England Journal of Medicine 316: 1429–35.

9

Diseases of the Respiratory System

Because the lungs are open to the external environment, the study of respiratory disease has wider horizons than the lungs or even the whole body. Structural, functional, immunological or microbiological changes within the lungs can be closely related to epidemiological, environmental, occupational, personal or social factors. In future, advances in molecular biology may reveal more fully the genetic basis of such conditions as asthma and cystic fibrosis.

Respiratory disease imposes its chief burden on the community not only through acute infections, but also through bronchial carcinoma – which caused more than 39 000 deaths in Great Britain in 1987 – and the long progress of morbidity caused by chronic bronchitis and emphysema. In the UK, the incidence of tuberculosis continues to fall but it remains of great importance worldwide. The general public is now more aware of asthma, following surveys indicating that up to 10% of British children may show some symptoms of the condition. Public concern about industrial air pollution is also increasing, but reduction in personal air pollution caused by smoking is the single most important factor in reducing respiratory disease.

APPLIED ANATOMY

UPPER RESPIRATORY TRACT

This includes the nose, nasopharynx and larynx. It is lined by vascular mucous membrane with ciliated epithelium which extends down to the terminal bronchioles. The cilia and the film of mucus covering them have the function of trapping inhaled particles including bacteria and carrying them upwards towards the pharynx. The *larynx* is not only the organ of voice production, but prevents nasal secretions and foreign material from reaching the lower respiratory tract. Like the large bronchi, it is richly supplied with receptors for the cough reflex.

LOWER RESPIRATORY TRACT

This includes the trachea, bronchi and lungs, forming a system of conducting airways leading to the alveoli, where gas exchange takes place. Knowledge of the pattern of branching of the lobar and segmental bronchi and the layout of the pulmonary lobes and segments (Fig. 9.1) is important to the understanding of bronchoscopic findings (p. 348) and normal and abnormal chest radiographs especially in conditions such as lobar pneumonia, lung abscess, lobar or segmental collapse and bronchial tumours (p. 398).

The acinus

The portion of lung supplied by a terminal bronchiole (of which there are some 64 000) is called an acinus and is the functional unit of lung tissue where gas exchange takes place. Each consists of branching respiratory bronchioles leading to clusters of alveoli. The alveoli are lined by flattened epithelial cells (Type I pneumocytes) and also contain Type II or granular pneumocytes which secrete pulmonary surfactant a phospholipid which by reducing surface tension prevents alveolar collapse.

The anatomical implications of the layout of the pleura and mediastinum are dealt with in the sections on pneumothorax (p. 414), pleural effusion (p. 410) and bronchial (p. 398) and mediastinal tumours (p. 402).

APPLIED PHYSIOLOGY

The interpretation of the results of such tests of pulmonary function as ventilatory capacity (p. 349), measurements of lung volumes (p. 349), gas transfer factor (p. 349) and the pressures of oxygen and carbon dioxide in arterial blood (p. 349) depends on understanding of the effects of disease on several physiological mechanisms including pulmonary ventilation and blood flow, gas exchange, and control of breathing. This knowledge is also important in analysing the nature and severity of abnormal lung function in respiratory failure (p. 350) and in conditions such as chronic bronchitis and emphysema (p. 391) and interstitial lung disease (p. 404). Rational oxygen (p. 352) and bronchodilator (p. 381) therapy also depends on such knowledge.

EXAMPLES OF ALTERED RESPIRATORY RESISTANCE

Elastic resistance
Increased
    Pulmonary fibrosis
    Pulmonary oedema
    Kyphoscoliosis
    Ankylosing spondylitis

Decreased
    Emphysema

Non-elastic resistance
Increased
    Asthma
    Emphysema
    Chronic bronchitis
    Tumours of major bronchi

VENTILATION, BLOOD FLOW AND DIFFUSION

The muscular effort of inspiration overcomes elastic resistance of the lungs and chest wall and non-elastic resistance, chiefly in the airways. In normal subjects, the large central airways contribute most of the resistance, and the peripheral airways contribute less despite their individually small calibre because of their large combined cross-sectional area. In disease, resistance of either kind may greatly increase and call into action accessory muscles of inspiration (sterno-mastoid and scaleni) or expiration (abdominals). Examples are listed in the information box (p. 342).

Fatigue developing in muscles working against abnormal loads or at a mechanical disadvantage can contribute to respiratory failure (p. 350).

The right ventricle pumps blood against the relatively low pulmonary vascular resistance. Increased resistance, due for example to thromboembolism (p. 323) or to destructive changes caused by chronic bronchitis and emphysema (p. 391), imposes an additional load

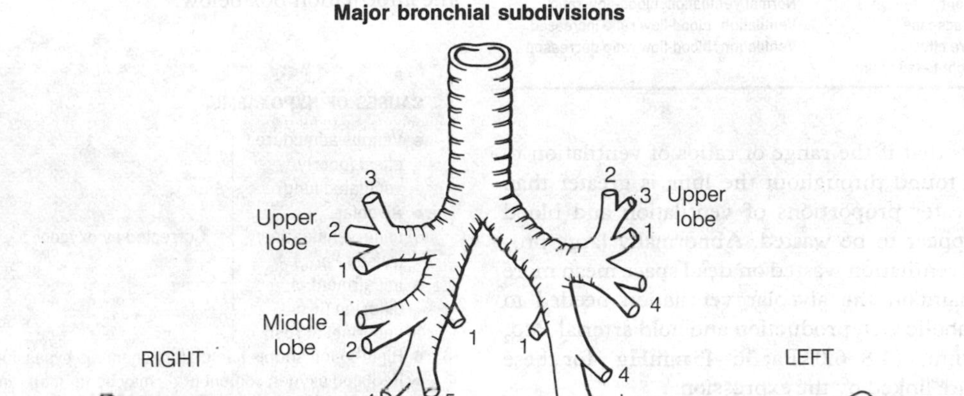

Major bronchial subdivisions

Lateral aspects of lung

Fig. 9.1 The major bronchial divisions and the fissures, lobes and segments of the lungs. The position of the oblique fissure is such that the left upper lobe is largely anterior to the lower lobe. On the right side the transverse fissure separates the upper from the anteriorly placed middle lobe which is matched by the lingular segment on the left side. The site of the lobe determines whether physical signs are mainly anterior or posterior. Each lobe is composed of two or more bronchopulmonary segments, i.e. the lung tissue supplied by the main branches of each lobar bronchus. BRONCHOPULMONARY SEGMENTS: **Right** *Upper lobe* 1. Anterior 2. Posterior 3. Apical *Middle lobe* 1. Lateral 2. Medial. *Lower lobe* 1. Apical 2. Posterior basal 3. Lateral basal 4. Anterior basal 5. Medial basal **Left** *Upper lobe* 1. Anterior 2. Apical 3. Posterior 4. Lingular. *Lower lobe* 1. Apical 2. Posterior basal 3. Lateral basal 4. Anterior basal.

resulting in right ventricular hypertrophy and eventually failure ensues.

Gas exchange

Gas exchange in the lungs is inefficient unless ventilation is distributed uniformly to different parts of the lungs and is matched by uniform distribution of blood flow. Because of the large number of gas-exchanging units in the lung it is convenient to assess inefficiency in terms of three compartments (Table 9.1).

Table 9.1 Three-compartment model of gas exchange

'Ideal compartment'	Normal ventilation : blood-flow ratio
Physiological deadspace	Ventilation : blood-flow ratio increased
Venous admixture effect (physiological right-to-left shunt)	Ventilation : blood-flow ratio decreased

It follows that if the range of ratios of ventilation to blood flow found throughout the lung is greater than normal, greater proportions of ventilation and blood flow will appear to be wasted. Abnormally large proportions of ventilation wasted on dead space mean more work to maintain the alveolar ventilation needed to match metabolic CO_2 production and hold arterial P_{CO_2} in normal limits (4.8–6.0 kPa; 36–45 mmHg), for these quantities are linked by the expression:

$$P_{CO_2} \alpha \frac{CO_2 \text{ production}}{\text{alveolar (useful) ventilation}}$$

This mechanism is, therefore, one of the causes of hypercapnia. Causes are listed in the information box below.

SOME CAUSES OF HYPERCAPNIA (RAISED $P_{a_{CO_2}}$)

Central
Brain-stem lesions
Central sleep apnoea

Neuromuscular
Peripheral neuropathy
Myasthenia gravis
Myopathies

Chest wall
Kyphoscoliosis
Ankylosing spondylitis
Trauma

Pulmonary
Chronic bronchitis
(and emphysema)

Hypercapnia is present if $P_{a_{CO_2}}$ exceeds 6 kPa (45 mmHg) at rest, but values of up to 6.5 kPa (50 mmHg) are seldom clinically important.

Blood flow wasted on perfusing poorly ventilated lung has the effect of a right-to-left shunt. Some of the pathological processes which produce this effect are shown in the information box (right).

PATHOLOGICAL PROCESSES CONTRIBUTING TO VENOUS ADMIXTURE

- Bronchial or bronchiolar obstruction
  Secretions, mucosal oedema, bronchoconstriction, tumour
- Destruction of elastic tissue
  Emphysema
- Pulmonary collapse, consolidation, fibrosis or oedema
- Chest-wall deformities

This mechanism is probably the most important cause of hypoxaemia in disease. The causes are listed in the information box below.

CAUSES OF HYPOXAEMIA

- Venous admixture effect (poorly ventilated lung)
- Alveolar underventilation (raised $P_{a_{CO_2}}$) } Corrected by oxygen
- Impairment of diffusion (less important at rest)
- Right-to-left shunts (circulatory channels bypassing lungs)
- Reduced oxygen content ($P_{a_{O_2}}$ may be normal) (anaemia; inactivated haemoglobin)

Hypoxaemia due to all these causes, except that due to congenital heart disease or vascular anomalies (where shunted blood does not pass through the alveoli), is reversed by giving oxygen. Hypoxaemia also occurs if the oxygen capacity of the blood is reduced as, for example, in anaemia or carbon monoxide poisoning.

The normal arterial P_{O_2} is over 12 kPa (90 mmHg) at the age of 20 and falls to around 11 kPa (82 mmHg) at 60. Above this age a further fall in P_{O_2} of up to 1.3 kPa (10 mmHg) may occur on lying down because of closure of small airways in the dependent regions of the lungs.

Maldistribution of ventilation and blood flow has, therefore, important effects on gas exchange.

Diffusion in the lungs

Oxygen and carbon dioxide move along the terminal airways and alveoli by molecular diffusion in the gas phase and move across the alveolar wall by diffusion in the liquid phase from a site of higher to one of lower partial pressure. It might be expected that thickening of the alveolar wall might impair diffusion, particularly of oxygen. However, most conditions which might have this effect can also cause maldistribution of ventilation and blood flow and analysis suggests that this remains the chief cause of hypoxaemia in these conditions.

If the area available for gas exchange is reduced (as in emphysema p. 394) or if the effective area is reduced by maldistribution and ventilation and perfusion, the overall ability of the lung to transfer gases will also diminish. Such a reduction may not be significant at rest, but may limit the amount of oxygen which can be taken up during exercise and so become a cause of hypoxaemia.

CONTROL OF BREATHING

Influences on the respiratory centre may be considered in two groups as shown in the information box below.

INFLUENCES ON THE RESPIRATORY CENTRE

Neural
Arising within the CNS and from receptors other than peripheral chemoreceptors

Chemical
Arising from chemoreceptors sensitive to composition of blood and CSF.

Their effects are summarised in Table 9.2. It follows that either hyper- or hypocapnia implies some alteration in respiratory control. In some patients with chronic bronchitis and chronic hypercapnia, relief of the concurrent hypoxaemia may, by removing one of the remaining stimuli to breathing, be followed by worsening of the hypercapnia.

REACHING A DIAGNOSIS IN RESPIRATORY DISEASE

The history and physical examination are as significant for reaching a diagnosis in respiratory disease as in disease in other systems. In several important conditions, however, notably pulmonary tuberculosis and bronchial carcinoma, the diagnosis can only be confirmed or excluded by more specialised procedures such as radiological, bacteriological or endoscopic examination.

THE HISTORY

The patient must always be asked about such symptoms as cough, sputum, haemoptysis, pain, breathlessness,

Table 9.2   Some influences on the respiratory centre

Stimulant	
Voluntary	Overbreathing
Upper brain stem lesions	Central neurogenic hyperventilation
Input from receptors	Pain; muscles and joints; pulmonary afferents
Increased Pa_{CO_2}	Via central and peripheral chemoreceptors
Increased arterial hydrogen ion concentration	Via peripheral chemoreceptors
Decreased Pa_{O_2} (<8 kPa at rest)	Via peripheral chemoreceptors
Pyrexia	
Depressant	
Voluntary	Breath-holding
Brain-stem lesions	
Sedative drugs (opiates; benzodiazepines)	
Hypothermia	

wheeze and nasal discharge. Because some respiratory diseases are related to present or past occupational hazards (p. 407), to contact with animals or birds (pp. 384 and 377) or to drug treatment (p. 377), a careful enquiry must be made into these aspects.

COMMON MANIFESTATIONS OF RESPIRATORY DISEASE

Cough. This common symptom has many forms. It is often worse at night or on waking and may be set off by changes in temperature or humidity or by exposure to irritants, such as cigarette smoke. Types of cough are given in Table 9.3.

Table 9.3   Types of cough (with some examples)

Freely productive	Bronchiectasis
Paroxysmal	Chronic bronchitis, asthma
Painful	Pneumonia with pleurisy
'Bovine' (lacking explosive element)	Recurrent laryngeal paralysis
Accompanied by stridor	Whooping cough; partial laryngeal or tracheal obstruction

Sputum. This has several characteristic appearances, which are summarised in Table 9.4. It should be noted that sputum appearing purulent macroscopically may contain either eosinophils or neutrophils on microscopic examination.

Table 9.4   Types of sputum

White	Mucoid
Grey	Mucoid (dust inhalation)
Black	Mucoid + coal dust (melanoptysis)
Yellow or green	Purulent
'Rusty'	Altered blood (pneumococcal pneumonia)
Pink frothy	Pulmonary oedema
Blood-stained	Haemoptysis

Haemoptysis. All grades of severity may occur, from slight blood-streaking to massive haemorrhage. Important causes are shown in the information box below.

CAUSES OF HAEMOPTYSIS

- Bronchial tumours (carcinoma, adenoma)
- Pulmonary infarction
- Bronchiectasis
- Pulmonary tuberculosis
- Mitral stenosis

Although haemoptysis is a common symptom of little prognostic importance in acute and chronic bronchitis, bleeding from the lower respiratory tract, however slight, is potentially serious and demands full investigation.

Chest pain. The common causes of chest pain (of respiratory origin) are given in Table 9.5.

Table 9.5   Varieties of chest pain in respiratory disease

Pleuritic	Unilateral, sharp, worse on deep inspiration (pleural inflammation; pulmonary infarction)
Tracheal	Central retrosternal, searing, worse on coughing (tracheitis)
Pain due to chest wall involvement by tumour	Constant; may have nerve root distribution

Pleural pain is thought to be due to stretching of inflamed parietal pleura; because it is maximal towards the end of inspiration patients may take shallow breaths and suppress cough to avoid it. Pleural pain may be referred to areas of skin supplied by the same spinal nerves as those from the inflamed area of pleura. Thus diaphragmatic pleurisy may present with shoulder pain in the territory of the supraclavicular nerves (C3 and 4).

Breathlessness. Some definitions and abnormal patterns of breathing are summarised in Table 9.6.

Table 9.6   Alterations in breathing

Hyperpnoea	Increased volume; appropriate to circumstances (e.g. exercise), normal sensations
Hyperventilation	Volume disproportionate to metabolic carbon dioxide production, associated sensations (e.g. tingling in fingers)
Tachypnoea	Increased rate
Dyspnoea	Breathing accompanied by conscious effort

Dyspnoea is a subjective sensation and the most common ways by which it may be produced are shown in Table 9.7. In mild heart or lung disease, dyspnoea is noticed only on effort. Its presence at rest is an indication that disease is severe or advanced. In conditions

Table 9.7   Some mechanisms of dyspnoea

Altered respiratory mechanics	
Increased airflow resistance	Asthma, bronchitis, emphysema
Increased lung stiffness	Pulmonary fibrosis
Lung reflexes	Pulmonary oedema, pulmonary embolism
Central mechanisms	Anxiety
Others	Anaemia, uraemia, low cardiac output

such as chronic bronchitis and emphysema, much of the respiratory reserve may have been lost before a sedentary patient complains of breathlessness, but in such patients measurements of ventilatory capacity will show that airflow obstruction is already established. Breathlessness must always be taken seriously, for although it is quite common in anxiety, it is an early manifestation of diseases such as allergic alveolitis (p. 384) or pulmonary thromboembolism (p. 323) at a stage when abnormalities may not be apparent clinically or radiologically. Tests of pulmonary function and objective assessment of exercise capacity are then of value.

Wheeze. This musical sound, best heard during expiration, is a characteristic symptom in diseases causing airflow obstruction and is usually associated with rhonchi on auscultation. It should be distinguished from *stridor* caused by obstruction of major airways (p. 399).

Finger clubbing. The causes of this important appearance are given in the information box below.

CAUSES OF FINGER CLUBBING

Respiratory
Bronchial carcinoma
Chronic intrathoracic suppuration (e.g. bronchiectasis, lung abscess; empyema)
Fibrosing alveolitis
Asbestosis

Non-respiratory
Cyanotic congenital heart disease
Infective endocarditis
Crohn's disease
Malabsorption syndrome
Hepatic cirrhosis
Familial trait

The earliest indication of finger clubbing is an abnormal degree of fluctuation at the bases of the nails; with more advanced clubbing there is also loss of nail angle, increased curvature of the nails and bulbous swelling of the fingertips. Clubbing may be associated with hypertrophic pulmonary osteoarthropathy (p. 399).

Clinical examination

It is important to relate the physical signs to both lateralised disease and generalised disease with airflow obstruction (Table 9.8).

Much can be gained from inspection of the chest wall and from noting the rate and character of the breathing, type and severity of cough and the amount and nature of sputum. For example timing a forced expiration may detect airflow obstruction, provoke cough and provide sputum for examination. Findings on palpation, percussion and auscultation should be thought of not in isolation but in relation to findings on the chest X-ray.

SPECIAL INVESTIGATIONS

IMAGING

The 'plain' chest radiograph

Many diseases, including bronchial carcinoma and pulmonary tuberculosis, cannot be detected at an early stage without an X-ray of the chest. A lateral film provides additional information about the nature and situation of a pulmonary, pleural or mediastinal abnormality. Comparison with previous radiographs may help to distinguish between a 'new' or progressive change which is thus potentially serious, and 'old' or static abnormalities which may be of no importance. In some diseases, such as chronic bronchitis and asthma, there is often no radiographic abnormality. In these diseases functional assessment (p. 379) may be of much more value in detecting abnormality.

Specialised techniques

Some specialised imaging techniques, with examples of their application, are listed in Table 9.9.

ENDOSCOPIC EXAMINATION

Laryngoscopy

The larynx may be inspected indirectly with a mirror or directly with a laryngoscope. Fibreoptic instruments allow a magnified view to be obtained.

Table 9.8 Summary of typical physical signs in the more common respiratory diseases

Pathological process	Movement of chest wall	Mediastinal displacement	Percussion note	Breath sounds	Vocal resonance	Added sounds
Consolidation as in lobar pneumonia	Reduction on affected side	None	Dull	High-pitched bronchial	Increased Whispering pectoriloquy	Fine crepitations early Coarse crepitations later
Collapse due to obstruction of major bronchus	Reduced on side affected	Towards lesion	Dull	Diminished or absent	Reduced or absent	None
Collapse due to peripheral bronchial obstruction	Reduced on side affected	Towards lesion	Dull	High-pitched bronchial	Increased Whispering pectoriloquy	None early-coarse crepitations later
Localised fibrosis and/or bronchiectasis	Slightly reduced on side affected	Towards lesion	Impaired	Low-pitched bronchial	Increased	Coarse crepitations
Cavitation (usually associated with consolidation or fibrosis)	Slightly reduced on side affected	None, or towards lesion	Impaired	'Amphoric' bronchial	Increased Whispering pectoriloquy	Coarse crepitations
Pleural effusion Empyema	Reduced or absent (depending on size) on side affected	Towards opposite side	Stony dull	Diminished or absent (occasionally bronchial)	Reduced or absent (occasionally increased)	Pleural rub in some cases (above effusion)
Pneumothorax	Reduced or absent (depending on size) on side affected	Towards opposite side	Normal or hyper-resonant	Diminished or absent (occasionally faint bronchial)	Reduced or absent	Tinkling crepitations when fluid present
Bronchitis: Acute Chronic	Normal or symmetrically diminished	None	Normal	Vesicular with prolonged expiration	Normal	Rhonchi, usually with some coarse crepitations
Bronchial asthma	Symmetrically diminished	None	Normal	Vesicular with prolonged expiration	Normal or reduced	Rhonchi, mainly expiratory and high-pitched
Bronchopneumonia	Symmetrically diminished	None	May be impaired	Usually harsh vesicular with prolonged expiration	Normal	Rhonchi and coarse crepitations
Diffuse pulmonary emphysema	Symmetrically diminished	None	Normal	Diminished vesicular with prolonged expiration	Normal or reduced	Expiratory rhonchi
Interstitial lung disease	Symmetrically diminished	None	Normal	Harsh vesicular with prolonged expiration	Usually increased	End-inspiratory crepitations uninfluenced by coughing

Table 9.9   Specialised imaging techniques in respiratory disease

Fluoroscopy (screening)	Determining diaphragmatic movement; guiding biopsy
Tomography (conventional or computed)	Determining location and character of lesions
Bronchography	Displaying all or part of the bronchial tree
Radionuclide scanning (perfusion and/or ventilation)	Revealing distribution of blood flow and ventilation
Angiography (including digital subtraction techniques)	Displaying the pulmonary vessels
Ultrasound	Delineating pleural effusions and lesions

Bronchoscopy

The trachea and larger bronchi are inspected by a bronchoscope of either flexible fibreoptic or rigid type. Structural changes, such as distortion or obstruction, can be seen. Abnormal tissue in the bronchial lumen or wall can be biopsied, and bronchial brushings, washings or aspirates can be taken for cytological or bacteriological examination. The range of direct vision is limited by the calibre of the sub-segmental bronchi, but peripheral lesions can sometimes be reached by flexible biopsy forceps directed under fluoroscopic control. Small biopsy specimens of lung tissue taken by forceps passed through the bronchial wall (transbronchial biopsy) may reveal sarcoid granulomata or malignant diseases, but are generally too small to be of diagnostic value in diffuse interstitial lung disease (p. 384 and p. 405).

Mediastinoscopy

In this surgical procedure the mediastinoscope is introduced through a small incision at the suprasternal notch to give a view of the upper mediastinum. Biopsy of some mediastinal nodes is possible which may be of value in obtaining a diagnosis and in determining whether a bronchial carcinoma has spread to the mediastinum and is, therefore, inoperable.

Skin tests

The tuberculin test (p. 366) and Kveim test (p. 409) may be of value in the diagnosis of tuberculosis and sarcoidosis respectively. Skin hypersensitivity tests are useful in the investigation of allergic disease (p. 376).

Immunological and serological tests

The presence of pneumococcal antigen (revealed by counter-immunoelectrophoresis) in sputum, may be of diagnostic importance. Exfoliated cells colonised by Influenza A virus (p. 355) can be detected by fluorescent antibody techniques. In blood, high or rising antibody titres to specific organisms (such as *Legionella*, *Mycoplasma*, *Chlamydia* or viruses) may eventually clinch a diagnosis suspected on clinical grounds. Precipitating antibodies may be found as a reaction to fungi such as *Aspergillus* (p. 373) or to antigens involved in allergic alveolitis (p. 384).

Microbiological investigations

Sputum, pleural fluid, throat swabs, blood and bronchial washings and aspirates can be examined for bacteria, fungi and viruses. In some cases, as when *M. tuberculosis* is isolated, the information is diagnostically conclusive but in other circumstances the findings must be interpreted in conjunction with the results of clinical and radiological examination.

Histopathological and cytological examination

Histopathological examination of biopsy material (obtained endoscopically, from pleural lymph node or lung biopsy) often allows a 'tissue diagnosis' to be made. This is of particular importance in suspected malignancy or in elucidating the pathological changes in interstitial lung disease (p. 405). Important causative organisms, such as *M. tuberculosis*, *Pn. carinii* or fungi may be identified in bronchial washings, brushings or transbronchial biopsies.

Cytological examination of exfoliated cells in sputum, pleural fluid or bronchial brushings and washings or of fine-needle aspirates from lymph nodes or pulmonary lesions (p. 400) can provide rapid evidence of malignancy. Cellular patterns in bronchial lavage fluid may help to distinguish pulmonary changes due to sarcoidosis (p. 409) from those caused by fibrosing alveolitis (p. 405) or allergic alveolitis (p. 384).

Haematological examination

Estimation of the total and differential white cell count may help to distinguish pyogenic infection from tuberculous or viral infection. In community-acquired pneumonia both leucocytosis and leucopenia imply a poorer prognosis. An increase in the eosinophil count may occur for a variety of reasons (p. 383). Estimates of lymphocyte subsets are used in the assessment of syndromes attributable to HIV.

FUNCTIONAL ASSESSMENT

The effects of disease on the function of the lungs are shown in the information box below.

> **FUNCTIONAL ASSESSMENT**
>
> *Impairment*
> Effect of disease on specific aspects of function (e.g. airflow obstruction)
>
> *Disability*
> Consequences of impairment (e.g. breathlessness)
>
> *Handicap*
> Effect of disability on everyday life (e.g. inability to climb stairs)

Most pulmonary function tests detect impairment and assess the effects of treatment or progress of the disease. The tests are listed in the information box below.

> **PULMONARY FUNCTION TESTS**
>
> ● Ventilatory capacity (FEV, and VC; PEF)
> ● Reversibility of airflow limitation
> ● Lung volumes
> ● Gas transfer factor (diffusing capacity)
> ● Arterial blood-gas analysis
> ● Exercise tests

Fewer tests, such as measurements of exercise tolerance, assess disability or handicap. Some tests require a high degree of skill and elaborate apparatus, but others are simple routine procedures which can be undertaken by any doctor without special training.

Table 9.10   Abbreviations used in pulmonary function testing

FEV,	Forced expiratory volume in one second
FVC	Forced vital capacity
VC	Vital capacity (forced or relaxed)
PEF	Peak (maximum) expiratory flow rate
TLC	Total lung capacity
FRC	Functional residual capacity
RV	Residual volume
T_{CO}	Gas transfer factor for carbon monoxide
D_{CO}	Diffusing capacity for carbon monoxide
K_{CO}	Transfer coefficient for carbon monoxide (T_{CO}/litre lung volume)

Measurements of ventilatory capacity

The forced expiratory volume in one second (FEV_1), forced vital capacity (FVC) and vital capacity (VC) are obtained from maximal forced and relaxed expirations into a recording spirometer and compared with predicted values based on age, sex and height and ethnic group. Typical patterns of abnormality known as *obstructive* and *restrictive* ventilatory defects are shown in Table 9.11.

Table 9.11   Patterns of abnormal ventilatory capacity

Test	Obstructive	Restrictive
FEV,	↓↓	↓
VC	↓ or normal	↓
FEV,/VC	↓	Normal or ↑

If an obstructive ventilatory defect is found, the response to bronchodilators in standard doses (salbutamol 200 mcg from pressurised aerosol) or larger doses (salbutamol 2.5 mg by nebuliser) can be measured. Reversibility of airflow obstruction is found in asthma (p. 379) and in some patients with chronic bronchitis.

Peak expiratory flow (PEF) can be measured during forced expiration by a gauge or meter which is simpler and cheaper than a spirometer. Reduced values indicate airflow obstruction, and serial measurements are of use in following circadian changes (p. 380) and responses to therapy or to occupational exposure to allergens or sensitising agents. PEF is of little value in restrictive ventilatory defects.

Even if no apparatus other than a watch and a stethoscope is available, forced expiration can still be used to detect airflow obstruction. Normal people can empty their chests from full inspiration in four seconds or less. Prolongation of forced expiratory time (FET) to more than six seconds indicates significant airflow obstruction.

Measurements of lung volumes

Normal landmarks and patterns of abnormality of lung volumes in obstructive and restrictive ventilatory defects are shown in Figure 9.2. The values are obtained either by diluting helium (a non-toxic, non-absorbed gas) into the gas in the lungs, or in a whole body plethysmograph.

Measurements of gas transfer factor

The gas transfer factor (diffusing capacity) may be thought of as the conductance of the lungs for the gas being studied. It forms a useful overall estimate of the ability of the lungs to exchange gases, and is of particular value in interstitial lung disease (p. 404), sarcoidosis (p. 409) and emphysema (p. 395). It is normally estimated by measuring the uptake of carbon monoxide from a single breath of a 0.3% mixture in air.

Arterial blood-gas analysis

Modern automatic analysers give a rapid direct read-out of Po_2, Pco_2 and hydrogen ion concentration in arterial blood, often supplemented by derived variables

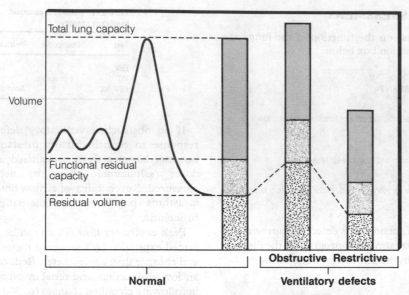

Volume

Total lung capacity

Functional residual capacity

Residual volume

Normal

Obstructive   Restrictive

Ventilatory defects

Fig. 9.2   Normal lung volumes and the changes which occur in obstructive and restrictive ventilatory defects.

(such as oxygen saturation and bicarbonate concentration) which may be of value in assessment of hypoxaemia or acid:base balance (p. 221). Such measurements are of particular value in the management of respiratory failure (p. 351) and asthma (p. 380) and adult respiratory distress syndrome (ARDS) (p. 353).

Ear or pulse oximeters allow continuous non-invasive measurement of arterial oxygen saturation, of value in assessing hypoxaemia and the effects of oxygen therapy.

Exercise tests

Exercise challenge is a self-evident test for detecting exercise-induced asthma (p. 379). Formal exercise tests, in which cardiac and respiratory responses to bicycle or treadmill exercise are measured in the laboratory, are of value in detecting exercise hypoxaemia and in assessing disability due to respiratory disease.

'Everyday' exercise tests, such as measurement of the distance the patient can walk in six minutes, require no complex apparatus and assist in the assessment of disability, handicap and the response to treatment.

RESPIRATORY FAILURE

DEFINITION AND CLASSIFICATION

The definition of respiratory failure is shown in the information box (right).

The mechanisms causing the two types of respiratory

RESPIRATORY FAILURE

Definition
$Pa_{O_2} < 8.0$ kPa (60 mmHg) and/or
$Pa_{CO_2} > 6.5$ kPa (50 mmHg)

Type I
Pa_{O_2} low, Pa_{CO_2} normal or low

Type II
Pa_{CO_2} raised, Pa_{O_2} low – 'ventilatory failure'

---

failure are those causing hypoxaemia and hypercapnia respectively and these have been summarised in the information boxes on page 344. Specific conditions causing each variety of respiratory failure are mentioned below.

ACUTE TYPE I RESPIRATORY FAILURE

Severe hypoxaemia with a normal or low Pa_{CO_2} can develop rapidly in many respiratory and cardiac disorders. Treatment is that of the underlying cause (e.g. pulmonary oedema (p. 353), pneumonia (p. 359)), adult respiratory distress syndrome (p. 353) and correction of hypoxaemia by administration of high concentrations of oxygen by oro-nasal mask. Young children may have to be treated in oxygen tents since few of them tolerate masks. Very ill patients may require artificial ventilation (p. 351).

CHRONIC TYPE I RESPIRATORY FAILURE

Chronic hypoxaemia without carbon dioxide retention has many causes, which include fibrosing alveolitis other types of interstitial lung disease (p. 405) and chronic pulmonary oedema. Treatment is that of the underlying disorder, combined with high concentration oxygen therapy. Such patients are rarely treated with artificial ventilation, since the prognosis is generally poor and aggressive therapy is usually considered to be ethically unjustified.

ACUTE TYPE II RESPIRATORY FAILURE

This type of respiratory failure is also known as asphyxia, and the causes and treatment of several varieties are summarised in Table 9.12. Acute retention of carbon dioxide in this type of respiratory failure also causes severe acute respiratory acidosis (p. 227).

Table 9.12   Treatment of acute Type II respiratory failure

Cause	Treatment
Upper airways obstruction Inhaled foreign body	Try to dislodge it by turning child upside down and forcibly compressing the thoracic cage or by Heimlich manoeuvre (p. 388) in adult. If ineffective, extract foreign body by laryngoscopy or bronchoscopy
Acute epiglottitis, laryngeal oedema, bilateral vocal cord paralysis	Treatment of cause. If medical treatment ineffective, tracheal intubation or tracheostomy
Severe acute asthma	Medical treatment (p. 382). If not rapidly effective, tracheal intubation and intermittent positive-pressure ventilation
Chest injuries Tension pneumothorax Massive haemothorax	Pleural decompression by intercostal tube Drainage of blood through intercostal tube. Thoracotomy if necessary for evacuation of clot and ligation of bleeding points
Flail chest	Tracheal intubation and intermittent positive-pressure ventilation. Fixation of rib and sternal fractures
Brain-stem and cervical cord lesions. Paralysis of respiratory muscles	Tracheal intubation and intermittent positive-pressure ventilation. Treatment of cause where possible
Poisoning with narcotic and other drugs	Measures to eliminate poison. Specific antidote (e.g. naloxone for opium alkaloids). Tracheal intubation and intermittent positive-pressure ventilation

CHRONIC TYPE II RESPIRATORY FAILURE

Causes and mechanisms. The most important cause is chronic bronchitis (p. 391), but Type II respiratory failure also occurs preterminally in other progressive respiratory diseases. Chronic hypercapnia leads to renal conservation of bicarbonate, which usually corrects the respiratory acidosis (p. 227), and restores arterial hydrogen ion concentration towards normal. Further episodes of hypercapnia, often precipitated by bronchial infection, will produce further acidosis, however. Hypercapnia also aggravates hypoxaemia (information box p. 344) and if severe may cause drowsiness which may proceed to coma. Associated right ventricular failure is usually made worse by hypoxaemia which aggravates pulmonary hypertension.

Management

Respiratory infection, with worsening airway obstruction and retained bronchial secretions, is the main factor responsible for exacerbations of Type II respiratory failure in patients with chronic lung disease. Treatment, therefore, requires the use of antibiotics and nebulised bronchodilators (p. 393), with particular emphasis on encouraging efficient cough in a patient who may be drowsy, and treating any oedema with diuretics. Loss of spontaneous cough or falling levels of consciousness may form an indication for the use of analeptics (e.g. an intravenous infusion of doxapram in doses of 1.5–4 mg/min/24 h), which may tide the patient over a period of hypoventilation. If these measures fail, mechanical ventilation must be considered. It is usually reserved for patients who were able to lead a fairly active life before the acute episode and in whom recovery in a day or two is a reasonable prospect.

Mechanical ventilation

Intermittent positive pressure ventilation (IPPV). Patients with both types of respiratory failure may have to be treated with IPPV through a cuffed endotracheal tube introduced through the mouth or nose under general anaesthesia. Positive end-expiratory pressure (PEEP) may be useful in some cases with Type I failure, to correct maldistribution of ventilation and blood flow. Powerful ventilators delivering a fixed volume are required for patients with Type II failure associated with airflow obstruction. Intubation also allows clearance of tracheobronchial secretions by suction or by fibreoptic bronchoscopy. If ventilation is required for more than a few days a tracheostomy should be performed and the endotracheal tube replaced by a cuffed tracheostomy tube.

The volume and oxygen concentration of the air supplied by the ventilator is adjusted to bring arterial Po_2 and Pco_2 towards normal values, and ventilatory assistance should be gradually reduced, if possible, as soon as the cause of respiratory failure has been successfully treated.

Continuous positive airway pressure (CPAP). This form of ventilatory support is delivered by a tight-fitting nasal or oro-nasal mask. It may be used in patients suffering from obstructive sleep apnoea (below), where the applied pressure prevents pharyngeal collapse.

Apparatus is also being developed to provide ventilatory support at night without intubation, and this may be of particular value to patients in whom chronic respiratory failure is the result of mechanical deformity, such as kyphoscoliosis (p. 416).

DISORDERS OF BREATHING DURING SLEEP – SLEEP APNOEA SYNDROMES

Obstructive sleep apnoea

Clinical features
Daytime sleepiness, sometimes uncontrollable, and loud snoring at night in a patient who is often obese suggest this syndrome. Studies using polysomnography indicate that apnoea and hypoxaemia follow obstruction of the upper airway due to pharyngeal closure, and in turn cause arousal with a loud snore. Deeper stages of sleep are not achieved and daytime sleepiness ensues.

Management
Continuous positive airway pressure (CPAP, above) prevents obstruction and relieves the symptoms. Some patients are benefited by reconstructive surgery (uvulo-pharyngoplasty).

Central sleep apnoea
In this ill-defined group of conditions, apnoea occurs without obstruction of the airway. A variety of neurological lesions including failure of respiratory drive has been suggested as the cause.

Symptomatic management in respiratory disease

Cough. Productive cough should normally be encouraged. Patients with bronchiectasis or lung abscess should perform postural drainage, and expectoration in those with tenacious sputum may be aided by hot drinks and inhalations of steam or nebulised saline.

Chest pain. For pleural pain mild analgesics are rarely adequate and most patients require pethidine, 50–100 mg by mouth or intramuscular injection, or even morphine, 10–15 mg i.m. Opiates must, however, be used with caution in patients with poor respiratory function.

Haemoptysis. A sedative (e.g. diazepam 2–5 mg 3 times daily) may be given to allay the anxiety almost always produced by this alarming symptom.

In very severe haemorrhage blood transfusion, aspiration of blood from the bronchial tree through a bronchoscope and, rarely, surgical intervention or embolisation of the bleeding vessel may be needed.

Airflow obstruction. In bronchitis and asthma this is treated by bronchodilators (p. 382) and in some cases by corticosteroids given by inhalation or as tablets (p. 382).

Oxygen therapy

Objective
The objectives of therapy are:

1. To overcome the reduced pressure and quantity of oxygen in the blood in hypoxaemia.
2. To increase the quantity of oxygen carried in solution in the plasma, even when the haemoglobin is fully saturated.

Benefits of oxygen
Many of the causes of hypoxaemia (information box p. 345) are corrected by increased concentrations of inspired oxygen, but right-to-left shunting, either through circulatory channels bypassing the lungs, or through parts of the lungs in which the alveoli are inaccessible to inspired oxygen, is less susceptible. The increased amount of dissolved oxygen carried by blood which has perfused alveoli with a high Po_2 can saturate the haemoglobin in small quantities of shunted blood; persistence of cyanosis when pure oxygen is breathed indicates that the shunt is larger than 20% of the cardiac output.

Adverse effects
Pure oxygen is both irritant and toxic if inhaled for more than a few hours. Premature infants develop retrolental fibroplasia and blindness if exposed to excessive concentrations. Pulmonary oedema and consolidation may occur in adults ventilated with high concentrations for several days. Pulmonary damage by oxygen is one of the possible mechanisms by which ARDS (p. 353) arises; if such patients require oxygen, they should receive the lowest concentration which corrects hypoxaemia.

Technique of administration
Oxygen is a drug which should be prescribed in writing, with clearly specified flow rates or concentrations. Administration should be continuous, though this may be

difficult in restless or confused patients. All oxygen-enriched gas mixtures carry an increased fire risk.

Oxygen masks. These are of two types:

1. Those designed to produce a high inspired concentration. An example is the MC mask, delivering about 60% O_2 when the flow rate is 4–6 l/min.
2. Those designed to produce O_2 enrichment and to prevent rebreathing of expired CO_2. Ventimasks, delivering 24, 28, 35 and 60% O_2, are of this type.

Nasal cannulae. Double cannulae fit into the nostrils and do not interfere with eating, drinking and the wearing of spectacles. At an oxygen flow rate of 2 l/min, the inspired concentration is around 30%. Cannulae are of particular use if oxygen is given for long periods.

Humidification. When MC masks are used, the oxygen should be humidified, either by passing it over warm water (as in the East-Radcliffe humidifier) or through a nebuliser. This is not necessary with Venti-masks or nasal cannulae, as a high proportion of atmospheric air is mixed with the oxygen.

ADULT RESPIRATORY DISTRESS SYNDROME (ARDS)

Aetiology
This is a serious syndrome complicating many disorders (Table 9.13) rather than a single disease entity.

Table 9.13   Causes of adult respiratory distress syndrome

Pneumonias	Viral, bacterial, tuberculous, fungal, *Pneumocystis carinii*, *Mycoplasma pneumoniae*
Inhaled toxic substances	Corrosive chemicals (ammonia, chlorine, nitrogen dioxide), oxygen in high concentration, smoke
Aspiration of irritant substances	Vomitus, water (fresh and salt), hydrocarbons
Systemic disorders	Shock of any cause, septicaemia, eclampsia, uraemia
Blood disorders	Disseminated intravascular coagulation, blood product transfusion, thrombocytopenic purpura
Lung emboli	Fat, air, amniotic fluid, X-ray contrast media
Lung trauma	Contusion, irradiation
Drugs	Diamorphine, methadone, thiazides, barbiturates
Miscellaneous	Acute pancreatitis, high altitude, increased intracranial pressure, cardiopulmonary bypass

Pathology
The alveolar epithelium and pulmonary capillary endothelium are damaged and the alveolar spaces become flooded with oedema fluid of high protein content (noncardiogenic pulmonary oedema).

Clinical features
This is characterised by dyspnoea, hypoxaemia and hypotension. Both lungs are usually affected and crepitations are heard in all areas, especially the bases. The chest X-ray shows rapidly progressive widespread 'fluffy' or 'soft' and sometimes homogeneous shadowing. Often the costophrenic angles remain clear in the early stages.

Management
Treatment is of the underlying cause and correction of the hypoxaemia keeping in mind possible adverse effects of oxygen therapy (p. 352). Many patients require assisted ventilation with positive end-expiratory pressure (PEEP) to maintain an adequate Pa_{O_2}. There is a high mortality in patients who require to be treated by ventilation.

INFECTIONS OF THE RESPIRATORY SYSTEM

Infections of the respiratory tract may be caused by viruses, bacteria or fungi. Viruses are frequently responsible for upper respiratory illnesses. Although viral infection is a relatively uncommon specific cause of pneumonia, it is often complicated by bacterial infection of the bronchi and lungs, as for example in influenza. The bacteria most frequently responsible for respiratory infection, including pneumonia, are *Streptococcus pneumoniae* often in association with *Haemophilus influenzae*, *Staphylococcus aureus*, various species of Gram-negative bacilli and *Legionella pneumophila*. Other organisms such as mycoplasma, coxiella and chlamydia are other but less common, causes of acute pneumonia. Pulmonary infection by *Mycobacterium tuberculosis*, atypical mycobacteria and fungi results in diseases of a more chronic type, which are described separately.

UPPER RESPIRATORY TRACT INFECTIONS

The vast majority of these illnesses, of which acute coryza is by far the most common, are caused by viruses (Table 9.14). Immunity is short-lived, and specific for each virus. The average person can, therefore, expect to have at least two or three attacks of coryza every year. Other viral infections include acute laryngitis and acute laryngotracheobronchitis. Bacterial infection is the usual cause of acute tonsillitis, otitis media and epiglottitis.

Table 9.14 Respiratory infections caused by viruses

Clinical syndrome	Usual cause (other causes in parentheses)
Epidemic influenza	Influenza A and B
'Flu-like' illness	Adenoviruses rhinoviruses. (Enteroviruses)
Sore throat	Adenoviruses. (Enteroviruses, parainfluenza viruses, influenza A and B in partially immune)
Common cold (Coryza)	Rhinoviruses. (Coronaviruses, enteroviruses, adenoviruses, respiratory syncytial virus)
'Feverish' cold	Rhinoviruses, enteroviruses. (Influenza A and B, parainfluenza viruses, respiratory syncytial virus)
Croup	Parainfluenza 1, 2, 3. (Rhinoviruses, enteroviruses)
Bronchitis	Rhinoviruses, adenoviruses. (Influenza A and B)
Bronchiolitis	Respiratory syncytial virus. (Parainfluenza 3)
Pneumonia	Influenza A and B. (Respiratory syncytial virus and parainfluenza viruses in adults)

Investigations

Most patients with upper respiratory tract infections recover rapidly and specific investigation is indicated only in the more severe illness. Viruses can be isolated from exfoliated cells collected on throat swabs, and viral infections may be identified retrospectively by serological tests. In sputum exfoliated cells colonised by certain viruses can be identified by the fluorescent antibody technique, allowing the pathogen to be rapidly defined. Culture of throat swabs and pharyngeal exudate may be helpful if streptococcal sore throat is suspected, and examination of the blood will identify infectious mononucleosis. Radiographic examination may be required to confirm the presence of chronic sinus infection.

ACUTE CORYZA (COMMON COLD)

Clinical features

The onset is usually sudden with a burning and tickling sensation in the nose accompanied by sneezing. The throat often feels dry and sore, the head feels 'stuffed' and there is a profuse watery nasal discharge (rhinorrhoea). These symptoms last for one to two days, after which, with secondary infection, the secretion becomes thick and purulent and impedes nasal breathing. However nasal allergy rather than viral infection is suggested in patients complaining of frequent attacks of sneezing and watery rhinorrhoea without systemic upset.

Complications

Coryza may lead to sinusitis which can become chronic, particularly in the maxillary sinuses, causing persistent discharge from the front and back of the nose often accompanied by nasal obstruction and headache. Other complications are infections of the lower respiratory

tract, occlusion of the Eustachian tubes causing deafness, and otitis media.

Management

In most cases symptoms are mild and do not require treatment. Paracetamol 0.5–1 g every 4–6 hours can be used to relieve systemic symptoms. Nasal decongestants such as oxymetazoline hydrochloride (0.05% solution – 0.15 ml instilled into each nostril every 8–12 h) are of value when nasal obstruction is troublesome but such preparations should only be used for short periods. Antibiotics are not necessary in uncomplicated acute coryza.

ACUTE LARYNGITIS

This usually occurs either as a complication of coryza or a manifestation of one of the infectious fevers, for example, measles. The laryngeal mucous membrane is swollen, congested and coated with mucus.

Clinical features

The throat is dry and sore. The voice is at first hoarse and then reduced to a whisper. Speaking may be painful. There is an irritating non-productive cough but the general upset is usually mild. In children the small laryngeal opening may be almost completely obstructed by oedema and viscid secretion, giving rise to stridor (croup).

Complications

Acute laryngitis usually clears up in a few days but frequently recurring episodes may predispose to chronic laryngitis. Downward spread of the infection may cause tracheitis, bronchitis or even pneumonia.

Management

The voice should be rested as much as possible. Inhalations of steam are helpful and paracetamol (0.5–1 g 4–6-h) can be used to relieve discomfort, pyrexia and systemic symptoms. Antibiotic therapy is of no value in simple acute laryngitis.

ACUTE LARYNGOTRACHEOBRONCHITIS (CROUP)

This illness, which is particularly serious in very young children because of the small calibre of their airways, may be caused by several viruses (Table 9.14).

Clinical features

The initial symptoms may be those of the common cold. These are followed by severe and sometimes violent cough which may be paroxysmal, accompanied by dyspnoea and stridor (croup), contraction of accessory muscles and indrawing of intercostal spaces. The child may be cyanosed and asphyxia may occur if appropriate treatment is not given.

Complications

Superinfections with bacteria, especially *Strep. pneumoniae* and *Staph. aureus*, may occur. The mucosa is intensely inflamed, the secretions are extremely tenacious and fibrinous casts of the bronchi may form.

Management

Inhalations of steam and humidified air are of value, but strong aromatic decongestants should be avoided. Clearing of secretions is of utmost importance and bronchoscopy, endotracheal intubation or tracheostomy may be required as life-saving measures in patients with severe respiratory obstruction. High concentrations of oxygen (p. 353) should be administered to all cyanosed patients and adequate hydration must be maintained. It is wise to give intravenous antibiotic therapy to seriously ill patients on the assumption that bacterial superinfection has occurred. The combined preparation of amoxycillin and clavulanic acid (Augmentin) 30 mg/kg i.v. 8-hourly, or intravenous erythromycin 25–50 mg/kg daily in divided doses are effective drugs which can also be given orally to less critically ill children.

ACUTE EPIGLOTTITIS

This is a rare but serious disease particularly in young children usually caused by bacterial infection almost always *Haemophilus influenzae*.

Clinical features

Fever and sore throat are the presenting features. Stridor develops rapidly because of inflammatory swelling of the epiglottis and surrounding submucosa. In acute epiglottitis, stridor and cough in the absence of hoarseness help to distinguish it from laryngeal causes of stridor.

Complications

Death from asphyxia may occur rapidly. Attempts to examine the throat using a tongue depressor or any instrument should be avoided when epiglottitis is suspected unless facilities for tracheal intubation or tracheostomy are immediately available because this may precipitate complete respiratory obstruction.

Management

In acute epiglottitis intravenous antibiotic therapy is essential. Amoxycillin/clavulanic acid (Augmentin) 30 mg/kg 8-hourly by slow i.v. injection or infusion of chloramphenicol 50–100 mg/kg daily in divided doses should be given as soon as the diagnosis is confirmed or even suspected. Tracheostomy may be necessary as a life-saving measure if complete obstruction of the upper airways occurs.

INFLUENZA

Influenza is a specific acute illness caused by a group of myxoviruses. It occurs in epidemics, and occasionally pandemics, often explosive in nature.

Aetiology

There are two common types of virus, A and B. At least four strains of influenza A, which is responsible for pandemics, have been identified. Influenza B is usually associated with smaller and less virulent outbreaks. The immunity which follows infection is type-specific and of relatively short duration. This causes problems in providing effective immunisation.

Clinical features

These are listed in the information box below.

CLINICAL FEATURES OF INFLUENZA

Incubation
24–48 h

Onset
Sudden pyrexia associated with headache, generalised aches and pains, anorexia, nausea and vomiting

Chest symptoms
Cough – harsh and unproductive

Clinical signs
Fauces hyperaemic. Usually no abnormalities on examination of chest

White cell count
Leucopenia

Course
When no complications acute symptoms subside within 3–5 days. Post-influenzal asthenia may persist for a few weeks

---

The disease may spread rapidly throughout a household or institution. During epidemics, the diagnosis is usually easy. Most sporadic cases are identifiable only as respiratory viral infections unless the virus is isolated, or demonstrated by the fluorescent antibody technique or if serological tests for specific antibodies are positive.

Complications

The disease may be complicated by tracheitis, bronchitis, bronchiolitis and bronchopneumonia. Secondary bacterial invasion by *Strep. pneumoniae*, *H. influenzae* and occasionally *Staph. aureus* may also occur.

Toxic cardiomyopathy may cause sudden death, especially when there is pre-existing cardiac disease. Encephalitis and post-influenzal demyelinating encephalopathy and peripheral neuropathy are rare complications. Post-influenzal asthenia and depression are common, often marked, and may last for several weeks.

Management

Bed rest is advisable until the fever has subsided. A mild analgesic such as paracetamol 0.5–1 g every 4–6 hours usually relieves the headache and generalised pains. Pholcodine 5–10 mg 3–4 times daily may be used to suppress unproductive cough. Specific treatment of complications such as bronchitis (below) and pneumonia (p. 362) may be necessary.

Prevention

Immunity is type-specific and if the antigenic constitution of a new strain can be detected early a specific vaccine may give about 70% protection. Annual winter vaccination is recommended for patients suffering from chronic pulmonary, cardiac or renal disease.

ACUTE BRONCHITIS

Aetiology

This condition is an acute inflammation of the trachea and bronchi caused by viruses and pathogenic bacteria such as *Strep. pneumoniae*, *H. influenzae* and rarely *Staph. aureus*. Bacterial infection is a common sequel of coryza, influenza, measles and whooping-cough. Other factors predisposing to bacterial infection include cold, damp, foggy and dusty atmospheres and cigarette smoking.

Clinical features

The first symptom is an irritating, unproductive cough accompanied by upper retrosternal discomfort or pain caused by tracheitis (Table 9.5). When the bronchi become involved there is also a sensation of tightness in the chest, and breathlessness with wheeze may be present. Respiratory distress may be particularly severe when acute bronchitis complicates chronic bronchitis and emphysema.

The sputum is at first scanty, mucoid, viscid and difficult to produce, and occasionally may be streaked with blood. A day or two later it becomes mucopurulent and more copious. As the infection extends down the bronchial tree there may be associated a pyrexia of 38–39°C and a neutrophil leucocytosis. In the vast majority of cases recovery takes place spontaneously over the next four to eight days without the patient ever becoming seriously ill. Occasionally breathlessness and cough increase, cyanosis appears and if the infection reaches the smaller bronchi and bronchioles ('bronchiolitis') the conditions becomes indistinguishable from bronchopneumonia.

Tracheitis without bronchitis produces no abnormal physical signs. In bronchitis there may be prolonged expiration accompanied by rhonchi and, in bronchiolitis, crepitations (crackles).

Management

In the early stages when cough is painful and unproductive the tough viscid secretion may be loosened by steam inhalation three or four times a day. Cough should be controlled at night by pholcodine 5–10 mg 6–8-hourly. If symptoms or signs of airflow obstruction are present salbutamol or terbutaline 200–500 µg 4–6-hourly should be given by inhalation. Antibiotic therapy is rarely necessary but patients who have signs of bronchiolitis should be treated with oral tetracycline or ampicillin 250–500 mg 4 times daily. Oxygen is seldom required in uncomplicated acute bronchitis.

THE PNEUMONIAS

Pneumonia is the term used to describe inflammation of the lungs. There are many different kinds of pneumonia, some common, others rare.

Aetiology

The pneumonias can be divided into primary and secondary as shown in the information box below.

Occasionally in some types of both primary and

AETIOLOGY OF THE PNEUMONIAS

Primary pneumonia
Disease caused by a specific pathogenic organism, e.g. *Streptococcus pneumonia*, *Staphylococcus aureus*, *Legionella pneumophila*, Gram-negative bacilli, mycoplasma, coxiella and chlamydia species

Secondary pneumonia
(Aspiration pneumonia)
Infection reached alveoli by aspiration from other parts of the respiratory tract because of pre-existing abnormality such as nasal sinus infection, bronchial infection or aspiration of secretions or vomitus during episodes of disordered consciousness (e.g. general anaesthesia, drunkenness). Organisms are often of low virulence

secondary pneumonia, prominent features are destruction of lung tissue by the inflammatory process, a high incidence of abscess formation and the subsequent development of pulmonary fibrosis and bronchiectasis. The term 'suppurative pneumonia' has been applied to this group of conditions (p. 362).

Investigation

Sputum

An attempt should always be made to establish a positive microbiological diagnosis, though this is not always possible particularly if antibiotics have been given before specimens are submitted for examination. Direct smear examination of sputum by Gram and Ziehl–Neelsen stains may give an immediate indication of possible pathogens and indicate what treatment should be prescribed. Culture (including anaerobic culture where indicated) and sensitivity testing should be carried out.

Where a microbiological diagnosis is essential, as in severely ill immunosuppressed patients, and a specimen of sputum cannot be obtained an attempt should be made to aspirate secretions or washings from the trachea or bronchi either by bronchoscopy or by inserting a needle through the cricothyroid membrane. Some patients can be induced to produce sputum by the administration of nebulised hypertonic saline. Transthoracic lung puncture has been advocated if the other techniques are unsuccessful but carries the risk of pneumothorax which may have lethal consequences in dangerously ill patients.

Blood culture

Blood culture should be performed in patients with severe pneumonia and may yield a positive result when sputum examination is negative, particularly in pneumococcal pneumonia.

Serological tests

Pneumococcal antigen may be detected in serum. Serological tests may be helpful in the diagnosis of mycoplasma, chlamydia, legionella and viral infections, specimens being examined at ten-day intervals. A fourfold rise of antibody titre suggests recent infection.

Nose and throat swabs

Swabs of the nose and throat, and post-nasal and bronchial aspirates, can be cultured for viruses or examined by immunofluorescence or electron microscopy.

Total and differential white blood count

The total white cell count is often below $5.0 \times 10^9/l$ in patients with viral infection. A high neutrophil polymorph leucocytosis favours bacterial infection but in overwhelming bacterial infections the total white cell count may be low.

Arterial blood-gas measurements

The Po_2 and Pco_2 and the hydrogen ion concentration or pH of arterial blood are of vital importance in all patients who are seriously ill and in those with a previous history of chronic respiratory disease.

Radiological examination

This is necessary for confirmation of the diagnosis and for the early detection of complications such as pleural effusion and empyema. Follow-up radiological examination is important because if a pneumonia fails to resolve it may be secondary to bronchial obstruction, e.g. by a carcinoma.

Differential diagnosis of pneumonia

The following conditions may be difficult to distinguish from pneumonia:

Pulmonary infarction

In pulmonary infarction pyrexia is less marked and is uninfluenced by antibiotics, frank haemoptysis is common, cough is inconspicuous and the source of an embolus can be identified in a few cases.

Tuberculous pleurisy with effusion

In this condition the correct diagnosis can usually be suspected from the insidious onset, the virtual absence of cough and sputum, the physical signs of pleural effusion, the absence of leucocytosis, failure of the pyrexia to respond to antibiotics, the radiological findings and the aspiration from the pleural space of serous fluid, in which lymphocytes predominate.

Pulmonary tuberculosis

Acute pulmonary tuberculosis can often simulate pneumonia. The patient is, however, seldom as acutely ill as in other primary pneumonias. It is uncommon for the respiratory rate to be markedly increased and the white blood count is seldom above $12.0 \times 10^9/l$. The diagnosis can usually be made by radiological examination, and the demonstration of tubercle bacilli puts it beyond doubt.

Pulmonary oedema

Pulmonary oedema may be difficult to distinguish from pneumonia. If fever is present, pneumonia is the more likely diagnosis but where there is any doubt, both an antibiotic and a diuretic should be given.

Inflammatory conditions below the diaphragm
These conditions such as cholecystitis, perforated duo-denal ulcer, acute appendicitis, subphrenic abscess, generalised peritonitis, acute pancreatitis and hepatic amoebiasis may occasionally be mistaken for pneumonia. A carefully taken history helps determine the site and nature of the primary disease. A high temperature and a rapid respiratory rate favour a diagnosis of pneumonia, whereas tenderness of the abdominal wall suggests that the primary lesion is below the diaphragm. Sometimes radiological exami-nation of the chest is necessary before the presence of pneumonia can be confirmed or excluded.

THE PRIMARY PNEUMONIAS

The organisms which cause primary pneumonias are listed in the information box below.

ORGANISMS CAUSING PRIMARY PNEUMONIA

- Most common
  Streptococcus pneumoniae
- Common
  Staphylococcus aureus, Legionella pneumophila, Mycoplasma pneumoniae
- Uncommon
  Haemophilus influenzae, Klebsiella pneumoniae, Streptococcus pyogenes, Pseudomonas aeruginosa
- Rare
  Coxiella burnetii, Chlamydia psittaci, Actinomyces israeli, viruses

---

PNEUMOCOCCAL PNEUMONIA

Pneumococcal pneumonia is characterised by homo-geneous consolidation of one or more lobes or segments. The disease occurs at all ages but most frequently in early and middle adult life. The highest incidence is in winter. It is usually a sporadic disease spread by droplet infection.

Clinical features
The onset is sudden, often with rigors, or with vomiting or a convulsion in children. The temperature rises in a few hours to 39–40°C. Loss of appetite, headache and aching pains in the body and limbs accompany the pyrexia. Localised chest pain of pleural type often develops at an early stage in the illness. Occasionally it may be referred to the shoulder or to the abdominal wall. There is a short, painful cough, dry at first but later productive of tenacious sputum which is char-acteristically rust-coloured and occasionally frankly

blood-stained. Breathing is rapid (30–40 per min in adults, 50–60 in children), and shallow when pleural pain is present. The pulse is rapid, the skin is hot and dry, the face is flushed, and central cyanosis may be observed in severe cases. Herpes labialis is often present. A marked neutrophil leucocytosis is char-acteristic. *Strep. pneumoniae* can usually be isolated from the sputum, and a positive blood culture may be obtained.

Physical signs in the chest
In the first 24–48 h of the illness there is diminution of respiratory movement, slight impairment of the per-cussion note and often a pleural rub on the affected side. At a variable time after the onset, generally within two days, signs of consolidation appear (p. 347), with breath sounds of high pitched bronchial type. When resolution begins, numerous coarse crepitations are heard, in-dicating liquefaction of the alveolar exudate. If a pleural effusion develops physical signs of fluid in the pleural space are usually found, but bronchial breath sounds can persist and the presence of an effusion may be suspected only from stony dullness on percussion and recurrence or persistence of pyrexia.

Radiological examination
X-rays show a homogeneous opacity localised to the affected lobe or segment appearing within 12–18 hours of the onset of the illness (Fig. 9.3A, p. 359). Radio-logical examination is particularly helpful if a complication such as pleural effusion or empyema is suspected.

Management
Most patients respond promptly to antibiotic treatment and recovery is usual within a week. Delayed recovery suggests either that some complication such as empyema has developed or that the diagnosis is incorrect.

Antibiotic treatment
When a clinical diagnosis of pneumonia is made, pro-vided the patient is not seriously ill, the initial treatment should consist of ampicillin or erythromycin, 500 mg 4 times daily, or co-trimoxazole 960 mg 2 times daily by mouth. Patients who are gravely ill and in whom a staphylococcal or a Gram-negative infection is con-sidered should receive, in addition to ampicillin by intravenous injection, antibiotics to which the causative organism is unlikely to be resistant, for example, fluc-loxacillin, 250–500 mg 6-hourly i.v. and gentamicin 2–5 mg/kg daily in divided doses 8-hourly i.v. If *Strep. pneumoniae* is isolated or no pathogenic organisms are

reported on culture, and the patient appears to be making satisfactory clinical progress flucloxacillin and gentamicin can be withdrawn and treatment with ampicillin, erythromycin or co-trimoxazole continued. In most cases of uncomplicated pneumococcal pneumomia a seven to ten-day course of treatment is usually adequate.

Treatment of pleural pain
It is important to relieve pleural pain in order to allow the patient to breathe normally and cough efficiently. Mild analgesics such as paracetamol are rarely adequate and most patients require pethidine 50–100 mg or morphine 10–15 mg by intramuscular or intravenous injection. Opiates, however, must be used with extreme caution in patients with poor respiratory function.

Oxygen
Oxygen should be administered to all hypoxaemic patients. High concentrations should be used in all patients who do not have hypercapnia or advanced obstructive airways disease.

Physiotherapy
Assisted coughing is important especially in patients who suppress cough because of pleural pain. The administration of analgesic drugs should be co-ordinated with physiotherapy to allow optimum patient co-operation.

STAPHYLOCOCCAL PNEUMONIA

Pneumonia due to *Staph. aureus* may occur either as a primary respiratory infection or as a blood-borne infection from a staphylococcal lesion elsewhere in the body, for example, osteomyelitis. The second condition is essentially one of pyaemic abscess formation in the

lungs and is much less common than staphylococcal pneumonia.

Primary staphylococcal pneumonia, although it occurs much less frequently than pneumococcal pneumonia, is a relatively common illness, especially as a complication of influenza. Staphylococcal infection must also be assumed when pneumonia develops in debilitated patients in hospital and in patients with cystic fibrosis. It may present as a lobar or segmental pneumonia, which may be difficult to distinguish clinically from a severe pneumococcal infection, or as a suppurative pneumonia (p. 362) with multiple lung abscesses which may persist as thin-walled cysts after the acute infection has subsided.

Management
Intravenous flucloxacillin 0.25–1 g every 6 hours or erythromycin 2–4 g daily in divided doses. In severe infections sodium fusidate 500 mg i.v. over 6 hours, 3 times daily should be administered as well as flucloxacillin or erythromycin. Antibiotic therapy often has to be given for 14 days or longer. Oral therapy can be substituted for intravenous (flucloxacillin and erythromycin) when pyrexia has subsided and the patient is obviously recovering.

KLEBSIELLA PNEUMONIA

Pneumonia due to *Kl. pneumoniae* is an uncommon disease with a high mortality. There is usually massive consolidation and excavation of one or more lobes, the upper lobes being most often involved, with profound systemic disturbance and the expectoration of large amounts of purulent sputum sometimes chocolate-coloured. The diagnosis is made by the radiological appearances of pulmonary suppuration often associated

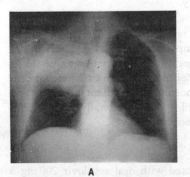
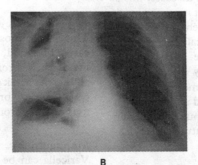
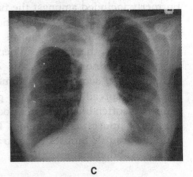

A   B   C

Fig. 9.3   Pneumonia right upper lobe. A. Dense consolidation seen above the transverse (horizontal) fissure. **B.** Klebsiella pneumonia right upper lobe. Consolidation and cavitation within a larger than normal upper lobe as indicated by ballooning down of the transverse fissure. **C.** Right upper lobe collapse.

with increase in size of the affected lobe and the isolation of the causative organism from sputum.

Management

Gentamicin 2–5 mg/kg i.v. daily in divided doses 8-hourly with peak and trough blood level monitoring, ceftazidime 1 g i.v. 8-hourly or ciprofloxacin 200 mg twice daily by intravenous infusion over 30–60 min. Treatment may have to be continued for 2 to 3 weeks.

LEGIONELLA PNEUMONIA (LEGIONNAIRES' DISEASE)

Legionnaires' disease is caused by a bacillus (*L. pneumophila*) which appears to be transmitted in water droplets often originating in infected humidifier cooling towers and perhaps from stagnant water in cisterns and showerheads. Epidemics traced to institutions such as hospitals receive much publicity but sporadic cases infected from unknown sources are common. It can be a serious and fatal illness, but most patients survive. Gastrointestinal symptoms, mental confusion, hyponatraemia and proteinuria often accompany the pneumonia and if present raise the suspicion of Legionella infection.

Management

Erythromycin 0.5–1 g 6-hourly (i.v. in severely ill). Rifampicin 600 mg twice daily by mouth or intravenous injection should be given in combination with erythromycin to all severely ill patients in whom the diagnosis has been confirmed or thought to be likely, e.g. during epidemics. At least 14 days of antibiotic treatment is usually required in Legionnaires' disease.

ACTINOMYCOSIS

Formerly included amongst the fungal diseases, this is now regarded as a bacterial infection. It is caused by *A. israeli*, an anaerobic organism which exists as a commensal in the mouth. When local defences are impaired, actinomycosis can cause cervicofacial, abdominal or, occasionally, pulmonary infection such as a widespread suppurative pneumonia (p. 362). Empyema, often bilateral and associated with persistent chest wall sinuses, may develop. The pus may contain 'sulphur grains'. Sinuses are also a feature of cervicofacial and abdominal infection.

Management

Benzylpenicillin 2–4 g i.v. 6-hourly. The duration of therapy depends upon response.

PNEUMONIA CAUSED BY VIRUSES AND OTHER ORGANISMS

Clinical features

A distinctive form of pneumonia may be produced by certain viruses, and also by unclassified organisms such as mycoplasma and chlamydia which have some features of viruses and bacteria. The clinical picture differs from that of the bacterial pneumonias in that fever and toxaemia usually precede respiratory symptoms by several days. Severe headache, malaise and anorexia are characteristic features in the early stages. The physical signs in the chest, if there are any, appear later and are seldom gross. The existence of a pulmonary lesion may not be recognised without a chest X-ray. The spleen may be palpable in the first week, the white blood count is generally normal and the pyrexia does not respond to penicillin. The diagnosis can often be confirmed by isolation of the causal organism or by serological tests.

The disease is often self-limiting. Pyrexia usually subsides by lysis after 5–10 days and complete recovery and radiographic resolution follow, the latter sometimes being slow. Very rarely death takes place from widespread extension of the pneumonia or from viral encephalitis.

Influenza, parainfluenza and measles

These illnesses are occasionally complicated by pneumonia (primary viral pneumonias) which are frequently complicated by bacterial infection. The combination of influenza and staphylococcal pneumonia is often fatal.

Varicella (chickenpox)

In adults pneumonia caused by varicella (chickenpox) virus is a serious complication of the disease and usually has characteristic radiographic features. The chest X-ray shows numerous miliary nodular shadows which may eventually calcify.

Respiratory syncytial virus

This is the most important respiratory pathogen of early childhood, especially in the first two months of life. It causes bronchiolitis and occasionally pneumonia, and carries a risk of mortality. The infant is fevered, and cough, wheezy breathing and occasionally an erythematous rash are prominent features.

Management

Varicella can be treated with oral acyclovir 200 mg 5 times daily for 5 days (half dose for children under age of two) or intravenous vidarabine 10 mg/kg daily for at least 5 days. These antiviral agents are usually reserved for the treatment of chickenpox in immuno-compromised patients. There are no specific treatments available for infections caused by the other viruses.

Chlamydia psittaci

This organism is the cause of psittacosis (ornithosis), a systemic illness contracted from infected birds. The pneumonia associated with it may be extensive and severe systemic upset and death are common. Headache is a prominent early symptom.

Management

Tetracycline 500 mg 4 times daily by mouth or 500 mg twice daily by intravenous infusion.

Mycoplasma pneumoniae

Outbreaks of pneumonia caused by this organism are common in barracks and institutions. Most cases occur in children and young adults. Maculo-papular rashes, haemolytic anaemia and meningo-encephalitis occur rarely.

Cold agglutinins (p. 723) can be demonstrated in a high proportion of cases. Antibodies can be detected and haemagglutination and complement-fixation tests are available for diagnosis.

Management

Tetracycline 500 mg 4 times daily or erythromycin 500 mg 4 times daily. In severe infections treatment should be given intravenously.

Coxiella burnetii

This organism causes *Q fever* which may be complicated by pneumonia and endocarditis.

Management

Tetracycline 500 mg 4-hourly by mouth.

THE SECONDARY PNEUMONIAS

This group, sometimes described as 'non-specific', bronchopneumonia and aspiration pneumonia, comprises a large number of different conditions. Their common features are the absence of any specific pathogenic organism in the sputum and the existence of some abnormality of the respiratory system. This predisposes to the invasion of the lung by organisms of relatively low virulence derived from the upper respiratory tract or from the mouth, for example, streptococci, certain types of pneumococci, *H. influenzae* and various species of anaerobic bacteria.

Infection may reach the lungs in various ways. Pus may be aspirated from an infected nasal sinus, or septic matter may be inhaled during tonsillectomy or dental extraction under general anaesthesia. Vomitus or the contents of a dilated oesophagus may enter the larynx during general anaesthesia, coma or even sleep and aspiration may also occur in patients with gastro-oesophageal reflux (p. 426). Pus from acute bronchitis, dilated bronchi or a lung abscess, may also be carried into the alveoli by the air stream or by gravity.

Ineffective coughing caused by post-operative or post-traumatic thoracic or abdominal pain, by debility or immobility, or by laryngeal paralysis may also predispose to the development of a secondary (aspiration) pneumonia.

Partial bronchial obstruction, as for example, by a tumour, is another potential cause of secondary pneumonia, because it allows infection derived from the upper air passages to become established in the inadequately drained portion of lung beyond the obstruction.

ACUTE BRONCHOPNEUMONIA

This type of secondary pneumonia is invariably preceded by bronchial infection, which accounts for the widespread patchy distribution of the lesion. It occurs most frequently at the extremes of life and may be described as 'hypostatic pneumonia' when it occurs in elderly or debilitated patients. In children, it is often a complication of measles or whooping cough, and in adults, of acute bronchitis or influenza. It is particularly common in patients with chronic bronchitis.

Pathology

There is acute inflammation of bronchi, especially the terminal bronchioles, which are filled with pus. Collapse and consolidation of the associated groups of alveoli follow. The lesions are distributed bilaterally in small patches which tend to become larger by confluence and are more often extensive in the lower lobes. There is interstitial oedema and compensatory emphysema around the collapsed alveoli.

Clinical features

After two or three days of acute bronchitis (p. 356), as bronchopneumonia develops, the temperature rises to a higher level, the pulse and respiration rates increase, and breathlessness and central cyanosis appear. There is generally a severe cough with purulent sputum. Pleural pain is uncommon, in contrast to pneumococcal pneumonia.

During the early stages the physical signs are those of acute bronchitis but crepitations later become more numerous. Radiological examination shows mottled opacities in both lung fields, chiefly in the lower zones. A neutrophil leucocytosis is present.

Course and complications

The disease has a more insidious onset than pneumococcal pneumonia and tends to run a more protracted course (up to ten days). Incomplete resolution may lead to bronchiectasis and replacement fibrosis (p. 396). Mortality is higher at the extremes of life especially if the disease supervenes on chronic bronchitis and emphysema or any debilitating illness.

Management

Ampicillin 250–500 mg 4 times daily by mouth or co-trimoxazole 960 mg every 12 hours are usually effective in acute bronchopneumonia. Control of pleural pain (p. 359), oxygen (p. 352) and physiotherapy may be required (p. 359).

BENIGN ASPIRATION PNEUMONIA

This type of secondary pneumonia is due to the aspiration of infected secretion into the lungs during the course of an upper respiratory infection such as coryza or sinusitis. The organisms causing the pneumonia, being derived from the upper respiratory tract, are generally of low virulence and the degree of systemic disturbance is usually slight. In fact, the symptoms are often no more severe than would be expected with an uncomplicated upper respiratory infection and the existence of pneumonia may be discovered only by chest X-ray.

Clinical features

The main features of this type of pneumonia are shown in the information box below.

CLINICAL FEATURES OF BENIGN ASPIRATION PNEUMONIA

Symptoms
Cough, purulent sputum and occasionally pleural pain in association with symptoms of an upper respiratory tract infection

Clinical signs
Low-grade pyrexia. Localised unilateral crepitations or no abnormalities on chest examination

White cell count
Moderate polymorphonuclear leucocytosis

Chest X-ray
Unilateral mottled opacity involving a single lobe or segment

---

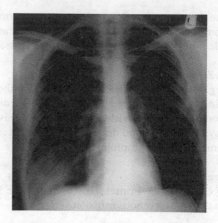

Fig. 9.4   Aspiration pneumonia right lower zone. Hazy shadowing in the right costophrenic area.

Management

There is usually rapid response to ampicillin 250–500 mg 4 times daily by mouth or to co-trimoxazole 960 mg every 12 hours.

SUPPURATIVE PNEUMONIA (INCLUDING PULMONARY ABSCESS)

Suppurative pneumonia is the term used to describe a form of pneumonic consolidation in which there is destruction of the lung parenchyma by the inflammatory process. Although microabscess formation is a characteristic histological feature of suppurative pneumonia, it is usual to restrict the term 'pulmonary abscess' to lesions in which there is a fairly large localised collection of pus, or a cavity lined by chronic inflammatory tissue, from which pus has escaped by rupture into the bronchus.

Suppurative pneumonia and pulmonary abscess may be produced by infection of previously healthy lung tissue with *Staph. aureus* or *Kl. pneumoniae*. These are, in effect, primary bacterial pneumonias associated with pulmonary suppuration. More frequently suppurative pneumonia and pulmonary abscess are forms of secondary pneumonia. They may develop after the inhalation of septic material during operations on the nose, mouth or throat under general anaesthesia, or of vomitus during anaesthesia or coma.

In such circumstances gross oral sepsis may be a predisposing factor. Bacterial infection of a pulmonary infarct or of a collapsed lobe may also produce a suppurative pneumonia or a lung abscess. The organisms isolated from the sputum may include *Strep. pneumoniae*, *Staph. aureus*, *Strep. pyogenes*, *H.*

influenzae, and in some cases anaerobic bacteria. In many cases, however, no pathogens can be isolated particularly when antibiotics have been given.

Clinical features
These are listed in the information box below.

CLINICAL FEATURES OF SUPPURATIVE PNEUMONIA

Onset
Acute or insidious

Symptoms
Cough productive of large amounts of sputum which is sometimes fetid and blood-stained. Pleural pain common
Sudden expectoration of copious amount of sputum occurs if abscess ruptures into a bronchus

Clinical signs
High remittent pyrexia. Profound systemic upset. Finger clubbing may develop quickly (10–14 days). Chest examination usually reveals signs of consolidation; signs of cavitation rarely found. Pleural rub common. Rapid deterioration in general health with marked weight loss can occur if disease not adequately treated

---

Radiological examination
There is a homogeneous lobar or segmental opacity consistent with consolidation or collapse. A large, dense opacity, which may later cavitate and show a fluid level is the characteristic finding when a frank lung abscess is present.

Management
In many patients oral treatment with ampicillin 500 mg 4 times daily or co-trimoxazole 960 mg twice daily is effective. If an anaerobic bacterial infection is suspected (e.g. from fetor of the sputum) oral metronidazole 400 mg 8-hourly should be added. Antibacterial therapy should be modified according to the results of microbiological examination of sputum. Prolonged treatment for 4 to 6 weeks may be required in some patients with lung abscess.

Physiotherapy is of great value especially when large abscess cavities have formed. It may not be possible to drain lower lobe cavities without postural coughing.

In most patients there is a good response to treatment and although residual fibrosis and bronchiectasis are common sequelae these seldom give rise to serious morbidity. Empyema (p. 412) may complicate the acute phase of the disease.

Prevention
Every precaution should be taken during operations on the mouth, nose and throat to prevent the inhalation of blood, tonsillar fragments and other material. Oral sepsis should be eradicated, especially if a general anaesthetic is contemplated.

PNEUMONIA IN THE IMMUNOCOMPROMISED PATIENT
Pulmonary infection is common in patients receiving immunosuppressive drugs and in those with diseases causing defects of cellular or humoral immune mechanisms. For example, patients with the acquired immune deficiency syndrome (AIDS) (p. 105) are susceptible to many types of pneumonia and pulmonary infection with *Pneumocystis carinii* is a common cause of death in patients with AIDS. The common pathogenic bacteria are responsible for the majority of lung infections in immunocompromised patients, but Gram-negative bacteria, especially *Pseudomonas aeruginosa* are more of a problem than Gram-positive organisms, even *Staph. aureus*. However, in such patients unusual organisms or those normally considered to be of low virulence or non-pathogenic may become 'opportunistic' pathogens. The protozoon *Pneumocystis carinii*, fungi such as *Aspergillus fumigatus*, viral infections, cytomegalovirus and herpes viruses, and infections with *M. tuberculosis* and other types of mycobacteria are all common causes of infection in patients with AIDS and in those being treated with immunosuppressive drugs.

Clinical features
Diagnosis is often very difficult because all the normally pathogenic organisms and the 'opportunists' tend to cause a similar clinical and radiological picture. The onset of disease, however, tends to be less rapid in *Pneumocystis carinii* and mycobacterial infections than with pathogenic bacteria. In *Pneumocystis carinii* pneumonia symptoms of cough and breathlessness can be manifestations of the disease days before the onset of systemic symptoms or even a chest X-ray abnormality.

Diagnosis
Open-lung biopsy offers the greatest chance of establishing a diagnosis if examination of sputum has not been of any diagnostic help or patients do not have sputum. This, however, is a major high-risk invasive procedure and should be reserved for patients in whom less invasive procedures fail to establish a diagnosis and in whom there has been no response to wide spectrum antibiotic treatment. Some patients who cannot produce sputum can be induced to do so by the inhalation of nebulised hypertonic saline. Fibreoptic bronchoscopy should be performed early since a diag-

nosis can often be established by examination of lavage fluid, bronchial brushings or transbronchial biopsies. Sputum, bronchial aspirates and bronchoalveolar lavage fluid should be examined for *Pneumocystis carinii*, bacteria, mycobacteria, fungi and viruses.

Management

Whenever possible treatment should be based on an established aetiological diagnosis. In practice, however, the cause of the pneumonia is frequently not known when treatment has to be started. A combination of antibiotics to provide a wide spectrum of antibacterial activity is often given (e.g. a third generation cephalosporin plus an antistaphylococcal antibiotic, or an antipseudomonal penicillin plus an aminoglycoside) and bronchoscopy is performed if there is no response to such treatment.

Treatment of Pneumocystis carinii *pneumonia*
Co-trimoxazole 120 mg/kg daily in divided doses by mouth, or 960 mg i.v. every 12 h. In patients who do not respond to high dose co-trimoxazole the use of inhaled or intravenous pentamidine should be considered.

NOSOCOMIAL PNEUMONIA

Pneumonia developing in hospital in a patient who has been admitted for more than 48 h should be considered to be hospital-acquired. The spectrum of pathogenic organisms involved is different from community-acquired pneumonia in which *Strep. pneumoniae* is common, and other pathogenic bacteria, *Mycoplasma pneumoniae*, and *Legionella pneumophila* have to be considered. In nosocomial pneumonia there is a predominance of Gram-negative bacteria such as pseudomonas species, *Escherichia* species and *Klebsiella* species. Infections caused by *Staph. aureus* are also common in hospital and anaerobic organisms are much more likely than in pneumonia acquired at home.

TUBERCULOSIS

Although tuberculosis is a problem of rapidly diminishing proportions in Western Europe and North America, it remains an important specific communicable disease in many countries. As the disease decreases in frequency there is a tendency for tuberculosis to be overlooked.

Aetiology

Three types of mycobacteria are responsible for disease in man as shown in the information box (right).

TYPES OF MYCOBACTERIA CAUSING DISEASE IN MAN

Myco. tuberculosis
Cause of most infections

Myco. bovis
Endemic in cattle. Spread to man by milk. Now rarely responsible for human disease in UK

Atypical or opportunistic mycobacteria
Rare compared with human type. Cause pulmonary and generalised infections in immunocompromised; cervical lymph node infection in children. Are primarily resistant in vitro to many drugs used for treatment of *M. tuberculosis*

Entry of the tubercle bacillus into the body or the alimentary or respiratory tract is not necessarily followed by a clinical illness, the development of which is dependent upon several other factors. Those of most practical importance are:

Age and sex. In Europe and America, tuberculosis used to affect predominantly the young people in the community, especially females, but there has been a radical change in the age and sex incidence. Most patients are now over the age of 45 years, males predominating.

Natural resistance. Susceptibility to tuberculosis is not inherited in the strict sense of the word, but the observation that certain races and even certain regional groups are more prone to develop the disease suggests that natural resistance varies between races and from region to region. The natural resistance of a community tends to rise as the period of exposure increases. Immigrants to Britain from Asia are more prone to have the disease than the indigenous population and also tend to have more florid types of tuberculosis.

Standard of living. The prevalence of tuberculosis diminishes as social and economic conditions improve. Poor housing with associated overcrowding increases the risk of massive infection or reinfection.

Conditions affecting individual patients. Diabetes mellitus, gastric surgery, silicosis and alcoholism all predispose to the development of tuberculosis as does AIDS and treatment with corticosteroids or immunosuppressive drugs.

Pathology

The initial *'primary' tuberculosis infection* usually occurs in the lung but occasionally in the tonsil or alimentary tract, especially the ileocaecal region. The primary infection differs from subsequent infections in that the primary focus in lung, tonsil or bowel is almost invariably accompanied by caseous lesions in the regional lymph nodes, such as the mediastinal, cervical or mesenteric groups respectively.

In most people the primary infection and the associated lymph node lesions heal and calcify. In a few, healing, particularly in lymph nodes, is incomplete and viable tubercle bacilli may enter the blood-stream. In consequence tuberculous lesions may develop elsewhere. 'Haematogenous' lesions of this kind are more common in the lungs, bones, joints and kidneys and lesions may develop months or even years after the primary infection.

Sometimes the primary infection does not heal. A pulmonary lesion, particularly when it occurs during adolescence or early adult life, may lead to progressive pulmonary tuberculosis. A tuberculous mediastinal lymph node, in children especially, may compress a lobar or segmental bronchus (rarely a main bronchus) and produce pulmonary collapse. Occasionally the node may ulcerate through the bronchial wall and discharge caseous material into the lumen with the production of acute tuberculous lesions in the related lobe or segment. Infection may also be carried by lymphatics from tuberculous mediastinal lymph nodes to the pleura or pericardium with the production of tuberculous pleurisy or pericarditis. Comparable complications may occur when the primary lesion is in the tonsil or gut, for example 'cold abscess' of the neck or tuberculous peritonitis.

Rarely a caseous tuberculous focus ruptures into a vein and produces acute dissemination throughout the body, a condition known as *acute miliary tuberculosis*. Meningitis often complicates this condition.

Progressive pulmonary tuberculosis may develop directly from a primary lesion or it may occur later following reactivation of an incompletely healed primary focus. Alternatively it may be the result of reinfection.

Post primary pulmonary tuberculosis is the term used to describe lung disease, the characteristic pathological feature of which is the tuberculous cavity, formed when the caseated and liquefied centre of a tuberculous pulmonary lesion is discharged into a bronchus. Extension of infection to the pleura causes tuberculous pleurisy, which is sometimes accompanied by effusion and is occasionally followed by the development of a tuberculous empyema. Blood-borne dissemination to other organs is uncommon in post-primary pulmonary tuberculosis.

Clinical features

The two groups of clinical features in tuberculosis are shown in the information box below.

CLINICAL FEATURES OF TUBERCULOSIS

Systemic effects
Anorexia, weight loss, lassitude, sleep sweats, evening pyrexia

Local effects
Cough, sputum and haemoptysis

PREVENTION

Mortality rates are no longer considered so important in the assessment of the success of control measures because of the very low rates now existing in some countries and the inaccuracy of certification in many countries where tuberculosis remains a major problem. Notification rates are of limited value because of the adoption of varying standards, but the annual recording of the number of smear-positive patients with pulmonary tuberculosis is a useful indication of the efficiency of preventative measures.

The tuberculin index

This is the percentage of positive reactors to tuberculin at a standard age, e.g. 5 or 13 years and is a useful indicator of disease prevalence.

Improvement in socio-economic conditions

This, mainly in respect of adequate housing, ventilation and nutrition may still be the most important control measure of all.

Case-finding

Mass radiography is an expensive method of case-finding and should in the UK be used in a selective manner concentrating on certain specific groups. The highest yield by far is from patients referred by general practitioners because of symptoms. Open access to chest radiography for general practitioners and minimum waiting time for patients are essential for success.

Sputum-smear examination (Ziehl-Neelsen stain or auramine-phenol fluorescent test) is an important method of case-finding in developing countries.

Contact examination achieves a high yield in case-finding. Efforts should be concentrated on the immediate examination of household contacts of sputum-smear positive patients especially contacts under 25 years of age.

Chemotherapy
Proper use of modern highly-effective chemotherapy, by rendering patients non-infectious rapidly, makes a very important contribution to the control of the disease.

Isolation of patients
Isolation is rarely considered necessary nowadays even in smear-positive patients, except where young children are at risk, provided the source case is being properly treated by chemotherapy.

BCG vaccination
This is carried out by the administration of freeze-dried vaccine, reconstituted at the time of use injected by the intradermal route (0.1 ml) at the junction of the upper and middle thirds of the upper arm. Complications such as local abscess formation and enlargement of regional lymph nodes are very rare. Bacille Calmette-Guérin (BCG) vaccine should not be given in the presence of immunodeficiency. The duration of protection is up to seven years. Vaccination reduces the incidence of pulmonary tuberculosis in young adults by 80% and minimises the risk of serious disseminated disease – miliary tuberculosis and tuberculous meningitis.

Policy in relation to BCG vaccination in a community depends upon the size of the problem locally. If the infection rate is very low (1% or less) mass vaccination is inappropriate on the grounds of cost and the fact that BCG interferes with the diagnostic value of the tuberculin test in such a situation. Where there are many positive tuberculin reactors, as occurs in communities with low living standards, vaccination of the newborn is usually indicated. Where infection rates are falling to low levels, vaccination at puberty, as is still performed in the UK, is practical.

Chemoprophylaxis
The concept of administering chemotherapy to individuals in order to try to prevent the development of tuberculosis is adopted in different communities with varying degrees of enthusiasm (p. 369).

Elimination of bovine infection
Although such infection is now extremely rare in Western countries constant vigilance will be required to ensure that it remains so.

Tuberculin test
With the Mantoux technique a solution of Old Tuberculin or purified protein derivative (PPD) tuberculin is injected intradermally on the flexor aspect of the forearm. The test is regarded as positive if, two to four days after the injection, there is a reaction consisting of a raised area of inflammatory oedema not less than 5 mm in diameter, with surrounding erythema.

The test should first be performed with one tuberculin unit (TU) in 0.1 ml of normal saline. If there is no reaction it should be repeated with 10 TU in the same volume of saline. In order to obtain accurate results it is essential to use freshly prepared dilutions of tuberculin. Differential tuberculin testing with antigens prepared with other mycobacteria, e.g. PPD-A (*Myco. avium*) or PPD-Y (*Myco. kansasii*) is often a satisfactory method of distinguishing atypical mycobacterial infection from tuberculosis.

The younger the patient the greater is the diagnostic significance of a positive tuberculin test. A repeatedly negative test over a period of six weeks from the onset of symptoms practically rules out tuberculosis except in the elderly, or after acute exanthemata, or in the later stages of miliary tuberculosis and tuberculous meningitis in patients taking immunosuppressive drugs. The tuberculin test is usually negative in patients with sarcoidosis.

Tuberculin testing is an essential part of the examination of family contacts. If positive it is of value as a diagnostic measure and if negative it indicates which of the contacts should be vaccinated with BCG. When large numbers of individuals are being tested, particularly children, a multiple puncture technique, which is quick and almost painless is preferable to the Mantoux test. A disposable tine test unit should be used for this purpose which has four prongs (tines) 2 mm in length mounted on a disc and coated with Old Tuberculin. If firmly pressed on the skin of the forearm it yields results as reliable as those obtained with the Heaf unit which, being difficult to sterilise, may carry some risk of transmitting viral infections.

The test should be read after three days and four grades of positivity are recognised (Table 9.15).

Table 9.15 Positive tine test grades

Grade
I   One or two faint papules
II Four discrete papules
III The area encircled by the papules is completely indurated
IV Any reaction which is greater than III, including central necrosis

Reactions in grades III and IV indicate infection with mammalian tubercle bacilli and a grade I reaction may indicate infection with atypical mycobacteria. The significance of a grade II reaction is uncertain. Individuals previously vaccinated with BCG usually have a positive reaction of Grade II or III.

MANAGEMENT

General principles

Antituberculosis chemotherapy

Specific chemotherapy is by far the most important measure in the treatment of all forms of tuberculosis and should be given to every patient with active disease.

Rest

Rest is unimportant except in a few specific circumstances and the majority of patients are now ambulant throughout treatment, many of them remaining at work. Immobilisation is necessary in certain forms of skeletal tuberculosis.

Isolation

Isolation of patients who are excreting tubercle bacilli and who are therefore potentially infectious has previously been an important principle. The observation made in Madras that the frequency of disease amongst contacts was no greater when the patient was being treated at home than in a sanatorium has led to the adoption of a policy whereby the majority of patients are treated wholly as out-patients. However, many authorities still prefer to isolate patients from contact with young children. An initial period of treatment in hospital, as distinct from isolation, may be recommended for patients who cannot be relied upon to take their drugs regularly and for those who present difficult therapeutic problems.

Surgical treatment

Pulmonary resection, nephrectomy or removal of superficial lymph nodes is rarely required, but drainage of an abscess from tuberculosis lymph nodes or of an empyema may be necessary. Surgical treatment of tuberculosis of the spine may be essential to prevent paraplegia.

Chemotherapy

Effective treatment of tuberculosis is based on detailed knowledge of the drugs available so that the most appropriate regimen for the individual patient can be devised.

In Britain, five drugs – rifampicin, isoniazid, ethambutol, streptomycin and pyrazinamide – are normally considered in the initial treatment of tuberculosis. Thiacetazone, which is cheap, is widely used in developing countries. Pyrazinamide is particularly useful in the treatment of tuberculous meningitis because it diffuses well into the cerebrospinal fluid. Apart from a few minor variations in dose the duration of treatment and the policy governing the use of antituberculosis drugs is the same for all forms of the disease.

These drugs should be used in once daily doses as shown in Table 9.16.

Adverse effects

In choosing a suitable drug regimen for individual patients it is important to bear in mind those side-effects which are particularly liable to cause serious

Table 9.16 Daily doses and side-effects of commonly used antituberculous drugs

Drug	Group	Dose	Side-effects
Rifampicin[1]	Children	10–20 mg/kg	Drug interactions, hypersensitivity hepatitis, vasculitis, fever, skin flushing, nausea and abdominal pain, breathlessness and wheeze (intermittent regimens only). Rifampicin should not be given again to any patient in whom it has caused vasculitis
	Adults weighing less than 50 kg and in the elderly	450 mg	
	Adults weighing more than 50 kg	600 mg	
Isoniazid	Children	3 mg/kg	Hypersensitivity, polyneuropathy, lack of mental concentration
	Adults	200–300 mg	
	Intermittent regimen	15 mg/kg[2]	
	Miliary/meningitis	10–12 mg/kg[2]	
Ethambutol	Children and adults: initial 8 weeks	25 mg/kg	Optic neuritis, hypersensitivity
	subsequently	15 mg/kg	
	In renal failure	According to serum levels	
Streptomycin sulphate	Children	30 mg/kg	Vestibular disturbance, hypersensitivity
	Adults under 40 years and weighing more than 45 kg	1 g	Deafness (rare)
	Adults 40–60 years or weighing less than 45 kg	0.75 g	
	Adults over 60 years or in patients with renal failure	According to serum levels	
	Intermittent regimens	0.75–1 g	
Pyrazinamide	Children and adults	20–35 mg/kg (max 2.5 g)	Hepatitis, gout, hypersensitivity

[1] Taken at least 30 minutes before breakfast.
[2] Plus pyridoxine 10 mg to prevent peripheral neuropathy.

chronic disability, such as vestibular disturbance due to streptomycin which accordingly must be prescribed with caution. Even in the relatively low dose recommended for ethambutol, a few patients develop optic neuritis and some are left with a permanent visual defect. This potential hazard must be taken into consideration whenever ethambutol is prescribed particularly in children.

Streptomycin and occasionally isoniazid, ethambutol and rifampicin may produce a hypersensitivity reaction, comprising pyrexia and an erythematous skin eruption which usually but not invariably develops two to four weeks after treatment is started. Rifampicin which colours the urine orange-pink is a potent liver enzyme inducer (p. 814) and should be used with appropriate caution when prescribed with other drugs such as oestrogens (e.g. oral contraceptives), warfarin, corticosteroids, oral hypoglycaemic drugs, phenytoin and digoxin. It should, if possible, be avoided in patients with liver disease. The principal adverse effects of the most commonly prescribed drugs are shown in Table 9.16.

Drug regimens

The 'short course' regimens shown in the information box below are virtually 100% effective in the treatment of tuberculosis.

SIX AND NINE-MONTH DRUG REGIMENS

Duration 6 months
Initial phase 2 months
    Ethambutol or streptomycin plus isoniazid plus rifampicin
    plus pyrazinamide
Continuation phase 4 months
    Isoniazid plus rifampicin

Duration 9 months
Initial phase 2 months
    Ethambutol or streptomycin plus isoniazid plus rifampicin
Continuation phase 7 months
    Isoniazid plus rifampicin

Any patient who cannot be trusted to take antituberculosis drugs regularly should be kept in hospital for the initial (two months) phase of treatment or be given supervised out-patient therapy. Thereafter for 10 months, the following should be given at home twice weekly (at 3 and 4-day intervals): streptomycin sulphate 1 g i.m., and isoniazid 15 mg/kg orally in a single dose, plus pyridoxine 10 mg. Pyridoxine is given to prevent peripheral neuropathy. This type of chemotherapy should be wholly supervised, the tablets being administered at the same time as the injection.

Inexpensive treatment regimens
In developing countries it is sometimes impossible for economic reasons to adhere to ideal chemotherapeutic regimens.

12-MONTH REGIMENS – INEXPENSIVE – REASONABLY EFFECTIVE

Twice weekly
Streptomycin 1 g i.m.
Isoniazid 15 mg/kg plus pyridoxine 10 mg orally

The effectiveness of this regimen is nearly 100% in the absence of primary drug resistance if daily treatment with standard doses of streptomycin and isoniazid can be afforded for the first 2–3 months.

Daily

Isoniazid 300 mg ⎱
                  ⎰ single doses by mouth
Thiacetazone 150 mg ⎰

Very cheap regimen which is 80–95% effective

Response to treatment
It is most unusual, even in advanced cases, for sputum cultures to remain positive for longer than six months if bacilli at the start of treatment are fully sensitive to the drugs used. Reliance must be placed on smear examination where facilities for sensitivity testing do not exist.

Drug-resistant tubercle bacilli
The treatment of patients infected with drug-resistant tubercle bacilli presents a problem requiring specialised knowledge. Additional drugs available for the treatment of such cases are: sodium aminosalicylate (PAS-5 g twice daily by mouth), ethionamide or prothionamide (0.75–1 g once daily by mouth), capreomycin (0.7–1 g i.m. once daily) and cycloserine (0.75–1 g once daily by mouth).

Corticosteroid drugs

These agents suppress the cell-mediated reaction induced by the tubercle bacillus and may promote a rapid dissemination of infection by interfering with tissue defence mechanisms. If, however, a corticosteroid drug is given in conjunction with effective antituberculous chemotherapy, it may exert a favourable influence on the course of the disease by reducing the severity both of the local inflammatory reaction and of the associated systemic disturbance. In acute pulmonary tuberculosis such treatment will rapidly relieve pyrexia and will often produce a dramatic improvement in the radiological appearances. The effect is temporary and ceases when the corticosteroid drug is withdrawn, but it may save the lives of patients with fulminating infection by enabling them to survive until antituberculous chemotherapy has had time to exert its influence. Prednisolone is given in a dose of 20 mg daily for 6–12 weeks.

Corticosteroid drugs in combination with chemotherapy may prevent or minimise the formation of fibrous tissue and be of value in tuberculosis affecting the pleura, pericardium, intrathoracic or superficial lymph nodes, the eye and meninges. Whenever there is evidence of ureteric obstruction, corticosteroids should be administered in addition to chemotherapy because such treatment significantly reduces the need for surgery.

Chemoprophylaxis
Chemoprophylaxis using isoniazid is listed in the information box below.

CHEMOPROPHYLAXIS OF TUBERCULOSIS

Isoniazid (5 mg/kg by mouth) daily for 1 year should be considered in:
- Non-BCG vaccinated tuberculin positive children under age 3 years – vulnerable in respect of miliary TB and TB meningitis
- Unvaccinated contacts who have recently become tuberculin positive
- Immunosuppressed patients
- Adolescents with high degree of tuberculin sensitivity

Isoniazid (5 mg/kg by mouth) daily for 6 weeks should be considered in:
- Infants of highly infectious patients – isoniazid resistant BCG vaccine can be used with isoniazid chemoprophylaxis

---

PRIMARY PULMONARY TUBERCULOSIS

The pathological features of this type of tuberculosis are outlined on page 364. The primary infection usually occurs in childhood. A history of contact with a case of active pulmonary tuberculosis is obtained in many instances.

Clinical features
In the vast majority of patients the primary infection produces no symptoms or signs and passes unnoticed unless routine radiological examination of the chest happens to be performed at the appropriate time or serial tuberculin tests show conversion from negative to positive.

In a few patients the primary infection produces a febrile illness which is generally mild and lasts for no more than 7 to 14 days. It is unusual for gross focal symptoms or signs to develop but a slight dry cough is occasionally present. The leucocyte count is normal but the ESR is raised.

The primary infection may be accompanied by erythema nodosum which is characterised by bluish-red, raised, tender, cutaneous lesions on the shins, and less commonly, on the thighs, and is associated in some patients with pyrexia and polyarthralgia. Erythema nodosum may be the first clinical indication of a tuberculous infection. The tuberculin reaction is always strongly positive in these patients and evidence of primary tuberculosis can usually be detected on the chest radiograph. Erythema nodosum is, however, seen in conditions other than primary tuberculosis, for example sarcoidosis, streptococcal infections and drug reactions.

Occasionally the primary pulmonary infection pursues a progressive course (p. 365). Symptoms and signs due to its complications may appear either during the course of the initial illness or after a latent interval of weeks or months. Such complications include pleurisy or pleural effusion (p. 410), lobar or segmental collapse (p. 390), acute miliary tuberculosis (p. 370), tuberculous meningitis (p. 884) and post-primary pulmonary tuberculosis (p. 370).

Investigations
The three most valuable diagnostic investigations in primary pulmonary tuberculosis are listed in the information box below.

INVESTIGATIONS IN PRIMARY TUBERCULOSIS

X-ray of chest
Children – unilateral hilar lymph node enlargement; the accompanying intrapulmonary lesion may or may not be seen
Adolescents and young adults – lymph node enlargement less conspicuous but pulmonary lesion more prominent

Tuberculin test
Extremely valuable in children. A positive test in a child who has not previously been vaccinated with BCG must be assumed to indicate active disease

Bacteriological examination
Sputum seldom available. If not, 3 laryngeal swabs or fasting gastric washings should be examined. Isolation of tubercle bacilli provides absolute proof of diagnosis.

Prognosis
Because primary pulmonary tuberculosis and its complications respond satisfactorily to antituberculous chemotherapy (p. 368), which should be given in every case, the prognosis is excellent.

MILIARY TUBERCULOSIS

The pathogenesis of this condition has already been described (p. 365). Hitherto it has occurred chiefly in children and young adults but with the changing age-structure of tuberculosis in many countries miliary tuberculosis is affecting persons in older age groups in whom it tends to take the form of an insidious illness – the 'cryptic' type – which is often difficult to diagnose. Before the introduction of chemotherapy the disease was invariably fatal but most treated patients now recover completely.

Clinical features

The disease may start suddenly or may be preceded by a few weeks of vague ill-health. In children and young adults systemic disturbance rapidly becomes profound. In particular there is a high pyrexia with drenching sweats during sleep. Marked tachycardia, loss of weight and usually progressive anaemia. Cough and breathlessness are only occasionally present. There may be no abnormal physical signs in the lungs, although widespread crepitations may be heard late in the disease. The liver is often enlarged and the spleen may be palpable. Choroidal tubercles may be visible on ophthalmoscopy but are rarely present in the elderly. Leucocytosis is usually absent or slight. If chemotherapy is not given death takes place within days or weeks.

'Cryptic' miliary tuberculosis

Diagnosis of this form of disseminated disease is shown in the information box below.

'CRYPTIC' MILIARY TUBERCULOSIS

Diagnosis often made at autopsy – often not suspected during life

Age group
Adults and elderly, particularly females

Symptoms
Chest symptoms *rare*. Lassitude, weight loss and general debility

Clinical signs
Choroidal tubercles *rare*. Chest usually normal. Liver and occasionally spleen may be enlarged. Low-grade pyrexia common

Chest X-ray
Usually *normal*

Blood
Neutropenia, pancytopenia and leukaemoid reaction quite common

---

Investigations

The diagnosis of acute miliary tuberculosis can be made with confidence only when radiological examination of the chest shows the characteristic 'miliary' mottling symmetrically distributed throughout both lung fields or when choroidal tubercles are seen. The diagnosis can often be suspected at an earlier stage by the symptoms, progressive clinical deterioration, persistent pyrexia and splenomegaly.

Bacteriological confirmation should be sought by culture of sputum, urine or bone marrow. A liver biopsy may be diagnostic in difficult cases. Although the tuberculin reaction is usually positive in young patients a negative result does not exclude acute miliary tuberculosis as tuberculin sensitivity is occasionally depressed in the later stages of the illness.

A therapeutic trial of chemotherapy with ethambutol and isoniazid in conventional doses (p. 367) is indicated in patients suspected to have the cryptic form of miliary tuberculosis. Clinical improvement is usually evident within 10 days if the diagnosis is correct.

Prognosis

Antituberculosis chemotherapy (p. 367) has reduced the mortality of miliary tuberculosis from 100% to virtually zero providing the diagnosis is made at an early stage.

POST-PRIMARY PULMONARY TUBERCULOSIS

Most of the morbidity and mortality from tuberculosis is caused by this form of the disease. The majority of cases in Western Europe and North America now occur in middle-aged and elderly subjects although in developing countries it is most prevalent in adolescence and early adult life.

The lesions are most frequently situated in the upper lobes. The disease is often bilateral and occasionally a whole lobe may be consolidated in acute pneumonic tuberculosis.

Clinical features

The onset of post-primary pulmonary tuberculosis is usually insidious, with the gradual development of general symptoms or cough and sputum. Sometimes a dramatic event such as haemoptysis, pleural pain or a spontaneous pneumothorax marks the onset but the diagnosis is now frequently made by radiography before any symptoms have appeared.

The respiratory symptoms are listed in the information box (p. 371).

At first no abnormal physical signs may be present

SYMPTOMS OF POST-PRIMARY TUBERCULOSIS

Cough
May be an early symptom but often not troublesome until a late stage

Sputum
Only when disease has reached an advanced stage. Mucoid at first; later purulent

Haemoptysis
Common when disease advanced. May be massive from a large vessel in a cavity wall; sometimes fatal

Breathlessness
Late symptom unless caused by pneumothorax when onset is acute

Pleural pain
Can be due to tuberculous pleurisy, but occasionally pneumothorax

but despite this an extensive lesion may be visible radiologically. The earliest physical signs consist of a few crepitations usually situated over one or other lung apex posteriorly. Ultimately physical signs of consolidation, cavitation and fibrosis may develop, and occasionally those of pleurisy with or without effusion, or spontaneous pneumothorax (Table 9.8, p. 347).

Radiological examination
This is of paramount importance for diagnosis in the early stages before physical signs appear and for assessment of the extent and progress of the disease.

The earliest radiological change is an ill-defined opacity or opacities usually situated in one of the upper lobes. In more advanced cases opacities are larger and

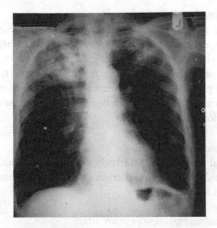

Fig. 9.5 Bilateral pulmonary tuberculosis. Upper zone shadowing more obvious on the right.

more widespread and may be bilateral. Occasionally there is a dense homogeneous shadow involving the whole lobe ('pneumonic tuberculosis'). An area or areas of translucency within the opacities indicates cavitation; very large cavities may be visible in some cases. The presence of cavitation in an untreated patient usually indicates that the disease is active. When fibrosis is marked the trachea and heart shadow are displaced towards the side of the lesion.

The radiological appearances of pleural effusion and pneumothorax, which may accompany those of pulmonary tuberculosis are described on pages 411 and 415.

Diagnosis
The grounds on which pulmonary tuberculosis should be suspected are listed in the information box below.

SYMPTOMS AND SIGNS WHICH SHOULD ALWAYS RAISE THE SUSPICION OF TB

- Persistent cough
- Haemoptysis
- Pleural pain not associated with an acute illness
- Spontaneous pneumothorax
- Lethargy
- Weight loss

The presence of any of these symptoms demands immediate radiological examination of the lungs and, if an abnormality is found, the examination of at least three specimens of sputum for tubercle bacilli. The diagnosis can readily be made by microscopical examination of sputum smears stained by the Ziehl–Neelsen method when bacilli are numerous, whereas the auramine-phenol fluorescent test is of value in the detection of small numbers of tubercle bacilli. Culture of sputum, or of bronchoalveolar lavage fluid, fasting gastric washings or laryngeal swabs if no sputum can be obtained, is necessary when smears are negative and is essential for the detection of drug resistance (p. 368). Cultural methods are thus of great practical value and should be used in the examination of every specimen if facilities permit.

In the vast majority of patients the diagnosis of pulmonary tuberculosis can be made with confidence by radiological examination of the chest and examination of the sputum. In some patients it is necessary to perform further radiological examination after a course of treatment with an antibiotic, such as ampicillin, in order to exclude an acute inflammatory cause for an abnormal X-ray shadow.

Complications

The complications are shown in the information box below.

COMPLICATIONS OF TUBERCULOSIS

Pleurisy
With or without pleural effusion

Pneumothorax
May follow rupture of cavity into pleural space

Empyema or pyopneumothorax
Serious complications of rupture of a tuberculous lesion into the pleural space

Tuberculous laryngitis
Usually only occurs in advanced pulmonary disease

Tuberculous enteritis
Follows swallowing heavily infected sputum in some patients with extensive pulmonary disease

Ischiorectal abscess
Consider TB in all cases. Tubercle bacilli can pass through rectal mucosa

Blood-borne dissemination
Uncommon complication of post-primary pulmonary disease except in the immunosuppressed

Respiratory failure and right ventricular failure
Late complications when disease has caused extensive pulmonary destruction and fibrosis

Fungal colonisation of cavities
Cavities which persist after antituberculosis treatment may become colonised with *Aspergillus fumigatus* and a ball of fungus (aspergilloma) may develop.

Prognosis

There has been a remarkable decline in the mortality from pulmonary tuberculosis with the advent of effective chemotherapy. Provided the tubercle bacilli are not initially drug-resistant and chemotherapy is used correctly, a fatal outcome is uncommon even if the disease has reached an advanced stage when it is first recognised. Late complications of respiratory failure and secondary infection with pyogenic bacteria or fungi can be prevented if pulmonary tuberculosis is diagnosed at a reasonably early stage and is efficiently treated.

NON-PULMONARY TUBERCULOSIS

Tuberculosis can affect any organ and tissue of the body.

Gastrointestinal tuberculosis

Tuberculous ulceration of the tongue can occur but is rare. Diarrhoea, malabsorption, intestinal obstruction and ascites can result from tuberculosis of the intestines and peritoneum. Peritoneal involvement is a common autopsy finding in patients who have died from undiagnosed disseminated disease.

Pericardium

Infection of the pericardial sac is uncommon but can give rise to pericardial effusion and tamponade (p. 327). Constrictive pericarditis can be a late result of infection and is the consequence of fibrosis and calcification.

Genito-urinary tuberculosis

Renal tuberculosis is a fairly common form of non-pulmonary tuberculosis but rarely gives rise to symptoms until the renal lesions are extensive. Haematuria and increased frequency of micturition can be caused by renal tuberculosis. Patients with 'sterile pyuria' should always be suspected of having tuberculosis and at least three early morning urine specimens should be examined.

Infection of the fallopian tubes was a common cause of infertility; it can also give rise to salpingitis and tubal abscess. Epididymal tuberculosis presents as a painless craggy swelling which subsequently can form a sinus.

Central nervous system tuberculosis

Tuberculous meningitis is an extremely serious form of infection which can be associated with miliary tuberculosis but can also present in the absence of generalised disease. Headache, neck stiffness, vomiting and disordered consciousness are features of the disease which can be fatal or result in permanent neurological deficit if not diagnosed and treated at an early stage. Cerebral tuberculomata are uncommon and may or may not present with focal neurological signs.

Lymph node tuberculosis

This is a very common manifestation of tuberculous disease, especially in Asians. Lymph node enlargement in any site can occur but cervical node involvement is most common. The enlargement of lymph nodes is usually painless. When caseation and liquefaction of the nodes occur the swellings become fluctuant and sinus formation is common.

Bone and joint tuberculosis

Skeletal infection is relatively common and can lead to vertebral collapse, pyarthrosis, osteomyelitis and 'cold' abscess formation.

Tuberculous infection in other sites

Destruction by infection of the adrenal glands can give rise to Addison's disease (p. 649). Tuberculous infection of the skin is referred to as lupus vulgaris and erythema nodosum can be a manifestation of primary tuberculosis. Phlyctenular kerato-conjunctivitis, iritis and choroiditis can occur in patients who have a tuberculous infection.

Management

Treatment of non-pulmonary tuberculosis
The principles of chemotherapy and duration of treatment are the same as for the treatment of pulmonary tuberculosis. Corticosteroid therapy is usually used in combination with specific antituberculosis treatment in most forms of non-pulmonary tuberculosis.

RESPIRATORY DISEASES CAUSED BY FUNGI

Most fungi encountered by man are harmless saprophytes but some species may, in certain circumstances, infect human tissue or promote damaging allergic reactions.

The term *mycosis* is applied to disease caused by fungal infection. Predisposing factors include metabolic disorders such as diabetes mellitus, toxic states, for example, chronic alcoholism, diseases in which immunological responses are disturbed such as AIDS, treatment with corticosteroids and immunosuppressive drugs, and radiotherapy. Local factors such as tissue damage by suppuration or necrosis and the elimination of the competitive influence of a normal bacterial flora by antibiotics may also facilitate fungal infection.

Diagnosis

The diagnosis of fungal disease of the respiratory system is usually made by mycological examination of sputum – microscopic examination of stained films for fungal hyphae being extremely important – supported by serological tests and in some cases by skin sensitivity tests.

ASPERGILLOSIS

Most cases of bronchopulmonary aspergillosis are caused by *Aspergillus fumigatus*, but other members of the genus (*A. clavatus, A. flavus, A. niger* and *A. terreus*) occasionally cause disease. The conditions associated with Aspergillus species are listed in the information box (right).

Intracavitary aspergilloma
Inhaled air-borne spores of *A. fumigatus* may lodge and germinate in damaged pulmonary tissue, and an

***

> **CLASSIFICATION OF BRONCHOPULMONARY ASPERGILLOSIS**
>
> ● Allergic asthma (p. 376)
> ● Allergic bronchopulmonary aspergillosis (asthmatic pulmonary eosinophilia) (p. 383)
> ● Extrinsic allergic alveolitis (p. 384)
> ● Intracavitary aspergilloma
> ● Invasive pulmonary aspergillosis

'aspergilloma' (a ball of aspergillus fungus) can form in any area of damaged lung in which there is a persistent abnormal space. The most common cause of such pulmonary damage is tuberculosis, but an aspergilloma can develop in an abscess cavity, a bronchiectatic space or even a cavitated tumour. Most, but not all, are caused by *A. fumigatus*.

Clinical features

An aspergilloma often produces no specific symptoms but may be responsible for recurrent haemoptysis which is often severe. The presence of a fungus ball in the lung can also give rise to non-specific systemic features such as lethargy and weight loss.

Radiological examination

The development of a fungal ball within a cavity produces a tumour-like opacity on X-ray. An aspergilloma can usually be distinguished from a peripheral bronchial carcinoma by the presence of a crescent of air between the fungal ball and the upper wall of the cavity. Aspergillomata may be multiple.

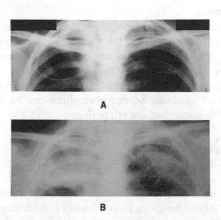

Fig. 9.6 Aspergillomata. A. Bilateral apical cavities **B.** Cavities now opaque due to formation of bilateral aspergillomata. Fungus ball clearly visible in left sided cavity.

Diagnosis

The diagnosis is usually suspected because of the chest X-ray findings. Serum precipitins to *A. fumigatus* can be demonstrated in virtually all patients. Sputum contains hyphal fragments on microscopy which are often only scanty, and is usually positive on culture. Less than 50% of patients exhibit skin hypersensitivity to extracts of *A. fumigatus*.

Management

Specific antifungal therapy is of no value. Surgical removal of the aspergilloma is indicated in patients who have massive haemoptysis and in whom thoracotomy is not contraindicated because of poor respiratory reserve caused by the initial disease leading to persisting pulmonary cavities, for example, tuberculosis, bronchiectasis.

Invasive pulmonary aspergillosis

Invasion of previously healthy lung tissue by *A. fumigatus* is uncommon but can produce a serious and often fatal disease which usually occurs in patients who are immunocompromised either by drugs or disease. The source of the infection can be an aspergilloma but this is by no means always so.

Clinical features

Spread of the disease throughout the lungs is usually rapid with the production of consolidation, necrosis and cavitation. There is grave systemic disturbance. The formation of multiple abscesses is associated with the production of copious amounts of purulent sputum which is often blood-stained.

Diagnosis

Invasive pulmonary aspergillosis should be suspected in any patient thought to have severe suppurative pneumonia (p. 362) which has not responded to antibiotic therapy. The diagnosis can be established by the demonstration of abundant fungal elements in stained smears of sputum. Serum precipitins can be demonstrated in some, but not all, patients.

Management

If the diagnosis is established at an early stage antifungal therapy can be successful. Amphotericin 0.25–1 mg/kg daily by slow intravenous infusion over 6 hours should be given in combination with flucytosine 150–200 mg/kg daily by mouth or by i.v. infusion, in 4 divided doses. The combination of flucytosine and amphotericin prevents resistance to flucytosine developing and allows a smaller daily dose of amphotericin to be used than would be possible if this drug was used on its own.

OTHER PULMONARY MYCOSES

Histoplasmosis

Histoplasmosis is caused by *Histoplasma capsulatum* or a variant, *Histoplasma duboisii* found in soil. Infection with these fungi is by inhalation of infected dust. Occasionally infection passes through the buccal or intestinal mucosa or through the skin. The disease attacks dogs, rats and mice, and the fungus multiplies in soil enriched by the droppings of chickens, pigeons and bats. Infection has proved a hazard for explorers of caves.

Histoplasma capsulatum. This is found in all parts of the United States of America, especially in the East Central states and less commonly in Latin America from Mexico to Argentina, in Europe, North, South and East Africa, Nigeria, Malaysia, Indonesia and Australia.

Pathology

The parasite in its yeast phase multiplies mainly in monocytes and macrophages and produces areas of necrosis in which the parasites may abound. From these foci the bloodstream may be invaded causing metastatic lesions in the liver, spleen and lymph nodes. Pulmonary histoplasmosis may produce pathological changes similar to those of tuberculosis.

Clinical features

The majority, perhaps 90% of pulmonary infections are benign producing no symptoms but more severe infections may closely simulate pulmonary tuberculosis, including the production of a primary complex with enlarged regional lymph nodes, multiple small discrete lesions and occasionally cavitation. Healed lesions may calcify.

The severity of the symptoms of histoplasmosis varies from, in the majority of cases, a slight fever of short duration like influenza, to a severe and prolonged pyrexial illness which ultimately proves fatal.

Diagnosis

In those areas where the disease occurs histoplasmosis should be suspected in every obscure infection in which there are pulmonary signs or where there are enlarged lymph nodes with or without hepatosplenomegaly.

Tissue is obtained by biopsy for impression smear, histology, culture and animal inoculation. Radiological examination in long-standing cases may show calcified lesions in the lungs, spleen or other organs. In the more acute phases of the disease single or multiple soft pulmonary shadows with enlarged mediastinal nodes may be seen.

Delayed hypersensitivity to the intradermal injection of histoplasmin develops in patients with either active or healed infections but is usually negative in the rapidly progressive form of the disease. Complement-fixing antibodies are detected within three weeks of the onset of an acute primary infection and increase in titre as the disease progresses. Precipitating antibodies may also be detected.

Management
Specific treatment with amphotericin is only indicated in severe infection. The dosage of 0.5 mg/kg given intravenously over a 6-hour period gradually increasing to a maximum of 1.0 mg/kg combined with an oral antifungal imidazole. Amphotericin treatment can be given on alternate days and may have to be continued for a prolonged period which will almost inevitably result in renal toxicity. Recovery from generalised histoplasmosis is rare.

Histoplasma duboisii. The fungus of African histoplasmosis is considerably larger than the classical *H. capsulatum*. It is found throughout East, Central and West Africa. This disease differs in several ways from *H. capsulatum* infection. The bones, skin, lymph nodes and liver develop granulomatous lesions or cold abscesses resembling tuberculosis but the lungs are seldom involved. The disease is treated in the same way as *H. capsulatum* infections.

Coccidioidomycosis
Coccidioidomycosis is caused by *Coccidioides immitis* and occurs in Southern United States, and in Central and South America. The disease is acquired by inhalation.

Pulmonary coccidioidomycosis has two forms: primary and progressive. *Primary coccidioidomycosis* behaves very much like primary tuberculosis or histoplasmosis and often does not produce recognisable symptoms. The *progressive* form of the disease is associated with marked systemic upset and respiratory symptoms, and signs of lobular pneumonia. In more chronic cases granulomatous lesions develop within the lungs and can be responsible for symptoms resembling chronic tuberculosis.

Management
Treatment with amphotericin or an antifungal imidazole may be effective.

Blastomycosis
North American blastomycosis is caused by *Blastomyces dermatitidis*. It also occurs in Africa. Systemic infection begins in the lungs and mediastinal lymph nodes and resembles pulmonary tuberculosis. Treatment is with amphotericin.

Cryptococcosis
Cryptococcosis is caused by *Cryptococcosis neoformans*. Its distribution is worldwide. It causes local gummatous-like tumours and granulomatous lesions in the lungs, bones, brain and meninges. Treatment is with amphotericin (p. 374) in combination with an oral antifungal imidazole. Surgical removal of localised pulmonary lesions may be necessary.

ALLERGIC DISEASES

Three types of allergic response are concerned in the production of respiratory disease. The anaphylactic response (p. 37) is associated with an immediate hypersensitivity reaction, the clinical manifestations of which include allergic rhinitis and bronchial asthma. The tuberculin test is the classical example of delayed hypersensitivity. The immune complex response possibly associated with a delayed hypersensitivity reaction may contribute to the production of allergic alveolitis. Both anaphylactic and immune complex reactions may be concerned in the production of some forms of pulmonary eosinophilia such as allergic bronchopulmonary aspergillosis.

ALLERGIC RHINITIS

This is a disorder in which there are episodes of nasal congestion, watery nasal discharge and sneezing. It may be *seasonal* or *perennial*.

Aetiology
Allergic rhinitis is due to an immediate hypersensitivity reaction in the nasal mucosa (p. 37). The antigens concerned in the seasonal form of the disorder are pollens from grasses, flowers, weeds or trees. Grass pollen is responsible for *hay fever* (*pollenosis*) the most common type of seasonal allergic rhinitis in Britain; this disorder is at its peak between May and July.

Perennial allergic rhinitis may be a specific reaction to

antigens derived from house dust, fungal spores or animal dander but similar symptoms can be caused by physical or chemical irritants, for example, pungent odours or fumes including strong perfumes, cold air and dry atmospheres. The term 'vasomotor' rhinitis is often used for this type of nasal problem because in this context the term 'allergic' is a misnomer.

Clinical features
In the seasonal type there are frequent sudden attacks of sneezing with profuse watery nasal discharge and nasal obstruction. These attacks last for a few hours and are often accompanied by smarting and watering of the eyes and conjunctival injection. In the perennial variety the symptoms are similar but more continuous and generally less severe. Skin hypersensitivity tests with the relevant antigen are usually positive in seasonal allergic rhinitis and are thus of diagnostic value; but these tests are less useful in perennial rhinitis.

Management
The following symptomatic measures, singly or in combination, are usually effective in both seasonal and perennial allergic rhinitis:

1. an antihistamine drug such as terfenadine 60 mg twice daily by mouth;
2. sodium cromoglycate nasal spray, one metered dose of a 2% solution into each nostril 4–6 times daily;
3. beclomethasone dipropionate or budesonide nasal spray, one or two metered doses of 50 µg into each nostril twice daily.

Patients failing to respond to these measures may obtain symptomatic relief from intramuscular injection of a long-acting corticosteroid preparation but this form of treatment should be reserved for occasional use in patients whose symptoms are very severe and interfere seriously with school, business or social activities. Vasomotor rhinitis is often difficult to treat, but may respond to ipratropium bromide administered from a metered dose inhaler 0.02 mg into each nostril 3 or 4 times daily.

Prevention
In the seasonal type an attempt should be made to reduce exposure to pollen, for example, by avoiding country districts and keeping indoors as much as possible with windows closed during the pollen season especially when pollen counts are reported to be high. Some patients with hay fever may obtain benefit from pre-seasonal hyposensitisation (p. 380) with grass pollen extract, but this therapy is now rarely used in Britain because of the risk of anaphylactic reaction. The prevention of perennial rhinitis consists of avoiding, as far as possible, exposure to any identifiable aetiological factors but this is often difficult or impossible.

BRONCHIAL ASTHMA

Bronchial asthma is characterised by paroxysms of breathlessness, chest tightness and wheezing, resulting from narrowing of the airways by a combination of muscle spasm, mucosal swelling and viscid bronchial secretion. These changes are thought to be manifestations of an inflammatory reaction within the bronchial wall involving mast cells, eosinophils and other cells. The airflow obstruction, which characteristically fluctuates markedly, causes mismatch of alveolar ventilation and perfusion and increases the work of breathing. Being more marked during expiration it also causes air to be 'trapped' in the lungs. A narrowed bronchus can no longer be effectively cleared of mucus by the act of coughing and many of the smaller bronchi become obstructed by mucus plugs. This is usually a conspicuous finding at autopsy. Death may occur from alveolar hypoventilation and severe arterial hypoxaemia culminating in cardiac arrest.

Aetiology

Early onset asthma (atopic)
It is common for asthma to have its onset in childhood and generally it occurs in atopic individuals who readily form IgE antibodies to commonly encountered allergens. Asthma in these individuals is often referred to as 'atopic' asthma. They can be identified by skin hypersensitivity tests (p. 380) which produce positive reactions to a wide range of common allergens. Other allergic disorders such as allergic rhinitis and eczema are often present, and a family history of these disorders and of 'early onset' asthma is common. It is unusual for a single allergen to be the sole cause of asthma.

The allergens responsible for asthma in atopic individuals generally enter the bronchi with the inspired air and are derived from organic material such as pollen, mite-containing house dust, feathers, animal dander and fungal spores. Previous exposures to these agents will have stimulated the formation of IgE and an anaphylactic antigen-antibody reaction in the bronchi may follow further exposure to specific allergen. This causes the release, from the cells in the bronchial wall, of pharmacologically active substances which provoke bronchial constriction and an inflammatory reaction of allergic type in the bronchial wall. Much less frequently similar effects may be produced by ingested allergens derived from certain foods such as fish, eggs, milk, yeasts and wheat, which presumably reach the bronchi via the bloodstream.

The previously held view that asthma could be explained solely by the release of mast cell mediators such as histamine, prostaglandins and leukotrienes must be modified. It is likely that several different cells are involved in the pathogenesis of asthma, including mast cells, macrophages and eosinophils. These cells probably produce a variety of mediators which inter-react in a complex way to produce a number of pathological effects which, together, contribute to bronchial hyper-responsiveness and the inflammatory reaction within the bronchial wall.

Eosinophil infiltration is a characteristic feature of asthmatic airways and differentiates asthma from other inflammatory conditions of the airways. These cells are capable of releasing a variety of mediators including leukotriene C_4, platelet-activating factor (PAF) and also basic proteins such as major basic protein and eosinophil cationic protein which are toxic to airway epithelium. Neural mechanisms may also be important contributors to bronchial hyper-responsiveness and asthma. Enhanced cholinergic and alpha-adrenergic responses or reduced beta-adrenergic responses have been proposed and many different neural peptides have been identified in human airways which have potent effects on airways function. Vaso-active intestinal peptide (VIP) is a potent relaxant of human airways and is a co-transmitter of acetylcholine in cholinergic nerves. Sensory neuropeptides such as substance P and neurokinins may also be involved in asthma. Damage to airway epithelium may expose unmyelinated C-fibre afferent nerves, which may then be triggered by inflammatory mediators such as bradykinin.

Asthma can, therefore, no longer be regarded as simple bronchoconstriction produced by contraction of bronchial muscle because it is known to be associated with an 'inflammatory' reaction which involves all the structures of the bronchial wall and not just the muscle. There is a close association between this bronchial inflammatory process and bronchial hyper-responsiveness. Compared with normal individuals asthmatic patients have an increased response to the inhalation of irritant substances such as histamine and methacholine. Airways narrowing can also be induced in patients with hyper-reactive airways by exercise, hyperventilation or the inhalation of cold air.

An immune complex allergic reaction may also be implicated in the pathogenesis of bronchial asthma particularly where antigens derived from fungi such as *A. fumigatus* are implicated. Acute attacks of asthma may be caused by drugs such as aspirin and beta-blockers and by exposure to chemical substances in the electronics, plastics and other industries (Table 9.17).

Late onset asthma (non-atopic)

Asthma can occur at any age in non-atopic individuals and because the majority of these patients are adults this type of asthma is often called late onset asthma. It would appear that external allergens play no part in the production of this form of the disease to which the term 'intrinsic asthma' is sometimes applied (Fig. 9.7).

Triggers of the asthmatic response

Allergens can trigger episodes of asthma in atopic patients but asthma is often aggravated by non-specific factors such as cold air, tobacco smoke, dust and acrid fumes, respiratory viral infection and emotional stress. In children and young adults, usually atopic subjects, asthma almost invariably follows strenuous exertion (*exercise-induced asthma*) or exposure to cold air.

Clinical features

Bronchial asthma may be either *episodic* or *chronic*, and although there is a good deal of overlap between these two syndromes the distinction is clinically useful par-

Table 9.17   Allergens and other substances liable to provoke attacks of asthma

Causative agent	Preventive measures	Efficacy
Pollens	Try to avoid exposure to flowering vegetation Keep bedroom windows closed	Low
Mites in house dust	Vacuum-clean mattress daily Shake out blankets daily Dust bedroom thoroughly	Doubtful
Animal dander	Avoid contact with dogs, cats, horses or other animals	High
Feathers in pillows or quilts	Substitute latex foam pillows and terylene quilts	High
Drugs (e.g. beta-blockers)	Avoid all preparations of relevant drugs	High
Foods	Identify and eliminate from diet	Low[1]
Industrial chemicals (e.g. isocyanates, epoxy resins)	Avoid exposure to chemical, or change occupation	High

[1] More effective in control of eczema.

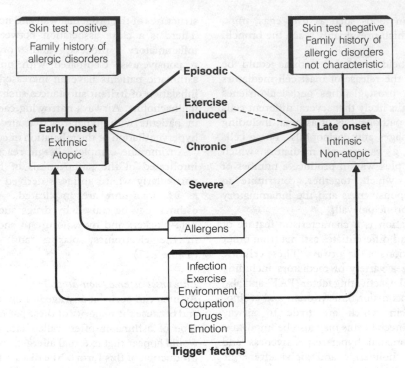

Fig. 9.7   Aetiology and types of asthma.

ticularly in terms of prognosis and management. In general atopic individuals tend to develop episodic asthma, and non-atopic individuals chronic asthma (Fig. 9.7).

Episodic asthma
In this form of the disease the patient has no respiratory symptoms between episodes of asthma. Paroxysms of wheeze and dyspnoea may occur at any time and can be of sudden onset. Episodes of asthma can be triggered by allergens, exercise, viral infections such as the common cold, or may be apparently spontaneous. Attacks may be mild or severe and may last for hours, days or even weeks.

Severe acute asthma
This term has replaced 'status asthmaticus' as the description of life-threatening attacks of asthma. The patient usually adopts an upright position fixing the shoulder girdle to assist the accessory muscles of respiration. There is often an unproductive cough which aggravates respiratory distress. The respiratory symptoms are accompanied by tachycardia, pulsus paradoxus (p. 254), sweating and, in severe cases, central cyanosis.

Chronic asthma
Symptoms of chest tightness, wheeze and breathlessness on exertion, together with spontaneous cough and wheeze during the night may be chronic unless controlled by appropriate therapy. Episodes of 'severe acute asthma' can occur, and cough productive of mucoid sputum with recurrent episodes of frank respiratory infection is common in this type of asthma which in adults may be difficult to distinguish from chronic bronchitis.

Physical signs in the chest
During an attack the chest is held near the position of full inspiration and the percussion note may be hyperresonant. Breath sounds when not obscured by numerous high pitched polyphonic expiratory and inspiratory rhonchi are vesicular in character with prolonged expiration. In very severe asthma airflow may be insufficient to produce rhonchi; a 'silent chest' in such patients is an ominous sign. There are usually no abnormal physical signs between attacks except in patients with chronic asthma who are seldom without expiratory rhonchi. Severe asthma persisting from childhood may cause a 'pigeon chest' deformity (p. 416).

Radiological examination

In an acute attack of asthma the lungs appear hyper-inflated. Between episodes the chest X-ray is usually normal. In long-standing cases the appearances may be indistinguishable from hyperinflation caused by emphysema and a lateral view may demonstrate a 'pigeon chest' deformity. Occasionally, when a large bronchus is obstructed by tenacious mucus, there is an opacity caused by lobar or segmental collapse.

A chest X-ray should be performed, if possible, in all patients with severe acute asthma to exclude pneumo-thorax, a rare but potentially fatal complication of the pulmonary hyperinflation produced by severe airflow obstruction in asthma. The chest X-ray may show mediastinal and subcutaneous emphysema in very severe disease.

Pulmonary function tests

Measurement of the forced expiratory volume in one second (FEV_1) and vital capacity (VC) or peak expiratory flow (PEF) provide a fairly reliable indication of the degree of airflow obstruction (p. 349), and can also be used to determine whether and to what extent it can be relieved by bronchodilator drugs or corticosteroids (Fig. 9.8), or to confirm that the obstruction is provoked by exercise (Fig. 9.9) or hyper-ventilation or occupational exposure (p. 377). Such tests have an important place in the diagnosis and treatment

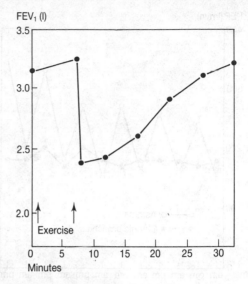

Fig. 9.9 **Exercise induced asthma:** serial recordings of forced expiratory volume in one second (FEV_1) in patient with bronchial asthma before and after 6 minutes of strenuous exercise. Note initial slight rise on completion of exercise, followed by sudden fall and gradual recovery.

of asthma. Serial recordings of PEF are useful in dis-tinguishing patients with chronic asthma from those with fixed or irreversible airflow obstruction associated with chronic bronchitis. In asthma there is usually a marked diurnal variation in PEF the lowest values being recorded in the mornings ('morning dipping') (Fig. 9.10). Serial PEF recordings are also invaluable in the assessment of a patient's response to corticosteroid drugs and in the long-term monitoring of patients with poorly controlled disease.

Arterial blood gas analysis

Measurements of arterial blood-gas pressures (Pa_{O_2} and Pa_{CO_2}) are indispensable in the management of patients with severe acute asthma.

Skin hypersensitivity tests

A prick is made in the skin with a fine needle through a drop of an aqueous extract of the substance to be tested. A positive reaction is indicated by the development of a wheal and flare, which begin to appear within a few minutes. Tests are usually performed with a group of common allergens known to cause bronchial asthma. It is seldom possible with these tests to identify one particular allergen as the cause of asthma in an in-dividual patient and their chief value is to distinguish atopic from non-atopic subjects.

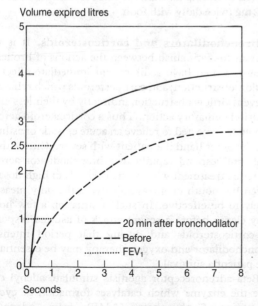

Fig. 9.8 **Reversibility test.** Forced expiratory manoeuvres before and 20 min after inhalation of a beta$_2$ adrenoreceptor agonist. Note the increase in FEV_1 from 1.0 to 2.5 litres.

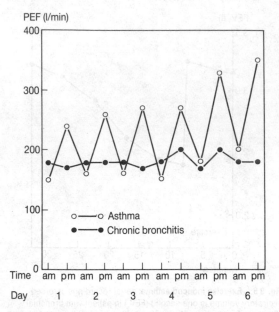

Fig. 9.10 'Morning dipping': serial recordings of peak expiratory flow (PEF) in patients with chronic bronchitis and asthma. Note sharp overnight fall (morning dip) and subsequent rise during the day in patient with asthma which does not occur in patient with chronic bronchitis.

Management

Avoidance of allergens

There are a few instances in which a single agent can be identified as the cause of attacks of asthma. These allergens include grass pollens, mites, animal dander, drugs, industrial chemicals such as isocyanates and certain articles of diet. The measures which can be taken to prevent or reduce exposure to these agents, and the degree of success likely to be achieved, are summarised in Table 9.17. The vast majority of asthmatic patients are hypersensitive to a wide range of allergens and attempts to avoid them all are impracticable.

Hyposensitisation

This is the only specific measure available for the prevention of damaging antigen-antibody reaction. It involves the subcutaneous injection of initially very small, but gradually increasing doses of extracts of allergens believed to be responsible for the patient's asthma. Hyposensitisation may be of some value when only a single allergen, such as grass pollen, house dust mite or animal dander is implicated but it is not without the risk of producing an acute anaphylactic reaction. This form of therapy has been abandoned in Britain because of the attendant risks. Hyposensitisation with a

mixture of allergens is irrational and cannot be recommended.

Drugs which control or suppress clinical manifestations of asthma

Sodium cromoglycate. Administered by inhalation. This has actions which include prevention of mediator release from mast cells. It seems to be of particular value in children with atopic asthma and should be given a trial of at least 4 weeks' duration in all such patients. If the drug is found to be effective regular inhalation of 20 mg in a dry powder by 'Spinhaler' or 5–10 mg from a metered dose inhaler 4 times daily may completely prevent recurrence of asthma in this group of patients. Sodium cromoglycate may be of value in some patients with non-atopic asthma but has no place in the management of severe asthma.

Nedocromil sodium. This is an anti-inflammatory drug with similar properties to those of sodium cromoglycate and is administered by inhalation from a metered dose inhaler in a dose of 4 mg 2 or 4 times daily.

Ketotifen. Taken by mouth it is claimed to have a similar mode of action, but is less effective than sodium cromoglycate or nedocromil sodium and has the serious disadvantage in some patients of causing drowsiness which may be a dangerous side-effect in patients driving cars or operating machinery. The recommended dose is 1–2 mg twice daily with food.

Bronchodilators and corticosteroids. It is important to distinguish between the actions of bronchodilators which have a direct and immediate effect on airflow obstruction, and corticosteroids which relieve or prevent airflow obstruction indirectly by their less rapid anti-inflammatory action. Thus a corticosteroid aerosol cannot be expected to relieve an acute episode of asthma. On the other hand if a patient with severe acute asthma does not respond rapidly to a bronchodilator aerosol systemic treatment with corticosteroids in high dosage, given by mouth or intravenously, is the only measure likely to be effective. In such a situation a few hours may elapse before a severe attack of asthma responds to corticosteroids and during that period intensive bronchodilator and oxygen therapy may be essential to the patient's survival.

Beta-adrenoreceptor agonists stimulate adenyl cyclase the enzyme which catalyses formation of cyclic-adenosine 5'-phosphate (AMP) from adenosine triphosphate (ATP). Basically, there are two types of beta-adrenoreceptors. Stimulation of beta$_1$-receptors produce effects on the heart, intestinal muscle and also lipolysis. Beta$_2$-receptors mediate the beta-adrenergic effects on smooth muscle in the bronchi, uterus and arteries supplying skeletal muscle. Selective beta$_2$-adrenoreceptor agonists have been developed and their duration of action compared with the non-selective drugs of this type (e.g. isoprenaline) has been increased by alterations being made in the chemical structures to make them resistant to the inactivation process mediated by catechol-o-methyl transferase.

The selective beta$_2$-adrenoreceptor agonists in common use (e.g. salbutamol and terbutaline) have a duration of action of 4–6 hours. The effects of beta$_2$-adrenoreceptor agonists are principally mediated by relaxation of bronchial muscle and they do not have any long lasting effect on bronchial inflammation or bronchial hyper-responsiveness. Indeed, it has been postulated that prolonged use of beta$_2$-agonists may make bronchial hyper-reactivity worse and that there may be a rebound increase in bronchial hyper-responsiveness after withdrawal of beta-agonist therapy. Corticosteroids do have a beneficial effect on bronchial inflammation and decrease bronchial hyper-responsiveness. The vast majority of patients with bronchial asthma respond to corticosteroid drugs but there are a few who are genuinely asthmatic but have little or no response to corticosteroids. These patients are difficult to treat and have been labelled 'cortico-steroid-resistant'.

There is considerable controversy about the relative efficacy of the various methods of administering bronchodilator drugs. In the case of selective beta$_2$-agonists such as salbutamol, terbutaline or fenoterol, the inhalation of an aerosol has clear advantages over oral administration because it reduces airflow obstruction more rapidly. Because the effective dose is much lower it is less liable to produce side-effects such as tremor and anxiety. Patients should be taught that failure to obtain the accustomed degree of relief from the inhalation of a bronchodilator means that the asthma is in a refractory phase and that a more potent form of treatment, such as a course of prednisolone by mouth is urgently required.

Methyl xanthine. Derivatives such as theophylline or aminophylline can be given by intravenous injection, mouth or suppository. There has been a revival of interest in the oral methyl xanthines since the introduction of sustained-release formulations which can maintain serum concentrations of theophylline at therapeutically effective but subtoxic levels. Treatment with sustained release oral methyl xanthine preparations should, whenever possible, be monitored by measure-ment of serum concentrations and may be of value in the prevention of troublesome nocturnal asthma.

Treatment of episodic asthma

Mild and infrequent episodes of asthma can be controlled by inhalation of a bronchodilator aerosol. When the episodes are more frequent treatment should be supplemented by regular prophylactic therapy with sodium cromoglycate (p. 380) or a corticosteroid by inhalation.

Treatment of exercise-induced asthma

This common phenomenon which occurs particularly in children and young adults can often be prevented by the inhalation of 2 metered doses of salbutamol or terbutaline a few minutes before exercise. Regular treatment with sodium cromoglycate or an inhaled corticosteroid may be necessary if treatment with a beta$_2$-adrenoreceptor agonist is not wholly effective.

Treatment of chronic asthma

Some form of suppressive treatment is necessary in all patients with chronic asthma. Sodium cromoglycate is worth a trial especially in children, but there is usually a better response to regular inhalation of a corticosteroid aerosol. The role of nedocromil sodium in the management of chronic asthma has not yet been determined. Corticosteroid aerosols are free from systemic unwanted effects in conventional doses, beclomethasone dipropionate (200 µg) or budesonide (200 µg) twice daily, but can cause oropharyngeal candidiasis and a husky voice in a few patients. In severe illness higher doses may be necessary in order to control symptoms, occasionally supplemented by a small maintenance dose of prednisolone given by mouth and/or by occasional short courses of prednisolone in higher dosage (40 mg daily for 7–10 days).

Supplementary treatment with oral prednisolone is required less frequently if the dose of inhaled corticosteroid aerosol is increased, e.g. to 1500 µg beclomethasone dipropionate per day, to 2000 µg budesonide per day. These doses should not be exceeded because systemic absorption will cause impairment of pituitary-adrenal function. When such higher doses of inhaled corticosteroids are used there is a greater likelihood of oropharyngeal candidiasis and effects on the voice (dysphonia). These effects and also some of the systemic effects can be decreased by the use of large-volume space systems or holding chambers (e.g. Nebuhaler or Volumatic). Most patients with chronic asthma also require to inhale a bronchodilator aerosol either regularly or periodically to control recurrences of symptoms. Oral bronchodilator drugs are seldom as effective as aerosols but slow release oral preparations of $beta_2$-adrenoreceptor agonists and methyl xanthines taken at night can be useful in preventing nocturnal symptoms.

Treatment of severe acute asthma

When an acute attack of asthma becomes severe and life-threatening a state of decreased responsiveness to inhaled $beta_2$-adrenoreceptor agonists occurs. All such patients should be admitted to hospital as quickly as possible and emergency admission schemes which eliminate the delays inherent in normal hospital admission procedures can do much to reduce the number of unnecessary deaths from severe acute asthma. It is equally important that the general practitioner should start effective treatment before the ambulance arrives.

Treatment of severe acute asthma at home

Bronchodilator therapy. Salbutamol (5 mg) or terbutaline (10 mg) by nebuliser or 10–20 doses of these drugs from the metered dose inhaler via a large-volume spacer device is administered. Alternatively salbutamol (250 µg) or terbutaline (250–500 µg) can be given by slow intravenous injection. Intravenous aminophylline can be given by a slow intravenous injection over 20 minutes in a dose of 5 mg/kg to patients who are not already taking a sustained-release methyl xanthine preparation by mouth.

Oxygen. Whenever possible high concentrations of oxygen should be given to all patients with severe asthma before, during and after administration of bronchodilator drugs because all have the potential to increase existing arterial hypoxaemia.

Corticosteroids. Hydrocortisone sodium succinate 200 mg i.v. or prednisolone 40 mg orally should be administered to all patients who do not respond promptly to the first dose of bronchodilator.

Treatment in the ambulance

Emergency admission to hospital should be arranged in an ambulance equipped to give oxygen and nebulised $beta_2$-agonist therapy.

Treatment of severe acute asthma in hospital

Oxygen. High concentrations of oxygen – 35–60% should be given to all patients (p. 353).

Nebulised $beta_2$-adrenoreceptor agonists. Salbutamol (5 mg) or terbutaline (10 mg) nebulised in oxygen should be administered immediately irrespect-

ive of any treatment given or taken prior to hospital admission. Treatment with nebulised salbutamol or terbutaline can be repeated within a few minutes if there is no response.

Nebulised ipratropium bromide. 0.5 mg together with salbutamol 5 mg or terbutaline 10 mg nebulised in oxygen is recommended for patients who do not respond to the first treatment with a nebulised beta-agonist within 15–30 minutes.

Intravenous aminophylline. This treatment is usually reserved for patients who do not respond rapidly to nebulised bronchodilator therapy. A loading dose of 5 mg/kg should be given by slow intravenous injection over 20 minutes and followed by a continuous infusion of 0.5 mg/kg/h. The loading dose should not be given to patients who have been given intravenous aminophylline prior to hospital admission or those taking a sustained-release methyl xanthine preparation.

Corticosteroids. Hydrocortisone sodium succinate 200–500 mg i.v. 4–6-hourly should be administered to all severely ill patients. Oral prednisolone in a loading dose of 40–60 mg and thereafter 20 mg 6-hourly can be used in those who are less severely ill.

The response to treatment must be assessed by continuous clinical observation of respiratory rate, heart rate, presence of pulsus paradoxus and patient distress. It is essential for arterial blood gas analysis to be performed on repeated occasions as indicated by the initial blood gas figures and response to therapy (p. 349). Most patients respond to treatment and only occasionally is it necessary to employ major resuscitative measures such as tracheal intubation and mechanical ventilation.

Home nebulisers

Nebulisers are of unquestionable value in the domiciliary treatment of young children unable to use other inhalation devices. Nebulised therapy allows them to be treated with inhaled bronchodilators and drugs such as sodium cromoglycate and inhaled corticosteroids which would not be possible without a home nebuliser.

Recently there has been an increase in the use of nebulisers for self-administration of bronchodilators by adult patients in their homes. Those who are hypoxaemic and do not have access to oxygen may be at some risk from this form of treatment. Furthermore, over-confidence in the efficacy of this treatment can lead to delay in seeking medical advice during an episode of severe asthma when prompt admission to hospital may be vital for survival. Doctors must, therefore, ensure that patients who are provided with nebulisers fully understand their potential dangers and how these can be avoided. This illustrates the important place of education of patients in the management of their disease. Such involvement and understanding is as necessary in asthma as it is in diabetes mellitus and many other diseases.

Prognosis

The prognosis of the individual attack is good except in severe acute asthma where there is occasionally a fatal outcome especially if treatment is inadequate or delayed. Spontaneous remission is fairly common in episodic asthma particularly in children but rare in chronic asthma which can lead to irreversible airflow obstruction. Seasonal fluctuations can occur in both types of asthma. Atopic subjects with episodic asthma are usually worse in the summer when they are more heavily exposed to antigens while chronic asthmatics are usually worse in winter months because of the increased frequency of viral infections.

PULMONARY EOSINOPHILIA

This term is applied to a group of allergic disorders of different aetiology in which lesions of the bronchi and/or the lungs produce a chest X-ray abnormality associated with an increase in the number of the eosinophil leucocytes in the peripheral blood. In some of these diseases the bronchi appear to be primarily affected although there may be secondary effects on lung tissue, while in others the pathological changes are confined to the lungs.

There is no satisfactory classification of this disparate group of disorders, but they can be divided into two main categories: pulmonary eosinophilia with asthma and pulmonary eosinophilia without asthma.

PULMONARY EOSINOPHILIA WITH ASTHMA

Although bronchial asthma could logically be included in this category it is not customary to do so and the term is normally restricted to patients with a severe allergic reaction in the bronchi which gives rise to the production of casts of inspissated mucus heavily infiltrated with eosinophils (asthmatic pulmonary eosinophilia). These casts frequently obstruct bronchi and produce lobar or segmental collapse (Fig. 9.13, p. 390). In some patients the allergic reaction extends to the collapsed lung tissue, but because lung biopsy is seldom indicated in patients with pulmonary eosinophilia the frequency of this complication is uncertain. There is evidence of dual anaphylactic and immune complex reactions in the bronchial wall; an antigen derived from a fungus, usually *Aspergillus fumigatus* is often the causal agent.

Clinical features

Chronic asthma is the dominant clinical manifestation but bronchi, usually in the upper lobes, become obstructed by casts with the production of lobar or segmental collapse, and there may be an associated mild febrile illness. In some patients the radiographic abnormality is peripheral and diffuse. When episodes of bronchial obstruction occur over a period of years, as they usually do, permanent damage to the bronchi and lungs occurs. Cast formation first produces dilatation of the larger bronchi (proximal bronchiectasis). At a later stage bacterial and possibly fungal infection in lung tissue beyond the bronchial obstruction causes extensive pulmonary fibrosis and distal bronchiectasis. These changes together with the associated chronic asthma, which seldom responds well to treatment, eventually cause respiratory failure, pulmonary hypertension and right ventricular failure.

Investigation

In many cases *A. fumigatus* can be isolated from sputum or bronchial casts. Skin tests with an *A. fumigatus* antigen are positive and precipitating antibodies can be detected in the serum. The total serum IgE is usually grossly elevated. Occasionally all investigations are negative and a causal antigen cannot be identified.

In advanced disease the chest radiograph shows extensive bilateral fibrosis and bronchiectasis predominantly affecting the upper lobes.

Management

Initially a short course of prednisolone 40 mg daily for 7–10 days may be followed by the expectoration of bronchial casts and clearing of pulmonary opacities presumably from relief of airflow obstruction. If not it may be necessary to extract the cast or casts by bronchoscopy in an attempt to avert permanent bronchopulmonary damage. Further occlusion of bronchi by mucus plugs can, in some cases, be prevented by a maintenance dose of prednisolone 5–10 mg per day, but in many patients this does not prevent development of bronchiectasis and progressive pulmonary fibrosis.

PULMONARY EOSINOPHILIA WITHOUT ASTHMA

The causes are shown in the information box (p. 384).

PULMONARY EOSINOPHILIA WITHOUT ASTHMA

Causes known
Helminths
   E.g. Ascaris, toxocara, filariae
Drugs
   Nitrofurantoin, para-aminosalicyclic acid, sulphasalazine, imipramine, chlorpropamide, phenylbutazone
Fungi
   E.g. *Aspergillus fumigatus*
Polyarteritis nodosa
   Rare

Cause unknown
Eosinophilic pneumonia (cryptogenic pulmonary eosinophilia)

The conditions shown above predominantly involve lung tissue of patients who do not have asthma although in a few cases this form of pulmonary eosinophilia may precede the development of bronchial asthma sometimes by many years. There is a cellular infiltrate chiefly consisting of eosinophil leucocytes in the alveoli and alveolar walls, to which the term eosinophilic pneumonia can be applied. This may be localised or diffuse and appears to be an immunological reaction of the lung to a variety of antigens. In some patients eosinophilic pneumonia, which may be severe and extensive, develops in the absence of any identifiable cause and is called cryptogenic pulmonary eosinophilia.

Clinical features

The clinical features vary widely in severity depending upon the aetiology and on the extent of pulmonary involvement. Many patients have only a trivial febrile illness the nature of which would have passed unrecognised in the absence of radiological and haematological investigations. Others, particularly those in whom the illness is an allergic reaction to worms (tropical pulmonary eosinophilia) or to drugs, may become gravely ill with high fever and severe breathlessness. In such patients the absolute eosinophil count in peripheral blood is high, often much higher than in pulmonary eosinophilia associated with asthma.

Management

If a cause is found or suspected it must be treated or removed. Helminthic infections should be eradicated and any drug likely to be responsible should be withdrawn. When the condition is due to filariae the patient should be given diethylcarbamazine in an initial oral dose of 1 mg/kg body weight, gradually increased over 3 days to 6 mg/kg daily in divided doses.

Eosinophilic pneumonia (cryptogenic pulmonary eosinophilia) usually responds dramatically to oral prednisolone 20 mg daily but because it is apt to recur after corticosteroid therapy is withdrawn a small maintenance dose may have to be continued for some months, or even for a few years.

EXTRINSIC ALLERGIC ALVEOLITIS

In this condition the inhalation of certain types of organic dust produces a diffuse immune complex reaction (p. 37) in the walls of the alveoli and bronchioles.

The pathogenic mechanisms concerned in the production of extrinsic allergic alveolitis are not fully understood. It is thought that the disease develops in sensitised individuals mainly through a Type III Arthus reaction although Type IV mechanisms are probably also important. When the antigen is inhaled the immune complexes formed in antibody excess are precipitated very rapidly. Deposition of these immune complexes results in complement activation, causing a localised inflammatory action in the alveolar walls. Immunofluorescence has shown IgG, IgA and complement to be fixed in the pulmonary tissues when biopsy specimens are examined in the acute stages. The presence of granulomas in the alveolar walls provides some evidence for a Type IV response to antigen being involved. Bronchoalveolar lavage fluid from patients with extrinsic allergic alveolitis usually shows an increase in the number of lymphocytes. In cryptogenic fibrosing alveolitis (p. 404) bronchoalveolar lavage fluid shows an increase in neutrophils and eosinophils.

Some of the agents which produce extrinsic allergic

Table 9.18 Examples of extrinsic allergic alveolitis

Agent	Source	Disease
Avian protein from pigeons and budgerigars	Pigeon loft or bird cage	Bird fancier's lung
Micropolyspora faeni Thermophilic actinomycetes	Mouldy hay Compost Mouldy sugar cane fibre	Farmer's lung Mushroom worker's lung Bagassosis
Aspergillus clavatus	Malting barley	Maltworker's lung
Coniosporium corticale	Bark of maple trees	Maple bark disease

alveolitis, their source, and the names applied to the resulting diseases are shown in Table 9.18. If patients with this disorder continue to be exposed to the relevant antigen for long periods they may eventually develop permanent pulmonary damage with severe respiratory disability.

Clinical features

Extrinsic allergic alveolitis should be suspected when a person regularly exposed to a heavy concentration of organic dust complains within a few hours of re-exposure to the same dust, of malaise, pyrexia, dry cough and breathlessness without wheeze or insidiously develops similar symptoms, particularly breathlessness, after constant exposure to antigen, as in some cases of bird fancier's lung.

Investigation

In the acute stage of the disease there may be end-inspiratory crepitations (crackles) audible over both lungs. The chest radiograph may show diffuse micro-nodular shadowing. Pulmonary function studies show a restrictive ventilatory defect with preservation of the FEV_1/VC ratio. The Pa_{O_2} is reduced and the Pa_{CO_2} is often below normal because of over-ventilation. Gas transfer is impaired.

The diagnosis of extrinsic allergic alveolitis can be confirmed serologically by a positive precipitin test or by more sensitive serological tests based on the ELISA technique. In some cases it may be necessary to prove the diagnosis by a positive provocation test in which the inhalation of the relevant antigen is followed after three to six hours by pyrexia and a reduction in VC and gas transfer factor.

Management

Mild forms of extrinsic allergic alveolitis rapidly subside when exposure to the antigen ceases. In acute cases prednisolone should be given for 3 to 4 weeks starting with oral prednisolone in a dose of 40–60 mg per day. Severely hypoxaemic patients may require high concentration oxygen therapy initially. Most patients recover completely, but the development of interstitial fibrosis causes permanent disability when there has been prolonged exposure to an antigen.

DISEASES OF THE LARYNX, TRACHEA AND BRONCHI

Acute infections have already been described (p. 354). Other disorders of the larynx include chronic laryngitis,

laryngeal tuberculosis (p. 372), laryngeal paralysis and laryngeal obstruction. Tumours of the larynx are relatively common. For detailed information on these conditions the reader should refer to a textbook of disease of the ear, nose and throat.

LARYNGEAL DISORDERS

CHRONIC LARYNGITIS

The common causes of this condition are listed in the information box below.

SOME CAUSES OF CHRONIC LARYNGITIS

- Repeated attacks of acute laryngitis
- Excessive use of the voice, especially in dusty atmospheres
- Heavy tobacco smoking
- Mouth-breathing from nasal obstruction
- Chronic infection of nasal sinuses

Clinical features

The chief symptom is hoarseness and the voice may be lost completely (aphonia). There is irritation of the throat and a spasmodic cough. The disease pursues a chronic course frequently uninfluenced by treatment, and in long-standing cases the voice is often permanently impaired.

Differential diagnosis

The causes of chronic hoarseness are listed in the information box below.

CAUSES OF CHRONIC HOARSENESS

Consider if hoarseness persists for more than a few days:
- Tumour of larynx
- Tuberculosis
- Laryngeal paralysis
- Inhaled corticosteroid treatment

These conditions must be considered in the differential diagnosis if hoarseness does not improve within a few weeks. In some patients a chest radiograph may bring to light an unsuspected bronchial carcinoma or pulmonary tuberculosis. If no such abnormality is found laryngoscopy should be performed, usually by a specialist in otolaryngology.

Management

The voice must be rested completely. This is particularly important in public speakers. Smoking should be prohibited. Some benefit may be obtained from frequent inhalations of medicated steam.

LARYNGEAL PARALYSIS

Aetiology
Paralysis is due to interference with the motor nerve supply of the larynx. It is nearly always unilateral and, by reason of the intrathoracic course of the left recurrent laryngeal nerve, usually left-sided. One or both recurrent laryngeal nerves may be damaged at thyroidectomy or by carcinoma of the thyroid. Rarely the vagal trunk itself is involved by tumour, aneurysm or trauma.

Clinical features
Hoarseness. This always accompanies laryngeal paralysis whatever its cause. Paralysis of organic origin is seldom reversible, but when only one vocal cord is affected hoarseness may improve or even disappear after a few weeks following a compensatory adjustment whereby the unparalysed cord crosses the midline and approximates with the paralysed cord on phonation.

'Bovine cough'. A characteristic feature of organic laryngeal paralysis is a cow-like cough which results from the loss of the explosive phase of normal coughing consequent upon the failure of the cords to close the glottis. Difficulty in bringing up sputum, which some patients experience, is also explained on the same basis. A normal cough in patients with partial loss of voice or aphonia virtually excludes laryngeal paralysis.

Stridor. This is occasionally present but is seldom severe except when laryngeal paralysis is bilateral.

Diagnosis
Laryngoscopy. This is necessary to establish the diagnosis of laryngeal paralysis with certainty. The paralysed cord lies in the so-called 'cadaveric' position, midway between abduction and adduction (Fig. 9.11).

Management
The cause of laryngeal paralysis should be treated if that is possible. In unilateral paralysis the voice may be improved by the injection of teflon into the affected vocal cord. In bilateral organic paralysis, tracheal intubation, tracheostomy or a plastic operation on the larynx may be necessary.

HYSTERICAL HOARSENESS AND APHONIA

Hoarseness or complete loss of voice may occur as a manifestation of hysteria. There are often clues in the history to suggest a diagnosis of hysteria but laryngoscopy may be necessary to exclude a pathological cause of the voice abnormality. In hysteria only the voluntary movement of adduction of the vocal cords is seen to be impaired.

Laryngeal obstruction
Laryngeal obstruction is more liable to occur in children than in adults because of the smaller size of the glottis. Some important causes are given in the information box below.

CAUSES OF LARYNGEAL OBSTRUCTION

- Inflammatory or allergic oedema, or exudate
- Spasm of laryngeal muscles
- Inhaled foreign body
- Inhaled blood clot or vomitus in an unconscious patient
- Tumours of the larynx
- Bilateral vocal cord paralysis
- Fixation of both cords in rheumatoid disease

Clinical features
Sudden complete laryngeal obstruction by a foreign body produces the clinical picture of acute asphyxia – violent but ineffective inspiratory efforts with indrawing of the intercostal spaces and the unsupported lower ribs, accompanied by cyanosis. Unrelieved, the condition progresses rapidly to coma and death within a few minutes. When, as in most cases, the obstruction is incomplete at first, the main clinical features are progressive breathlessness accompanied by stridor and cyanosis. There is indrawing of the intercostal spaces and lower ribs on both sides with each inspiratory effort. In such cases the great danger is that complete laryngeal obstruction may occur at any time and result in sudden death.

Management
Transient attacks of laryngeal obstruction due to exudate and spasm, which may occur with acute laryngitis in children (p. 354) and with whooping cough, are potentially dangerous but can usually be relieved by the inhalation of steam.

Laryngeal obstruction from all other causes carries a high mortality and demands prompt treatment. The following measures may have to be employed.

The relief of obstruction by mechanical measures
When a foreign body is known to be the cause of the obstruction in children it can often be dislodged by

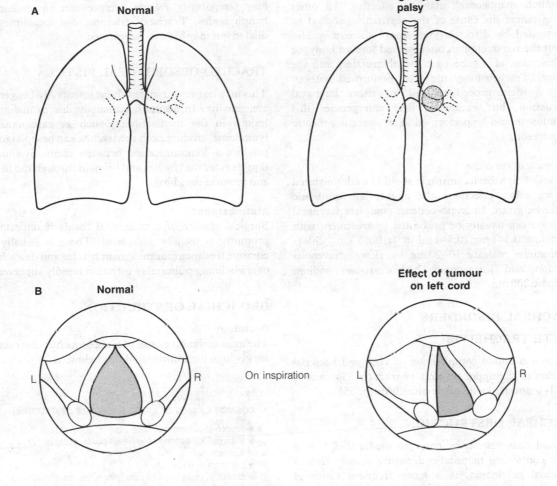

Fig. 9.11   Laryngeal paralysis caused by left hilar tumour. A. Radiological views of the lung. The position of the tumour is shown on the right-hand diagram. **B.** Laryngoscopic view of cords showing normal movement on the left and paralysis of the left cord on the right-hand side. Note that the paralysed left cord is in the cadaveric position (between inspiration and phonation) in both circumstances.

turning the patient head downwards and squeezing the chest vigorously. In adults this is often impossible, but a sudden forceful compression of the upper abdomen (Heimlich manoeuvre) may be effective. In other circumstances the cause of the obstruction should be investigated by direct laryngoscopy which may also permit the removal of an unsuspected foreign body, or the insertion of a tube past the obstruction into the trachea. Tracheostomy must be performed without delay if these procedures fail to relieve laryngeal obstruction, but except in dire emergencies this operation should be performed in an operating theatre by a surgeon.

Treatment of the cause
In cases of diphtheria, antitoxin should be administered and for other infections the appropriate antibiotic should be given. In angio-oedema complete laryngeal occlusion can usually be prevented by treatment with adrenaline 0.5–1 mg (0.5–1 ml of 1:1000) i.m., chlorpheniramine maleate 10–20 mg by slow intravenous injection and intravenous hydrocortisone sodium succinate 200 mg.

TRACHEAL DISORDERS

ACUTE TRACHEITIS

This is a common complication of viral and bacterial infection of the upper respiratory tract (p. 354), and is usually associated with acute bronchitis (p. 356).

TRACHEAL OBSTRUCTION

External compression by enlarged mediastinal lymph nodes containing metastatic deposits, usually from a bronchial carcinoma, is a more frequent cause of tracheal obstruction than the uncommon primary benign or malignant tumours. Rarely the trachea may be compressed by an aneurysm of the aortic arch, or in children by tuberculous mediastinal lymph nodes. Tracheal stenosis is an occasional complication of tracheostomy, prolonged intubation or trauma.

Clinical features
Stridor can be detected in every patient with severe tracheal narrowing. Endoscopic examination of the trachea should be undertaken without delay to determine the site, degree and nature of the obstruction.

Management
Localised tumours of the trachea can be resected, but reconstruction after resection may present complex technical problems. Laser therapy and radiotherapy are alternatives to surgery. The choice of treatment depends upon the nature of the tumour and the general health of the patient. Radiotherapy or chemotherapy may temporarily relieve compression by malignant lymph nodes. Tracheal strictures can sometimes be dilated but may have to be resected.

TRACHEO-OESOPHAGEAL FISTULA

This may be present in new-born infants as a congenital abnormality. In adults it is usually due to malignant lesions in the mediastinum, such as carcinoma or lymphoma, eroding both the trachea and oesophagus to produce a communication between them. Swallowed liquids enter the trachea and bronchi through the fistula and provoke coughing.

Management
Surgical closure of a congenital fistula if undertaken promptly is usually successful. There is usually no curative treatment for malignant fistulae and death from overwhelming pulmonary infection rapidly supervenes.

BRONCHIAL OBSTRUCTION

Aetiology
The most common causes of large bronchus obstruction are given in the information box below.

COMMON CAUSES OF LARGE BRONCHUS OBSTRUCTION

- Bronchial carcinoma or adenoma
- Enlarged tracheobronchial lymph nodes, malignant or tuberculous
- Inhaled foreign bodies
- Bronchial casts or plugs consisting of inspissated mucus or blood clot
- Collections of mucus or mucopus retained in the bronchi as a result of ineffective expectoration

---

Rarer causes of bronchial obstruction include congenital bronchial atresia, fibrous bronchial stricture (often post-tuberculous), aortic aneurysm, giant left atrium and pericardial effusion.

Clinical features
The manifestations of obstruction of a large bronchus depend on whether the obstruction is complete or partial, on the presence or absence of secondary infection, and the effect on pulmonary function. The clinical features also vary with the cause of the obstruction.

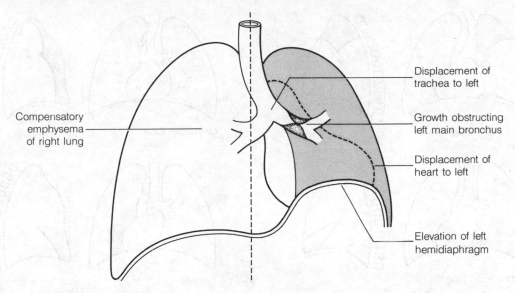

Compensatory
emphysema
of right lung

Displacement of
trachea to left

Growth obstructing
left main bronchus

Displacement of
heart to left

Elevation of left
hemidiaphragm

Fig. 9.12   Collapse of the left lung—effects on neighbouring structures.

Complete obstruction

When a large bronchus is completely obstructed, the air in the lung, lobe or segment it supplies is absorbed, the alveolar spaces close and the affected portion of lung tissue becomes collapsed and solid. The percussion note over the collapsed lung or lobe is dull, and the breath sounds are absent or diminished. Radiological examination shows displacement of the trachea and/or heart shadow towards the side of the lesion, elevation of the diaphragm on the same side and a dense pulmonary opacity of characteristic size, shape and position (Fig. 9.12).

If the collapse involves a smaller portion of lung (for example, the right middle lobe or a bronchopulmonary segment), displacement of the mediastinum may not occur and abnormal physical signs may be difficult to detect, but a characteristic radiographic opacity will be present (Fig. 9.13).

Partial obstruction

A situation occasionally arises if a large bronchus is partially obstructed in which there is less resistance to airflow through the narrowed bronchus during inspiration than during expiration when the obstruction may become temporarily complete. This differential between inspiratory and expiratory airflow, which is increased by coughing, results in over-distension of the lung, lobe or segment supplied by the partially obstructed bronchus (obstructive emphysema). The percussion note over such a lesion is resonant or hyper-resonant, and the breath sounds are diminished . A

chest radiograph shows hypertranslucency of the affected part of lung, and on fluoroscopic examination the mediastinum can be seen to move towards the opposite side of the chest during expiration because the volume of the affected lung then exceeds that of the contralateral lung.

Secondary infection

Whenever a bronchus is narrowed bacterial infection of the lung tissue it supplies is inevitable and this may occur even when the degree of obstruction is insufficient to cause collapse. This explains why pneumonia may be the first clinical manifestation of a bronchial carcinoma. The infection is usually of low virulence but in some cases severe pulmonary suppuration leading to abscess formation occurs.

Impaired pulmonary function

This is unlikely to produce symptoms unless a main or lobar bronchus is involved, or the patient's overall pulmonary function is so poor that obstruction of a smaller bronchus critically diminishes the respiratory reserve. Sudden occlusion of a main or lobar bronchus by mucus or mucopus occurring as a post-operative complication may cause severe breathlessness and hypoxaemia.

Clinical features related to the cause of the obstruction

Tumours. Bronchial obstruction by a carcinoma usually produces pulmonary collapse at an early stage and seldom causes obstructive emphysema. Pulmonary

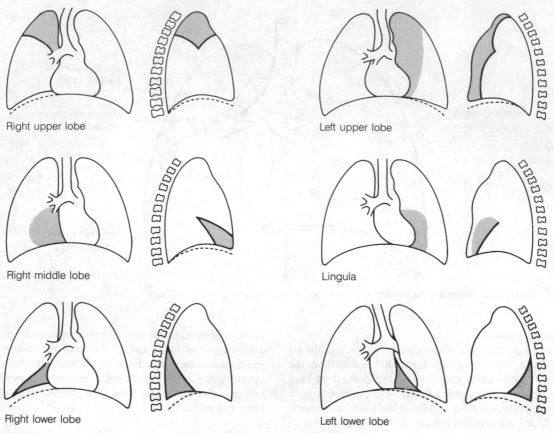

Right upper lobe

Left upper lobe

Right middle lobe

Lingula

Right lower lobe

Left lower lobe

Fig. 9.13 Radiological features of lobar collapse caused by bronchial obstruction. The dotted line represents the normal position of the diaphragm.

infection is common and this may be complicated by empyema. The degree of exertional breathlessness produced by a bronchial carcinoma is directly related to the size of the bronchus it obstructs. The rate of growth of a bronchial adenoma (p. 402) is much less rapid than that of a carcinoma. Complete bronchial obstruction and pulmonary collapse are, therefore, later developments in the presence of an adenoma, and obstructive emphysema, caused by partial bronchial obstruction, may be observed during the intervening period.

Enlarged tracheobronchial lymph nodes. Enlarged lymph nodes by compressing or invading the bronchial wall, may produce the same clinical manifestations of bronchial obstruction of a tumour within the lumen and in bronchial carcinoma both types of lesion may co-exist. Bronchial obstruction by enlarged lymph nodes in Hodgkin's disease and other forms of lymphoma is less common than in bronchial carcinoma presumably because these are less invasive types of tumour.

In some children with primary tuberculous infection large caseous tracheobronchial lymph nodes may compress and erode lobar or segmental bronchi, occasionally even a main bronchus (p. 369).

Foreign bodies. An inhaled foreign body generally lodges in the right main, intermediate or lower bronchus as these bronchi are almost directly in line with the trachea. Children, more often than adults, inhale foreign bodies such as nuts (usually peanuts), peas, beans and small pieces of pens or toys. Adults on the other hand, are more likely to inhale fragments of tooth during extractions under general anaesthesia and articles of food.

When a foreign body becomes impacted in a bronchus it first produces either obstructive emphysema or lobar collapse. A persistent low-pitched rhonchus (fixed rhonchus) may be audible all over the chest if the bronchial lumen is not totally occluded. Within a few days pathogenic bacteria carried into the respiratory tract with the foreign body give rise to a suppurative pneumonia in the collapsed lobe. At this stage there is often a high temperature, cough productive of purulent sputum, and pleural pain. On clinical examination there may be a pleural rub and physical signs of either collapse or consolidation. Radiological examination shows either obstructive emphysema or usually collapse/consolidation. The chest X-rays may also detect and locate a radio-opaque foreign body.

Bronchial casts or plugs. These may consist of either inspissated mucus or blood clot. Plugs of mucus may cause bronchial obstruction in patients with asthma or pulmonary eosinophilia (p. 383). Secondary bacterial infection of the collapsed lung may occur but is seldom severe. Bronchial obstruction by blood clot frequently follows severe haemoptysis but as this complication is usually recognised and treated at an early stage, secondary bacterial infection of collapsed lung tissue seldom occurs.

Retained secretions. A main, lobar or segmental bronchus may be obstructed by retained mucus or mucopus when a patient is unable to cough effectively because of chest pain, muscular weakness or debility, e.g. following an upper abdominal or thoracic operation, or an injury to the chest wall. Secondary bacterial infection of the collapsed lung tissue supervenes at an early stage.

Investigation and treatment of bronchial obstruction

The cause of the bronchial obstruction can be discovered by bronchoscopic examination, and in the case of tumour and tuberculosis histological confirmation of the diagnosis can often be obtained by biopsy. Foreign body can be extracted by bronchoscopy or bronchotomy. Bronchial casts, plugs or secretions which cannot be dislodged by postural coughing should be removed through a bronchoscope. In other forms of bronchial obstruction the treatment is that of the primary condition.

CHRONIC BRONCHITIS AND EMPHYSEMA

Chronic bronchitis and emphysema are pathologically distinct but they frequently co-exist and it may be difficult or impossible to determine the relative importance of each condition in the individual patient. Generalised airflow obstruction is the dominant feature of both diseases.

Chronic bronchitis and emphysema are often grouped together and can be regarded as forming a spectrum with 'pure' chronic bronchitis at one end and 'pure' emphysema at the other (p. 394). For descriptive purposes, however, it is convenient to deal with them separately, with emphasis on their similarities and differences, and on the relationships which frequently exist between them.

CHRONIC BRONCHITIS

Definition
This is clinical and is based on the history. A patient can be assumed to have chronic bronchitis if sputum has been coughed up on most days on at least three consecutive months for more than two successive years, providing other causes of productive cough such as bronchiectasis and untreated chronic asthma have been excluded.

Aetiology
Chronic bronchitis develops in response to the long-continued action of various types of irritant on the bronchial mucosa. The most important of these is cigarette tobacco smoke, but others include dust, smoke and fumes occurring as specific occupational hazards or as part of a general atmospheric pollution in industrial cities and towns. Infection is sometimes a precipitating factor in the onset of chronic bronchitis but its main role is in aggravating the established condition. Exposure to dampness, sudden changes in temperature and to fog may cause exacerbations of chronic bronchitis.

Chronic bronchitis occurs most commonly in middle and late adult life and is much more common in smokers than in non-smokers, and in urban than in rural dwellers.

Strep. pneumoniae and/or *H. influenzae* can be isolated from sputum in most patients at some time particularly during exacerbations associated with purulent sputum.

Pathology
In all cases there is hypertrophy of the mucus-secreting glands and an increase in the number of goblet cells in the bronchi and bronchioles with a consequent decrease in ciliated cells. There is, therefore, less efficient transport of the increased mucus in the airways. Mucosal oedema and permanent structural damage of the airway walls reduces the calibre of the air passages. A major proportion of airflow obstruction in chronic bronchitis is irreversible unlike the airflow obstruction in chronic asthma. Air is 'trapped' in the alveoli because the degree of obstruction is greater during expiration. Over-distension of the alveoli results and disruption of their walls may occur (emphysema, p. 394).

Clinical features

The disease generally starts with repeated attacks of productive cough, usually after colds during the winter months, which show a steady increase in severity and duration with successive years until cough is present all the year round. Wheeze, breathlessness and tightness in the chest are also common complaints, especially in the morning, before the excessive bronchial secretions are cleared by coughing. Sputum may be scanty, mucoid and tenacious and occasionally streaked with blood. Frankly purulent sputum is indicative of bacterial infection which often occurs in these patients.

Breathlessness is caused by airflow obstruction and is aggravated by infection, excessive cigarette smoking and adverse atmospheric conditions. Clinically apparent airflow obstruction is not a feature of all patients but when it does occur it worsens the prognosis.

Variable numbers of inspiratory and expiratory rhonchi, mainly low and medium pitched, are audible in most patients. Crepitations which usually, but not always, disappear after coughing may be audible over the lower lobes. Physical signs attributable to emphysema may co-exist (p. 394)

Investigations

Radiological examination

Chronic bronchitis produces no characteristic abnormality in the chest radiograph but features suggesting emphysema (p. 395) may be prominent in some patients. Bronchography shows various irregularities of bronchial outline, calibre and branching, but this is not a routine investigation.

Pulmonary function tests

Ventilatory capacity. The forced expiratory volume in one second (FEV_1) is reduced and the ratio of FEV_1 to vital capacity (VC) is also subnormal. Peak expiratory flow (PEF) is also reduced and, in contrast to asthma, serial measurements usually do not show circadian variation (Fig. 9.10, p. 380).

Lung volumes. An increase in residual volume (RV), functional residual capacity (FRC) and total lung capacity (TLC), with decreased VC and increased RV/TLC ratio is found when pulmonary hyperinflation is present.

Gas transfer. This may be normal or mildly reduced; severe reduction is correlated with the presence of emphysema (p. 395).

Arterial blood gas measurement. Reduction in Pa_{O_2} reflects disturbance of distribution of pulmonary ventilation and blood flow. If generalised alveolar underventilation supervenes in the later stages of the disease, there is a rise in Pa_{CO_2} and a further fall in Pa_{O_2}. Hypoxaemia becomes more severe during sleep and some patients have periods of marked hypoventilation which cause profound falls in Pa_{O_2}. These may be factors in the production of pulmonary hypertension.

Exercise tests. Simple tests of exercise tolerance, such as the distance walked in six minutes, are valuable estimates of everyday disability.

Complications

Type I and II respiratory failure. This is recognised from the changes in arterial gas pressures (see above). Type I respiratory failure (p. 350) occurs in patients with mild to moderate disease; acute or chronic Type II respiratory failure is a common complication in patients with severe airflow obstruction associated with chronic bronchitis.

Secondary polycythaemia. This occurs in many patients as a consequence of prolonged hypoxaemia but rarely requires therapy, although venesection may be performed if the haematocrit exceeds 60%.

Pulmonary hypertension and right ventricular failure. The increase in pulmonary artery pressure is due both to vasoconstriction mediated by the effect of hypoxia on pulmonary arterioles and to destruction of the pulmonary vascular bed. Because any increase in the degree of airflow obstruction aggravates hypoxia, bacterial infection in the respiratory tract, oedema of the bronchial mucosa, over-secretion of bronchial mucus and spasm of the bronchial muscles are all liable to increase the pulmonary arterial pressure and may precipitate right ventricular failure (cor pulmonale). Similarly falls in arterial oxygen saturation occurring during sleep (p. 352) may also contribute.

Course and prognosis

Chronic bronchitis is usually a progressive disease, punctuated by acute exacerbations and remissions and eventually causing respiratory and cardiac failure. Some patients die within a few years of the onset of symptoms; others survive for many years with gradually diminishing respiratory reserve.

A productive cough continues in some patients but severe airflow obstruction does not occur. Their prognosis is very much better than those who have airflow obstruction.

Management

Reduction of bronchial irritation

It is of extreme importance that bronchial irritation should be reduced to a minimum. The patient who smokes should be urged to stop completely and permanently. Dusty and smoke-laden atmospheres should be avoided, which may involve a change of occupation.

Treatment of respiratory infection

Respiratory infection must be treated promptly because it aggravates breathlessness and may precipitate Type II respiratory failure in patients with severe airflow obstruction. Purulent sputum is treated with oral oxytetracycline or ampicillin in a dose of 250 mg 4 times daily or co-trimoxazole 960 mg twice daily. A 5–10-day course of treatment is usually effective and the sputum becomes mucoid. Well informed, reliable patients can be given a supply of one of these drugs and be permitted to start a course of treatment on their own initiative when the need arises.

Because the vast majority of bacterial infections in chronic bronchitis are caused by *Strep. pneumoniae* or *H. influenzae* bacteriological examination of sputum is essential only when the response to empirical treatment is unsatisfactory and the sputum remains purulent. In that event a change of antibiotic, guided by the results of bacterial sensitivity tests, will be indicated. Continuous suppressive antibiotic treatment is not advised as it is apt to promote the emergence of drug-resistant organisms within the respiratory tract.

Bronchodilator therapy

Bronchodilators are much less effective in chronic bronchitis than in bronchial asthma but should be given to all patients with reversible airflow obstruction. Regular treatment with an inhaled beta$_2$-adreno-receptor agonist (salbutamol 200 mcg or terbutaline 500 mcg, 4–6 hourly) may be sufficient in patients with mild to moderate disease. The anticholinergic bronchodilator drug ipratropium bromide in a dose of 36–72 mcg 6 hourly should be added in patients with more severe airflow obstruction. Theophylline therapy often has little measurable effect on the airways obstruction associated with chronic bronchitis but it will improve quality of life in some patients.

Symptomatic measures

These may be required to control unproductive cough during the night. An unproductive nocturnal cough is often less troublesome if the patient sleeps in a warm bedroom. A hot drink or the inhalation of steam helps to liquefy sputum and make it easier to cough up. The so-called expectorant cough mixtures and drugs which claim to reduce sputum viscosity are of little or no value. Cough suppressants are usually contraindicated.

Hospital treatment of severe exacerbations

Antibiotic treatment

Oral or intravenous ampicillin 500 mg 6-hourly or oral cotrimoxazole 960 mg 12-hourly are effective in most patients. Antistaphylococcal treatment should also be given during influenza epidemics (p. 359).

Bronchodilator therapy

Nebulised salbutamol (5 mg) or terbutaline (10 mg) 4–6 hourly plus nebulised ipratropium bromide (0.5 mg 6-hourly is given to all patients with airflow obstruction during the initial treatment of severe exacerbations.

Diuretic therapy

Frusemide 40–120 mg daily or bumetanide 1–5 mg daily by mouth is administered to all oedematous patients. Intravenous therapy may be necessary if right ventricular failure is gross.

Oxygen therapy

Controlled low-concentration oxygen therapy (p. 353) monitored by arterial blood gas measurements is essential in patients with uncompensated Type II respiratory failure and right heart failure.

'Respiratory stimulants'

Drugs which stimulate the 'respiratory centre' may sometimes be of value in patients with profound respiratory acidosis. An intravenous infusion of doxapram hydrochloride 1.5–4 mg per minute should be administered, the dose being monitored to the patient's response.

Mechanical ventilation

Assisted ventilation is rarely justified in patients with severe chronic bronchitis but may be necessary in a few patients with severe uncompensated Type II respiratory failure whose respiratory function was relatively good prior to the exacerbation.

Physiotherapy

Assisted expectoration is of value in patients who are drowsy because of CO_2 retention (carbon dioxide narcosis), but of less importance in patients who are fully alert.

Long-term domiciliary oxygen therapy

Long-term low concentration oxygen therapy (2 l/min

by nasal cannulae) decreases pulmonary hypertension and prolongs life in hypoxaemic chronic bronchitic patients who have developed right heart failure. The most efficient way of providing oxygen in this way is by an oxygen concentrator. Low-concentration oxygen should be administered for 15 hours or more per 24 hours.

Prevention

Stopping smoking is the most important preventative measure. The control of atmospheric pollution in urban areas and the increased use of measures to prevent the inhalation of dust by industrial workers will also help to reduce the prevalence of chronic bronchitis.

EMPHYSEMA

The word 'emphysema' means 'inflation' in the sense of unnatural distension with air. Although normally confined to the lungs (pulmonary emphysema) air may, for example, enter the mediastinum (mediastinal emphysema) following the rupture of over-distended alveoli into the interstitial tissues of the lung in patients with severe bronchial asthma, or following rupture of the oesophagus. If a large amount of air escapes rapidly into the mediastinum, it may produce cardiac tamponade (p. 327), but in most patients it tracks harmlessly upwards into the soft tissues of the neck where it imparts a characteristic crackling sensation to the palpating fingers (subcutaneous emphysema). Penetrating wounds of the chest wall may also cause subcutaneous emphysema, and when a spontaneous pneumothorax is treated by pleural decompression with an intercostal tube (p. 415) widespread subcutaneous emphysema is an occasional alarming but not serious complication.

Pulmonary emphysema

Definition

Emphysema is defined pathologically as dilation of the air spaces lying beyond the terminal bronchioles.

The definition therefore covers a wide variety of pathological processes ranging from overdistension of otherwise normal alveoli in conditions such as bronchial asthma to the widespread disruption of the alveolar walls which occurs in the more serious forms of pulmonary emphysema. There is a close association between the latter and chronic bronchitis but the physical signs and radiological changes attributable to 'emphysema' may be more conspicuous in some cases of chronic bronchitis than in others.

Aetiology

Emphysema in young adults may be associated with genetically determined alpha$_1$-antitrypsin deficiency (p. 498). It is believed that connective tissue in the lung is digested by proteolytic enzymes normally inhibited by alpha$_1$ antitrypsin. This type of emphysema is rare. Most patients do not have alpha$_1$-antitrypsin deficiency; the disease is caused by cigarette smoking and usually associated with chronic bronchitis. Inhalation of cigarette smoke causes alveolar macrophages to accumulate around the terminal bronchioles and smoke damages the macrophages allowing release of their endogenous proteolytic enzymes. Leucocytes in the peripheral parts of the lung may also release enzymes such as elastase as a consequence of contact with cigarette smoke. The end result of these processes is destruction of alveolar walls by 'digestion'.

Pathology

In some cases generalised destruction of the alveolar walls ('panacinar' emphysema) is the dominant lesion. Where emphysema occurs together with a major component of chronic bronchitis, it is 'centrilobular' or 'centriacinar', and principally affects those alveoli which are most closely related to the respiratory bronchioles.

Clinical syndromes of emphysema and chronic bronchitis

Although the two types of emphysema develop in different ways, factors such as bacterial infection, alveolar over-distension and distortion of the airways may eventually blur their features. Two distinctive clinical patterns, however, have been recognised. In one (the 'blue and bloated' type) cough and sputum, infective exacerbations, cyanosis with arterial hypoxaemia and hypercapnia and right ventricular failure with peripheral oedema predominate. In the other (the 'pink and puffing' type) disabling exertional dyspnoea may antedate by many years the onset of respiratory and cardiac failure and cough and cyanosis are not prominent. A mixed syndrome of chronic bronchitis and emphysema is, however, much more commonly seen than either of the two individual syndromes, and computed tomography studies (p. 396) do not support the original supposition that the pathological changes of bronchitis predominated in the 'blue and bloated' type and those of emphysema in the 'pink and puffing'.

Clinical features

Most patients with pulmonary emphysema complain of exertional breathlessness but because other causes of airflow obstruction, such as chronic bronchitis and bronchial asthma, often co-exist it is seldom possible to assess the contribution of emphysema per se to the production of this symptom. There is a progressive increase in respiratory disability but the tempo of deterioration varies widely from one patient to another.

Clinical abnormalities found in the advanced stages of any chronic condition causing airflow limitation (including chronic bronchitis, emphysema and chronic asthma) are given in the information box below.

CLINICAL ABNORMALITIES FOUND IN PATIENTS WITH ADVANCED AIRFLOW OBSTRUCTION

- A reduction in the length of the trachea palpable above the sternal notch
- Tracheal descent during inspiration
- Contraction of the sterno-mastoid and scalene muscles on inspiration
- Excavation of the suprasternal and supraclavicular fossae during inspiration
- Jugular venous filling during expiration
- Indrawing of the costal margins during inspiration
- An increase in the antero-posterior diameter of the chest relative to the lateral diameter

---

These signs of generalised abnormality contrast with the signs of lateralised disease (Table 9.8 p. 347). Purselip breathing is characteristic of emphysema and is assumed to be adopted by patients to aid expiration by breathing out against a resistance in an attempt to prevent air trapping.

The physical signs in the chest are caused by pulmonary hyperinflation (Table 9.8). Chest expansion is symmetrically diminished as are the breath sounds. There is decreased cardiac dullness.

Investigations

Radiological examination
A diagnosis of emphysema is suggested if the following abnormalities are present:

1. bullae
2. unusually translucent lung fields, with loss of peripheral vascular markings
3. a low flat diaphragm
4. prominence of the pulmonary arterial shadows at both hila.

It is rarely possible to make a confident diagnosis of emphysema from the chest X-ray unless obvious bullae are visible. In the late stages of the disease, when pulmonary hypertension and right ventricular failure supervene, there is enlargement of the main pulmonary artery and of the heart which is visible on the conventional chest X-ray.

Computed tomography (CT)
CT scanning can detect emphysema with certainty but this investigation is not yet routinely used for diagnostic purposes.

Pulmonary function tests

Ventilatory capacity. Measurements of FEV_1 and VC show an obstructive defect with reduced FEV_1/VC ratio. Peak expiratory flow is reduced and serial measurements show no circadian variation (Fig. 9.10).

Lung volumes. Total lung capacity (TLC), residual volume (RV) and RV/TLC ratio are increased.

Transfer factor for carbon monoxide. The transfer factor and transfer co-efficient for carbon monoxide are usually severely reduced in gross emphysema, in contrast to the relatively normal values often found in chronic bronchitis or chronic asthma with a comparable degree of severity of airflow obstruction.

Arterial blood gas measurements. Relatively normal blood gas pressures tend to be maintained at rest for a longer period in emphysema than in chronic bronchitis but hypoxaemia may occur on exercise. Eventually Type I and Type II respiratory failure develop.

Complications

Pulmonary bullae. These may be single or multiple, large or small and can develop in emphysematous lung tissue regardless of the primary pathology. Bullae are inflated thin-walled spaces created by rupture of alveolar walls. They are usually situated subpleurally and commonly occur along the anterior borders of the lungs. A subpleural bulla may rupture and cause spontaneous pneumothorax. In other circumstances bullae may increase progressively in size and eventually become so large that they interfere with pulmonary ventilation (Fig. 9.14).

Respiratory failure and right heart failure. These are generally late complications in patients in whom emphysema predominates.

Weight loss. Profound weight loss leading to emaciation is seen in some patients. The reason for this is not well understood although impaired testosterone secretion has been found in some cases. Many emphysematous patients are unnecessarily investigated for other causes of weight loss.

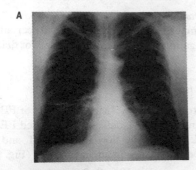

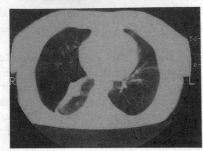

Fig. 9.14   **Large emphysematous bulla occupying the right upper and mid zone. A.** The X-ray shows the position of the bulla with compression of lung tissue beneath it. **B.** CT scan of patient shown in A. Large emphysematous bulla seen in right lung with compression of lung tissue posteriorly.

Management

There is no specific remedy for generalised emphysema but considerable benefit may be obtained from the treatment of associated chronic bronchitis (p. 393). *Respiratory failure* (p. 350) and *right heart failure* (p. 288) are late complications and require treatment as they occur.

Psysiotherapy

Physiotherapy may aid relaxation of cervical muscles and help patients to exhale slowly and steadily through pursed lips. Physiotherapy may also be necessary to encourage expectoration. Regular mild exercise has been shown to increase mobility even in severely disabled patients.

Surgical treatment of giant bullae

Surgical ablation of giant bullae may allow relatively normal lung tissue compressed by the bullae to expand and may bring about a dramatic improvement in pulmonary function.

Heart and lung transplantation

Young patients with severe emphysema due to alpha₁ antitrypsin deficiency may be candidates for trans-plantation of lungs and heart or of both lungs if facilities exist.

Prognosis

Progressive increase in exertional breathlessness is the rule unless the patient stops smoking at an early stage of the illness. Respiratory and right heart failure are usually late complications but when they develop death usually ensues within a few years.

BRONCHIECTASIS

Aetiology and pathogenesis

Bronchiectasis, the term used to describe abnormal dilatation of the bronchi, may be produced in different ways. It may be acquired, or less commonly, congenital. The causes are listed in the information box below.

CAUSES OF BRONCHIECTASIS

Congenital
Ciliary dysfunction syndromes, cystic fibrosis, primary hypogammaglobulinaemia

Acquired
Children
Pneumonia (whooping cough and measles), primary tuberculosis, foreign body

Adults
Suppurative pneumomia, pulmonary tuberculosis, pulmonary eosinophilia, bronchial tumours

---

Bronchiectasis is usually secondary to severe bacterial infection in childhood often as a complication of whooping cough or measles.

Bronchiectasis may be due to bronchial distension resulting from the accumulation of pus beyond a lesion obstructing a major bronchus, such as a tuberculous hilar lymph node, an inhaled foreign body or a bronchial carcinoma. Recurrent infection and chronic obstruction by viscid mucus are both factors in causing bronchiectasis in cystic fibrosis (p. 479). Rarely, it may be the result of congenital dysfunction of the cilia, which is a feature of, for example, Kartagener's syndrome (bronchiectasis, sinusitis and transposition of the viscera). Because of the many different causes of bronchiectasis no precise age incidence can be stated.

Pathology

The bronchiectatic cavities may be lined by granulation tissue, squamous epithelium or normal ciliated epithelium. There may also be inflammatory changes in the deeper layers of the bronchial wall and hypertrophy of the bronchial arteries. Chronic inflammatory and fibrotic changes are usually found in the surrounding lung tissue.

Clinical features

Bronchiectasis may involve any part of the lungs but the more efficient drainage by gravity of the upper lobes usually produces less serious symptoms and complications than when bronchiectasis involves the lower lobes.

The three groups of clinical features that occur in more severe cases are shown in the information box below.

SYMPTOMS OF BRONCHIECTASIS

Due to accumulation of pus in dilated bronchi
Chronic productive cough usually worse in mornings and often brought on by changes of posture. Sputum often copious and persistently purulent in advanced disease

Due to inflammatory changes in lung and pleura surrounding dilated bronchi
Fever, malaise and increased cough and sputum volume when spread of infection causes pneumonia, which is frequently associated with pleurisy. Recurrent pleurisy in the same site often occurs in bronchiectasis

Haemoptysis
Can be slight or massive and is often recurrent. Usually associated with purulent sputum or an increase in sputum purulence. Can, however, be the only symptom in so-called 'dry bronchiectasis'

General health
When disease is extensive and sputum persistently purulent a decline in general health occurs with weight loss, anorexia, lassitude, sleep sweating and failure to thrive in children. In these patients finger clubbing is common

---

Physical signs in the chest may be unilateral or bilateral and are usually basal. If the bronchiectatic cavities are dry without lobar collapse there may be no abnormal physical signs. In the presence of large amounts of secretion numerous coarse crepitations will be heard over the affected areas. When collapse is present the character of the physical signs depends on whether or not the proximal bronchi supplying the collapsed lobe are patent (Table 9.8).

Investigations

Bacteriological and mycological examination of sputum
This is necessary in all patients but is especially important in bronchiectasis associated with cystic fibrosis and in any patient who has received repeated antibiotic courses.

Radiological examination
Bronchiectasis, unless very gross, is not usually apparent on the conventional chest X-ray. In advanced disease the cystic bronchiectatic spaces may be visible. Abnormalities produced by associated pulmonary infection and/or collapse are evident. A diagnosis of bronchiectasis can only be made with certainty by bronchography.

Assessment of ciliary function
A screening test can be performed in patients suspected of having a ciliary dysfunction syndrome by assessing the time taken for a small pellet of saccharin placed in the anterior chamber of the nose to reach the pharynx, when the patient can taste it. This time should not exceed 20 minutes and is greatly prolonged in patients with ciliary dysfunction. It is possible to assess ciliary function by measuring ciliary beat frequency using biopsies taken from the nose. Whenever possible the ciliary ultrastructure should also be determined by electron microscopy.

Management

Postural drainage
The aim of this measure is to keep the dilated bronchi emptied of secretions. Efficiently performed it is of great value both in reducing the amount of cough and sputum and in preventing recurrent episodes of bronchopulmonary infection. In its simplest form, postural drainage consists of adopting a position in which the lobe to be drained is uppermost thereby allowing secretions in the dilated bronchi to gravitate towards the trachea from which they can readily be cleared by vigorous coughing. 'Percussion' of the chest wall with cupped hands aids dislodgement of sputum and a number of mechanical devices are available which cause the chest wall to oscillate thus achieving the same effect as postural percussion and chest wall compression. The optimum duration and frequency of postural drainage depends on the amount of sputum but 5–10 minutes once or twice daily is a minimum for most patients.

Antibiotic therapy
The policy governing the use of antibiotics in most patients with bronchiectasis is the same as that in chronic bronchitis (p. 393). Some, especially those with cystic fibrosis, present difficult therapeutic problems because of secondary infection with bacteria such as staphylococci and Gram-negative bacilli, in particular pseudomonas species. In these circumstances it may prove necessary to use oral ciprofloxacin (250–750 mg twice daily) or ceftazidime by intravenous injection or infusion (100–150 mg/kg daily in 3 divided doses). The

bronchi of some patients with cystic fibrosis also become colonised by *Aspergillus fumigatus*.

Surgical treatment

It is essential to obtain bronchograms demonstrating exactly the extent of the bronchiectasis if surgery is being considered. For this purpose all segments of both lungs must be outlined. Pulmonary function should also be carefully assessed. Unfortunately many of the patients in whom medical treatment proves unsuccessful are also unsuitable for resection either because the bronchiectasis is too extensive or frequently because most of the symptoms are due to co-existing chronic bronchitis. The most favourable cases for surgical resection are children and young adults in whom the bronchiectasis is unilateral and confined to a single lobe or part of a lobe. Resection of areas of bronchiectatic lung has no role in the management of the progressive forms of bronchiectasis, for example those associated with ciliary dysfunction or cystic fibrosis. However, heart-lung transplantation has been successful in a few patients with cystic fibrosis who were disabled by bronchiectasis.

Prognosis

The disease is progressive when associated with ciliary dysfunction and cystic fibrosis and inevitably causes respiratory failure and right ventricular failure. Prognosis has greatly improved in cystic fibrosis with recent developments in the control of bronchial sepsis and a better maintenance of nutrition, and many patients now survive into adult life. Heart-lung transplantation offers the possibility of long-term survival for a minority. In other patients prognosis is relatively good if postural drainage is performed regularly and antibiotics are used judiciously.

Prevention

Because bronchiectasis commonly starts in childhood following measles, whooping cough or a primary tuberculous infection, it is essential that these conditions receive adequate prophylaxis and treatment. The early recognition and treatment of bronchial obstruction is particularly important. It is likely that the numbers of

Table 9.19 Common cell types of bronchial carcinoma

	Percentage
Squamous	50%
Small cell	25%
Adenocarcinoma	15%
Large cell	10%

children born with cystic fibrosis will rapidly decline in the future following the recent advances in the field of genetics.

INTRATHORACIC TUMOURS

TUMOURS OF BRONCHUS AND LUNG

Bronchial carcinoma is by far the most common malignant pulmonary tumour. Benign tumours are rare. A primary carcinoma of any organ, but particularly of breast, kidney, uterus, ovary, testes and thyroid may give rise to pulmonary metastatic deposits as may an osteogenic or other sarcoma.

BRONCHIAL CARCINOMA

Bronchial carcinoma accounts for more than 50% of all male deaths from malignant disease. It is more common in men than women although the gap between the sexes is now narrowing, and occurs most frequently between the ages of 50 and 75 years.

Aetiology

Cigarette smoking is responsible for most cases of bronchial carcinoma and the increased risk is directly proportional to the amount smoked and to the tar content of the cigarettes. For example, the death rate from the disease in heavy cigarette smokers is 40 times that in non-smokers. The incidence is slightly higher in urban than in rural dwellers presumably because of atmospheric pollution. There is a higher incidence of bronchial carcinoma in pulmonary fibrosis induced by the inhalation of asbestos (asbestosis).

Pathology

Bronchial carcinomas arise from the bronchial epithelium or mucous glands. The common cell types are listed in Table 9.19.

When the tumour obstructs a large bronchus it causes pulmonary collapse and infection and symptoms arise early. A tumour of a peripheral bronchus may, however, attain a very large size without producing symptoms. Such a tumour, which is usually of the squamous type, may undergo central necrosis and cavitation when it may have similar radiographic features to a lung abscess (p. 363).

Bronchial carcinoma may involve the pleura either directly or by lymphatic spread. It may also extend into the chest wall and cause severe pain by invading the intercostal nerves or the brachial plexus. The tumour or its lymph node metastases may spread into the mediastinum where the phrenic and left recurrent laryngeal nerves may be affected. Lymphatic spread may occur to supraclavicular ('scalene') as well as to the mediastinal lymph nodes. Blood-borne metastases occur most commonly in liver, bone, brain, adrenals and skin. Even a small primary tumour may cause widespread metastatic deposits. A carcinoma of the small cell type has often spread beyond the lung by the time of diagnosis.

Clinical features

Symptoms due to tumour in the bronchus

Cough. This is the most common early symptom. Sputum is purulent if there is secondary bacterial infection. The bronchial carcinoma itself does not produce sputum, but patients often have associated chronic bronchitis which is also caused by cigarette smoking.

Haemoptysis. This is a common symptom of carcinomas arising in large central bronchi but is less frequent in peripheral tumours. Repeated slight haemoptysis is a common and characteristic feature. Centrally situated tumours can invade large pulmonary vessels causing massive haemoptysis, which is often fatal.

Breathlessness. This may occur early when the tumour obstructs a large bronchus resulting in collapse of a lobe or lung. A large pleural effusion may also cause breathlessness of rapid onset.

Stridor. This develops when spread of the tumour to the subcarinal and paratracheal glands causes compression of the main bronchi and lower end of the trachea.

Infection distal to bronchial carcinoma

Bronchial obstruction often causes distal infection because there is interference with bronchial drainage. This permits the development of pneumonia which may either be slow to respond to treatment or recurs at the same site (p. 361). A lung abscess can develop in infected lung distal to a bronchial tumour (p. 364).

Spread to pleura and chest wall

Pleural pain is a frequent symptom which is usually due to malignant invasion of the pleura but may follow infection distal to a bronchial carcinoma. Pain in the chest wall or in an upper limb with a nerve root distribution may be present if the tumour involves intercostal nerves or the brachial plexus. A bronchial car-

Table 9.20 Mediastinal invasion – structures involved and clinical manifestations

Structures involved	Clinical manifestations
Left recurrent laryngeal nerve	Hoarse voice and 'bovine' cough
Superior vena cava (obstruction)	Non-pulsatile distension of neck veins. Oedema and cyanosis of head, neck, hands and arms. Dilated anastomotic veins on chest wall.
Oesophagus	Dysphagia, initially for solids.
Phrenic nerve	Paralysis of a hemidiaphragm may cause breathlessness, but more often is an X-ray finding
Pericardium	Cardiac tamponade
Trachea	Stridor

cinoma in the apex of the lung may cause Horner's syndrome. The combination of pain in the shoulder and arm plus ipsilateral Horner's syndrome is often referred to as Pancoast's syndrome.

Spread to the mediastinum

Mediastinal structures are involved by spread to mediastinal lymph glands or by direct extension of the tumour mass. Evidence of mediastinal spread almost invariably means that the tumour is inoperable. Ways in which tumour invasion of the mediastinum can present are shown in Table 9.20.

Distant blood-borne metastatic spread

The presenting feature of the disease may be from blood-borne metastases, for example focal neurological signs, fits, personality change, jaundice, bone pain or skin nodules which may be tender. Lassitude, anorexia and weight loss are relatively late symptoms in bronchial carcinoma and usually indicate the presence of extensive metastatic spread.

Clubbing of the fingers

Digital clubbing is often seen and some patients present with the features of hypertrophic pulmonary osteoarthropathy (HPOA). In this syndrome there is pain, which may be severe, usually in the wrists and ankles but also in the knees and shins. The distal parts of the long bones of the wrists and ankles may be exquisitely tender to touch and pitting oedema is often present over the anterior aspect of the shin. Finger clubbing is present in most patients and is usually gross. X-rays of the painful bone shows subperiosteal new bone formation. HPOA is most frequently associated with bronchial carcinoma but can occur with other tumours and has been described in association with cystic fibrosis.

Digital clubbing and hypertrophic pulmonary osteoarthropathy are examples of non-metastatic extrapulmonary manifestations of bronchial carcinoma.

Paraneoplastic syndromes associated with bronchial carcinoma

These are listed in the information box below.

NON-METASTATIC EXTRA-PULMONARY MANIFESTATIONS OF BRONCHIAL CARCINOMA

Endocrine
Inappropriate secretion of antidiuretic hormone (ADH)
Ectopic ACTH secretion
Hypercalcaemia
Carcinoid syndrome
Gynaecomastia

Neurological
Polyneuropathy
Myelopathy
Cerebellar degeneration

Other
Digital clubbing
Hypertrophic pulmonary osteoarthropathy
Nephrotic syndrome
Myasthenia
Polymyositis and dermatomyositis

Finger clubbing and hypertrophic pulmonary osteoarthropathy can also be regarded as paraneoplastic, or non-metastatic syndromes. Two of the endocrine syndromes, inappropriate ADH secretion and ectopic ACTH secretion (p. 644) are associated with small cell carcinoma. Hypercalcaemia is usually caused by a squamous carcinoma. Associated neurological syndromes (p. 903) may occur with any type of bronchial carcinoma but perhaps most often with small cell tumours.

Physical signs in the chest

Examination is usually normal unless significant bronchial obstruction has been produced, or spread to the pleura or mediastinum has taken place. A tumour obstructing a large bronchus produces the physical signs of collapse or occasionally obstructive emphysema. Pulmonary infection beyond an obstructing tumour gives rise to pneumonia that usually responds slowly to treatment; an underlying bronchial carcinoma is suspected from the relative absence of physical signs usually associated with pneumonia (p. 358). Involvement of the pleura produces the physical signs of pleurisy (p. 410) or of pleural effusion (p. 411). Occasionally a massive tumour may cause the signs of a large pleural effusion.

Investigation

The conditions which radiological examination can reveal are shown in the information box (right).

Bronchoscopy

Inspection of the intrabronchial portion of the tumour and removal of tissue for pathological examination is

---

RADIOLOGICAL EXAMINATION REVEALING PRESENTATIONS OF BRONCHIAL CARCINOMA

Unilateral hilar enlargement
Central tumour. Hilar glandular involvement. Peripheral tumour in apical segment of a lower lobe can look like an enlarged hilar shadow on the straight X-ray

Peripheral pulmonary opacity
Usually irregular but well circumscribed. May have irregular cavitation within it. Can be very large (Fig. 9.15A, B)

Lung, lobe or segmental collapse
Usually caused by tumour within the bronchus causing occlusion. Whole lung collapse can be produced by compression of main bronchus by enlarged lymph glands

Pleural effusion
Usually indicates tumour invasion of pleural space; very rarely a manifestation of infection in collapsed lung tissue distal to a bronchial carcinoma

Broadening of mediastinum, enlarged cardiac shadow, elevation of a hemidiaphragm
Manifestations of mediastinal invasion. If a raised hemidiaphragm is caused by phrenic nerve palsy screening will show it to move paradoxically upwards when patient sniffs

Rib destruction
Direct invasion of the chest wall or blood-borne metastatic spread can cause osteolytic lesions of the ribs

---

possible in about two-thirds of patients. If abnormal tissue is not visible at bronchoscopy bronchial washings can be taken from the lung segment in which the tumour is shown to be on radiological examination.

Cytology

Cytological examination of sputum, bronchial brushings or bronchial washings for malignant cells is a valuable diagnostic measure. Percutaneous needle aspiration biopsy under screening is a useful method of obtaining a positive cytological diagnosis in peripheral tumours. The diagnosis can often be confirmed by needle aspiration when metastatic spread has occurred to lymph nodes, skin or liver.

Other investigations

Scalene node biopsy, mediastinoscopy or pleural biopsy may be required in some patients. CT scanning of the thorax, barium swallow, ultrasound examination of the liver, radionuclide bone scanning and examination of bone marrow trephine biopsies may be used in the 'staging' of bronchial carcinoma (p. 237).

Management

Curative treatment is almost exclusively achieved by surgical resection. Unfortunately the majority of

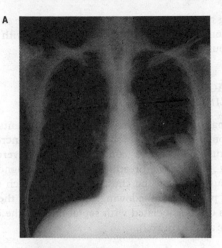

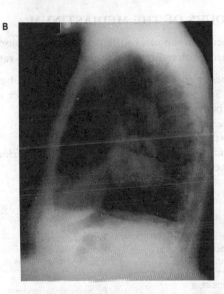

Fig. 9.15   Large cavitated bronchial carcinoma. A. Posterior-anterior (PA) view **B.** Lateral view of A showing tumour in the right lower zone.

patients present with evidence of tumour spread at the time of diagnosis and can only be offered palliative therapy. Radiotherapy, and in some cases chemotherapy, can relieve distressing symptoms.

Surgical treatment
Regrettably, few patients are suitable for surgery. Even if after investigation the tumour appears to be localised to the lung the results of surgical resection are poor in undifferentiated and poorly differentiated tumours. By contrast the five-year survival rate after resection of squamous carcinoma can be as high as 50%.

Staging of the tumour (p. 237) is essential prior to surgical resection and it is also important to assess pulmonary function because many patients have poor function from associated chronic bronchitis. These patients have a high risk of post-operative complications and surgical resection is usually not considered (if their pulmonary function is very poor).

Radiotherapy
Radiotherapy is much less effective than surgery in the curative treatment of bronchial carcinoma. It is of greatest value in the palliation of distressing complications such as superior vena caval obstruction, recurrent haemoptysis and pain caused by chest wall invasion or by skeletal metastatic deposits. Obstruction of the trachea and main bronchi can also be relieved temporarily by radiotherapy. Undifferentiated tumours (e.g. small cell) or poorly differentiated tumours are usually more susceptible to radiotherapy than well differentiated tumours especially adenocarcinoma. Radiotherapy is used in conjunction with chemotherapy in the treatment of small cell carcinoma.

Chemotherapy
The treatment of small cell carcinoma with combinations of cytotoxic drugs, sometimes in combination with radiotherapy, can increase the median survival of patients with this highly malignant type of bronchial carcinoma from 3 months to well over a year. Different combinations of chemotherapeutic agents, adjuvant therapy and radiotherapy have and are being assessed in order to improve the prognosis of patients with small cell lung cancer. The combination of vindesine and etoposide (vindesine $3 \, mg/m^2$ (maximum $5 \, mg$) by bolus i.v. on day 1 and etoposide $120 \, mg/m^2$ by i.v. on days 2 and 3 is a widely used regimen; 6 pulses of this treatment at 3-week intervals) has minimal toxicity except for alopecia and is effective in 50% or more of patients. Many combinations of chemotherapeutic agents have been used in the past for more aggressive treatment of this disease. The combination of doxorubicin hydrochloride, cyclophosphamide and etoposide is probably as effective as any other combination.

The use of combinations of chemotherapeutic drugs requires considerable medical skill and expertise and it is recommended that such treatment should only be given under the supervision of clinicians experienced in such treatment. In general, chemotherapy has very little effect on non-small cell bronchial cancers.

Laser therapy
Laser treatment via a fibreoptic bronchoscope is essentially palliative, the aim being to destroy tumour

tissue occluding major airways to allow re-aeration of collapsed lung. The best results are achieved in tumours of the main bronchus.

Prognosis

The overall prognosis in bronchial carcinoma is very poor. Less than 10% of patients survive five years after diagnosis. The best prognosis is with well-differentiated squamous tumours which have not met-astasised and are amenable to surgical treatment.

BRONCHIAL ADENOMA

This is an uncommon tumour occurring in a younger age group than carcinoma and affecting equally females and males. Although classified as a benign tumour it possesses some of the properties of a malignant growth and may eventually metastasise. There are two histo-logical types of bronchial adenoma, the relatively more common bronchial carcinoid and the rare cylindroma (adenoid cystic carcinoma) which often arises at the tracheal bifurcation.

Clinical features

A bronchial adenoma may produce symptoms over several years. Recurrent haemoptysis due to the vas-cularity of tumour is common as is recurrent broncho-pulmonary infection distal to bronchial obstruction caused by the adenoma. Very rarely, and usually when metastatic spread has occurred, the bronchial adenoma may give rise to the carcinoid syndrome (p. 458). The physical signs are usually those of collapse. The tumour may be suspected if the patient is young and symptoms have been present over a prolonged period; but con-firmation of the diagnosis can only be made by broncho-scopy, biopsy and histology.

Management

Treatment is by resection of the pulmonary lobe or segment containing the tumour along with the bronchus from which it arises. Occasionally when surgical resection is not possible local removal of tumour tissue from the bronchial lumen or laser therapy may be an alternative.

SECONDARY TUMOURS OF THE LUNG

Blood-borne metastatic deposits in the lungs may be derived from many primary tumours (p. 398). The secondary deposits are usually multiple and bilateral. Often there are no respiratory symptoms and the diag-nosis is made by radiological examination. Breathless-ness may be the only symptom if a considerable amount

of lung tissue has been replaced by metastatic tumour. Occasionally haemoptysis occurs in patients with meta-static pulmonary malignant disease.

PULMONARY LYMPHATIC CARCINOMATOSIS

Lymphatic infiltration may develop in patients with carcinoma of the breast, stomach, bowel, pancreas or bronchus. This grave condition causes severe and rapidly progressive breathlessness. The diagnosis is often suggested by the chest radiograph which shows diffuse pulmonary shadowing radiating from the hilar regions often associated with septal lines in the costo-phrenic angles (p. 262).

TUMOURS OF THE MEDIASTINUM

The mediastinum can be divided into four major com-partments with reference to the lateral chest X-ray:

1. *Superior mediastinum* – above a line drawn between the 5th dorsal vertebral body and the upper end of the body of the sternum
2. *Anterior mediastinum* – in front of the heart
3. *Posterior mediastinum* – behind the heart
4. *Middle mediastinum* – between the anterior and posterior compartments.

COMMON MEDIASTINAL MASSES

Superior mediastinum
Retrosternal goitre
Vascular lesions:
    Persistent left superior
    vena cava
    Prominent left subclavian
    artery
Thymic tumours
Dermoid cysts
Lymphomas
Aortic aneurysm

Anterior mediastinum
Retrosternal goitre
Dermoid cysts
Thymic tumours
Lymphomas
Aortic aneurysm

Pericardial cysts
Hernias through the
diaphragmatic foramen of
Morgagni

Posterior mediastinum
Neurogenic tumours
Paravertebral abscesses
Oesophageal lesions
Aortic aneurysm
Foregut duplications

Middle mediastinum
Bronchial carcinoma
Lymphomas
Sarcoidosis
Bronchogenic cysts
Hiatus hernias

BENIGN TUMOURS AND CYSTS

The conditions in this category include intrathoracic goitre, vascular lesions, benign thymic tumours, dermoid cysts, pericardial cysts, diaphragmatic hernias, neurogenic tumours and developmental cysts. These may compress but do not invade vital structures. The diagnosis is usually made by chance when radiological examination of the chest is undertaken for some other reason. The tumour may cause dyspnoea by compression of lung tissue or occasionally by narrowing of the trachea if it becomes very large. A benign tumour in the upper part of the thorax occasionally compresses the superior vena cava. A dermoid cyst very occasionally ruptures into a bronchus.

MALIGNANT TUMOURS

Included in this category are mediastinal lymph node metastases, lymphomas, leukaemia, malignant thymic tumours and mediastinal sarcoma. Aortic and innominate aneurysms have destructive features resembling those of malignant mediastinal tumours. All these conditions, except lymph node malignancies, are uncommon. The distinguishing feature of this group of tumours is their power to invade as well as to compress mediastinal structures, bronchi and lungs. As a result even a small malignant tumour can produce symptoms although as a rule the tumour has attained a considerable size before this happens. The structures which may be invaded or compressed and the symptoms and signs produced in each case are outlined in the information box below.

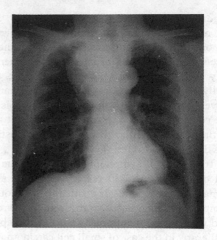

Fig. 9.16   Large mass extending from right upper mediastinum— intrathoracic goitre.

SYMPTOMS AND SIGNS PRODUCED BY MALIGNANT INVASION OF THE STRUCTURES OF THE MEDIASTINUM
Trachea and main bronchi   Stridor, breathlessness, paroxysmal cough, pulmonary collapse
Oesophagus   Dysphagia, oesophageal displacement or obstruction on barium swallow examination
Phrenic nerve   Diaphragmatic paralysis
Left recurrent laryngeal nerve   Paralysis of left vocal cord giving rise to hoarseness and bovine cough
Sympathetic trunk   Horner's syndrome
Superior vena cava   Superior vena caval obstruction (p. 399)
Pericardium   Pericarditis and/or pericardial effusion

Investigation

Radiological examination

A benign mediastinal tumour generally appears as a sharply circumscribed opacity situated mainly in the mediastinum but often encroaching on one or both lung fields (Fig. 9.16). A malignant mediastinal tumour seldom has a clearly defined margin and often presents as a general broadening of the mediastinal shadow. Fluoroscopic examination of the hemidiaphragms and oesophagus (barium swallow) should be undertaken in all suspected cases of mediastinal tumour.

CT scanning

CT scanning of the thorax is a useful investigation for mediastinal tumours and has virtually replaced conventional tomography in the investigation of these lesions.

Bronchoscopy

Bronchoscopy should be carried out in most patients because bronchial carcinoma is such a common primary cause of mediastinal tumour.

Mediastinoscopy

If enlarged lymph nodes are suspected in the anterior mediastinum tissue from these nodes can be removed for histological examination by this technique.

Surgical exploration

An exact diagnosis cannot be made in some patients without surgical exploration of the chest and removal for histological examination of part or all of the tumour.

Management

Benign mediastinal tumours should be removed surgically once they are discovered because they will produce symptoms sooner or later. Some of them, particularly cysts, may become infected while others, especially neural tumours, may become malignant. The operative mortality is low providing there is not a relative contra-indication to surgical treatment such as co-existing cardiovascular disease, chronic obstructive airways disease or extreme age.

The treatment of lymphoma and leukaemia is described on p. 741 and 730 respectively. A malignant thymoma usually responds dramatically to radiotherapy and lymph node metastases from bronchial carcinoma respond well though temporarily to radiotherapy or to chemotherapy in the case of small cell carcinoma. Complications such as superior vena caval obstruction and tracheal obstruction can also be treated with radiotherapy or a combination of radiotherapy and chemotherapy.

PULMONARY FIBROSIS AND RELATED DISEASES

The three main types of pulmonary fibrosis are shown in the information box below.

TYPES OF PULMONARY FIBROSIS

Replacement fibrosis
Replacement of lung by destructive processes such as pulmonary suppuration or infarction. TB a common cause. Often associated with bronchiectasis

Focal fibrosis
Reaction to inhaled solid inanimate particles – pneumoconiosis

Interstitial fibrosis
Diffuse – end result of the interstitial lung diseases

If pulmonary fibrosis is extensive it will cause exertional breathlessness and hypoxaemia, and this is more likely to occur in focal and interstitial fibrosis than in replacement fibrosis. On the other hand the physical signs and radiological changes will usually be more conspicuous in replacement fibrosis which generally produces gross localised abnormalities.

INTERSTITIAL LUNG DISEASE

This term is applied to a group of pulmonary diseases which have the following features in common:

1. thickening of alveolar walls by oedema, cellular exudate or fibrosis;
2. increased stiffness of the lungs (reduced compliance), associated with exertional breathlessness;
3. maldistribution of pulmonary ventilation and perfusion and a gas transfer defect leading to hypoxaemia (particularly on exercise), hyperventilation and hypocapnia.

Aetiology

Interstitial lung disease is caused by several different pathological processes which all give rise to similar symptoms, physical signs, radiological changes and disturbances of pulmonary function. They are thus worthy of collective consideration. The information box below contains some causes of interstitial lung disease.

CAUSES OF INTERSTITIAL LUNG DISEASE

- Chronic pulmonary oedema e.g. secondary to mitral valve disease
- Extrinsic allergic alveolitis
- Cryptogenic fibrosing alveolitis and fibrosing alveolitis associated with connective tissue disorders
- Pulmonary damage following radiotherapy to the lungs
- Drugs, e.g. bleomycin (p. 242), busulphan (p. 735), methotrexate (p. 239), amiodarone (p. 275), gold (p. 775), nitrofurantoin (p. 579), paraquat
- Sarcoidosis (p. 409)
- Asbestosis (p. 408)
- Idiopathic pulmonary haemosiderosis

FIBROSING ALVEOLITIS

Fibrosing alveolitis exemplifies many of the typical features of interstitial lung disease. It may be a manifestation of one of the connective tissue disorders such as rheumatoid disease or it may occur as an isolated pulmonary abnormality (cryptogenic fibrosing alveolitis).

Cryptogenic fibrosing alveolitis is probably not a single disease entity but a group of diseases with similar pathological changes. Pathologically, cryptogenic fibrosing alveolitis is characterised by cellular infiltration and thickening of alveolar walls in the presence of large mononuclear cells in alveolar spaces. There is a variable degree of fibrosis and in most cases progressive fibrosis occurs. It is known that, whatever the cause, alveolar macrophages and neutrophils are 'activated' and produce cellular chemotactic and activating factors. It has been suggested that the release of oxidants from neutrophils, and to a lesser extent eosinophils and alveolar macrophages, is one of the mechanisms of tissue injury. Alveolar macrophages are probably involved in the production of fibrosis by their release of fibronectin and alveolar macrophage-derived growth factors.

Clinical features

Progressive exertional breathlessness is usually the presenting symptom often accompanied by persistent dry cough. In most patients there is gross clubbing of the fingers and toes. Chest expansion is poor but hyperventilation is usually a striking feature. Numerous bilateral end-inspiratory crepitations (crackles) are audible on auscultation particularly over the lower zones posteriorly.

Radiological examination

The chest X-ray shows diffuse pulmonary opacities which are usually most obvious in the lower zones. The hemidiaphragms are high and the lungs appear small. In advanced disease the chest X-rays may show 'honeycomb lung' in which diffuse pulmonary shadowing is interspersed with small cystic translucencies. 'Honeycomb lung' is also a characteristic feature of rare diseases such as histiocytosis X and tuberous sclerosis (Fig. 9.17).

Pulmonary function tests

These show a restrictive ventilatory defect with proportionate reduction in FEV_1 and VC (p. 349). The carbon monoxide transfer factor is low and there is an overall reduction in lung volume. In early disease there is arterial hypoxaemia on exercise; later arterial hypoxaemia and hypocapnia are present at rest.

Bronchoalveolar lavage and lung biopsy

Bronchoalveolar lavage fluid usually contains increased numbers of neutrophils and eosinophils. Transbronchial biopsy is often of no help because the small size of the biopsy specimens does not allow the pathologist to differentiate between fibrosing alveolitis and other forms of pulmonary fibrosis. Open lung biopsy is rarely necessary except in a few patients with atypical X-ray changes.

Diagnosis

The diagnosis can usually be made with confidence from the history, clinical findings, chest X-ray, pulmonary function test abnormalities and in some cases the bronchoalveolar lavage fluid cell counts. Serological tests for antinuclear and rheumatoid factors may be positive even in patients without evidence of a connective tissue disorder.

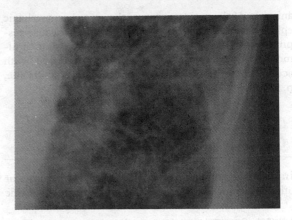

Fig. 9.17   Honeycomb lung.

Management

Treatment with corticosteroids is effective in about 30% of patients but is of little value or no value in the remainder, few of whom survive for more than five years. A trial of prednisolone is indicated in most patients with progressive disease and should be given in a daily dose of 40–60 mg for 6–8 weeks. Assessment of response to this treatment is by repeat measurement of lung volumes, transfer factor and chest X-ray. Prednisolone should be withdrawn rapidly over a few weeks if there is no response. Should objective evidence of improvement be demonstrated the dose can be reduced gradually to a maintenance dose of 10 or 12.5 mg daily. In patients in whom it is not possible to reduce the dose of prednisolone below 15 or 20 mg daily without evidence of relapse, azathioprine in a dose of 1.5–2 mg/kg daily should be added in an attempt to reduce the dose of prednisolone to levels which are less likely to give side-effects.

Prognosis

The rate of progression of pulmonary changes varies considerably from death within a few months to survival with minimal symptoms for many years. Occasionally the disease process may 'burn out', but in the majority of patients the disease is progressive, even in those who have responded to treatment. Single lung transplantation may improve the outlook for some patients.

IDIOPATHIC PULMONARY HAEMOSIDEROSIS

This is a rare disease of unknown cause in which spontaneous haemorrhage into the lungs causes recurrent episodes of pyrexia, haemoptysis and iron-deficiency anaemia. If the patient survives the acute haemorrhagic episodes, interstitial fibrosis may eventually cause respiratory failure and pulmonary hypertension. Pulmonary haemorrhage may also be associated with acute glomerulonephritis (Goodpasture's syndrome, p. 570).

OCCUPATIONAL LUNG DISEASE

In certain occupations the inhalation of dusts, fumes or other noxious substances may give rise to specific pathological changes in the lungs. The nature of each substance, the occupation in which the hazard occurs, the description of each disease and the pathological changes produced in the lungs are summarised in Table 9.21.

The injurious substances can be broadly divided into three main groups which are summarised in Table 9.22

It is important to take a detailed occupational history, past as well as present, because a diagnosis of occupational lung disease can be easily overlooked and the patients may be eligible for compensation. It must be emphasised that in many types of pneumoconiosis a long period of exposure to dust is required before radio-

Table 9.21   Causes and effects of occupational lung disease

Cause	Occupation	Description of disease	Characteristic features
Mineral dusts:			
Coal dust	Coal mining	Coal-worker's pneumoconiosis	
Silica	Gold mining	Silicosis	Focal and interstitial fibrosis
	Iron and steel industries		Centrilobular emphysema
	Metal grinding		Progressive massive fibrosis
	Stone dressing		
	Pottery		
Asbestos	Manufacture of fireproof and insulating materials	Asbestos-related disease	Asbestos bodies
	Shipbreaking		Interstitial fibrosis
			Pleural plaques and effusion
			Bronchial carcinoma
			Pleural mesothelioma
Iron oxide	Arc welding	Siderosis	Mineral deposition only
Tin dioxide	Tin ore mining	Stannosis	
Beryllium	Aircraft and atomic energy industries	Berylliosis	Granulomata
			Interstitial fibrosis
Organic dusts:			
Cotton, flax or hemp dust	Textile industries	Byssinosis	Acute bronchiolitis
			Bronchoconstriction
Fungal spores from mouldy hay, straw or grain, mushroom compost, bagasse, etc.	Agriculture and related industries	Farmer's lung	Extrinsic allergic alveolitis
		Maltworker's lung	
		Mushroom worker's lung	
		Bagassosis	
Gases and fumes:			
Irritant gases (ammonia, chlorine, phosgene, sulphur and nitrogen dioxide)	Various industries (accidental exposure)		Acute pulmonary oedema
Cadmium	Welding and electroplating		Chronic bronchitis and emphysema
Isocyanates, e.g. toluene diisocyanate	Manufacture of plastic foam, paints and adhesives		Bronchial asthma
	Paint-spraying of vehicles in motor industry		Eosinophilic pneumonia
			Alveolitis
Platinum salts	Platinum refining		Bronchial asthma
	Laboratory work involving platinum compounds		
Acid anhydride and amine hardening agents (including epoxy resin curing agents)	Manufacture of epoxy resins		Bronchial asthma
	Manufacture of adhesives		
	Moulding of resins and plastics		
Rosin (colophony) used in soldering fluxes	Electronics industry		Bronchial asthma
Biological substances:			
Proteolytic enzymes, e.g. *Bacillus subtilis*, pancreatic extracts, papain	Detergent manufacturing		Bronchial asthma
	Pharmaceutical industry		
	Food processing		
Animal and insect excreta	Animal laboratories		Bronchial asthma
	Farming		
	Flour milling		
Grain dust contaminated by mites and fungal spores	Combine harvesting		Bronchial asthma
	Handling of stored grain		

Table 9.22   Injurious substances in the principal bronchopulmonary disorders

Substances	Disorders
Gases and fumes	Airways obstruction; emphysema; pulmonary oedema
Mineral dusts	Pneumoconiosis; bronchial carcinoma; mesothelioma
Organic dusts	Allergic alveolitis; airways obstruction

logical changes appear which may precede symptoms for several years. Notes on diagnosis and claims for benefits in pneumoconiosis, occupational asthma and other related occupational diseases in Britain are contained in Government pamphlets (p. 416). New industrial processes are constantly being introduced and it is necessary to remain alert to the possibility that they may be associated with new occupational lung diseases.

DISEASES CAUSED BY MINERAL DUSTS (PNEUMOCONIOSIS)

Aetiology

The dust particles, after inhalation, are conveyed by macrophages from the bronchial mucosa to minute foci of lymphoid tissue throughout the lungs. There the irritation produced by solution of the particles in tissue fluid may initiate widespread pulmonary fibrosis. The fibrogenic capacities of mineral dusts vary, silica being markedly fibrogenic whereas iron is almost inert. The most important types of pneumoconiosis are coalworkers pneumoconiosis, silicosis and asbestosis.

COALWORKERS PNEUMOCONIOSIS

The disease follows prolonged inhalation of coal dust. The condition is subdivided into simple pneumoconiosis and progressive massive fibrosis for clinical purposes and for certification. It must be emphasised that for certification purposes in Britain the diagnosis rests at present on radiological and not clinical features.

Simple coalworkers pneumoconiosis

This is categorised radiologically into three grades, depending on the size and extent of the nodulation present. It does not progress if the miner leaves the industry.

Progressive massive fibrosis

In this form of the disease, large dense masses, single or multiple, occur mainly in the upper lobes. These may be irregular in shape and may cavitate. Tuberculosis may be a complication. The disease can be disabling,

may shorten life-expectancy and progress even after the miner leaves the industry.

Cough and sputum from associated chronic bronchitis are frequently present. The sputum may be black (melanoptysis). Progressive breathlessness on exertion occurs in the later stages and respiratory and right ventricular failure supervene as terminal events. There may be no abnormal physical signs in the chest but where present they are those of chronic obstructive airways disease.

Antinuclear factor is present in the serum of about 15% of patients with coalworkers pneumoconiosis. Rheumatoid factor is present in some patients in whom rheumatoid arthritis coexists with rounded fibrotic nodules 0.5–5 cm in diameter. These are mainly in the periphery of the lung fields and the association is known as *Caplan's syndrome*. This syndrome may also occur in other types of pneumoconiosis.

SILICOSIS

This disease is becoming rare as the standards of industrial hygiene improve. It is caused by the inhalation of fine free crystalline silicone dioxide (silica) dust or quartz particles. It occurs in the occupations shown in the information box below.

OCCUPATIONS ASSOCIATED WITH SILICOSIS

- Mining – coal, tin, gold, other minerals
- Quarrying
- Dressing of sandstone and granite
- The pottery and ceramics industry
- Manufacture of silica blocks and abrasive soaps
- Iron and steel industries
- Sand-blasting
- Metal grinding
- Boiler scaling

Silica is a most fibrogenic dust and causes the development of hard nodules which coalesce as the disease progresses. Tuberculosis may modify the silicotic process with ensuing caseation and calcification. The radiological features are similar to those seen in coalworkers pneumoconiosis though the changes tend to be more marked in the upper zones. The hilar shadows may be enlarged and 'egg-shell' calcification in the hilar lymph nodes is a distinctive feature but does not occur in all patients. The disease progresses even when exposure to dust ceases. The patient should, therefore, be removed from the offending environment as soon as possible. Clinical features are similar to those of coalworkers pneumoconiosis.

ASBESTOS-RELATED DISEASES OF THE LUNGS AND PLEURA

The main types of the fibrous mineral, asbestos, are chrysotile (white asbestos), which accounts for 90% of the world's production, crocidolite (blue asbestos) and amosite (brown asbestos). Exposure occurs in the following occupations: mining and milling of the mineral; manufacturing processes involving asbestos, (e.g. pipe lagging and spraying limpet asbestos); demolition and shipyard workers, including those who may work alongside them, e.g. joiners, painters and electricians.

Four forms of disease related to inhalation of asbestos are recognised and are given in the information box below.

PLEURO-PULMONARY DISORDERS CAUSED BY INHALATION OF ASBESTOS

- Benign pleural plaques
- Benign pleural effusion
- Progressive pulmonary fibrosis (asbestosis)
- Malignant disease of the pleura (mesothelioma)

Of these only asbestosis and mesothelioma qualify for industrial injury benefit in Britain.

Benign pleural plaques
These areas of pleural thickening do not produce clinical symptoms and are usually identified on routine chest X-ray. They are often calcified and in the early stage are best seen on oblique films. They are most commonly observed on the diaphragm and anterolateral pleural surfaces.

Benign pleural effusion
This is considered to be a specific asbestos-related entity and may be associated with pleural pain, fever and leucocytosis. The pleural liquid may be blood-stained and differentiation of this benign condition from a malignant effusion caused by mesothelioma can be difficult. The disease is self-limiting but may cause considerable pleural fibrosis which sometimes leads to breathlessness.

Asbestosis
Pulmonary fibrosis caused by the inhalation of asbestos fibres is characterised by increasing exertion/breathlessness. Finger clubbing is usually present and end-inspiratory crepitations (crackles) are audible over the lower zones of both lungs.

The radiological changes are usually confined to the lower two-thirds of the lung fields and comprise mottled shadows with some streaky opacities and sometimes 'honeycombing'. The cardiac silhouette often appears 'shaggy'.

The most important physiological abnormalities are a reduced carbon monoxide transfer factor, decreased lung volumes and a restrictive ventilatory defect.

Respiratory and right ventricular failure eventually supervene. The incidence of bronchial carcinoma is much increased, and is at least ten fold in persons suffering from asbestosis who also smoke.

The diagnosis is usually easy to establish from the history of exposure to asbestos, the clinical features of end-inspiratory crepitations and finger clubbing, the pulmonary function test abnormalities and the chest X-ray which also often show pleural plaques. Open lung biopsy may be required to confirm the diagnosis but is not without risk and should not be undertaken solely for the purposes of allowing patients to claim benefit.

Mesothelioma of the pleura
This malignant tumour of the pleura is usually caused by exposure to asbestos which may be trivial. Blue asbestos is thought to be the most potent cause of mesothelioma. Clinical presentation is frequently with chest pain. A pleural effusion, often blood-stained, may develop and cause breathlessness. A diagnosis can be confirmed histologically by pleural biopsy in some patients, but tumour masses may later develop in the chest wall at the site of the biopsy. Thoracotomy is seldom justified as a diagnostic procedure in patients with suspected mesothelioma. There is no curative treatment and chest wall pain is often difficult to control.

Management
No specific treatment is available. In the later stages treatment is required for associated conditions such as chronic bronchitis and respiratory failure, pulmonary tuberculosis or malignant pleural effusions.

Prevention
Improvements of standards of industrial hygiene are now enforced by law in many countries; such measures as wearing respirators, damping dust and efficient ventilation systems are already proving effective in a number of industries.

DISEASES CAUSED BY ORGANIC DUSTS

BYSSINOSIS

In byssinosis the initial lesion is an acute bronchiolitis

associated with symptoms and signs of generalised airflow obstruction which tend to be worse after the weekend break ('Monday fever'), but eventually become continuous. There is no radiological abnormality. Recovery usually follows removal from exposure to the dust hazard. Smokers have a greater incidence of byssinosis than non-smokers and smoking should be discouraged in all workers at risk. In chronic disease the treatment is similar to that for patients with chronic obstructive bronchitis (p. 393).

HUMIDIFIER FEVER

Humidifier fever is a disease with a similar pattern of symptoms to byssinosis because fever and breathlessness may be a problem at the beginning of the week but subside towards the weekend. It is thought to be caused by water-borne microorganisms including amoebae from contaminated humidifiers in air conditioning systems.

Other diseases caused by organic dusts are forms of asthma or extrinsic allergic alveolitis, described on pages 377 and 384.

SARCOIDOSIS

Sarcoidosis is a multi-system granulomatous disease. It is associated with imbalance between subsets of T lymphocytes and other disturbances of cell-mediated immunity, but the relationship between these phenomena and sarcoidosis has not been explained. The lesions are histologically similar to tuberculous follicles apart from absence of caseation and tubercle bacilli, but there is no convincing evidence that the disease is caused by any of the mycobacteria. Chronic beryllium poisoning produces a disease which mimics sarcoidosis both pathologically and clinically but exposure to beryllium is now extremely uncommon and such cases are rare. Histological changes resembling those of sarcoidosis are occasionally seen in individual organs, such as lymph nodes, in conditions such as carcinoma and fungal infections, but these localised 'sarcoid reactions' are not associated with systemic sarcoidosis.

Pathology

The mediastinal and superficial lymph nodes, lungs, liver, spleen, skin, eyes, parotid glands and phalangeal bones are most frequently involved. The characteristic histological feature consists of non-caseating epitheloid follicles which usually resolve spontaneously, but in some patients, the production of fibrous tissue is stimulated which may have grave effects on local structure and function. Sarcoidosis is seldom fatal and then only when it affects vital organs such as the lungs, the heart or the central nervous system. Calcium metabolism may be disturbed causing hypercalcaemia and, rarely, nephrocalcinosis and renal failure.

Clinical features

Sarcoidosis may present in a subacute or chronic form. The three stages of pulmonary changes and extra-pulmonary manifestations are shown in the information boxes below and on page 410.

PULMONARY CHANGES IN SARCOIDOSIS

Stage I
X-ray shows bilateral hilar enlargement, usually symmetrical; paratracheal nodes often enlarged

Spontaneous resolution usually within one year in majority of cases. Often asymptomatic, but may be associated with erythema nodosum and arthralgia

Stage II
X-ray shows a combination of hilar glandular enlargement and pulmonary opacities which are often diffuse, but not always

Patients usually asymptomatic. Spontaneous improvement occurs in majority

Stage III
X-ray shows diffuse pulmonary shadows without evidence of hilar adenopathy. Evidence of pulmonary fibrosis may be present or develop.

Disease less likely to resolve spontaneously. Pulmonary fibrosis can cause breathlessness, pulmonary hypertension and cor pulmonale

---

Investigations

Skin sensitivity to tuberculin is depressed or absent in most patients, and the Mantoux reaction is, therefore, a useful 'screening' test; a strongly positive reaction to one TU virtually excludes sarcoidosis. Although the diagnosis can often be made with a fair measure of confidence from the clinical and radiological features and the tuberculin test it should, if possible, be confirmed histologically by biopsy of a superficial lymph node or of a skin lesion when these are present. Transbronchial lung biopsy frequently confirms the diagnosis. Bronchoalveolar lavage usually yields fluid with an increased proportion of lymphocytes.

The Kveim test is also a helpful diagnostic procedure provided a potent antigen can be obtained from human sarcoid tissue. The antigen (0.1 ml) is injected intra-

---

EXTRA-PULMONARY MANIFESTATIONS OF SARCOIDOSIS

Eyes
Phlyctenular conjuctivitis; uveitis; iridocyclitis; lacrimal gland involvement

Skin
Erythema nodosum, cutaneous 'sarcoïds' (skin papules), infiltration of scars; lupus pernio – red/blue infiltration of nose, cheeks and ear lobes.

Salivary glands
Parotid gland enlargement. Can cause facial palsy. May be associated with eye involvement and fever ('uveoparotid fever')

Heart
Myocarditis; conduction defects

Kidneys
Nephrocalcinosis

Liver and spleen
Enlargement caused by granulomatous infiltration. Usually asymptomatic. Hypersplenism rarely

Nervous system
Cerebral, meningeal, cranial and peripheral nerve involvement

Bones and joints
Arthralgia; arthritis; phalangeal cysts

---

dermally and a small nodule develops about four weeks later when the test is positive, biopsy of which reveals typical sarcoid follicles. The development of a positive Kveim test is suppressed by corticosteroid therapy.

There is also an elevation of the plasma level of angiotensin-converting enzyme which although not specific for sarcoidosis may be valuable in the assessment of disease activity and response to treatment.

In Stage 3 sarcoidosis assessment of disease progression is by repeated measurement of lung volumes, carbon monoxide transfer factor and serial chest radiographs.

Management
Stage 1 and Stage 2 usually resolve spontaneously and treatment is seldom required but occasionally patients with persistent erythema nodosum, pyrexia and arthralgia, or iridocyclitis require oral corticosteroid therapy for a short period.

Stage 3 pulmonary sarcoidosis and sarcoidosis involving the eyes or other vital organs usually needs to be treated with corticosteroids which may have to be continued for several years. Sarcoidosis usually responds rapidly to prednisolone 20–40 mg daily for 4 weeks; thereafter the disease is usually suppressed by a maintenance dose of 7.5–10 mg daily, or 20 mg daily on alternate days.

DISEASES OF THE PLEURA AND CHEST WALL

PLEURISY

Pleurisy is not a diagnosis but simply the term used to describe the result of any disease process involving the pleura and giving rise to pleuritic pain or evidence of pleural friction. It is usually secondary to bacterial infection in the underlying lung but may also occur in association with Coxsackie B a viral infection which primarily involves the intercostal muscles and is known as '*Bornholm disease*'. Pleurisy is a common feature of pulmonary infarction and may be an early manifestation of pleural invasion in pulmonary tuberculosis or by a pulmonary tumour.

Clinical features
Pleural pain is the characteristic symptom. On examination rib movement is restricted and the breath sounds may be diminished on the affected side. A pleural rub is present in many cases particularly when the patient takes a deep breath. It is not heard when the breath is held except near the pericardium where a so-called pleuropericardial rub may be present. The other clinical features depend upon the nature of the disease causing the pleurisy. There may be complete clinical recovery or an effusion may develop, depending upon the underlying cause.

Every patient must have a chest X-ray but a normal radiograph does not exclude a pulmonary cause for the pleurisy. A preceding history of a few days of cough, purulent sputum and pyrexia is presumptive evidence of a pulmonary infection which may not have been severe enough to produce a radiographic abnormality or which may have resolved before the chest X-ray was taken.

Management
The primary cause of pleurisy must be treated. The symptomatic treatment of pleural pain is described on p. 359.

PLEURAL EFFUSION

This term is used when serous fluid accumulates in the pleural space. The condition of purulent effusion or empyema is described on p. 412. The passive transudation of fluid into the pleural cavity *hydrothorax* occurs in cardiac failure, nephrotic syndrome, decompensated cirrhosis of the liver and severe malnutrition.

The most common causes of pleural effusion are shown in the information box (p. 411).

COMMON CAUSES OF PLEURAL EFFUSION

- Pneumonia
- Tuberculosis
- Malignant disease
- Pulmonary infarction

Pleural effusion, often bilateral, may also be a manifestation of rheumatoid disease, systemic lupus erythematosus and lymphoma. Inflammatory lesions below the diaphragm including subphrenic abscess, amoebic liver abscess and pancreatitis occasionally produce a pleural effusion. The cause of the majority of pleural effusions can be identified if a careful history is taken and comprehensive clinical examination performed.

Where the cause is obscure a lead may be given by enquiry regarding travel abroad, occupation, for example exposure to asbestos, contact with tuberculosis, or causes of thromboembolism such as oral contraception, recent immobilisation or operation. Detailed investigations as described below may, however, be necessary.

Clinical features

The symptoms and signs of pleurisy often precede the development of effusion but the onset in some patients may be insidious. Breathlessness is the only symptom related to the effusion and the severity depends on the size and rate of accumulation of the fluid. The physical signs in the chest are those of fluid in the pleural space (p. 347).

Investigations

Radiological examination

The chest X-ray shows a dense uniform opacity in the lower and lateral parts of the hemithorax shading off above and medially into translucent lung. Occasionally the fluid is localised below the lower lobe the appearances simulating an elevated hemidiaphragm. A localised opacity is seen when the effusion is loculated, for example, in an interlobar fissure.

Ultrasonography

This investigation is valuable to differentiate between a loculated pleural effusion and pleural tumour and also helps to localise an effusion prior to aspiration and pleural biopsy.

Pleural aspiration and pleural biopsy

Absolute proof that an effusion is present can be obtained only by the aspiration of fluid. Pleural biopsy is

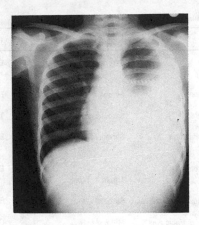

Fig. 9.18   Large left pleural effusion. When chest X-rays are taken in the upright position and there are no pleural adhesions a pleural effusion produces uniformly dense shadowing with a concave upper margin which extends up towards the axilla.

always indicated whenever a diagnostic aspiration of pleural fluid is performed because the chances of obtaining a diagnosis from pleural biopsy material are much greater than by examination of the pleural liquid alone. A pleural biopsy needle should be inserted through an intercostal space at the area of maximum dullness on percussion and at the site of maximum radiological opacity as shown by postero-anterior and lateral films, or at a site determined by ultrasound. At least 50 ml of fluid should be withdrawn, aliquots being placed in separate containers for microbiological examination including culture for tuberculosis, cytological examination and biochemical examination. Whenever there is a strong suspicion of tuberculosis a large volume of pleural liquid should be submitted to the laboratory for examination. Pleural biopsies should be taken after pleural liquid has been aspirated for diagnostic purposes.

The appearance of the fluid is – straw coloured, blood-stained, purulent or chylous. The protein content gives an indication as to whether the effusion is an exudate ($> 30\,g/l$) or a transudate ($< 30\,g/l$). The predominant cell type (neutrophil, eosinophil, lymphocyte, red blood cell) provides useful information, and fluid should always be examined for malignant cells.

There is a high amylase level in effusions secondary to acute pancreatitis and a high concentration of cholesterol in most chronic rheumatoid effusions.

Other investigations

Estimation of the total and differential peripheral blood leucocyte count, a tuberculin test, and examination of

Table 9.23 Pleural effusion: main causes and features

	Appearance of fluid	Type of fluid	Predominant cells in fluid	Other diagnostic features
Tuberculous	Serous, usually amber coloured	Exudate	Lymphocytes (occas. polymorphs)	Positive tuberculin test Isolation of *Myco. tuberculosis* Positive pleural biopsy (80%)
Malignant disease	Serous, often blood-stained	Exudate	Serosal cells and lymphocytes Often clumps of malignant cells	Positive pleural biopsy (40%) Evidence of malignant disease elsewhere
*Cardiac failure	Serous, straw-coloured	Transudate	Few serosal cells	Other evidence of left heart failure Response to diuretics
*Pulmonary infarction	Serous or blood-stained	Exudate	Red blood cells Eosinophils	Contralateral evidence of infarction Source of embolism Factors predisposing to venous thrombosis
*Rheumatoid disease	Serous Turbid if chronic	Exudate	Lymphocytes (occas. polymorphs)	Rheumatoid arthritis Rheumatoid factor in serum Cholesterol in chronic effusion. Low glucose
*Systemic lupus erythematosus	Serous	Exudate	Lymphocytes and serosal cells	Other manifestations of SLE ANF or anti-DNA in serum
Obstruction of thoracic duct	Milky	Chyle	None	Chylomicrons

* Effusion often bilateral.

the sputum for tubercle bacilli and malignant cells should be routine in most situations. A chest X-ray may disclose an underlying pulmonary lesion and indicate its nature. If the lung is obscured by a massive effusion the radiograph should be repeated after a large volume of fluid has been aspirated. Other investigations which may be of help include bronchoscopy, biopsy or aspiration of the scalene lymph node, thoracoscopy and serological tests for antinuclear and rheumatoid factors.

The main diagnostic features and more important causes of pleural effusion are shown in Table 9.23.

Management
Aspiration of pleural fluid may be necessary to relieve breathlessness. It is inadvisable to remove more than 1 litre on the first occasion because pulmonary oedema occasionally follows the aspiration of larger amounts. A pneumothorax, usually hydropneumothorax, may be produced even by a careful operator and a chest radiograph must always be taken after the procedure.

Treatment of the underlying cause, for example, heart failure, pneumonia, pulmonary embolism and subphrenic abscess will often be followed by resolution of the effusion. However certain conditions require special measures as detailed below.

Post-pneumonic pleural effusion
Pleural effusions complicating pneumonia may require aspiration to ensure that an empyema has not developed, and to prevent pleural thickening.

Tuberculous pleural effusion
Patients with tuberculous effusions should always receive antituberculosis chemotherapy (p. 367). Aspiration is required initially if the effusion is large and

causing breathlessness. The addition of prednisolone 20 mg daily by mouth for 4–6 weeks will promote rapid absorption of the fluid and obviate the need for further aspiration and may prevent fibrosis.

Malignant effusions
Effusions caused by malignant infiltration of the pleural surfaces re-accumulate rapidly. To avoid the distress of repeated aspirations, an attempt should be made to obliterate the pleural space (pleurodesis) by the injection of substances into the pleural fluid which produce an inflammatory reaction and extensive pleural adhesions. The agents most frequently used are inactivated *Corynebacterium parvum*, tetracycline and mustine hydrochloride.

EMPYEMA

The term empyema is used to describe the presence of pus in the pleural space. The pus may be as thin as serous fluid or so thick that it is difficult to aspirate even through a wide-bore needle. Microscopically neutrophil leucocytes are present in large numbers. The causative organism may or may not be isolated from the pus. An empyema may involve the whole pleural space or only part of it ('loculated' or 'encysted' empyema) and is almost invariably unilateral.

Aetiology
Empyema is always secondary to infection in a neighbouring structure usually the lung. The principal infections liable to produce empyema are the bacterial pneumonias and tuberculosis. Other causes are infection of a haemothorax and rupture of a subphrenic abscess through the diaphragm. Empyema has become

a relatively rare disease because pulmonary infection can now be so readily controlled by antibacterial therapy.

Pathology

Both layers of pleura are covered with a thick, shaggy inflammatory exudate. The pus in the pleural space is often under considerable pressure and if the condition is not adequately treated there may be rupture into a bronchus from which pus is expectorated, or through an intercostal space with the formation of a sub-cutaneous abscess or sinus. A bronchopleural fistula is produced and a pyopneumothorax is formed when an empyema ruptures into a bronchus.

The only way in which an empyema can heal is by apposition of the visceral and parietal pleural layers with obliteration of the empyema space by organisation of the intervening exudate. This cannot occur unless re-expansion of the collapsed lung is secured at an early stage by removal of all the pus from the pleural space. Re-expansion of the lung cannot take place if:

1. there is delay in treatment or inadequate drainage and the visceral pleura becomes grossly thickened and rigid;
2. the pleural layers are kept apart by air entering the pleura through a bronchopleural fistula;
3. if disease in the lung, such as bronchiectasis, bronchial carcinoma or pulmonary tuberculosis, renders it incapable of re-expansion.

In all these circumstances an empyema tends to become chronic and healing may not take place without recourse to major thoracic surgery.

Clinical features

An empyema should be suspected in patients with pulmonary infection if there is a recurrence of pyrexia despite the continued administration of a suitable anti-biotic. In other cases the illness produced by the primary infective lesion may be so slight that it passes unrecognised and the first definite clinical features are due to the empyema itself.

Once an empyema has developed two separate groups of clinical features are found. These are shown in the information box (right).

Investigation

Radiological examination

The appearances are indistinguishable from those of pleural effusion. When air is present in addition to pus (pyopneumothorax) a horizontal 'fluid level' marks the interface of liquid and air if the film is taken in the erect position.

CLINICAL FEATURES OF EMPYEMA

Systemic features
Pyrexia; usually high and remittent
Rigors, sweating, malaise and weight loss
Polymorphonuclear leucocytosis; usually high

Local features
Pleural pain; breathlessness; cough and sputum usually because of underlying lung disease; copious purulent sputum if empyema ruptures into a bronchus (bronchopleural fistula)

Clinical signs of fluid in the pleural space

Aspiration of pus

This confirms the presence of an empyema. A wide bore needle is inserted through an intercostal space over the area of maximum dullness on percussion. The position of the empyema should have previously been confirmed whenever possible by postero-anterior and lateral radiographs or by ultrasonography.

Bacteriological examination of pus

This may help to determine the cause of the empyema. The pus is frequently sterile in post-pneumonic patients where intensive treatment with antibiotics has been given. The distinction between tuberculous and non-tuberculous disease can usually be made from the radiological changes in the lungs or by the isolation of tubercle bacilli from pus.

Management

Treatment of non-tuberculous empyema

1. *Acute* When the patient is acutely ill and the pus is thin in consistency:
   (a) An intercostal tube should be inserted into the most dependent part of the empyema space and connected to a water seal drain system.
   (b) An antibiotic to which the organism causing the empyema is sensitive should be given.

   An empyema can often be aborted if these measures are started early enough and the organisms are drug-sensitive. If, however, the intercostal tube is not providing adequate drainage, which can happen when the pus thickens and clots, a short segment of rib is resected, the empyema cavity cleared of pus and clot, and a wide-bore tube inserted to allow pro-longed drainage.
2. *Chronic.* If the diagnosis is made before any drainage procedure is carried out it may be feasible to resect the empyema sac *in toto*, provided the patient is fairly fit and the underlying lung is

healthy. 'Decortication' may be required if open drainage has been performed, and re-expansion of the lung is prevented by gross thickening of the visceral pleura. This procedure allows the lung to re-expand and obliterate the pleural space.

Treatment of tuberculous empyema

Antituberculosis chemotherapy must be started immediately and the pus in the pleural space should be aspirated through a wide-bore needle until it ceases to re-accumulate. In many patients no other treatment is necessary but surgery is occasionally required to ablate a residual empyema space.

SPONTANEOUS PNEUMOTHORAX

Aetiology

The two chief causes of spontaneous pneumothorax are:

1. rupture of a subpleural emphysematous bulla or pleural bleb, or of the pulmonary end of a pleural adhesion;
2. rupture of a subpleural tuberculous focus into the pleural space.

The first cause is very much more common in Britain. Other conditions such as staphylococcal lung abscess, pulmonary infarction and bronchial carcinoma rarely give rise to spontaneous pneumothorax.

Pathology

There are three types of spontaneous pneumothorax (Fig. 9.19):

1. *Closed*. The communication between pleura and lung seals off as the lung deflates and does not reopen. The air is gradually absorbed and the lung re-expands (Fig. 9.19A).
2. *Open*. The communication is generally with a bronchus (bronchopleural fistula) and does not seal off when the lung collapses. The air pressure in the pleural space approximates to atmospheric pressure both on inspiration and expiration and the lung cannot re-expand. Moreover the large bronchial communication facilitates the transmission of infection from the air passages into the pleural space and empyema is a common complication. The term 'open' is also applied to a pneumothorax resulting from a penetrating wound of the chest wall (Fig. 9.19B).
3. *Tension (valvular)*. The communication between pleura and lung persists but is small and acts as a one-way valve which allows air to enter the pleural space during inspiration and coughing but prevents

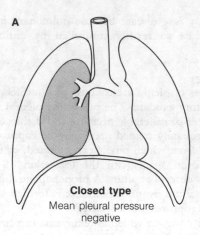

Closed type
Mean pleural pressure
negative

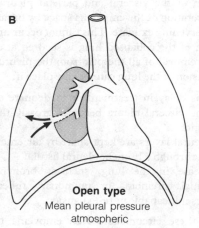

Open type
Mean pleural pressure
atmospheric

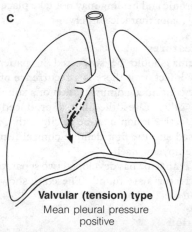

Valvular (tension) type
Mean pleural pressure
positive

Fig. 9.19   Types of spontaneous pneumothorax. A. Closed type. **B.** Open type. **C.** Valvular (tension) type.

it from escaping. Very large amounts of air may be trapped in the pleural space and the intrapleural pressure may rise to well above atmospheric levels. This causes not only compression of the underlying deflated lung but also mediastinal displacement towards the opposite side with consequent compression of the opposite lung (Fig. 9.19C).

Clinical features

The onset is usually sudden, with pain or a feeling of tightness on the affected side of the chest that may be aggravated by deep breathing. The patient becomes increasingly breathless and in severe cases cyanosed. Physical signs in the chest are of air in the pleural space (p. 347) but when the pneumothorax is small and localised there may be no abnormal signs and it may be revealed only by an X-ray.

Closed spontaneous pneumothorax

Breathlessness which is seldom severe gradually abates over the course of a few days. Progressive spontaneous absorption of the air takes place and re-expansion of the lung is complete within two and four weeks depending upon the initial size of the pneumothorax. Pleural infection is uncommon in this type of pneumothorax.

Open spontaneous pneumothorax

This usually follows rupture of an emphysematous bulla, or a small pleural bleb, or a tuberculous cavity, or a lung abscess into the pleural space. The onset is similar to that of the closed type but breathlessness does not improve and, when the cause is tuberculosis or lung abscess, pyrexia and systemic disturbance soon ensue. There are the physical and radiological signs of air and fluid in the pleural space. Acid-fast bacilli can be isolated from the pleural fluid in tuberculosis.

Tension pneumothorax

A tension or valvular pneumothorax produces the most dramatic clinical picture. Breathlessness is rapidly progressive and is accompanied by central cyanosis. Death may occur from asphyxia within a few minutes, but usually the course of events is less rapid and medical attention can be obtained in time to avert a fatal outcome.

Recurrent spontaneous pneumothorax

Recurrence of pneumothorax is not uncommon especially in patients with emphysematous bullae. Subsequent incidents are usually on the same side.

Radiological examination

The chest X-ray shows a sharply defined edge of the deflated lung which may be more easily seen, when the pneumothorax is small, on a film taken in expiration. There is complete translucency between this and the chest wall with no lung markings. The degree of pulmonary deflation varies. Radiographs also show the degree of mediastinal displacement and give information regarding the presence or absence of pleural fluid and underlying pulmonary disease.

Management

Closed spontaneous pneumothorax

The patient is asymptomatic or only has slight breathlessness when the pneumothorax is small and no treatment is required but radiographic observation should be continued until re-expansion of the lung is complete. If the pneumothorax is large and there is breathlessness it is essential to employ more active measures. Rapid and complete re-expansion of the lung is obtained by inserting a catheter into the pleural cavity through an intercostal space and connecting it to a water-seal drainage system or a non-return (Heimlich) valve. In this type of pneumothorax evacuation of air can be attempted using a syringe and needle, a three-way tap and an underwater-seal system.

Specific chemotherapy should be started immediately if a tuberculous aetiology is suspected. The fluid may be drained through the catheter, if a pleural effusion develops, by suitable posturing or aspirated with a needle and syringe.

Open spontaneous pneumothorax

There is a large bronchopleural fistula and pleural infection can rapidly supervene. Such patients are less amenable to medical treatment and the expertise of a thoracic surgeon is often required.

Tension pneumothorax

This constitutes an acute medical emergency. An intercostal catheter is immediately connected to a water-seal drainage system. Symptomatic relief is prompt and dramatic. A wide-bore plastic cannula should be used instead of an intercostal catheter if suitable equipment or medical expertise for this procedure is not immediately available. This should be attached to a length of tubing, the end of which should be placed underwater in a bottle or basin.

Recurrent spontaneous pneumothorax

Recurrent pneumothorax, particularly if bilateral, should be treated by obliteration of at least one pleural space. This can be achieved by introduction of an irritant substance such as kaolin, or by pleural abrasion or parietal pleurectomy at thoracotomy.

DEFORMITIES OF THE CHEST WALL

THORACIC KYPHOSCOLIOSIS

Abnormalities of alignment of the dorsal spine and its consequent effects on thoracic shape may be caused by:

1. congenital abnormality
2. vertebral disease including tuberculosis, osteoporosis and ankylosing spondylitis
3. trauma
4. neuromuscular disease such as poliomyelitis.

Simple kyphosis causes less pulmonary embarrassment than kyphoscoliosis.

Kyphoscoliosis, if severe, restricts and distorts expansion of the chest wall causing maldistribution of the ventilation and blood flow in the lungs. Patients with severe deformity may develop Type II respiratory failure, pulmonary hypertension and right ventricular failure, survival beyond middle age is uncommon. The tempo of deterioration is often accelerated by bacterial infection in the bronchi and lungs.

PECTUS CARINATUM

Pectus carinatum (pigeon chest) is almost always caused by severe asthma during childhood. Very occasionally this deformity can be produced by rickets or occurs without any obvious explanation.

PECTUS EXCAVATUM

In pectus excavatum (funnel chest) the body of the sternum, usually only the lower end, is curved backwards. The heart is displaced to the left and may be compressed between the sternum and the vertebral column but only rarely is there associated disturbance of cardiac function. The deformity may restrict chest expansion and reduce vital capacity. The impairment of cardiac or pulmonary function is seldom sufficient to warrant surgical correction but an operation may be indicated for cosmetic reasons.

FURTHER READING

Brewis R A L, Gibson G J, Geddes D M (eds) 1990 Textbook of Respiratory Medicine. Bailliere Tindall, Eastbourne. A new multi-author reference text

Cotes J E 1979 Lung function: assessment and application in medicine, 4th Edn. Blackwell Scientific Publications, Oxford. A comprehensive review of methods and an excellent source of normal values

Crompton G K 1990 In: Munro J, Edwards C R (eds) Macleod's Clinical Examination, 8th Edn. Churchill Livingstone, Edinburgh. For information about examination of the respiratory system

Department of Health and Social Security NI 238 1982 Clinical notes on occupational asthma: a disease prescribed under the industrial injuries scheme. DHSS, London

Department of Health and Social Security NI 226 1989 Pneumoconiosis and other prescribed respiratory diseases: notes on diagnosis and claims for industrial injuries scheme benefits. DHSS, London

Horne N W 1990 Modern drug treatment in tuberculosis, 7th Edn. Chest, Heart and Stroke Association, London. All the essential information in concise form

James D G, Studdy P R 1981 A colour atlas of respiratory diseases. Wolfe, London. Fine illustrations of a somewhat limited range of conditions

Parkes W R 1990 Occupational lung disorders, 3rd Edn. Butterworth, London. A detailed account which has become a classic

Seaton A, Seaton D, Leitch A G 1990 Crofton and Douglas's Respiratory Diseases, 4th Edn. Blackwell Scientific Publications, Oxford. An established and detailed reference work

Periodicals

American Review of Respiratory Disease. American Thoracic Society, New York. A prestigious journal with excellent 'state of the art' reviews

Thorax. British Medical Association, London. A wide-ranging medical and surgical journal with valuable editorial reviews

10

Diseases of the Alimentary Tract and Pancreas

THE ALIMENTARY TRACT

The alimentary tract is a co-ordinated structure with the function of ingesting and absorbing nutrients and excreting unabsorbed and waste products. It should not be regarded as a series of separate organs, since the role of each component is closely related to that of other parts of the tract.

THE CONTROLLING AND CO-ORDINATING MECHANISMS

Cellular function of the gastrointestinal tract is controlled by chemical messengers which may be hormones, or amino acids or their derivatives, amines or peptides. For example, the secretion of acid by the stomach is stimulated mainly by the release of gastrin and by the vagus nerves, but many other enteric hormones probably have smaller roles to play. A peptide system is an important component of the autonomic nervous system. The nerves contain mediators such as vasoactive intestinal peptide, substance P and encephalins.

MOTILITY

Oesophagus. The upper oesophageal sphincter is formed by the striated cricopharyngeus muscle which exerts constant tone to keep the sphincter closed except during swallowing. Once the upper oesophageal sphincter relaxes, peristalsis sweeps along the length of the body of the oesophagus. The lowest few centimetres of the oesophagus form the lower oesophageal sphincter. This has a high resting tension which prevents reflux of gastric contents into the oesophagus. Normally the sphincter relaxes when the peristaltic wave arrives. The sphincter is controlled by nervous and hormonal mechanisms.

Stomach. The normal tonic contraction of the fundus is inhibited by the arrival of food probably by means of a centrally mediated vagal reflex. The gastric slow wave controls the frequency and direction of antral peristalsis which is responsible for the thorough mixing of the gastric contents and their progressive emptying into the duodenum. Chemoreceptors for fat and acid and osmoreceptors in the duodenal mucosa control gastric emptying by means of local reflexes and the release of secretin, cholecystokinin and other enteric hormones.

Small intestine. Here the co-ordination is due to the slow wave in the interstitial cells of Cajal. It is the pacemaker which dictates the times at which any given segment of the gut can contract. The frequency of the slow wave in the duodenum is greater than in the ileum, thus enabling the proximal bowel to override more distal areas. By this means contractions are co-ordinated both to mix and propel the small bowel content so that all nutrients can be exposed to the absorptive cells. It is thought that the myenteric plexus and the enteric hormones determine the local response to the slow wave so that contraction may or may not occur depending on the state of affairs in the lumen at any one time.

Colon. Two main types of contraction occur which may be associated with two different functions. First, there is segmentation which consists of contraction rings forming and disappearing over long periods: these produce a slow mixing of faeces but no propulsion, thus facilitating the absorption of water and electrolytes. Second, propulsion occurs through 'mass movement,' a peristaltic wave which occurs several times a day. This action carries out the second function of the colon, namely the elimination of faeces. All activity in the colon is increased after eating, and defecation is more likely to occur postprandially. The enteric hormones may be responsible for this activity.

SECRETION

Gastric secretion. The vagus stimulates acid and pepsin secretion by a direct effect on the parietal and peptic cells and it also initiates the release of gastrin from the antrum. More sustained output of this hormone is produced by a rise in pH and by ingested protein. The parietal cell has receptors for gastrin, acetylcholine (vagal stimulation) and for histamine (the H_2-receptor). Each receptor has a secondary messenger system within the parietal cell, but the proton pump H^+ K^+ adenosine triphosphatase is the final common pathway for acid secretion. Mechanisms are also required to turn off gastric secretion once digestion within the stomach is complete. These are largely the same as those which slow gastric emptying, i.e. the release of secretin and other enteric hormones and also the presence of a low pH in the gastric antrum which inhibits the further release of gastrin.

THE ABSORPTIVE SYSTEM (see also p. 444)

The area for absorption in the small intestine is increased several hundredfold by the presence of villi and microvilli. Under normal circumstances nutrients are transported from the absorptive cell by the lymphatic system (e.g. fat and fat-soluble vitamins) or by the portal venous system (e.g. amino acids and hexoses).

DEFENCE MECHANISMS

Cell turnover. The epithelial cells of the gastro-intestinal tract are constantly renewed so that, for example, the epithelial surface of the small intestine is replaced every 48 hours.

Production of mucus. Mucus producing cells are present throughout the gastrointestinal tract and mucus has a protective function. In the stomach, the mucous layer on the surface of the epithelium contains bicarbonate ions which form part of the barrier to gastric acid.

Immunological system. The lamina propria of the stomach and intestines contains many lymphocytes and plasma cells. Some of these cells synthesise secretory IgA which is resistant to digestion by intestinal enzymes and has a role in protecting mucosal surfaces from bacterial invasion.

THE SYMPTOMS OF ALIMENTARY DISEASE

Pain. This is often the most important symptom of gastrointestinal disease. It must be analysed in relation to its main site, radiation, character, severity, duration, frequency, times of occurrence, aggravating and relieving factors and any associated phenomena.

Loss of appetite (anorexia). This may have a local cause such as carcinoma of the stomach but may also be a feature of any debilitating disease or of a psychological disturbance.

Waterbrash. This is the sudden filling of the mouth with saliva which is produced as a reflex response to a variety of symptoms from the upper gastrointestinal tract, e.g. peptic ulcer pain.

Vomiting. This may occur in any acute disorder of the alimentary tract including intestinal obstruction. Numerous other conditions may also be responsible, for example, meningitis, uraemia, migraine, drugs such as digoxin or morphine and particularly in the child, infection. The type, timing and related features of the vomiting are important diagnostically. Sudden vomiting without preceding nausea may be due to direct stimulation of the vomiting centre in the medulla and thus be an indication of intracranial disease. Vomiting in the morning may be due to pregnancy, alcoholism or anxiety. Vomiting of large quantities of food and secretions late in the day or night indicates gastric outlet obstruction. Vomiting which relieves pain is often due to a peptic ulcer. The complaint of persistent vomiting without loss of weight is nearly always indicative of psychological disturbance.

Heartburn. This is a burning retrosternal sensation usually due to inflammation of the oesophagus as in reflux oesophagitis. Sometimes dysmotility of the oesophagus produces a similar sensation.

Regurgitation. This is the appearance of previously swallowed food in the mouth without vomiting. It usually has an acid or bitter taste because of the presence of gastric juice or bile but not in patients with obstruction in the oesophagus.

Dysphagia, i.e. difficulty in swallowing. This is discussed on page 424.

Flatulence. This is often due to excessive swallowing of air (aerophagy). Under normal circumstances a small amount of air is swallowed with food, drink and saliva. Some of this gas may be expelled as a belch. The remainder passes into the intestine. Some will be absorbed but the nitrogen, will be expelled per rectum. Most of the colonic gas is the consequence of bacterial action in food residues in the lower small intestine and colon. A plain radiograph of the abdomen shows that gas is normally present in the stomach and colon but that very little is seen in the small intestine.

Constipation. In Britain fewer than 20% of people have less than one bowel motion per day and only 4% have a bowel movement less frequently than 3 times a week. These latter should be regarded as constipated. In addition, if the stool is hard and difficult to pass the patient should be regarded as constipated whatever the frequency of bowel movement.

Diarrhoea. In contrast, less than 1% of the population have more than three bowel movements daily and this should be regarded as abnormal, that is, particularly if the stool is not formed. When the stool is liquid or semi-formed it is considered to be diarrhoea whatever the frequency of bowel movement. The diet in Western countries is low in roughage; where a high residue diet is usual, more than three bowel movements daily may be normal. An explanation must be found for any change in bowel habit.

Loss of weight. This may be due to a reduced intake of food because of anorexia, nausea or vomiting, to malabsorption of nutrients or to the loss of protein from a diseased bowel as in ulcerative colitis. Carcinoma is the most important alimentary cause of loss of weight.

INVESTIGATION OF THE ALIMENTARY TRACT

RADIOLOGICAL EXAMINATION

Plain radiographs

These show the normal soft tissue shadows due to the liver, spleen and kidneys and also abnormal shadows. Gas in the intestine acts as a contrast medium so that the distribution of the bowel within the abdomen can be assessed. In obstruction there may be an excessive amount of gas and fluid in the bowel above the obstruction and films with the patient erect will demonstrate fluid levels. Finally, areas of opacification due to stones or to calcification in the liver, pancreas, cysts or blood vessels may provide important diagnostic information.

A chest radiograph will show the diaphragm. Free gas under the diaphragm indicates a perforation but may also be seen for the first few days following a laparotomy. Gas with a fluid level may be associated with a subphrenic abscess. Pulmonary lesions, from which pain may be referred to the abdomen, can also be identified.

Barium studies

These will demonstrate a break in the continuity of the outline of the gut, abnormalities in the appearance of the mucosa and disorders of motility.

The barium swallow and meal examination. Because pharyngeal swallowing is rapid video

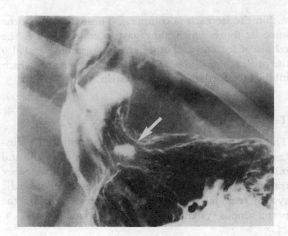

Fig. 10.1   Hiatus hernia with an ulcer (arrow) in the herniated portion of the stomach. (Courtesy Dr G.M. Fraser.)

recording or rapid sequence films are often necessary. The oesophagus is studied while barium is being swallowed so that it is seen distended with barium. Mucosal films are taken immediately after the barium has passed through the area. The procedure may demonstrate a disorder of motility, a filling defect caused by a tumour or varices, a stricture, a diverticulum or a hiatus hernia (Fig. 10.1).

The mucosa of the stomach is usually examined by a double-contrast study in which a small amount of barium is used together with the introduction of gas to distend the stomach. An ulcer is usually seen face on as a small collection of barium with radiating folds of mucosa (Figs 10.4 and 10.5). It may also appear as a projection beyond the normal outline while tumours cause filling defects. Small cancers can be detected by irregularity in the mucosal pattern. Observation of the motility of the stomach may indicate an inert area caused by infiltrating carcinoma. The duodenal cap is examined by studying its contours when it is completely filled with barium, and its mucosal pattern when it is distended with gas and the mucosa coated with barium.

Small bowel meal. When disease of the small intestine is suspected, barium is observed during its passage through the small intestine and radiographs are taken at intervals. The outline of the barium may indicate structural abnormalities such as diverticula or strictures. When there is malabsorption, excess secretions may cause the barium to clump and flocculate.

Barium enema. This procedure is uncomfortable and sometimes exhausting, particularly in the elderly or in those with cardiac disease in whom arrhythmia may be induced. Barium enema must always have been preceded by digital examination of the rectum and preferably also by sigmoidoscopy a few days earlier. The colon must be meticulously cleared of faeces by means of laxatives followed by a cleansing enema just before the barium enema. Barium alone or, for double-contrast examination, barium and air, is run into the bowel through a self-retaining catheter. Radiographs are taken with the colonic mucosa coated with barium and the lumen distended with air. In this way the colonic mucosa can be studied in detail and polyps or small tumours identified (Fig. 10.20). In inflammatory bowel disease mucosal abnormalities are readily recognised (Fig. 10.12). In some patients there will be a reflux of barium into the terminal ileum which can be outlined.

IMAGING STUDIES

Ultrasonography. This non-invasive technique which can be used safely in pregnancy is of great value in assessing the abdomen. It can be used in the diagnosis of liver, pancreatic and gallbladder disease, to identify ascites and also to define a variety of gut disorders.

Computed tomography (CT) and magnetic resonance imaging (MRI). CT is an important technique for defining certain intra-abdominal diseases particularly those involving inaccessible organs or regions. Thus it is used in the diagnosis and management of pancreatitis and pancreatic cancer, and in diagnosing diseases of the retroperitoneal space and lymph nodes. It is also of importance in assessing the spread of tumour, e.g. gastric cancer so that decisions can be made on whether surgery should be palliative or curative. MRI has not yet proven to be superior to CT for any intra-abdominal diagnostic problem.

Radionuclide scanning. This is used for examining the liver and spleen and for detecting the approximate site of gastrointestinal haemorrhage.

ENDOSCOPY

It is not difficult to examine the whole of the oesophagus, stomach, duodenum and colon with fibreoptic instruments. Endoscopic instruments can also be used for the therapeutic procedures which would otherwise require laparotomy such as removal of a polyp.

Rigid instruments are used to examine the rectum and lower pelvic colon (sigmoidoscope) and occasionally the oesophagus (oesophagoscope).

Upper alimentary tract

It is usual to carry out the procedure with the patient under sedation, often as an out-patient. After a 12-hour fast the pharynx is anaesthetised with a spray or gargle. The instrument is passed with the assistance of the patient in swallowing, and the procedure, whilst uncomfortable, should be no more so than any other intubation. Possible complications are perforation of the oesophagus or stomach whilst passing the instrument or during biopsy, the inhalation of secretions, cardiac arrhythmias or arrest, and the transmission of infections. All these are rare when appropriate precautions are used but resuscitation and after-care facilities must be available in endoscopy units.

Where possible, the oesophagus, stomach and duodenum are all inspected at the same examination, because the presence of one lesion does not exclude another and double lesions are not uncommon, e.g. oesophagitis and duodenal ulcer. This is particularly important when endoscopy is carried out in patients with haematemesis or melaena because there may be more than one source of bleeding.

Oesophagoscopy. This should be performed when there is dysphagia or when barium examination suggests a tumour or stricture. Other indications include suspected oesophagitis, varices or a motility disorder. Therapeutic procedures that can be carried out include dilatation of a stricture and injection of sclerosing material into oesophageal varices to control bleeding.

Gastroscopy. This is always indicated when a gastric ulcer has been demonstrated on barium studies so that biopsies can be taken to exclude malignancy; subsequent healing of the ulcer should also be confirmed. Gastroscopy is also necessary following a haematemesis, when there is upper abdominal pain or dyspepsia, and in the investigation of patients with symptoms after gastric surgery because the appearances are difficult to define radiologically.

Endoscopic retrograde cholangiopancreatography (ERCP). At duodenoscopy the ampulla of Vater is cannulated with a fine bore catheter passed through the shaft of the instrument and radio-opaque dye is injected into the biliary and pancreatic ducts. The procedure is of great value in patients suspected of having pancreatic disease because distortion or obstruction of the ductal system may indicate a diagnosis of chronic pancreatitis or pancreatic carcinoma. It is of value in the diagnosis of pancreas divisum (p. 479). Obstruction or distortion of the common bile duct by a stone or a tumour can also be demonstrated and sphincterotomy can be performed to allow removal of stones.

Lower alimentary tract

Proctoscopy and sigmoidoscopy. These simple procedures should always be carried out in patients with symptoms referable to the lower bowel or anus. Both terms are inaccurate because proctoscopy visualises the anal canal and only 2–3 cm of the rectum, and sigmoidoscopy examines the rectum and the lower few centimetres of the pelvic colon. It is usual to carry out the procedures without preparation but if the rectum contains faeces endoscopy is repeated after the bowel has been emptied. Digital examination of the rectum should always precede endoscopy and the instruments should be warmed and well lubricated. Proctoscopy is used for the demonstration and injection of haemorrhoids. Sigmoidoscopy is necessary for the diagnosis of polyps, cancer of the rectum, ulcerative proctitis or colitis and Crohn's disease of the large bowel. Biopsy of the mucosa or lesion may also be taken.

Colonoscopy. The fibreoptic colonoscope permits inspection of the entire colon but the procedure is time-consuming and occasionally difficult. More often a short colonoscope (flexible sigmoidoscope) is used to examine the sigmoid and left colon where most lesions will be found. The bowel must be carefully prepared. During colonoscopy it is possible to take a biopsy of suspicious lesions and polyps can be removed using a diathermy snare.

OTHER INVESTIGATIONS

Biopsy

The biopsy of lesions is an essential part of each endoscopic procedure. Biopsy of the small intestine is indicated if malabsorption is suspected and is carried out by means of the Crosby capsule.

Secretory studies

The pentagastrin test. The acid output is measured in response to pentagastrin, a synthetic pentapeptide which exerts the biological effects of gastrin. Preparation consists of an overnight fast and H_2-receptor antagonist drugs must be stopped for at least 48 hours before the test. The fasting contents of the stomach are aspirated and their volume measured; then the secretions are collected continuously for one hour. This is termed the 'basal acid output'. Then pentagastrin is given subcutaneously and the secretions are collected for a further hour. The acid output in this hour is termed the 'maximum acid output'.

The pentagastrin test is helpful because:

1. a large volume of fasting juice indicates obstruction of the gastric outlet;
2. a very high basal acid output suggests that the patient has the Zollinger-Ellison syndrome (p. 438);
3. in patients with peptic ulcer it provides a preoperative base line;
4. achlorhydria can be demonstrated.

The insulin test. This is used after gastric surgery to indicate the completeness of vagotomy.

Bacteriological studies

The malabsorption syndrome may be due occasionally to bacterial colonisation of the small intestine. When this is suspected, secretion can be obtained for bacteriological studies by passing a fine sterile tube into the upper small intestine. A mercury bag attached to the tip of the tube ensures that the tube moves rapidly to the correct site. The patient should not be receiving antibiotics.

Motility studies

Barium examination gives a poor demonstration of the motility of the oesophagus, stomach and small intestine. The isotope ^{99m}Technetium sulphur colloid incorporated into a solid or liquid bolus can be used to measure transit down the oesophagus. Radioactive markers incorporated into solid food and liquids are also used to measure emptying of the stomach. Small intestinal motility can be estimated by giving a non-absorbable carbohydrate and hydrogen gas excreted in the breath is then measured. Motility can be studied more accurately by measuring the pressure changes in the lumen of the organ but only in the case of the oesophagus is this manometry of diagnostic value.

Examination of the stool

In malabsorption the stool may be pale and frothy; in the irritable bowel syndrome it may be like pellets or ribbon with or without mucus. In mild ulcerative disease of the colon there may be flecks of blood in the mucus. Inspection of the stool is sufficient to diagnose fresh bleeding from the lower alimentary tract while the loss of over 60 ml of blood from a site proximal to the ascending colon will produce a black tarry stool.

Tests for occult blood using the guaiac test or immunological techniques detect small amounts in the stool and are performed for several successive days because bleeding from the gastrointestinal tract is often intermittent. Specimens obtained on the fingerstall at rectal examination can be readily examined.

Microscopic examination is of value particularly in distinguishing amoebic dysentry and other parasitic diseases.

DISEASES OF THE MOUTH

DISORDERS OF THE TEETH

Mastication of food to a soft pulp is a prerequisite for good digestion. The teeth should be inspected to determine if they are healthy, present in adequate numbers and in correct apposition in the upper and lower jaws to allow efficient mastication. If dentures are worn it should be ascertained if they are comfortable and efficient. Bacteraemia may have its source in gingivitis or an apical abscess. It is particularly liable to occur after dental manipulation and may cause endocarditis in patients with valvular disease of the heart. All patients should be advised to consult a dentist regularly in order to conserve the teeth and to prevent or treat foci of infection in the mouth.

STOMATITIS

The mouth harbours a population of commensal microorganisms which normally is controlled by a reasonable standard of oral hygiene; if this is neglected the bacterial population may proliferate and cause stomatitis. This may also occur when resistance to the commensal population is lowered by disease especially in the compromised host. Stomatitis may also be due to nutritional deficiencies or other factors.

Ulcerative stomatitis (Vincent's infection)
This occurs mainly in adults with malnutrition and poor dental hygiene. Ulcers with ragged necrotic margins occur especially on the gums, but may involve the palate, the lips, or the inner aspects of the cheeks; the ulcers are covered by a grey slough surrounded by an erythematous margin. A stained smear shows many spirochaetes and fusiform bacilli; these organisms are present in small numbers in the normal commensal population of the mouth and the condition may be regarded as an endogenous infection due to impairment of host resistance. The condition is infectious, so that

the patient's food vessels and cutlery should be sterilised.

The acute phase responds to local treatment with metronidazole (200 mg t.i.d. for 4 d), or to penicillin. Necrosis of the gums may occur, so that when the acute phase has been controlled it is important that proper dental treatment is undertaken.

Candidiasis
The fungus *Candida albicans* (p. 147) is a normal commensal in the mouth but it may proliferate to cause *thrush* in babies, in the aged and particularly in debilitated or compromised patients. Thrush is also common in those receiving prolonged treatment with oral antibiotics. White patches appear on the tongue and buccal mucosa and may enlarge and coalesce to form an easily detached membrane; there is little surrounding inflammation. In severe infection, the lower pharynx and oesophagus may be affected, causing dysphagia, or the fungus may spread to the lungs.

Thrush may be treated by gentian violet mouth wash 3 times a day for 4 days or by nystatin tablets (500 000 units) retained in the mouth for as long as possible, and given 4 times daily for at least 4 days.

Stomatitis due to deficiency of nutritional factors
This may arise directly from an insufficient intake or indirectly as a result of impaired absorption of vitamins, especially niacin, riboflavin, folic acid, and vitamin B_{12}. When the deficiency is acute and severe, the tongue is red, raw and painful. When the deficiency is chronic and less severe the tongue appears moist and unduly clean because of atrophy of the papillae. Angular stomatitis often accompanies glossitis, especially in the case of gross iron deficiency. In severe vitamin C deficiency the gums become swollen and spongy and bleed readily.

Aphthous ulceration
This is a common recurrent condition characterised by painful superficial ulceration in the mouth. The lesion begins as an indurated erythematous area followed in a day or so by ulceration. The ulcers are often multiple and may recur over several weeks. The aetiology is unknown and the patient is usually healthy otherwise. Emotional stress may precipitate an attack, and in some women ulcers tend to recur in cyclical fashion during the premenstrual phase. Severe chronic aphthous ulceration may be found in association with Crohn's disease, ulcerative colitis or coeliac disease.

Hydrocortisone hemisuccinate lozenges (2.5 mg t.i.d.) may be effective in the early phase of lesions. Pain can be reduced with topical anaesthetics and secondary infection controlled with tetracycline mouth washes.

Other forms of stomatitis

An allergic reaction to chemicals in toothpaste, dentures, foodstuffs and many drugs, especially antibiotics, can cause stomatitis. A characteristic blue-black punctate line may be seen where the gum margins adjoin the teeth in lead poisoning. Skin diseases such as lichen planus, pemphigus and erythema multiforme involve the mouth, sometimes before being seen on the skin.

DISEASES OF THE TONGUE

In health the tongue is moist with only a slight white fur on the dorsum. The papillae are readily seen. Mouth breathing causes a dry tongue, but otherwise dryness of the tongue is an indication of dehydration. The tongue may be coated with whitish-yellow fur in persons who smoke excessively but in general, the presence of fur on the tongue has little clinical significance.

Glossitis. It may be a prominent feature of stomatitis resulting from nutritional deficiency.

Geographical tongue. This is the name given to a chronic migrating superficial glossitis; it looks odd but has no clinical significance.

Glossodynia. This is a persistently painful tongue which appears normal on inspection and, unlike true glossitis, is not exacerbated by hot liquids; the symptom is usually psychogenic. A bad taste in the mouth may be caused by local disease in the oropharynx and by some drugs; when these causes can be excluded the symptom is usually neurotic in origin.

Syphilis. This may occur as a primary chancre, in the secondary stage as 'mucous patches', or in the tertiary stage as painless gummatous ulcers.

Leukoplakia. This is a chronic condition characterised by white, firm, smooth patches beginning at the side of the tongue and later spreading over the dorsum. In the early stages the tongue is not painful but later the patches are split by fissures with resultant tenderness. The significance of leukoplakia is that it may precede the development of carcinoma, and a biopsy of such lesions should always be undertaken.

Carcinoma. In the mouth and tongue this is often related to excessive consumption of tobacco and alcohol and poor oral hygiene. It must be considered in all cases of chronic ulcer of the tongue; if any doubt exists biopsy should be carried out.

DISEASES OF THE SALIVARY GLANDS

Xerostomia (dryness of the mouth). This may be due to dehydration or may be caused by anticholinergic or antidepressant drugs; commonly it is due to anxiety. Xerostomia is one of the features of Sjögren's syndrome (p. 768). Excessive salivary secretion may be a response to irritation or inflammation in the mouth, e.g. oral sepsis.

Parotitis. This may be due to the virus of mumps or to bacterial infection of the gland. The latter tends to develop during severe febrile illnesses and after major abdominal operations if adequate attention is not given to oral hygiene and to the prevention of dehydration and infection. Its treatment consists of the parenteral administration of penicillin and surgical drainage if abscess formation has occurred.

Sarcoidosis. This is another cause of enlargement of the parotid glands.

Salivary calculi. These occur occasionally in the submandibular gland or its duct. They cause pain and swelling brought on by eating. Infection of the gland is a complication. Stones in the duct can be felt in the floor of the mouth and can be removed by incision over the duct. Stones in the gland may require excision of the gland.

A 'mixed' salivary tumour. This presents as a slow, painless enlargement of one salivary gland. The tumour is essentially of epithelial origin but may contain stromal elements and shows a variable degree of malignancy. It is treated either by excision or excision and radiotherapy.

DISEASES OF THE OESOPHAGUS

DYSPHAGIA

Because the only function of the oesophagus is the transmission of food from the mouth to the stomach, most diseases of the oesophagus as well as disease of some related structures may cause difficulty in swallowing (dysphagia).

AETIOLOGY OF DYSPHAGIA

Oral (painful mastication)
Stomatitis
Aphthous ulceration
Moniliasis
Herpes Simplex
Tonsilitis
Oral malignancy

Pharyngeal
Following cerebrovascular accident
Bulbar and pseudobulbar palsy
Motor neurone disease
Syringomyelia
Myasthenia gravis
Pharyngeal malignancy
Pharyngeal diverticulum

Oesophagus
Peptic oesophagitis ± stricture
Carcinoma (including carcinoma of cardia)
Motility disorders (achalasia, diffuse spasm)
Dermatomyositis
Chagas' Disease
Webs and rings: sideropenic dysphagia, lower oesophageal ring
Moniliasis, herpes simplex
Mediastinal mass lesion:
    Goitre
    Bronchogenic carcinoma
    Aortic aneurysm
    Dilated left atrium
Foreign bodies

Aetiology

Painful diseases of the oral cavity
These include stomatitis, tonsillitis, severe aphthous ulceration or carcinoma of the tongue.

Pharyngeal dysphagia
This is due to neurological conditions such as pseudobulbar palsy or myasthenia gravis and occurs immediately after swallowing is attempted. Because of the neurological deficit, tracheal aspiration occurs causing coughing and laryngissmus, with an ever present risk of aspiration pneumonia. Management of this distressing condition usually requires nasogastric feeding. Pharyngeal carcinoma may cause difficulty in initiating swallowing.

Oesophageal dysphagia
This is recognised as a sensation, sometimes painful, of food sticking in the oesophagus. Relief is obtained by regurgitation or the patient may sip liquids until obstruction is relieved and the impacted bolus moves onwards.

Congenital abnormalities. Atresia, in which the oesophagus ends blindly at about the level of the tracheal bifurcation, occurs occasionally and requires urgent surgery in the new born.

Oesophagitis ulceration and stricture. The commonest cause of oesophagitis is acid-peptic digestion of the mucosa due to gastro-oesophageal reflux. When severe the inflammatory response involves the whole thickness of the oesophageal wall so that eventually a stricture may develop due to fibrosis. Oesophagitis and stricture formation occur occasionally due to ingestion of corrosives such as bleach or caustic soda, or due to bile reflux after total gastrectomy. Unusual causes of oesophagitis include herpes viral infection and candidiasis in immunocompromised patients. A variety of drugs given as tablets or capsules may impact in the oesophagus especially in the elderly causing local ulceration.

Carcinoma. Carcinoma (see p. 429) of the oesophagus or of the cardia of the stomach.

Motility disorders. Primary motility disorders of the oesophagus such as achalasia and oesophageal spasm (p. 428) may cause dysphagia. Motility may also be impaired when the oesophagus is affected in connective tissue disorders such as scleroderma (p. 429).

Webs and rings. Sideropenic dysphagia (Plummer-Vinson syndrome) is a very rare condition associated with iron deficiency anaemia glossitis and koilonychia. A thin web of degenerated epithelial cells forms in the post cricoid area and causes intermittent dysphagia to solids. The web is difficult to detect on barium examination or at endoscopy, but the dilatation caused by the passage of the endoscope is usually sufficient to relieve symptoms. The condition occurs usually in post-menopausal women. Treatment is with iron replacement. A membrane known as a lower oesophageal ring may form at the lower end of the oesophagus, causing dysphagia. The cause is unknown, and treatment is by dilatation.

Extrinsic disease. Dysphagia may result from compression of the oesophagus by a goitre or by a mediastinal mass such as bronchogenic carcinoma, malignant lymph nodes, aneurysm of the aorta or dilatation of the left atrium.

Investigation

The exclusion of malignant disease is essential in any patient who complains of dysphagia. Barium swallow and oesophagoscopy are essential Where the disorder appears to be one of function rather than structure, as for example in achalasia or systemic sclerosis, then manometry can give additional information.

GASTRO-OESOPHAGEAL REFLUX; REFLUX OESOPHAGITIS

Several mechanisms operate to prevent reflux of gastric contents into the oesophagus. The most important is the lower oesophageal sphincter; this is not an anatomical entity but a physiological zone of high pressure which is maintained just above the gastro-oesophageal junction. Because it is situated below the diaphragm the physiological effect of the sphincter is reinforced by intra-abdominal pressure; and moreover the oblique entry of the oesophagus to the stomach ensures that the intra-abdominal oesophagus is closed when the stomach is distended. The latter two mechanisms are lost when the oesophago-gastric junction 'slides' through the diaphragm when a hiatus hernia develops, so making gastro-oesophageal reflux more likely to occur. It is important to appreciate that a hiatus hernia facilitates gastro-oesophageal reflux but does not directly cause it. Gastro-oesophageal reflux occurs to some degree in all individuals, but the re-fluxed material is cleared by secondary peristaltic waves in the oesophagus and acid is neutralised by swallowed saliva. When the anti-reflux mechanisms fail, persistent exposure of the lower oesophagus to acid and pepsin, or bile, results in oesophagitis.

Peptic oesophagitis occurs most frequently in middle-aged and elderly women of whom 50% will have a hiatus hernia. Table 10.1 lists some of the factors associated with or promoting gastro-oesophageal reflux.

Clinical features

Heartburn is the characteristic symptom. It is felt as a deeply placed 'burning' pain behind the sternum, often radiating to the throat; patients may indicate their discomfort with upward movements of the fingers over the chest. It occurs after meals and characteristically is brought on by bending and by lifting or straining due to an increase in the intra-abdominal pressure. It may also occur on lying down in bed at night preventing sleep and is then relieved by sitting up. No other pain of alimentary origin is so closely related to posture as that of reflux oesophagitis.

Regurgitation of gastric content to the mouth may occur during bending, after a large volume meal, or at night and may cause tracheal aspiration with coughing or laryngismus or aspiration pneumonia. There may be pain on swallowing (odynophagia). Transient dys-

Table 10.1   Factors promoting gastro-oesophageal reflux

Factor	Mechanism
Hiatus hernia Surgical procedures involving lower end of oesophagus e.g. cardiomyotomy, vagotomy	Impaired efficiency of lower oesophageal sphincter (LOS)
Pregnancy Obesity Ascites Heavy lifting and straining Abdominal constriction e.g. by surgical corsets	Increase in intra-abdominal pressure
Cigarette smoking Alcohol Fatty foods Caffeine	Reduction in LOS pressure
Impaired gastric emptying e.g. by gastric outlet obstruction, anticholinergic drugs, fatty foods. Large volume meals	Increased gastric content available for reflux

phagia for solids is usually due to spasm; persistent dysphagia suggests the development of a stricture.

Occasionally oesophagitis is symptomless, presenting with iron deficiency anaemia due to blood loss.

In long-standing oesophagitis the inflamed squamous mucosa may change to columnar type. This effect, termed Barrett's mucosa, is considered potentially pre-malignant, because it is associated with an increased incidence of adenocarcinoma of the oesophagus. Oesophageal ulcers may occur also in the transformed mucosa.

The diagnosis of oesophagitis and the presence of stricture or Barrett's mucosa is made on the visual and biopsy findings at endoscopy. The presence of a hiatus hernia is shown by a barium meal (Fig. 10.1) and an ulcer in the hiatus hernia can be revealed by endoscopy or barium studies. Some patients have symptoms of oesophagitis, yet have minimal or no endoscopic or biopsy evidence, and here the perfusion of acid into the oesophagus may be useful diagnostically by reproducing the symptoms. In those patients with chest pain which might be either cardiac or oesophageal, a resting ECG and exercise stress testing is indicated. If these are negative the possibility of oesophageal dysmotility should be investigated with barium swallow followed by oesophageal motility studies. When a patient with gastro-oesophageal reflux develops angina-like chest pain, it is often because the refluxed material initiates abnormal motility in the oesophagus.

Management

General measures

A number of factors are known to promote gastro-oesophageal reflux, many of which can be modified or altered by practical measures which the patient can undertake. Their importance should be explained and emphasised (Table 10.1). Much the most important are obesity and cigarette smoking. Weight reduction and stopping smoking alone will relieve symptoms in about 75% of patients. Meals should be of small volume and alcohol, fatty foods and caffeine avoided. Heavy lifting, stooping and bending at the waist should be avoided as far as possible especially after meals. The head of the bed should be elevated to 15°, and late night meals avoided to reduce reflux during sleep.

Medical treatment
Individual episodes of heartburn are promptly relieved by antacids, liquid preparations being best. Regular dosage of antacids taken one and three hours after meals will reduce the frequency of heartburn (10–15 ml of antacid suspension).

When symptoms are severe, or if oesophagitis is present, histamine$_2$-receptor antagonists should be used to reduce acid and pepsin secretion. Cimetidine (400 mg) or ranitidine (150 mg) should be given 2–4 times daily with meals and before bedtime. Treatment should be continued for at least 6 weeks if oesophagitis is present. Indeed treatment may be required lifelong since gastro-oesophageal reflux not associated with obesity or smoking is likely to become a permanent condition. A new drug, omeprazole (20 mg orally daily for 8 weeks), powerfully inhibits gastric secretion and induces healing in oesophagitis and in oesophageal ulcer.

Various alginate preparations are available which form a gel on the surface of the gastric contents preventing reflux in the upright position. Preparations are given in the same way as for conventional antacids. Dopamine receptor antagonist drugs (metoclopramide, domperidone) increase the contraction of the lower oesophageal sphincter as well as promoting gastric emptying, and are occasionally useful; metoclopramide may cause troublesome extrapyramidal side-effects. The dose is 10 mg orally 3 times daily.

Oesophageal strictures are treated by dilatation carried out at endoscopy and the procedure may be repeated as often as necessary. A semi-liquid diet will be required pending dilatation, and permanent treatment with H$_2$-receptor antagonists is advisable.

Anaemia will usually respond to oral iron; blood transfusion may be required rarely.

Surgical treatment
This is indicated if severe symptoms persist despite adequate medical therapy. The aim of surgery is to return the lower oesophageal sphincter to the abdomen and to construct an additional valve mechanism should a sliding hiatus hernia be present. Most oesophageal strictures can be treated by dilatation at endoscopy followed by further dilatation as necessary. However, a small proportion cannot be helped in this way and surgical resection of the stricture is necessary. This is associated with significant morbidity and mortality, particularly in the aged.

SLIDING HIATUS HERNIA

Aetiology
The aetiology of the sliding hiatus hernia is unknown. Obesity, pregnancy and occasionally ascites by increasing the intra-abdominal pressure may be aetiological factors. The condition is common, occurring in up to 33% of normal adults and 50% of aged individuals. The majority of individuals with a hiatus hernia have no symptoms and the hernia is of no clinical significance. In a minority however the hiatus hernia appears to facilitate gastro-oesophageal reflux. However the exact mechanisms responsible for this effect are not fully understood and the relationship between the sliding hiatus hernia and oesophageal reflux is not always clear.

Clinical features
The only symptoms that can be convincingly associated are those of gastro-oesophageal reflux (p. 426). There is no evidence of increased gastric acid secretion in patients with a sliding hiatus hernia.

Investigation
The diagnosis is made either by a barium swallow which will demonstrate the presence of the gastro-oesophageal junction within the thorax, or by endoscopy.

Management
A sliding hiatus hernia does not require treatment on its own account. However, when gastro-oesophageal reflux is severe, and is not adequately controlled by medical treatment, surgical repair of the hernia should be considered. This involves repair of the diaphragmatic defect, and fixing the stomach in the abdominal cavity (fundoplication) combined with an anti-reflux procedure.

It is most important that the presence of a sliding hiatus hernia is not used as an explanation for unrelated upper gastrointestinal symptoms.

PARA-OESOPHAGEAL HERNIA

In this less common hernia (20% of all hiatus hernia) the gastro-oesophageal junction is placed normally but the greater curve of the stomach herniates through the oesophageal hiatus.

Clinical features

These include retrosternal pain while eating, relieved by standing or walking around; gastric ulceration at the site of herniation, and bleeding. Dysphagia may occur but heartburn is rare.

Management

Surgical correction of the hernia is necessary.

DIVERTICULUM OF THE OESOPHAGUS

A traction diverticulum. This is most commonly situated in the anterior wall of the oesophagus just below the level of the tracheal bifurcation. It is due to chronic inflammation, usually tuberculosis, in adjacent lymph nodes. By the time the diverticulum is discovered, often accidentally during barium swallow, the disease in the lymph nodes has healed. It is seldom that diverticulum itself causes symptoms and surgical treatment is rarely necessary.

A pharyngeal pouch. This develops at the site of the inferior constrictor of the pharynx probably as a result of inco-ordination of the cricopharyngeus muscle and causes dysphagia due to forward displacement of the oesophagus. There is swelling and gurgling in the neck on swallowing. The patient may present with recurrent attacks of stridor, or inhalation of contents of the sac may lead to pneumonia. The pouch is removed surgically.

ACHALASIA OF THE CARDIA (ACHALASIA; CARDIOSPASM)

Although apparently confined to the lower end where there is failure of the sphincter to relax, this is in fact a motility disorder of the whole oesophagus which shows progressive atony and dilatation. The cause is probably a failure of nerve conduction due to diminution in the number of ganglion cells. Chagas' disease (American trypanosomiasis, p. 163) produces similar changes.

Clinical features

Dysphagia may at first be intermittent but later is always present. It is caused both by solids and liquids and may be localised behind the lower end of the sternum. Retrosternal pain occurs in some patients. In

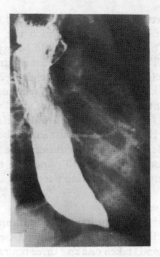

Fig. 10.2   Achalasia of cardia. (Courtesy of Dr D.H. Cummack.)

the initial stages, the patient continues to eat a normal diet but food accumulates in the capacious non-contractile oesophagus. Later the retained food cannot be expelled into the stomach and weight loss ensues. Inhalation of food and secretions may occur at night and cause recurrent pulmonary infection.

Investigation

A chest radiograph may be sufficient to show a dilated oesophageal outline, perhaps with a fluid level behind the heart shadow. There is absence of the usual gas shadow in the fundus of the stomach. A barium swallow shows the dilated atonic oesophagus coming to a smooth pointed termination (Fig. 10.2). While the appearances are typical, they are not diagnostic because they can be mimicked by a carcinoma at the lower end of the oesophagus or in the cardiac portion of the stomach. Treated or untreated, patients with achalasia have an increased liability to carcinoma of the oesophagus which makes initial endoscopy essential and periodic review after treatment desirable.

Oesophagoscopy is always required. Cleansing of the oesophagus is necessary and this may involve repeated lavage and aspiration at oesophagoscopy. Once the oesophagus is clean it can be inspected and biopsies taken if necessary. Motility studies which show reduced motility in the body of the organ and failure of the lower oesophageal sphincter to relax (p. 422) are of value in establishing the diagnosis and in determining the severity of the lesion.

Management

This may be by dilatation or cardiomyotomy. In the first a hydrostatic or pneumatic bag is positioned at the level of the diaphragm and then distended forcibly so as to weaken the lower oesophageal sphincter. One or more dilatations may be required to bring about adequate swallowing.

Failure of hydrostatic dilatation or inability to introduce the dilator are indications for operation, which takes the form of cardiomyotomy (Heller's operation). Here the muscle at the lower end of the oesophagus, and for some distance above and below, is slit to expose but not to penetrate the mucosa. The operation is relatively effective and safe, even in the elderly, but both dilatation and cardiomyotomy may be complicated by reflux oesophagitis, or occasionally by oesophageal perforation.

DIFFUSE SPASM OF THE OESOPHAGUS

In this condition there is muscular hypertrophy of the lower two-thirds of the oesophagus; Auerbach's plexus is normal, but there are degenerative changes in the vagus nerves.

The main symptom is pain precipitated by eating, by hot and cold liquids or by emotional stress. The pain is retrosternal and there may be radiation to the back, neck or arms, thus mimicking angina pectoris. The pain may or may not be accompanied by dysphagia. The diagnosis is established by barium swallow which shows a hold-up of barium in the oesophagus due to multiple unco-ordinated contractions. The appearance resembles a 'corkscrew'. Manometry shows strong unco-ordinated contractions.

Treatment involves education in eating in a relaxed atmosphere with adequate mastication. Any emotional stress should receive attention. Nitroglycerine, hydralazine or nifedipine may all relieve pain in some patients. Since most patients are over the age of 60, the physician has to persist with medical management but in the occasional younger patient, an extended cardiomyotomy may be required.

CARCINOMA OF THE OESOPHAGUS

There are wide geographical variations in the incidence of this tumour; it is very common around the Caspian Sea and some parts of Southern Africa. In Europe and the USA, alcohol and tobacco are important aetiological factors. In other parts of the world, chewing various noxious substances contributes.

In Western communities, the average age of patients with carcinoma of the oesophagus is between 60 and 70 years. The most frequent site is the lower third of the oesophagus; it is less common in the middle third and least common in the upper third. The lesion is usually ulcerative and it extends circumferentially and longitudinally in the wall of the oesophagus, often producing stenosis. Direct invasion of surrounding structures and involvement of related lymph nodes is common by the time of diagnosis. Squamous carcinoma is most frequent. Of the 10–20% of adenocarcinomas, the majority probably arises in Barrett's columnar epithelium, the remainder invading the lower oesophagus from the stomach.

Clinical features
Progressive dysphagia is typical. It starts with the 'sticking' of solid food, at first intermittently and then regularly and proceeds to difficulty with semisolids and eventually with liquids. There is discomfort, not amounting to pain, at the site of the obstruction which is usually well localised by the patient. The development of symptoms occupies some months so that by the time the patient first attends, weight loss is already a feature and there may be metastases in lymph nodes, liver and the mediastinum.

Investigation
Obstruction and an irregular narrowing of the oesophagus, seen at barium swallow, are highly suggestive of the diagnosis (Fig. 10.3). At the lower end it may not be possible to distinguish between carcinoma of the oesophagus and achalasia of the cardia. Oesophagitis and a benign stricture may also simulate carcinoma.

Oesophagoscopy and biopsy should always be performed. Repeated biopsy may be required to obtain positive confirmation of the diagnosis particularly when stricture formation prevents further insertion of the oesophagoscope or the biopsy forceps. In these circumstances the passage of a brush through the narrowed area dislodges cells which can be examined for malignancy.

Management
The choice lies between palliation and radical measures. The chances of cure seldom exceed 10%. In squamous carcinoma, particularly of the upper and middle thirds, high voltage radiotherapy is the treatment of choice in those centres possessing the necessary facilities. Otherwise, and with tumours of the lower third, oesophagogastrectomy offers the best hope. There is the possibility that a combined approach of surgery with pre-operative radiotherapy may lead to enhanced survival.

Extensive tumours that are unsuitable for radical surgery or for intensive radiotherapy are treated palliatively, occasionally by bypass surgery, but more often by endoscopic insertion of a permanent tube into the

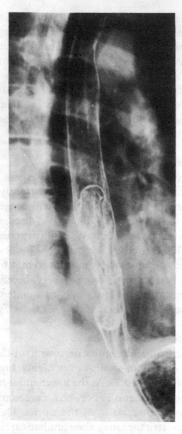

Fig. 10.3 Carcinoma of the oesophagus. (Courtesy of Dr G.M. Fraser.)

oesophagus. This allows liquids to be taken and is effective in relieving the patient of that most distressing problem – the inability to swallow saliva.

In some centres endoscopic laser therapy is available for tumour ablation. Treatment can be repeated as necessary and gratifying palliation with restoration of swallowing can be achieved. Hazards include perforation and bleeding.

DISEASES OF THE STOMACH AND DUODENUM

PEPTIC ULCER

The term 'peptic ulcer' refers to an ulcer in the lower oesophagus, stomach or duodenum, in the jejunum after surgical anastomosis to the stomach, or rarely in the ileum adjacent to a Meckel's diverticulum. Ulcers in the stomach or duodenum may be acute or chronic; both penetrate the muscularis mucosae but the acute ulcer shows no evidence of fibrosis. Erosions do not penetrate the muscularis mucosae.

Although the incidence of peptic ulcer is decreasing in many Western communities, it still affects, at some time, approximately 10% of all adult males. The male to female ratio for duodenal ulcer varies from 4:1 to 2:1 in different communities whilst that for gastric ulcer is 2:1 or less. Variations in the incidence of gastric and duodenal ulcer occur between different countries and between different parts of the same country; the incidence of peptic ulcer is higher in Scotland than in Southern England due to a preponderance of duodenal ulcers in Scotland. Peptic ulcer is becoming more common in many developing countries. There is growing evidence that cigarette smoking prevents healing of gastric and duodenal ulcers and may be a factor contributing to their development.

Aetiology of chronic ulceration

Heredity
Patients with peptic ulcer often have a family history of the disease; this is particularly so with duodenal ulcers which develop below the age of 20 years. Gastric and duodenal ulcers are inherited as separate disorders; thus the relatives of gastric ulcer patients have three times the expected number of gastric ulcers, and duodenal ulcer relatives have three times the expected number of duodenal ulcers.

Acid-pepsin versus mucosal resistance
The immediate cause of peptic ulceration is digestion of the mucosa by acid and pepsin of the gastric juice but the sequence of events leading to this is unknown. Digestion by acid and pepsin cannot be the only factor involved because the normal stomach is obviously capable of resisting digestion by its own secretions. The concept of ulcer aetiology may be written as 'acid plus pepsin versus mucosal resistance'. Some factors which affect this balance can be identified.

Gastric hypersecretion. Ulcers occur only in the presence of acid and pepsin; they are never found in achlorhydric patients such as those with pernicious anaemia. On the other hand, severe intractable peptic ulceration nearly always occurs in patients with the Zollinger-Ellison syndrome which is characterised by very high acid secretion. Acid secretion is more important in the aetiology of duodenal than gastric ulcer because patients with duodenal ulcer, as a group, secrete more hydrochloric acid than normal individuals.

Mucosal resistance. Several mechanisms protect the gastric mucosa from hydrogen ions secreted into the lumen of the stomach. The surface epithelial cells secrete bicarbonate which creates an alkaline milieu at the surface of the mucosa; this bicarbonate secretion is under the influence of mucosal prostaglandins. The tight junctions between the epithelial cells and their surface lipoprotein layer provide a mechanical barrier. The normal turnover of epithelial cells and gastric mucus also has a protective function. Collectively, all these mechanisms can be described as the 'gastric mucosal barrier'. Its integrity is important in preventing gastric ulcer and some of these mechanisms may also operate in the duodenum.

Factors reducing mucosal resistance. Several drugs, particularly those used in rheumatoid arthritis, will disrupt the gastric mucosal barrier. When aspirin is in solution at a pH below 3.5 it is undissociated and fat-soluble, so that it is absorbed through the lipoprotein membrane of the surface epithelial cells; during absorption it damages the membrane and the tight junctions. It also inhibits prostaglandin synthesis thus reducing bicarbonate secretion by the surface epithelial cells. Aspirin has been shown to be an important aetiological factor in gastric ulcer in Australia. There is also a relationship between aspirin ingestion and acute bleeding from the upper gastrointestinal tract.

Reflux of bile and intestinal secretions into the stomach occurs more frequently in patients with gastric ulcers than in normal individuals or patients with duodenal ulcer, due presumably to a poorly functioning pyloric sphincter. Bile damages the gastric mucosal barrier, predisposing the mucosa to ulceration. The organism *Helicobacter pylori* can be identified in the antral mucosa in 90% of cases of duodenal ulcers and in the body or antral mucosa of about 60% of cases of gastric ulcer. These strong associations suggest that the organism may play an aetiological role in chronic peptic ulcer, the issue is undecided (p. 441).

Aetiology of acute and stress ulcers

Many of the factors described above also contribute to the development of acute ulcers. Aspirin is particularly important. Acute peptic ulcers developing after head injury, burns, severe sepsis, surgery or trauma are termed *stress ulcers*. Gastric hypersecretion is the usual cause of acute ulcer after head injury, while the reflux of duodenal contents and mucosal ischaemia may be responsible factors after burns or shock.

Pathology

Chronic gastric ulcer is usually single; 90% are situated on the lesser curve within the antrum or at the junction between body and antral mucosa. Chronic duodenal ulcer is usually in the first part of the duodenum just distal to the junction of pyloric and duodenal mucosa; 50% are on the anterior wall. Gastric and duodenal ulcers coexist in 10% of all patients with peptic ulcers. More than one peptic ulcer is found in 10–15% of patients. Acute ulcers or erosions are frequently multiple, and are more widely distributed.

Clinical features

Peptic ulcer disease is a chronic condition with a natural history of spontaneous relapse and remission lasting for decades if not for life. Although they are different diseases duodenal and gastric ulcers share common symptoms which will be considered together.

The commonest presentation is that of recurrent abdominal pain which has three notable characteristics – localisation to the epigastrium, relationship to food, and episodic occurrence.

Epigastric pain. Pain is referred to the epigastrium and is often so sharply localised that the patient can indicate its site with two or three fingers – the 'pointing sign'.

Hunger pain. Pain occurs intermittently during the day, often when the stomach is empty, so that the patient identifies it as 'hunger pain' and obtains relief by eating.

Night pain. Pain wakes the patient from sleep and may then be relieved by food, a drink of milk or antacids; this symptom when present is virtually pathognomonic for ulcer.

Pain relief. Pain is relieved by food, milk or antacids and by belching and vomiting. The effect of vomiting is so striking that many patients learn to induce vomiting for pain relief.

Episodic pain ('periodicity'). Characteristically pain occurs in 'on again/off again' episodes, lasting one to three weeks at a time, three or four times in a year. Between episodes the patient feels perfectly well. To begin with episodes may be quite brief and infrequent lasting only for a few days at a time, once or twice per year; as the natural history evolves, however, episodes of pain become more frequent and last longer. In temperate climates seasonal variations may be noted, with an increased frequency of symptoms during winter and spring. Although the factors responsible for relapse and remission and seasonal variations, are not known, there is no doubt that relapses occur more frequently in smokers than in non-smokers.

Other symptoms that occur, especially during

episodes of pain, include waterbrash (excessive salivation), heartburn, loss of appetite and vomiting. Occasional vomiting occurs in about 40% of ulcer subjects: persistent vomiting, occurring daily suggests the possibility of outlet obstruction.

In 30% of patients the history is less characteristic. This is especially true in elderly subjects under treatment with non-steroidal anti-inflammatory drugs (NSAIDs). In these patients pain may be absent or so slight that it is experienced only as a vague sense of epigastric unease. Occasionally the only symptoms are anorexia and nausea, or a sense of undue repletion after meals. Sometimes the ulcer is completely 'silent' presenting for the first time with anaemia from chronic undetected blood loss, or as an abrupt haematemesis or as acute perforation.

GASTRIC ULCER VS DUODENAL ULCER

It is difficult to distinguish between gastric and duodenal ulcer on symptoms alone. Age and sex however are important discriminators. Gastric ulcer tends to occur over age 40, and affects the sexes equally while duodenal ulcer occurs predominantly in male subjects between the ages of 20 and 50. In general gastric ulcer runs a less remittent course than duodenal ulcer so that episodes tend to last longer and pain may occur daily for

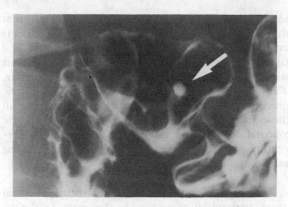

Fig. 10.5   Duodenal ulcer. (Courtesy of Dr G.M. Fraser.)

long periods at a time. In contrast to duodenal ulcer, the pain of gastric ulcer is not consistently relieved by antacids and may be provoked rather than relieved by food; heartburn and night pain are less common, and anorexia and nausea are more common in gastric ulcer.

Investigation

The diagnosis can be confirmed by barium meal examination or at endoscopy. Endoscopy is the preferred investigation because it is more accurate and has the enormous advantage that suspicious lesions can be biopsied. At least 10% of gastric ulcers may be malignant therefore endoscopy and biopsy are mandatory when a gastric ulcer is detected on barium examination. Moreover in gastric ulcer disease endoscopy must be repeated after suitable treatment to confirm that the ulcer has healed and to obtain further biopsies if it has not.

In contrast endoscopy is not essential for the management of duodenal ulcer, but because the clinical history is unreliable endoscopy is generally required for a firm diagnosis. Unless symptoms persist it is not necessary to repeat an endoscopy to confirm healing after treatment of duodenal ulcer.

Ulcer symptoms in young subjects can be safely treated without investigation, and endoscopy can be deferred until symptoms recur. However ulcer-like symptoms occurring for the first time in a patient over age 40 should always be investigated, preferably by endoscopy.

Management

The aims of treatment are to relieve symptoms and induce ulcer healing in the short term, and to prevent relapse in the long term. While the majority of ulcers will heal in 4–6 weeks of treatment, the prevention of

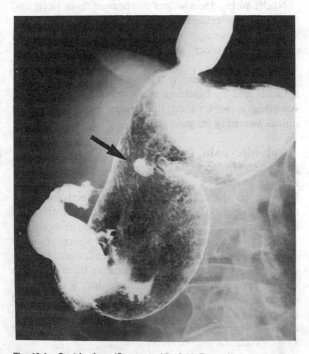

Fig. 10.4   Gastric ulcer. (Courtesy of Dr G.M. Fraser.)

Table 10.2   Drugs used in the management of peptic ulcer

	Short-term treatment	Maintenance treatment	Side-effects
Cimetidine	800 mg at night or 400 mg b.d.	400 mg at night	Delays elimination of warfarin, phenytoin and theophylline and should not be used concurrently with these drugs. Rarely causes confusion in the elderly, and gynaecomastia in males – both effects reversible on stopping the drug
Ranitidine	300 mg at night, or 150 mg b.d.	150 mg at night	Reversible confusion
Nizatidine	300 mg at night, or 150 mg b.d.	150 mg at night	Sweating, urticaria, somnolence. (All rare, none serious)
Famotidine	40 mg at night or 20 mg b.d.	20 mg at night	Headache, dizziness, dry mouth. (All rare, none serious)
Pirenzepine	50 mg b.d.	Not recommended	Dry mouth, blurred vision
Bismuth chelate (Tri-potassium di-citrato bismuthate)	240 mg b.d.	Not recommended	Blackens tongue, teeth and faeces. Risk of Bismuth toxicity with prolonged use
Sucralfate	2 grams b.d.	Not recommended	Reduces absorption of warfarin, phenytoin, tetracycline, digoxin
Misoprostol	200 micrograms 4 times daily	Not recommended	Abortefacient activity. Avoid use in women of child bearing age. Diarrhoea
Omeprazole	20 mg once daily	Not recommended	Delays elimination of diazepam, phenytoin, warfarin. Induces significant hypergastrinemia

Antacids are prescribed principally for symptomatic relief and dosage varies with the preparations used. Calcium compounds cause constipation, magnesium compounds cause diarrhoea and prolonged overdosage of either may rarely lead to hypercalcaemia or hypermagnesaemia. Aluminium compounds block absorption of digoxin tetracycline and dietary phosphate. Most antacids have a high sodium content which may exacerbate congestive heart failure or ascites.
Note: The doses recommended for gastric and duodenal ulcer are the same. Duodenal ulcer should be treated for 4–6 weeks, and gastric ulcer for 6–8 weeks.
   Cimetidine, ranitidine, famotidine and nizatidine are used in the management of peptic oesophagitis, in the doses recommended for maintenance treatment listed above, but given 2–4 times per day. The dose of omeprazole used for peptic oesophagitis is 20 mg per day.
   Except for antacids and sucralfate all the drugs listed should be avoided during pregnancy and lactation.

relapse can be achieved only with maintenance treatment for years if not for life, or by surgery.

The discovery of the H_2-receptor antagonist drugs revolutionised the treatment of peptic ulcer. The therapeutic effect of the H_2-receptor antagonists is due to their capacity to inhibit acid and pepsin secretion by the stomach; other ulcer healing agents are now available which induce their effects by different mechanisms. While all the currently available drugs satisfactorily relieve symptoms and induce ulcer healing, none of them alter the natural history of the disease. The short and long-term treatment of ulcer will be considered separately.

The recommended dose of the drugs used in the treatment of peptic ulcer, and their side-effects, are given in Table 10.2.

Short-term management

General measures. Cigarette smoking undoubtedly exacerbates the course of peptic ulcer disease and should be strongly discouraged. Aspirin and the nonsteroidal anti-inflammatory drugs (NSAIDs) should be avoided because of their injurious effects on the gastroduodenal mucosa. Alcohol in moderation is not harmful, and no special dietary advice is required.

Antacids. These are now prescribed mainly for symptomatic relief and are widely used for self-

medication. Given in sufficiently large doses for 4–6 weeks antacids will induce ulcer healing; however many patients find the side-effects and the inconvenience of frequent dosing unacceptable.

Many preparations are available varying in neutralising capacity, side-effects, palatability and cost. Sodium bicarbonate is the quickest acting and is widely used for self-medication. However it is readily absorbed with the risk of alkalosis so that its use should be discouraged and it should not be prescribed.

The majority of antacids are based on combinations of calcium, aluminium and magnesium, all of which cause side-effects (Table 10.2).

Antacids are available in tablet and liquid forms; although tablet forms are more convenient to take, they are probably less effective than liquid preparations.

Histamine H_2-receptor antagonist drugs. The H_2-receptor antagonist drugs available include the long established agents cimetidine and ranitidine and newer drugs such as famotidine and nizatidine; several others are under development. Although they differ in chemical structure, pharmacological properties and cost, for practical purposes the H_2-receptor antagonist drugs are all equally effective in ulcer treatment when prescribed in recommended doses.

They may be prescribed in twice daily doses or as a single larger dose at night (see Table 10.2); night time dosing is more convenient and improves patient compliance. Whether taken twice daily or at night symptoms remit promptly, often within days of starting treatment. Ulcer healing takes longer, but about 80% of duodenal ulcers will have healed after 4 weeks. Treatment should be prolonged for 6–8 weeks in patients who persist in smoking, and in patients who have had a recent major complication such as haematemesis or perforation.

Gastric ulcers heal more slowly than duodenal ulcers so that treatment should be prolonged for 6 weeks. It is important to confirm ulcer healing by further endoscopy. If the ulcer persists biopsies should be taken to confirm that it is benign, and treatment continued until healing is complete as determined by repeated endoscopy. If a gastric ulcer has not healed after 12 weeks treatment with a H_2-antagonist type drug omeprazole should be tried or surgical treatment considered.

Worldwide experience suggests that cimetidine and ranitidine are safe drugs but the long-term safety of famotidine and nizatidine has not yet been established.

Pirenzepine. This is a tricyclic compound which preferentially blocks muscarinic receptors in the stomach, so reducing gastric secretion. It is less effective in healing ulcers than the H_2-receptor antagonists.

Prostaglandin analogues. Prostaglandins exert complex effects on the gastroduodenal mucosa. In low doses they protect against injury induced by noxious agents such as aspirin, an effect which is designated as 'cytoprotection'; at higher doses acid secretion is inhibited and bicarbonate and mucus secretion are stimulated. A synthetic analogue now available (misoprostol) induces ulcer healing when given in doses that inhibit acid secretion. It should not be prescribed in women of child bearing age.

Omeprazole. This is a substituted benzimidazole compound that specifically inhibits the proton pump hydrogen-potassium ATP-ase in the parietal cell. It is the most powerful inhibitor of gastric secretion yet discovered so that a single dose induces prolonged achlorhydria, with a reciprocal increase in gastrin production. In experimental animals omeprazole produces a marked degree of hypergastrinaemia which causes hyperplasia of the ECL cells of the gastric mucosa and the formation of carcinoid tumours. Because of these potential effects omeprazole is not recommended for clinical use except in the special circumstances of Zollinger Ellison syndrome, severe oesophagitis or oesophageal ulcer, and peptic ulcers unresponsive to other forms of medical treatment.

Modest hypergastrinaemia occurs in proportion to the degree of acid reduction achieved by vagotomy or the use of drugs such as the H_2A antagonists or pirenzepine.

Colloidal bismuth compounds. Tri-potassium di-citrato bismuthate is an ammoniacal suspension of a complex colloidal bismuth salt. It precipitates in acid conditions binding with proteins in the ulcer base to form a coat which protects against further acid-pepsin digestion. In addition it exerts a powerful antimicrobial effect against *Helicobacter pylori*. It seems likely that *H. pylori* plays a role in the causation of duodenal ulcer, so that the ulcer healing properties of bismuth salts may be due to their antimicrobial effects. Moreover there is suggestive evidence that the rate of duodenal ulcer relapse is lower after treatment with bismuth salts than it is after other drugs. Because of the risk of toxicity, bismuth salts should not be used for maintenance treatment, and treatment courses should be limited to two per year.

Sucralfate. This is a basic aluminium salt of sucrose octasulphate which forms an adherent complex with proteins in the ulcer slough, protecting it from further digestion. The drug is not absorbed and has no known systemic effects.

Other drugs. Carbenoxolone sodium accelerates the healing of both gastric and duodenal ulcers. However because of its aldosterone-like effects it may cause sodium retention, hypokalaemia and hypertension and it is no longer recommended.

Choice of drug. The H_2-receptor antagonist drugs are considered the treatment of choice because they are safe and effective. Sucralfate and tri-potassium di-citrato bismuthate are acceptable alternatives for short-term therapy, and, if it can be firmly established that treatment with the bismuth salt is associated with a lower relapse rate than the other drugs discussed, it may become a first-line treatment; it is not suitable for long-term treatment. Carbenoxolone and pirenzepine and the currently available prostaglandin analogues are not recommended because of side-effects.

Long-term management
The natural tendency of gastric and duodenal ulcers to recur is not altered once ulcer healing has been induced by any of the short-term 'treatments' discussed above and indeed 80% will recur within 12 months. Further management depends upon a number of factors including the rate of relapse, the occurrence of compli-

cations, the age of the patient and the presence of other serious medical conditions.

Intermittent treatment

In the majority of patients symptomatic relapse occurs less than four times per year. In these patients each relapse can be treated with a 4-week course with one of the ulcer healing agents described. This form of 'intermittent' treatment is satisfactory for most patients.

Maintenance treatment

Clinical trials have established that continuous maintenance treatment with small doses of H_2-receptor antagonists will prevent ulcer relapse; as many as 80% of patients remain ulcer free for as long as treatment is maintained. Maintenance treatment should be considered:

1. When symptomatic relapse occurs frequently (more than four per year) interfering with employment or the quality of life;
2. When there is a history of life-threatening complications such as repeated bleeding or perforation;
3. When the risk of future complications or ulcer operation must be avoided if at all possible – for example in elderly subjects or patients with another Serious condition such as respiratory, cardiac, renal or hepatic impairment. In such patients maintenance treatment should be considered for life.

Long-term maintenance treatment with H_2-receptor antagonists is safe and effective. The effects and safety of long-term maintenance treatment with other ulcer healing agents is unknown; bismuth salts should not be used for maintenance therapy because of the risk of bismuth toxicity.

Surgical treatment

This has much to offer the patient with intractable peptic ulceration. It can relieve severe or persistent symptoms and prevent complications. While in many patients the assessment of the disability is straightforward, in those in whom anxiety or depression is present, the decision becomes difficult. Elective surgery should be considered in the following circumstances:

1. When the ulcer relapses after several courses of cimetidine or other ulcer-healing drugs; when relapse occurs during maintenance therapy; or more rarely when the ulcer fails to heal at all, particularly when symptoms interfere with the enjoyment of life or reduce the capacity to work. The indications for surgery are strengthened if the ulcer has developed in adolescence or young adult life, if there is a strong family history, or if there has been a previous complication such as haemorrhage or perforation. Finally some patients fail to comply with medical therapy or express reservations about prolonged therapy, both points being in favour of elective surgical treatment.
2. When there is an ulcer which has produced gastric outlet obstruction, or an hour-glass stomach because of fibrosis.
3. In a recurrent ulcer following previous gastric surgery.

There is no single, ideal operation suitable for all ulcers and all patients. For a gastric ulcer, the operation of choice is partial gastrectomy preferably with a Billroth I anastomosis, in which the ulcer itself and the ulcer-bearing area of the stomach is resected (Fig. 10.6).

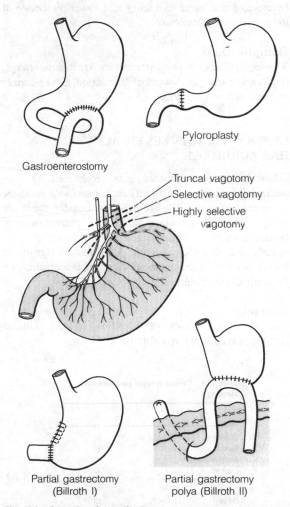

Gastroenterostomy

Pyloroplasty

Truncal vagotomy
Selective vagotomy
Highly selective vagotomy

Partial gastrectomy (Billroth I)

Partial gastrectomy polya (Billroth II)

Fig. 10.6 Operations for peptic ulcer.

For duodenal ulcer the acid secretory capacity of the stomach may be reduced by vagotomy which eliminates nervous stimulation (Fig. 10.6). At truncal vagotomy the main nerves are divided and thereafter gastric emptying may be retarded so that a drainage operation such as pyloroplasty or gastroenterostomy has to be added. A drainage procedure is also required in selective vagotomy in which vagal innervation to the small intestine, pancreas and biliary tree is preserved.

The aim of highly selective vagotomy is to denervate only the acid-producing area of the stomach while leaving intact the vagal supply of the antrum and pylorus. Gastric emptying is thus not impaired and a drainage procedure is not required unless there is stenosis from ulcer scarring. The avoidance of a drainage procedure markedly reduces the incidence of post-cibal syndromes and in particular dumping (p. 439). Vagotomy is preferred to partial gastrectomy because of the lesser mortality and lower incidence of long-term complications.

Complications

The complications of peptic ulcer are haemorrhage, perforation and gastric outlet obstruction. Ulcer-cancer is discussed on page 443.

UPPER GASTROINTESTINAL HAEMORRHAGE

Gastroduodenal haemorrhage is recognised by *haematemesis* (vomiting of blood) and/or *melaena* (passage of altered blood in the stools), and usually there are symptoms of hypovolaemia. Upper gastrointestinal bleeding carries a mortality that may reach 30% in elderly and shocked patients. A history of significant blood loss within the previous 48 hours is an indication for immediate admission to hospital.

Aetiology

The common causes of bleeding in the United Kingdom are shown in Table 10.3.

Table 10.3   Causes of upper gastrointestinal bleeding

	%
Duodenal ulcer	40
Gastric ulcer	17
Acute erosions	12
Varices	10
Mallory-Weiss	5
Cancer	3
Other	13

Erosions are usually caused by the ingestion of aspirin either alone or in combination with alcohol or by non-steroidal anti-inflammatory drugs. In some patients the stomach shows petechiae, multiple erosions and areas of confluent mucosal bleeding; this appearance is called *acute haemorrhagic gastritis*. The usual presentation of stress ulcer, caused by burns or head injury, is with haematemesis and melaena.

Clinical features

In severe bleeding from whatever cause, the patient complains of weakness, faintness, nausea, and sweating: these symptoms are followed by haematemesis or melaena. Haematemesis and melaena occur together with a sudden large bleed whereas melaena alone indicates that bleeding is slower and less in amount. If blood remains in the stomach it becomes partially digested and appears brown and granular in the vomit or gastric aspirate, like 'coffee grounds'. Blood passing through the intestinal canal is also altered in appearance, so that the faeces become black and sticky, (a melaena, or 'tarry' stool) but in severe bleeding, transit may be so rapid that the blood in the rectum is bright red.

The patient may be shocked or restless and disorientated because of cerebral anoxia. These signs may be absent in the young patient in whom compensatory mechanisms are more effective. The haemoglobin level will not alter until haemodilution occurs which may not take place for some hours, nor be complete for some days. A reduced haematocrit on admission to hospital suggests chronic bleeding prior to the acute episode. A raised urea with a normal serum creatinine indicates a blood loss of at least one litre. There is no simple laboratory procedure which will give a reliable estimate of the amount of blood loss until haemodilution is complete and in ordinary circumstances the assessment of the degree or rate of bleeding depends on clinical judgement. Serial recordings of the pulse rate and blood pressure give some indication, but for a more accurate assessment in patients who continue to bleed, measurement of central venous pressure is necessary. In patients with severe bleeding a record of urinary output by catheterisation is helpful.

Investigation

On admission there should be joint assessment by the physician and surgeon and in large centres the management of gastroduodenal bleeding can with advantage be centralised in a single unit. The diagnosis and bleeding status should be established at the outset. Urgent endoscopy is necessary to show the source of the bleeding, whether it is continuing or whether it is likely to recur.

The bleeding status is ascertained by passage of a nasogastric tube which should be aspirated at half-hourly intervals and the quantity and type of aspirate recorded.

Management

Blood is taken and stored for cross matching on every patient even if immediate transfusion is not indicated. Urgent treatment of hypovolaemic shock requires rapid and adequate blood replacement. Guidelines for transfusion are given in the information box below.

GUIDELINES FOR TRANSFUSION

Transfusion is required
- If the patient is clinically shocked
- If the pulse rate is consistently > 100/minute
- If the systolic pressure is < 100 mm Hg
- If the haemoglobin is < 10 dl

Whole blood should be given as soon as it is available; until then, a colloidal solution such as dextran can be used. Transfusion must keep pace with the estimated loss. This may be difficult in the elderly patient who is liable to develop cardiac or renal failure or cerebral anoxia and in whom coronary blood supply may also be impaired leading to angina or even myocardial infarction.

The injection of drugs such as diazepam to control restlessness and anxiety is to be preferred to morphine which may itself cause vomiting.

Subsequent management depends on the initial response and on the site and cause of bleeding. In general, emergency surgery should be advised in patients over the age of 50 in whom there is continued or recurrent bleeding from a gastric or duodenal ulcer. Conversely operation is unlikely to be necessary in such patients under the age of 30 or in patients with erosions in whom conservative management, including cimetidine or ranitidine, will usually suffice. The greatest risks are in the shocked and elderly with continued severe bleeding and when operation is delayed too long.

Because of the risks associated with emergency surgery, endoscopic methods for the control of upper gastrointestinal bleeding are being developed and seem promising. Techniques by which coagulating electrodes, heater probes, laser energy or injection of sclerosant materials can be applied to a bleeding lesion under vision at endoscopy are under investigation. All these techniques require that the lesion is accessible to endoscopic instrumentation and that the vessel responsible for bleeding can be identified; hazards include perforation and rebleeding.

The need for surgery does not disappear once the crisis is over. Early elective operation may still be indicated in patients with chronic ulcers which have bled, in those requiring continued treatment with salicylates, non-steroidal analgesics or corticosteroids, and in patients whose occupation or residence makes supervision difficult. In general, excision of the bleeding gastric ulcer, or exposure and suture of the duodenal ulcer coupled in either case with vagotomy is safer than partial gastrectomy which should be reserved for the complicated case in expert hands.

Bleeding from oesophageal varices secondary to portal hypertension can be extremely severe and demands special management (p. 526).

ACUTE PERFORATION OF A PEPTIC ULCER

The contents of the stomach escape into the peritoneal cavity when free perforation occurs. If perforation occurs without loss of contents, as in the accidental perforation of the empty stomach at gastroscopy, few symptoms are produced and the accident may even pass unnoticed. It follows that the symptoms of perforation are those of peritonitis and they are in proportion to the extent of peritoneal soiling. Occasionally the symptoms of perforation appear and rapidly subside; presumably the perforation has then closed spontaneously, or more commonly the ulcer has perforated locally into an area confined by adhesions to adjacent structures. Perforation occurs more commonly in duodenal than in gastric ulcers, and usually in ulcers on the anterior wall. About one-quarter of all perforations occur in acute ulcers.

Clinical features

Although perforation may be the first sign of ulcer, usually there is a history of recurrent epigastric pain. The most striking symptom is sudden, severe pain; its distribution follows the spread of the gastric contents over the peritoneum. Thus, initially the pain may be referred to the upper abdomen, but it quickly becomes generalised; shoulder tip pain may occur as a result of irritation of the diaphragm. The pain is accompanied by shallow respiration due to limitation of diaphragmatic movements and by shock. The abdomen is held immobile, and there is generalised 'board-like' rigidity. Intestinal sounds are absent, and liver dullness to percussion may decrease due to the presence of gas under the diaphragm. Vomiting is common. After some hours the symptoms improve though the abdominal rigidity remains. This period of improvement may deceive the clinician examining the patient for the first time. After this temporary improvement, the patient's condition deteriorates as general peritonitis follows the initial peritoneal irritation.

A radiograph of the upper abdomen in the erect position may help to establish the diagnosis because free gas within the peritoneal cavity, if in sufficient amount, will show as a translucent crescent between the liver and diaphragm. Where doubt remains, an emergency gastrografin meal may confirm that perforation has occurred.

Management and prognosis

After initial treatment of the patient for shock, the acute perforation should be treated surgically either by simple closure, or occasionally in the case of perforation of a chronic ulcer by closure combined with vagotomy and drainage. More than half the patients who have a simple closure will eventually require a further elective operation for recurrence of ulcer symptoms, and for this reason some surgeons recommend a definitive procedure for the ulcer at the time of operation.

Acute perforation carries a mortality of about 5%. The outlook is poorest in elderly patients, when a large perforation results in extensive peritonitis or when operation is delayed.

GASTRIC OUTLET OBSTRUCTION

An ulcer in the region of the pylorus may lead to gastric outlet obstruction. This may be due to fibrous stricture or to oedema or spasm produced by the ulcer; frequently it is a combination of all three. Gastric outlet obstruction may also be caused by carcinoma of the antrum and by a rare condition, adult hypertrophic pyloric stenosis. The syndrome of gastric outlet obstruction is loosely described as 'pyloric stenosis', even when the cause is chronic duodenal ulcer; here the stenosis is distal to the pylorus which itself may be seen radiologically to be greatly dilated.

Clinical features

Symptoms of obstruction are usually preceded by a long history of duodenal ulceration. Without such symptoms a patient with gastric outlet obstruction is likely to have a pyloric carcinoma. When the cause is a peptic ulcer, the symptoms change and nausea and vomiting become prominent. Vomiting produces such striking relief that a patient may start to eat immediately after the stomach has been emptied. If the obstruction progresses, the stomach dilates so that, eventually, surprisingly large amounts of gastric content may be vomited. Articles of food which have been eaten 24

hours or more previously may be recognised in the vomit. The loss of gastric contents results in water and electrolyte depletion. The blood urea may be raised because of dehydration. Alkalosis develops if large amounts of hydrochloric acid are lost, as occurs particularly in obstruction due to duodenal ulcer.

Physical examination shows evidence of wasting and dehydration, and there may be signs of tetany (p. 642). A succussion splash may be elicited four hours or more after the last meal or drink. In normal persons splashing occurs for less than an hour after meals because gastric emptying is rapid. Visible gastric peristalsis is diagnostic of gastric outlet obstruction and the abdomen should be inspected for its presence.

Investigation

Aspiration of the stomach contents will confirm the diagnosis if the volume is in excess of 100 ml after fasting overnight or if the aspirate contains food residue, or is foul.

Barium meal shows:

1. an increase in the fasting residue of the stomach,
2. dilatation of the stomach with or without excessive peristalsis,
3. a lesion at or near the pylorus, and
4. delayed gastric emptying.

Endoscopy may demonstrate the cause of the obstruction and its degree.

Management

The stomach is washed out to remove all food debris and then aspirated 2–4 hourly for 3–4 days at which point, if the volume of aspirate has decreased, it may be possible to allow fluids by mouth. Dehydration and metabolic alkalosis must be treated. A multivitamin preparation should be given by injection to all but the mildest cases. The majority of patients will be greatly improved by these methods; the volume of the gastric aspirate steadily declines, and the size of the stomach returns to near normal. Relief of obstruction by conservative measures provides an opportunity to complete investigation and to render the patient as fit as possible for subsequent elective surgery.

ZOLLINGER-ELLISON SYNDROME (GASTRINOMA)

This is a rare disorder in which severe peptic ulceration occurs due usually to an adenoma or hyperplasia of the islets of the pancreas secreting large amounts of gastrin which stimulates the parietal cells of the stomach excessively. Tumours may also be located in the stomach or duodenum. The tumour may be benign or malignant. The acid output may be so great that the 'acid tide' may reach the upper small intestine, reducing the luminal pH to 2 or less; at this pH, pancreatic lipase is inactivated and bile acids may be precipitated, causing diarrhoea and steatorrhoea. Excessive gastric secretion results in large volumes on aspiration under 'basal' conditions. Pentagastrin does not increase the secretory rate much above 'basal' values, since the stomach is already continuously secreting at or near maximal rates.

Clinical features

The ulcers are often multiple and severe and may occur in unusual sites such as the jejunum or the oesophagus. The history is usually short and bleeding and perforation are common. The syndrome may present in the form of severe recurrent ulceration following a standard operation for peptic ulcer, the underlying cause not having been recognised.

Investigation

About one-third of the patients have multiple endocrine neoplasia Type 1 (MEN I) involving parathyroid, pituitary and pancreas.

The diagnosis should be suspected in all patients with unusual or severe peptic ulceration, especially if the barium meal examination shows abnormally coarse gastric mucosal folds. It may be confirmed by finding very high levels of gastrin in the circulation.

Management

Theoretically the condition should be cured by removing the tumour, but this may not be possible because of its size or diffuse nature. In these circumstances it is necessary to eliminate, or very greatly reduce, acid secretion so that the ulcers may heal. In most patients continuous therapy with omeprazole is effective, but larger doses than those used to treat duodenal ulcer are required. In unresponsive patients, total gastrectomy is necessary.

LATE COMPLICATIONS FOLLOWING GASTRIC SURGERY

Although most operations carried out for the relief of peptic ulcer are successful, 10% of patients will develop complications months or years afterwards. Some of these, such as anaemia and nutritional impairment, develop insidiously, so that patients who have had an operation on the stomach should be reviewed at least once a year.

Recurrent ulcer ('stomal' ulcer). When this occurs after surgery for duodenal ulcer, it is usually due to insufficient reduction of the secretory capacity of the stomach because of incomplete vagotomy or inadequate gastrectomy. A *jejunal ulcer* develops just distal to the jejunogastric anastomosis, because the jejunal mucosa is more susceptible to acid-pepsin digestion than gastric or duodenal mucosa. About 15% of patients develop recurrent ulcer after highly selective vagotomy but the operation has the virtue of being free from the side-effects associated with resection, truncal vagotomy or drainage procedures.

After months or years of freedom following the operation, ulcer pain recurs or the patient may present with melaena or severe anaemia without any dyspeptic symptoms. Occasionally, perforation occurs. Rarely a jejunal ulcer penetrates the colon causing a *gastro-jejunal-colic fistula*. Bacterial contamination of the small bowel follows causing diarrhoea, malabsorption and wasting. The fistula can be demonstrated by barium enema.

Recurrent ulcer uncomplicated by perforation or fistula is best diagnosed by endoscopy which will also reveal the occasional ulcer due to an unabsorbed suture which can be removed endoscopically. Recurrent ulcer can be treated by H_2-receptor antagonists or omeprazole but if this fails, a more radical surgical procedure may be necessary.

Biliary gastritis. This is the result of reflux of bile into the stomach through a drainage stoma. It may be symptomless and observed only on routine post-operative endoscopy. There may be epigastric discomfort, nausea, heartburn or vomiting of bile. Reduction in fluid intake, the eating of meals dry, avoidance of alcohol and stopping smoking may bring relief. Drugs are of little value but some patients have symptoms due to delayed gastric emptying which are helped by metoclopramide or domperidone (p. 442). Revisional surgery may be required if dietetic measures fail and when there is a mechanical cause for the reflux.

Post-cibal syndromes. These are mainly associated with gastrectomy and have become less frequent with the more general adoption of operations in the vagus.

1. *The small stomach syndrome.* Discomfort and distension with meals leads to diminished intake and weight loss or failure to regain weight. High energy small meals and, in some cases, revisional surgery are indicated.

2. *Dumping syndrome.* After a meal and particularly after hot sweet foods, there is a feeling of intense

drowsiness with weakness and nausea; there may also be flushing and palpitations. The syndrome usually improves with time. The ingestion of small dry meals with the avoidance of fluids at meal times is often of value. Occasionally further surgery may be necessary.

3. *Hypoglycaemia*. Rarely, one or two hours after a meal, the patient experiences attacks of weakness, tremor and faintness. The hypoglycaemia responsible for these symptoms can be relieved by glucose or barley sugar. Guar gum has also been used successfully in some patients.

Diarrhoea. This may occur after any operation on the stomach, but especially after truncal vagotomy when most patients report some looseness of the stools. Moderate or severe diarrhoea occurs in about 10% and is characteristically episodic, several watery stools being passed daily for several days. A striking feature is the sense of urgency associated with the diarrhoea; defecation may be precipitate, and the patient becomes worried because of the fear of soiling. Loperamide (1 tablet 3 times daily or more frequently) or codeine (30–60 mg 3 times daily) should be tried. Mild steatorrhoea is common after all ulcer operations and does not require treatment.

Anaemia. It is a common sequel to operations on the stomach, particularly partial gastrectomy, due to inadequate absorption of iron, or to recurrent minor blood loss from gastritis or oesophagitis. Its incidence increases in the first 10 years as the stores of iron are exhausted. The occurrence of anaemia reflects the adequacy of postoperative supervision, because it is preventable by and responds to the administration of iron. Megaloblastic anaemia may also occur (p. 711) from vitamin B_{12} or folate deficiency.

Nutritional impairment and osteomalacia. In a small proportion of patients there is some nutritional impairment following gastric surgery, and this increases with the extent of any resection. Severe weight loss is its most common manifestation. There may also be malabsorption with steatorrhoea and osteomalacia which may develop for the first time 15 to 20 years after partial gastrectomy, and may present as bone pain or as a pathological fracture. Treatment is described on page 69.

GASTRITIS

Gastritis signifies an acute or chronic inflammation of the stomach. Knowledge of the changes that occur in the gastric mucosa has been obtained by direct studies of the gastric mucosa in patients with gastrostomies, by gastroscopic observation and by histological examination of specimens removed at operation, biopsy or autopsy. There is poor agreement between these three approaches, so that the classification of gastritis is difficult. If histological specimens are examined, it is very rare to find a normal stomach completely free from any signs of inflammation. In this sense 'gastritis' is almost an invariable finding in adults. However, there are gross departures from this 'normal' state of affairs, even if they do not give rise to symptoms. For these reasons the condition is best defined in histological terms as acute or chronic gastritis.

ACUTE GASTRITIS

This is most commonly caused by the ingestion of aspirin, anti-inflammatory drugs and probably alcohol. It is also caused by the regurgitation of bile into the stomach, especially after gastric surgery. Macroscopically, there is engorgement of the mucosa with oedema and erosions or an acute haemorrhagic gastritis (p. 436). Microscopically there is loss of the surface epithelium, hyperaemia and some infiltration with inflammatory cells.

Clinical features
Acute gastritis may be asymptomatic. In some patients, there is anorexia, nausea, epigastric pain and heartburn. If gastritis persists, a slow loss of blood may lead to anaemia. The condition is diagnosed by gastroscopy.

Management
Drug consumption should be reviewed with a view to omitting or reducing drugs which are known to cause gastric mucosal damage. Alcohol should be avoided.

CHRONIC GASTRITIS

The classification is histological; there are three stages which are progressive over many years. In *chronic superficial gastritis*, the mucosa is normal in thickness and there is patchy infiltration of lymphocytes and plasma cells. In *atrophic gastritis* there is a reduction of the specialised cells in the glands of the body and of mucous cells in the pyloric glands. There is epithelial metaplasia and an infiltrate of lymphocytes and plasma cells. In *gastric atrophy* the thickness of the mucosa is reduced, metaplasia is common but round cell infiltration is slight.

Type A gastritis (chronic fundal gastritis)
In pernicious anaemia and other autoimmune dis-

orders, chronic gastritis affecting the body mucosa is due to an immunological process and circulating antibodies to parietal cells and intrinsic factor are frequently found. Chronic gastritis is common in peptic ulcer, gastric cancer and after gastric surgery. In these instances, the gastritis is thought not to be immunological.

Type B gastritis (chronic antral gastritis)

Gastritis localised to the antrum is almost always associated with the presence of *Helicobacter pylori*, a bacillus specially adapted for survival in the hostile environment of the gastroduodenal mucosa. It can be identified in biopsy material lying in close apposition to the epithelial cells of the antrum, protected from acid peptic digestion by the overlying layer of mucus. It is present, associated with antral gastritis in almost 90% of patients with duodenal ulcer and in about 60% of patients with gastric ulcer. It is found also in areas of gastric metaplasia that commonly occur in the duodenal mucosa close to a duodenal ulcer. The strong association of *H. pylori* with antral gastritis on the one hand and duodenal ulcer on the other hand suggests that the organism must play a causative role in both conditions. An alternative view is that *H. pylori* occurs merely as a secondary invader of already damaged epithelium and has no clinical importance. The former view is favoured.

Clinical features

The condition may be asymptomatic or present with features similar to peptic ulceration. Its importance lies in its association with the disorders noted above.

Investigation

The diagnosis may be suspected from the absence of mucosal folds at barium meal examination or from the gastroscopic appearances. However, the diagnosis is confirmed only by gastric biopsy.

Management

Bismuth compounds (Table 10.2) may be used for antral gastritis. Symptomatic relief may be obtained from antacids. No treatment is known to stimulate regeneration of the mucosa.

NON-ULCER DYSPEPSIA (SYNONYMS: FUNCTIONAL DYSPEPSIA; NERVOUS DYSPEPSIA; NON-ORGANIC DYSPEPSIA)

Dyspepsia is a term commonly used as a collective description for a variety of alimentary symptoms; the term 'ulcer dyspepsia', for example, is often used as an

---

SYMPTOMS INCLUDED IN THE TERM DYSPEPSIA

- Upper abdominal pain which may or not be related to food
- Gastro-oesophageal regurgitation and heartburn
- Anorexia nausea and vomiting
- Early repletion or satiety after meals
- A sense of abdominal distension or 'bloating'
- Flatulence (burping, belching) and aerophagy

---

inclusive term for the symptoms of peptic ulcer. The symptoms are listed in the information box above.

Although dyspepsia is most commonly associated with organic disease of the upper alimentary tract such as peptic oesophagitis, peptic ulcer or gastric carcinoma, symptoms such as anorexia, nausea and vomiting with or without upper abdominal pain may be due to many other causes. These are included in the information box below.

OTHER CAUSES ASSOCIATED WITH DYSPEPSIA

- Other organic disease of the digestive system
  Pancreatic disease
  Crohn's disease
  Colon cancer etc
- Systemic disease
  Cardiac renal or hepatic failure
  Extra-abdominal malignancy such as lung carcinoma
- Medication
  Non-steroidal anti-inflammatory drugs (NSAIDs)
  Digoxin
  Analgesics
  Antibiotics
- Alcohol abuse
- Pregnancy
- Psychiatric disorders
  Depressive illness
  Anxiety neurosis

When all such causes are excluded there remains a large group of patients who complain of persistent dyspepsia for which no cause can be found. Such patients are considered to have *non-ulcer* or *functional dyspepsia*, and it is believed that the symptoms are generated by disturbances in the motor function of the alimentary tract, analogous to the motility disturbances that occur in the Irritable Bowel Syndrome (p. 477); indeed the symptoms of both disorders may be present suggesting a generalised motility disorder.

'Flatulent dyspepsia' is often used as a collective term for symptoms such as early satiety, flatulence, bloating and belching with or without abdominal pain. These symptoms are almost always due to functional disorder, sometimes due to organic disease such as Crohn's disease and rarely to biliary disorders (p. 540).

Aetiology

Although the exact cause is not known it is generally agreed that the ultimate cause may be a combination of psychological, neurological and gut peptide factors. Patients are usually young (< 40 years) and women are affected twice as commonly as men.

Clinical features

Abdominal pain is associated with a variable combination of other 'dyspeptic' symptoms the commonest being nausea and bloating after meals. Morning symptoms are characteristic and pain or nausea may occur on waking. Direct enquiry may elicit symptoms suggestive of colonic dysmotility such as pellet-like stools or a sense of incomplete rectal evacuation on defaecation.

Generally the problem is to exclude peptic ulcer disease; in older subjects intra-abdominal malignancy is the prime concern. Features that distinguish functional dyspepsia from organic disease are listed in the information box below.

DISTINGUISHING FEATURES OF FUNCTIONAL DYSPEPSIA

- Pain/discomfort is not episodic but tends to occur daily for long periods at a time.
- Pain may persist throughout the entire day from morning to night, unaffected by food antacids or bowel movement; food may provoke pain.
- Pain is diffuse, described by sweeping movements of the hands over the abdomen, and may be referred to more than one site.
- Night pain, waking the patient from sleep, is rare.
- When vomiting occurs it brings no relief from pain, and the patient cannot eat for hours afterwards; by contrast vomiting almost always relieves pain in ulcer subjects and they can eat almost immediately.

There are no diagnostic signs, apart perhaps from inappropriate tenderness on abdominal palpation. Symptoms appear disproportionate to clinical well-being and there is no weight loss. Patients may appear anxious and distraught. It is often possible to detect associated psychological factors. Many patients are self-admitted 'worriers', concerned about finance, employment or family affairs. Older subjects may be fearful of developing cancer. Often there is a history of previous psychotropic medication or a personal or family history of 'nerves'.

A drug history should be taken and the possibility of a depressive illness should be considered. In young women pregnancy should be ruled out before radiological studies are undertaken.

Alcohol abuse should be suspected when nausea and retching are prominent especially in the mornings. The detection of spider naevi or a palpable liver are suggestive and the findings of abnormal liver function tests or a raised mean corpuscular volume (MCV) in the blood count support the diagnosis.

Investigation

The history will often suggest the diagnosis, but especially in older subjects a barium meal or endoscopy should be carried out to resolve doubt. A blood count, sedimentation rate and tests for faecal occult blood should be carried out to help exclude organic disease.

Management

The most important element is explanation and reassurance. Possible psychological factors should be explored making the concept of psychological influences on gut function seem respectable and acceptable to the patient.

Cigarette smoking and alcohol abuse should be discouraged, and sensible dietary advice may be necessary.

Drug treatment is not especially successful, but merits trial. Antacids are sometimes helpful. Prokinetic drugs such as metaclopramide (10 mg t.i.d.) or domperidone (10–20 mg t.i.d.) may be given before meals if nausea, vomiting or bloating are prominent. Metaclopramide may induce extrapyramidal side-effects including Tardive dyskinesia in young subjects. H_2-receptor antagonist drugs may be tried if night pain or heartburn are troublesome. Pirenzepine (50 mg b.d.) is sometimes helpful.

When symptoms can be associated with an identifiable cause of stress (e.g. impending marriage or divorce, financial or employment difficulties, etc.) they may resolve with appropriate counselling. In many cases however symptoms may persist or recur over a lifetime so that if major psychological difficulties are identified, formal psychotherapy should be considered.

CARCINOMA OF THE STOMACH

The incidence of this tumour varies considerably in different parts of the world – it is frequent in Japan but relatively uncommon in the USA. Its incidence is falling in many countries. Japanese immigrants to America have a lower incidence than in Japan indicating the possible importance of environmental factors such as trace elements in water, or differences in methods of food preparation. It has been suggested that nitrites, often used as preservatives in food, can be converted to the carcinogens nitrosamines in the milieu of the stomach. Patients with pernicious anaemia have an increased risk of developing gastric cancer and this may extend to gastric atrophy from other causes. In particular there is an increased incidence of cancer of the stomach after partial gastrectomy or gastroenterostomy.

Pathology

Almost 60% of all gastric cancers occur at the pylorus or in the antrum; the lesion does not spread to the duodenum. Such growths may produce symptoms of obstruction to the gastric outlet. Cancer of the body of the stomach occurs in 20–30% of cases and often produces a fungating ulcerating mass. In 5–20% of cases, the tumour is cardiac and produces dysphagia. Least common is a diffuse infiltrating scirrhous lesion spreading throughout the body of the stomach and producing the 'leather-bottle stomach'.

Gastric dysplasia is the term applied to precancerous lesions of the stomach; it is recognised by cytological changes in the epithelial cells. *Early gastric cancer* is defined as cancer confined to the mucosa or mucosa and submucosa regardless of the presence of lymph node metastasis. The lesion may be represented only by a depressed area with obliteration or distortion of the mucosal folds, by irregular ulceration on an elevated base, or by a small polypoid lesion. Such changes can be seen and a biopsy taken during gastroscopy at a stage when the cancer is potentially curable.

The tumour is an adenocarcinoma of intestinal or diffuse type. The intestinal type has well-defined cells and a clear margin and it is this type which has shown a fall in incidence in several countries. The diffuse type consists of clusters of cells which spread widely within the mucosa. The tumour spreads by extension through the stomach wall, by lymphatic permeation and by embolism via the portal vein to the liver and thence to the systemic bloodstream.

Gastric carcinoma may present as a malignant ulcer, and whether it is then the result of malignant transformation of a benign ulcer is debatable. A chronic peptic ulcer rarely becomes malignant and malignant ulcers, however long they have been present, have always been malignant. The problem in the individual patient is to decide whether a chronic gastric ulcer is benign or malignant.

Clinical features

Loss of appetite, slight nausea and discomfort after meals occurring for the first time in middle age should always arouse suspicion. If the diagnosis is to be made early such patients require careful investigation. Unfortunately, the majority of patients have advanced gastric carcinoma before they seek advice. In some there have been no symptoms; in others symptoms have been present for 6 months or even a year. Dyspepsia, which is at first vague, becomes troublesome with increasing anorexia and nausea, discomfort or pain, vomiting and weight loss. There may be cachexia and pallor, a mass may be palpable or peristalsis visible. The abdomen may be distended by ascites from peritoneal metastases. Sometimes it is acanthosis nigricans (p. 236) or the presence of metastases in the liver, pelvis or scalene lymph nodes which first brings the patient to the physician.

Carcinoma of the stomach should always be considered as a cause of unexplained iron deficiency anaemia in the middle-aged person or as an uncommon cause of haematemesis or melaena. Tumours at the cardia may cause dysphagia, and tumours at the gastric outlet may cause vomiting. In the infiltrating type of tumour, diarrhoea may occur because of rapid emptying from the stomach.

Investigation

Early curable cancer is usually missed by a barium meal examination unless a double-contrast study is carried out to show distortion of the mucosal pattern. The only method of establishing a positive diagnosis is by gastroscopy and biopsy of suspicious areas. These procedures are also necessary to distinguish malignant from benign gastric ulceration. The commonest appearance at barium meal is a filling defect in the antrum or body of the stomach (Fig. 10.7). In the rare diffuse infiltrating carcinoma, the radiograph is that of a rigid tube through which the barium pours rapidly into the intestine. If dysphagia is the presenting symptom, a lesion in the cardia will probably be found, but symptomless lesions in this area can be easily missed. Exfoliative cytology is sometimes used for diagnosis.

Management

The curative treatment is gastrectomy, but it is usually only at laparotomy that the possibility of resection can be decided. About one-third of patients coming to operation are found to have tumours capable of removal; in the remainder it is possible to perform only a palliative procedure. This is worthwhile if pyloric obstruction is present even if there are secondary deposits; such an operation relieves distressing vomiting and gives the patient some comfort.

A total gastrectomy may be required for tumours involving the upper part of the stomach. Careful preoperative treatment is essential including, the restoration of fluid and electrolyte balance and the correction

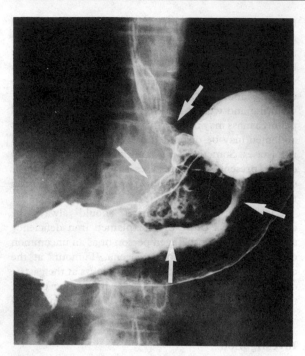

Fig. 10.7 Carcinoma of the stomach. (Courtesy of Dr G.M. Fraser.)

of anaemia. Every effort should be made to improve nutrition, if necessary by parenteral or enteral feeding.

A small proportion of patients with cancer of the stomach obtain worthwhile remission with cytotoxic drugs.

Prognosis

The prognosis in carcinoma of the stomach is poor and has shown little improvement in the last 40 years. After an apparently successful resection, the 5-year survival rate is in the region of 20%. The overall 5-year survival rate is 5%. However for early gastric cancer, the 5-year survival rate is 85%. Thus, pending an entirely new approach to the problem, the only means currently available by which the prognosis can be improved is the detection of gastric cancer when it is at a curable stage; this requires a vigorous approach to the problem of dyspepsia in the middle-aged, including careful radiological and endoscopic examination and the critical follow-up of doubtful abnormalities.

MALIGNANT ASCITES

Carcinoma of the stomach and other intra-abdominal tumours, including carcinoma of the colon and ovary, may be associated with the exudation of fluid into the peritoneal cavity. This follows the deposition of malignant cells on the peritoneal surface and is a sign of gross spread of the disease. The fluid is rich in protein and its sediment contains malignant cells which may be identifiable on microscopy.

Treatment is palliative. Relief of abdominal distension can be obtained by paracentesis, whilst instillation of an antimitotic agent such as methotrexate may slow the rate of reaccumulation.

DISEASES OF THE SMALL INTESTINE

NORMAL ABSORPTION AND ITS MEASUREMENT

FAT

The digestion and absorption of fat takes place predominantly in the duodenum and upper jejunum. Dietary fat occurs largely in the form of insoluble long-chain triglycerides which are emulsified mechanically in the stomach and by detergents, mainly bile acids, in the small intestine. Bile acids are re-absorbed by the terminal ileum, returned to the liver and re-excreted in the bile – an enterohepatic circulation. Pancreatic lipase hydrolyses the triglycerides to monoglyceride and fatty acids. Pancreatic bicarbonate is required to maintain the optimum pH for this hydrolysis and for the next step in fat absorption, the solubilisation of the mono-glycerides and fatty acids by bile acids. This consists of their incorporation into micelles which orientate the fatty acid and monoglyceride in such a way that they can be presented to the intestinal mucosal cell for absorption (Fig. 10.8). After absorption by the enterocyte the monoglycerides are re-esterified with fatty acids to form triglycerides which are coated with phospholipid and protein to form chylomicrons or converted into very low density lipoproteins. Both chylomicrons and the lipoproteins leave the cell via the lymphatic system and are transported into the blood.

CARBOHYDRATE

Dietary carbohydrate is in the form of starch (60%), lactose (10%) and sucrose (30%). These are digested by saccharidases to glucose, galactose and fructose. Glucose and galactose are absorbed into the cell by active transport mechanisms, the process requiring sodium ions and energy. The fructose molecule is too large to move across the cell membrane by simple diffusion and it is thought that its absorption might be facilitated by a carrier.

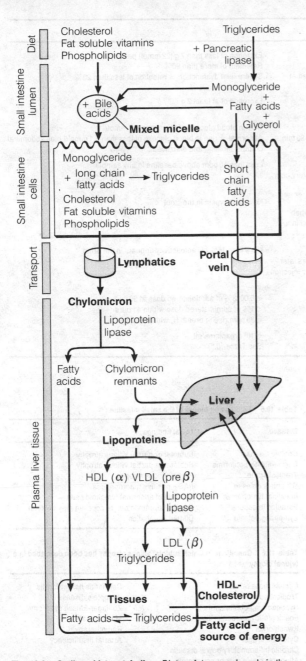

Fig. 10.8 Outline of fat metabolism. Dietary fat occurs largely in the form of long-chain triglycerides which are hydrolysed by pancreatic lipase to monoglyceride and fatty acids which are then made soluble and absorbed as micelles. In the cells of the small intestine monoglycerides and fatty acids are re-esterified into triglycerides which are coated with phospholipid and protein to form chylomicrons to be transported by the lymphatics to the blood. Their metabolism thereafter is described on page 489.

PROTEIN

Initial hydrolysis of dietary protein molecules is performed by gastric pepsin and pancreatic enzymes. Further hydrolysis of peptides occurs at the brush border and a mixture of peptides and amino acids is absorbed into the cell. A large amount of protein enters the lumen of the gastrointestinal tract each day, derived from sources other than dietary such as various secretions, desquamated cells and the exudation of plasma proteins. These are absorbed by the same mechanisms as dietary protein.

VITAMINS

The fat soluble vitamins A, D and K are incorporated into micelles and are then absorbed by passive diffusion, mainly in the proximal jejunum.

Folic acid is absorbed by an active process throughout the length of the small intestine.

Vitamin B_{12} is bound to gastric intrinsic factor and to a lesser extent to 'R' protein. It proceeds along the intestine to the terminal ileum where B_{12} binds to a specific receptor and is absorbed.

MALABSORPTION

A number of disorders result in malabsorption of one or more of the essential nutrients, electrolytes, minerals or vitamins. Some or all of the following features may ensue: diarrhoea, abdominal pain and distension, loss of weight, anaemia, or other evidence of specific deficiency. However, some patients complain only of vague ill-health, and the diagnosis may not be made for many years.

Aetiology

Malabsorptive disorders can be classified according to whether the primary disturbance is within the intestinal lumen due to insufficiency of digestive enzymes or bile acids, or within the intestinal mucosa. The classification is listed in the information box (p. 446).

Investigation

The commonly used absorption tests are detailed in Table 10.4. In addition low serum levels of folate, iron, calcium and vitamin B_{12} are often used to infer malabsorption of these substances.

The barium follow-through examination is helpful in two ways. It may show non-specific features such as dilated loops with flocculation and segmentation of barium and it may show specific structural abnor-

Table 10.4   Tests for malabsorption

		Normal
Fat	*Measurement of fat in a 5-day collection of stool*	Excretion of less than 7 g (22 mmol) per day
	SeHCAT test	Retention of more than 90%
	This synthetic bile acid is given orally and its retention measured at 7 days by whole body counting	Severe ileal dysfunction = retention of less than 20%
Carbohydrate	*Xylose absorption test*	Excretion of at least 2 g
	5 g xylose is given orally, and the urine is collected for 5 hours	
	Lactose tolerance test	Rise in blood glucose of more than 1.1 mmol/l
	50 g lactose is given orally, and blood samples are taken every 20 min for 2 hours	Abnormal = rise in blood glucose of less than 1.1 mmol/l plus abdominal cramps, bloating and diarrhoea
	Hydrogen breath test	Less than 10 ppm above baseline in any sample
	50 g lactose is given orally and breath hydrogen is measured every hour for 4 hours (see below)	
Protein	*Faecal clearance of endogenous α_1-antitrypsin*	No α_1-antitrypsin in the stool
	This normal serum protein is excreted unchanged in the stool when there is any protein loss into the stool and is therefore measured in a 3-day collection of stool	
Vitamins	*Vitamin B_{12} absorption*	More than 16% of radioactivity appears in the urine
	0.5 μg of radiolabelled vitamin B_{12} is given orally followed 2 hours later by 1000 μg of non-radioactive vitamin B_{12} given by intramuscular injection. Urine is collected for 24 hours	
Breath tests	^{14}C-Xylose	< 0.0013% of administered dose at 30 min
	Cholyl-^{14}C-glycine	< 1% of administered dose within 4 hours
	Lactose H_2 (50 g orally)	< 20 ppm rise in breath H_2 within 3 hours
Small intestinal culture		< 10^5 organisms/ml
Small intestinal biopsy		(See Table 10.5)

CLASSIFICATION OF MALABSORPTIVE DISORDERS

Disorders of intraluminal digestion
Pancreatic insufficiency
   chronic pancreatitis
   cystic fibrosis
   carcinoma of the pancreas
Deficiency of bile acids
   interruption of the enterohepatic circulation of bile acids due to resection or disease of the terminal ileum
   colonisation of the small intestine with bacteria which deconjugate bile acid which reduces their efficiency (stagnant loop syndrome)
Uncoordinated gastric emptying which delivers gastric chyme too quickly to the intestine
   gastroenterostomy
   partial gastrectomy

Disorders of transport in the intestinal mucosa
Generalised mucosal abnormalities. The mucosa is abnormal histologically
   coeliac disease
   tropical sprue
   lymphoma
   Whipple's disease
   radiation enteritis
Malabsorption of specific substances. The mucosa is normal histologically
   lactose deficiency

Table 10.5   Findings on biopsy of the small intestine

Disease	Usual findings
Coeliac disease	Subtotal or partial villous atrophy
Dermatitis herpetiformis	Subtotal or partial villous atrophy
Tropical sprue	Partial villous atrophy
Whipple's disease	PAS – positive macrophages
Intestinal lymphomas	Infiltrate of abnormal lymphoid cells
Parasitic infections	Giardia, strongyloides or coccidia may be seen
Lymphangiectasia	Dilated lymphatics

Table 10.6   Conditions in which subtotal villous atrophy has been described in a jejunal biopsy

Coeliac disease	Dermatitis herpetiformis
Tropical sprue	Whipple's disease
Hypogammaglobulinaemia	Zollinger-Ellison syndrome
Eosinophilic gastroenteritis	Mastocytosis
Kwashiorkor	Radiotherapy
Cytotoxic drugs	Arterial insufficiency
Chronic inflammatory bowel disease	
Allergy to cow's milk or soy protein	
Infections with bacteria, viruses or giardia in children	

malities which can cause malabsorption, e.g. Crohn's disease (p. 452), diverticula (p. 464) or strictures.

Biopsy of the jejunum with a Crosby capsule or of the duodenum via an endoscope is important in making the diagnosis of coeliac disease and valuable diagnostic information may be found in other disorders (Tables 10.5 and 10.6). If the intestinal biopsy is normal, pancreatic function tests may be necessary.

COELIAC DISEASE

Aetiology

Coeliac disease is characterised by an abnormal mucosa in the small intestine induced by a component of the gluten protein of wheat. Barley, rye and probably oats are also injurious. Local immunological responses to the gluten component are responsible for the damage to the mucosa. Antibodies to gliadin are found in the peripheral blood and splenic atrophy is common. The disease shows a high association with the histocompatibility antigens B8 DR3, DR7 and DQ2 and a family history of the disorder may be obtained in up to a quarter of patients.

Incidence

The incidence of the disease in Great Britain is 1 in 2000 to 1 in 8000, but may be higher because many cases remain undiagnosed.

Pathology

The mucosa of the normal small intestine has finger-like or leaf-like villi (Fig. 10.9A) which are seen as

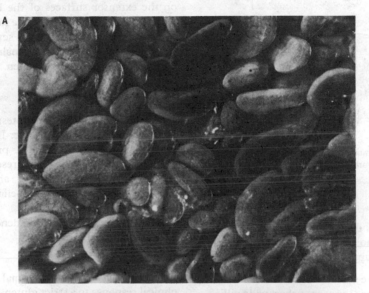

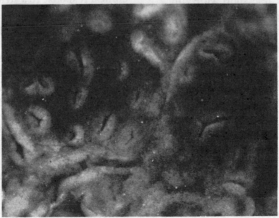

Fig. 10.9 Jejunal mucosa. A. Normal. Dissecting microscopy. The surface shows finger and leaf forms of villi. **B. Subtotal villous atrophy.** Dissecting microscopy. The crypts open directly onto the surface which appears flat.

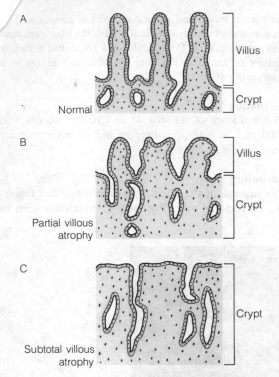

Fig. 10.10 Pathology of the mucosa at the duodenojejunal flexure.
A. Partial villous atrophy. **B.** Partial villous atrophy. **C.** Subtotal villous atrophy.

histological sections in Figure 10.10. In coeliac disease the mucosa at the duodeno-jejunal flexure is always abnormal and the abnormality extends distally for a variable distance. The appearance is either that of:

1. convolutions, like the surface of the cerebrum, which, when sectioned, appear as short wide villi ('partial villous atrophy' Fig. 10.10)
2. a totally flat mucosa which is termed 'subtotal villous atrophy' (Fig. 10.9**B** and Fig. 10.10).

In addition, the height of the epithelial cells is reduced and there is an increase in the number of plasma cells in the lamina propria. The appearance may be patchy. All these histological features return towards normality during treatment with a gluten-free diet.

Clinical features
The disease usually presents in children under 2 years old and within 6 months of starting cereals. The child ceases to thrive and becomes fractious and irritable. The stools become voluminous and pale and the abdomen distended. As the disorder progresses growth is retarded and anaemia develops.

Less commonly the disorder may manifest for the

first time in adult life and occasionally even in the elderly when the presenting symptoms range from those of a mild anaemia and listlessness of long duration to a florid malabsorptive state developing rapidly over a period of weeks. The commonest features are diarrhoea, weight loss and anaemia, usually due to combined deficiency of folate and iron. There may be peripheral neuropathy, evidence of vitamin deficiency or hypo-proteinaemia, oedema from hypoprothrombinaemia, and bone pain and tetany due to hypocalcaemia secondary to vitamin D deficiency. Other clinical features are finger-clubbing, glossitis, angular stomatitis, skin pigmentation, dermatitis herpetiformis, amenorrhoea and infertility.

Dermatitis herpetiformis consists of itchy red papules on the extensor surfaces of the body together with a jejunal mucosa which shows the same features as coeliac disease but the changes are less severe.

On examination features of malnutrition and anaemia are common and the abdomen may be slightly dis-tended and tympanitic.

Lymphoma
Lymphoma of the small intestine is a recognised complication of coeliac disease. In contrast to primary lymphoma of the intestine it primarily involves the jejunum. The complication presents with a return of weight loss, diarrhoea and abdominal pain after previous good control of the coeliac disease; obstruction or perforation may occur.

There is an increased incidence of gastrointestinal carcinoma in coeliac disease.

Investigation
In adults, an abnormal jejunal biopsy and a good clinical response to a strict gluten-free diet are sufficient for the diagnosis to be made. In children more strict diagnostic criteria are applied because there are other common causes of subtotal villous atrophy such as milk-protein intolerance, giardiasis and following gut viral infections. An initial biopsy is followed by a gluten-free diet and once the biopsy returns to normal as indicated by a second biopsy a gluten challenge (an oral load of gluten) is given followed by a further biopsy.

In untreated coeliac disease, tests of carbohydrate, fat and vitamin absorption are frequently abnormal but return to normal after treatment with a gluten-free diet. These tests are not essential for diagnosis but indicate deficiencies which often require treatment during the initial weeks of the diet.

Management
A gluten-free diet must be taken indefinitely. This

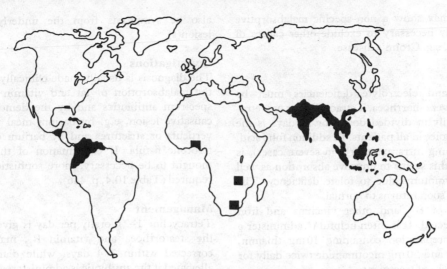

Fig. 10.11   The geographical distribution of tropical sprue showing areas principally affected by the disease.

requires the exclusion of wheat, rye, oats and barley, and imposes severe restrictions which must be fully explained to the patient. Booklets, produced by Coeliac Societies in many countries containing diet sheets and recipes for gluten-free flour, are of great value in this respect. Initially frequent dietary counselling is required to make sure the diet is being observed. Mineral and vitamin supplements are also given when indicated but are seldom necessary if a strict gluten-free diet is adhered to.

TROPICAL SPRUE

Tropical sprue is the malabsorption occurring in a patient in or from the tropics, in the absence of other intestinal disease or parasites. Its manifestations resemble those of coeliac disease.

Aetiology

The prevalence of sprue in certain well-defined tropical countries and localities, and its epidemiological pattern, including occasional epidemics suggest that an infective agent may be involved. The disease occurs mainly in the West Indies and in Asia, including Sri Lanka, Southern India, Malaysia and Indonesia (Fig. 10.11).

Pathology

The changes closely resemble those of coeliac disease although partial villous atrophy rather than subtotal villous atrophy is the usual lesion. Mild changes in the jejunal mucosa are common in asymptomatic indigenous peoples, without gross malabsorption,

throughout the tropics (tropical enteropathy), and for this reason the diagnosis of tropical sprue is made on a combination of clinical and laboratory findings as well as the jejunal histology.

Clinical features

There is diarrhoea, abdominal distension, anorexia, fatigue and weight loss. In visitors to the tropics the onset of severe diarrhoea may be sudden and accompanied by fever. When the disorder becomes chronic the features of megaloblastic anaemia from folic acid malabsorption and subsequent deficiency are common. Remissions and relapses may occur. There may be oedema, glossitis and stomatitis. On investigation it is usual to find several of the abnormalities listed in the information box below.

LABORATORY FINDINGS IN TROPICAL SPRUE

- Steatorrhoea
- Xylose malabsorption
- Vitamin B_{12} malabsorption
- Megaloblastic anaemia
- Hypoalbuminaemia
- Partial villous atrophy on jejunal biopsy

The differential diagnosis in the indigenous population in the tropics, is from other infective, usually parasitic, causes of diarrhoea. The important differential diagnosis in visitors to the tropics is from giardiasis (p. 457) and a barium follow-through examination, which may show a non-specific malabsorptive pattern, is only necessary to exclude other causes of malabsorption, e.g. Crohn's disease.

Management

Dehydration and electrolyte deficiencies must be corrected in severe diarrhoea. Tetracycline or oxytetracycline, 1 g daily in divided doses for 28 days is the treatment of choice in all patients. In addition folic acid, 5 mg daily (10 mg intramuscularly in severe cases), is given because this seems to improve absorption as well as relieving symptoms due to folate deficiency. The jejunal mucosa soon returns to normal.

Deficiencies of B_{12} and other vitamins and iron should be corrected. It is often helpful to administer a multivitamin preparation containing 10 mg thiamin, 5 mg riboflavin and 50 mg nicotinamide twice daily for the first few weeks of treatment.

STAGNANT LOOP SYNDROME

This term is used to describe the intestinal abnormality associated with bacterial overgrowth in the small intestine and causing steatorrhoea and vitamin B_{12} malabsorption both of which are improved by oral broad spectrum antibiotics.

Aetiology

The normal duodenum and jejunum contain less than 10^4/ml organisms which are usually derived from the saliva. The count of coliform organisms never exceeds 10^3/ml. In the stagnant loop syndrome there may be 10^8–10^{10} organisms/ml and these are organisms which are normally found only in the colon. The stagnant loop syndrome is predisposed to by conditions which impair the normal physiological mechanisms controlling bacterial proliferation in the intestine, for example gastric acidity which acts as a barrier to orally ingested bacteria, intestinal motility which clears bacteria, and antibodies to bacteria in the intestinal juice which control bacteria. Finally bacterial proliferation is predisposed to by structural abnormalities which deliver colonic bacteria to the small intestine (fistulas) or which provide a secluded haven away from the main peristaltic stream (Table 10.7).

Clinical features

The patient presents with diarrhoea and/or steatorrhoea with anaemia due to vitamin B_{12} deficiency. These arise because of deconjugation of bile acids and utilisation of vitamin B_{12} by bacteria. There is also malabsorption of protein and carbohydrate. There may also be symptoms from the underlying intestinal lesion(s).

Investigations

The diagnosis is usually made clinically by reversal of the malabsorption of fat and vitamin B_{12} by broad spectrum antibiotics and by the demonstration of a causative lesion, e.g. by barium meal for jejunal diverticula or strictures and by barium enema for enterocolic fistula. If confirmation of the diagnosis is thought to be necessary, more sophisticated tests are required (Table 10.4, p. 446).

Management

Tetracycline 1–2 g orally per day is given and usually the steatorrhoea and vitamin B_{12} malabsorption is corrected within 3–4 days, while diarrhoea can be alleviated if the antibiotic is administered for 7–10 days every 4–6 weeks. Surgical resection is advocated when the abnormality is localised, for example stricture or fistula.

SOME SPECIFIC CAUSES OF STAGNANT LOOP SYNDROME

Jejunal diverticula

Clinical features

These are often seen on barium follow-through examinations in patients over the age of 50 years. The diverticula are usually asymptomatic but in addition to stagnant loop syndrome they may occasionally cause acute or chronic gastrointestinal bleeding or colicky abdominal pain. Obstruction and perforation may also occur.

Management

Surgery is avoided unless there is acute bleeding, obstruction or perforation.

Diabetic diarrhoea

This may result from diabetic autonomic neuropathy (p. 689) which disturbs small intestinal motility. Diarrhoea may also be due to stagnant loop syndrome, to pancreatic insufficiency or to coeliac disease which is more common in diabetes.

Clinical features

The patient complains of intermittent, watery diarrhoea which is often severe and may occur at night.

Management

Treatment is with tetracycline for stagnant loop

Table 10.7 Causes of stagnant loop syndrome

Cause	Mechanism
Gastric surgery	Reduction in acid Duodenal blind loop after Polya operation
Jejunal diverticula	Diverticula act as blind loop
Enterocolic fistulas e.g. in Crohn's disease	Delivery of colonic bacteria to small intestine via the fistula
Strictures, e.g. in Crohn's disease	Delay of the faecal stream
Extensive bowel resection	Proximity of remaining small intestine to the colon
Diabetic autonomic neuropathy	Abnormal small intestinal motility
Scleroderma	Abnormal small intestinal motility
Hypogammaglobulinaemia	Lack of antibody in the intestine

syndrome and diphenoxylate, 5 mg 3 times daily orally or loperamide, 6–8 mg daily orally for diarrhoea. Clonidine, an α_2-adrenergic agonist may also be of value.

Progressive systemic sclerosis (scleroderma)
In this condition the circular and longitudinal layers of the intestinal muscle are fibrosed and motility is abnormal.

Clinical features
Malabsorption due to stagnant loop syndrome is common. The patient may also present with intestinal pseudo-obstruction in which the clinical and radiographic features of obstruction are present but there is no mechanical cause of obstruction. There are other causes of pseudo-obstruction which are primarily disorders affecting the intestinal smooth muscle or the autonomic nervous system of the gut.

Acquired hypogammaglobulinaemia
This rare disorder is characterised by a lack of IgA IgG and IgM antibodies in the serum and secretions including the jejunal fluid.

Clinical features
Diarrhoea is common because of stagnant loop syndrome and giardiasis.

Investigations
The diagnosis is made on the low serum immunoglobulin concentrations and a jejunal biopsy which shows nodular lymphoid hyperplasia; frequently giardia are seen.

Management
Treatment consists of repeated courses of antibiotic and antigiardia therapy (p. 458) but many patients require parenteral replacement therapy with gammaglobulin to control intestinal and respiratory infections.

INTESTINAL RESECTION

Resection of the small intestine, sometimes extensive, may be necessary in Crohn's disease and in vascular insufficiency with gangrene. The main results and their causes are shown in Table 10.8.

Table 10.8 Consequences of small intestinal resection including ileal resection

	Cause
Diarrhoea	Bile acids cannot be absorbed and enter the colon where they have a purgative effect The remaining small intestine may act as a stagnant loop Fat malabsorption
Steatorrhoea	Insufficient bile acids in the upper small intestine because of their loss in the stool; fat malabsorption and fatty acid diarrhoea
Gallstones	Supersaturated bile because of diminished bile acid pool
Oxalate nephrolithiasis	Increased absorption of oxalate because calcium, which normally binds to oxalic acids, binds instead to the excess fatty acids in the intestine

Clinical features
There is severe diarrhoea with fluid and electrolyte loss in the postoperative period following extensive resections. Even when the resection involves only the terminal ileum, diarrhoea can be severe.

Investigations
The degree of ileal insufficiency can be tested by the measurement of vitamin B_{12} absorption and SeHCAT retention.

Management

Parenteral fluids and feeding may be necessary initially in the post-operative period together with the antidiarrhoeal agents loperamide (6–8 mg daily orally) and diphenoxylate (5 mg 3 times daily, orally). Subsequent oral feeding should be accompanied by attempts to reduce gastrointestinal secretions so as to reduce the volume of diarrhoea. H_2-receptor antagonists such as cimetidine, 400 mg twice daily or ranitidine 150 mg twice daily, will reduce the volume of gastric secretion and an elemental diet provides some of the nutritional requirements with minimal stimulation of digestive secretions. Cholestyramine given in a dose of 4 g orally at mealtimes acts to bind bile acids in the intestine and so prevents their cathartic effect in the colon. Supplements of calcium and all the vitamins are necessary.

CROHN'S DISEASE

This disease is characterised by localised areas of non-specific, granulomatous inflammation of the bowel. It was formerly termed regional ileitis or enteritis. However, the eponymous designation 'Crohn's disease' is preferable because the alimentary tract can be affected anywhere from the mouth to the anus, the sites most commonly involved being, in order of frequency, terminal ileum and right side of colon, colon alone, terminal ileum alone, ileum and jejunum. The term 'inflammatory bowel disease' comprises Crohn's disease and ulcerative colitis (p. 467). Crohn's disease of the colon has many similarities to ulcerative colitis and is considered mainly on page 467.

Epidemiology

In Western communities the disease has an incidence of 5–10 per 100 000 per year and a prevalence of 50 per 100 000 and is becoming more common. It affects both sexes equally and it is most common between the ages of 10 and 40 years though it can occur at any age.

Aetiology

The cause of Crohn's disease is unknown but several potential factors have been considered and these are listed in the information box below.

POSSIBLE AETIOLOGICAL FACTORS IN CROHN'S DISEASE

- Infective agents
- Oral contraceptives
- Diet, particularly sugar
- Smoking
- Abnormal immunological responses

In addition, genetic factors are important because a family history is common and furthermore, ulcerative colitis also occurs more commonly in families where Crohn's disease is present.

Pathology

The macroscopic features of Crohn's disease at different sites in the gastrointestinal tract are shown in Table 10.9.

Table 10.9   Macroscopic features of Crohn's disease at different sites

Site	Appearance
Common	
Small intestine	Narrowing, ulceration and cobblestone appearance of terminal ileum
	Strictures of jejunum and ileum
Large intestine (p. 467)	Diffuse involvement resembling ulcerative colitis
	Short segments of disease
	Strictures
	Proctitis alone
Anus	Chronic fissures
	Fistula
	Ulceration
Less common	
Duodenum	Ulceration
	Thickened folds
	Narrowing
	Stricture
Stomach	Thickening of antrum which may resemble carcinoma
Mouth	Aphthous-like ulcers
Uncommon or rare	
Oesophagus	Ulcers
	Thickened folds of epithelium
Skin	Ulceration in perineum, genitalia or abdominal wall

Characteristically the entire wall of the bowel is oedematous and thickened. There are deep ulcers which often appear as linear fissures so that the mucosa between them is described as 'cobblestoned'. The deep ulcers may penetrate through the bowel wall to initiate abscesses or fistulas. Fistulas may develop between adjacent loops of bowel or between affected segments of bowel and the bladder, uterus or vagina and may appear in the perineum.

Characteristically the changes are patchy; even when a relatively short segment of bowel is affected, the inflammatory process is interrupted by islands of normal mucosa, the change from the affected part being abrupt. A small lesion separated in this way from a major area of involvement is referred to as a 'skip' lesion. The mesenteric lymph nodes are enlarged and the mesentery thickened.

The microscopic features of Crohn's disease are of great importance because they allow confirmation of the diagnosis to be made on rectal and colonoscopic biopsies (see also Table 10.9). Non-caseating granulomas are characteristic of Crohn's disease. They consist of focal aggregates of epithelioid histiocytes and may be surrounded by lymphocytes and contain giant cells. Lymphoid aggregates or microgranulomas are also seen and when these are near to the surface of the mucosa, they often ulcerate to form tiny aphthous-like ulcers.

Clinical features

Crohn's disease is a chronic disorder with unpredictable exacerbations and remissions. The quality of life is diminished as determined by professional and personal activities but overall mortality is only twice that in the general population.

The presentation and symptoms depend in part on the site and extent of the bowel affected. The presentations which may be confused with other diseases are given in Table 10.10.

Table 10.10   Presentations of Crohn's disease which may be confused with other diseases

Presentation	Other diseases
Terminal ileitis	Confused with acute appendicitis, Yersinia enteritis
Stomach and duodenal Crohn's	Confused with peptic ulceration
Colonic or rectal Crohn's	Confused with ulcerative colitis or proctitis

Crohn's disease of the small intestine or ileum and right colon (ileocolitis) has a spectrum of features which may be considered together.

Pain is the commonest symptom and may be due either to peritoneal involvement, or obstruction, or both. Because the terminal ileum and right side of the colon are most commonly affected, pain occurs most frequently in the right lower quadrant and may be associated with local tenderness or guarding. A mass is palpable by abdominal and frequently rectal examination, being formed of inflamed loops of bowel bound together, possibly including an abscess. It may be of any size. Colicky pain, which is usually situated in the mid or lower abdomen suggests obstruction, and may be associated with nausea and vomiting and excessive borborygmi. Indeed, recurrent episodes of colic due to attacks of subacute obstruction are a prominent feature in the life history of a patient with Crohn's disease.

Exacerbations of pain may be accompanied by diarrhoea and fever. The diarrhoea is seldom as severe as in ulcerative colitis. The stools may be formed or loose, and rarely contain frank blood, mucus or pus unless the colon is involved. Steatorrhoea and malabsorption of other substances are common. Their cause is multifactorial (see the information box (right)).

CAUSES OF MALABSORPTION IN CROHN'S DISEASE

Fat
Reduction in absorptive surface due to
   Extensive disease
   Resection of bowel
Bacterial colonisation of the small intestine due to
   Strictures
   Fistulas from the colon
Interruption of the enterohepatic circulation of bile acids due to
   Disease of the terminal ileum
   Resection of the terminal ileum

Vitamin D
Due mainly to the interruption of the enterohepatic circulation of bile acids

Protein
Protein-losing enteropathy is common due to loss of protein through the ulcerated mucosa

Carbohydrate
Lactose deficiency is common due to damage to the mucosa

Vitamin B$_{12}$
Due to disease or resection of the terminal ileum

Most patients suffer from malnutrition and weight loss, contributing factors being reduced food intake because of anorexia, malabsorption and increased catabolism. Malabsorption of iron, folic acid and vitamin B$_{12}$ commonly leads to anaemia. In children growth retardation may be the principal presentation. In patients with chronic diarrhoea, sodium, potassium and water depletion are common and deficiency of magnesium and zinc may occur.

A diagnostic feature, when present, is the occurrence of anal lesions such as oedematous skin tags or perianal abscesses and fistulas; they are more common when the colon is affected.

As in ulcerative colitis (p. 467) complications outside the gastrointestinal tract occur and these are listed in the information box (p. 454).

Urinary tract problems may occur because an inflammatory mass obstructs a ureter leading to hydronephrosis; an ileovesical fistula may develop.

On examination of the abdomen, tenderness and fullness in the right iliac fossa are common and there may be a mass.

Intra-abdominal complications

Abscess is common following slow penetration of the intestine by an ulcer. It may discharge into the intestinal lumen or elsewhere into the intestine, bladder or vagina to create a fistula. Ileovesical fistula may lead to recurrent urinary infections, symptoms of cystitis, and pneumaturia may be noticed in males. Free per-

EXTRAINTESTINAL MANIFESTATIONS OF INFLAMMATORY BOWEL

Hepatic	*Ocular lesions*
Fatty change	Uveitis
Pericholangitis	Episcleritis
Granulomas	Conjunctivitis
Cirrhosis	
Amyloidosis	*Haematological disease*
Abscess	Autoimmune haemolytic
Gallstones	anaemia
Carcinoma of the biliary tree	Thrombosis
Sclerosing cholangitis	
	Vasculitis
Skin	
Erythema nodosum	*Bronchopulmonary disease*
Pyoderma gangrenosum	
	Cardiovascular disease
Aphthous stomatitis	
	Renal disease
Arthritis	Urolithiasis
Ankylosing spondylitis	Pyelonephritis
Seronegative arthritis	Amyloidosis
Clubbing of the fingers	

foration of the intestine may occur. There is an increased incidence of carcinoma of the intestine in those segments affected by Crohn's disease.

Investigation

The extent of the disease is assessed by barium meal and follow-through, and barium enema examination which may show alteration of the mucosal pattern, deep ulceration or the pathognomonic 'string sign' due to marked narrowing of a segment of affected bowel (Fig. 10.12). In long-standing cases there may be stricture for-

mation. The lesions tend to be discontinuous along the length of the bowel. Endoscopy of the stomach and duodenum is performed if the barium studies indicate any abnormality in these organs. Sigmoidoscopy and colonoscopy are usually required when the radiological abnormalities extend into the colon and indeed they may detect rectal and colonic abnormalities when the barium enema is normal. Biopsies of the rectum and/or colon often confirm the diagnosis by showing granulomas even when the mucosa is macroscopically normal. Similarly, biopsies or excision of perianal skin tags may show granulomas. Another helpful investigation is the use of white cells labelled with ^{111}In or ^{99m}Tc to locate areas of active disease by scanning.

Blood tests may show a moderate anaemia (normochromic, normocytic, or hypochromic) a raised erythrocyte sedimentation rate (ESR), a leucocytosis, abnormal liver function tests and hypoproteinaemia. Malabsorption of vitamin B_{12} can be confirmed by a Schilling test (p. 712) and when there has been intestinal resection, the absorption of SeHCAT (23-selena-25-homotaurocholate, the taurine conjugate of a synthetic bile acid) can be used to indicate whether the enterohepatic circulation of bile acids has been interrupted.

Differential diagnosis

The other common diseases in the ileocaecal region are appendicitis, appendix abscess and mesenteric adenitis. It may be impossible to decide between these possibilities in an acutely ill patient and a laparotomy may be necessary. Less commonly infections such as yersinia, tuberculosis and actinomycosis, and lymphoma may mimic Crohn's disease.

Ulcerative colitis may be difficult to distinguish from Crohn's disease if only the large bowel is diseased. The distinctive features of Crohn's disease are fistula and stricture formation but when these are absent differentiation from ulcerative colitis may depend on demonstration of the extent and location of the disease and ultimately on biopsy. The possibility of carcinoma, either in association with or as a complication of Crohn's disease or ulcerative colitis, requires consideration.

Ileocaecal tuberculosis may be indicated by evidence of tuberculosis elsewhere, for example, on the chest radiograph. A 'negative' tuberculin test is common in patients with Crohn's disease whereas it is often strongly positive in tuberculosis. Carcinoma in the caecal region may sometimes be confused with Crohn's disease. Caecal amoebiasis (p. 156), actinomycosis (p. 360) and lymphoma of the ileum or colon are rarer conditions to be considered in the differential diagnosis.

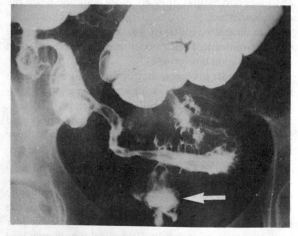

Fig. 10.12 Crohn's disease of the ileum showing marked narrowing and a fistula between the ileum and the bladder (arrow). (Courtesy of Dr G.M. Fraser.)

Management

Diet and nutrition

It is essential to restore and maintain the patient's nutritional status. This is particularly difficult but of considerable importance in children. Great care and encouragement are needed to ensure that the patient takes a high-protein, high-energy diet, if necessary by providing supplemental dietary preparations. Enteral feeding by nasogastric tube can be tolerated for prolonged periods even in the young. In addition to improving nutrition the inflammatory process may possibly benefit and the symptoms of partial obstruction may be relieved. Enteral feeding is particularly useful in the preoperative preparation of patients especially in those with external fistulas. Total parenteral nutrition may occasionally be required in very severely ill patients. In addition plasma or blood transfusion may be used to correct anaemia or severe hypoproteinaemia.

A low-fat diet or milk-free diet may improve symptoms which are due to steatorrhoea or lactose deficiency and a low-residue diet is often of value for colic and subacute obstruction. When bacterial colonisation is suspected as the cause of steatorrhoea, intermittent courses of oral antibiotics are indicated using either metronidazole and/or broad spectrum antibiotics. Supplements of iron, folic acid, calcium, zinc, vitamins D and B_{12} and electrolytes, especially potassium, will be required when deficiencies occur.

Drugs

Diarrhoea may be helped by appropriate dietary management and by treatment with corticosteroids. Diarrhoea can be treated with oral doses of di-phenoxylate 5 mg or loperamide 2 mg 3 times daily. Corticosteroids are beneficial when there is extensive active disease which does not improve with the general medical measures outlined above. However, they do not alter the long-term course of the disease. Prednisolone is given in a dose of 40–60 mg daily in divided doses for 1 or 2 weeks depending on response, and the dose gradually reduced thereafter to 10–20 mg daily for 4 to 6 weeks and then withdrawn. The drug therapy is shown in the information box (right).

Every effort should be made to stop steroids but this may be difficult in the occasional patient because of an early relapse when the dose is reduced.

Surgical treatment

Although episodes of subacute obstruction can usually be managed by nasogastric suction and intravenous feeding, a surgical operation may be necessary if such

---

DRUG THERAPY FOR CROHN'S DISEASE

- Diphenoxylate
  5 mg orally 3 times daily
- or Loperamide   } for diarrhoea
  2 mg orally 3–4 times daily
- or Codeine phosphate 30 mg orally 3–4 times daily
- or Prednisolone 40–60 mg orally daily for 1–2 weeks then reduce to 10–20 mg daily for 4–6 weeks and discontinue
- Sulphasalazine 2 gm b.d. for colonic disease only – long-term maintenance
- Azathioprine 2 mg/kg BW orally for those who fail to respond to steroids
- Metronidazole 400 mg twice daily for perineal Crohn's disease

---

attacks occur frequently. The majority of patients will require surgery at some time and often multiple operations are necessary. As the disease is multicentric extensive resections cannot eradicate it and the principle of surgery is to use only minimal resections for strictures and fistulas. Surgery may also be necessary for abscess, perforation and for extensive and severe involvement of the colon.

LACTOSE INTOLERANCE

Aetiology

This is due to a deficiency of the enzyme lactose which is normally present in the brush border of the small intestinal mucosa. Lactose cannot be hydrolysed and so it passes into the colon where it is fermented by bacteria causing discomfort and diarrhoea. In primary lactose deficiency the intestinal biopsy is normal; the deficiency is racial, being common in Blacks, Asians and South Americans. Primary deficiency is an uncommon cause of diarrhoea in Western communities because the lactose deficient individual learns to avoid milk. On the other hand secondary lactose deficiency is common in conditions associated with an abnormal intestinal biopsy, for example coeliac disease, tropical sprue and Crohn's disease of the small intestine; it also occurs transiently after gastrointestinal infections particularly giardiasis and viral gastroenteritis.

Clinical features

The patient complains of colic, abdominal distension, increased flatus and sometimes diarrhoea after ingesting milk or milk products. The diagnosis is suggested by an improvement in symptoms on lactose withdrawal. Useful investigations include the hydrogen breath test and the measurement of lactose activity in a jejunal biopsy specimen.

Management

A lactose free or a lactose-restricted diet is recommended depending on the severity of the symptoms.

PROTEIN-LOSING ENTEROPATHY

This term is used when there is excessive loss of protein into the lumen of the gastrointestinal tract, the loss being sufficient to cause hypoproteinaemia. Protein-losing enteropathy occurs in many gastrointestinal disorders but is most common in those with ulceration of the intestine, for example inflammatory bowel disease (Table 10.11). In some other disorders, e.g. Ménétrier's disease and intestinal lymphangiectasia, the consequences of protein loss are the presenting features.

Table 10.11 Diseases producing protein-losing enteropathy

Diseases of the stomach	e.g. Ménétrier's disease
Disorders of intestinal lymphatics	Intestinal lymphangiectasia, primary or secondary
Inflammatory disease of the gut	Inflammatory bowel disease Parasitic infections Blind loop syndrome
Tumours	Gastric, small intestinal, colonic, familial polyposis
Coeliac disease Tropical sprue Radiation enteritis Collagen-vascular disease Whipple's disease Allergic gastroenteropathy Constrictive pericarditis	

Clinical features

The patient has peripheral oedema and hypoproteinaemia in the presence of normal liver function, in that there is no evidence of failure of hepatic synthesis of plasma proteins, no evidence of proteinuria, and no cardiac failure.

Investigations

The diagnosis is confirmed by measurement of the faecal clearance of endogenous α_1-antitrypsin.

Management

Treatment is that of the underlying condition.

INTESTINAL LYMPHANGIECTASIA

A congenital malunion of the lymphatics causes impaired drainage of the intestinal lymphatics, and the lymph, which contains protein and fat, is discharged into the lumen of the intestine. The condition presents with oedema of the lower limbs and investigation shows hypoalbuminaemia, lymphocytopenia and steatorrhoea. The diagnosis is confirmed by intestinal biopsy which shows greatly dilated lymphatics and by lymphangiography in which a radio-opaque dye is introduced into the lymphatic system via lymphatics in the feet.

RADIATION DAMAGE TO THE INTESTINES

Radiation enteritis, colitis and proctitis are common after radiotherapy to the abdomen for malignancy.

Pathology

The rectum, sigmoid colon and terminal ileum are most frequently involved. Acute radiation damage causes an acute inflammation with crypt abscess formation. Over subsequent months and years the bowel may become fibrotic and stenotic. The underlying lesion appears to be damage to the endothelial cells of the submucosal arterioles. An endarteritis develops which causes ischaemia, atrophy of the mucosa, and ulceration which can lead to fistulas and abscesses.

Clinical features

In the acute phase which occurs within days of the commencement of radiotherapy there is abdominal pain and diarrhoea. When the rectum or colon is the main site of injury blood and mucus occur in the stool. Small intestinal injury (enteritis) is associated with nausea, colic and watery diarrhoea. The chronic phase commences 6–12 months after radiotherapy and the patient may have one or more of the problems listed in the information box below.

CHRONIC COMPLICATIONS OF RADIATION DAMAGE TO THE INTESTINE

- Proctitis
- Proctocolitis
- Small intestinal strictures
- Fistulas
  - Rectovaginal
  - Colovesical
  - Enterocolonic
- Obstruction due to strictures
- Malabsorption due to:
  - damage to terminal ileum
  - stagnant loop syndrome

On examination there is often evidence of weight loss and malnutrition and it can be difficult to decide whether this is due to recurrence of a tumour or from the radiation damage. There are no specific findings on examination of the abdomen.

Investigation

In the acute phase, the rectal changes at sigmoidoscopy resemble those of ulcerative proctitis (p. 468). The extent of the lesion is determined by sigmoidoscopy, colonoscopy and barium enema. Characteristically there are ulcers with surrounding telangiectasia. The mucosa may be granular. Barium follow-through examination is used to seek structural changes such as strictures and fistulas in the small intestine. A 5-day stool is collected to detect steatorrhoea and the absorption of vitamin B_{12} and SeHCAT is tested to determine whether the terminal ileal function is abnormal.

Management

There is no specific treatment. Diarrhoea in the acute phase is treated with codeine phosphate, diphenoxylate or loperamide in standard dosage (see information box p. 455).

The drug therapy recommended for ulcerative colitis may bring improvement for chronic disease of the colon and rectum. Antibiotics may be required for stagnant loop syndrome and nutritional supplements are usually necessary when malabsorption is present.

Surgery is to be avoided because the injured intestine is difficult to resect and anastomose, but may be necessary when obstruction supervenes.

WHIPPLE'S DISEASE

This rare disease is important because it is curable. There is characteristically infiltration of the intestinal mucosa and other organs with macrophages which stain positively with periodic acid-Schiff (PAS) stain. Electron-microscopy shows numerous bacilliform bodies indicating that the disease is probably caused by an organism which has yet to be defined.

Clinical features

The patient presents with malabsorption and steatorrhoea consequent upon the infiltration of macrophages which interfere with lymph flow and thus restrict the absorption of nutrients. There is polyarthritis, fever, weight loss, abdominal pain and respiratory symptoms. On examination lymphadenopathy, anthropathy, skin pigmentation and abdominal distension and tenderness may be identified.

The diagnosis is made by jejunal biopsy.

Management

Treatment consists of antibiotic for 1 year, tetracycline 1 g per day being the drug of choice. Relapses occur and the patient must be followed-up permanently.

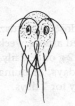

Fig. 10.13 Giardia intestinalis. Vegetative form (14 × 7 μ); cystic form (8 × 12 μ).

GIARDIASIS

Infection with the flagellate *Giardia intestinalis* (Fig. 10.13), known also as *G. lamblia*, is worldwide but commonest in the tropics.

It particularly affects children, tourists to endemic areas and immunosuppressed individuals, and may be a commensal in some individuals. The cysts remain viable in water for up to 3 months and infection occurs by ingesting contaminated water or by the faecal oral route. The flagellates attach to the mucosa of the duodenum and jejunum and cause inflammation and partial villous atrophy.

Clinical features

After an incubation period of 1–3 weeks, there is diarrhoea, abdominal pain, weakness, anorexia, nausea and vomiting. On examination there may be abdominal distension and tenderness. These features usually last for only a few days but in some individuals they may continue for weeks or months. In such patients investigation often reveals steatorrhoea, malabsorption of xylose and vitamin B_{12}, lactose intolerance and partial villous atrophy. Thus, in persons returning from the tropics with diarrhoea, it may be confused with tropical sprue, and in residents of Western communities it must be considered in the differential diagnosis of other causes of malabsorption such as coeliac disease or Crohn's disease of the small intestine.

Diagnosis

Diarrhoeal stools are obtained at 2–3-day intervals on three separate occasions and examined for cysts within an hour of collection; or they can be placed in a fixative and examined later.

The diagnosis is made most easily on examination of duodenal or jejunal fluid. Thus if endoscopy is being performed for upper gastrointestinal symptoms it is important to remember the possibility of giardiasis and to aspirate juice for microscopic examination. Alternatively, if a jejunal biopsy is obtained, giardia are usually seen on the surface of the epithelium.

Management

Treatment is with a single dose of tinidazole 40 mg/kg in the range 0.5–2 g, repeated after 1 week. Alternative therapies are metronidazole 2 g once daily for 3 days or 200 mg 3 times a day for 7 days, or quinacrine hydrochloride 100 mg 3 times a day for 7 days.

TRAVELLERS' DIARRHOEA

Aetiology

Pathogens which may be responsible for Travellers' diarrhoea are shown in the information box below. Commonly, no organism is identified.

SOME CAUSES OF TRAVELLERS' DIARRHOEA

- Enterotoxigenic *Esch. coli*
- Vibrio parahaemolyticus
- Campylobacter
- Shigella
- V. cholera – El Tor biotype
- Rota and Norwalk virus

Clinical features

An attack of diarrhoea lasting 2–5 days affects the traveller, particularly when visiting developing countries. The onset is usually abrupt and the stool is watery. Abdominal cramps, anorexia and vomiting are common and there may be fever. Examination of the abdomen usually shows no abnormality but there may be diffuse tenderness.

Management

The disorder resolves spontaneously and the use of antibiotics is discouraged because they lead to the emergence of resistant organisms. Antidiarrhoeal agents are also best avoided as the infection may last longer when they are given. Dehydration should be avoided by the use of oral rehydration supplements in children, but in adults, such measures are not usually required.

Table 10.12 Lymphomatous tumours of the small intestine

	Features
Primary	Commonly in the ileum
Secondary	The intestine is involved as part of a generalised lymphomatous process which began elsewhere in the body
In coeliac disease	Commonly in the jejunum and multicentric
Immunoproliferative (α-heavy chain disease)	Multicentric

Prevention

Doxycycline 100 mg per day is probably prophylactic for a few weeks but is not effective over longer periods. Bismuth subsalicylate 60 ml 4 times a day has also been recommended for prophylaxis.

TUMOURS OF THE SMALL INTESTINE

LYMPHOMA

Lymphomatous tumours which involve the small intestine are shown in Table 10.12.

The condition tends to occur in children or young adults. There is abdominal pain, fever and weight loss and some patients have diarrhoea and steatorrhoea. On examination there may be an abdominal mass due to enlarged glands and oedema from protein losing enteropathy. The diagnosis is suspected on barium follow-through examination but the radiographic findings may be confused with Crohn's disease. Staging is performed as with other lymphomas and this provides important information on optimal treatment and prognosis. Treatment involves a combination of surgery, abdominal radiotherapy and chemotherapy.

CARCINOMA

Adenocarcinoma arises predominantly in the duodenum or jejunum. It may be associated with coeliac disease, Crohn's disease or some of the multiple polyposis syndromes (familial polyposis, Gardner's syndrome). There is abdominal pain, weight loss, bleeding leading to iron deficiency anaemia, obstruction or intussusception. The diagnosis is made on barium follow-through examination. The treatment is surgical.

Leiomyosarcomas occur at any level in the small intestine but their presentation and treatment are similar to adenocarcinoma.

BENIGN TUMOURS

These are usually adenomas, leiomyomas or lipomas. Many are asymptomatic but they may present with abdominal pain, obstruction or bleeding and are diagnosed by barium follow-through examination.

CARCINOID TUMOURS

This tumour occurs at many sites in the gastrointestinal tract but is most common in the appendix, the ileum and the rectum. In the appendix, carcinoids are almost always benign, but may lead to appendicitis.

Carcinoids in the small intestine are multiple in 20%

of cases and show low-grade malignancy with metastases to the abdominal lymph nodes and the liver.

The term 'carcinoid syndrome' refers to the systemic symptoms produced when the secretory products of the neoplastic enterochromaffin cells which comprise the tumour are released into the systemic circulation. These do not usually reach the systemic circulation until they are produced by liver metastases. Serotonin (5HT) is released, and its metabolite 5-HIAA appears in the urine. Many kinins and hormones are also released and these cause diarrhoea and peripheral symptoms. The clinical features are shown in the information box below. The diagnosis is made by measuring urinary 5-HIAA in a 24-hour collection of urine.

CLINICAL FEATURES OF THE CARCINOID SYNDROME

- Symptoms due to:
    Local invasion of the bowel
    Hepatic metastases
- Flushing ⎫
- Diarrhoea ⎬ Often precipitated by food, alcohol or exercise
- Right heart valve lesions
- Facial telangiectasia
- Hepatomegaly due to metastases

Management

The treatment of a carcinoid tumour is surgical resection. The treatment of patients with carcinoid syndrome is palliative because hepatic metastases have usually occurred. Surgical removal of the primary tumour is attempted, and the hepatic metastases are excised if possible. A variety of pharmacological agents are available which block some of the affects of serotonin, kinins and other secretory products. The most promising are the long-acting somatostatin analogues.

ACUTE ABDOMEN

Acute abdomen is the term used to define a group of abdominal conditions in which prompt surgical treatment must be considered to treat perforation, peritonitis and vascular and other catastrophies. Some important causes are listed in the information box (right).

Clinical features

The history depends on the underlying condition. Abdominal pain is the most prominent symptom. Visceral abdominal pain is experienced in that region of the abdominal wall innervated by spinal nerves with the same segmental origin as the sympathetic nerves of the

---

CAUSES OF ACUTE ABDOMEN

Important causes
Acute appendicitis (p. 461)
Cholecystitis (p. 541)
Acute pancreatitis (p. 480)
Perforated peptic ulcer (p. 437)
Diverticular disease (p. 464)
Acute vascular insufficiency (p. 463)
Intestinal obstruction and strangulation (p. 462)

Other causes
Congenital
    Meckel's diverticulum
Vascular
    Ruptured aortic aneurysm
Gynaecological
    Ruptured ectopic pregnancy
    Ruptured ovarian cyst
    Acute salpingitis
Infective
    Acute mesenteric adenitis
    Terminal ileitis due to *Yersinia*

---

obstructed or inflamed viscus (Fig. 10.14). Parietal abdominal pain results from irritation of the parietal peritoneum innervated by spinal nerves supplying the overlying abdominal wall. Thus, parietal pain is localised to the area of abdomen affected.

Abdominal tenderness, muscle guarding and rigidity are signs of peritonitis. Inflammation of the diaphragmatic peritoneum is suggested by shoulder-tip pain and hyperaesthesia. Inflammation of the pelvic peritoneum

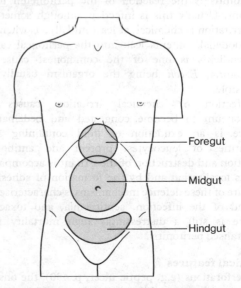

Fig. 10.14 **Site of appreciation of abdominal colic according to the area of gut involved.**

may produce tenderness which is detected on rectal examination.

Other clinical features are described with the appropriate diseases.

Medical conditions which may simulate the acute abdomen include pleurisy and pneumonia and myocardial infarction, all of which may cause upper abdominal pain. The former are detected by careful examination of the chest together with a *chest radiograph*. When the latter is suspected an *electrocardiograph* is necessary.

There are a number of less common conditions which may simulate an acute abdomen which are listed in the information box below.

MEDICAL CONDITIONS WHICH MAY MIMIC ACUTE ABDOMEN

- Diabetes mellitus
    Severe ketoacidosis
- Acute porphyria
- Henoch-Schonlein purpura
- Irritable bowel syndrome
- Arteritis
    e.g. in systemic lupus erythematosis
- Herpes zoster
- Acute infections
    e.g. gastroenteritis, tonsilitis, otitis media
- Genitourinary diseases

PERITONITIS

Peritonitis is the reaction of the peritoneum to an irritant. Usually this is infection although sometimes the irritation is chemical, at least initially, as when bile or duodenal contents leak into the peritoneal cavity. Appendicitis is one of the commonest causes of peritonitis, *E. coli* being the organism usually responsible.

Infection or chemical irritation causes the peritoneum to become congested and oedematous. There is an exudation of fluid containing large quantities of leucocytes, protein and antibodies. Dilution and destruction of the irritant is accompanied by its localisation and by the formation of adhesions. Failure of these defence mechanisms is characterised by spread of the infection, septicaemia, and toxaemia. There is still a distressingly high mortality from generalised peritonitis.

Clinical features

In perforations (e.g. peptic ulcer, p. 430), the onset is sudden with severe abdominal pain, vomiting, tenderness, rigidity and shock. Reflex guarding and muscle rigidity occur in relation to the area of peritoneum which is inflamed. Pelvic peritonitis is associated with tenderness on rectal examination. These initial severe features gradually decrease; the patient appears to have improved and the diagnosis can be missed. Subsequently paralytic ileus develops, fluid collects in the peritoneal cavity, and there is increasing distension, the rigidity lessens, the tenderness remains and toxaemia develops.

When peritonitis is secondary to inflammation of a viscus, such as appendicitis, the initial signs are those of the underlying disease, later to be replaced by the features of peritonitis. Only the history of the onset will be a guide to the probable cause in advanced peritonitis.

Management

Shock is common in diffuse peritonitis and resuscitation must be undertaken before surgical intervention. Blood cultures are obtained and parenteral treatment with an appropriate antibiotic and metronidazole is commenced. The surgical treatment of established peritonitis is by removal of the contaminating source such as in appendicitis, or perforated bowel or gallbladder, together with peritoneal toilet and lavage.

General peritonitis may resolve completely, but often inflammation localises to form an abscess at the primary site, in the subphrenic region or in the pelvis. Persistence of fever, or continued elevation of pulse rate, white blood count and ESR, should lead to efforts to locate such residual loci of infection, for example by ultrasonography.

Pelvic abscess

This usually follows the localisation of a general peritonitis and forms in the lower part of the peritoneal cavity in front of the rectum. The abscess may irritate the bladder causing frequency of micturition or involve the bowel causing diarrhoea with the passage of mucus and a feeling of incomplete emptying. It is evident on rectal or vaginal examination as a tender mass, which may discharge rectally or vaginally. Treatment with metronidazole (400 mg 3 times daily) is usually effective.

Subphrenic abscess

The localisation of pus between diaphragm and liver on the right side or between the diaphragm and the liver, spleen and stomach on the left is a complication of peritonitis most commonly following perforation of the stomach, duodenum or gallbladder, or after an operation on these organs. There are signs of persistent infection. There may be dullness at the base of the lung and tenderness and slight oedema over the lower ribs posteriorly. Diagnosis is aided by ultrasonography or a radiograph of the diaphragmatic region which may show elevation of the diaphragm with a fluid level below or an effusion above. Treatment is by drainage either at laparotomy or by insertion of a drain under ultrasound control.

LESS COMMON FORMS OF PERITONITIS

Granulomatous peritonitis

This is caused by talc and occasionally starch used as surgical glove powder. Symptoms and signs of peritonitis begin within weeks of operation. Unfortunately a laparotomy may be required to exclude other causes of peritonitis.

Primary, spontaneous peritonitis

There is no recognisable source for peritonitis and it is assumed that bacteria enter the peritoneal cavity via the genital tract or during bacteraemia. The organisms involved are pneumococci, haemolytic streptococci or gonococci.

Tuberculous peritonitis

Although rare in Britain it is still relatively common elsewhere notably in tropical countries. Peritonitis is secondary to a tuberculous focus in the abdomen, usually in a mesenteric lymph node.

The disease is characterised by wasting, malaise and gradually increasing abdominal distension and tenderness. Masses caused by matted omentum and loops of bowel may be palpable. The abdomen contains a straw coloured fluid from which tubercle bacilli may be cultured. The fluid shows a protein concentration greater than 2.5 g/100 ml and large numbers of lymphocytes. Diagnosis may also be made by biopsy of granulomas seen at laparotomy or laparoscopy.

In the adult, the condition may be confused with advanced malignant disease and an unnecessarily hopeless prognosis given. The response to anti-tuberculous chemotherapy (p. 367) is good and often dramatic.

ACUTE APPENDICITIS

Acute appendicitis is more common in young people. It is usually obstructive, the lumen of the appendix being narrowed by swelling of lymphoid tissue in its wall or by stricture from previous inflammation. Obstruction is made complete by impaction of a faecolith causing gangrene, perforation and a local abscess or generalised peritonitis. Another outcome is the formation of an oedematous inflammatory appendix mass.

Clinical features

The classical history is the sudden onset of vague central abdominal pain followed within a few hours by a shift of the pain to the right iliac fossa where it becomes localised to McBurney's point, that is situated one-third of the distance along a line from the anterior superior iliac spine to the umbilicus. There is nausea and malaise. There may be vomiting but this is seldom severe and is often absent. The pulse rate is increased. In the early stages there is little elevation of temperature and the occurrence of rigors and a high fever make the diagnosis of appendicitis unlikely. There is tenderness and guarding in the right iliac fossa progressing to rigidity as peritonitis develops. Rectal examination may disclose tenderness in the right side of the pelvis.

The 'classical' history and findings account for less than 50% of patient presentations. Because of variations in its anatomical position the inflamed appendix may simulate other diseases of the abdomen. The patient may present with diarrhoea or with urinary or gynaecological symptoms and other causes of acute abdomen may be mimicked. The differential diagnosis is shown in the information box below.

DIFFERENTIAL DIAGNOSIS OF ACUTE APPENDICITIS

- Non-specific mesenteric lymphadenitis
- Terminal ileitis
    Yersinia infection
    Crohn's disease
- Meckel's diverticulum
- Irritable bowel syndrome
- Salpingitis or ovarian disease
- Perinephric abscess or acute cholecystitis when the appendix is retrocaecal

---

Investigations

The diagnosis is made on clinical findings and further investigations other than a white blood count and abdominal X-ray are unnecessary.

Management

The diseased appendix should be removed as early in the acute stage as possible. Attempts to temporise in the belief that mild forms of appendicitis can be distinguished from severe are dangerous because the condition is notoriously deceptive. Even in the absence of obvious peritonitis the acute case should receive intraoperative antibiotic cover with rectal metronidazole and where there is obvious peritonitis, the systemic administration of ampicillin and metronidazole.

A conservative policy is acceptable only when a clearly defined appendix mass is present without generalised abdominal signs. Not all patients presenting with an appendix mass require antibiotics. Some need no more than rest, restriction of diet and the avoidance of purgatives. Others in whom there is more marked local tenderness, with low-grade fever and malaise, benefit from ampicillin (0.25–1 g orally 6-hourly) and metronidazole (400 mg orally 8-hourly). Once the mass has subsided, probably within 2 to 3 weeks, the appendix should be removed.

MECKEL'S DIVERTICULUM

This remnant of the vitelline duct which occurs in about 2% of the population is found on the anti-mesenteric border of the ileum about 50 cm from the ileocaecal valve. It may contain gastric mucosa which may secrete acid to cause mucosal ulceration and bleeding. It may cause obstruction or inflammation and so present as an acute appendicitis.

INTESTINAL OBSTRUCTION

Intestinal obstruction may be complete or incomplete, acute or chronic, intermittent or continuous. The most important issue to decide is whether the obstruction is *simple* or associated with *strangulation*. The latter occurs when there is interference with the intestinal blood supply as when the bowel is trapped or twisted. Urgent relief is required if gangrene, perforation and peritonitis are to be avoided.

A simple classification is provided in the information box (right).

Mechanical causes will in general require surgical relief while paralytic ileus may respond to conservative measures.

Clinical features

Pain. The pain of mechanical obstruction is colicky and the distribution reflects the region of gut obstructed. Episodes of pain are accompanied by borborygmi. The advent of constant severe pain with abdominal tenderness is indicative of strangulation. Paralytic obstruction is characterised by a dull constant pain in an abdomen which is ominously silent.

Vomiting. This is copious in high obstruction and may be late or absent in obstructions of the lower small bowel or colon.

Distension. This may be absent or confined to some loops of the bowel which can be seen as ridges across the

---

CAUSES OF INTESTINAL OBSTRUCTION

Mechanical obstruction
Luminal obstruction (obturation)
  Faecal impaction
  Gallstone ileus
  Worms, e.g. ascariasis
Intrinsic lesions of the bowel wall
  Tumours of the large intestine*
  Strictures
    e.g. Crohn's disease
  Intussusception
Extrinsic compression
  Adhesions*
  Hernias*
  Volvulus

Strangulation obstruction

Paralytic ileus
  Peritonitis
  Postoperative
  Vascular

* Common in Western communities

---

abdomen in the thin patient forming the so-called ladder pattern. Diffuse distension is late and may indicate chronic large bowel obstruction or paralytic ileus.

Bowel movements. In complete obstruction neither faeces nor flatus is passed. In high obstruction, the bowels may move unaided or with enemas because of residual contents below the obstruction, while in large bowel obstruction spurious diarrhoea may be due to the discharge of faecal-stained mucus.

Physical examination. A careful examination is vital. The seven points to be assessed are listed in the information box below.

Investigation

Plain radiographs taken in the erect and supine

CHECK LIST ON EXAMINATION FOR SUSPECTED OBSTRUCTION

- Is there evidence of inguinal or femoral hernias?
- Are there scars from previous operations?
- Is the abdomen distended, especially caecal distension?
- Is the abdomen tender?
- Is there a mass present?
- Are bowel sounds increased and tinkling (mechanical obstruction) or absent (paralytic ileus)?
- Is the rectum empty on rectal examination or is there faecal impaction?

positions will reveal the diagnosis in most cases by revealing gaseous distension and fluid levels. However gas may not be seen with high intestinal obstruction and in such patients a barium contrast study is performed of the upper gastrointestinal tract. A barium enema is indicated when large bowel obstruction is suspected. Barium examination is contraindicated if the clinical evidence suggests perforation and Gastrografin should be used instead.

Management

A surgical opinion is necessary if intestinal obstruction is suspected even if non-operative measures are to be used. The mainstays of treatment are decompression by gastrointestinal suction and the intravenous replacement of fluids and electrolytes. Once resuscitation has restored any disturbance of the circulatory state, urgent surgery is performed for hernia, mechanical obstruction of the large bowel and strangulation. An initial conservative approach is adopted for paralytic ileus, obstruction due to adhesions and postoperative obstruction. In addition sigmoid volvulus which is usually recognised on the plain radiograph can often be treated at sigmoidoscopy by the insertion of a soft rubber tube into the twisted loop.

ISCHAEMIA OF THE ALIMENTARY TRACT

Aetiology

The intestines are supplied by the coeliac, superior mesenteric and inferior mesenteric arteries. The superior mesenteric, which supplies the mid-gut, has poor collateral support from the other two arteries. It follows that intestinal ischaemia is usually due to sudden or slow occlusion of the superior mesenteric artery. However, ischaemia may also arise from obstruction to the venous outflow from the intestine, or from a reduction in blood flow due to shock or cardiac failure, without evidence of obstruction to the arterial or venous supply. The usual causes of blockage of the superior mesenteric artery are atheroma, thrombosis due to blood diseases, and embolism. Most cases of intestinal ischaemia occur in the elderly and in those with cardiac failure or arrhythmias.

ACUTE INTESTINAL FAILURE

This term describes the consequences of acute obstruction of the superior mesenteric artery. A variable length of the small intestine undergoes necrosis of the superficial epithelium and over several hours this progresses to gangrene. There may be a prodromal period of episodic or chronic abdominal pain often related to meals. This progresses to more severe abdominal pain, vomiting, watery and later bloody diarrhoea. Signs of peritonitis and hypovolaemic shock develop.

The diagnosis is essentially clinical but is assisted by the finding of a leucocytosis of up to 20 000–30 000/mm³. The findings on a plain abdominal radiograph are usually non-specific. Arteriography may be used to confirm the diagnosis provided it does not delay the urgent vascular surgery necessary to prevent gangrene. Unfortunately extensive resection of the small intestine is necessary in many patients and the overall mortality is 50%.

ISCHAEMIC COLITIS

Occlusion of the inferior mesenteric artery leads to ischaemia of the left colon particularly when blood flow in the superior mesenteric artery is also reduced.

The patient presents with colicky lower abdominal pain, nausea, vomiting and diarrhoea with the passage of blood and mucus. On examination there is tenderness and guarding on the left side of the abdomen and particularly in the left iliac fossa. Bowel sounds are usually present. In some patients the episode is transient; in others there may be persistent bleeding and pain suggesting progression to stricture formation. About 10% of patients progress to shock with generalised abdominal pain indicative of peritonitis secondary to gangrene.

Investigations

Several investigations are helpful. Leucocytosis is common. Sigmoidoscopy usually shows a normal rectal mucosa but blood may be seen descending from above. A plain radiograph of the abdomen shows 'thumb printing' at the splenic flexure and descending colon which are indentations of the bowel wall from submucosal haemorrhage and oedema.

A double-contrast barium enema usually demonstrates the characteristic distribution of maximal involvement at the splenic flexure and sigmoid colon. The mucosal features are 'thumb printing' and ulceration. Stricture develops in up to 50% of patients and is demonstrated by a barium enema repeated after 2–3 weeks.

Management

Most cases resolve with conservative management. Surgery is necessary when there are signs of peritonitis or when symptomatic stricture develops.

CHRONIC INTESTINAL ISCHAEMIA

This occurs when there is a gradual reduction of blood flow in the superior mesenteric artery with resulting impairment of the normal postprandial increase in blood flow to the small bowel. There is abdominal pain ('abdominal angina') some 30 minutes after each meal and the patient is afraid to eat and loses weight. The condition is rare.

DISEASES OF THE LARGE INTESTINE

The main functions of the large bowel are the removal of water from the intestinal contents, the storage of faeces, and their evacuation at controlled intervals. Continence depends on training, on the function of a sphincter mechanism in the anal canal and on rectal sensation whereby the need to defecate is appreciated.

The anal canal is sensitive to pain and touch, as is well demonstrated by the severe pain caused by fissures and inflamed haemorrhoids. The rectum is insensitive to painful stimuli so that the injection of a sclerosing agent for the treatment of haemorrhoids is painless. Rectal 'sensation' implies an ability to appreciate distension and contraction.

In addition to the clinical examination which includes a digital examination of the rectum, endoscopy, stool examination and radiological investigation are important aids to diagnosis.

DIVERTICULAR DISEASE

Though diverticula occur throughout the gastrointestinal tract, they are most common in the large bowel of middle-aged or elderly subjects. The presence of diverticula is known as *diverticulosis*; when they are inflamed the condition is known as *diverticulitis*. Such inflammation occurs almost exclusively in colonic diverticula. Because it is often difficult to separate the two conditions on clinical or radiological evidence, they are grouped together under the term 'diverticular disease'.

Aetiology
In diverticulosis the muscular coat of the bowel is often greatly thickened, suggesting that the diverticula have formed as a result of increased intracolonic pressure. Manometric measurements support this view. It can be shown that pressure in the bowel is high and that there is an area of spasm or failure to relax at the rectosigmoid junction.

Dietary factors may be at least partly responsible.

Diverticulosis is rare in areas of the world such as Africa and Asia where the usual diet is one of high residue; by contrast the incidence is increasing in Western countries where natural fibre is removed from the diet in the processes of food refining. Moreover there is evidence that intracolonic pressures vary with the bulk of faecal residue, a high faecal residue being associated with a low intraluminal pressure and vice versa.

Incidence
The incidence in Western communities is between 5 and 10% and in those over the age of 60 it is 30%, though only a small proportion of patients have symptoms.

Pathology
The pelvic colon is most commonly involved. Its muscle wall is thickened but the diverticula themselves are pouchings of the mucosa and have no muscle coat (Fig. 10.15). It is not clear how they become inflamed. Radiological examination frequently shows the presence of a faecolith in a diverticulum, and it may be that faeces collect because of the inability of the diverticulum to contract. Faecal retention may then cause a local inflammatory reaction which may resolve spon-

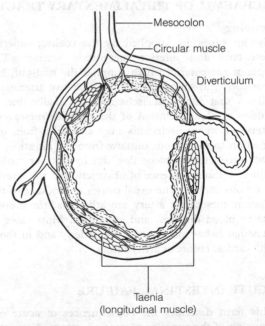

Fig. 10.15 The human colon in diverticulosis. The colonic wall is weak between the taeniae. The blood vessels that supply the colon pierce the circular muscle and weaken it further by forming tunnels. Diverticula usually emerge through these points of least resistance.

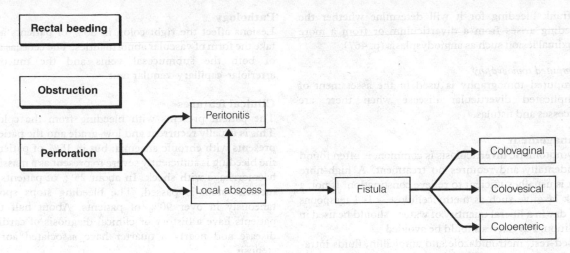

Fig. 10.16   Complications of diverticulitis.

taneously or progress to cause perforation, local abscess formation, fistula and peritonitis. When there are repeated attacks of diverticulitis, the bowel wall becomes thickened with narrowing of the lumen leading eventually to obstruction.

Clinical features

Pain or discomfort felt in the left iliac fossa is a common complaint and there may be associated local tenderness. Acute diverticulitis can give rise to severe pain, guarding and rigidity on the left side, the signs of peritonitis and obstruction being combined. Change of bowel habit, either increasing constipation or constipation alternating with diarrhoea, is frequent. Complications are shown in Figure 10.16.

On examination, the thickened tender colon may be palpable in the left iliac fossa and a mass may be present in those patients who have developed diverticulitis, with or without abscess formation.

Investigation

Sigmoidoscopy is necessary to exclude cancer of the rectum or lower sigmoid colon. Usually there are no positive features apart from possible discomfort and tenderness at the rectosigmoid junction.

Barium enema examination

This shows characteristic sacs along the contour of the gut in diverticulosis (Fig. 10.17). After evacuation barium frequently remains in the diverticula which are clearly outlined. The barium enema is postponed for 2–3 weeks in acute diverticulitis until the inflammation has settled when narrowing, rigidity and loss of normal haustration of a segment of colon can be identified.

Evidence of fistula or abscess formation may be seen. Whether or not there are diverticula present, the main diagnostic difficulty is to distinguish the appearances from those of carcinoma; radiological differentiation may be impossible and cancer and diverticular disease may coexist.

Flexible sigmoidoscopy

Flexible sigmoidoscopy is used to inspect the affected segment of bowel for visual evidence of cancer and biopsies are taken. Colonoscopy is indicated when there

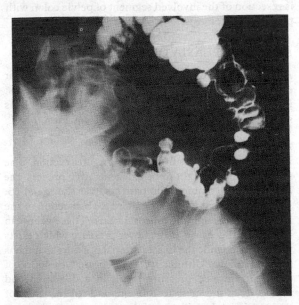

Fig. 10.17   Diverticular disease of the sigmoid colon. (Courtesy of Dr G.M. Fraser.)

is frank bleeding for it will determine whether the bleeding arises from a diverticulum or from a more proximal lesion such as angiodysplasia (p. 467).

Computed tomography
Computed tomography is used in the assessment of complicated diverticular disease when there are abscesses and fistulas.

Management
Asymptomatic diverticulosis is common, is often found accidentally and requires no treatment. A high-fibre diet is usually sufficient to relieve constipation. If not, a bulk laxative such as methylcellulose – 1–4 teaspoons per day in a liberal quantity of water – should be used in addition. Purgatives should be avoided.

Bed-rest, metronidazole and ampicillin, fluids intravenously and orally, or even cessation of feeding and nasogastric suction may be required during an attack of acute diverticulitis. Most subside spontaneously but a few require emergency surgery which will probably take the form of a temporary defunctioning proximal colostomy to be followed later by local resection. However, many centres now prefer resection and primary anastomosis. An emergency partial colectomy may be required for acute bleeding.

Elective surgery is indicated after recovery from an acute attack in those patients who have developed obstructive features, in those who have complications such as fistula, and in those in whom the possibility of carcinoma cannot be excluded. The treatment of choice is resection of the involved segment of pelvic colon with primary anastomosis.

ANGIODYSPLASIA OF THE COLON

Angiodysplasia of the colon, also known as vascular ectasia of the colon, is recognised as one of the most important causes of bleeding from the colon. It is second only to diverticular disease in frequency.

Aetiology
Ectasias probably result from venous obstruction. The mechanism is thought to be a degenerative process, the lesions being commoner in patients over the age of 65. It is thought that with aging there is obstruction of the blood flow through the mucosal veins. These veins can be occluded because of the lower pressure which exists within them while the higher arterial pressure maintains arterial inflow. Ultimately, the repeated episodes of transient elevated pressure result in a dilatation and tortuosity of the submucosal veins and subsequently of the venules and capillaries of the mucosal units draining into the veins.

Pathology
Lesions affect the right colon in 80% of patients and take the form of vascular abnormalities. The ectasias are of both the submucosal veins and the mucosal arteriolar-capillary-venular unit.

Clinical features
The patient presents with bleeding from the colon. This is usually recurrent and low-grade and the patient presents with chronic anaemia; but in 15% of patients the bleeding is sufficiently severe to present as a massive haemorrhage with shock. In about 25% of patients, a melaena stool is passed. The bleeding stops spontaneously in over 90% of patients. About half the patients have a history or clinical diagnosis of cardiac disease and nearly a quarter have associated aortic stenosis.

The diagnosis is established by colonoscopy or angiography. If the patient is actively bleeding, abdominal scintigraphy using either technetium-99m sulphur colloid or technetium-99m labelled red cells. A barium enema has only a small role to play in the diagnosis. Colonoscopy will demonstrate vascular ectasias which can be seen as small dilated vessels, spiders or venous tufts on the mucosal surface. The vascular ectasia and telangectasia may not be evident in patients who are anaemic or shocked.

Management
In most patients, haemostasis occurs spontaneously and blood replacement is only necessary for the shocked or the anaemic patient. Colonic ablation may be used to treat the ectasias and a variety of technologies have been used to obliterate the identified vascular ectasia. Transcatheter embolisation of bleeding vessels has also been used. Right hemicolectomy is widely used to treat those patients who have bled from ectasia in the right colon, identified either by colonoscopy or angiography but in whom the bleeding has either not been stopped or the vessels have not been adequately ablated. Because up to 80% of the bleeding occurs in the right colon, the risks of subsequent bleeding remain relatively low.

HAEMORRHAGE FROM THE LOWER GASTROINTESTINAL TRACT

The usual causes of bleeding from the lower gastrointestinal tract are shown in the information box (p. 467).

With bleeding from the proximal colon or ileum, the blood may appear as melaena. Bleeding may also occur from haemorrhoids or anal fissures but the patient's description of the bleeding usually allows them to be distinguished.

CAUSES OF BLEEDING FROM THE LOWER GASTROINTESTINAL TRACT

Common
Carcinoma of the left colon
Diverticular disease
Angiodysplasia

Less common
Ulcerative colitis and proctitis

Ischaemic colitis
Polyps

Rare
Arteriovenous malformations
Solitary ulcer
Meckel's diverticulum

Investigation

Rectal examination and sigmoidoscopy will detect most causes of bleeding from the ano-rectal region. If blood is coming from above the rectum, conservative measures are instituted until bleeding has stopped, to be followed by colonoscopy which is the investigation of choice for it may detect angiodysplasia and other vascular lesions which cannot be seen by barium enema examination. In addition some of these lesions can be treated successfully by electrocoagulation during colonoscopy. Occasionally, the site of bleeding can be detected by radionuclide scanning with ^{99m}Tc-labelled red cells.

If bleeding continues, angiography of the superior and inferior mesenteric arteries can be performed to detect the bleeding site which might then be treated by embolisation through the arterial catheter. The appropriate segment of the colon can be resected if the bleeding fails to stop.

ULCERATIVE COLITIS

Aetiology

There are no known aetiological factors. Changes in colonic mucus and the metabolism of arachidonic acid in the colon have been postulated. Many immunological abnormalities have been described but are likely to be secondary to colonic damage. However, circulating immune complexes may be responsible for the development of arthritis and uveitis. Although individual attacks of colitis often appear to be precipitated by stressful life experiences, psychological factors are not otherwise considered important in aetiology. The burden of frequent or uncontrollable bowel evacuation may induce profound psychological disturbances such as anxiety and depression and feelings of helplessness. These traits are a consequence of the disease rather than its cause and generally decrease or disappear during remission. Genetic factors are important. A family history is often found and such families have an increased incidence of Crohn's disease and ankylosing spondylitis.

Incidence

Ulcerative colitis has an incidence rate of 5–10 per 100 000 and a prevalence rate of about 80 per 100 000 in Western communities. It occurs equally in males and females and can occur at any age but especially between the ages of 10 and 40.

Pathology

The disease always involves the rectum (proctitis) and may also involve a variable part of the colon or the entire colon; but the colonic disease is always continuous with that in the rectum in contrast to Crohn's disease which is often discontinuous.

In the early stages the mucosa is haemorrhagic and granular; thereafter ulceration develops. The ulcers may be superficial or penetrate deeply, spreading longitudinally beneath the mucosa. The mucosa may slough in parts in severe disease to expose granulation tissue; the mucosa that remains becomes oedematous, hyperplastic and raised, giving the appearance of pseudopolyposis. In *acute fulminant disease* the bowel, especially the transverse colon, may be greatly dilated (*toxic dilatation*) and the bowel wall becomes thin and may rupture. In long-standing disease the colon is shortened and generally narrowed with a lack of haustrations. Strictures are uncommon compared to Crohn's disease and anal lesions such as fissure and fistula are also less severe and less common.

The important microscopic features are listed in Table 10.13 where they are compared to those of

Table 10.13 Microscopic features of the large intestine in ulcerative colitis and Crohn's disease

Ulcerative colitis	Crohn's disease
The inflammation is mucosal and submucosal	The inflammation is transmural
Granulomas absent	Granulomas present in bowel and lymph nodes
Crypt abscesses common	Crypt abscesses infrequent
Width of the mucosa is normal or reduced	Width of mucosa is normal or increased
Loss of goblet cells	Normal population of goblet cells

Crohn's disease of the colon. The lamina propria is uniformly infiltrated with lymphocytes and plasma cells whilst polymorphs accumulate around ulcerated areas. Crypt abscesses consist of a collection of polymorphs in a crypt.

In 10–20% of patients it is not possible to distinguish ulcerative colitis from Crohn's disease of the colon from histological criteria. The term *colitis intermediate* has been used for such cases.

In a small proportion of patients with chronic ulcerative colitis and Crohn's disease of the colon, multicentric precancerous lesions can be found on histological examination. Some of these are invisible to the naked eye and thus surveillance for cancer (p. 473) depends upon multiple biopsies taken at colonoscopy.

Clinical features

Ulcerative colitis and Crohn's disease of the colon have many clinical similarities and both will be considered here.

The first attack is often the most severe and thereafter the disease is characterised by exacerbations and re-missions although a minority of patients develop chronic symptoms. The clinical features and the management are largely determined by the extent to which the colon is involved, the severity of the inflam-mation and the duration of the disease.

The principal symptom is diarrhoea with loose bloody stools containing mucus and pus; defecation is often accompanied by lower abdominal discomfort although severe pain is uncommon. Tenesmus may occur because of proctitis. Tenderness may be present on palpation of the colon, especially in the left iliac fossa; when peritoneal irritation is present it signifies that the serosa is involved in the inflammatory process.

In severe ulcerative colitis or Crohn's colitis, there is exhausting diarrhoea and dehydration. *Toxic dilatation* represents the most serious complication with tachycardia, a high swinging temperature and abdominal distension and tenderness. The patient is at grave risk of dying from colonic perforation.

In chronic colitis the bowel is permanently damaged by fibrosis and behaves as a rigid tube incapable of absorbing fluid properly or of acting as a faecal reservoir. There is no toxaemia, but the patient lives in chronic ill-health and with persistent diarrhoea.

The symptoms may be trivial when the disease is confined to the rectum, and consist of loose motions and perhaps blood-streaking of the stool. A severe proctitis will cause tenesmus, frequent small loose stools, and bleeding and mucus per rectum, but systemic dis-turbance is absent. Paradoxically, in distal colitis spasm

may result in constipation with retention of faeces in the proximal colon and small hard stools.

Relapse is often associated with emotional stress, intercurrent infection or the use of antibiotics. There is no special risk to the patient during pregnancy in either ulcerative colitis or Crohn's colitis.

Cancer of the colon in chronic colitis occurs with an increased frequency in patients with extensive or total colitis of more than 10 years' duration and an early age of onset. The onset of cancer is usually impossible to detect clinically.

Stricture of the colon, anal fissure, abscess and fistula occur in ulcerative colitis but are much less common than in Crohn's colitis.

Many systemic complications occur (see information box, p. 454) and are common to both ulcerative colitis and Crohn's colitis except sclerosing cholangitis which is much more common in ulcerative colitis.

Investigations

The patient is often anaemic from blood loss and there may be a leucocytosis and a raised ESR. In severe disease there are electrolyte disturbances, and protein loss from the colon may lead to hypoalbuminaemia. Sometimes tests of liver function are abnormal. The stool should be cultured for pathogenic bacteria and a search of the mucus made for amoebae to exclude an infective cause for the colitis. Blood cultures are required if septicaemia is suspected.

Sigmoidoscopy

This is essential in most patients. In ulcerative colitis, the mucosa appears engorged and hyperaemic and the normal vascular pattern is obliterated. In severe disease spontaneous bleeding will be seen; in less severe involvement the mucosa appears intact and bleeds only when it is gently rubbed while in mild cases the only abnormality is the absence of the normal vascular pattern. In colitis due to Crohn's disease the rectal mucosa shows focal inflammation and ulceration with the intervening mucosa appearing normal or oedematous; but in some patients the appearance is indistinguishable from that of ulcerative proctitis. Biopsies are always taken.

Plain radiograph of the abdomen

This is essential in the diagnosis of suspected toxic dilatation and is also of value at the initial presentation as the colon will usually contain sufficient air to outline an abnormal mucosal pattern.

Barium enema and colonoscopy

The double-contrast barium enema will demonstrate

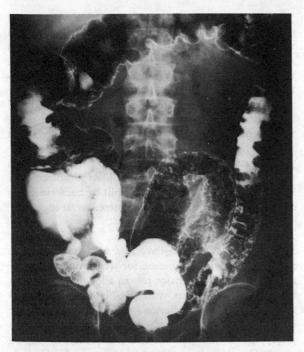

Fig. 10.18   Severe ulcerative colitis with deep ulcers and pseudopolyps affecting mainly the sigmoid colon. (Courtesy of Dr G.M. Fraser.)

Table 10.14   Conditions which must be differentiated from ulcerative and Crohn's colitis

Infective	Non-infective
Salmonellosis	Ischaemic colitis
Shigellosis	Radiation proctitis and colitis
Campylobacter gastroenteritis	Diffuse lymphoma
Haemorrhagic colitis due to *E. coli*	Vasculitides
Gonorrhoeal proctitis	Cathartic colon
Chlamydial proctitis	
Proctitis due to herpes simplex	
Pseudomembranous colitis	
Amoebiasis	
Other parasitic infections	

the severity and extent of the disease. The earliest radiological change is a granular appearance of the colonic mucosa. In more severe disease ulceration and pseudopolyps will be seen (Fig. 10.18). In long-standing disease there may be shortening of the colon with narrowing of the lumen. Some of these features may be seen in Crohn's colitis but in addition the disease is often discontinuous, the ulcers are deeper and the ileum is narrow and irregular. Colonoscopy is frequently used to assess the extent and severity of colitis because barium enema may underestimate these. In addition colonoscopic biopsies are important in distinguishing ulcerative colitis and Crohn's disease from each other and from other diseases which may cause colitis. Barium enema should not be performed in acute cases and where toxic dilatation is suspected because of the risk of perforation.

Differential diagnosis
A large number of diseases may cause inflammation of the colon and rectum (Table 10.14). Many of these are infective and their occurrence in homosexuals and in patients with acquired immunodeficiency syndrome (AIDS) makes it essential that these possibilities are kept in mind. The infective conditions are diagnosed visually (e.g. membranes seen coating the mucosa in pseudomembranous colitis, or amoebae seen microscopically in fresh stools), on biopsy (e.g. herpes simplex) or culture of stool. The non-infective conditions are suspected from the history (abuse of laxatives or previous irradiation) or radiological features.

Medical management

General measures
Admission to hospital is required for patients with severe bowel symptoms, especially when there are general disturbances such as weight loss, anaemia, fever or tachycardia. Such patients may require intense supportive treatment either until the disease remits or as a preparation for surgery. Parenteral nutrition through a central venous line allows correction of nutritional deficiencies in the severely wasted patient and will do much to hasten recovery after operation. The measures should include the correction of dehydration and electrolyte deficiencies especially hypokalaemia; blood and plasma infusions to correct anaemia and hypoproteinaemia; and a high-protein, low-residue diet.

Blood cultures should be taken initially and repeated throughout the course of the illness if fever persists. Gram-negative bacteria are the commonest organisms involved; if septicaemia is suspected parenteral administration of broad spectrum antibiotics is necessary. However, antibiotics have no place in the primary management of ulcerative colitis; indeed a broad spectrum antibiotic may precipitate a relapse. Candidosis of the mouth and upper pharynx is common, especially in ill patients on corticosteroids and must be treated (p. 423). There is no satisfactory drug for controlling diarrhoea. Codeine phosphate (30 mg 3 or 4 times daily) or loperamide (2 mg 4 times daily) may be helpful in the chronic illness, but these drugs must be avoided in severely ill patients because they may precipitate toxic dilatation of the colon.

Corticosteroids

There is no specific treatment for ulcerative colitis but corticosteroids are very effective in inducing remission.

Local treatment. The preparations commonly used are prednisolone-21-phosphate or betamethasone. When sigmoidoscopic examination confirms that only the rectum is involved topical treatment with corticosteroid suppositories is all that is required; the patient is instructed to insert one, 2 times daily retaining the material for as long as possible. Corticosteroid suppositories inserted twice per day can be used in distal proctitis.

Topical treatment with corticosteroid enemas used once or twice daily may also be administered for distal colitis when symptoms are mild – not more than 4 stools per day with intermittent bleeding and little or no systemic upset. When symptoms are more severe, patients with distal colitis may require systemic corticosteroids. Systemic or local treatment may be continued for 3–6 weeks, the duration being judged from the sigmoidoscopic appearances and the clinical response.

Systemic treatment. Prednisolone is given in doses of between 40–60 mg daily by mouth for 3–6 weeks depending on the response. In severe disease corticosteroids may have to be administered intravenously as hydrocortisone (100–200 mg 6-hourly). The usual contraindications to the use of these drugs must be observed and supplements of potassium salts should be given. Used in this way, corticosteroids will induce remission in the majority of patients, the dose being reduced at weekly intervals as improvement takes place. Corticosteroids give rise to a sense of well-being and improve appetite, so that the problem of persuading the patient to eat sufficient food is often solved. Intramuscular or subcutaneous injections of long-acting corticotrophin may be marginally more effective in treating relapses but are seldom used.

Sulphasalazine

This is less effective than corticosteroids but may be used in mild or moderately severe attacks in doses of 2–4 g daily. However, its principal value is that it reduces the liability to relapse so that once remission has been induced by corticosteroids all patients with colitis should be maintained on a small dose of sulphasalazine (0.5 g q.i.d.) for 1–2 years or longer. Sulphasalazine is a combination of 5-aminosalicylic acid which is the active agent linked to sulphapyridine acting as a 'carrier'. The compound is broken down by bacterial action in the colon, liberating 5-aminosalicylic acid which is believed to act locally. Side-effects attributed to the sulphapyridine moiety include nausea, headache, rashes, reversible sterility in the male, and very rarely haemolytic anaemia and agranulocytosis.

Oral 5-ASA is not effective because it is absorbed from the small intestine and therefore does not reach the colon. Several preparations have been developed which deliver 5-ASA to the colon without using sulphapyridine as carrier. Mesalazine uses 5-ASA with an enteric coating and azodisalicylate joins 2 molecules of 5-ASA by an azo bond which is split by bacteria in the colon. 5-ASA may also be administered as an enema.

Azathioprine

In a dose of 2.5 mg/kg/day, this may be helpful in patients with chronic disease for whom surgery is inappropriate. It has a major role in allowing the dose to be reduced in patients with troublesome side-effects from corticosteroids. Serious side-effects may occur including suppression of the bone marrow with pancytopenia and patients must be carefully supervised. The drug is used more frequently for Crohn's disease than ulcerative colitis.

Surgical management

If the appropriate medical measures are carried out assiduously the majority of patients with proctitis or moderately severe colitis will pass into remission. In severe forms of ulcerative colitis, or where there is toxic dilatation of the colon or perforation, and in the occasional patient with severe haemorrhage, emergency surgical treatment is required. A proctocolectomy is performed but in some urgent circumstances surgery will be restricted to a colectomy with ileostomy, the rectum and distal colon being removed at a later stage when the crisis is over.

Acute ulcerative colitis which fails to respond to medical treatment, or which relapses frequently in spite of adequate treatment, is an indication for proctocolectomy. This operation is also indicated in chronic illness, or when the disease burns out but leaves a permanently damaged bowel, perhaps with stricture formation. Long-standing disease carries a risk of carcinoma and accordingly total bowel involvement, with activity extending over more than 10 years, should lead to serious consideration of proctocolectomy especially when precancerous lesions are detected during surveillance.

At all stages of the disease, the timing of and preparation for surgery are important and require a joint medical and surgical approach. In emergency situations, intensive preoperative replacement of blood, fluid and electrolytes is needed and operation is performed as soon as the patient is fit to withstand surgery. In less urgent situations, the timing of surgery depends on the degree of improvement in the patient's general condition to be expected from preoperative medical measures.

Whenever possible, in addition to a full explanation of ileostomy and its management with a demonstration of the actual appliance to be used, the patient should have the opportunity before operation of meeting someone with an established ileostomy. Modern surgical techniques and the range of ileostomy appliances available make for easy management of the stoma and allow the patient to live an almost normal life with little restriction of physical activity. To be kept in touch with advances in techniques of ileostomy care, patients should join an ileostomy association or be enrolled in a stoma therapy clinic.

When the rectum is not grossly involved it may be preserved and ileorectal anastomosis performed. In selected patients ileo-anal anastomosis with formation of an ileal pouch can be used. Such methods are gaining in acceptance because of the avoidance of a stoma but are only used to treat ulcerative colitis and not Crohn's colitis.

A summary of therapeutic measures required for colitis of varying severity is listed in the information box below.

MANAGEMENT OF ULCERATIVE AND CROHN'S COLITIS

Severe disease
Hospitalisation
Parenteral fluid, nutrition and blood
Systemic corticosteroids
Surgery for non-response and toxic dilatation

Mild disease or proctitis
Corticosteroid enemas
Oral sulphasalazine

Chronic disease
Oral corticosteroids
Azathioprine
Surgery for chronic ill health

Disease in remission
Oral 5-aminosalicylic acid preparation
Surveillance for cancer of colon after 10 years

Prognosis

In population studies on ulcerative colitis one quarter to a half of patients have proctitis and one quarter have or develop extensive colitis. Life expectancy is normal in patients with proctitis; a third have only one attack, the remainder follow a chronic relapsing course with more extensive disease, there is an increased mortality in the first year, but thereafter mortality is probably no greater than in the general population.

Similar population studies have not been performed for Crohn's colitis but surgery is more commonly necessary and the mortality rate is twice that expected in the general population.

PSEUDOMEMBRANOUS COLITIS

Aetiology
Diarrhoea is quite common in patients receiving antibiotics. In a small proportion of these the diarrhoea is due to proliferation of *C. difficile* when the normal colonic flora is altered or suppressed. Many antibiotics have been implicated.

Pathology
Characteristically the rectum and colon show a membrane of fibrin and polymorphs which is adherent to eroded mucosa.

Clinical features
The patient presents with profuse, watery diarrhoea usually whilst receiving antibiotics. The presenting and radiological features mimic those of acute ulcerative colitis (p. 467) although blood in the stool is present only in severe cases.

Investigation
The diagnosis is made on the rectal appearance at sigmoidoscopy, the histological features of the rectal biopsy and the presence in the stool of a toxin produced by the organism.

Management
The offending antibiotic should be stopped. The patient should be isolated, and supportive therapy as for ulcerative colitis (p. 469) is given. The treatments of choice are oral vancomycin 500 mg or bacitracin 20 000 U every 6 hours for 14 days.

POLYPS OF THE LARGE INTESTINE

The types of polyps found in the large intestine are shown in Table 10.15. Some of the multiple forms may also involve the small intestine and the stomach.

NEOPLASTIC POLYPS

These polyps are classified histologically into tubular adenoma, tubular-villous adenoma and villous

Table 10.15 Classification of benign colonic polyps

Type	Solitary	Multiple
Neoplastic	Adenoma	Familial polyposis
Hamartomatous	Juvenile Peutz-Jegher's	Juvenile polyposis Peutz-Jegher's syndrome
Inflammatory	Benign lymphoid polyp	Benign lymphoid polyposis Inflammatory polyposis in colitis (p. 467)
Metaplastic	Multiple metaplastic polyps	

adenoma, the risk of malignancy being greater in the latter two and greatest in the villous form. The risk of malignancy is also related to size and all polyps of diameter greater than 1 cm must be regarded with suspicion.

Polyps are mostly asymptomatic and may be found incidentally on barium enema (Fig. 10.18, p. 469) or they may cause bleeding, discharge of mucus or intussusception. Occasionally, because of its mobility, a polyp may prolapse through the anus to appear as a red, cherry-like mass.

Polyps may be detected by a double-contrast barium enema but preferably by colonoscopy which is more accurate and permits removal of the smaller tumours.

Management

Polyps in the rectum can be removed at sigmoidoscopy. Polyps in the colon can usually be treated at colonoscopy. Most polyps are pedunculated and both the stalk and the polyp are removed and then examined for malignant changes. If the polyp is malignant and there is infiltration beyond the stalk it is usual practice to resect that portion of the colon from which the polyp originated.

Patients who have had more than three polyps removed should have further colonoscopies every 1–2 years to detect recurrences. Colonoscopy at 1 and 3 years after polypectomy is sufficient if only 1–3 polyps were present.

FAMILIAL ADENOMATOUS POLYPOSIS (FAP)

This condition has an incidence of 1 in 24 000 and it is transmitted by autosomal dominant inheritance. It is characterised by thousands of small polyps diffusely scattered over the mucosal surface of the colon and rectum. These appear at adolescence and become malignant in about 15 years; the patient often dies from carcinomatosis before the age of 40. The disease is recognised by radiological and colonoscopic examination of the colon in patients and these procedures are used on members of affected families from adolescence to diagnose the polyps. Prevention of carcinoma means removal of the colon and rectum with permanent ileostomy, although symptomless members of the family may find ileorectal anastomosis with diathermy removal of rectal polyps and periodic surveillance more acceptable. A variant of the FAP genetic disorder is Gardner's syndrome in which exostoses (particularly mandibular) and congenital retinal hyperplasia are prominent.

OTHER FORMS OF BENIGN TUMOURS

These exist in single or multiple forms (Table 10.16). The multiple forms tend to be associated with gastrointestinal malignancy. Juvenile polyps nearly always present with bleeding. In the Peutz-Jegher's syndrome, polyps are present throughout the gastrointestinal tract and there is melanin pigmentation at the mucocutaneous junctions.

Other polypoid lesions which may occur in the colon are lipomas, carcinoids (p. 473) and leiomyomas.

Table 10.16 Gastrointestinal polyposis syndrome

	Familial polyposis (includes Gardner syndrome)	Peutz-Jeghers syndrome	Turcot syndrome	Cronkhite-Canada syndrome	Cowden's disease
Oesophegal polyps	–	–	–	+	+
Gastric polyps	+	+ +	–	+ + +	+ + +
Small intestinal polyps	+	+ + +	–	+ +	+ +
Colonic polyps	+ + +	+ +	+ + +	+ + +	+
Other features	Osteomas, soft tissue tumours, congenital retinal pigment hyperplasia	Pigmentation of lips, fingers	Malignant central nervous tumours	Hair loss, hyperpigmentation, nail dystrophy	Multiple congenital abnormalities, Orocutaneous hamartomas, thyroid tumours, breast hypertrophy

– Absent
+ Occasionally present
+ + Present
+ + + Frequently present

CARCINOMA OF THE COLON AND RECTUM

Carcinoma of the large intestine is the most common malignant tumour of the alimentary tract in most Western communities and has an incidence approaching 40 per 100 000. It is rare in Africa and Asia. The variation in incidence of the disease between different countries has led to speculation that dietary factors and differences in bacterial flora of the bowel may be of aetiological significance. Diseases known to be clearly associated with colonic carcinoma are long-standing ulcerative colitis and familial polyposis, but in the majority of patients the cancer arises from a malignant transformation of a benign adenomatous polyp.

Pathology

In communities with a high incidence of large bowel cancer, the distribution of tumours is shown in Figure 10.19. Concomitant (synchronous) multiple tumours are present in 2% of patients and the risk of a second cancer is higher in those who also have adenomatous polyps.

Macroscopically the tumour may be proliferative and fungating, ulcerative and infiltrating, polypoidal or encircling as a 'string' stricture. Perforation may occur at the site of the tumour leading to peritonitis, localised abscess or a fistula.

Spread occurs directly into and through the bowel wall, by lymphatics and by the bloodstream through both portal and systemic circulations. Colonic carcinoma is capable of direct implantation on exposed surfaces, such as a suture line or area of trauma in the bowel. Metastases most commonly involve the liver.

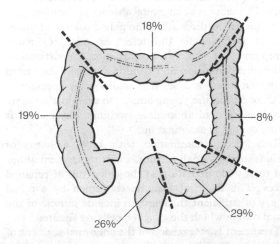

Fig. 10.19   Distribution of cancer of the large intestine.

Table 10.17   Dukes' classification of large bowel cancer

Stage	Definition	% of cases	Prognosis (5-year survival)
A	Spread not beyond muscularis No lymph node metastases	4	80%
B	Spread is beyond muscularis into pericolic tissues but no lymph node metastases	28	58%
C	Spread to lymph nodes	27	36%
D	Metastases present	41	6%

Tumours are classified by the Dukes' system which has important prognostic implications (Table 10.17).

Clinical features

Symptoms vary depending on the site of the carcinoma. In tumours of the left colon bleeding is common and obstruction is early. Tumours of the right colon present with anaemia, cachexia and alteration of bowel habit but obstruction is late because of the relatively fluid nature of the bowel contents. As a consequence left-sided tumours tend to be diagnosed earlier. Some patients may present with perforation and caecal carcinoma may mimic acute appendicitis.

Change in bowel habit, anaemia, weight loss and sometimes excessive borborygmi, abdominal distension and colicky pains indicating subacute obstruction, all point to a large bowel tumour. Some, however, are relatively symptomless until the patient presents as an emergency with obstruction.

Carcinoma of the lower rectum will almost always cause early bleeding with mucus discharge; later there is tenesmus and a feeling of incomplete emptying of the bowel. Obstruction is a feature of tumours of the pelvi-rectal junction but not the rectum proper which is capacious and distensible.

The findings on physical examination range from no obvious abnormality to the signs of advanced malignancy with cachexia and signs of extra-colonic spread. A mass may be palpable. Rectal tumours may be palpated on digital examination. Fresh blood in the stool should always suggest the possibility of a tumour of the rectum or pelvic colon. Occult blood is found in the stool if an ulcerating lesion is present higher in the colon.

Investigation

In most communities the initial investigations are a rigid sigmoidoscopy which will detect approximately one third of tumours followed by a double-contrast barium enema examination. A barium enema will demonstrate advanced cancer as a filling defect or

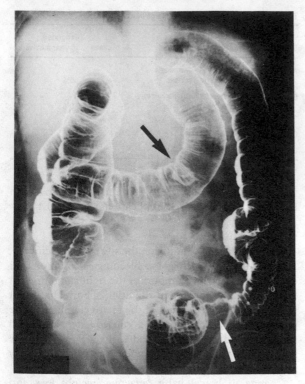

Fig. 10.20   Carcinoma of the sigmoid colon and a polyp in the transverse colon. (Courtesy of Dr G.M. Fraser.)

stricture (Fig. 10.20). However the barium enema is not as accurate as colonoscopy in detecting small tumours and polyps and thus in many centres, flexible sigmoidoscopy and colonoscopy have become the investigations of choice. There is a tendency for carcinomas of the caecum to be missed because the filling with barium may be incomplete and the colonoscopy may not reach the area in a small proportion of cases. When caecal cancer is suspected, a barium follow-through examination may help to define the tumour.

Computed tomography is a valuable technique to search for hepatic metastases prior to surgery so that appropriate treatment can be planned.

Management
The treatment of choice is resection of the tumour as a one-stage procedure. If there is no colonic obstruction, or if it can be overcome by enemas, time should be spent in preparing the bowel by washouts and antibiotics. Anaemia should be corrected by preoperative transfusion.

Carcinoma of the rectum may require total removal of the rectum with permanent colostomy and for this the patient requires preoperative explanation of colostomy and its management. However, advances in suture techniques allow preservation of continuity in many more patients by means of a colo-rectal or colo-anal anastomasis. In addition, some centres are instituting local treatment of rectal cancers with irradiation, electrocoagulation or laser therapy in order to avoid colostomy.

Hepatic secondary tumour can sometimes be treated by resection in the hope of cure and the symptoms from multiple metastases can be palliated with hepatic artery ligation, embolisation and infusion chemotherapy.

Screening for colon cancer
Successful treatment depends on early diagnosis and operation before spread has occurred and before obstruction renders the surgeon's task more complicated. Screening programmes utilising occult blood tests and regular endoscopy have been instituted in an attempt to diagnose the tumour at an early stage. To date there is no evidence that they have increased the survival rate. However regular surveillance is justified in those patients with a strong family history of colon cancer, patients with ulcerative colitis (p. 467) and those with a family history of familial polyposis.

MEGACOLON

Megacolon is a condition characterised by dilatation of the colon and obstinate constipation. The patients may be separated into two groups, congenital (Hirschsprung's disease) and acquired megacolon.

HIRSCHSPRUNG'S DISEASE

This is a familial disorder with an incidence of 1 in 5000. The cause is a congenital absence of the myenteric nerve plexus in the wall of the pelvic colon and upper rectum. Occasionally the defect extends proximally. Symptoms of colonic obstruction (constipation, abdominal distension and vomiting) usually date from birth, but in a few cases the condition may present in childhood or in the young adult. On examination there may be persistent abdominal swelling. The rectum is empty on digital examination.

Radiological examination with small amounts of barium shows a small rectum, a narrow segment above and then wide dilatation of the colon full of retained faeces. The diagnosis can be confirmed by a rectal biopsy of sufficient thickness to include muscle of the bowel wall in which the ganglion cells are situated.

Treatment is by excision of the abnormal segment of colon and rectum.

Table 10.18 Megacolon in the adult

	Cause
Psychogenic megacolon	Disregard for urge to defaecate; antidepressant drugs
Prolonged laxative abuse	Degeneration of myenteric plexus
Neurological disorders	Interruption of sensory and/or motor nerve supply
Smooth muscle disorders, e.g. scleroderma	Degeneration of colonic smooth muscle
Metabolic disorders, e.g. hypothyroidism	Delay in colonic transit

ACQUIRED MEGACOLON

This may present in childhood when its usual cause is the withholding of stool during the toilet training period. It is distinguished from Hirschsprung's disease by the presence of the urge to defaecate and the presence of stool in the rectum. It responds to osmotic laxatives.

Acquired megacolon has several causes in the adult (Table 10.18). Abnormalities of sphincter muscle, pelvic floor and innervation are recognised in some patients.

Radiologically, acquired megacolon usually shows no narrowed segment and the dilatation extends down to the anus. The rectum is full of faeces.

Most patients can be managed conservatively by treatment of the cause where identifiable, by high-residue diets, laxatives and perhaps saline enemas. The response will depend on the underlying pathogenesis. In a few patients colonic resection has been used as a last resort in the relief of obstinate constipation.

CONSTIPATION

This may be defined as less than 3 motions per week or as difficult or painful defaecation. The causes are classified in the information box (right) according to their frequency.

In addition constipation is extremely common in the irritable bowel syndrome (p. 477) but here it is recognised in the context of the other clinical features.

Constipation is a common complaint and initially it is important to determine if there is true constipation. The normal bowel habit of many individuals is less than one stool per day; this does not constitute constipation. The clinical approach to true constipation is based on the possible causes (see information box (right)). Information about constipation is shown in the information box (right).

Management

A classification of laxatives is shown in Table 10.19. However, most constipation is simple and can be

Table 10.19 Laxatives

	Use
Chemical – anthracine and phenylmethane derivatives, e.g. bisacodyl	Elderly or bed-bound individuals Preoperative preparation
dioctyl sodium sulphosuccinate	Preoperative preparation
Saline laxatives	Radiological preparation
Hydrophilic agents ('bulk laxatives') e.g. methylcellulose	Routinely used in chronic constipation especially in individuals who cannot tolerate dietary roughage

---

CAUSES OF CONSTIPATION

- Inadequate diet and lifestyle ('simple constipation'), e.g. Lack of fibre and exercise
- Drugs
  Analgesics
  Anti-inflammatory agents
  Antacids
  Antidepressants
  Diuretics
  Iron and many more
- Psychiatric and neurological disorders
  Ignoring call to stool
  Physical disability
- Organic diseases of the anus, rectum and colon
- Disorders of intestinal motility which may be secondary to metabolic problems
  Hypothyroidism
  Disease of the colonic muscle or nervous plexuses (e.g. scleroderma)

IMPORTANT INFORMATION IN A CONSTIPATED PATIENT

- Is the constipation of recent origin? If so a full G.I. investigation is needed in those over 30 years old
- Is the diet well-balanced and containing fibre?
- What drugs is the patient receiving – particularly opiates, antacids, psychotropic agents?
- Are laxatives being used?
- Are there any psychiatric, neurological or systemic diseases?

treated with an increase in roughage in the diet, e.g. bran plus an adequate fluid intake and exercise.

LAXATIVE ABUSE SYNDROMES

The prolonged consumption of chemical laxatives may lead to degeneration of the myenteric plexus of the colon. The patient complains of increasing constipation despite large doses of laxatives. A barium enema demonstrates a 'cathartic colon' which has a featureless mucosa, loss of haustration and pseudostrictures. When the patient has used prolonged anthraquinone purgatives, sigmoidoscopy may show a brown or black mucosa termed *melanosis coli*. Treatment of constipation is very difficult. The aim is to replace chemical laxatives with saline and then bulk laxatives, but many patients do not respond.

Surreptitious laxative abuse may occur particularly in women who complain of diarrhoea, abdominal discomfort and tiredness. They strongly deny taking laxatives and may continue even during investigation in hospital. Electrolyte disturbances are common and there may be malabsorption due to the effect of laxatives on the small intestine.

ANAL CONTINENCE AND INCONTINENCE

Continence depends upon an intact internal sphincter, external sphincter and puborectalis muscles and their afferent and efferent innervation. The more usual causes of incontinence are shown in the information box below.

CAUSES OF INCONTINENCE

- Damage to the innervation of pelvic floor muscles during childbirth
- Anorectal disease
  Haemorrhoids
  Rectal prolapse
  Inflammatory bowel disease
- Neurological and psychiatric disease
  Spina bifida
  Spinal trauma
  Senile dementia
- Faecal impaction
- Congenital abnormalities of the anorectal region

Management

This is usually very difficult. A reduction in stool volume by the use of loperamide (6–8 mg daily) or lomotil (5 mg 3 times daily) may help all patients.

Thereafter, the use of electrophysiological tests to detect activity in the muscles of continence often identifies the main problem. Repair operations can sometimes be instituted when the primary abnormality is identified as muscle damage.

FUNCTIONAL DISORDERS OF THE GASTROINTESTINAL TRACT

A functional disorder is one for which no structural, infective or biochemical cause can be found. Functional disorders of the gastrointestinal tract are extremely common and the most important are listed in the information box below.

FUNCTIONAL DISORDERS OF THE GASTROINTESTINAL TRACT

- Complaints of bad taste (cacogeusia) or offensive breath (halitosis)
- Globus hystericus
- Non-cardiac chest pain originating in the oesophagus
- Psychogenic vomiting
- Non-ulcer dyspepsia (functional dyspepsia)
- Functional biliary pain including some patients with post-cholecystectomy syndrome
- Irritable bowel syndrome

While it can be readily shown that the blood flow as well as the secretory and motor activities of the gastrointestinal tract are influenced by emotion, the mechanisms by which psychological distress elicits a symptomatic response from the gut are poorly understood. When psychological problems are obvious, as in anxiety or depressive states, or in the response to a stressful life experience, their relationship to symptoms can be readily confirmed. Often, however, the underlying mechanism is a long-standing emotional conflict and the connection between such problems and physical symptoms is much more difficult to establish.

Psychological disturbances can induce a great variety of individual symptoms. Anxious or stressed patients may complain of a dry mouth, a sensation of a lump in the throat, anorexia, nausea or vomiting, aerophagy with belching, abdominal pain or discomfort, constipation or diarrhoea, or excessive flatus. Depressed patients commonly complain of a bad taste in the mouth, or of nausea and vomiting especially on waking. Although symptoms may occur singly and are occasionally bizarre, some common patterns occur.

GLOBUS HYSTERICUS

Globus hystericus describes the sensation of a lump in the throat which is independent of swallowing and indeed may be relieved by swallowing food or drink. It occurs most frequently in tense, anxious individuals, but before accepting a psychogenic basis it is necessary to exclude organic disease by a barium swallow and endoscopy.

PSYCHOGENIC VOMITING

Psychogenic vomiting may occur in anxiety neurosis. Usually it commences on wakening, or immediately after breakfast; only rarely does it occur later in the day. The disorder is probably a reaction to awakening and facing up to the worries of everyday life; in the young it can be due to school phobia. There may be retching alone or the vomiting of gastric secretions or food. Although psychogenic vomiting may occur regularly over long periods, there is little or no weight loss and this is of value in distinguishing it from vomiting due to organic disease of the alimentary tract. Early morning vomiting also occurs in pregnancy, alcohol abuse and depression.

In all patients it is essential to assess and, if possible, alleviate the underlying psychological disturbance. Tranquillisers and antiemetic drugs (e.g. metoclopramide 10 mg 3 times daily; domperidone 10 mg 3 times a day, prochlorpexazine 5–10 mg 3 times daily) have only a secondary place in management.

NON-ULCER DYSPEPSIA (see p. 441)

THE IRRITABLE BOWEL SYNDROME

Aetiology

One of the commonest disorders of the alimentary tract is that of long-standing dysfunction associated with abdominal pain for which no organic cause can be found. Bowel habit is disturbed by diarrhoea or constipation occurring alone, or alternating. Some forms of this irritable bowel syndrome have in the past been called *spastic colon* and *idiopathic or nervous diarrhoea*.

Whilst it is generally accepted that disturbed motility in the colon forms the basis of the symptoms consistent changes which would be helpful diagnostically have not been found. Disturbances of motility have also been demonstrated in the small intestine, stomach, lower oesophagus and bladder and these help to explain the widespread nature of the symptoms.

Although the aetiology of the irritable bowel syndrome is uncertain, psychological disturbances, especially anxiety, are frequent; patients are often tense, conscientious individuals who worry excessively about family or financial affairs. Some relate the onset of their symptoms to an attack of infective diarrhoea; in others certain foods may precipitate symptoms.

Clinical features

The syndrome is most frequent in women between the ages of 20 and 40 years. The commonest symptom is pain referred to the left or right iliac fossa or the hypogastrium, sometimes varying in site. Pain often occurs in attacks usually relieved by defecation and sometimes provoked by food, and may be severe. Bowel habit is variable. Almost all patients at some time, notice pellet like or ribbon like stools with or without mucus. Diarrhoea may be painless and characteristically occurs in the morning, and almost never at night. An urge to defecate after meals may be the consequence of an exaggerated gastrocolic reflex. Other symptoms include abdominal distension, a sensation of incomplete emptying of the rectum, excessive flatus and audible borborygmi. There may be dyspepsia, heartburn, frequency and dysuria.

Investigation

Although the diagnosis is usually suggested by the history alone, organic bowel disease has to be excluded, especially in patients developing symptoms for the first time over the age of 40 years. Sigmoidoscopy may be required to exclude an organic lesion of the rectum or rectosigmoid junction. The mucosa appears normal in the irritable bowel syndrome but the bowel may show marked motor activity, contracting and relaxing quite unlike the normal inert bowel. In appropriate circumstances a barium enema may be indicated to exclude organic disease. There are no diagnostic radiological features in the irritable bowel syndrome. The possibility of lactose intolerance, hyperthyroidism or alcohol excess should not be overlooked in patients whose principal complaint is painless diarrhoea.

Management

The patient must first be reassured that no organic disease is present as anxiety may precipitate or aggravate the condition and there is sometimes an underlying fear of cancer. An explanation for the symptoms must be offered and this is best based upon a simple description of intestinal motility and its disorder, spasm, which can cause pain. In patients with persistent or troublesome symptoms, measures designed to modify the intestinal dysmotility are required. For constipation and pain, the patient should be encouraged to increase the roughage content of the diet and one of the bulk laxatives such as methylcellulose should be prescribed in a dose sufficient to ensure normal bowel movement. It is important that the patient should stop chemical laxatives.

For pain and diarrhoea an anticholinergic drug such as dicyclomine (10 mg 3 times daily) or an anti-spasmodic such as mebeverine hydrochloride (135 mg 3 times daily) may be tried. For patients with painless diarrhoea, improvement is commonly obtained with some dietary restriction, particularly the avoidance of fresh fruits and salads. Codeine phosphate (30 mg 3–4 times daily) and loperamide (6–8 mg daily) are useful drugs which act quickly and can be carried by the patient to use either in emergency or before any event which is known to precipitate diarrhoea.

THE PANCREAS

DISEASES OF THE PANCREAS

The pancreas produces exocrine secretions which are important to digestion and also endocrine secretions concerned with the regulation of carbohydrate metabolism. The exocrine tissue, composed of acinar cells grouped in lobules and drained by a duct system, forms almost the entire mass of the gland. The exocrine secretion is discharged into the intestine through the pancreatic duct, which usually enters the duodenum together with the common bile duct at the sphincter of Oddi; in about 10% of individuals, however, the main outflow of the pancreatic juice reaches the duodenum by a separate duct.

The endocrine tissue is composed of specialised cells collected together in the small islets of Langerhans scattered throughout the gland, and accounts for only 1% of the mass of the pancreas. The A cells produce glucagon, the B cells insulin and the D cells gastrin, somatostatin and pancreatic polypeptide.

Pancreatic juice is an alkaline secretion which is isotonic with plasma, the main cations being sodium and potassium while the main anion is bicarbonate which is produced by the cells lining the duct system. The juice also contains enzymes which digest carbohydrate, fat and protein, the main ones being amylase, lipase and trypsin. These enzymes are synthesised by the acinar cells; they all require an alkaline medium for optimal efficiency, so that theoretically digestion may be impaired if the bicarbonate content of the pancreatic juice is reduced.

Exocrine pancreatic secretion is stimulated partly through the autonomic nervous system and partly through hormonal mechanisms, particularly secretin and cholecystokinin in response to food. Over 24 hours, 1–3 litres of pancreatic juice is secreted.

INVESTIGATION OF THE PANCREAS

Once pancreatic disease is suspected ultrasonography and computed tomography are the key investigative methods to demonstrate the size, shape and position of the pancreas, and tumours, cysts, oedema, inflammatory changes and dilated ducts. These techniques also play an important role in guiding the biopsy needle into the pancreas to confirm a diagnosis of pancreatic cancer. Plain radiographs have a more limited role and barium studies are rarely used.

Endoscopic retrograde cholangiopancreatography (ERCP) has a defined role in the differentiation of pancreatic cancer and chronic pancreatitis and will also define intrapancreatic cysts and duct strictures which may be an indication for surgical resection.

Tests of pancreatic exocrine function are used to demonstrate exocrine insufficiency when diarrhoea or steatorrhoea is present in chronic pancreatitis or cystic fibrosis. Exocrine function may be measured directly by passing a tube into the second part of the duodenum and collecting the secretory output of the gland in response to exogenous stimulation (secretin-chole-cystokinin test) or endogenous stimulation by a meal (Lundh test). In the *secretin-cholecystokinin test* the hormones are injected intravenously and pancreatic secretions are collected for 1 hour. Measurements are made of the volume of secretion and the concentration of bicarbonate and amylase or lipase. A special double lumened tube allows gastric and pancreatic secretions to be collected separately to prevent neutralisation of pancreatic bicarbonate by gastric hydrochloric acid. The *Lundh test* is simpler. A tube is passed into the duodenum and a liquid meal of fixed composition is given orally. The duodenal aspirate is collected by syphonage and the concentration of trypsin and amylase is recorded. Both tests detect the presence of established pancreatic insufficiency but usually give no information as to the cause.

There is a variety of simple non-invasive tests of pancreatic function such as the *bentiromide* and *pancreolauryl tests* which depend upon the cleavage of an orally given marker by pancreatic enzyme and its excretion in the urine. Alternatively, serum trypsin-like immunoreactivity or serum isoamylase determinations may be made. When normal values for these tests are obtained, pancreatic insufficiency is excluded.

CONGENITAL ABNORMALITIES

PANCREAS DIVISUM

This occurs in 10% of the population and results from a failure of the dorsal and ventral pancreas to unite; consequently most of the pancreas is drained through the accessory papilla which is proximal to the papilla of Vater. There is an unresolved debate whether such patients are more prone to pancreatitis.

ANNULAR PANCREAS

The ventral pancreas surrounds the second part of the duodenum and can constrict it causing obstruction soon after birth or in adult life. The diagnosis is made by barium studies or endoscopy and the treatment is surgical bypass of the constriction.

ECTOPIC PANCREATIC TISSUE

This may occur in the gastric antrum or duodenum and takes the form of a smooth nodule. It is usually asymptomatic.

CYSTIC FIBROSIS

This disease is transmitted as an autosomal recessive with an incidence in Caucasian populations from 1 in 1500 to 1 in 15 000 live births. The basic abnormality probably lies in the movement of electrolytes across the cell membrane.

Pathology

The pathological findings and the clinical features result from the obstruction by abnormal, viscid secretions, of ducts or passages in the respiratory tract, salivary glands, digestive and biliary tracts, pancreas and genitourinary tracts. These changes, as they affect the alimentary tract, are summarised in Table 10.20.

Clinical features

Increasing numbers of patients are surviving to adulthood because of better treatment of respiratory infection. The respiratory problems become progressively more important in the adolescent and adult and determine the fate of the individual; by contrast malabsorption is less troublesome. Nevertheless frequent, offensive stools are still common. There may be bronchiectasis, recurrent spontaneous pneumothorax, recurrent haemoptysis, pulmonary fibrosis and right ventricular failure. Liver disease also increases in importance in adolescents and adults and portal hypertension often develops. Females with cystic fibrosis may become pregnant but males are nearly always infertile.

Investigations

Whilst the diagnosis is often strongly suspected from the clinical findings it should be confirmed by a sweat test which is based upon the quantitative pilocarpine iontophoresis technique. Sweating is stimulated over a

Table 10.20 Alimentary tract features of cystic fibrosis

Pathological changes	Clinical features
Pancreas	
Blockage of ducts	Recurrent pancreatitis
Eventual fibrosis and atrophy	Pancreatic exocrine insufficiency
	Steatorrhoea
	Peptic ulcer
Intestine	
Blockage of the lumen with thick mucus	Meconium ileus causing neonatal obstruction
Blockage of the lumen with mucofaeculent masses	Meconium ileus equivalent causing childhood obstruction
Liver and biliary tract	
Congenital abnormalities of the gallbladder	Obstructive neonatal jaundice
	Cholecystitis
Blockage of the cystic biliary ducts	Biliary cirrhosis and portal hypertension
Gallstones	
Intrahepatic bile duct obstruction	

Table 10.21   Complications of acute pancreatitis and their causes

Complication	Cause
Systemic	
Shock and renal failure	Loss of fluid into the pancreas and surrounding tissues
Respiratory failure	Shock lung syndrome
Diabetes mellitus	Destruction of pancreatic tissue
Hypocalcaemia	Sequestration of calcium in areas of fat necrosis
Subcutaneous fat necrosis	Release of pancreatic lipase
Pancreatic	
Abscess	Infection of necrotic pancreatic tissue
Pseudocyst	Collection of pancreatic debris and secretions
Gastrointestinal	
Haemorrhage	Gastric and duodenal erosions Necrosis of duodenal wall
Intestinal ileus	Local inflammation due to spread of pancreatic enzymes
Obstruction to the duodenum	Mechanical compression from the pancreatic mass
Obstructive jaundice	Compression of the common bile duct

small area of skin of the inner forearm by pilocarpine iontophoresis, the sweat being collected on a gauze pad of known weight covered by a plastic square and sealed at the edges with waterproof adhesive tape. After 1 hour the pad is removed, weighed and the sweat eluted and analysed for sodium and chloride. In children, chloride values greater than 60 mmol/l are diagnostic. In the adult, diagnosis is based upon a sweat sodium greater than 70 mmol/l on 2 occasions.

A number of other investigations may be required to evaluate the complications listed in Table 10.21.

In adolescence and adulthood occasional patients have borderline values for sweat sodium. In these patients the demonstration of pancreatic insufficiency by a test of exocrine function supports the diagnosis. The measurement of faecal fat excretion is important in assessing the response to treatment.

Management

Optimal treatment in the adolescent and adult depends on a team approach to complicated respiratory, nutritional and hepatobiliary problems. Many centres have now established special clinics for such patients with appropriate specialist care.

Patients with cystic fibrosis need 120–150% of recommended daily energy allowance because of malabsorption and the catabolism induced by acute and chronic respiratory infections. Nutritional counselling and supervision are therefore very important with the use of high energy supplements and snacks. Fat restriction is not advised because it limits calorie intake. Supplements of fat-soluble vitamins are required.

All patients with pancreatic insufficiency require oral pancreatic enzyme supplements. The dose of up to 30

capsules per day is titrated to reduce steatorrhoea to a point at which stool frequency and offensiveness are reduced. Gastric acid neutralisation with antacid or H_2-receptor antagonists are often indicated to ensure a neutral pH in the duodenum which is necessary for the proper functioning of the pancreatic enzyme supplements.

ACUTE PANCREATITIS

This is an acute condition typically presenting with abdominal pain, and usually associated with raised pancreatic enzymes in blood or urine due to inflammatory disease of the pancreas. In Western communities it has an incidence of 5–10 per 100 000.

Aetiology

In Britain about 50% of cases are associated with biliary disease and about 20% with alcoholism while in about 20% no cause can be identified. Alcoholism accounts for a much higher proportion in some countries especially the USA and South Africa. The risk factors are listed in the information box below.

RISK FACTORS FOR ACUTE PANCREATITIS

- Alcohol
- Gallstones
- Local obstructive factors
  Duodenal diverticulum
  Stenosis of the papilla of Vater
  Carcinoma in the head of the pancreas
- Drugs
  Azathioprine
- Infections:
  Mumps
- Hyperlipoproteinaemia
- Major surgery or procedures:
  ERCP
- Diffuse vascular diseases
- Hypercalcaemia
- Fulminant hepatic failure
- Abdominal trauma

The pancreas secretes the digestive enzymes as proenzymes which are activated in the intestinal lumen. Acute pancreatitis may result when activation occurs in the pancreatic duct system or even in the pancreatic acinar cells. In pancreatitis associated with gallstones the passage of a gallstone down the common bile duct precipitates the attack by allowing duodenal contents including bile to reflux into the pancreatic duct system. The precise events are not understood. Under normal circumstances digestive and lysosomal enzymes are separated within the acinar cell. It is possible that contact between them activates the digestive enzyme to cause acute pancreatitis and this may explain the mechanism of action of some of the risk factors such as drugs and infections.

Pathology

The pancreas shows oedema, necrosis of the acinar and duct cells and an infiltration with inflammatory cells. With progression the entire pancreas may become an inflammatory mass with haemorrhage into and around it. The release of enzymes leads to fat necrosis both in the pancreas and in the peritoneal cavity. Pancreatic secretions may subsequently collect to form one or more pseudocysts which have no epithelial lining and are lined with granulation and fibrous tissue. A pseudocyst communicates with a pancreatic duct and thus it may increase in size because of continued pancreatic secretion. A pancreatic abscess may form when the pseudocyst or the inflammatory mass becomes infected by bacteria.

Clinical features

The onset is usually sudden with severe pain in the epigastrium or right hypochondrium. It often occurs within 12–24 hours following a large meal and alcohol. The pain is usually persistent and radiates most frequently through to the back, to either shoulder or to one of the iliac fossae before spreading to involve the whole abdomen. Nausea and vomiting are common. In severe cases profound shock supervenes and there is tachycardia, hypotension, cardiac arrhythmias and renal failure. An increased respiratory rate and hypoxia are common. Many other serious complications may arise either in the first few days or weeks of the disease (see Table 10.21, p. 480).

Despite the severity of the pain there may be little or no guarding of the abdominal muscles at first. Later the upper abdomen becomes tender and rigid as peritoneal irritation increases and the initial shock passes off. The condition may simulate acute cholecystitis (with which it may coexist) and myocardial infarction. The disease may be recognised for the first time at laparotomy, the patients having been diagnosed as perforated peptic ulcer or acute appendicitis.

Pancreatic abscess

This presents 2–5 weeks after the onset of acute pancreatitis. The patient deteriorates with further abdominal pain, fever and weight loss. On examination there is abdominal tenderness but a palpable mass is uncommon.

Pancreatic pseudocyst

This develops 1–2 weeks after the onset of acute pancreatitis. There is abdominal pain, nausea and vomiting and weight loss. On examination there is often a smooth, round, tender mass in the upper abdomen. Frequently there is obstruction to the duodenum and common bile duct.

Pancreatic ascites

Pancreatic ascites refers to ascites resulting from pancreatic duct disruption or from leaking of a pancreatic pseudocyst in patients with acute or chronic pancreatitis. The secretions may track into the mediastinum and as a result, a pleural effusion may develop. The ascites presents with abdominal pain and an increase in girth.

Investigations

Amylase activity

Serum amylase activity is elevated on the first day of the disease and thereafter falls rapidly because of renal clearance. Urinary amylase activity measured on a 24-hour collection of urine may be helpful when the serum level is not diagnostic. A persistently raised serum amylase suggests the development of pseudocyst or pancreatic abscess or a non-pancreatic cause (Table

Table 10.22   Non-pancreatic causes of a raised serum amylase activity

Other causes of acute abdomen	
Intestinal obstruction with gangrene	Like acute pancreatitis the rise is
Cholecystitis	short-lived, but is rarely above 1200 u/l
Ruptured ovarian cyst	
Perforated duodenal ulcer	
Abnormal amylase	
Macroamylasaemia	The elevation is persistent
Raised salivary amylase in alcoholics	

10.22). Very high levels of amylase activity also occur in ascitic fluid in pancreatic ascites and in pleural effusion secondary to pancreatic ascites.

Plain radiographs

Whilst changes may be seen on a plain radiograph of the abdomen, these are often non-specific. However, the plain radiograph is used to diagnose ileus or obstruction secondary to acute pancreatitis. A plain radiograph of the chest often shows a left pleural effusion, collapse or consolidation of the lung.

Imaging

Ultrasound scanning and computed tomography are used to confirm the diagnosis and are vital in

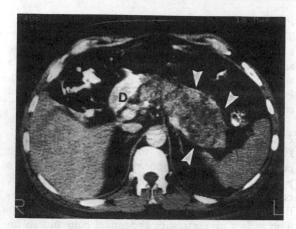

Fig. 10.21 Acute pancreatitis. This CT shows a large oedematous pancreas, particularly the body and tail (arrows). Duodenal loop = D.

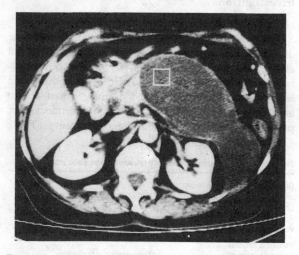

Fig. 10.22 Pancreatic pseudocyst. The cyst appears homogeneous.

monitoring the progress of the disorder and in detecting the development of pseudocyst, abscess and haemorrhage. The procedures are complementary. Computed tomography best indicates the degree of damage to the pancreas itself, is helpful in defining haemorrhage into and around the pancreas, and it identifies gas which is an important sign of pancreatic abscess formation. Ultrasonography is suited to the identification and serial assessment of pseudocysts, the assessment of biliary obstruction and the identification of gallstones.

Laparotomy
This may be performed when a condition requiring surgery such as a perforated duodenal ulcer cannot be excluded. The diagnosis is then made on the appearance of the pancreas and the absence of any other acute intra-abdominal condition.

Management
The reduced mortality from acute pancreatitis in recent years is due to an understanding of the complications which may arise and the application of effective supportive therapy.

The immediate requirements are the energetic treatment of shock and of respiratory failure and the relief of pain. A central venous line is used to monitor the need for fluid replacement, and to guard against overloading the circulation. Serial arterial oxygen pressures should be recorded because if respiratory failure becomes a major factor, endotracheal intubation and positive pressure ventilation will be required. The bladder is catheterised so that urinary output can be measured. Intravenous saline, plasma, plasma expanders or whole blood may be required in large volumes as determined by the clinical response, urinary output and central venous pressure. Oral feeding is withheld until pain, tenderness, fever and leucocytosis have resolved; parenteral alimentation is necessary in all but the milder cases. Gastric intubation and aspiration are used for symptomatic benefit.

Pain is best relieved by intravenous or intramuscular administrations of pethidine (100 mg); morphine should be avoided because of its undesirable effect of causing spasm of the sphincter of Oddi. Ileus is almost inevitable in the acute phase and nasogastric suction is continued until distension is relieved and active peristalsis has returned. When obstruction continues a Gastrografin meal will indicate if the duodenum is obstructed. Haemorrhage from the upper gastrointestinal tract is investigated and treated; bleeding into a cyst or the peritoneal cavity can be confirmed by computed tomography. Selective arteriography and therapeutic embolisation may be necessary to control haemorrhage.

Surgery
This is necessary for a pancreatic abscess and when there is cholecystitis the gallbladder should be drained or removed. If the diagnosis of acute pancreatitis is made when laparotomy is undertaken for diagnostic uncertainty no direct surgical intervention should be attempted unless there is cholecystitis. Surgical resection of the pancreas may be attempted when there is severe necrosis of the entire pancreas but the mortality rate is high.

Once the attack of acute pancreatitis has subsided it is essential to identify cholelithiasis and obstructive causes of pancreatitis (see Table 10.21, p. 480) in order to prevent further attacks.

Pseudocysts

These are treated conservatively for 4–6 weeks because many will resolve spontaneously. However surgery is necessary when there is rapid enlargement or persistent obstruction to the duodenum or common bile duct. The cyst is drained into the stomach or intestine. Surgical resection of the damaged pancreas is usually necessary for pancreatic ascites.

Prognosis

This depends upon the severity of the attack. Overall, the mortality is 10–20%. Patients with haemorrhagic pancreatitis have a mortality of over 50% whereas when there is only oedema of the pancreas, the mortality is less than 5%. Of the deaths, 75% occur in the first week.

CHRONIC PANCREATITIS

Chronic pancreatitis is defined as a continuing inflammatory disease of the pancreas, characterised by irreversible morphological change and typically causing pain and/or permanent impairment of function.

Aetiology

The majority of cases of chronic pancreatitis in the Western world occur as a result of a persistent high alcohol consumption. It is possible that a small number result from cholelithiasis. It is rare for acute attacks of pancreatitis to proceed to chronic pancreatitis. Chronic pancreatitis may occasionally be caused by stenosis or disease of the sphincter of Oddi and rarely the condition may be familial. In some parts of the tropics, chronic pancreatitis is common and malnutrition may be an aetiological factor. Chronic pancreatitis is common in cystic fibrosis (p. 479).

Pathology

Plugs of protein and calcium carbonate crystals form in the ducts and these progress to stones which in turn lead to duct obstruction and dilatation. On microscopy the pancreas shows fibrosis around the ducts and acina which are gradually replaced. By contrast, there is usually preservation of the islets of Langerhans. The end result of these changes is an atrophic pancreas with dilated cystic ducts, retention cysts and calcification.

Clinical features

The disease is most common in males between the ages of 35 and 45 years. Nearly all patients present with abdominal pain. Recurrent attacks occur at intervals of several weeks or months often within a few hours to two days of an alcoholic bout. In contrast to acute pancreatitis the pain may begin gradually and persist for days or weeks. Pain is located in the epigastrium, right or left subcostal areas or around the umbilicus; characteristically it may radiate to the back between T10 and T12 and relief may be obtained by crouching forward or leaning forward over a chair. Weight loss is common due to malnutrition secondary to pancreatic pain, steatorrhoea and diabetes mellitus. Diarrhoea is common.

Diabetes mellitus develops in about a fifth of patients and steatorrhoea in a third and may occasionally be the presenting feature. Both these complications are more likely when the pancreas is calcified. Jaundice may arise from obstruction to the common bile duct by fibrosis within the pancreas and such obstruction is a possible cause of abdominal pain. Pseudocysts may develop and cirrhosis is common.

On examination there may be diffuse tenderness in the upper abdomen and features of malnutrition and weight loss.

Investigation

A variety of investigations may be used in chronic pancreatitis (Table 10.23 and Fig. 10.23). They may be conveniently classified into radiographic and imaging techniques which demonstrate the structural changes in the gland, and function and metabolic studies which indicate whether the function of the gland is inadequate for normal physiological processes.

Table 10.23 Investigations for chronic pancreatitis

Investigation or test	Use or indication
Plain radiograph of the abdomen	Calcification of pancreas
Ultrasonography and computed tomography	To demonstrate atrophy and calcification, temporary enlargement in acute attacks and stricture of the common bile duct
ERCP	For planning surgery
N-benzoyl-l-tyrosyl-p-amino benzoic acid test	A normal test excludes pancreatic insufficiency
Secretin/CCK stimulation test	To confirm pancreatic insufficiency
Glucose tolerance test	To demonstrate diabetes mellitus
5-day stool collection for fat excretion	To demonstrate steatorrhoea as the cause of diarrhoea and as a basis for monitoring treatment
Liver function tests	Raised serum alkaline phosphatase may indicate biliary obstruction

Management

Pancreatic extracts are indicated when there is loss of weight, diarrhoea or abdominal discomfort; an average of 10 000–12 000 lipase units per meal is given (usually

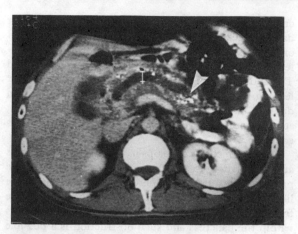

Fig. 10.23   Chronic pancreatitis. There is a large dilated pancreatic duct shown by a marker. Calcification is shown by an arrow.

5–6 tablets or capsules). The effectiveness of this therapy is assessed by improvement in symptoms and a reduction in faecal fat. In patients who respond poorly, antacids and H_2-receptor antagonists prevent the inactivation of the pancreatic extract by gastric acid. The diet should be normal and nutritious. Fat may be restricted to 25% of total calories except in the case of cystic fibrosis. Supplements of fat-soluble vitamins are often required. For diabetes, oral hypoglycaemic agents are usually of no value; the patient is managed with diet and insulin.

The treatment of pain is often difficult. Abstinence from alcohol is absolutely essential for it reduces the frequency and sometimes the severity of pain. Some authorities believe that therapy with pancreatic extracts reduces the frequency and severity of pain and that these should be tried even if they are not required for reasons of malabsorption. The use of analgesics (aspirin, paracetamol) is often indicated especially before meals in order to counteract the postprandial increase in pain. Failing these, opiate analgesics may have to be used and occasionally percutaneous coeliac plexus block may be necessary. Addiction to the analgesic drugs can be a problem.

Surgery should be contemplated for the relief of intractable pain. Drainage of the pancreatic duct into the small bowel or removal of part or most of the pancreas, are the most usual procedures. Surgery is also necessary for pseudocysts and for biliary obstruction. The ultimate result is so dependent on the alcoholic's ability to stop drinking that an operation is not worthwhile in the patient who cannot abstain.

Prognosis
Over a 10-year period, approximately one third of patients will obtain relief from pain without surgical treatment, pain will stabilise in one third and will worsen in one third. A fifth will develop diabetes mellitus and a third steatorrhoea. There is an increased mortality with only 50% survival at 7–10 years.

CARCINOMA OF THE PANCREAS

Incidence
The incidence of carcinoma of the pancreas is increasing in many Western countries and in males in the USA has reached 15 per 100 000. It is more common in males than in females and it occurs most frequently in the seventh decade.

Aetiology
Aetiological factors are smoking, high dietary fat and occupational exposure in chemical and metal industries.

Pathology
Ductal adenocarcinoma is by far the commonest tumour and is located in the head of the pancreas in about 60% of patients, the body or tail in 20% and in a combination of sites in the remainder. Tumours of the ampulla of Vater obstruct the common bile duct; they should be amenable to surgery and have a better prognosis. Islet cell carcinoma (p. 485), cystadenocarcinoma and papillary cystic neoplasms are rare forms of pancreatic cancer but are important because they have a better prognosis than adenocarcinoma.

Clinical features
All cancers of the pancreas are advanced by the time they cause symptoms apart from carcinoma of the ampulla which may bleed into the duodenum, or cause jaundice at a relatively early stage. Epigastric pain is common, but occasionally it may be absent throughout the course of the disease. The pain is variable in type but is characteristically dull and boring and radiates through to the back. It is often intensified by eating and by lying supine, especially at night. Pain may be relieved by crouching forward. Other symptoms include anorexia, nausea, discomfort and sometimes vomiting. Weight loss is common. The symptoms of diabetes mellitus may occasionally be the presenting feature.

Other clinical features depend largely on the site of the growth. In the majority of cases with involvement of the head of the pancreas, jaundice is the presenting feature and may be painless and progressive. Gastrointestinal haemorrhage and diarrhoea due to steatorrhoea may occur.

A large firm liver eventually develops. An abdominal

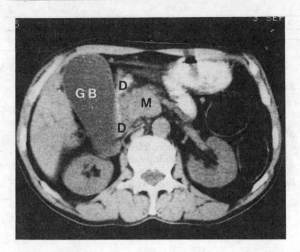

Fig. 10.24   Carcinoma of the head of the pancreas (M) which is causing a dilated gallbladder (GB) and a displaced duodenal loop (D).

mass is present in one-quarter of all patients and occasionally a distended gallbladder is palpable or ascites can be detected. Jaundice may not appear when the lesion affects mainly the body and tail of the pancreas.

Investigation

Pancreatic cancer is suspected from the clinical features, a raised serum alkaline phosphatase, a diabetic glucose tolerance test and a barium meal or endoscopy which may show distortion or displacement of the stomach or duodenum with possible invasion by tumour. Ultrasonography is a good initial screening test for pancreatic disease but computed tomography (Fig. 10.24) is the preferred method for confirming the diagnosis and deciding upon operability. In a minority of patients, it is impossible to distinguish cancer from chronic pancreatitis. Fine-needle aspiration biopsy performed percutaneously under guidance with ultrasound, computed tomography or ERCP are helpful in such patients. Duodenoscopy is important in detecting cancer of the ampulla. It is important to emphasise that all these investigations will detect only advanced cancer and as yet there is no means of making an earlier diagnosis.

Management

A Whipple operation which is a curative resection is rarely possible because most patients have extensive disease, are elderly and too ill. The procedure consists of removal of the duodenum and head of the pancreas and is only attempted when tumour is confined to the head of the pancreas. Thus, in the majority of patients only palliative measures are considered. The aim of surgical palliation is to relieve or prevent obstructive jaundice by anastomosing the gallbladder to the jejunum (cholecystojejunostomy). Gastroenterostomy is usually carried out to prevent duodenal obstruction. Alternatively relief of obstructive jaundice may be achieved by the insertion of a stent along the obstructed bile duct via an endoscope in the duodenum and this is becoming the favoured palliative approach. Relief of pain is very important. Initially oral methadone 5–10 mg may be used but the use of systems for the continuous delivery of morphine, or blockade of the coeliac ganglion may be necessary.

Prognosis

Mean survival is 14 months after resection and 5 months after palliative surgery. Of all patients with this cancer, less than 10% survive for 1 year and 5-year survival is rare.

PERIAMPULLARY TUMOURS

These arise from the papilla of Vater, from the terminal parts of the pancreatic or common bile ducts or from the duodenal mucosa adjacent to the papilla. Usually the tumour is an adenocarcinoma.

Most patients present with obstructive jaundice and half also have pain. Less common presentations are with iron deficiency anaemia due to bleeding from the tumour, or acute pancreatitis. The diagnosis is usually made at duodenoscopy. Computed tomography is used to assess the resectability of the tumour. The treatment is Whipple resection or transduodenal excision. The importance of the tumour lies in its relatively good prognosis in comparison with carcinoma of the pancreas. On average 40% of patients survive for 5 years.

ISLET CELL TUMOURS

These tumours which arise from the islet cells of the pancreas may be benign or malignant. The majority produce an excess of insulin (p. 678) or gastrin (Zollinger-Ellison syndrome, p. 438). The remainder are termed 'non-functioning' because they do not release any physiologically active hormone. The tumour usually presents with pain and jaundice and it is diagnosed by the same methods as pancreatic cancer. In contrast to pancreatic cancer there is a 40% survival at 5 years.

FURTHER READING

Bateson M C, Bouchier I A D 1988 Clinical investigations in gastroenterology. Kluwer Academic Publishers, London. A guide to the more widely used tests of function for trainees and clinicians with no special expertise in gastroenterology

Bouchier I A D et al 1984 Textbook of Gastroenterology. Bailliere Tindall, London. A major text with an emphasis on clinical gastroenterology

Clinics in gastroenterology. Saunders, London. A series of specialist volumes consisting of three numbers annually and each dealing with a specific disorder of the alimentary tract. Recommended for selective reading and as a reference library to current practice

Macleod J, Munro J 1986 Examination of the alimentary system. In: Clinical examination, 7th Edn. Churchill Livingstone, Edinburgh. Complementary to this chapter and designed to be read in conjunction with it

Shearman D J C, Finlayson N D C 1989 Diseases of the gastrointestinal tract and liver, 2nd Edn. Churchill Livingstone, Edinburgh. A new textbook primarily for clinicians

Sleisenger M H, Fordtran J S 1989 Gastrointestinal disease, 4th Edn. Saunders, London. The most complete reference text from the USA containing extensive bibliographies to each chapter

Books and journals dealing also with hepatobiliary disease are listed on page 546

11

Diseases of the Liver and Biliary System

HEPATOBILIARY ANATOMY, PHYSIOLOGY AND INVESTIGATION

ANATOMY

The liver lies in the right-upper quadrant of the abdomen and is the largest organ in the body (1200–1500 g). It descends 1–3 cm in inspiration and can normally be palpated in adults below the right costal margin during deep inspiration. Light percussion from above (fifth rib) and from below (epigastrium) in the right midclavicular line helps to determine liver size and is mainly of value in revealing a small liver. Auscultation over the liver may reveal an arterial bruit due to hepatocellular carcinoma or acute alcoholic hepatitis or a rub due to perihepatitis, and auscultation between the xiphisternum and umbilicus may reveal a venous hum due to collateral vessels in portal hypertension.

Traditionally, the liver has been divided into right and left lobes by the falciform ligament, the fissure of

the ligamentum teres and the fissure of the ligamentum venosum, but advances in hepatic surgery have determined a more useful division into right and left *hemilivers* separated by the course of the middle hepatic vein lying roughly on a line between the inferior vena cava and the gallbladder bed and passing through the porta hepatis (Fig. 11.1). The right and left hemilivers are further subdivided into a total of eight segments in accordance with further subdivisions of the hepatic vasculature. Each segment is in turn made up of histological units known as *lobules*, and each lobule comprises a central vein, radiating sinusoids (p. 491) separated from one another by liver cell (hepatocyte) plates containing the biliary canaliculi, and peripheral portal tracts. This histological unit has no functional significance. The portal tracts comprise the main connective tissue stroma of the liver. They originate in the porta hepatis, divide progressively as they branch out into the liver parenchyma, and contain branches of the hepatic artery and portal vein, the bile ducts (below) and the main hepatic lymphatics draining to the nodes in the porta hepatis. The branches of the hepatic vein contain little connective tissue, and they unite progressively to form three main veins which enter the inferior vena cava. Lymphatics are associated with the hepatic veins.

The biliary tract begins in the biliary canaliculi, which are integral parts of the hepatocytes, and the intrahepatic bile ducts derived from them join progressively to form the right and left hepatic ducts. These ducts join as they emerge from the liver to form the common hepatic duct which then forms the common bile duct by joining the cystic duct. The common bile duct is approximately 5 cm long and has a thin-walled wide-lumened proximal part and a thick-walled narrow-lumened distal part surrounded by the choledochal sphincter. The distal common bile duct usually joins the pancreatic duct before it enters the duodenum. The gallbladder is a pear-shaped sac lying under the right hemiliver with its fundus anteriorly behind the tip of the ninth costal cartilage. Its body and neck pass posteromedially towards the porta hepatis and the cystic duct then joins it to the common hepatic duct. The cystic duct mucosa has prominent crescentic folds (valves of Heister) giving it a beaded appearance on cholangiograms.

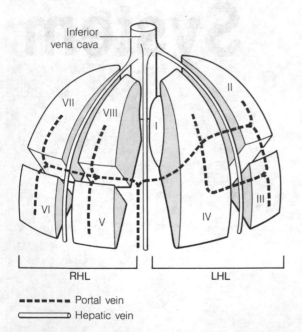

Fig. 11.1 Schematic representation of the liver. It shows the division of the liver into four hepatic sectors making up a right hemiliver (RHL) and a left hemiliver (LHL) by the three main hepatic veins, and the subdivision of these sectors into eight hepatic segments (I–VIII) by the branches of the portal vein. The caudate lobe (I) is a separate hepatic segment with independent portal venous supply and hepatic venous drainage.

EXAMPLES OF LIVER FUNCTIONS

Nutrient metabolism
Carbohydrate
Protein
Fat

Protein synthesis
Albumin
Coagulation factors (and inhibitors except von Willebrand factor)
Complement factors
Transferrin
Haptoglobin
Ceruloplasmin
Protease inhibitors (α-antitrypsin)
α-Fetoprotein

Metabolism and excretion
Exogenous material
  Drugs
  Alcohol
  Copper
Endogenous material
  Bilirubin
  Hormones

Storage
Vitamins (vit. A, vit. B_{12} folate)
Minerals (iron)

PHYSIOLOGY

The liver performs a wide variety of functions, and these are listed in the information box above. These various functions are subserved by a unique blood supply including arterial and venous blood which flows to a system of highly permeable capillaries (sinusoids). The liver also has important immunological functions. The biliary tract conveys bile to the duodenum.

FUNCTIONAL ANATOMY

The functional unit of the liver is the *hepatic acinus* which comprises a group of hepatocytes receiving blood from single terminal branches of the hepatic artery and portal vein in a terminal portal tract. The anatomy of the hepatic acinus is almost the reverse of the hepatic lobule (p. 488), as the blood passing through the sinusoids of the acinus drains to branches of the hepatic veins located on its periphery. All hepatocytes appear capable of performing the many metabolic functions of liver cells, but under physiological conditions the metabolic activities of individual hepatocytes vary in relation to their location in the acinus. This may be determined by the microenvironment created for the hepatocyte by the composition of the blood in the adjacent sinusoids.

CARBOHYDRATE METABOLISM

The main function of the liver in carbohydrate metabolism is the maintenance of the blood glucose concentration. Hepatocytes are rich in membrane receptors for insulin, and as a result the liver takes up a half or more of glucose absorbed during feeding, thereby preventing marked hyperglycaemia. The glucose taken up is stored as glycogen or metabolised to glycerol and fatty acids. Fructose and galactose can also be used for glycogen synthesis. Glucose derived from the breakdown of glycogen or from gluconeogenesis is released into the blood during fasting. Glycogen stores (70–80 g) suffice for some 24 hours of fasting, but thereafter gluconeogenesis, particularly from amino acids, becomes the main source of glucose.

PROTEIN METABOLISM

Dietary proteins enter the portal vein as amino acids and most of the straight chain amino acids are taken up by the liver. The liver utilises amino acids for endogenous hepatic protein and plasma protein synthesis and for the production of urea. A substantial proportion of the amino acids is released into the blood for the use of other tissues. During fasting, amino acids, including those reaching the liver from extrahepatic tissues, are used more for gluconeogenesis while endogenous protein synthesis, urea production and aminoacid release to the blood are suppressed. All the plasma albumin and most of its globulins, other than the gammaglobulins, are produced in the liver (see information box, left).

LIPID METABOLISM

Most dietary fat enters the body in chylomicrons. Triglyceride is removed from the chylomicrons by lipoprotein lipase in the blood, the fatty acids released are taken up by adipose tissue, and the chylomicron remnants are removed by the liver. Triglyceride taken up by the liver is broken down to 2-carbon fragments which may be used in many metabolic processes. Free (non-esterified) fatty acids, liberated into the blood from adipose tissue, are also taken up by the liver and used similarly. Among these processes is the formation of lipid aggregates containing triglyceride, phospholipid and cholesterol which are combined with a variety of apoproteins to form lipoproteins which are released into the blood. These lipoproteins are the very low density lipoproteins (VLDL), later converted to intermediate density lipoproteins (IDL) and low density lipoproteins (LDL) in the blood, which transport triglyceride from the liver to other tissues as a source of energy or for storage in adipose tissue, and the high density lipoproteins (HDL) which transport triglyceride from other tissues to the liver. The density of lipoproteins is determined by their relative protein and lipid content, with higher density lipoproteins containing more protein and less lipid.

The liver synthesises more cholesterol than any other organ, and this can be incorporated into lipoproteins, converted into bile acids (below), or excreted into the bile. In biliary obstruction of any severity the serum lipid concentration increases, largely due to the formation of an abnormal lipoprotein known as lipoprotein X.

BILIRUBIN

Unconjugated bilirubin is produced from the catabolism of haem after removal of its iron component. Some 425–510 μmol (250–300 mg) is produced daily, and most is derived from haemoglobin breakdown by Kupffer cells in the liver and other macrophages in the spleen and bone marrow. The rest is formed from catabolism of other haem-containing proteins, particularly myoglobin, cytochrome enzymes and free haem in the liver, and ineffective erythropoiesis in the marrow. Bilirubin normally present in the blood is almost all unconjugated and, as it is not water-soluble, it is bound to albumin and does not pass into the urine. It is taken up by hepatocytes, conjugated with glucuronic acid by the enzymes of the smooth endoplasmic reticulum (p. 514) to form bilirubin mono- and diglucuronide which renders it water-soluble, and excreted into the bile (Fig. 11.2). The uptake and ex-

cretion of bilirubin by hepatocytes into the bile is probably carrier-mediated.

Conjugated bilirubin is not absorbed in the small intestine. Bacteria in the terminal ileum and colon reduce it to a group of colourless chromogens (stercobilinogen) most of which are excreted in the stool (100–200 mg/d). Some are absorbed from the gut and pass to the liver where most are re-excreted in the bile; a small amount (4 mg/d) passes through the liver and is excreted in the urine where it is known as urobilinogen. Urobilinogen and its oxidation product urobilin in the urine are identical, respectively, with stercobilinogen and its oxidation product, stercobilin, in the faeces.

BILE ACIDS

Cholic and chenodeoxycholic acids, the *primary bile acids*, are produced in the liver from cholesterol and are conjugated with glycine or taurine. They are secreted into the bile, where they generate bile flow (p. 492), and they are carried in the bile to the duodenum. Most conjugated bile acids are conserved in the jejunal and ileal lumen and are actively reabsorbed in the terminal ileum, but glycine-conjugated chenodeoxycholate may be absorbed from the jejunum. The absorbed bile acids pass to the liver and are almost completely re-excreted in the bile. Small amounts reach the colon where bacterial deconjugation and dehydroxylation result in the production of *secondary bile acids*, deoxycholic acid from cholic acid, and lithocholic acid from chenodeoxycholic acid. Most of the secondary bile acids are excreted in the faeces, but small amounts are absorbed, reach the liver where they are conjugated with glycine or taurine, and are excreted in the bile (Fig. 11.3). This

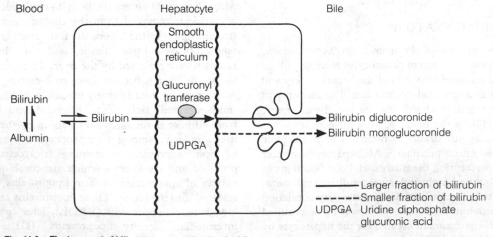

Fig. 11.2 The transport of bilirubin from the blood to the bile.

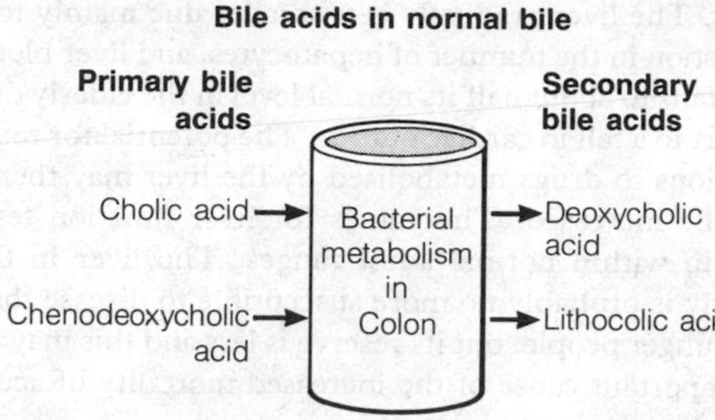

Bile acids in normal bile

Primary bile acids

Cholic acid →

Chenodeoxycholic acid →

Bacterial metabolism in Colon

Secondary bile acids

→ Deoxycholic acid

→ Lithocolic acid

Fig. 11.3   Bile acids in normal bile.

enterohepatic circulation allows large amounts of bile acid to be delivered to the intestine daily from a relatively small total bile acid pool owing to almost complete reabsorption and to frequent recycling of bile acids passing through the bowel. At any time about 85% of the bile acid pool is either in the gallbladder (fasting) or in the intestinal lumen (feeding). Synthesis of new bile acid compensates only for that lost in the faeces. The hepatic capacity for bile acid synthesis is limited, and large losses from the bowel cannot be replaced. Little bile acid reaches the systemic circulation normally, but the amount increases in liver disease.

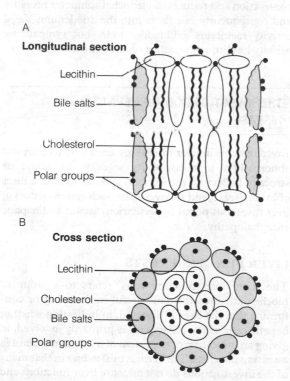

A

Longitudinal section

Lecithin

Bile salts

Cholesterol

Polar groups

B

Cross section

Lecithin

Cholesterol

Bile salts

Polar groups

Fig. 11.4   The structure of mixed micelles in bile.

Bile acids, as they enter bile, combine with cholesterol and phospholipids to form mixed micelles (Fig. 11.4). In the small intestine, provided the bile acid concentration remains sufficient to maintain the micellar state, this greatly increases the efficiency of fat absorption. Insufficiency of bile acids results in poor absorption of dietary fat and fat-soluble vitamins, notably vitamins A, D and K. Such deficiency may result from impaired synthesis in chronic liver disease, biliary obstruction, small intestinal overgrowth of bacteria capable of deconjugating and dehydroxylating bile acids (p. 450), and loss of bile acids into the colon in disease of the terminal ileum or after its resection. In this last instance, the bile acids interfere with colonic water and electrolyte metabolism causing choleretic diarrhoea, while their absence from the small intestine can result in steatorrhoea.

VITAMINS AND MINERALS

Vitamins A, D and B_{12} are stored in large amounts; vitamin K and folate are stored in smaller amounts which soon disappear if dietary intake is deficient. The liver can convert tryptophan to nicotinic acid (p. 62) and can activate vitamins by phosphorylation of thiamin (p. 60), by 25-hydroxylation of vitamin D (p. 66) and by the production of tetrahydrofolate. Vitamin K is required by hepatocytes for converting the fully synthesised procoagulants of factors II (prothrombin), VII, IX and X into active coagulation factors. The liver stores iron as ferritin and haemosiderin and excretes excess copper into the bile (p. 532).

HORMONES

The liver is an important site of hormone action and of hormone degradation. Some hormones such as insulin, glucagon, growth hormone, glucocorticoids, oestrogens and parathormone are catabolised mainly in the liver.

DRUG AND ALCOHOL METABOLISM

The hepatic metabolism of drugs (p. 514) and alcohol (p. 529) is considered elsewhere.

BLOOD SUPPLY AND LYMPHATIC DRAINAGE

The hepatic artery and the portal vein supply about 1.5 l of blood/minute to the liver, and both vessels are distributed throughout the liver in the portal tracts. The hepatic artery supplies about 25% of the total liver blood flow and about 50% of the total oxygen supply. The portal venous pressure is normally 3–5 mmHg and portal blood flow varies considerably, but autoregulation of blood flow by the hepatic artery ensures that the total liver blood flow remains constant. The hepatic arterial and portal venous blood flows into the hepatic sinusoids, which are devoid of basement membranes and lined by fenestrated endothelial cells making them highly permeable capillaries. All the plasma constituents pass through the sinusoidal walls into the space of Disse, which is the interstitial space of the liver. The sinusoids contain the phagocytic Kupffer cells, and the space of Disse contains unique stellate (Ito) cells responsible for vitamin A storage. Lymph flow is considerable, as about half the lymph flowing through the thoracic duct comes from the liver.

MONONUCLEAR PHAGOCYTE (RETICULOENDOTHELIAL) FUNCTION

The functions of the liver include the activities of about 15% of its cells which are not hepatocytes. Foremost among these are the Kupffer cells, derived from blood monocytes, which have important immunological functions. They constitute the largest single mass of mononuclear phagocytes in the body and account for about 80% of the phagocytic capacity of this system. They phagocytose damaged and ageing red blood cells, bacteria, viruses, antigen-antibody complexes and endotoxin and produce numerous substances involved in inflammatory and immune reactions (p. 28). They also take up antigenic material, but unlike macrophages elsewhere in the body they do not produce processed antigen and thus prevent antigen from eliciting immunological responses. These cells therefore seem capable of preventing undesirable immunological responses, and this may be particularly important in relation to antigens which gain repeated access to the body from the gut.

AGE AND THE LIVER

The liver begins to function early in fetal life, but many functions require several weeks or months of postnatal development before their full functional capacities are reached. Examples of limited functional capacity at birth include reduced ability to transport bilirubin across the liver cell and to conjugate bilirubin, limited capacity to synthesise and secrete bile acids into bile, which may in turn limit bile flow (below), and limited ability to synthesise coagulation factors.

Changes in the liver occur only slowly in adult life, but significant changes have occurred in those over 70 years. The liver gradually gets smaller due mainly to a reduction in the number of hepatocytes, and liver blood flow falls to about half its normal level in the elderly due in part to a fall in cardiac output. The potential for toxic reactions to drugs metabolised by the liver may therefore be increased. The values for liver function tests remain within normal adult ranges. The liver in the elderly is probably no more susceptible to disease than in younger people, but its reserve is less and this may be an important cause of the increased mortality of acute liver diseases in older people.

BILE

The liver secretes 1–2 litres of bile daily, and the hepatocytes provide the driving force for bile flow by creating osmotic gradients of bile acids which form micelles in bile (bile acid dependent bile flow) and of sodium (bile acid independent bile flow). Common bile duct pressure is maintained by rhythmic contraction and relaxation of the choledochal sphincter and this pressure exceeds gallbladder pressure in the fasting state so that bile normally flows into the gallbladder where it is concentrated some ten-fold by resorption of water and electrolytes. Cholecystokinin released from the duodenal mucosa during feeding causes gallbladder contraction and reduces choledochal sphincter pressure and consequently bile flows into the duodenum. Vagal activity maintains gallbladder tone, but sympathetic activity has little or no effect on the gallbladder.

THE INVESTIGATION OF HEPATOBILIARY DISEASE

Investigations in liver disease are used to detect hepatic abnormality, to measure its severity, to define its structural effect on the liver, to look for specific causes of liver disease, and to investigate such consequences of liver disease as portal hypertension, ascites and hepatic encephalopathy.

LIVER FUNCTION TESTS

The term 'liver function tests' refers to a group of biochemical investigations useful in revealing or confirming that the liver is diseased, in indicating whether hepatic cells or the biliary tree is primarily involved, in giving an indication of the extent of liver damage, and in assessing progress. The term is misleading in that many of the investigations do not measure liver functions and most liver functions are not tested in clinical practice;

Table 11.1 Liver function tests used to assess liver disease

Measurement	Fluid	Assessment
Bilirubin	Plasma Urine	Transport
Aminotransferases	Plasma	Hepatocellular damage
Alkaline phosphatase	Plasma	Biliary obstruction
Gamma-glutamyl transferase	Plasma	Enzyme induction
Proteins (total and albumin)	Plasma	Synthesis
Coagulation tests		Synthesis

Note: Bilirubin detected in the urine identifies unconjugated hyperbilirubinaemia and indicates hepatobiliary disease. Alanine aminotransferase is more specific for liver damage than aspartate aminotransferase.

however, the term has become generally accepted. Liver function tests are variably abnormal in patients with liver disease and therefore a group of tests is usually done (Table 11.1). It is important to realise that there are no patterns of abnormality indicative of specific diagnoses and that normality of all the commonly used tests does not prove that the liver is normal.

BILIRUBIN

Hyperbilirubinaemia may be due to increased concentrations of unconjugated or conjugated bilirubin. Estimates of both unconjugated and conjugated bilirubin in the blood are seldom necessary and are inaccurate when the total plasma bilirubin is less than 70 µmol/l (4 mg/dl).

Unconjugated hyperbilirubinaemia without any abnormality of other liver function tests may result from increased bilirubin production, as in haemolysis or ineffective erythropoiesis (p. 716), or from inability to transport bilirubin across the liver, as in Gilbert's syndrome (p. 503). Except in the newborn, the hyperbilirubinaemia rarely exceeds 100 µmol/l (6 mg/dl), and there is no bilirubin in the urine as the normal plasma albumin can bind about 400 µmol/l of unconjugated bilirubin. Conjugated bilirubin is also found in the blood in unconjugated hyperbilirubinaemia, but it does not exceed 20% of the total plasma bilirubin and is insufficient to cause bilirubinuria. Conjugated hyperbilirubinaemia without any abnormality of other liver function tests, as in the Dubin–Johnson syndrome (p. 504), is accompanied by bilirubinuria but is rare.

Hyperbilirubinaemia in hepatobiliary disease is predominantly conjugated, bilirubinuria is present, and other tests of liver function are almost always abnormal. The plasma bilirubin in parenchymal liver disease varies widely depending on the severity of the disease and its activity. Very high concentrations occur most frequently in biliary tract obstruction, with sustained high levels in malignant disease and a tendency to fluctuating levels where obstruction is caused by gallstones. The plasma bilirubin reflects the depth of jaundice and repeated estimations may be useful in following the progress of disease.

Urine tests

Simple, sensitive, inexpensive dip-stick tests for bilirubin and urobilinogen in the urine are available. Bilirubin is not found in the urine of normal persons as virtually all the plasma bilirubin is unconjugated and bound to albumin. Thus, absence of bilirubinuria in a jaundiced patient points to unconjugated hyperbilirubinaemia (above), while bilirubinuria implies a conjugated hyperbilirubinaemia and points to hepatobiliary disease. An excess of urine urobilinogen occurs in haemolytic diseases due to increased biliary excretion of bilirubin leading to increased urobilinogen formation, and in any cause of hepatic dysfunction including pyrexia and cardiac failure due to reduced biliary re-excretion of urobilinogen. No urobilinogen is found in the urine in complete biliary obstruction. Increased amounts of urobilinogen are found in the urine in haemolytic diseases and with any cause of hepatic dysfunction, but in practice urine urobilinogen tests are of no value in liver disease.

ENZYMES

Liver cells contain many enzymes which may be released into the blood in various pathological processes. Measurement of their activity in the blood may give evidence of hepatobiliary disease. In practice, maximal information may be obtained by measuring the activity of relatively few enzymes. None of the enzymes is specific to the liver and alternative origins should be considered, particularly where abnormalities have been found incidentally in patients with no clinical evidence of liver disease.

Aminotransferases

Alanine aminotransferase (ALT), a cytoplasmic enzyme, and aspartate aminotransferase (AST), present both in cytoplasm and mitochondria, are the two important aminotransferases. Normal plasma contains low activities of both enzymes, the source of which is unknown. Neither enzyme is specific to the liver, but ALT occurs in much higher concentration in the liver than elsewhere and consequently increased serum ALT activity reflects hepatic damage more specifically. ALT and AST are liberated into the blood whenever liver cells are damaged and increased plasma enzyme activity is a very sensitive index of hepatic damage. Plasma ALT and AST activity test the integrity of liver cells. The highest activities are caused by any form of acute liver damage, but they have no prognostic significance in acute or chronic liver disease.

In viral hepatitis there is greatly increased activity even in the prodromal phase, and maximal levels of 10 to 100 times the normal value are usually reached early in the jaundiced phase, after which activity falls rapidly. Equally high activity occurs in acute hepatic damage due to drugs, in acute circulatory failure, and in exacerbations of chronic active hepatitis. Most patients (80%) with infectious mononucleosis or cytomegalo-viral infection have an acute hepatitis with serum aminotransferase activity raised 2 to 10 times but few develop jaundice. Hepatic damage due to paracetamol produces particularly high activities of 100 to 500 times the normal value. Plasma aminotransferase activity in alcoholic hepatitis is usually increased less than fivefold. Patients with cirrhosis generally show only modest elevations of serum aminotransferase. In obstructive jaundice, activity may rise up to fivefold, but greater increases are unusual unless cholangitis is present.

Alkaline phosphatase

This enzyme is situated principally in the canalicular and sinusoidal membranes of liver cells. Blood normally contains alkaline phosphatase derived mainly from bone and liver, and to a lesser extent intestine; in pregnancy additional activity of placental origin is found. When hepatocytes are damaged little alkaline phosphatase is liberated into the blood, most probably coming from cells which are killed. Consequently, plasma alkaline phosphatase activity does not usually rise more than two-fold in acute or chronic hepato-cellular disease. In biliary tract obstruction at any level new alkaline phosphatase is synthesised in the hepato-cyte membrane, much of which escapes into the blood. A greatly increased plasma alkaline phosphatase activity is, therefore, the main indicator of biliary obstruction though it provides no information about the site of that obstruction. The alkaline phosphatase activity has no prognostic significance in liver disease.

Sometimes a raised plasma alkaline phosphatase activity is found incidentally and is the sole abnor-mality. Hepatobiliary disease may be present, but it is important to ensure that the alkaline phosphatase does not have an extrahepatic origin before investigating the liver further. This may be done by finding increased plasma activities of enzymes more specific for the liver, such as γ-glutamyl transferase or 5' nucleotidase, or by electrophoretic separation of the isoenzymes of alkaline phosphatase. Increased osteoblastic activity from bone

is the main alternative origin of a raised plasma alkaline phosphatase and occurs in adolescents when it may increase about two- to three-fold, in Paget's disease, rickets, hyperparathyroidism, and metastatic tumour in bone. Myelomatosis is not associated with much bone repair and the plasma alkaline phosphatase is not usually raised. During the third trimester of pregnancy, alkaline phosphatase of placental origin may increase the serum activity two- to three-fold.

Enzyme combinations

Serum aminotransferase and alkaline phosphatase activities may be considered relative to one another. Large increases of aminotransferase activity and small increases of alkaline phosphatase activity favour hepatocellular damage; small increases of aminotrans-ferase activity and large increases of alkaline phospha-tase activity favour biliary obstruction (Table 11.2). It

Table 11.2   Relation of plasma aminotransferase and alkaline phosphatase activity in patients with jaundice due to acute viral hepatitis and biliary obstruction

Enzyme combination		Diagnostic likelihood	
Aminotransferase	Alkaline phosphatase	Viral hepatitis	Biliary obstruction
> ×6	< ×2.5	90%	10%
< ×6	> ×2.5	10%	80%
Other combinations		No clear separation	

is important that these patterns do not separate the two diagnostic groups absolutely and other combinations give much poorer separation.

Gamma-glutamyl transferase (γ-GT)

This is a microsomal enzyme which is distributed widely in body tissues. Increased plasma γ-GT activity is a sensitive index of liver abnormality. The highest activities occur in biliary obstruction but marked increases also occur in acute parenchymal damage from any cause. Gamma-GT measurements give little in-formation in patients with liver disease beyond that provided by transferase and alkaline phosphatase measurements. Plasma γ-GT activity is also increased by microsomal enzyme-inducing agents such as alcohol and various drugs (Table 11.3). Increased γ-GT activity is used to detect and follow alcohol abuse in patients with little or no other abnormality of liver function provided they are not taking enzyme-inducing drugs. Increased γ-GT activity due to alcohol implies prolonged intake of more than about 60 g alcohol daily; unfortunately, normal γ-GT activity does not exclude prolonged intake above that level.

Table 11.3   Drugs causing hepatic microsomal enzyme induction and increased plasma γ-glutamyl transferase activity

Barbiturates	Griseofulvin
Carbamazepine	Meprobamate
Diphenylhydantoin	Primidone
Glutethimide	Rifampicin

PLASMA PROTEINS

Albumin

This is synthesised solely in the liver. In chronic liver disease, especially cirrhosis, the plasma albumin concentration is frequently low. Impaired albumin synthesis can be the cause but other factors such as malnutrition, fever and the dilutional effect of fluid retention with ascites can be important. Low plasma albumin concentrations usually detect patients with more severe liver damage, and a falling concentration is a bad prognostic sign especially when there is no ascites. Albumin has a long half-life in the blood (20–26 days) and changes in concentration occur slowly. Thus, even in severe acute hepatitis, the plasma albumin remains normal unless the illness continues for many weeks.

Globulins

It is characteristic of chronic liver disease that hyperglobulinaemia occurs in addition to hypoalbuminaemia, and once established it tends to persist. It may also be found irrespective of changes in the plasma albumin concentration in prolonged viral hepatitis or chronic active hepatitis. The causes of hyperglobulinaemia are not fully understood; increases in gammaglobulins are prominent and probably reflect an increased activity of the immune system, to which many factors may contribute. In those with hypoalbuminaemia it may represent a response to a reduced colloid osmotic pressure in the plasma. Individual plasma immunoglobulins are variably increased, IgG mainly in chronic active hepatitis and cryptogenic cirrhosis, IgA mainly in alcoholic liver disease, and IgM in primary biliary cirrhosis. Variations, however, are so frequent that Ig measurements are of limited diagnostic value in liver disease.

Plasma protein electrophoresis

The commonest changes in the electrophoretic pattern of the plasma proteins in cirrhosis are a decreased albumin and an increased gammaglobulin peak. There is some relation between the electrophoretic pattern and particular forms of liver disease, but this is not precise enough to be of diagnostic value.

COAGULATION FACTORS

The liver synthesises all the coagulation factors, and requires vitamin K to activate factors II, VII, IX and X. Reduced plasma concentrations of coagulation factors occur in liver damage, which is most readily recognised by prolongation of the prothrombin time. The prothrombin time depends on factors I, II, V, VII and X, and it prolongs when the plasma concentration of any of these factors falls below 30% of normal. This occurs in severe liver damage and in prolonged biliary obstruction which reduces vitamin K absorption. The prothrombin time can therefore be used as a liver function test provided that vitamin K is given first (above). Furthermore, as the normal half-lives of these factors in the blood are short (5–72 hours), prothrombin time changes occur relatively quickly when liver damage occurs, allowing the test to be used in acute and chronic liver disease. The prothrombin time is a most valuable prognostic guide in acute hepatitis, such as viral hepatitis, and an abnormal value indicates severe damage; an increasing prothrombin time indicates a progressively worse prognosis.

BROMSULPHTHALEIN (BSP) CLEARANCE

Estimation of BSP clearance from the blood is a sensitive test for hepatic dysfunction but is rarely used. It remains of value in the diagnosis of the rare Dubin–Johnson syndrome (p. 504); blood concentrations of BSP are measured 45 minutes and 120 minutes after injection and a higher value at 120 minutes confirms the diagnosis.

SEROLOGICAL TESTS

HEPATITIS A VIRUS ANTIGENS AND ANTIBODIES

Only one antigen has been found associated with the hepatitis A virus (HAV), and individuals infected with the HAV make an antibody to this antigen (anti-HAV). Anti-HAV is found in the blood early in the clinical illness, and certainly by the time jaundice develops. It is very important in diagnosis because HAV viraemia occurs only transiently in the incubation period. HAV excretion in the stools occurs for only 7–10 days after the onset of the clinical illness. The virus cannot be grown readily. The mere presence of the antibody is not enough for diagnosis as HAV infection is common in all communities and antibody to it persists for years after infection. It is anti-HAV of IgM type, indicating a primary immune response, which is diagnostic of a recent infection; titres of this antibody fall to low levels after about 3 months. Anti-HAV (IgG) measurements can be used to determine the necessity for giving immune serum globulin to those travelling abroad and in studies of the prevalence of hepatitis A virus infection.

HEPATITIS B VIRUS ANTIGENS AND ANTIBODIES

The hepatitis B virus contains several antigens to which infected persons can make immune responses (Fig. 11.5); these antigens and their antibodies are important in identifying hepatitis B viral infection (Table 11.4).

Table 11.4   Interpretation of main investigations used in the serological diagnosis of hepatitis B virus infection

Interpretation	HBsAg	Anti-HBc		Anti-HBs
		IgM	IgG	
Incubation period	+	+	−	−
Acute hepatitis				
Early	+	+	−	−
Established	+	+	+	±
Established (occasional)	−	+	+	−
Convalescence (3–6 months)	−	+	+	+
Post-infection				
> 1 year	−	−	+	+
Uncertain	−	−	+	−
Chronic infection				
Usual	+	±	+	−
Occasional	−	−	+	−
Immunisation without infection	−	−	−	+

Note: + = positive; − = negative; ± = present at low titre or absent. HBsAg: surface antigen; Anti-HBc: antibody to core antigen; Anti-HBs: antibody to surface antigen.

Acute infection

The hepatitis B surface antigen (HBsAg) is a reliable marker of hepatitis B virus infection, and a negative test for the HBsAg makes hepatitis B virus infection very unlikely but not impossible (Fig. 11.5). It appears in the blood late in the incubation period and before the prodromal phase of acute type B hepatitis; it may be present for only a few days, disappearing even before jaundice has developed, but it usually last for 3–4 weeks and may persist for up to 3 months. It should therefore be sought as soon as possible in acute hepatitis. Antibody to HBsAg (anti-HBs) usually appears after about 3 months and persists for many years or perhaps permanently. Anti-HBs implies either that infection has occurred at some time (in which case anti-HBc (below) is usually also present) or that the individual has been vaccinated.

The hepatitis B core antigen (HBcAg) is not found in the blood, but antibody to it (anti-HBc) appears early in

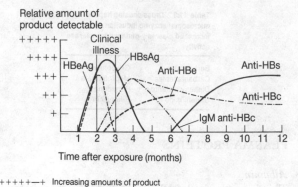

++++++—+   Increasing amounts of product

Fig. 11.5   Serological responses to hepatitis B virus infection (HBsAG = hepatitis B surface antigen; anti-HBs = antibody to HBsAg; HBeAg = hepatitis Be antigen; anti-HBe = antibody to HBeAg; anti-HBc = antibody to hepatitis B core antigen).

the illness and rapidly reaches a high titre which then subsides gradually and persists. Anti-HBc is initially of IgM type and IgG antibody appears later. Anti-HBc (IgM) can sometimes reveal an acute hepatitis B viral infection when the HBsAg has disappeared and before anti-HBs has developed (Fig. 11.5). The hepatitis Be antigen (HBeAg) appears only transiently at the outset of the illness and is followed by the production of antibody (anti-HBe). The HBeAg reflects active replication of the virus in the liver.

Chronic infection

Chronic hepatitis B virus infection (p. 516) is marked by the presence of the HBsAg and anti-HBc (IgG) in the blood. Rarely, anti-HBc (IgG) alone is the sole evidence of chronic infection. Usually, the HBeAg or anti-HBe is also present; the HBeAg is thought to indicate continued active replication of the virus in the liver while anti-HBe implies that replication is occurring at a much lower level or that the viral DNA has become integrated into the hepatocyte DNA.

DELTA VIRUS

This virus contains a single antigen (delta antigen) to which infected individuals make an antibody (anti-delta). Delta antigen appears in the blood only transiently, and in practice diagnosis depends on detecting anti-delta. Simultaneous infection with the hepatitis B virus and delta virus followed by full recovery is associated with the appearance of low titres of anti-delta of IgM type within a few days of the onset of the illness. This antibody generally disappears within about 2 months but persists in a few patients. Superinfection of patients with chronic hepatitis B virus infection leads to the production of high titres of anti-delta, initially IgM and later IgG. Such patients may then develop chronic infection with both viruses, in which case anti-delta titres plateau at high levels.

NON-A, NON-B VIRUSES (HEPATITIS C VIRUS)

There are probably several non-A, non-B hepatitis viruses (p. 509). One has been described recently and has been named the hepatitis C virus (HCV). Antibody to a polypeptide component of the virus (anti-HCV) appears in the blood 4–6 months after infection, and an assay for this antibody is likely to be available generally soon.

OTHER VIRUSES

Cytomegalovirus and the Epstein–Barr virus (infectious mononucleosis) are occasional causes of acute hepatitis, and infection can be detected by serological tests.

AUTOANTIBODIES

Three autoantibodies in the blood are important in liver disease: antinuclear antibody, antismooth muscle antibody and antimitochondrial antibody. These autoantibodies are all heterogenous and can be found in apparently healthy people, particularly in women and in older people. Antinuclear antibodies occur in about 5% of healthy people and antismooth muscle antibody in 1.5%, but antimitochondrial antibody is rare being found in about 0.01%. Autoantibody titres in such healthy people are usually low. Antinuclear and antimitochondrial antibodies also occur in connective tissue diseases and in autoimmune diseases, including various thyroid disorders and pernicious anaemia, while antismooth muscle antibody has been reported in infectious mononucleosis and in a variety of malignant diseases. In liver disease, antismooth muscle antibody and to a lesser extent antinuclear antibody may occur transiently and at low titre in acute viral hepatitis. The autoantibodies are, however, more important in chronic liver disease where they are present for long periods and at relatively high titres (Table 11.5). They are found particularly in chronic active hepatitis, cryptogenic cirrhosis and primary biliary cirrhosis, and until recently they were not thought to have any diagnostic specificity. However, the antimitochondrial antibody detected in most clinical laboratories is now known to be very strongly associated with primary biliary cirrhosis, and patients with connective tissue or autoimmune diseases found to have this antibody usually prove to have

Table 11.5 Approximate occurrence of antinuclear (ANA), antismooth muscle (SMA) and antimitochondrial (AMA) antibodies in chronic liver diseases not associated with chronic hepatitis B virus infection

Disease	Autoantibodies		
	ANA (%)	SMA (%)	AMA (%)
Chronic active hepatitis	80	70	25
Primary biliary cirrhosis	25	35	95
Cryptogenic cirrhosis	40	30	25

Note: Patients with AMA frequently have cholestatic liver function tests and may have primary biliary cirrhosis (see text).

primary biliary cirrhosis as well. Antimitochondrial antibody found in a patient with cholestasis, is of particular value in indicating the presence of primary biliary cirrhosis. Antimitochondrial antibody occurs in primary biliary cirrhosis in 95% or more of patients and in less than 1% of those with large bile duct obstruction. A rare form of chronic active hepatitis is associated with liver-kidney microsomal (LKM) antibodies, and in this condition other autoantibodies are not usually found.

None of these autoantibodies damages liver tissue, and they are therefore unlikely to have aetiological importance.

BIOCHEMICAL TESTS

Biochemical tests can be of value in identifying the nature of hepatic disease or its cause.

Ferritin
The serum ferritin concentration is important in the diagnosis of haemochromatosis as it reflects the total body iron. The serum ferritin concentration is almost always above 1000 µg/l in haemochromatosis; a normal serum ferritin excludes haemochromatosis as the cause of chronic liver disease and serum ferritin measurements are used to assess the results of venesection therapy. The serum ferritin, however, cannot establish a diagnosis of haemochromatosis on its own because increased concentrations occur in alcoholic liver disease albeit usually at levels below 1000 µg/l.

Iron binding capacity saturation
The plasma iron binding capacity exceeds 60% in haemochromatosis. The serum ferritin is now generally preferred in diagnosing haemochromatosis, but iron binding capacity saturation remains useful in detecting iron overload in the relatives of patients.

Caeruloplasmin

This is a copper-containing globulin produced by the liver. The serum caeruloplasmin concentration in Wilson's disease is low and may be undetectable. Concentrations in the low normal range occur rarely, particularly during active disease, in the terminal stages, or during pregnancy or oestrogen (oral contraceptives) therapy. Low serum concentrations also occur in fulminant hepatic failure, in any advanced and severe chronic liver disease, in protein-losing enteropathy, and malabsorption. Increased serum concentrations occur in pregnancy, when oestrogens are taken, in a wide variety of inflammatory and neoplastic diseases including acute and chronic hepatitis, and in any form of biliary obstruction.

Copper

Concentrations of copper in the liver are very high in Wilson's disease and in any condition associated with chronic cholestasis such as primary biliary cirrhosis. This excess of copper cannot be shown reliably histologically, especially in Wilson's disease, and has to be measured chemically. The serum copper concentration in Wilson's disease is low (unless fulminant hepatic failure occurs, when it is very high) and the urinary copper excretion is high. Wilson's disease can also be diagnosed by showing failure of incorporation of radioactive copper (^{64}Cu) into caeruloplasmin, but this is rarely required and is difficult to do because ^{64}Cu has a very short half-life.

Alpha$_1$-antitrypsin

This is an α_1-globulin produced by the liver which comprises 90% of the α_1-globulin peak seen on serum electrophoresis. It is a component of the protease inhibitor (Pi) system which inhibits the activity of protease enzymes. Its production is inherited through a system of co-dominant alleles each determining the synthesis of a form of α_1-antitrypsin named in accordance with its electrophoretic behaviour. The main forms of α_1-antitrypsin are PiM (medium), PiS (slow) and PiZ (very slow). PiMM is the normal phenotype giving normal serum α_1-antitrypsin concentrations, while the phenotype PiZZ gives low serum α_1-antitrypsin concentrations and is associated with liver disease (p. 533) and pulmonary disease (p. 394).

Alpha-fetoprotein

This is made mainly by the fetal liver production falling to low levels after birth. The reappearance of substantial serum concentrations in adult life and increasing concentrations in chronic liver disease suggest strongly that a hepatocellular carcinoma has developed.

Table 11.6   Diseases associated with increased serum α-fetoprotein concentration

Adults
Neoplastic
Hepatocellular carcinoma[1]
Other carcinomas (very rare)
   Stomach
   Pancreas
   Gallbladder
   Bile ducts
   Lungs
Non-neoplastic
Viral hepatitis
Chronic hepatitis (esp. chronic active)
Cirrhosis

Children
Neoplastic
Hepatoblastoma[1]
Gonadal teratoblastoma[1]
Non-neoplastic
Biliary atresia
Neonatal hepatitis
Indian childhood cirrhosis
Tyrosinosis
Ataxia telangiectasia

Pregnancy
Neural tube defects[2]
Fetal distress

[1] α-Fetoprotein frequently and greatly increased.
[2] α-Fetoprotein also increased in amniotic fluid.

Some increase in serum α-fetoprotein occurs in about 90% of patients with hepatocellular carcinoma, but moderate increases can occur in several other conditions (Table 11.6).

INVESTIGATIVE PROCEDURES IN HEPATOBILIARY DISEASE

Investigative procedures are designed to determine the site and nature of structural lesions in the liver and biliary tree, and they should be used only when there is clinical or biochemical evidence of hepatobiliary disease. They range from the less invasive but less specific to the more specific but more invasive, and from those which examine the liver as a whole to those which look at only a part of it. Imaging is the best way of starting investigation, and ultrasound has emerged as the most generally useful method.

IMAGING

This can identify and localise disease but often cannot make specific diagnoses, which require further investigations as outlined in Figure 11.6.

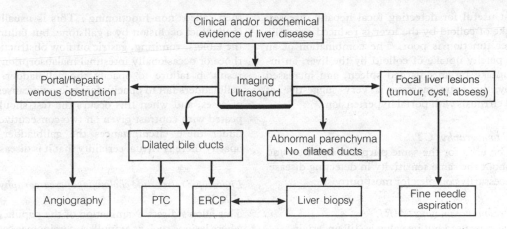

Fig. 11.6 **Investigative procedures in liver disease.** Suggested sequence for identifying structural lesions in the liver and biliary tract. ERCP = endoscopic retrograde cholangio-pancreatography; PTC = percutaneous transhepatic cholangiography.

Ultrasonography

This requires a skilled operator but is safe and comfortable for the patient and can be repeated. It detects gallstones down to 5 mm diameter with great accuracy, and reveals gallbladder tumours and thickening due to cholecystitis (Fig. 11.7). It is the most important initial investigation in obstructive jaundice as dilation of the bile ducts implies mechanical obstruction in a large duct, and it may be possible to determine the site of the obstruction and sometimes its causes (Fig. 11.8). Normal bile ducts in a patient with obvious jaundice make a mechanical cause unlikely. Ultrasound can also

be used to identify focal liver diseases including tumours, abscesses and cysts, provided they are more than about 2 cm in diameter, and can identify generalised parenchymal conditions such as fatty change and cirrhosis without being able to make a specific diagnosis. Ultrasound has become increasingly important for examining the portal vein and the splenic vein particularly in portal hypertension and portal venous obstruction, and Doppler ultrasound allows portal blood flow to be studied. The hepatic veins can be studied in a similar way.

Radionuclide imaging

This has the advantage of simplicity and is usually performed with technetium (^{99m}Tc) sulphur colloid which is taken up by the monocyte-macrophage system.

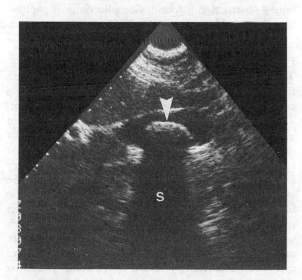

Fig. 11.7 **Ultrasound of the gallbladder showing stone in the gallbladder.** Stone (arrow) with acoustic shadow (S).

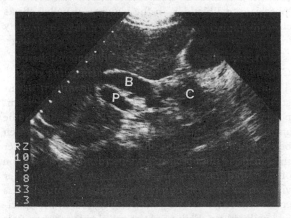

Fig. 11.8 **Carcinoma of the pancreas** (C) with dilated common bile duct (B). The portal vein (P) is posterior to the bile duct.

It is most useful for detecting focal hepatic diseases. The uptake of colloid by the liver is reduced generally when liver function is poor. The combination of an impaired patchy uptake of colloid by the liver, an increased uptake by an enlarged spleen, and increased uptake by the bone marrow is very suggestive of advanced cirrhosis with portal hypertension.

Computed tomography (CT)
This can be used for the same purposes as ultrasound and has about the same sensitivity in detecting disease. It is unnecessarily complex for most purposes.

Magnetic resonance imaging (MRI)
This can also be used but its value is still uncertain.

Cholescintigraphy
This is a safe method of imaging the biliary tract using ^{99m}Tc-labelled imidodiacetic acid derivatives. It is particularly useful in the diagnosis of acute cholecystitis where failure to visualise the gallbladder is found in almost 100% of patients and probably results from a blocked cystic duct.

RADIOLOGY

Radiological procedures can be used to investigate the biliary tract and the hepatic vasculature, and to look for oesophageal varices which imply the presence of portal hypertension.

Plain abdominal radiograph
A plain radiograph shows about 20% of gallstones, and can show the soft tissue mass of an inflamed gallbladder or gas in the biliary tree when a biliary-enteric fistula is present. Calcification in the gallbladder wall occurs in 'porcelain' gallbladder, in the pancreas usually reflects chronic pancreatitis and in the liver occurs occasionally in lesions such as cysts, tumours or areas of infarction.

Cholecystography
This is used to diagnose gallbladder disease and demonstrate gallbladder function. Iodine-containing compounds are given orally which are excreted in the bile and concentrated in the gallbladder which then becomes radio-opaque. Hyperbilirubinaemia greater than 35 µmol/l (2 mg/dl) interferes with biliary excretion of the contrast agent sufficiently to prevent gallbladder visualisation. Non-opaque gallstones and the much less common adenomas show as filling defects in the opacified gallbladder. Failure of the gallbladder to opacify is frequent in gallbladder disease, and the gallbladder is then called 'non-functioning'. This is usually due to cystic duct occlusion by a gallstone, but failure to take the tablets, vomiting, gastric outflow obstruction, diarrhoea or occasionally intestinal malabsorption will also result in failure to opacify the gallbladder. Normal gallbladders fail to opacify for unknown causes in 20% of cases, and when this occurs the test should be repeated with contrast given on two consecutive days. If under these circumstances the gallbladder fails to opacify there is virtual certainty that it is diseased.

Endoscopic retrograde cholangiopancreatography (ERCP)
This allows direct examination of the papilla of Vater, where lesions such as ampullary carcinomas can be seen and biopsied, and radiological examination of the biliary tree and pancreatic duct by injection of contrast into these systems. It is valuable for determining the nature of cholestasis of unknown cause and for investigating pain which may be of biliary or pancreatic origin. The procedure is also used to carry out papillotomy at the papilla of Vater which allows stones to be removed from the common bile duct with balloon catheters or wire baskets. This is sometimes done urgently in patients with cholangitis or pancreatitis due to gallstones who are not responding to therapy. Stents can also be passed through malignant strictures to allow biliary drainage, and occasionally benign biliary strictures can be dilated. Complications of ERCP include pancreatitis in about 1–3% of cases and cholangitis which can be prevented by broad-spectrum antibiotics such as cefotaxime (1 g 8-hourly i.v.) when large duct biliary obstruction is found. Complications of papillotomy include bleeding and duodenal perforation.

Percutaneous transhepatic cholangiography (PTC)
This involves passing a fine-bore (Chiba) needle into the liver under radiological control and injecting contrast material directly into an intrahepatic bile duct. The technique is useful for investigating cholestasis of unknown cause as bile ducts dilated because of mechanical obstruction of a large bile duct can almost always be entered. Excellent delineation of the biliary tract is obtained, but the pancreatic duct cannot be examined and stones cannot be removed from the biliary tract. Stents can be passed through malignant strictures, particularly those in the hepatic hilum which are not easily treated by ERCP. Complications are uncommon, but bleeding and bile leakage from the liver can occur. Accordingly, blood coagulation should be checked as for liver biopsy before the procedure and facilities for surgery should be available.

Operative cholangiography

This should be carried out during operations on the biliary tract by injecting contrast into the cystic duct or the common bile duct.

T-tube cholangiography

This can be carried out when a T-tube has been left in the common bile duct at choledochotomy. When stones are found in the common bile duct the T-tube can be left in place for 8–12 weeks to allow its track to mature after which the stones can be removed through the track with a wire (Burhenne) basket.

Arteriography

Hepatic arteriography is most useful for localising focal liver lesions, particularly tumours, and is essential in planning hepatic surgery. Hepatocellular carcinomas are usually highly vascular in contrast to metastatic-tumours which usually show low vascularity. Highly vascular metastatic tumours occur occasionally and include renal, thyroid, carcinoid, islet-cell and chorion carcinomas and sarcomas.

Portal venography

This is most useful in investigating portal hypertension of unknown cause. It is also essential prior to portal-systemic shunt surgery, though such surgery is now done relatively infrequently. Portal venography is performed most safely by studying the venous phase following superior mesenteric arteriography. Spleno-portography and transhepatic portography are more invasive and are much less used. Digital vascular imaging (DVI) can be used to examine the portal vein but the quality of the imaging is variable.

Hepatic venography

This is most important in the diagnosis of the Budd–Chiari syndrome (p. 534) and undertaken by passing a catheter into the hepatic veins via the inferior vena cava.

Portal pressure

This can be measured by passing needles or catheters into the spleen, the portal vein or the hepatic parenchyma, but these methods are all invasive and are rarely used. The pressure recorded by a catheter wedged in a hepatic vein (wedged hepatic venous pressure) reflects the portal venous pressure via the hepatic sinusoids, and this less disturbing procedure is most widely used for measuring the portal venous pressure. The portal venous pressure is calculated as the difference between the wedged hepatic venous pressure and the free hepatic venous pressure and is normally 3–5 mmHg.

Varices

The presence of varices in the oesophagus and stomach can be demonstrated by barium swallow and meal examination. They establish the presence of portal hypertension.

ENDOSCOPY

Upper gastrointestinal endoscopy is superior to barium examination in the diagnosis of oesophageal varices but small varices cannot always be differentiated easily from mucosal folds. Endoscopy is the only means of diagnosing the congestive gastropathy of portal hypertension. Choledochoscopy is useful for identifying common bile duct stones at operation.

PARACENTESIS

Analysis of ascites provides useful information. The fluid in cirrhosis is clear, the protein content usually below 30 g/l, and in the absence of infection there are less than 250 polymorphonuclear leucocytes/mm^3. Blood-stained ascites is usually due to malignant disease, and milky (chylous) ascites to obstruction of the cisterna chyli. Ascitic protein concentrations above 30 g/l occur most often in peritoneal infection, especially tuberculosis, peritoneal tumour, hepatic venous obstruction and ascites associated with pancreatic disease. Amylase activity is high in ascites caused by pancreatitis. Infections, such as spontaneous bacterial peritonitis (p. 529) or tuberculosis, can be identified by ascites polymorphonuclear leucocyte counts above 250/mm^3 and by bacteriological examination. Ascites cytology can show malignant cells, but negative examinations do not exclude malignant disease.

LIVER BIOPSY

This is performed with a special needle, usually through an intercostal space, using local analgesia. It requires a co-operative patient who will stop breathing when the biopsy is taken. The haemostatic mechanisms must be intact as indicated by a prothrombin time not more than 4 seconds longer than the control value and a platelet count not less than 100×10^9/l (100 000/mm^3). The patient remains in bed for 24 hours after the procedure, regular pulse and blood pressure measurements must be recorded, and blood for transfusion (2 units) should be available. The main complications are abdominal and/or shoulder pain, bleeding and, rarely, biliary peritonitis which usually occurs when there is obstruction of a large bile duct. Liver biopsy is a relatively safe procedure but should never be undertaken lightly as the mortality rate is about 0.05%.

Liver biopsies can be carried out in patients with defective haemostasis if this can be corrected with fresh frozen plasma and platelets or if the biopsy is obtained by the transjugular route or percutaneously under radiological control with subsequent plugging of the needle track with gelfoam.

Biopsy yields only a small sample of liver and consequently the best results are obtained in patients with diffuse liver disease. The procedure is essential in the diagnosis of chronic hepatitis and in separating the persistent, aggressive and lobular forms. It can also be important in establishing a diagnosis of cirrhosis in which it may indicate a cause such as alcohol abuse or haemochromatosis. Other investigations are now preferred in cholestasis (p. 505), as the histological differentiation of obstruction of a large bile duct from other liver diseases is sometimes difficult and there is an increased risk of biliary peritonitis following biopsy in cholestasis. Biopsy is not usually required in acute hepatitis for the diagnosis can normally be made on other grounds but it may be needed in atypical cases. Focal disease, particularly malignancy, is only diagnosed accurately if the site of the disease in the liver is first identified by some other method such as ultrasound or laparoscopy. Operative liver biopsy may sometimes be valuable, as in the staging of lymphoma.

LIVER ASPIRATION

This technique using fine-bore needles (20–22 gauge) usually guided by ultrasound has become the initial method of choice for investigating focal liver lesions such as tumours, abscesses and cysts. This can be done with minimal discomfort or risk provided the haemostatic mechanisms are satisfactory. Aspirated material can be examined cytologically, histologically and bacteriologically.

LAPAROSCOPY

Laparoscopy can be performed under local analgesia or general anaesthesia. Modern laparoscopes of relatively small size provide an excellent view of the anterior and superior surfaces of the liver as well as some of its inferior aspects and the gallbladder. The spleen, the prominent blood vessels of portal hypertension and evidence of peritoneal disease may also be seen. Biopsies can be taken directly from diseased areas, which is valuable in focal disorders, especially malignant disease. The main contraindications are haemostatic abnormalities, marked ascites and previous surgery which may have caused adhesions.

LIVER DISEASES

JAUNDICE

Jaundice refers to the yellow appearance of the skin, sclerae and mucous membranes resulting from an increased bilirubin concentration in the body fluids. It is detectable when the plasma bilirubin exceeds 50 µmol/l (3 mg/dl). Internal tissues and body fluids are coloured yellow but not the brain as bilirubin does not cross the blood-brain barrier other than in the immediate neonatal period. Pathological mechanisms giving rise to jaundice are listed in the information box (left).

HAEMOLYTIC JAUNDICE

This results from increased destruction of red blood cells or their precursors in the marrow causing increased bilirubin production (p. 716). Jaundice due to haemolysis is usually mild because a healthy liver can excrete a bilirubin load 6 times greater than normal before unconjugated bilirubin accumulates in the plasma. Exceptions to this occur in the newborn when the hepatic bilirubin transport mechanism is immature and in patients with liver disease.

MECHANISMS PRODUCING JAUNDICE

- Haemolysis
- Impaired hepatic bilirubin transport
- Hepatocellular damage
- Cholestasis (impaired bile flow)

Clinical features

These are detailed elsewhere (p. 717). There are no stigma of liver disease other than jaundice. Increased excretion of bilirubin and hence stercobilinogen leads to normal coloured or dark stools, and increased urobilinogen excretion causes the urine to turn dark on standing as urobilin is formed. Pallor due to anaemia and splenomegaly due to excessive reticuloendothelial activity are usually present.

Investigation

The plasma bilirubin is usually less than 100 μmol/l (6 mg/dl) and the liver function tests are otherwise normal. There is no bilirubinuria because the hyperbilirubinaemia is dominantly unconjugated. Evidence of haemolytic anaemia is also present (p. 716).

Management

This is detailed elsewhere (p. 717).

CONGENITAL NON-HAEMOLYTIC HYPERBILIRUBINAEMIA

Gilbert's syndrome is the only common form of congenital non-haemolytic hyperbilirubinaemia. All other forms are very rare (Table 11.7). In adults they have an excellent prognosis, need no treatment, and are clinically important only because they may be mistaken for more serious liver disease.

GILBERT'S SYNDROME

This common benign condition is usually first recognised in adolescents or young adults. It is more common in men (male:female ratio 4:1) and occurs in about 5% of the population.

Aetiology

The aetiology is varied but it can be inherited as an autosomal dominant. The main cause of the unconjugated hyperbilirubinaemia is a deficiency of hepatic glucuronyl transferase; in some patients uptake of unconjugated bilirubin from the plasma may be impaired; in others mild haemolysis not detectable by conventional laboratory tests is present.

Clinical features

Gilbert's syndrome generally presents as mild jaundice, occasionally noted after viral hepatitis from which there has been a complete recovery, or is found incidentally. Many patients have no symptoms; others suffer episodes of malaise, anorexia and upper abdominal pain, the last occasionally severe, with increases in the jaundice. These episodes may be related to infection, fatigue or fasting. Physical examination shows mild jaundice but is otherwise normal.

Investigations

Investigations indicate hyperbilirubinaemia, generally below 100 μmol/l (6 mg/dl), with no abnormality of other liver function tests. Estimations of unconjugated bilirubin are unreliable when the plasma bilirubin is below 70 μmol/l (p. 493) and are generally unnecessary as failure to find bilirubin in the urine points to unconjugated hyperbilirubinaemia (p. 493). The peripheral blood count, reticulocyte count and plasma haptoglobin concentration are normal giving no evidence of overt haemolysis. Liver biopsy is normal and should be performed only if there is clinical or biochemical evidence suggesting liver disease.

Management

No treatment is necessary.

HEPATOCELLULAR JAUNDICE

Hepatocellular jaundice results from inability of the liver to transport bilirubin into the bile as a result of liver cell damage. Bilirubin transport across the hepatocytes may be impaired at any point between uptake of unconjugated bilirubin into the cells and transport of conjugated bilirubin into the canaliculi. In addition, swelling of cells and oedema resulting from the disease itself may cause obstruction of the biliary canaliculi. In hepatocellular jaundice the concentrations in the blood of both unconjugated and conjugated bilirubin increase, perhaps because of the variable way in which bilirubin transport is disturbed.

Acute parenchymal liver diseases, usually due to the hepatitis viruses or to drugs, are common causes. Prolonged alcohol abuse and chronic hepatitis or cirrhosis irrespective of cause also cause hepatocellular jaundice. The severity of jaundice, the other clinical features and the investigation and treatment vary with the underlying disease and are considered later in this chapter.

CHOLESTATIC JAUNDICE

Cholestasis is a failure of bile flow, and its cause may lie anywhere between the hepatocyte and the duodenum. The causes are listed in the information box (p. 505).

Jaundice becomes progressively severe in unrelieved cholestasis because conjugated bilirubin is unable to enter the bile canaliculi and passes back into the blood,

Table 11.7 Congenital non-haemolytic hyperbilirubinaemia

| Syndrome | Inheritance | Age of presentation | Hyperbilirubinaemia | | Bilirubinuria | Liver | | Histology | Cholecystography | Bromsulphthalein excretion | Prognosis | Treatment |
			Type	Severity		Defect(s)						
Gilbert's	Autosomal dominant	Young adult (any)	Unconjugated	Mild	No	Glucuronyl transferase reduced. Others occasional. Mild haemolysis. Defective bilirubin uptake		Normal	Normal	Normal	Normal life span	None. Phenobarbitone occasionally
Crigler–Najjar – Type I	Autosomal recessive	Neonate	Unconjugated	Very severe	No	Glucuronyl transferase absent		Normal	—	—	Rapid death (kernicterus)	None
– Type II	Autosomal dominant	Neonate	Unconjugated	Severe	No	Glucuronyl transferase greatly reduced		Normal	—	—	Can survive to adulthood	Phenobarbitone. Ultraviolet light. Liver transplant
Dubin–Johnson	Autosomal recessive	Any	Conjugated	Mild	Yes	Canalicular excretion of organic anions (e.g. bilirubin, cholecystographic contrast agents) reduced		Black deposits (melanin)	Gallbladder not visualised	Normal at 45 min. Secondary rise at 120 min	Normal life span	None
Rotor	Autosomal dominant	Any	Conjugated	Mild	Yes	Defective bilirubin uptake. Reduced intrahepatic binding		Normal	Gallbladder not visualised	Abnormal at 45 min. No secondary rise at 120 min	Normal life span	None

CAUSES OF CHOLESTASIS

Hepatocyte (canalicular) cholestasis
Drugs*
Alcohol*
Viral hepatitis
Chronic active hepatitis
Cirrhosis
Severe bacterial infections
Postoperative
Hodgkin's lymphoma
Pregnancy
Idiopathic recurrent cholestasis

Biliary obstruction
Intraluminal
    Stones*
    Cystic fibrosis (tenacious secretions)
    Parasites
Carcinoma
    Pancreas*
    Bile duct*
    Peripapillary
        pancreas,
        bile duct,
        duodenum
Benign tumours
    Periampullary adenoma
    Biliary papilloma
Metastatic tumours
    Intrahepatic*
    Lymph nodes (e.g. in porta hepatis)
Strictures
    Trauma (usually surgical)
    Stones
    Primary sclerosing cholangitis
Biliary cirrhosis
    Primary*
    Secondary
Choledochal cyst
Pancreatitis
Duodenal ulcer

* More common causes.

and also because there is a failure of clearance of un-conjugated bilirubin arriving at the liver cells.

Aetiology

Cholestasis may be due to failure of the hepatocytes to generate bile flow, to obstruction to bile flow in the bile ducts in the portal tracts, or to obstruction to bile flow in the extrahepatic bile ducts between the porta hepatis and the papilla of Vater. Causes of cholestasis can operate at more than one of these levels, and those confined to the extrahepatic bile ducts may be amenable to surgical correction.

Clinical features

Clinical features in cholestatic jaundice include those due to cholestasis itself and to the development of cholangitis consequent on biliary obstruction. These features are listed in the information box below.

CLINICAL FEATURES IN CHOLESTATIC JAUNDICE

Cholestasis
Early features
    Jaundice
    Dark urine
    Pale stools
    Pruritus
Late features
    Xanthelasma and xanthomas
    Malabsorption
        Weight loss
        Steatorrhoea
        Hepatic osteodystrophy
        Bleeding tendency

Cholangitis
Fever
Rigors
Pain
    Biliary infection
    Hepatic abscess

Jaundice is very variable; it may be static or fluctuate, and if it is prolonged and severe it can give the skin a greenish appearance. The stools are pale or clay-coloured due to deficiency of pigments derived from bilirubin and to steatorrhoea consequent on bile salt deficiency. The urine is dark from the renal excretion of conjugated bilirubin. Some patients have generalised pruritus and accessible parts of the body may show scratch marks. Lipid deposits can develop in the skin in prolonged cholestatic jaundice. Most of these are xanthelasmas on the eyelids but occasionally xanthomas also occur. Prolonged cholestasis can cause marked mal-absorption leading to weight loss, severe steatorrhoea, a haemorrhagic tendency due to vitamin K deficiency, and hepatic osteodystrophy following calcium and vitamin D deficiency. Eventually clinical and bio-chemical evidence of biliary cirrhosis and hepato-cellular failure occur. Cholangitis due to infection in biliary obstruction causes fever with or without rigors, and coincident pain and hepatic tenderness may indicate the development of a hepatic abscess. Clinical features in cholestatic jaundice also include those which point to a likely cause for the condition (Table 11.8). None of these features is pathognomonic of a particular cause, but each is more likely in some diseases than in others.

Investigation

Investigations in individual patients are determined by

Table 11.8 Underlying causes of cholestatic jaundice related to clinical features

Clinical feature	Causes
Jaundice	
Static or increasing	Carcinoma
Fluctuating	Stone
	Stricture
	Pancreatitis
	Choledochal cyst
Abdominal pain	Stone
	Pancreatitis
	Choledochal cyst
Cholangitis	Stone
	Stricture
	Choledochal cyst
Abdominal scar	Stone
	Stricture
Irregular hepatomegaly	Hepatic carcinoma
Palpable gallbladder	Carcinoma below cystic duct (usually pancreas)
Abdominal mass	Carcinoma
	Pancreatitis (cyst)
	Choledochal cyst
Occult blood in stools	Papillary tumour

Note: Each of the diseases listed here can give rise to almost any of the clinical features shown. The more likely causes of each clinical feature are given.

the clinical findings, but where there is no obvious cause for cholestasis initial efforts are directed to identifying a large duct biliary obstruction (Fig. 11.5). Ultrasonography should be carried out in all cases, and tests for the antimitochondrial antibody should be performed. ERCP is the best investigation if the biliary tract is dilated, particularly when the dilatation extends to the lower common bile duct, and PTC is used only if ERCP is unavailable. ERCP may also be appropriate when ultrasonography does not show dilated bile ducts, if there are no clinical clues to the cause of cholestasis or if a condition such as sclerosing cholangitis which does not necessarily cause biliary dilatation is suspected as when ulcerative colitis is also present. Liver biopsy would be preferred if evidence of liver disease such as spider telangiectasias was present.

Management
This depends on the underlying cause of the cholestasis.

UNUSUAL FORMS OF CHOLESTASIS

Cholestasis of pregnancy
This is probably caused by an inherited susceptibility of the patient's liver cells to oestrogens; the condition is sometimes precipitated by oral contraceptives. Pruritus is the dominant symptom and jaundice occurs in about a half of patients. Itching almost always starts in the third trimester of pregnancy and remits within about 2 weeks of delivery. Pruritus can be relieved with cholestyramine (p. 534). No harm comes to the fetus,

but the condition tends to recur in subsequent pregnancies.

Benign recurrent intrahepatic cholestasis
This is a rare condition in which episodes of cholestasis lasting from 1–6 months occur starting in adolescence or early adult life. Genetic factors are probably important as more than one family member may be affected. Episodes start with pruritus and painless jaundice develops later. Liver function tests show the pattern of cholestasis (p. 494), and liver biopsy shows cholestasis during an episode but is normal between episodes. Treatment is required to relieve pruritus (p. 534) and the long-term prognosis is good.

ACUTE PARENCHYMAL LIVER DISEASE

Aetiology
In acute parenchymal liver disease (acute hepatitis) there is sudden widespread liver damage in which variable numbers of hepatocytes undergo necrosis. These episodes are due mainly to hepatitis viruses or drugs. The causes are listed in the information box (p. 507).

Pathology
The pathology in acute parenchymal liver damage depends on the cause of the damage. Lesions in acute virus hepatitis and in most instances of acute damage due to drugs are similar. Cell damage throughout the liver is the dominant abnormality particularly in centrilobular areas, though individual lobules are variably affected. Damaged hepatocytes have a swollen granular appearance, while dead ones become shrunken and deeply stained, sometimes losing their nuclei to form eosinophilic bodies. These bodies, originally described in yellow fever (Councilman bodies), are strong indicators of acute hepatitis. The lobules may be infiltrated with mononuclear cells. Polymorphonuclear leucocytes and fatty change are not seen. The portal tracts are enlarged and contain a predominantly mononuclear cell infiltrate. More severe damage is accompanied by collapse of the reticulin framework particularly between the central veins and portal tracts which become linked to one another; this is known as bridging or subacute hepatic necrosis. Very severe damage results in destruction of whole lobules (massive necrosis) and is the lesion underlying most instances of fulminant hepatic failure. Cholestasis is occasionally prominent. Less commonly, the main histological abnormality is fatty change. This occurs in damage due to carbon tetrachloride, tetracycline and a number of

CAUSES OF ACUTE PARENCHYMAL LIVER DAMAGE

Viral infections
Hepatitis A virus
Hepatitis B virus
Delta virus
Hepatitis C virus
Non-A, non-B viruses
Cytomegalovirus
Epstein–Barr virus
Herpes simplex virus
Yellow fever virus

Post-viral infection
Reye's syndrome (aspirin association)

Non-viral infections
Leptospirae (usually icterohaemorrhagiae)
Toxoplasma gondii
Coxiella burneti

Drugs
See p. 513

Poisons
Mushrooms (Amanita phalloides)
Carbon tetrachloride

Metabolic
Wilson's disease
Fatty change of pregnancy

Ischaemic
Shock
Severe cardiac failure or tamponade
Budd–Chiari syndrome

there is a polymorphonuclear leucocytosis and protein, blood and casts are found in the urine. The diagnosis is made by demonstrating a rise in specific antibodies, and leptospires may be isolated from the blood or urine. The development of *cholestatic hepatitis* can cause confusion with other causes of cholestasis, especially obstruction of a major bile duct. Features of an acute hepatitis at the onset of the illness, absence of features common in biliary obstruction (information box, p. 505), high plasma transaminase activity, a negative antimitochondrial test and lack of biliary dilatation on ultrasonography favour cholestatic hepatitis, but liver biopsy may be required.

VIRAL HEPATITIS

Viral hepatitis is almost always caused by one or other of the hepatitis viruses; hepatitis due to other viruses accounts for only about 1–2% of cases. All these viruses give rise to illnesses which are similar in their clinical and pathological features and which are frequently anicteric or asymptomatic. The information box (left) lists the causes.

Aetiology, epidemiology and prevention
Viral hepatitis is caused by four main agents (Table 11.9).

HEPATITIS A VIRUS

The hepatitis A virus (HAV) may belong to the picornavirus group of enteroviruses and it can be cultured though this is only done for research purposes. It is highly infectious and is spread by the oral-faecal route. Infected persons excrete viruses in the faeces for about 2 weeks before the onset of illness and for 5–7 days thereafter. Children are most commonly affected and conditions of overcrowding and poor sanitation facilitate spread. In occasional outbreaks water, milk and shellfish have been the vehicles of transmission. Though faeces is the usual source, uncommonly infection can be spread by blood and by homosexual activity, especially in men. The sources in the community appear to be persons incubating or suffering from the disease. A carrier state, analogous to that for hepatitis B virus, does not occur.

Infection in the community is prevented best by improving social conditions, especially overcrowded and unhygienic situations. Individuals can be protected from infection for about 3 months by immune serum globulin provided this is given very soon after exposure

other toxins. Rarely, severe fatty degeneration of the liver is encountered in pregnancy or as a metabolic disturbance in Reye's syndrome in children (p. 511). Alcohol also causes fatty change but is not a cause of acute parenchymal liver damage (p. 530).

Differential diagnosis
Most patients with acute parenchymal liver disease are suffering from *viral hepatitis* which may be suggested by previous contact with a jaundiced person, travel to areas where viral hepatitis is endemic, parenteral drug abuse, a history of transfusion with blood or blood products or other exposure to blood. *Drug-induced hepatitis* must always be considered and enquiry should include drugs and herbal remedies taken by the patient (p. 515). *Wilson's disease* should be thought of in young patients who have had recurrent acute hepatitis of unknown cause or where haemolysis is present (p. 532), and *fatty liver of pregnancy* considered in the third trimester of pregnancy (above). Hepatic damage due to *circulatory causes* is recognised from associated shock, cardiac failure or tamponade. *Weil's disease* (p. 140) may cause severe jaundice and in contrast to viral hepatitis

Table 11.9 Features of the main hepatitis viruses

	A	B	Delta	Non-A, non-B Epidemic[1]	Non-A, non-B Post-transfusion[2]	Non-A, non-B Sporadic[2]
Virus						
Group	Enterovirus	Hepadna	Incomplete virus	—	Flavivirus	Flavivirus
Nucleic acid	RNA	DNA	RNA	RNA	RNA	RNA
Size (diameter)	27 nm	42 nm	35 nm	27 nm	—	—
Particles in blood	No	Yes	Yes	—	—	—
Incubation (weeks)	2–4	4–20	6–9	3–8	short (1–4) long (6–12)	—
Spread						
Faeces	Yes	No	No	Yes	—	No
Blood	Uncommon	Yes	Yes	No	Yes	Yes
Saliva[3]	Yes	Yes	Yes	?	—	?
Sexual	Uncommon	Yes	Yes	?	—	?
Vertical	No	Yes	Yes	No	—	Yes
Chronic infection	No	Yes (5–10%)	Yes	?	Yes (> 10%)	Yes (> 10%)
Prevention						
Active	No	Vaccine	Prevented by	No	No	No
Passive	Immune serum globulin	Hyperimmune serum globulin	prevention of hepatitis B virus infection	No		No

[1] Hepatic E virus.
[2] Hepatitis C virus.
[3] All body fluids are potentially infectious, though some (e.g. urine) are lowly infectious.

to the virus. Its use can be considered for those at particular risk such as close contacts, the elderly, those with other major disease and perhaps pregnant women. Prevention can be effective in an outbreak of hepatitis, for example in a school or nursery, as injection of those at risk prevents secondary spread, for example to families. Persons travelling to endemic areas can be protected by immune serum globulin for about 3 months. The protective effect of immune serum globulin is attributed to its anti-HAV content.

HEPATITIS B VIRUS

The hepatitis B virus is the only hepadna virus causing infection in humans. It cannot yet be grown but can be transmitted to certain primates, such as the chimpanzee, in which it replicates. It comprises a capsule and a core containing DNA and a DNA polymerase enzyme. The virus and an excess of its capsular material circulate in the blood, where it can be identified (p. 496). Humans are the only source of infection. Individuals incubating or suffering from acute hepatitis are highly infectious for at least as long as the HBsAg is in the blood. Asymptomatic individuals and some patients with chronic liver disease have chronic infections and may carry the virus for life. These individuals are most infectious when markers of continuing viral replication such as HBeAg, viral DNA or DNA polymerase are present in the blood, and are least infectious when they are absent and anti-HBe is present.

Blood is the main source of infection and spread may follow transfusion of infected blood or blood products or injections with contaminated needles, a mode of spread most common among parenteral drug abusers who share needles. Blood and blood products used for transfusion are no longer a major source of infection provided that donor blood is tested for the virus, and less than 10% of all post-transfusion hepatitis is now attributable to the hepatitis B virus. Only products such as albumin solutions and gammaglobulin which are pasteurised are free of risk. Tattooing or acupuncture can also spread this disease if inadequately sterilised needles are used.

The hepatitis B virus can also cause sporadic infections which cannot be attributed to parenteral modes of spread. The means of non-parenteral transmission are uncertain, but the discovery of the HBsAg or viral DNA in body fluids such as saliva, urine, semen and vaginal secretions suggests many mechanisms. Close personal contact seems necessary for transmission of infection, and sexual intercourse, especially in male homosexuals, is an important route. The virus may be spread from mother to child; transmission at or soon after birth seems more likely than transplacental spread.

Hepatitis B vaccines containing HBsAg are available capable of producing active immunisation in 95% of normal individuals. Recombinant vaccines have reduced the high cost of plasma-derived vaccines and will be used most in future. Vaccines give quite a high degree of protection and should be used particularly in those at special risk of infection who are not already immune as evidenced by anti-HBs in the blood. Those

AT RISK GROUPS MERITING HEPATITIS B VACCINATION

Parenteral drug abuse

Homosexuals (male)

Close contacts of infected individuals
Newborn of infected mothers
Regular sexual partners

Chronic haemodialysis

Medical/nursing personnel
Dentists
Surgeons/obstetricians
Accident and emergency departments
Intensive care
Liver units
Endoscopy units
Oncology units

Laboratory staff handling blood

at special risk of infection are listed in the information box above. The vaccine is ineffective in those already infected by the hepatitis B virus.

Type B hepatitis can be prevented or minimised by the intramuscular injection of hyperimmune serum globulin prepared from blood containing anti-HBs. This should be given within 24 hours, or at most a week, of exposure to infected blood in circumstances likely to cause infection; these include accidental needle puncture, gross personal contamination with infected blood, oral ingestion or contamination of mucous membranes, or exposure to infected blood in the presence of cuts and grazes. Vaccine can be given together with hyperimmune globulin (active-passive immunisation).

DELTA VIRUS

The delta virus is an RNA-containing partial virus which has no independent existence; it requires the hepatitis B virus for replication and has the same sources and modes of spread as that virus. It can infect individuals simultaneously with the hepatitis B virus, or it can superinfect those who are already chronic carriers of the hepatitis B virus. Simultaneous infections give rise to acute hepatitis which is often severe but which is limited by recovery from the hepatitis B virus infection. Infections in individuals who are chronic carriers of the hepatitis B virus can cause acute infection with spontaneous recovery, and occasionally simultaneous cessation of the chronic hepatitis B virus infection occurs. Chronic infection with the hepatitis B virus and the delta virus can also occur, and this frequently causes progressive chronic hepatitis and eventually cirrhosis.

Delta virus has a world-wide distribution but is endemic in parts of the Mediterranean basin, Africa and South America. It is transmitted mainly by close personal contact and occasionally by vertical transmission from mothers who also carry the hepatitis B virus in endemic areas and by parenteral drug abuse outside endemic areas.

NON-A, NON-B HEPATITIS VIRUSES HEPATITIS C AND E VIRUSES

Non-A, non-B hepatitis is caused by several viruses, and they can transmit infection and confer specific immunity in humans and chimpanzees. The modes of transmission in humans are probably similar to those of the hepatitis B virus. Non-A, non-B hepatitis is now the cause of 90% of post-transfusion hepatitis in developed countries, and it also accounts for up to 25% of sporadic acute viral hepatitis. All blood products capable of transmitting hepatitis B can transmit non-A, non-B hepatitis, and coagulation factor concentrates have proved a particular problem. Recently a non-A, non-B hepatitis virus has been described and named the hepatitis C virus. Serological tests (p. 497) show that HCV infection is common in post-transfusion hepatitis and in drug addicts and contributes to sporadic acute viral hepatitis. The non-A, non-B viruses can cause chronic infection but the contribution of these viruses to chronic liver disease is unknown. Prevention is not possible but the frequency of post-transfusion hepatitis should be reduced with increasing availability of serological assays for the hepatitis C virus. Immune serum globulin, useful in type A hepatitis, may prevent or ameliorate non-A, non-B hepatitis.

An epidemic water-borne form of non-A, non-B hepatitis has also now been recognised (hepatitis E virus). It is associated with excretion of viral particles in the stool and the appearance of antibodies in the blood during recovery.

OTHER VIRUSES

Cytomegalovirus and Epstein-Barr virus infection causes abnormal liver function tests in most patients, and occasionally icteric hepatitis occurs. Herpes simplex is a rare cause of hepatitis in adults most of whom are immunocompromised, and yellow fever virus causes hepatitis in parts of the world where it is endemic.

Clinical features

Prodromal symptoms usually precede the development of jaundice by a few days to 2 weeks. They are the common manifestations of an acute infectious disease and include chills, headache and malaise. Gastrointestinal symptoms may be prominent; anorexia and distaste for cigarettes are frequent, and nausea, vomiting and diarrhoea may follow. A steady upper abdominal pain, occasionally severe, occurs as a result of stretching of the peritoneum over the enlarged liver. Initially physical signs are scanty; the liver is usually tender though not readily palpable, enlarged cervical lymph nodes may be found, and splenomegaly may occur, particularly in children. Patients with hepatitis B virus infection often have arthralgia during the prodrome, and occasionally a 'serum sickness syndrome' with skin rashes (including urticaria) and polyarthritis occurs.

Dark urine and a yellow tint to the sclerae herald the onset of jaundice. As obstruction to the biliary canaliculi develops, the jaundice deepens, the stools become paler, the urine darker, and the liver more easily palpable. At this time the appetite often improves and gastrointestinal symptoms diminish in intensity. Thereafter the jaundice usually recedes, the stools and urine regain their normal colour, the liver enlargement regresses, and in the course of 3–6 weeks the majority of patients recover.

Mild illnesses may run an anicteric course recognised by known contact with a definite case or by the association of vague gastrointestinal complaints or malaise with bilirubinuria and biochemical evidence of hepatic dysfunction.

Investigations
A plasma aminotransferase activity exceeding 400 units/l, even before jaundice develops, is the most striking abnormality. The plasma bilirubin is variably modestly or markedly elevated, the alkaline phosphatase activity rarely exceeds 250 units/l unless marked cholestasis develops, and the albumin concentration is normal. Prolongation of the prothrombin time is a reliable indication of severe liver damage, and changes in the prothrombin time are a good guide to prognosis. Bilirubinuria is an early finding, occurring in the prodromal phase and usually continuing into the convalescent period. Mild proteinuria may be present. The white cell count is normal or low in uncomplicated cases, sometimes with a relative lymphocytosis; this is of some value in differentiation from Weil's disease (p. 507). Serological tests can identify the particular virus causing the illness (p. 495). Non-A, non-B hepatitis is diagnosed by excluding hepatitis A, hepatitis B, cytomegalovirus and Epstein–Barr virus infection. Differential diagnosis is discussed on page 507.

Complications
Many complications can occur but in practice serious complications are uncommon. The complications are listed in the information box below.

COMPLICATIONS OF ACUTE VIRAL HEPATITIS

- Fulminant hepatic failure
- Relapsing hepatitis
    Biochemical
    Clinical
- Cholestatic hepatitis
- Posthepatitis syndrome
- Hyperbilirubinaemia (Gilbert's syndrome)
- Aplastic anaemia
- Connective tissue disease
- Renal failure
- Henoch–Schönlein purpura
- Papular acrodermatitis
- Chronic hepatitis
- Cirrhosis (hepatitis B and non-A, non-B viruses)
- Hepatocellular carcinoma

Fatalities are rare and are attributable to the development of *fulminant hepatic failure* (p. 511). Return of symptoms and signs of acute hepatitis during recovery are characteristic of *relapsing hepatitis* and occur in 5–15% of patients. Asymptomatic 'biochemical' relapses with increases of plasma aminotransferase activity are even more common. Relapsing hepatitis does not imply a worse prognosis because it resolves spontaneously. *Cholestatic viral hepatitis* can develop from the onset or during the course of the illness, with more severe jaundice of a clinically and biochemically obstructive type which may follow a prolonged course. Liver biopsy shows the features of hepatitis with prominent cholestasis and no evidence of chronic liver damage. This cholestatic illness may continue for many months but the prognosis is good.

Debility for 2–3 months is common following clinical and biochemical recovery. Sometimes, particularly in anxious patients, there may be prolonged malaise, anorexia, nausea and right hypochondrial discomfort without clinical or biochemical evidence of liver disease. This syndrome, which may be exacerbated by too frequent clinical and biochemical assessment, is known as the *posthepatitis syndrome* and is not due to liver disease.

Chronic hepatitis and cirrhosis develop when chronic hepatitis B virus infection with or without delta virus superinfection or chronic non-A, non-B virus infection occurs. Chronic hepatitis B virus infection is also associated with hepatocellular carcinoma. *Unconjugated hyperbilirubinaemia* is sometimes found after acute viral hepatitis. Most instances are probably due to pre-existing Gilbert's syndrome but occasional cases can be attributed to the viral infection.

Systemic complications are rare and include *aplastic anaemia*. This seems most common after non-A, non-B virus infection and may not become apparent for up to a year after the hepatic illness. Other complications are mostly related to hepatitis B virus infection and include *connective tissue disease*, particularly polyarteritis nodosa, and *renal damage* such as glomerulonephritis. *Henoch-Schönlein purpura* and *papular acrodermatitis* have been reported in children.

Management

There is no specific treatment for acute viral hepatitis. Only more severely affected patients require care in hospital so that developing fulminant hepatic failure can be detected at an early stage.

Bed-rest. When symptoms are marked, bed-rest should be advised the patient rising to the toilet if desired. Thereafter younger patients may be up and about, taking care only to avoid exhaustion. For those in whom the risks of hepatitis are greater, bed-rest should be continued until symptoms and signs have disappeared and liver function tests have returned substantially towards normal. These patients include those over 50 years, the pregnant, and patients with other major disease.

Diet. A nutritious diet containing 2000–3000 kcal daily is given. This is often not tolerated, initially owing to anorexia and nausea, in which case a light diet supplemented by fruit drinks and glucose is usually acceptable. The content of the diet is dictated largely by the patient's wishes; however, a good protein intake should be encouraged. If vomiting is severe, intravenous fluid and glucose may be required.

Drugs. Drugs should be avoided especially in severe hepatitis because many are metabolised in the liver. This applies especially to sedative and hypnotic agents. Alcohol must be avoided during the illness and should not be taken in the ensuing 6 months. Oral contraceptives may be resumed after clinical and biochemical recovery. The posthepatitis syndrome is treated by reassurance.

Prognosis

The overall mortality of acute viral hepatitis is about 0.5%. Very few otherwise well patients under 40 years old die, but mortality reaches about 3% in patients over 60 years. Hepatitis B virus, delta virus and non-A, non-B virus infections account for most fatalities, and morbidity and mortality can be high in patients with other serious diseases and in pregnant women.

FULMINANT HEPATIC FAILURE

Fulminant hepatic failure is a rare syndrome in which hepatic encephalopathy, characterised by mental changes progressing from confusion to stupor and coma, results from sudden severe impairment of hepatic function. The syndrome is defined further as occurring within 8 weeks of onset of the precipitating illness, in the absence of evidence of pre-existing liver disease, to distinguish it from those instances in which hepatic encephalopathy represents a deterioration in chronic liver disease.

Aetiology

Any cause of acute liver damage can produce fulminant hepatic failure providing it is sufficiently severe (see information box p. 507). Acute viral hepatitis is the commonest cause, drugs (p. 515) being the next most frequent. Otherwise fulminant liver failure occurs occasionally in pregnancy, in Wilson's disease, following shock or from poisons such as amanita phalloides, and rarely in extensive malignant disease in the liver.

Reye's syndrome

This is a rare acute encephalopathy in which cerebral oedema and severe fatty degeneration of the liver develop after an infectious illness such as influenza or chickenpox which has often been treated with aspirin. It occurs primarily in children and adolescents, but adults are affected occasionally.

Pathology

Extensive parenchymal necrosis is the most common lesion (p. 506). In fatal cases, less than 30% of the liver cells appear viable histologically and often few such cells are seen. Severe fatty degeneration is characteristic of fulminant hepatic failure caused by drugs such as tetracycline, pregnancy and Reye's syndrome.

Clinical features

Cerebral disturbance (encephalopathy) is the cardinal manifestation of fulminant hepatic failure. Its causes are uncertain (p. 522), but cerebral oedema is a particularly important factor. The earliest features are reduced alertness and poor concentration progressing through behavioural abnormalities such as restlessness, aggressive outbursts and mania, to drowsiness and coma. Confusion, disorientation, inversion of sleep rhythm, slurred speech, yawning, hiccoughing and convulsions may occur. A flapping 'hepatic' tremor (asterixis) of the extended hands is characteristic. Cerebral oedema is likely when unequal or abnormally reacting pupils, fixed pupils with spontaneous respiration, hyperventilation, profuse sweating, local or general myoclonus, focal fits or decerebrate posturing is present. Papilloedema does not occur or is a late sign.

More general symptoms include weakness, nausea and vomiting. Right hypochondrial pain is only an occasional feature. Examination shows jaundice which develops rapidly and is usually deep in fatal cases. Jaundice is not seen in Reye's syndrome, and death occasionally occurs before it develops in other causes of fulminant hepatic failure. Fetor hepaticus, a sweet musty odour to the breath, may be present (p. 525). The liver may be enlarged initially but later becomes impalpable; disappearance of hepatic dullness on percussion indicates much shrinkage and a bad prognosis. Splenomegaly is uncommon and never prominent. Ascites and oedema occur in patients surviving a week or more and may be a consequence of fluid therapy. Other features are related to the development of complications which are considered below in the management of the condition.

Investigations

The plasma bilirubin reflects the degree of jaundice. Initially, plasma aminotransferase activity is high, as in acute viral hepatitis, but with progression of damage activity falls; this investigation has diagnostic but not prognostic significance. Alkaline phosphatase activity is variable. The prothrombin time rapidly becomes prolonged as coagulation factor synthesis fails; this is the laboratory test of greatest prognostic value, a progressive and marked prolongation carries a poor prognosis. Plasma albumin concentration remains normal unless the course is prolonged. Increased plasma and urine amino acids are characteristic but are not generally measured. White blood cell counts vary, leucocytosis occurring even in the absence of infection. The urine contains protein, bilirubin and urobilinogen.

Liver biopsy is contraindicated because of the severe haemostatic deficiency and because it rarely gives information required for management. Viral causes are sought serologically. Wilson's disease should always be considered (p. 532).

Management

There is no specific treatment, but certain measures should be instituted as soon as encephalopathy occurs. The patient's life is sustained in the hope that hepatic regeneration will take place or that liver transplantation can be undertaken. There should be close observation so that complications (see information box p. 513) can be corrected promptly. The observations are listed in the information box below.

OBSERVATIONS IN FULMINANT HEPATIC FAILURE

Neurological
Conscious level
Pupils – size, equality, reactivity
Fundi – for papilloedema
Plantar responses

Cardiorespiratory
Pulse
Blood pressure
Central venous pressure
Respiratory rate

Fluid balance
Input – oral, intravenous
Output – hourly urine output, 24-hour sodium output
       – vomiting, diarrhoea

Temperature

Blood analyses
Peripheral blood count (including platelets)
Urea, sodium, potassium, CO_2, calcium, magnesium
Glucose (2-hourly in acute phase)
Prothrombin time

Infection surveillance
Cultures – blood, urine, throat, sputum, cannula sites
Chest radiograph

Encephalopathy. This is treated by withdrawing all nitrogen intake, by reducing the nitrogen-producing colonic flora with neomycin (1 g orally 4–6-hourly), and by increasing faecal output with lactulose (p. 523). Enemas can be used to empty the colon if tests for stool blood are positive. Electroencephalography may be used to follow the course of the encephalopathy. Sedative drugs must be used with very great care, restlessness and excitement being controlled where necessary with the smallest possible dose of diazepam or midazolam given intravenously. The benzodiazepine antagonist flumazenil should be available.

Cerebral oedema. This is a frequent cause of death and is difficult to diagnose as it often develops rapidly and rarely causes papilloedema. It can present as a sudden respiratory arrest. The appearance of any one of the indicators of cerebral oedema given above indicates the need for treatment. Mannitol 20% (1 g/kg body weight) should be infused intravenously over half an hour, and the dose repeated if the clinical signs are not reversed. Most patients need two doses (range 1–4) for any one episode of cerebral oedema. Intracranial pressure can be monitored but the placement of an intracranial pressure sensor in the presence of severely impaired blood coagulation is risky.

Nutrition. Calories are provided as glucose (300 g/d) either orally or by nasogastric tube or into a large central vein as a 10–20% solution. The blood glucose should be measured 2-hourly in the severe phase because potentially fatal hypoglycaemia often occurs; its treatment may require large amounts of glucose. Estimations can be made simply by using dip-stick tests, but checks using laboratory methods should also be made. Capillary blood is used for dip-stick tests, and precautions to avoid infection, particularly wearing gloves, should be taken in obtaining samples. Fluid and electrolyte therapy depends on maintenance of accurate fluid balance records and on daily measurements of plasma urea, sodium, potassium and bicarbonate. Saline is used cautiously to avoid sodium overload, and treatment is made easier by knowledge of the 24-hour urine sodium output. Potassium deficiency, which occurs readily, should be corrected.

Cardiorespiratory function. Patients have poor vasomotor control and correction of abnormalities by intravenous infusion of fluid, colloid and blood requires regular recording of pulse, blood pressure, hourly urine output, and if possible central venous pressure. Careful respiratory supervision is also needed, as respiratory failure requires early assisted ventilation.

Haemorrhage. Impaired haemostasis, due mainly to failure of coagulation factor production, can result in bleeding from any site. Bruising and purpura are common. Gastrointestinal bleeding from gastric erosions is frequent and can be prevented by H_2 receptor-blocking drugs (cimetidine 50 mg i.v. hourly or ranitidine 50 mg i.v. over 2 h, every 8 h).

Infection. This is common and serious. As fever and leucocytosis may result solely from the liver disease itself, they are no guide and regular blood, urine and throat cultures and chest radiographs should be undertaken. Prophylactic antibiotics should not be used. If infection is strongly suspected, broad-spectrum antibiotics such as cefotaxime intravenously and metronidazole by suppository may be given once specimens have been taken for culture.

Renal failure. This can develop and may require dialysis.

Other measures. Many special treatments including corticosteroids, exchange transfusion, plasmapheresis, charcoal haemoperfusion and haemodialysis with special dialysis membranes have been advocated, but they are of no proven value. Liver transplantation can be very successful and should be considered as soon as a patient develops encephalopathy.

Prognosis

The prognosis of fulminant hepatic failure is closely related to the encephalopathy. When minor signs only are present and drowsiness is not prominent, some two-thirds of patients survive. Once coma develops, only 10–20% of patients survive. The prognosis is worse with increasing age and, perhaps, when due to certain agents such as halothane. Death usually occurs within a week in fatal cases. Life-threatening complications, some amenable to conservative therapy, may arise in the course of the illness. Complications are listed in the information box below.

COMPLICATIONS OF FULMINANT HEPATIC FAILURE

- Encephalopathy
- Cerebral oedema
- Respiratory failure
- Hypotension
- Hypothermia
- Infection
- Bleeding
- Pancreatitis
- Renal failure
- Metabolic
  - Hypoglycaemia
  - Hypokalaemia
  - Hypocalcaemia
  - Hypomagnesaemia
  - Acid-base disturbance

Those who recover from fulminant hepatic failure usually regain normal hepatic structure and function.

DRUGS, TOXINS AND THE LIVER

The liver is the main organ in which drugs are metabolised and consequently is important in determining the effects of drugs in the body. Liver disease may alter the capacity of the liver to metabolise drugs and unexpected toxicity may occur when patients with liver disease are given drugs in normal doses. Drugs themselves can damage the liver and there is increasing recognition of the many forms of hepatic damage attributable to drugs.

HEPATIC DRUG METABOLISM

Hepatic drug metabolism involves the conversion of fat-soluble (non-polar) drugs into water-soluble (polar) metabolites which can be excreted in the bile if they are relatively large molecules or in the urine if they are relatively small. This conversion is mediated by a group of mixed-function oxidase enzymes, the best known of which is cytochrome P_{450} located in the smooth endoplasmic reticulum of the liver cells. Drugs which are already highly polar undergo little or no metabolic change. Two types of reaction take place during hepatic drug metabolism:

Type I

Type I reactions mainly involve oxidation or reduction and usually increase the polarity of drugs. They have very variable effects on pharmacological activity, as they can produce or reduce drug activity or leave it unchanged.

Type II

Type II reactions involve conjugation, usually with glucuronide, sulphate or glutathione, and lead to the production of highly polar metabolites with no pharmacological activity. These metabolites are excreted in the bile or urine. Several factors alter the rate at which drugs are metabolised by the mixed-function oxidase enzymes, including *genetic factors*, *nutritional factors*, *induction or inhibition of the enzymes*, and the *number of drugs* given simultaneously.

Drug metabolism varies considerably between individuals mainly because of genetic factors. Nutritional factors are also important as malnutrition reduces enzyme activity and reduces the rate of drug metabolism. Certain factors, especially drugs, can increase enzyme activity (enzyme induction) or inhibit enzyme activity in the liver, and they can alter the rate of drug metabolism significantly (Table 11.10). Drugs metabolised by these enzymes compete with one another for enzyme sites, and the rate of metabolism of an individual drug is reduced when another drug is given simultaneously.

Factors other than hepatic enzyme activity affect drug metabolism by the liver, the most important of these being *hepatic blood flow*. The ability of the liver to extract drugs from the blood as it flows through the sinusoids varies considerably. Some drugs are so highly extracted that liver blood flow is the dominant factor determining the rate of their elimination from the blood. These drugs are said to have a high first-pass clearance by the liver, and their rate of metabolism is greatly reduced by any reduction in hepatic blood flow or diversion of blood through or past the liver. This effect is most striking for highly extracted drugs given by mouth, for all drugs absorbed from the intestine normally flow to the liver in the portal vein. The rate of removal from the blood of lowly extracted drugs is dependent mainly on the rate of their metabolism in the liver cells. Other factors affecting the rate of removal of a drug from the blood includes its *volume of distribution* in the body and the extent of its *binding to plasma proteins* as these in turn partly determine its availability to the liver cells.

DRUG THERAPY IN LIVER DISEASE

Drug therapy is particularly likely to produce undesirable effects in liver disease because of impaired hepatic metabolism and because portal-systemic shunting of blood diverts drugs away from the liver when portal hypertension is present. There is no way of predicting which patients will suffer undesirable effects, and overcaution can easily deprive patients of useful therapy. Rather, certain general principles should be observed. Drugs should only be used where they are clearly indicated, smaller than usual doses should be given initially, frequency of administration should be determined from effects, and particular care should be exercised in patients with poor liver function, signs of portal hypertension or a previous portal-systemic shunt operation (Table 11.11). Particular precautions in

Table 11.10 Drugs increasing or decreasing mixed-function oxidase enzyme activity in the liver

Increased activity (Enzyme induction)	Decreased activity
Alcohol (ethanol)	Cimetidine
Barbiturates	Isoniazid
Carbamazepine	Ketoconazole
Diphenylhydantoin	Propoxyphene
Ethanol	
Griseofulvin	
Primidone	
Rifampicin	

Table 11.11 Factors indicating the need for caution in drug therapy in patients with liver disease

Clinical	Investigation
Jaundice	Hypoalbuminaemia
Ascites	Prolonged prothrombin time
Encephalopathy	Oesophageal varices
Fetor hepaticus	
Palpable spleen	
Malnourished	

patients with varices (p. 524), ascites (p. 527) or encephalopathy (p. 522) are given elsewhere.

HEPATOTOXICITY OF DRUGS

Liver damage due to drugs is so common that the possibility should be considered whenever liver damage occurs rather than trying to remember lists of hepatotoxic drugs. Acute liver damage due to drugs is well recognised but other forms of hepatotoxicity have become recognised increasingly in recent years. These manifestations are listed in the information box below.

MANIFESTATIONS OF DRUG HEPATOTOXICITY

Acute hepatic damage
Acute hepatitis
Cholestatic hepatitis
Cholestasis

Abnormal liver function tests

Hepatic fibrosis

Chronic hepatitis

Cirrhosis

Hepatic vascular damage
Sinusoidal dilatation/peliosis hepatis
Budd–Chiari syndrome
Veno-occlusive disease
Hepatoportal sclerosis

Neoplasia
Adenoma
Hepatocellular carcinoma
Haemangioma/haemangiosarcoma

Acute hepatic damage

Acute hepatic damage is the best recognised form of drug-induced liver injury. Such damage may be *dose-related and predictable*, or it may be *unrelated to dose and unpredictable or idiosyncratic*. Predictable drug hepatotoxicity is mediated biochemically, though its occurrence and severity can be modified by factors affecting the drug metabolising enzymes such as alcohol (p. 529) or nutritional status (above).

Paracetamol in therapeutic doses is mainly conjugated to produce glucuronide and sulphate, but a small amount is metabolised to potentially toxic intermediates which are conjugated with glutathione to form mercapturic acid which is not toxic. Paracetamol in large doses produces toxic intermediates in amounts sufficient to deplete glutathione stores and damage the liver. Alcoholic individuals can suffer increased liver

damage because alcohol increases the activity of the drug-metabolising enzymes.

Unpredictable or idiosyncratic drug hepatotoxicity has usually been attributed to immunological injury and may be associated with autoantibody production as in halothane hepatitis. However, in most patients evidence for immunological injury is scanty or indirect, and unpredictable drug hepatotoxicity is increasingly being attributed to biochemical mechanisms for example in halothane hepatitis and in isoniazid hepatitis.

Clinical features. These usually develop within about 3 months of starting treatment. Jaundice is often present and the illness is usually indistinguishable from acute viral hepatitis. Cholestatic features (p. 505) can be prominent with certain drugs and biliary obstruction may be suspected particularly where this is associated with upper abdominal pain as in erythromycin toxicity.

Liver function tests. These show high transaminase activity reflecting hepatitis, and variably increased alkaline phosphatase activity reflecting cholestasis. A few drugs cause almost pure cholestasis. Diagnosis depends on relating the illness to taking the offending drug and on excluding other causes for the illness. Procedure for diagnosis is listed in the information box below.

THE DIAGNOSIS OF ACUTE DRUG-INDUCED LIVER DISEASE

- Consider the possibility of a drug
- Tabulate drugs taken
  Prescribed by doctor
  Self-administered
- Relate drugs to the onset of the illness
- Look for pre-existing liver disease
  Clinical examination
  Previous liver investigations
- Consider alternative causes
  Viral hepatitis – serological tests
  Biliary disease – cholecystogram
              – ultrasound
- Observe the effects of stopping the suspected drugs
- Liver biopsy
  Suspected pre-existing liver disease
  Failure to improve
- Challenge tests with drugs – never (hardly ever)

Abnormal liver function tests

Abnormal liver function tests are usually found incidentally and, even when due to a drug, may resolve in spite of continued therapy. The need to withdraw a drug suspected of causing abnormal liver function tests depends on the severity of the abnormalities, whether or not they become worse, and the importance of the drug to the patient.

Chronic liver disease

Drugs can cause chronic hepatitis, hepatic fibrosis and cirrhosis, and this should be suspected whenever chronic liver disease develops in a patient receiving long-term drug therapy. Recognition of drug-induced chronic liver disease depends on excluding other known causes of liver disease and is usually not helped by liver biopsy, as the histological abnormalities caused by drugs are variable and non-specific. Indeed, the histological features can mimic those of more common forms of liver disease, for example amiodarone causes appearances indistinguishable from alcoholic damage. Clinical and biochemical evidence of disease may not occur until liver damage is very advanced as with methotrexate which causes hepatic fibrosis; patients receiving long-term treatment with methotrexate require occasional liver biopsy. Recognition of drug-induced chronic liver disease is important because drug withdrawal leads to improvement and full recovery occurs provided that cirrhosis has not developed.

Hepatic vascular damage

This is an uncommon form of liver damage usually caused by oestrogens, androgens, anabolic agents or drugs used in the chemotherapy of neoplastic disease. Oral contraceptives occasionally cause ·hepatic vein thrombosis, and chemotherapeutic agents can cause occlusion of the central hepatic veins giving rise to features identical to the Budd–Chiari syndrome and veno-occlusive disease (p. 534). Peliosis hepatis (blood-filled cysts) and sinusoidal dilatation are usually asymptomatic but can cause intraperitoneal bleeding or portal hypertension, and damage to portal veins in the terminal portal tracts can cause portal hypertension.

Neoplastic changes

Oestrogens, androgens and anabolic agents occasionally cause neoplastic changes. Oral contraceptives have been associated with development of hepatic adenomas, and the other agents may induce malignant tumours.

HEPATIC TOXINS

Alcohol is the most common environmental hepatotoxin (p. 529). Others include the amatoxins in mushrooms (usually *A. phalloides*) which can cause fulminant hepatic failure, pyrollizidine alkaloids in several plants used to make teas which are associated with veno-occlusive disease (p. 534), aflatoxins in fungi which can cause acute liver damage and possibly hepatocellular carcinoma, and occasionally material used in herbal remedies. Industrial hepatotoxins rarely cause liver damage if proper precautions are taken. They include carbon tetrachloride, which causes liver failure due to fatty change, and vinyl chloride, which induces periportal fibrosis and portal hypertension, and rarely hepatic tumours.

CHRONIC PARENCHYMAL LIVER DISEASE

Chronic hepatitis and cirrhosis are the two main forms of chronic parenchymal liver disease. They are closely related because some forms of chronic hepatitis progress to cirrhosis.

Aetiology

There are numerous causes of chronic parenchymal liver disease and these are listed in the information box below.

CAUSES OF CHRONIC LIVER DISEASE

Infection
Hepatitis B virus
Delta virus
Non-A, non-B viruses (Hepatitis C virus)

Toxins
Alcohol
Drugs

Biliary obstruction
Primary biliary cirrhosis
Secondary biliary cirrhosis
    Stricture
    Stone
    Neoplasm

Metabolic diseases
Haemochromatosis
    Primary
    Secondary
Wilson's disease
Alpha,-antitrypsin deficiency
Fibrocystic disease

Nutritional
Intestinal bypass surgery (obesity)

Hepatic congestion
Budd–Chiari syndrome
Veno-occlusive disease
Cardiac failure

Unknown cause
Chronic active hepatitis
Cryptogenic cirrhosis

The most common are alcohol, hepatitis B virus infection, chronic active hepatitis and primary biliary cirrhosis. No cause can be found in 30% of patients (cryptogenic cirrhosis). Haemochromatosis accounts for about 5% of patients; all other causes are rare.

Alcohol. The mechanism whereby alcohol damages the liver is unknown, but it is now accepted as a direct liver toxin in man (p. 529).

Infection. Chronic hepatitis B virus infection is an important cause of chronic liver disease though its incidence shows marked geographic variation. Failure to recover from hepatitis B virus infection is probably due to a deficient immune response, and the severity of subsequent chronic liver disease is related to the activity of viral replication in the liver. Superinfection with delta virus increases the chances of progressive chronic hepatitis in such patients. The non-A, non-B viruses can cause chronic infection and are likely causes of chronic liver disease. The hepatitis A virus does not cause chronic liver disease.

Immunological factors. Some patients with chronic liver disease of unknown cause have abnormal serum autoantibodies (p. 497). Though the autoantibodies themselves are not cytotoxic, their presence suggests that liver damage may be produced by abnormal immune mechanisms. Lymphocytes sensitised to liver cells are currently favoured as the mediators of liver damage.

Metabolic disorders. These include the excess hepatic deposition of iron in haemochromatosis and of copper in Wilson's disease. Alpha$_1$ antitrypsin deficiency may cause chronic liver disease in children or in adults, but most other metabolic conditions involving the liver manifest themselves first in childhood, e.g. glycogen storage disease and fibrocystic disease (cystic fibrosis).

Drugs. Chronic hepatitis and cirrhosis occur in some patients on long-term drug treatment (p. 516).

Cholestasis. Prolonged obstruction anywhere in the biliary system can cause cirrhosis. In primary biliary cirrhosis there is obstruction from damage to interlobular bile ducts. Cirrhosis from large-duct obstruction may occur with biliary strictures or in sclerosing cholangitis but not with neoplastic lesions because survival is too short.

Congestion. Prolonged hepatic congestion can eventually cause cirrhosis. This is rare as death usually occurs before cirrhosis develops. Congestion may be due to hepatic venous outflow obstruction (p. 534) or chronic heart failure.

Malnutrition. Malnutrition is probably not primarily responsible for cirrhosis though it often occurs secondarily in patients with cirrhosis. Permanent liver damage is not found in marasmus or kwashiorkor but malnutrition may be important in cirrhosis following intestinal bypass surgery for gross obesity.

Pathology

Chronic hepatitis

Two main types of chronic hepatitis are recognised histologically. Their names (persistent hepatitis and aggressive hepatitis) are easily confused with the clinical syndromes they underlie (respectively chronic persistent hepatitis and chronic active hepatitis). A third type of chronic hepatitis (lobular hepatitis) has become recognised increasingly.

Persistent hepatitis. There is an infiltration of chronic inflammatory cells confined to the portal tracts which may be expanded or show short fibrous septa extending into the parenchyma. Changes in the hepatocytes are absent or slight; there may be small foci of liver cell necrosis with inflammatory cell infiltration (spotty necrosis) and sometimes the residual changes of viral hepatitis. Lobular architecture is normal and cirrhosis rarely develops.

Aggressive hepatitis. This is the histological process underlying the clinical condition chronic active hepatitis, both the portal tracts and the parenchyma are involved, lobular architecture becomes distorted, and cirrhosis often develops. The portal tract infiltration of mononuclear cells extends irregularly into the surrounding parenchyma and the swollen liver cells become isolated in the inflammatory cell infiltrate. This process of hepatocyte destruction, called 'piecemeal necrosis', leads to septum formation linking portal tracts and central veins. The ensuing disruption of lobular architecture is accompanied by the development of regenerative nodules and eventually cirrhosis. Changes in the rest of the parenchyma are variable and resemble persistent hepatitis. These changes do not occur diffusely and may be more advanced in some areas than others.

Lobular hepatitis. In this the histological features are identical to those of acute viral hepatitis.

Cirrhosis

The changes in cirrhosis affect the whole liver but not necessarily every lobule. They include gradually progressive widespread death of liver cells associated with inflammation and fibrosis leading to loss of the normal lobular liver architecture. Destruction of the liver architecture causes distortion and loss of the normal hepatic vasculature with the formation of portal-systemic vascular shunts, and in the formation of nodules rather than lobules as surviving hepatocytes proliferate. The evolution of cirrhosis is gradual and progressive, and consequently cirrhotic livers have an infinitely variable appearance limiting the usefulness of anatomical classifications. The current classification includes *micronodular cirrhosis* (previously called portal, septal, nutritional, monolobular or Laënnec's cirrhosis), characterised by regular connective tissue septa, regenerative nodules approximating in size to the original lobules (1 mm in diameter) and involvement of every lobule; and *macronodular cirrhosis* (previously called posthepatitic or postnecrotic cirrhosis) in which the connective tissue septa vary in thickness and the nodules show marked differences in size with large ones containing histologically normal lobules. *Mixed cirrhosis* shows features of both micronodular and macronodular cirrhosis. None of these types of cirrhosis is static, and micronodular cirrhosis tends to become macronodular gradually.

CHRONIC HEPATITIS

Gradually resolving acute hepatitis must not be confused with chronic hepatitis. There is no certain way to avoid this either by clinical assessment or investigation, including liver biopsy, during the first 6 months of the illness. Accordingly, a diagnosis of chronic hepatitis should only be made firmly once liver disease has been present on clinical or other grounds for at least 6 months and a liver biopsy has then been done. Furthermore, the main chronic hepatitis syndromes are not clearly separated from one another, and patients with intermediate illnesses are encountered.

CHRONIC PERSISTENT HEPATITIS (CPH)

Chronic persistent hepatitis is a mild illness comprising fatigue, poor appetite, fatty food intolerance and upper abdominal discomfort, especially over the liver. The condition may be asymptomatic and recognised only because of a previous episode of acute hepatitis or because of biochemical tests undertaken for other reasons. Examination is usually normal but may show slight hepatomegaly. There are no features of chronic liver disease.

The plasma bilirubin is normal or slightly raised, the plasma aminotransferase is raised variably, and the alkaline phosphatase is normal. Plasma albumin and globulin concentrations are normal. One or other of the causes of chronic liver disease may be present, but autoantibodies are not found in the blood. Liver biopsy shows persistent hepatitis (above).

Differentiation should be made from the post-hepatitis syndrome (p. 510), Gilbert's syndrome (p. 503), and from sclerosing cholangitis associated with ulcerative colitis or Crohn's disease (p. 544). The prognosis is usually excellent. The patient should be reassured, and no treatment is required. Rarely, progression to chronic active hepatitis or cirrhosis may occur.

CHRONIC ACTIVE HEPATITIS (CAH)

Chronic active hepatitis is more serious than chronic persistent hepatitis or chronic lobular hepatitis, because the underlying liver damage is more severe and progressive. The clinical illness in CAH varies considerably from being mild and even asymptomatic to being florid and severe. Increasing awareness has led to recognition of milder forms of the disease.

Autoimmune CAH

This form of CAH occurs most often in women, particularly in the second and third decades of life, and produces the most florid forms of the disease though it can also be mild.

Clinical features

The onset is usually insidious with fatigue, anorexia and jaundice. In about a quarter of patients the onset is acute, resembling viral hepatitis but normal resolution does not occur. Other features include fever, arthralgia and epistaxis. Amenorrhoea is the rule.

On examination, the general health is at first good. Jaundice is mild to moderate or occasionally absent, but signs of chronic liver disease, especially spider telangiectasia and hepatosplenomegaly, are usually present. Sometimes a 'Cushingoid' face with acne, hirsutism and pink cutaneous striae, especially on the thighs and abdomen, are present. Bruises may be seen. Though liver disease usually dominates the clinical syndrome, many *associated conditions* occur in florid CAH emphasising its essentially systemic nature. These include migrating polyarthritis of large joints, a variety of rashes, most non-specific but including inflammatory papules and urticaria, lymphadenopathy, thyroid disorders such as Hashimoto's thyroiditis, thyrotoxicosis and myxoedema, Coombs-positive haemolytic anaemia, pleurisy, transient pulmonary infiltrates, ulcerative colitis and glomerulonephritis. Some patients have Sjögren's syndrome (p. 768).

Investigations
Liver function tests vary with the activity of the disease. Active inflammation is reflected by the plasma aminotransferase, and the severity of liver damage by the plasma albumin concentration and the prothrombin time. Aminotransferase activity is often increased more than 10 times in relapses of florid disease, and hypoalbuminaemia and marked hyperglobulinaemia are common. Hyperglobulinaemia is due mainly to marked increases of IgG. The plasma bilirubin reflects the degree of jaundice but usually does not exceed 100 µmol/l (6 mg/dl). The plasma alkaline phosphatase activity reflects the degree of intrahepatic cholestasis. Antinuclear antibodies are found in half the patients, smooth muscle antibodies in two-thirds, and antimitochondrial antibodies in a quarter. Liver biopsy shows aggressive hepatitis with or without cirrhosis (p. 517).

Differential diagnosis
Differentiation from acute viral hepatitis can be impossible when CAH presents with an acute exacerbation. An acute hepatitis showing unremitting activity (plasma aminotransferase activity increased at least tenfold, or increased at least five-fold with plasma gamma-globulin increased at least twice for at least 10 weeks) is likely to be due to CAH, but the diagnosis cannot be considered certain until a liver biopsy is examined at least 6 months after the onset.

Management
Treatment with corticosteroids is life-saving in autoimmune CAH particularly during exacerbations of active symptomatic disease. Initially, prednisolone 30 mg/d is given orally and the dose reduced gradually as the patient and liver function tests improve. Maintenance therapy is required for at least 2 years after liver function tests have become normal, and withdrawal of treatment should not be considered unless a liver biopsy is also normal. Side-effects from prednisolone are uncommon at a maintenance dose of 10 mg/d or less; azathioprine 50–100 mg/d orally may be added to the therapy to allow the dose of prednisolone to be reduced to this level. Treatment reduces the 5-year mortality to about 10%. Corticosteroids are less important in asymptomatic CAH with mild activity.

Prognosis
The disease occurs in exacerbations and remissions, and most patients eventually develop cirrhosis and its complications (p. 520). Hepatocellular carcinoma is uncommon. About half the patients die of liver failure within 5 years if no treatment is given.

CAH due to hepatitis B virus infection
This form of CAH occurs most often in men over 30 years of age. It may come to attention when an episode of acute viral hepatitis fails to resolve, but more often there is no history of an acute episode and the disease is found by chance or when features of cirrhosis develop.

Clinical features
Symptoms are usually non-specific and examination often reveals little of note. Hepatomegaly is the most common abnormality, jaundice is slight or absent, and fewer than a third of patients have spider telangiectasia or splenomegaly at presentation. Systemic features other than arthralgia are uncommon.

Investigations
These show moderate increases of plasma bilirubin and aminotransferase activity and minor increases of alkaline phosphatase. Hypoalbuminaemia occurs with more advanced liver damage, and hyperglobulinaemia is not marked. Serology shows hepatitis B virus infection, the HBeAg is usually present, and delta virus superinfection may be found. Autoantibody tests give negative results. Liver biopsy shows aggressive hepatitis with or without cirrhosis, and hepatitis B virus antigens can be found in hepatocytes using special stains. Hepatocytes containing HBsAg may have a ground glass appearance in H & E stains.

Prognosis
The progression of the disease is slow but usually relentless, particularly in patients with delta virus superinfection, leading eventually to cirrhosis. Remission can occur spontaneously, usually with loss of the HBeAg and appearance of anti-HBe (p. 496). Hepatocellular carcinoma is liable to develop in the long term.

Management
Interferon can be given for active disease (HBeAg).

CAH due to other causes
These forms of CAH can be due to a variety of causes, or no cause can be found in which case they are often assumed to be due to non-A, non-B hepatitis virus infection. The clinical and biochemical features vary

considerably. It is important to detect disease due to drugs, which usually remits on withdrawal of the drug, and to Wilson's disease, which requires specific treatment (p. 532).

CHRONIC LOBULAR HEPATITIS (CLH)

Chronic lobular hepatitis is an uncommon condition in which relapses and remissions of acute hepatitis occur over a period exceeding 6 months. The illness is initially indistinguishable from acute viral hepatitis in about half the patients and is initially insidious in the other half. Jaundice and hepatomegaly can be found in relapses but signs of chronic liver disease (below) are rare. Liver function tests show the features of an acute hepatitis and about half the patients have hyperglobulinaemia though hypoalbuminaemia is rare. The disease is associated with hepatitis B virus or non-A, non-B virus infection in some patients and with antinuclear, smooth muscle and antimitochondrial antibodies in others. Liver biopsy shows the features of acute viral hepatitis. Most patients need no treatment, but those with active disease and autoantibodies respond well to corticosteroids as for autoimmune CAH. The prognosis is good as progression to cirrhosis does not occur.

CIRRHOSIS OF THE LIVER

Hepatic cirrhosis can occur at any age and often causes prolonged morbidity. It manifests itself particularly in younger adults and is an important cause of premature death.

Clinical features

These vary greatly and include any combination of the manifestations described below. None is related specifically to particular causes of cirrhosis though florid spider telangiectasia, gynaecomastia and parotid enlargement are more common in alcoholic cirrhosis, and pigmentation is most striking in haemochromatosis and in cirrhosis associated with prolonged cholestasis. Autopsy experience shows that cirrhosis may be entirely asymptomatic, and in life it may be found incidentally at surgery or with minimal features such as isolated hepatomegaly. Frequent complaints include weakness, fatigue, muscle cramps, weight loss and non-specific digestive symptoms such as anorexia, nausea, vomiting, upper abdominal discomfort and gaseous abdominal distension. Otherwise, clinical features are due mainly to hepatic insufficiency and portal hypertension. They are listed in the information box (right).

Hepatomegaly is common in cirrhosis, but progressive hepatocyte destruction and fibrosis reduce liver size

---

CLINICAL FEATURES OF HEPATIC CIRRHOSIS

Hepatomegaly

Jaundice

Ascites

Circulatory changes
Spider telangiectasia
Palmar erythema
Cyanosis

Endocrine changes
Loss of libido
Hair loss
Men
  Gynaecomastia
  Testicular atrophy
  Impotence
Women
  Breast atrophy
  Irregular menses
  Amenorrhoea

Haemorrhagic tendency
Bruises, purpura
Epistaxis
Menorrhagia

Portal hypertension
Splenomegaly
Collateral vessels
Fetor hepaticus

Hepatic (portal-systemic) encephalopathy

Other features
Pigmentation
Clubbing
Low-grade fever

---

as the disease progresses. The liver is often hard, irregular and painless. *Jaundice* is usually mild when it appears first and is due primarily to failure to excrete bilirubin. Mild haemolysis occurs in cirrhosis but is not important in the development of jaundice. *Ascites* results from inadequate sodium and water excretion (p. 528). Jaundice and ascites are signs of advanced liver damage and are late signs of cirrhosis. Cirrhosis is associated with an increased peripheral blood circulation and a reduced visceral circulation which becomes more marked as the disease progresses. *Palmar erythema* is a consequence of these changes and it can be seen early in the disease, but it is of limited diagnostic value as it occurs in any condition associated with a hyperdynamic circulation as well as in some normal people. *Spider telangiectasia* are due to associated arteriolar changes and comprise a central arteriole, from which small vessels radiate and which occasionally raises the skin surface (Fig. 11.9). They vary in size from 1–2 mm to 1–2 cm in diameter, they are usually found only on the

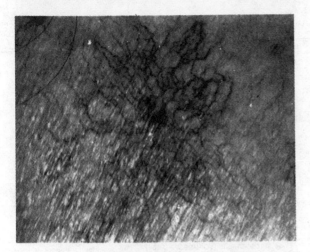

Fig. 11.9   Large spider telangiectasia with central arteriole and radiating capillaries in a patient with hepatic cirrhosis.

parts of the body above the nipples, and they can occur early in the disease. One or two small spider telangiectasia can be found in about 2% of healthy people and they can occur transiently in greater numbers in the third trimester of pregnancy, but otherwise they are strong indicators of liver disease. Pulmonary arteriovenous shunts also develop leading to hypoxaemia and eventually to *central cyanosis*, but this is a late feature. Endocrine changes are noticed more readily in men who show loss of *male hair distribution* and *testicular atrophy*. *Gynaecomastia* is infrequent and occurs most often in alcoholic liver disease, but can also be due to drugs such as spironolactone. *Easy bruising* becomes more frequent as cirrhosis advances and *epistaxis* is common, sometimes severe, and can mimic upper gastrointestinal bleeding if much blood is swallowed. *Splenomegaly*, *collateral vessels* and *fetor hepaticus* are features of portal hypertension which occurs in more advanced disease (p. 524). Evidence of hepatic encephalopathy also becomes increasingly common with advancing disease (p. 522). Non-specific features of chronic liver disease include *pigmentation*, *clubbing* of the fingers and toes and *low-grade fever*. *Dupuytren's contracture* is traditionally associated with cirrhosis, especially that due to alcohol, but the evidence for the association is weak.

Investigations

Biochemical investigations are used to assess the activity and severity of liver disease (p. 492). The plasma transaminase reflects the activity of the disease which is usually low in established cirrhosis. Transaminase activity can be much higher during the evolu-

tion of cirrhosis, particularly that caused by chronic active hepatitis (p. 518). The plasma alkaline phosphatase reflects the severity of cholestasis and is highest in biliary forms of cirrhosis. The plasma bilirubin and albumin concentrations and the vitamin K corrected prothrombin time reflect the severity of liver damage. All these tests may be normal in patients with well-compensated inactive disease (p. 492). Biochemical and serological tests are also used to determine the nature of the disease causing the cirrhosis (p. 505). Imaging is required for assessing the structural effects of the disease on the liver and is particularly useful in identifying complications such as hepatocellular carcinoma, portal hypertension and ascites (p. 498). Liver biopsy establishes the diagnosis of cirrhosis and may show the cause, but it is only needed when clinical observation and less invasive investigations have not established the diagnosis.

Differential diagnosis

This is listed in the information box below.

DIFFERENTIAL DIAGNOSIS OF CIRRHOSIS RELATED TO PRESENTATIONS

Hepatomegaly
Focal lesions
  Carcinoma
    Primary (cirrhosis)
    Secondary
  Other malignant disease
  Abscess (p. 537)
  Cysts (p. 538)
Infiltration
  Myeloproliferative diseases
  Lymphoproliferative diseases
  Sarcoidosis
  Amyloidosis
Congestion
  Cardiac failure
  Constructive pericarditis
  Budd–Chiari syndrome (p. 534)
  Veno-occlusive disease (p. 535)
Tropical
  Malaria
  Schistosomiasis
  Kala azar

Splenomegaly
Portal hypertension (cirrhosis)
Myeloproliferative disease
Lymphoproliferative disease

Jaundice (p. 502)

Gastrointestinal bleeding (p. 525)

Ascites (p. 527)

Encephalopathy (p. 522)

Complications

Cirrhosis is associated with the development of several important complications which have serious effects on the prognosis of the disease. These complications are listed in the information box below.

COMPLICATIONS OF HEPATIC CIRRHOSIS

- Portal hypertension
- Ascites
- Hepatic (portal-systemic) encephalopathy
- Renal failure
- Infection
- Hepatocellular carcinoma

Portal hypertension (p. 524), *ascites* (p. 527) and *hepatocellular carcinoma* (p. 535) are considered elsewhere, as they may be due to or associated with conditions other than cirrhosis.

HEPATIC (PORTAL-SYSTEMIC) ENCEPHALOPATHY

Hepatic encephalopathy is a neuropsychiatric syndrome caused by liver disease. It occurs most often in patients with cirrhosis but is also seen in more acute form in fulminant hepatic failure.

Aetiology

Hepatic encephalopathy is generally regarded as due to a biochemical disturbance of brain function because it is reversible and rarely shows marked pathological changes in the brain. *Liver failure and shunting of portal blood* past the liver directly to the systemic circulation are the two general factors underlying hepatic encephalopathy and the balance between them varies in different patients. Some degree of liver failure, however, is a constant factor, as portal-systemic shunting of blood rarely causes encephalopathy if the liver is normal. Little is known of the *biochemical neurotoxins* causing encephalopathy, but they are thought to be nitrogenous substances produced mainly in the gut, at least in part by bacterial action, which are normally metabolised by the healthy liver so that they do not enter the systemic circulation. Ammonia has long been considered an important factor and much recent interest has centred on the false neurotransmitter α-aminobutyric acid; both are produced in the intestine. Additional putative substances include other false neurotransmitters such as octopamine, amino acids, mercaptans and fatty acids. Some factors precipitate hepatic encephalopathy by increasing the availability of these substances, in addition the brain in cirrhosis may be sensitised to other factors such as drugs able to precipitate hepatic encephalopathy. (See the information box below.)

FACTORS PRECIPITATING HEPATIC ENCEPHALOPATHY

- Uraemia
  Spontaneous
  Diuretic induced
- Drugs
  Sedatives,
  Antidepressants
  Hypnotics
- Gastrointestinal bleeding
- Excess dietary protein
- Constipation
- Paracentesis (volumes >3–5 l)
- Hypokalaemia
- Infection
- Trauma (including surgery)
- Portal-systemic shunts
  Surgical
  Spontaneous (large)

Disruption of the function of the blood-brain barrier is more a feature of fulminant hepatic failure where it leads to cerebral oedema.

Pathology

Chronic or recurrent hepatic encephalopathy causes marked hypertrophy and hyperplasia of cerebral astrocytes and to a lesser extent oligodendrocytes especially in the cerebral cortex. More severe changes are very rare, but neuronal degeneration and demyelination occur in rare instances of chronic hepatic encephalopathy.

Clinical features

The clinical features include changes of intellect, personality, emotions and consciousness with or without neurological signs, and when an episode develops acutely a precipitating factor may be found such as one of those listed in the information box (above). The earliest features are very mild, but as the condition becomes more severe, apathy, inability to concentrate, confusion, disorientation, drowsiness, slurring of speech and eventually coma develop. Convulsions sometimes occur. Examination usually shows a flapping tremor (asterixis), inability to perform simple mental arithmetic or draw objects such as stars, and, as the condition progresses, hyper-reflexia and bilateral extensor plantar responses. Hepatic encephalopathy should not be diagnosed when focal neurological signs are found, though these do occur rarely. Fetor hepaticus is usually present but is more a sign of liver failure and portal-systemic shunting than of hepatic encephalopathy.

Investigations

The diagnosis can usually be made clinically, but when doubt exists an electroencephalogram shows diffuse slowing of the normal alpha waves with eventual development of delta waves. The arterial ammonia is usually increased but this investigation is of little or no value as increased concentrations occur in the absence of hepatic encephalopathy.

Differential diagnosis

Hepatic encephalopathy needs to be differentiated mainly from other causes of confusion and coma unassociated with lateralising neurological signs. Head injury leading to *subdural haematoma* with headache and fluctuating consciousness is particularly important, and where this possibility exists computed tomography of the head should be carried out. *Drunkenness* can also be deceptive, but the plasma ethanol generally exceeds 30 mmol/l in the drunk and 50 mmol/l in the very drunk or comatose. Alcoholic patients with *delirium tremens* are usually alert rather than drowsy and are nervous, tremulous, confused and hallucinating, while those with *Wernicke's encephalopathy* are disoriented and show marked loss of recent memory capacity, confabulation, ophthalmoplegia and ataxia of the limbs. Young patients with liver disease and neuropsychiatric features may have *Wilson's disease*. *Primary psychiatric diseases* may need to be considered, and *hypoglycaemia* should be excluded when an encephalopathy has had an acute onset.

Management

Episodes of encephalopathy are common in cirrhosis and are usually readily reversed until the terminal stages occur. The principles are to treat or remove precipitating causes (see information box p. 522), to reduce or eliminate protein intake, and to suppress production of neurotoxins by bacteria in the bowel. *Dietary protein* is eliminated or reduced below 20 g/d and glucose (300 g/d) is given orally or parenterally in severe cases. As encephalopathy improves, dietary protein is increased by 10–20 g/d on alternate days to an intake of 40–60 g/d which is usually the limit in cirrhotic patients. *Lactulose* (15–30 ml 3 times daily) is a disaccharide which is taken orally, reaches the colon intact to be metabolised by colonic bacteria. The dose is increased gradually until the bowels are moving twice

daily. It produces an osmotic laxative effect, reduces the pH of the colonic content thereby limiting colonic ammonia absorption, and promotes the incorporation of nitrogen into bacteria. *Lactitol* has been introduced as a rather more palatable alternative to lactulose with a less explosive action on the bowels. *Neomycin* (1–4 g/4–6-hourly) is an antibiotic which acts by reducing the bowel flora. It can be used in addition to or as an alternative to lactulose if diarrhoea becomes troublesome. Neomycin is poorly absorbed from the bowel but sufficient gains access to the body to require care when uraemia is present; it is less desirable than lactulose for long-term use. Ototoxicity is the main deleterious effect.

RENAL FAILURE

Renal failure consequent on liver failure can occur in cirrhosis. The kidneys themselves are intrinsically normal and renal failure is thought to result from a diminished renal blood flow. The condition is called *functional renal failure* of cirrhosis or the *hepatorenal syndrome*. It occurs in advanced cirrhosis, almost always with ascites, and uraemia is characterised by the absence of proteinuria or abnormal urinary sediment, a urine sodium excretion below 10 mmol/day, and a urine/plasma osmolality ratio greater than 1.5. It is important to exclude hypovolaemia by measuring the central venous pressure and giving colloidal solutions such as plasma protein solution or salt-poor albumin to maintain the pressure at 0–5 cm of water and to ensure the best possible renal blood flow by giving low-dose dopamine (1–2 µg/kg/min) and thereafter using diuretic drugs. Uraemia and endogenous protein breakdown should be limited by restricting protein intake to 20 g/day and giving 300 g of carbohydrate/day. Recovery depends ultimately on improvement of liver function but in chronic liver disease this seldom occurs. Accordingly, the prognosis is very poor.

INFECTION

Cirrhosis predisposes to bacterial infection, and this susceptibility increases as the disease progresses. Several factors contribute including poor nutrition, alcohol abuse and cellular and humoral immune deficiencies caused by cirrhosis itself. *Infection should be suspected in any patient whose condition deteriorates for no obvious reason*, and while infections can occur anywhere, *bacteraemia, spontaneous bacterial peritonitis* (p. 529) *and infection with unusual or occasionally multiple organisms is common*.

Management

No treatment can reverse cirrhosis or even ensure that no further progression occurs, but medical therapy can promote improved general health and alleviate symptoms. The main objectives are to detect treatable causes, to prevent and correct malnutrition, to manage chronic cholestasis (p. 534) and to treat complications (see information box p. 522). Liver transplantation should be considered in all patients with advanced liver damage.

Aetiological factors

Treatable conditions such as alcohol abuse, drug ingestion, haemochromatosis and Wilson's disease should always be sought. Relief of biliary obstruction will prevent secondary biliary cirrhosis.

Nutrition

In the absence of encephalopathy or ascites, a high energy (3000 kcal/d), protein-rich (80–100 g/d) diet should be advised. Fat intake need not be restricted where cholestasis is not a feature. Alcohol must be forbidden. When a good diet is taken, vitamins and other supplements are not required.

Drug therapy

Patients with cirrhosis are liable to develop toxic reactions to drugs owing to their unpredictable ability to metabolise drugs, and drugs are used with special care (p. 514).

Liver transplantation

Liver transplantation is now an established treatment for liver failure in patients with chronic liver disease, and provided transplantation is performed before the terminal stage of the illness, two-thirds or more of patients are alive a year after the operation with a good prognosis thereafter. Accordingly, transplantation should always be considered once signs of liver failure responding poorly to medical treatment have developed and before the malnutrition of chronic liver failure is established. Transplantation is applicable to all forms of chronic liver disease, but primary biliary cirrhosis is a particularly important subgroup and a steadily rising plasma bilirubin is a useful indicator of the likely need for transplantation. Contraindications to transplantation include continuing alcoholism, the development of hepatocellular carcinoma, hepatobiliary and extrahepatic infection, and coincident disease of the heart, lungs and kidneys.

Prognosis

The overall prognosis in cirrhosis is poor and only 25% of patients survive 5 years from diagnosis. This is because many patients present with serious complications carrying a high mortality (see information box p. 522), and those who present in other ways or who survive more than 6 months from presentation do much better. The prognosis is also more favourable where the cause of cirrhosis can be corrected, as in alcohol abuse, haemochromatosis and Wilson's disease. Laboratory tests give only a rough guide to prognosis in individual patients. Deteriorating liver function as evidenced by jaundice, ascites or encephalopathy indicates a poor prognosis unless a treatable cause such as infection is found. Increasing plasma bilirubin, falling plasma albumin, marked hypoalbuminaemia (below 25 g/l), marked hyponatraemia (below 120 mmol/l) not due to diuretic therapy, and a prolonged prothrombin time are all bad prognostic signs. The course of cirrhosis is uncertain, as unforeseen complications may lead to death unexpectedly.

PORTAL HYPERTENSION

Portal hypertension is a condition characterised by prolonged elevation of the portal venous pressure (normally 2–5 mmHg). Patients developing clinical features or complications of portal hypertension usually have portal venous pressures above 12 mmHg.

Aetiology and pathogenesis

Portal venous pressure is determined by the portal blood flow and by the portal vascular resistance. Increased vascular resistance is almost always the main factor producing portal hypertension, irrespective of its cause, and consequently the causes of portal hypertension are classified in accordance with the main sites of obstruction to blood flow in the portal venous system. These causes are listed in the information box (p. 525).

Extrahepatic portal vein obstruction is frequently the cause of portal hypertension in childhood and adolescence, while *cirrhosis* causes 90% or more of portal hyertension in adults in most countries. *Schistosomiasis* is the most common cause of portal hypertension in the world but it is infrequent outside endemic areas. Increased portal blood flow contributes to portal hypertension but is never the dominant factor. Increased portal vascular resistance leads to a gradual reduction in the flow of portal blood to the liver and simultaneously to the development of collateral vessels allowing portal blood to bypass the liver and enter the systemic circulation directly. Collateral vessel formation is widespread but occurs particularly in the gastrointestinal tract, especially the oesophagus, stomach and rectum, in the anterior abominal wall, and in the renal, lumbar,

CAUSES OF PORTAL HYPERTENSION ACCORDING TO SITE OF PORTAL VENOUS OBSTRUCTION

Extrahepatic
Sepsis*
    Umbilical
    Portal pyaemia
Umbilical vein transfusion
Thrombotic diseases
Oral contraceptives
Pregnancy
Abdominal trauma
Biliary surgery
Secondary – cirrhosis
Malignant disease
    Pancreas
    Liver
Pancreatitis
Congenital
Unknown* (50–75%)

Intrahepatic presinusoidal
Schistosomiasis*
Myeloproliferative/lymphoproliferative disease
Congenital hepatic fibrosis
Drugs
Vinyl chloride
Sarcoidosis
Idiopathic

Intrahepatic parenchymal
Cirrhosis*
Budd–Chiari syndrome
Veno-occlusive disease
Cystic liver disease
Partial nodular transformation of the liver
Secondary malignant disease

* Common causes.

ovarian and testicular vasculature. Virtually all the portal blood normally flows through the liver, but as collateral vessel formation progresses a half or more, and occasionally almost all, can be shunted directly to the systemic circulation.

Clinical features

The clinical features of portal hypertension result principally from portal venous congestion and from collateral vessel formation. *Splenomegaly* is a cardinal finding, and a diagnosis of portal hypertension is unlikely when splenomegaly cannot be shown clinically, on an abdominal radiograph or by ultrasonography. The spleen is rarely enlarged more than 5 cm below the left costal margin in adults, but much more marked splenomegaly can occur in childhood and adolescence. *Hypersplenism* is common and thrombocytopenia is the most common feature. Platelet counts are usually

around $100 \times 10^9/l$, and counts below $50 \times 10^7/l$ are rare. Leucopoenia occurs occasionally, but anaemia can hardly ever be attributed to hypersplenism. *Collateral vessels* may be visible on the anterior abdominal wall and occasionally several radiate from the umbilicus to form a caput medusae. Rarely, a large umbilical collateral vessel has a blood flow sufficient to give a venous hum on auscultation (Cruveilhier–Baumgarten syndrome). The most important collateral vessels occur in the oesophagus and stomach, where they can cause severe bleeding (p. 526). Rectal varices also cause bleeding and are often mistaken for haemorrhoids, which are no more common in portal hypertension than in the general population. *Fetor hepaticus* results from portal-systemic shunting of blood which allows mercaptans to pass directly to the lungs.

Investigations

Radiological and endoscopic examination of the upper gastrointestinal tract can show varices which establishes the presence of portal hypertension but not its cause. Imaging particularly ultrasonography can show features of portal hypertension and sometimes the cause such as liver disease or portal vein thrombosis. Portal venography demonstrates the site and often the cause of portal venous obstruction and is performed prior to surgical therapy. Portal venous pressure measurements are rarely needed but can be used to confirm portal hypertension and to differentiate sinusoidal and presinusoidal forms. These investigative methods are considered elsewhere (p. 501).

Complications

These are listed in the information box below.

COMPLICATIONS OF PORTAL HYPERTENSION

- Variceal bleeding
    Oesophageal
    Other (rare)
- Congestive gastropathy
- Hypersplenism
- Ascites
- Renal failure
- Hepatic encephalopathy

Gastrointestinal bleeding from varices or from congestive gastropathy is the main complication. Hypersplenism is rarely sufficiently severe to be clinically significant and portal hypertension is only one factor contributing to ascites (p. 528) and to renal failure (p. 523).

VARICEAL BLEEDING

Variceal bleeding almost always occurs from oeso-phageal varices within 3–5 cm of the oesophagogastric junction. Large varices, high portal pressure and liver failure are general factors predisposing to bleeding, and drugs capable of causing mucosal erosion, such as sali-cylates and other non-steroidal anti-inflammatory drugs, can precipitate bleeding. Variceal bleeding is often severe, and recurrent bleeding usually occurs if preventive treatment is not given. Bleeding from varices other than those in the oesophagus is comparatively uncommon and usually occurs from gastric or rectal varices or varices on intestinal stomas.

General management

The first priority in acute bleeding from oesophageal varices is to restore the circulation with blood and plasma because shock reduces liver blood flow and causes significant deterioration of liver function. Oeso-phageal varices should be confirmed as the source of bleeding as soon as acute bleeding has been controlled because about a quarter of patients with varices are bleeding from some other lesion, especially acute gastric erosions. Several treatments are available to stop acute variceal bleeding and to prevent its recurring and these are listed in the information box below.

TREATMENTS TO STOP OESOPHAGEAL VARICEAL BLEEDING AND TO PREVENT RECURRENT BLEEDING

Local measures
Sclerotherapy
Balloon tamponade
Oesophageal transection

Reduction of portal pressure
Vasopressin
Terlipressin

Prevention of recurrent bleeding
Sclerotherapy
Portal-systemic shunt surgery
   Unselective
   Selective
Propranolol

Reduction of portal venous pressure

Vasopressin. This constricts the splanchnic arterioles and reduces portal pressure and portal blood flow. It is given intravenously in a dose of 20 units in 100 ml of 5% glucose over 15 minutes, repeated if necessary 3–4 times at hourly intervals, or by intravenous infusion 0.4 unit/minute until bleeding stops, or for 24 hours and then 0.2 unit/minute for a further 24 hours. Abdominal colic, evacuation of the bowels and facial pallor from general arteriolar constriction indicate that vasopressin is active, and absence of these suggests an inert prepara-tion. Vasoconstriction also occurs generally and can cause angina, arrhythmia and even myocardial infarc-tion. Nitroglycerin can be given sublingually or intra-venously to combat these effects, but vasopressin should not be used in patients with ischaemic heart disease.

Terlipressin. This is an alternative to vasopressin with certain advantages. Terlipressin itself is not active, but vasopressin is released from it over several hours in amounts sufficient to reduce the portal pressure without producing systemic, including cardiac, effects. It is given in a dose of 2 mg intravenously every 6 hours until bleeding stops and then 1 mg every 6 hours for a further 24 hours. Investigations of the efficacy of vasopressin in variceal bleeding have given variable results, and vaso-pressin and terlipressin should be regarded only as adjuncts to other therapies.

Local measures

The measures used to control acute variceal bleeding include sclerotherapy, balloon tamponade and oeso-phageal transection. Emergency portal-systemic shunt surgery has a mortality of 50% or more and is virtually never used.

Sclerotherapy. This is the most important initial treatment and is undertaken if possible at the time of diagnostic endoscopy. It stops variceal bleeding in 80% of patients and can be repeated if bleeding recurs. Active bleeding at endoscopy may make sclerotherapy hazardous, and in such circumstances bleeding should be controlled by balloon tamponade prior to sclero-therapy.

Balloon tamponade. This is effected with a Sengstaken tube possessing two balloons which exert pressure respectively in the fundus of the stomach and in the lower oesophagus. Current modifications such as the Minnesota tube incorporate sufficient lumens to allow material to be aspirated from the stomach and from the oesophagus above the oesophageal balloon. The tube can be passed through the nose or the mouth under sedation, but the mouth is preferred because bleeding from the nose can be severe when the tube is removed. The presence of the tube in the stomach should be checked by hearing air injected into the gastric lumen enter the stomach during upper abdominal auscultation and radiologically, and gentle traction is used to maintain pressure on the varices. The gastric balloon only should be inflated initially as this alone will usually control bleeding, and if the oesophageal balloon needs to be used it should be deflated for about 10 minutes every 3 hours to avoid oesophageal mucosal damage. Balloon tamponade will almost always stop oesophageal variceal bleeding, and continued bleeding is usually due to an improperly placed tube or another source of bleeding. However, bleeding is stopped only for as long as tamponade is continued, and essentially the treatment allows time to apply other more definitive forms of therapy.

Oesophageal transection. Transection of the varices can be performed relatively easily with a stapling gun though it carries some risk of subsequent oesophageal stenosis. The operation is used when bleeding cannot be controlled by sclerotherapy and balloon tamponade.

Prevention

Recurrent variceal bleeding is the rule rather than the exception in patients who have had bleeding from oesophageal varices, and treatment to prevent this is needed.

Sclerotherapy. This is the most widely used method for preventing recurrent oesophageal variceal bleeding. Varices are injected with a sclerosing agent as soon as practicable after bleeding, and injections are repeated every 1–2 weeks thereafter until the varices are obliterated. Regular follow-up is necessary to allow treatment of any recurrence of varices. The treatment is not free of risk as injections can cause transient chest or abdominal pain, fever, transient dysphagia and occasionally oesophageal perforation. Oesophageal strictures may develop. However, mortality is low, even those with poor liver function can be treated, and recurrent bleeding is largely prevented. Prolongation of life has been claimed but this remains to be proven.

Portal-systemic shunt surgery. This was previously the treatment of choice because such shunts effectively prevent bleeding provided the shunt remains patent. However, follow-up of patients showed that they often suffered troublesome hepatic encephalopathy. It was thought that the earlier operations such as the portacaval shunt were *unselective* and diverted all the portal blood away from the liver and accordingly, *selective shunts*, particularly the distal splenorenal (Warren) shunt which decompresses the varices while preserving much of the portal blood flow to the liver, have been developed. The distal splenorenal shunt prevents re-bleeding, induces much less encephalopathy,

and is currently the favoured operation. However recent data suggest that this procedure has the same tendency to hepatic encephalopathy as unselective shunts. In practice, portal-systemic shunts are reserved for patients in whom sclerotherapy has not been successful and are offered only to those with good liver function.

Propanolol (usually 80–160 mg/d). This reduces the portal venous pressure in portal hypertension and has been used to prevent recurrent variceal bleeding. However, tests of its efficacy have given conflicting results and it has not yet been accepted generally as an effective treatment.

Prophylaxis of initial variceal bleeding
Portal-systemic shunts, sclerotherapy and propranolol have all been used to try to prevent initial bleeding from varices and none has been consistently successful. Consequently, treatment to prevent initial variceal bleeding is not generally given.

CONGESTIVE GASTROPATHY

Long-standing portal hypertension causes chronic gastric congestion recognisable at endoscopy as multiple areas of punctate erythema. These areas may become eroded causing bleeding from multiple sites. Acute bleeding can occur, but repeated minor bleeding causing recurrent iron-deficiency anaemia is more common. Anaemia may be prevented by oral iron supplements but repeated blood transfusions often become necessary. Reduction of the portal pressure using propranolol is the best available means of reducing blood loss, and sufficient propranolol (usually 80–160 mg/d) to reduce the resting heart rate by 20% should be given. Congestive gastropathy is often restricted to the gastric antrum, but few patients are fit enough to undergo antrectomy.

ASCITES

Ascites refers to the accumulation of free fluid in the peritoneal cavity. Cirrhosis is a common cause of ascites, but there are many other causes to be considered even in a patient with chronic liver disease.

Clinical features

Ascites causes abdominal distension with fullness in the flanks, shifting dullness on percussion, and a fluid thrill when a lot of ascites is present. These signs do not appear until the ascites volume exceeds a litre even in thin patients, and much larger volumes can be hard to detect in the obese. Associated features consequent on ascites include distortion or evertion of the umbilicus, herniae, abdominal striae, divarication of the recti and occasionally meralgia paraesthetica and scrotal oedema. Pleural effusions can be found in about 10% of patients, usually on the right side. Most are small and found on chest radiographs, but occasionally massive hydrothorax occurs. Pleural effusions, particularly on the left side, should not be assumed to be due to the ascites.

Investigation
Ultrasonography is the best means of confirming ascites, demonstrating ascites in the obese, or detecting small amounts. Abdominal radiographs can show ascites, but they are insensitive and non-specific. Paracentesis reveals ascites but is most useful in obtaining ascitic fluid for analysis, if necessary under ultrasonic guidance. The appearance of the ascites can point to the underlying cause (Table 11.12). The ascites protein

Table 11.12   Appearances and causes of ascites

Cause	Appearance
Cirrhosis	Clear Straw-coloured Light green
Malignant disease	Bloody
Infection	Cloudy
Biliary communication	Heavy bile staining
Lymphatic obstruction	Milky white (chylous)

Note: Milky white chylomicrons pass into supernatant on centrifugation.

concentration is used to separate ascites due to transudation ($<25\,g/l$) from ascites due to exudation ($>25\,g/l$), but it is now recognised that ascites protein concentrations are very variable in most diseases. However, protein concentrations below $25\,g/l$ are compatible with ascites due to cirrhosis. Ascites amylase activity above $1000\,u/l$ identifies pancreatic ascites, and low ascites glucose concentrations suggest malignant disease or tuberculosis. Cytological examination can reveal malignant cells, and polymorphonuclear leucocyte counts above $250/mm^3$ strongly suggest infection. Laparoscopy can also be valuable in detecting peritoneal disease.

Diagnosis
Ascites is caused by malignant disease, cirrhosis or cardiac failure in the great majority of patients, but the presence of cirrhosis does not necessarily mean that this is the cause of the ascites. This is particularly so when liver function is good or when there is no evidence of

portal hypertension, and in such patients a complication of cirrhosis, such as hepatocellular carcinoma or portal vein thrombosis, should be sought or an independent cause of ascites considered. Ascites associated with hypoalbuminaemia may be due to the nephrotic syndrome (p. 562) or to protein-losing enteropathy (p. 456) rather than to cirrhosis. Ascites with a protein concentration above $25\,g/l$ raises the possibility of infection, especially tuberculosis, hepatic venous obstruction, pancreatic ascites and rarely hypothyroidism.

ASCITES DUE TO CIRRHOSIS

Pathogenesis
Liver failure and portal hypertension in cirrhosis cause general sodium and water retention in the body with localisation of fluid in the peritoneum owing to the high venous pressure in the mesenteric circulation. The means whereby this occurs are unknown, and two general theories have been put forward. One explanation postulates a loss of fluid into the peritoneum as ascites develops with renal retention of sodium and water to compensate for this ('underfilling theory'), while the other postulates a primary renal retention of sodium and water with eventual overspill of fluid into the peritoneum ('overflow theory'). The mechanisms for sodium retention remain poorly understood but include activation of the renin-angiotensin system with secondary aldosteronism, increased sympathetic nervous activity, alteration of atrial natriuretic hormone secretion and altered activity of the kallikrein-kinin system.

Management
Successful treatment of ascites relieves discomfort but does not prolong life, and if over-vigorous can produce serious disorders of fluid and electrolyte balance, and as a consequence hepatic encephalopathy (information box p. 522). Treatment aims to reduce body sodium and water by restricting intake, promoting urine output, and if necessary removing ascites directly. The rate of loss of sodium and water is most easily measured by regular weighing, and as no more than 900 ml can be mobilised from the peritoneum daily, the body weight should not fall by more than 1 kg daily if fluid depletion in the rest of the body is to be avoided.

Sodium and water
Restriction of dietary sodium intake is essential to achieving negative sodium balance in patients with ascites. Restriction to 40 mmol/day initially may be adequate, but restriction to 20 mmol/day is necessary in

more severe ascites and requires close dietetic supervision. Drugs containing relatively large amounts of sodium and drugs promoting sodium retention such as non-steroidal analgesic agents must be avoided. Restriction of water intake to 0.5–1.0 l/day is necessary only if the plasma sodium falls below 130 mmol/l. A few patients will have a satisfactory diuresis on this treatment alone.

Diuretic drugs
Most patients require diuretic drugs in addition to sodium restriction. Spironolactone (100–400 mg/d) is the drug of choice for long-term therapy because it is a powerful aldosterone antagonist, but unfortunately it can cause painful gynaecomastia. Some patients will also require powerful loop diuretics, though these can cause fluid, electrolyte and renal function disorders. Diuresis is improved if patients are at bed rest while the diuretics are acting, perhaps because renal blood flow increases in the horizontal position.

Paracentesis
Paracentesis of 3–5 l over 1–2 hours has always been used for immediate relief of cardiorespiratory distress due to gross ascites, but it has previously been regarded as a hazardous treatment for ascites itself. Paracentesis of 3–5 l of ascites with the replacement of 40 g of salt-poor albumin intravenously daily has been found to be a safe and effective treatment for ascites and can be used when sodium restriction and diuretic drug therapy fails.

LeVeen shunt
The LeVeen shunt is a long tube with a non-return valve running subcutaneously from the peritoneum to the internal jugular vein in the neck which allows ascitic fluid to pass directly to the systemic circulation. There are several complications associated with its use, including infection, superior vena caval thrombosis, pulmonary oedema, bleeding from oesophageal varices and disseminated intravascular coagulopathy, but it can be very effective in patients with ascites resistant to other treatment who are not terminally ill.

Prognosis
Ascites is a serious development in cirrhosis as only 10–20% of patients survive 5 years from its appearance. The outlook is not universally bad, however, and is best in those with well-maintained liver function and where the response to therapy is good. The prognosis is also better where a treatable cause for the underlying cirrhosis is present (p. 516) or where a precipitating cause for ascites such as excess salt intake is found.

SPONTANEOUS BACTERIAL PERITONITIS (SBP)

Patients with cirrhosis are very susceptible to infection of ascitic fluid (SBP) as part of their general susceptibility to infection. SBP usually starts suddenly with abdominal pain, rebound pain, absent bowel sounds and fever in a patient with obvious features of cirrhosis and ascites. Hepatic encephalopathy also occurs, and in about a third of patients encephalopathy and fever are the main features because abdominal signs are mild or absent. Paracentesis may show cloudy fluid, and an ascites leucocyte count above $250/mm^3$ confirms infection. The source of infection cannot usually be determined but most organisms obtained on ascites and blood culture are of enteric origin and E. coli is the organism isolated most frequently. SBP needs to be differentiated from other intra-abdominal emergencies, and the finding of multiple organisms on culture should arouse suspicion of a perforated viscus. Treatment is started immediately with a broad spectrum of antibiotics such as cefotaxime (1 g i.v. 8-hourly) and metronidazole (1 g rectally 8-hourly). The prognosis is poor, and most patients die in spite of vigorous treatment.

ALCOHOLIC (ETHANOLIC) LIVER DISEASE

Alcohol is the most common cause of liver disease although it is entirely preventable.

Metabolism
Alcohol is metabolised almost exclusively in the liver. It is first converted to acetaldehyde, mainly by the mitochondrial enzyme alcohol dehydrogenase but also by the mixed-function oxidase enzymes of the smooth endoplasmic reticulum (p. 514). Alcohol is a powerful inducer of the mixed-function oxidases, increasing their activity and thereby increasing ability to metabolise alcohol and many drugs metabolised by these enzymes (p. 514). Acetaldehyde is converted in turn to acetate by acetaldehyde dehydrogenase, and acetate is metabolised by the Krebs cycle enzymes.

Pathogenesis
The hepatic lesions of alcoholic liver disease (below) are attributable directly to alcohol. The risk of developing alcoholic liver disease is related directly to the amount of alcohol of any kind ingested and becomes apparent at daily intakes above 40 g in men and 20 g in women. More than five years of drinking and usually more than ten years is required to produce alcoholic cirrhosis, and a steady daily intake is more hazardous than intermittent drinking.

The mechanisms whereby alcohol produces individual liver lesions are poorly understood. Fatty change is attributed to an increased production and decreased use of fatty acids in the liver cells following the conversion of alcohol to acetaldehyde by alcohol dehydrogenase. The development of alcoholic hepatitis, fibrosis and cirrhosis is much more obscure. Biochemical mechanisms involving the production of toxic metabolites, called adducts, during the conversion of acetaldehyde to acetate and immune reaction to liver cells altered by alcohol may be involved in these forms of liver damage.

Pathology

Alcohol causes several different lesions in the liver which can occur together in any combination.

Fatty change. This is the most common lesion and may affect from a few to almost all hepatocytes. It is regarded as readily reversible when alcohol is withdrawn, but it nevertheless reflects a severe metabolic derangement.

Alcoholic hepatitis. This is much more common than the severe clinical illness also called alcoholic hepatitis and is characterised by foci of necrotic hepatocytes infiltrated and surrounded by polymorphonuclear leucocytes. Related hepatocytes may be pale and swollen, and some contain dense eosinophilic masses called Mallory's hyaline. Alcoholic hepatitis is often a precursor of cirrhosis.

Mallory's hyaline. This is not pathognomonic of alcohol abuse as it occurs in other liver diseases such as primary biliary cirrhosis, Wilson's disease and liver damage due to some drugs such as amiodarone.

Central hyaline sclerosis. This is characterised by fibrosis around central veins and is a sign of severe alcohol abuse. It is often a prelude to cirrhosis and portal hypertension.

Cirrhosis. This is usually initially micronodular (p. 518), often with active inflammation in fibrous septae and marked pericellular fibrosis, and later becomes macronodular.

Mild siderosis. This is common in alcoholic liver disease.

Clinical features

Alcoholic liver disease manifests as a clinical spectrum ranging from non-specific symptoms with few or no physical abnormalities to advanced cirrhosis. The ready availability of laboratory investigations can also reveal alcoholic liver damage in patients with other diseases or in asymptomatic people undergoing medical examination. This spectrum is often divided into four syndromes, but in reality these overlap considerably and the various pathological changes can coexist in the same liver. The clinical syndromes are listed in the information box below.

CLINICAL SYNDROMES OF ALCOHOLIC LIVER DISEASE

Fatty liver
Non specific symptoms
Hepatomegaly

Hepatitis
Severe illness
Malnutrition
Jaundice
Hepatomegaly
Ascites
Encephalopathy

Cholestasis
Jaundice
Abdominal pain
Hepatomegaly (often tender)

Cirrhosis (p. 518)

Investigations

Investigations aim to establish alcohol abuse, exclude alternative causes of liver disease, and assess the severity of liver damage. The clinical history from the patient, relatives and friends is most important in establishing alcohol abuse, its duration and its severity. Biological markers of alcohol abuse suggest and support the history of alcohol abuse, and the most universally used of these are peripheral blood macrocytosis in the absence of anaemia and increased plasma γ-glutamyl transferase (p. 494). Absence of these markers does not exclude alcohol abuse. Unexplained rib fractures on a chest X-ray are also associated with alcohol abuse. Investigation of the extent of liver damage (p. 492) and possible alternative causes are given elsewhere (p. 495).

Management

Cessation of alcohol intake is the most important treatment and without this all other therapies are of limited value. Lifelong abstinence is the best advice and is essential for those with more severe liver damage. Good nutrition is also important and feeding via a fine-bore nasogastric tube may be needed in severely ill patients. Treatment for complications such as encephalopathy

(p. 523), ascites (p. 528) and variceal bleeding (p. 526) may be required.

Prognosis

The most important prognostic factor is the patient's ability to *stop drinking alcohol*, for general health and longevity are improved when this occurs irrespective of the form of alcoholic liver disease. Alcoholic fatty liver has a generally good prognosis and usually disappears after about 3 months of abstinence. Alcoholic hepatitis has a significantly worse prognosis because about a third of patients die in the acute episode if liver function is poor as evidenced by a prothrombin time sufficiently prolonged to preclude liver biopsy. Patients may progress to cirrhosis after recovery particularly if drinking continues. Alcoholic cirrhosis often presents with a serious complication such as variceal bleeding (p. 525) or ascites (p. 528), and only about a half of patients survive 5 years from presentation. Most who survive the initial illness and who become abstinent survive beyond 5 years.

HAEMOCHROMATOSIS

Haemochromatosis is a condition in which the total body iron is increased with the excess iron deposited in and damaging several organs including the liver. It may be primary or secondary to other diseases.

HEREDITARY (PRIMARY) HAEMOCHROMATOSIS

This is a disease in which the total body iron reaches 20–60 g (normal 4 g). Iron is deposited widely in the body. The important organs involved are the liver, pancreatic islets, endocrine glands and heart. In the liver, iron deposition occurs first in the periportal hepatocytes extending later to all hepatocytes. The gradual development of fibrous septa leads to the formation of irregular nodules, and finally regeneration results in macronodular cirrhosis. An excess of liver iron can occur in alcoholic cirrhosis but this is generally mild by comparison with haemochromatosis.

Aetiology and pathology

Hereditary haemochromatosis is caused by an increased absorption of dietary iron. This inability to limit iron absorption is inherited as an autosomal recessive associated with the HLA-B3, B7 and B14 histocompatibility antigens. Homozygotes alone develop the disease, but other factors must also be important as at least 90% of patients are male. Iron loss in menstruation and pregnancy may protect females.

Clinical features

The disease usually presents in men aged 40 years or over with manifestations of hepatic cirrhosis (p. 520), especially hepatomegaly, diabetes mellitus or heart failure. Leaden-grey skin pigmentation due to excess melanin occurs especially in exposed parts, axillae, groins and genitalia, hence the term 'bronzed diabetes'. Impotence, loss of libido, testicular atrophy and arthritis with chondrocalcinosis due to calcium pyrophosphate deposition are also common. Increasingly, early clinical features are being recognised particularly tiredness, fatigue and arthropathy.

Investigation

The serum ferritin is greatly increased and the plasma iron is increased with a highly saturated plasma iron binding capacity (p. 497). Computed tomography may show features suggesting excess hepatic iron. The diagnosis is confirmed by liver biopsy which shows heavy iron deposition and hepatic fibrosis which may have progressed to cirrhosis. The iron content of the liver can be measured directly.

Management

Treatment is by weekly venesection of 500 ml (250 mg iron) until the serum iron is normal; this may take 2 years or more. Thereafter venesection is continued as required to keep the serum ferritin normal. Other therapy includes that for cirrhosis and diabetes mellitus. Other first-degree family members should be investigated by measurement of the serum ferritin and plasma iron binding capacity saturation and any with asymptomatic disease treated.

Prognosis

Hereditary haemochromatosis has a good prognosis compared with other forms of cirrhosis, as three-quarters of patients are alive 5 years after the diagnosis. This is probably because liver function is usually well preserved at diagnosis and improves with therapy. Hepatocellular carcinoma is the main cause of death occurring in about a third with cirrhosis irrespective of therapy.

SECONDARY HAEMOCHROMATOSIS

Many conditions, including chronic haemolytic disorders, sideroblastic anaemia, other conditions requiring multiple blood transfusion (generally over 150 l), porphyria cutanea tarda, dietary iron overload (p. 56) and occasionally alcoholic cirrhosis, are associated with widespread secondary siderosis. The features are similar to haemochromatosis, but the history and clinical findings point to the true diagnosis. Some patients are heterozygotes for the primary haemochromatosis gene and this may contribute to the development of iron overload.

WILSON'S DISEASE (HEPATO-LENTICULAR DEGENERATION)

This is a rare but important condition in which the total body copper is increased with excess copper deposited in and damaging several organs.

Aetiology and pathology

Wilson's disease is inherited as an autosomal recessive leading to abnormal copper metabolism. Normally, dietary copper is absorbed from the stomach and proximal small intestine and is rapidly taken into the liver where it is stored and incorporated into caeruloplasmin which is secreted into the blood. The accumulation of excessive copper in the body is ultimately prevented by its excretion, the most important route being via the bile. The precise nature of the metabolic defect in Wilson's disease is unknown, but it results in a failure of biliary copper excretion causing accumulation in the body. There is almost always also a failure of synthesis of caeruloplasmin though occasional patients with Wilson's disease have a normal plasma caeruloplasmin concentration. The amount of copper in the body at birth is normal, but thereafter it increases steadily and the organs most affected are the liver, the basal ganglia of the brain, the eyes, the kidneys and the skeleton.

Clinical features

Symptoms usually arise between the ages of 5 and 30 years. Hepatic disease occurs predominantly in childhood and early adolescence, while neurological damage causes basal ganglion syndromes (p. 872) in later adolescence. These manifestations can occur alone or simultaneously. Other manifestations include haemolysis, renal tubular damage and osteoporosis, but these are virtually never presenting features.

Kayser–Fleischer rings

These are the most important single clinical clue to the diagnosis and they can be seen in most patients presenting in or after adolescence albeit sometimes only by slit-lamp examination. Appearances indistinguishable from Kayser–Fleischer rings are rarely found in other forms of chronic active hepatitis and cirrhosis. Kayser–Fleischer rings are characterised by greenish-brown discolouration of the corneal margin appearing first at

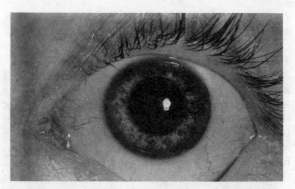

Fig. 11.10   Kayser-Fleischer rings at the junction of the cornea and sclera in a patient with Wilson's disease.

the upper periphery (Fig. 11.10). They eventually disappear with treatment.

Liver disease

This can manifest in many ways which are not specific. Episodes of acute hepatitis which are sometimes recurrent can occur, especially in children, and may progress to fulminant hepatic failure. Chronic persistent hepatitis and chronic active hepatitis can also develop, and eventually cirrhosis with liver failure and portal hypertension. *Recurrent acute hepatitis of unknown cause, especially accompanied by haemolysis, or chronic liver disease of unknown cause in a patient under 40 years old suggests Wilson's disease.*

Investigation

A low serum caeruloplasmin (p. 498) is the best single laboratory clue to the diagnosis. However, advanced liver failure from any cause can reduce the serum caeruloplasmin, and occasionally the serum caeruloplasmin is normal in Wilson's disease. Other features of a disordered copper metabolism should therefore be sought; these include a low serum copper concentration, a high urine copper excretion (p. 498), and a very high hepatic copper content (p. 498). Patients with Wilson's disease fail to incorporate radioactive copper into caeruloplasmin, but this test is almost never needed.

Management

The copper-binding agent penicillamine is the drug of choice in Wilson's disease. The dose given must be sufficient to produce cupriuresis and most patients require 1.5 g/day (range 1–4 g). The dose can be reduced once the disease is in remission, but treatment must continue for life and care must be taken to ensure that reaccumulation of copper does not occur. Young women should continue to take the drug during pregnancy. Serious toxic effects of penicillamine are rare in Wilson's disease. If they do occur, trientine dihydrochloride (1.2–2.4 g/d) is the next drug of choice. Liver transplantation is needed for deteriorating fulminant hepatic failure and for advanced cirrhosis with liver failure.

Prognosis
The prognosis of Wilson's disease is excellent provided treatment is started before there is irreversible damage; the long-term complication of hepatocellular carcinoma does not occur as it does in haemochromatosis. Siblings of patients with Wilson's disease must be investigated and treatment should be given to any who have the disease even if it is asymptomatic.

ALPHA₁-ANTITRYPSIN DEFICIENCY

Alpha₁-antitrypsin (A1AT) is an α_1-globulin protease inhibitor produced by the liver (p. 498). Several forms of A1AT are produced, and one of these (PiZ) cannot be secreted into the blood by the liver cells owing to its chemical structure. Homozygous individuals (PiZZ) have low plasma A1AT concentrations, though globules containing A1AT are found in the liver, and this form of A1AT deficiency is associated with hepatic and pulmonary (p. 394) disease. Liver disease includes cholestatic jaundice in the neonatal period (neonatal hepatitis) which can resolve spontaneously, chronic hepatitis and cirrhosis in adults, and in the long term the development of hepatocellular carcinoma. There are no clinical features distinguishing liver disease due to A1AT deficiency from other causes of liver disease, and the diagnosis is made from the low plasma A1AT concentration and the PiZZ phenotype. A1AT-containing globules can be demonstrated in the liver but this is not necessary for making the diagnosis. Occasionally patients with liver disease and minor reductions of plasma A1AT concentrations have A1AT phenotypes other than PiZZ, such as PiMZ or PiSZ, but the relation of these to the course of the liver disease is uncertain. No treatment other than that for any chronic liver disease is available and the patients are advised strongly to abandon cigarette smoking.

BILIARY CIRRHOSIS

Biliary cirrhosis results from prolonged obstruction anywhere between the small interlobular bile ducts and the papilla of Vater.

PRIMARY BILIARY CIRRHOSIS

This disease affects predominantly women, usually in middle age. The ready availability of diagnostic tests has shown that it is a relatively common form of cirrhosis.

Aetiology and pathology
The cause of primary biliary cirrhosis is unknown but immune reactions causing liver damage are suspected. Autoantibodies and immune complexes are found in the blood, cellular immunity is impaired, and abnormal cellular immune reactions have been described. The primary pathological lesion is a chronic granulomatous inflammation damaging and destroying the interlobular bile ducts, and progressive inflammatory damage with fibrosis spreading from the portal tracts to the liver parenchyma which eventually leads to cirrhosis and its complications (p. 522).

Clinical features
Pruritus is the commonest initial complaint and may precede jaundice by months or even years. The cause is unclear and although bile salts are implicated their role is unproved. Jaundice is occasionally a presenting feature but pruritus is usually also present. Although there may be abdominal discomfort, the abdominal pain, fever and rigors which are often a feature of large bile duct obstruction do not occur. Diarrhoea from malabsorption of fat, and pain and tingling in the hands and feet due to lipid infiltration of peripheral nerves occasionally occur. Bone pain or fractures because of osteomalacia from malabsorption or osteoporosis (hepatic osteodystrophy) can be prominent and distressing features in advanced disease.

Initially patients are well nourished but considerable weight loss can occur as the disease progresses. Scratch marks may be found. Jaundice is only prominent late in the disease and can become intense. Xanthomatous deposits occur in a minority especially around the eyes, in the hand creases and over the elbows, knees and buttocks. Hepatomegaly is virtually constant, and splenomegaly becomes increasingly common as portal hypertension develops. The complications of liver failure and portal hypertension arise as the disease progresses (p. 522).

Associated diseases
Autoimmune and connective tissue diseases occur with increased frequency in primary biliary cirrhosis, particularly the sicca syndrome (p. 768) and thyroid diseases.

Asymptomatic disease

Asymptomatic primary biliary cirrhosis has become recognised increasingly owing to the ready availability of liver function tests and autoantibody tests. This condition is found particularly in patients with the associated diseases mentioned above.

Investigations

Liver function tests show the pattern of *cholestasis* (p. 494) The *antimitochondrial antibody* is present in over 95% of patients, and when it is absent histological evidence for the diagnosis is needed and cholangiography by endoscopic retrograde cholangiopancreatography (ERCP) (p. 500) is required to exclude other biliary disease. The antinuclear and smooth muscle antibodies may be present, and autoantibodies found in associated diseases may also be found. Ultrasound examination shows no sign of biliary obstruction (p. 498), and liver biopsy is required only in doubtful cases.

Management

No specific therapy is available. Corticosteroids, azathioprine and penicillamine have all been tried, but none is effective and all may have serious adverse effects.

Transplantation should always be considered once liver failure has developed. Treatment may be needed for the consequences of cholestasis particularly for pruritus, malabsorption and cholangitis.

Pruritus

This is the main symptom demanding relief. It is best achieved with the anion-binding resin cholestyramine, which reduces the bile acids in the body by binding them in the intestine and increasing their excretion in the stool. A dose of 4–16 g/day orally is used. The powder is mixed in orange juice and the main dose (8 g) is taken with breakfast when maximal duodenal bile acid concentrations occur. Cholestyramine may bind other drugs in the gut (e.g. anticoagulants) which should therefore be taken one hour before the binding agent.

Cholestyramine is sometimes ineffective, especially in complete biliary obstruction. Terfenadine, an antihistamine (60 mg b.d.), or ultraviolet therapy may help in such patients. Methyltestosterone (25 mg/d sublingually) or, for women, norethandrolone (10 mg t.i.d.) may also be effective, though both reversibly increase cholestasis at the canalicular membrane and jaundice worsens.

Malabsorption

Prolonged cholestasis is associated with steatorrhoea and malabsorption of fat-soluble vitamins and calcium. Steatorrhoea can be reduced by limiting fat intake to 40 g/d. Monthly injections of vitamin K_1 (10 mg), vitamin D (calciferol 1 mg/d; alfacalcidol 1 µg/d orally) and calcium supplements should also be given, the last as effervescent calcium gluconate (2–4 g/d). This preparation, however, contains much sodium and, where there is fluid retention, calcium gluconate alone should be used.

Cholangitis

This requires treatment with antibiotics, which can be given continuously if attacks occur frequently.

SECONDARY BILIARY CIRRHOSIS

This develops after prolonged large duct biliary obstruction due to gallstones, bile duct strictures and, occasionally, sclerosing cholangitis (p. 544), Carcinomas rarely cause secondary biliary cirrhosis as survival is limited. There is chronic cholestasis with episodes of ascending cholangitis or even liver abscess (p. 537). Finger clubbing is common and xanthomas and bone pain may develop. Cirrhosis, ascites and portal hypertension are late features.

HEPATIC VENOUS OUTFLOW OBSTRUCTION

Obstruction to hepatic venous blood flow can occur in the small central hepatic veins, in the large hepatic veins, in the inferior vena cava or in the heart. The clinical features depend on the cause and on the speed with which obstruction develops, but congestive hepatomegaly and ascites are features in all patients.

BUDD–CHIARI SYNDROME

Aetiology and pathology

This is an uncommon condition in which obstruction occurs in the larger hepatic veins and sometimes the inferior vena cava. The cause cannot be found in about a half of patients, but in the others thrombosis due to haematological diseases, especially polycythemia vera, pregnancy and oral contraceptives, obstruction due to tumours particularly carcinomas of the liver, kidneys or adrenals, congenital venous webs and occasionally inferior vena caval stenosis are the main causes. Hepatic congestion mainly in the centrilobular areas, is the main consequence initially; centrilobular fibrosis develops later and eventually cirrhosis in those who survive long enough.

Clinical features

Sudden venous occlusion causes the rapid development of upper abdominal pain which is often severe, marked ascites and occasionally fulminant hepatic failure. More gradual occlusion causes gross ascites and often upper abdominal discomfort. Hepatomegaly, often with tenderness over the liver, is almost always present. Peripheral oedema occurs only when there is inferior vena cava obstruction. Features of cirrhosis (p. 520) and portal hypertension (p. 525) develop in those who survive long enough.

Investigation

Liver function tests vary considerably depending on the presentation and can show the features of acute hepatitis (p. 494) when the onset is rapid. Ascitic fluid analysis typically shows a protein concentration above 25 g/l in the early stages but is often lower later in the disease. Ultrasound examination may reveal obliteration of the hepatic veins and reversed flow in the portal vein. Isotope imaging may show preservation of the caudate lobe, as it often has a separate venous drainage not involved in the disease. Hepatic venography shows occlusion of the hepatic veins and any inferior vena cava involvement, and liver biopsy demonstrates centrilobular congestion with fibrosis depending upon the duration of the illness.

Management

Predisposing causes should be removed or treated as far as possible, and where recent thrombosis is suspected treatment with streptokinase followed by heparin and oral anticoagulation are considered. Ascites is treated medically initially but often has limited success, in which case a LeVeen shunt (p. 529) or a portal-systemic shunt can be used. Direct surgical treatment of the venous obstruction is rarely possible but occasionally a web can be resected or an inferior caval stenosis dilated. Progressive liver failure is an indication for liver transplantation.

Prognosis

The prognosis is generally poor, particularly, when the onset is sudden; a third to two-thirds of patients die within a year and few live more than 5 years. Some patients survive to develop cirrhosis.

VENO-OCCLUSIVE DISEASE

Widespread occlusion of central hepatic veins is the characteristic of this condition. Pyrollizidine alkaloids in Senecio and Heliotropium plants used to make teas are the best known causes, but cytotoxic drugs and hepatic irradiation are increasingly recognised causes. The clinical features, investigation and management of veno-occlusive disease are similar to the Budd–Chiari syndrome (above).

CARDIAC DISEASE

Hepatic damage due primarily to congestion is always present in cardiac failure from any cause, but the clinical features are usually dominated by the cardiac disease. Occasionally the hepatic features are more prominent.

Acute hepatitis

Rapidly developing cardiac failure sometimes causes a syndrome suggesting an acute hepatitis. This occurs most often following myocardial infarction, decompensation of any chronic myocardial disease or cor pulmonale, or rapidly developing cardiac tamponade. The patient is generally very ill with an enlarged tender liver, with or without jaundice, and liver function tests showing an acute hepatitis. The correct diagnosis is made by recognising that the cardiac output is low, the jugular venous pressure is high, and other signs of cardiac disease are present.

Ascites

Cardiac failure sometimes causes hepatomegaly and ascites disproportionate to peripheral oedema mimicking ascites due to liver disease. A high ascites protein concentration may suggest hepatic venous outflow obstruction. Constrictive pericarditis (p. 328) is particularly likely to mislead, as a normal heart size points away from heart disease. A raised jugular venous pressure is the most important single clue to the diagnosis. Rarely, long-standing cardiac failure and hepatic congestion cause cardiac cirrhosis, and this is suggested by hard irregular hepatomegaly or a palpable spleen due to portal hypertension.

Management

The treatment of these patients is that of the underlying causative disease.

TUMOURS OF THE LIVER

HEPATOCELLULAR CARCINOMA (HEPATOMA)

Hepatocellular carcinoma is the principal primary malignant liver tumour. Its incidence shows great geographic variation, being common in Africa and Southeast Asia but rare in temperate climates.

Aetiology

Chronic hepatitis B virus infection has emerged as the most important cause world-wide and chronic carriers of the virus have a much increased risk of the disease (p. 496). *Aflatoxin* contamination of foods may also be important in tropical countries (p. 516). *Cirrhosis* and *male sex* are the main factors related to hepatocellular carcinoma in temperate climates. Cirrhosis is present in 80% of cases and may be of any type, but hepatocellular carcinoma appears most commonly in haemochromatosis and alcoholic cirrhosis, dominantly male diseases, and rarely in primary biliary cirrhosis, which mainly affects women. Other aetiological factors include exposure to toxins such as thorotrast and arsenic which usually produce angiosarcomas but which may also cause hepatocellular carcinomas. Oestrogens, androgens and anabolic steroids may cause adenomas or, rarely, hepatocellular carcinomas.

Pathology

Macroscopically, the tumour may comprise a single mass or multiple nodules or occasionally be diffusely invasive. Microscopically, the tumour is made up of trabeculae of well-differentiated cells resembling hepatocytes. Bile secretion by tumour cells may be seen and is diagnostic. Intravascular invasion and growth is often a feature and may occur into the portal vein or the inferior vena cava. Spread is mainly to regional lymph nodes, the lungs and bones. Deterioration in a patient with cirrhosis should always lead to suspicion of hepatocellular carcinoma.

Clinical features

These include weakness, anorexia, weight loss, fever, abdominal pain, a large irregular liver or an abdominal mass, and ascites. Hepatocellular carcinomas are vascular and a bruit may be heard over the liver or intra-abdominal bleeding may occur. Metabolic abnormalities include polycythaemia, hypercalcaemia, hypoglycaemia and porphyria cutanea tarda. Liver function tests give variable non-specific results. A greatly increased or rising serum α-fetoprotein is virtually diagnostic (p. 498). Imaging almost always reveals one or more filling defects and the diagnosis is confirmed by liver aspiration or biopsy.

Management

Surgical removal requires a tumour confined to one lobe in the absence of cirrhosis and is rarely feasible, but the possibility should always be considered. Chemotherapy has been disappointing but can provide palliative therapy. Liver transplantation has been abandoned owing to the frequent recurrence of tumour in the transplanted liver or the lungs.

Prognosis

The outlook is very poor. Surgery alone gives prolonged survival, but only about 10% of patients are suitable for this therapy. Few patients survive beyond a year.

FIBROLAMELLAR HEPATOCELLULAR CARCINOMA

This rare variant differs from other hepatocellular carcinomas in that it occurs in young adults, equally in males and females, and is not associated with cirrhosis or hepatitis B virus infection. It usually presents with pain due to bleeding into the tumour, which may later cause intrahepatic calcification, or intraperitoneally. The serum α-fetoprotein is usually normal, and biopsy shows large polygonal malignant hepatocytes in a dense fibrous tissue stroma. Two-thirds of tumours are resectable and transplantation is worthwhile where there is no spread beyond the liver. Two thirds of patients survive beyond 5 years.

OTHER PRIMARY TUMOURS

These are rare; they include haemangioendothelial sarcomas and cholangiocarcinoma (p. 545).

SECONDARY MALIGNANT TUMOURS

These are common and usually originate from carcinomas in the bronchus, breast, abdomen or pelvis. They may be single or multiple. Peritoneal dissemination frequently results in ascites.

Clinical features

The primary neoplasm is asymptomatic in about half the patients. Hepatomegaly may suggest cirrhosis, but splenomegaly is rare. There is usually rapid liver enlargement with fever, weight loss and jaundice. A raised alkaline phosphatase activity is the commonest biochemical abnormality but the liver function tests may be normal. Ascitic fluid has a high protein content and may be blood-stained, and cytology sometimes reveals malignant cells. Imaging (p. 498) usually reveals filling defects, and the diagnosis is confirmed by liver aspiration or biopsy.

Management

Every effort should be made to detect resectable secondary tumours, as improvements in the techniques of hepatic resection now probably improve survival and give the best palliation, particularly for relatively slow-growing tumours such as colonic carcinomas. Patients with hormone-producing tumours such as gastrinomas, insulinomas and glucagonomas, and lymphomas may benefit from chemotherapy. Unfortunately, palliative treatment to relieve pain is all that is available for most patients.

BENIGN TUMOURS

Hepatic adenomas are rare vascular tumours which may present as an abdominal mass or with abdominal pain or intraperitoneal bleeding. They are more common in women and may be caused by oral contraceptives, androgens and anabolic steroids. Haemangiomas are the commonest benign liver tumours but they rarely cause symptoms.

LIVER ABSCESS

Liver abscesses are either pyogenic or amoebic, and both have similar clinical features.

PYOGENIC ABSCESS

Pyogenic liver abscesses are uncommon but important because they are potentially curable, inevitably fatal if untreated, and readily overlooked.

Aetiology and pathology
Infection can reach the liver in several ways as is shown in the information box below. Abscesses are most common in older patients and result from ascending infection due to biliary obstruction (cholangitis),

---

SOURCES OF BACTERIAL INFECTION OF THE LIVER

- Biliary obstruction (cholangitis)
- Haematogenous
  Portal vein
    Mesenteric infections
  Hepatic artery
    Bacteraemia (any source)
- Direct extension
- Trauma
  Penetrating
  Non-penetrating
- Infection of primary liver lesion
  Tumours
  Cysts

---

whereas abscesses in young adults consequent on suppurative appendicitis, which were previously most common, are now rare. Immunocompromised patients are particularly likely to develop liver abscesses. Abscesses vary greatly in size, single lesions are more common in the right liver, and multiple abscesses are usually due to infection in biliary obstruction. Many bacteria can cause liver abscesses. *E. coli* and various streptococci are the most common organisms, anaerobes including streptococci and *Bacteroides* can often be found, and several organisms are present in a third of patients.

Clinical features
Patients are generally ill with fever, sometimes rigors, and weight loss. Abdominal pain is the commonest symptom and is usually in the right upper quadrant sometimes with radiation to the right shoulder. The pain may be pleuritic. Hepatomegaly is found in more than half the patients and tenderness can usually be elicited by gentle percussion over the organ. Mild jaundice may be present and is severe only when large abscesses cause biliary obstruction. Abnormalities are present at the base of the right lung in about a quarter of patients. Atypical presentations are common and explain the frequency with which the diagnosis is made only at autopsy. This includes particularly patients with gradually developing illnesses which may not include abdominal pain, with pyrexia of unknown cause, and with clinical features pointing to an underlying cause such as colonic diverticular disease or to metastatic abscesses.

Investigations
Liver imaging, usually by ultrasound is the most revealing investigation and shows 90% or more of symptomatic abscesses. Needle aspiration at ultrasound examination confirms the diagnosis and provides pus for culture. A leucocytosis is frequent, plasma alkaline phosphatase activity is usually increased, and the serum albumin is often low. The chest radiograph may show a raised right diaphragm and collapse or effusion at the base of the right lung. Blood culture should always be done as it may reveal the causative organism.

Management
This includes antibiotics and drainage of the abscess. Pending the results of culture of blood and pus from the abscess, treatment should commence with a combination such as ampicillin, gentamicin and metronidazole. Aspiration or drainage with a catheter placed in the abscess under the guidance of ultrasound is increasingly

preferred to surgical drainage but the latter may be required for those which fail to respond.

Prognosis
The mortality of liver abscesses is about 50% and failure to make the diagnosis is the commonest cause of death because untreated abscesses are invariably fatal. Older patients and those with multiple abscesses also have a higher mortality.

AMOEBIC ABSCESSES

Amoebic liver abscesses occur particularly in endemic areas, but they can occur anywhere in the world. Amoebic infections are considered elsewhere (p. 155).

HEPATIC NODULES

Liver diseases characterised primarily by hepatic nodules which are not neoplastic are rare, and three types are usually recognised. Neoplastic nodules such as adenomas and the nodules occurring in cirrhosis are not included with these diseases.

Nodular regenerative hyperplasia of the liver
This disease is characterised by small hepatocyte nodules throughout the liver unassociated with fibrosis. It occurs in older people and has been associated with many conditions such as connective tissue disease and haematological diseases and with immunosuppressive and corticosteroid drugs. The condition usually presents as an abdominal mass or occasionally because of portal hypertension. Diagnosis is made by liver biopsy. Liver function is good and the prognosis is very favourable, but hepatocellular carcinoma occurs occasionally.

Focal nodular hyperplasia of the liver
This usually takes the form of a single subcapsular liver nodule, yellow-brown in colour and with central fibrosis. It is almost always asymptomatic and found by chance, but intraperitoneal bleeding is a rare complication.

Partial nodular transformation of the liver
Nodules in this condition are restricted to the perihilar region of the liver where they can cause portal hypertension. The rest of the liver is normal and liver function is excellent. The diagnosis can be made finally only by pathological examination of the liver as needle liver biopsy is normal.

FIBROPOLYCYSTIC DISEASE

Fibropolycystic diseases of the liver and biliary system constitute a heterogeneous group of rare disorders, some of which are inherited. They are not distinct entities as combined lesions occur.

Adult hepatorenal polycystic disease
The kidneys are the organs predominantly affected in this condition, which is inherited as an autosomal dominant (p. 597). Hepatic cysts which do not communicate with the biliary system are present in over half the patients with renal cysts. Hepatic cysts can occur alone and cysts are also found in other organs. Cerebrovascular aneurysms sometimes develop too.

Hepatic cysts are often discovered by chance because complications are rare, but these include pain or jaundice from cyst enlargement, haemorrhage into cysts, or cyst infection. Portal hypertension and bleeding from varices are very rare.

Diagnosis is best made by ultrasonography. Resection of a large cyst or groups of cysts is only required if symptoms are troublesome and the prognosis is excellent as liver function is good. Cholangiocarcinoma is a rare complication.

Congenital hepatic fibrosis
This is characterised by broad bands of fibrous tissue linking the portal tracts in the liver, abnormalities of the interlobular bile ducts, and sometimes a lack of portal venules. The renal tubules may show cystic dilatation (medullary sponge kidney, p. 598), and eventually renal cysts may develop. The condition can be inherited as an autosomal recessive. Liver involvement causes portal hypertension with splenomegaly and bleeding from oesophageal varices that usually presents in adolescence or in early adult life. The prognosis is good because liver function remains good. Treatment is required for variceal bleeding (p. 526) and occasionally cholangitis (p. 544). Patients can present during childhood with renal failure if the kidneys are severely affected.

Choledochal cyst
This term applies to cysts anywhere in the biliary tree. The great majority cause diffuse dilatation of the common bile duct (Type I), but others take the form of biliary diverticula (Type II), dilatation of the intraduodenal bile duct (Type III) and multiple biliary cysts (Type IV). The last type merges with Caroli's syndrome. Recurrent jaundice, recurrent abdominal pain and an abdominal mass are typical but these occur in only a minority of patients. Prolonged biliary obstruc-

tion predisposes to cholangitis, liver abscess and eventually biliary cirrhosis, and there is an increased incidence of cholangiocarcinoma. Excision is the treatment of choice if this is possible, otherwise a biliary bypass operation is performed.

Caroli's syndrome

This is very rare and is characterised by segmental saccular dilatations of the intrahepatic biliary tree. The whole liver is usually affected, and extrahepatic biliary dilatation occurs in about a quarter of patients. Recurrent attacks of cholangitis (p. 543) occur and may cause hepatic abscesses. Complications include biliary stones and cholangiocarcinoma. Antibiotics are required for episodes of cholangitis, and occasionally localised disease can be treated by segmental liver resection.

Non-parasitic cysts

Most non-parasitic liver cysts are congenital in origin and the majority are solitary. They rarely communicate with the biliary tree. Features include abdominal pain, nausea or vomiting if cysts become big enough, and they may be palpable. Jaundice occasionally results from biliary compression, and infection, haemorrhage and rupture are other rare complications. Other non-parasitic hepatic cysts include traumatic and neoplastic cysts.

Parasitic cysts

These are caused by *Echinococcus granulosus* infection (p. 172). These cysts have an outer layer derived from the host, an intermediate laminated layer, and an inner germinal layer. They can be single or multiple. Chronic cysts become calcified. The cysts may be asymptomatic or may cause abdominal pain or a mass. There is a peripheral blood eosinophilia, X-rays may show calcification, imaging shows the cyst(s), and serological tests are positive. Rupture or secondary infection of cysts can occur, and other organs may be involved. Surgical removal of the intact cyst after sterilisation with alcohol or formalin is necessary.

GALLBLADDER AND BILIARY DISEASES

GALLSTONES

Gallstone formation is the commonest disorder of the biliary tree and it is unusual for the gallbladder to be diseased in the absence of gallstones.

Pathology

Gallstones are conveniently classified into cholesterol or pigment stones. Cholesterol stones are the commonest type of gallstone encountered in industrialised countries whereas pigment stones are found more frequently in developing countries. In the Western world about 75% of stones are of the cholesterol variety, the remainder being pigment stones. Gallstones also contain varying quantities of calcium salts, calcium bilirubinate, carbonate, phosphate and palmitate, determining the degree of radio-opacity.

Epidemiology

The prevalence of gallstones is uncertain because most gallstones are asymptomatic. Probably about 15–20% of the adult population in Britain are affected, the frequency being greater than 40% in those over the age of 60 years. In those under 40 years there is a 3:1 female preponderance whereas in the elderly the sex ratio is about equal. Gallstones are common in North America, Europe and Australia and are less frequent in India, the Far East and Africa. In developed countries the incidence of symptomatic gallstones appears to be increasing and they occur at an earlier age.

Risk factors for cholesterol stones are shown in Table 11.13. There has been much debate over the role

Table 11.13 Risk factors for cholesterol gallstones

Increased age	Obesity
Female sex	Cystic fibrosis
Increased parity	
Oestrogen therapy	Gastric surgery
Clofibrate therapy	Parenteral nutrition

of diet in cholesterol gallstone disease and an increase of cholesterol, fat, calories, refined carbohydrate or lack of dietary fibres have all been blamed. At present the best data support an association between simple refined sugar in the diet and gallstones.

Aetiology

Cholesterol gallstones

Cholesterol is held in solution in bile by its association with bile acids and phospholipids to form a mixed micelle; biliary lipoproteins may also have a role in solubilising cholesterol. In gallstone disease the liver produces bile which contains an excess of cholesterol either because there is a relative reduction in the quantity of bile salts or a relative increase in the amount of cholesterol. Such bile which is supersaturated with cholesterol is termed 'lithogenic'. Defective bile salt synthesis, excessive intestinal loss of bile salts, oversensitive bile salt feedback, excessive cholesterol secretion and abnormal gallbladder function have all been implicated in the formation of saturated bile. However, the basic mechanism for the formation of supersaturated bile in the majority of patients with cholesterol gallstone disease is unknown. Factors influencing biliary lipid composition are shown in Table 11.14.

Table 11.14   Factors influencing biliary lipid composition

Factor	Cholesterol saturation
Age	↑
Clofibrate	↑
Oestrogen/Progesterone	↑
Dietary cholesterol	↑
Refined carbohydrate	↑
Brief fast	↑
Alcohol	↓
Chenodeoxycholic acid	↓
Ursodeoxycholic acid	↓

Factors initiating crystallisation of cholesterol in bile (nucleation factor) are also important as patients with cholesterol gallstones have gallbladder bile which forms cholesterol crystals more rapidly than equally saturated bile from patients who do not form gallstones. Both pronucleating and antinucleating factors have been described. Cholesterol-phospholipid vesicles are present in human hepatic and gallbladder bile, and function as a second carrier for cholesterol. Under certain conditions such vesicles are capable of nucleating cholesterol, from which crystal deposition and stones form. Factors stabilising the vesicles, and factors which are responsible for precipitation of cholesterol from these vesicles are probably critical in the formation of gallstones.

Pigment stones

Comparatively little is known about the mechanism of formation of pigment stones. The brown crumbly pigment stone is almost certainly the consequence of infection in the biliary tree. These are commonly found in the Far East where infection of the biliary tree allows bacterial beta-glucuronidase to hydrolyse conjugated bilirubin to its free form which then precipitates as calcium bilirubinate. The mechanism of pigment gallstone formation in the Western world is not satisfactorily explained. Haemolysis does play a role in some circumstances, for example the increased prevalence of calcium bilirubinate stones in cirrhosis is related to an underlying haemolytic tendency and ileal disease or resection may be a cause.

Biliary sludge

The term 'biliary sludge' describes bile which is in a gel form that contains numerous crystals or microspheroliths of calcium bilirubinate granules and cholesterol crystals as well as glycoproteins. This is thought to be the mechanism whereby many cholesterol stones form. Biliary sludge is formed frequently under normal conditions, but then either dissolves or is cleared by the gallbladder and only in about 15% of patients does it persist to form cholesterol stones.

Natural history

The great majority of gallstones are asymptomatic and remain so. Less than 10% of all gallstone sufferers develop clinical evidence of gallstone disease. Why this should be is not adequately explained. It is clear however that patients do not die because of the presence of gallstones, and the risk of major complications from gallstone disease is low. The great majority of patients with gallstones never require a cholecystectomy.

Clinical features

Symptomatic gallstones manifest either as biliary pain or cholecystitis. If a gallstone becomes acutely impacted in the cystic duct the patient will experience pain. The term 'biliary colic' is a misnomer because the pain does not rhythmically increase and decrease in intensity as in colic experienced in intestinal and renal disease. Instead the pain is of sudden onset and is sustained for about an hour; its continuation for more than 6 hours suggests that a complication such as cholecystitis or pancreatitis has developed. Pain is felt in the epigastrium or right upper quadrant radiating to the interscapular region or the tip of the right scapula, but other sites include the left upper quadrant, the epigastrium and the lower chest, and in these positions it can be confused with intrathoracic disease, oesophagitis, myocardial infarction or dissecting aneurysm.

Fatty food intolerance, 'dyspepsia' and flatulence are not symptoms of gallstones. 'Gallstone dyspepsia' is a misnomer and not an indication of cholecystectomy.

Complications

Occlusion of the cystic duct for any prolonged period of time will result in acute cholecystitis. In this circumstance the pain is more persistent and there is associated fever and tenderness. Other complications include chronic cholecystitis, and hydrops of the gallbladder, in which there is slow distension of the gallbladder from continuous secretion of mucus. If this material becomes infected an empyema develops. Calcium may be secreted into the lumen of the hydropic gallbladder causing limey bile and if calcium salts are precipitated in the gallbladder wall the radiological appearance of a 'porcelain' gallbladder results.

Gallstones will migrate to the common bile duct in 10–20% of patients and cause biliary colic, but choledocholithiasis may be asymptomatic. Rarely fistulas may develop between the gallbladder and the duodenum or colon or stomach, and a fistulous tract may arise between the common bile duct and adjacent organs. Air will be seen in the biliary tree on plain abdominal X-rays. If a stone is larger than 2.5 cm in diameter it may impact either at the terminal ileum or occasionally in the duodenum or sigmoid colon. The resultant intestinal obstruction may be followed by 'gallstone ileus'.

Cancer of the gallbladder is rare although it is recognised more frequently in an ageing population. It is usually undiagnosed until a cholecystectomy is performed for gallstone disease. In over 95% of patients who have cancer of the gallbladder there are accompanying gallstones.

Management

The management of gallstones depends on whether they are causing symptoms. Asymptomatic gallstones found incidentally are not usually treated because the majority will never give symptoms. Symptomatic gallstones are best treated surgically (p. 542), but they can also be fragmented in the gallbladder, removed from the common bile duct mechanically or dissolved (see the information box below). Medical dissolution of gallstones can be achieved using the naturally-occurring bile acids chenodeoxycholic acid and ursodeoxycholic acid. Radiolucent gallstones in a gallbladder that opacifies on oral cholecystography, stones not larger than 15 mm in diameter, and moderate symptomatology are the features which suggest that drug therapy may be useful. Success can be expected in between 70 and 75% of patients by careful selection of those who are not obese and by ensuring that bile becomes unsaturated in cholesterol during therapy. Non-responders are probably patients who have radiolucent pigment stones which do not respond to chenodeoxycholic or ursodeoxycholic acid.

The optimal dose of chenodeoxycholic acid is 13–15 mg/kg/day but obese patients need doses as large as 18–20 mg/kg/day. Because chenodeoxycholic acid therapy may be associated with mildly disturbed liver biochemistry and diarrhoea, it is being replaced by ursodeoxycholic acid, which is given in a dose of 8–13 mg/kg/day. Another popular regimen is a combination of chenodeoxycholic acid and ursodeoxycholic acid daily each in a dose of 7.5 mg/kg. Extracorporeal shock wave lithotripsy using shock waves generated by a variety of techniques has been introduced, with the advantage of being non-invasive and safe, but at present it is expensive. As in the case of oral bile salt therapy, only 30% of all patients with gallbladder disease are suitable for lithotripsy. Before and after shock-wave therapy it is advisable to give oral bile salt therapy to dissolve fragments of stones which remain.

NON-SURGICAL TREATMENT OF GALLSTONES

- Chenodeoxycholic acid
- Ursodeoxycholic acid
- Endoscopic sphincterotomy
- Extracorporeal lithotripsy

ACUTE CHOLECYSTITIS

Aetiology and pathology

Acute cholecystitis is almost always associated with obstruction of the gallbladder neck or cystic duct by a gallstone. Occasionally obstruction may be by mucus, a worm or a tumour. In 10% of patients no obstruction can be identified and the term 'acute acalculus cholecystitis' is used. The pathogenesis is unclear, but possibly the initial inflammation is chemically induced. This follows gallbladder mucosal damage which releases phospholipase, converting biliary lecithin to lysolecithin, a recognised mucosal toxin. At the time of surgery approximately 50% of cultures of the gallbladder contents are sterile.

Clinical features

The cardinal feature is pain in the right upper quadrant but also in the epigastrium, the right shoulder tip or interscapular region. It usually lasts for more than an hour but differentiation between biliary colic and acute cholecystitis may be difficult and features suggesting cholecystitis include restlessness, pallor, sweating and vomiting.

Examination shows right hypochondrial tenderness, rigidity worse on inspiration (Murphy's sign), and a gallbladder mass may be palpable. Fever is present and rigors may occur. Leukocytosis is common except in the elderly patient where the signs of inflammation may not be marked. Jaundice occurs in 20–25% of patients even though there are no stones in the common bile duct, and may represent oedematous pressure on the common hepatic duct. Minor increases of plasma transaminase and amylase activity (p. 481) may be encountered.

If the patient is untreated the inflammation may resolve only to recur. On the other hand the inflammation may progress to an empyema or perforation and peritonitis.

Acute cholecystitis in elderly people is a particular hazard as the disease tends to be severe, may have few localising clinical signs and a high frequency of empyema and perforation. The mortality rate in elderly patients may reach about 10%.

Differential diagnosis

This is from other causes of severe upper abdominal pain, including perforated peptic ulcer, acute pancreatitis and a retrocaecal appendicitis. Myocardial infarction and a right basal pneumonia should always be considered. Occasionally there may be confusion with renal colic, herpes zoster, epidemic myalgia, pleurisy and acute intermittent porphyria.

Investigation

Plain radiographs of the abdomen and chest may show gallstones and detect perforation of a viscus, fistulation of a gallstone into the intestine (p. 541) and pneumonia. Ultrasonography detects gallstones and gallbladder thickening due to cholecystitis, and cholescintigraphy if available shows cystic duct obstruction. The plasma amylase should be measured to detect pancreatitis (p. 481) which may be a complication due to gallstones. The peripheral blood count often shows a leucocytosis.

Management

This consists of bed-rest, relief of pain, antibiotics and maintenance of fluid balance. Severe pain is relieved using morphine 10–15 mg intramuscularly and increased tone of the choledochal sphincter may be minimised by the concurrent use of atropine 0.6 mg intramuscularly. Less severe pain can be relieved by pethidine 100 mg or pentazocine 30 mg intramuscularly. Effective relief of pain may require repeated doses of analgesic every 2–3 hours. Nasogastric aspiration is required only when there is persistent vomiting, in which case fluid must be given intravenously. Systemic antibiotics are required in the elderly, patients with jaundice, and those who are febrile. A cephalosporin such as cefotaxime (1 g 8-hourly i.v.) is the antibiotic of choice, and metronidazole (1 g 8-hourly by suppository) is usually added in severely ill patients.

Surgical treatment

Patients with acute cholecystitis require cholecystectomy. Two options are available: early cholecystectomy or delayed (interval) cholecystectomy. Early cholecystectomy, in which the patient is operated on within 2 or 3 days of the diagnosis, is gaining in popularity for the mortality is no higher than for the interval operation, readmission to hospital is not needed and recurrent acute cholecystitis before operation is prevented. The older interval approach entails treating the patient medically in hospital for 10–15 days, after which the patient is discharged to be readmitted 2–3 months later for an elective cholecystectomy. While there are many technical advantages in undertaking early cholecystectomy, the operation must be performed by an experienced surgeon. Peroperative cholangiography or choledochoscopy is routine in all patients undergoing cholecystectomy.

Emergency surgical intervention is occasionally required if the patient's condition deteriorates, if there is generalised peritonitis, an inflammatory mass in the right hypochondrium, gas present in the gallbladder wall or lumen, or evidence of intestinal obstruction.

ACUTE ACALCULUS CHOLECYSTITIS

This condition occurs in between 8 and 10% of patients with cholecystitis, presents in the same way as acute calculous cholecystitis, and is treated identically. It can occur following trauma and after surgical operations.

ACUTE EMPHYSEMATOUS CHOLECYSTITIS

This is a severe, fulminant form of cholecystitis that is caused by a mixed infection including gas-forming organisms. Elderly males and patients with diabetes mellitus are at particular risk. The condition manifests with marked pain, shock and a rapid deterioration in the clinical condition of the patient. Gas may be recognised radiologically in the gallbladder lumen or its wall, or in the bile ducts. Urgent cholecystectomy is required once the patient's clinical condition has been stabilised, but the mortality exceeds 20%.

POSTCHOLECYSTECTOMY SYNDROME

Symptoms following cholecystectomy occur in 12–68% of patients depending on how the condition is defined, how actively symptoms are sought, and the indications for cholecystectomy. When cholecystectomy is performed for acute calculous cholecystitis at least 70% of patients remain symptom-free. Postcholecystectomy symptoms occur most frequently in women, in patients who have a history longer than 5 years prior to cholecystectomy, and in patients in whom the operation was undertaken for non-calculous gallbladder disease. The information box below summarises some of the more common causes of postcholecystectomy symptoms.

CAUSES OF POSTCHOLECYSTECTOMY SYMPTOMS

Immediate post-surgical
Trauma
Bleeding
Biliary peritonitis
Abscess
Fistula

Biliary
Common bile duct stones
Benign stricture
Tumour
Cystic duct sump syndrome
Papillary disorders
    Dysfunction
    Stenosis

Extrabiliary
Flatulent dyspepsia syndromes
Peptic ulcer
Pancreatic disease
Hiatus hernia
Irritable bowel syndrome
Functional abdominal pain

The usual complaints include right upper quadrant pain, flatulence, fatty foods intolerance, and occasionally jaundice and cholangitis. Liver function tests may be abnormal and sometimes show cholestasis. Ultrasonography is used to detect biliary obstruction, and retrograde cholangiopancreatography is usually needed. Other investigations which may be required include barium studies of the gastrointestinal tract, pancreatic function tests, cholescintigraphy and a liver biopsy. If all of these tests are unhelpful the question of a psychiatric illness should be considered.

Management depends on demonstrating a cause. Frequently no intraabdominal disease is found and the patient is managed with advice regarding a low fat diet, the use of antacid preparations, and treatment for the irritable bowel syndrome (p. 477) depending on the nature of the symptoms which the patient is presenting.

CHRONIC CHOLECYSTITIS

Chronic inflammation of the gallbladder is almost invariably associated with gallstones. The condition may be asymptomatic. The usual symptoms are those of recurrent attacks of upper abdominal pain, often at night and following a heavy meal. The clinical features are similar to those of acute calculous cholecystitis but milder. The patient may recover spontaneously or following analgesia and antibiotics; if untreated the symptoms recur. Patients are advised to undergo a cholecystectomy.

CHOLEDOCHOLITHIASIS

Stones in the common bile duct occur in 10–15% of patients with gallstones. These secondary stones account for more than 80% of common bile duct stones, migrate from the gallbladder, and are similar in appearance and chemical composition to the stones found there. Primary bile duct stones may develop many years after a cholecystectomy and represent the accumulation of biliary sludge consequent upon dysfunction of the sphincter of Oddi. In Far Eastern countries where bile duct infection is common, primary common bile duct stones are thought to follow bacterial infection in the biliary tree secondary to parasitic infections with *Clonorchis sinensis*, *Ascaris lumbricoides* or *Fasciola hepatica*. A stone in the common bile duct can cause partial or complete bile duct obstruction which may be complicated by secondary bacterial infection, cholangitis, liver abscess and septicaemia.

Clinical features
Choledocholithiasis may be asymptomatic or manifest as recurrent abdominal pain with or without jaundice. The pain is usually in the right upper quadrant and fever, pruritus and dark urine may be present. Painless jaundice is uncommon. Physical examination may show the scar of a previous cholecystectomy; if the gallbladder is present it is usually small, fibrotic and impalpable.

Investigations
Liver function tests show a cholestatic pattern and bilirubinuria is present. Occasionally these tests are normal. If cholangitis is present the patient will have a leukocytosis. The most convenient method of demon-

strating obstruction to the common bile duct is by ultrasonography which will demonstrate dilated extra- and intra-hepatic bile ducts together with gallstones, but it is not always successful in indicating the cause of the obstruction. Endoscopic retrograde cholangiography has the advantage that not only can a diagnosis be made of obstruction and its cause, but common bile duct stones can be removed. Percutaneous transhepatic cholangiography may also be used but it is less satisfactory.

Management

Patients require stone removal either surgically or by endoscopic sphincterotomy. Cholangitis requires intravenous fluids and broad-spectrum antibiotics such as cefotaxime and metronidazole (p. 542). Blood cultures should be taken before the antibiotics are administered.

Biliary drainage and the removal of the gallstones can be achieved either at choledochotomy or using endoscopic techniques. Following endoscopic retrograde cholangiography a sphincterotomy is performed and the stones removed or left to pass spontaneously. Increasingly this technique is used as the first approach for the removal of stones, particularly in patients over the age of 60 years. Endoscopic sphincterotomy and stone extraction is successful in over 90% of patients and has a low morbidity and mortality. Less commonly used techniques include solvent infusions via a T-tube or a nasobiliary catheter, and extracorporeal lithotripsy.

Surgical treatment of choledocholithiasis is performed less frequently because of the higher morbidity and mortality compared with an endoscopic sphincterotomy. Before exploring the common bile duct an accurate diagnosis of choledocholithiasis should be confirmed by intraoperative cholangiography or choledochoscopy. If gallstones are found a supraduodenal exploration is undertaken and following removal of the stones a T-tube is inserted into the common bile duct. Once the stones have been removed steps should be taken to ensure that complete clearance of the biliary tree has been achieved and again choledochoscopy or cholangiography will be required.

RECURRENT PYOGENIC CHOLANGITIS (ASIATIC CHOLANGIOHEPATITIS)

This disease occurs in Hong Kong, Korea and South East Asia. Biliary sludge, calcium bilirubinate concretions and stones accumulate in the intrahepatic bile ducts with secondary bacterial infection. The patients present with recurrent attacks of upper abdominal pain, fever and evidence of cholestatic jaundice. Investigation

of the biliary tree demonstrates that both the intra- and extrahepatic portions are filled with soft biliary mud. Eventually the liver becomes scarred and liver abscess develops. The condition is difficult to manage and requires drainage of the biliary tract with extraction of stones, antibiotics and, in certain patients, partial resection of damaged areas of the liver.

SCLEROSING CHOLANGITIS

In this rare disease there is fibrotic obliteration of the intra- or extrahepatic bile duct system, which may be primary or secondary in type. Primary sclerosing cholangitis has no known cause but is often associated with ulcerative colitis and occasionally with retroperitoneal fibrosis or a variety of autoimmune disorders. In secondary cholangitis there is an underlying disorder of the biliary tree causing the fibrotic state, for example retained bile duct stones or strictures following surgery.

Clinical features

The patient presents with jaundice which may be fluctuating, intermittent fever, pruritus and right upper quadrant pain. Eventually jaundice is constant. Other features include anorexia, weight loss and rarely bleeding from oesophageal varices. The illness lasts for 5–15 years with the patient finally succumbing to liver failure with or without infection.

Investigation

Biochemical tests demonstrate cholestasis with elevation of the serum bilirubin and alkaline phosphatase. The prothrombin time may be prolonged. Ultrasonography may not show biliary abnormality as the thickened fibrotic ducts are not dilated, and diagnosis is best made by endoscopic retrograde cholangiography which typically shows narrowed, irregular obstruction and 'beading' of the extra- and intrahepatic bile ducts. The disease may affect the whole of the biliary system or may be confined to the extra- or intrahepatic portion of the bile ducts. The diagnosis may also be made by a percutaneous transhepatic cholangiogram. At liver biopsy a typical whorled appearance of bile ducts may be seen. Bile duct tissue obtained at the time of laparotomy may demonstrate the characteristic lymphocytic cell infiltrate with plasma cells and giant cells. The main differential diagnosis is from a cholangiocarcinoma and this can be extremely difficult.

There is no specific treatment; but antibiotics are needed during episodes of cholangitis. Corticosteroids and other immunosuppressive drugs are of no value.

Biliary drainage may be attempted which can be either extrabiliary using a T-tube, or by placing silicone stents in the common bile duct. Liver transplantation is required when secondary biliary cirrhosis leads to liver failure.

BILIARY DYSKINESIA

There are patients with right upper quadrant discomfort who do not have gallstones and the term 'biliary dyskinesia' has been introduced to describe the condition of some of these patients.

Clinical features

In many the mechanism appears to be gallbladder dysmotility either because of excessive contraction or hypofunction of the gallbladder. Biliary dyskinesia has also been related to abnormality of function of the sphincter of Oddi or to stenosis of the papilla of Vater.

The diagnosis is established by showing the absence of gallstones and undertaking evocative tests to demonstrate that contraction of the gallbladder is associated with pain or the papilla is stenosed. Endoscopic retrograde cholangiopancreatography, endoscopic manometry, intraoperative manometry and radiomanometry are all used in an attempt to define this disorder more clearly. Identification of a true syndrome of biliary dyskinesia remains controversial and the treatment is uncertain. The introduction of endoscopic sphincterotomy has resulted in many of these patients being treated with a sphincterotomy at the time of endoscopic assessment of the condition.

CHOLESTEROLOSIS OF THE GALLBLADDER

In this condition lipid deposits in the submucosa and epithelium appear as multiple yellow spots on the pink mucosa – 'strawberry gallbladder'. The condition is asymptomatic but may occasionally present with right upper quadrant pain. Radiologically the features are those of small fixed filling defects on cholecystography or ultrasonography and the radiologist can usually differentiate between gallstones and cholesterolosis. The condition is usually diagnosed at cholecystectomy; if the diagnosis is made radiologically, cholecystectomy is indicated.

ADENOMYOMATOSIS OF THE GALLBLADDER

In this condition there is hyperplasia of the muscle and mucosa of the gallbladder. The projection of patches of mucous membrane through weak points in the muscle coat produces 'Rokitansky-Aschoff' sinuses. There is much disagreement over whether adenomyomatosis is a cause of right upper quadrant pain and other gastrointestinal symptoms. It may be diagnosed by oral cholecystography when a halo or ring of opacified diverticula can be seen around the gallbladder. Other appearances include deformity of the body of the gallbladder or marked irregularity of the outline. Then gallstones may be present. Localised adenomyomatosis in the region of the gallbladder fundus causes the appearance of a 'phygian cap'. Most patients are treated by cholecystectomy although in the absence of gallstones other diseases in the upper gastrointestinal tract must be excluded.

CHOLEDOCHAL CYST

This condition is considered on p. 538.

TUMOURS OF GALLBLADDER AND BILE DUCT

CARCINOMA OF THE GALLBLADDER

This is a rare tumour occurring more often in females and is usually encountered above the age of 70. More than 90% of such tumours are adenocarcinomas; the remainder are anaplastic or rarely squamous tumours. Gallstones are usually present and may be important in the aetiology of the tumour.

The condition is usually diagnosed at surgery for gallstone disease. Occasionally it may manifest as repeated attacks of biliary pain and later persistent jaundice and weight loss. A gallbladder mass may be palpable in the right hypochondrium. Tests of liver biochemistry show cholestasis, and gallbladder calcification may be found on X-ray. The tumour may be diagnosed on ultrasonography. The treatment is surgical excision but it has frequently extended beyond the wall of the gallbladder into the liver and surrounding tissues and palliative management is usually all that can be offered. Survival is generally short.

CHOLANGIOCARCINOMA

This uncommon tumour arises anywhere in the biliary tree from the small intrahepatic bile ducts to the papilla of Vater. The majority are adenocarcinomas and three morphological variants are described – papillary, nodular or the diffuse variety where the duct wall is thickened over an extensive area. The last type of lesion is difficult to differentiate from sclerosing cholangitis.

The cause of cholangiocarcinoma is unknown but it may be associated with gallstones or ulcerative colitis and the disease may present either some years after proctocolectomy or as a presenting feature with ulcerative colitis only being discovered subsequently.

The cancer is classified into three anatomical areas: the upper third comprising the common hepatic duct and the confluence of hepatic ducts, the middle third and the lower third between the upper border of the duodenum and the papilla of Vater. Tumours in the upper third have the worst prognosis and are the most difficult to treat. These tumours usually arise at the junction of the right and left hepatic ducts and are difficult to diagnose.

The patient presents with jaundice which may be intermittent. Half the patients have upper abdominal pain and weight loss. Presentation with recurrent jaundice following an inappropriate cholecystectomy should not occur if intraoperative cholangiography is performed at the time of cholangiography.

The diagnosis is made by endoscopic cholangiography or percutaneous transhepatic cholangiography prior to surgery.

Tumours in the mid and low common bile duct can be excised. Upper third and high cholangiocarcinomas

pose major problems in management. Occasionally a resection is possible; otherwise palliative tubal drainage will be necessary. Local intrabiliary irradiation may be helpful.

CARCINOMA AT THE PAPILLA OF VATER

Nearly 40% of all adenocarcinomas of the small intestine arise in relationship to the papilla of Vater and present with pain, anaemia, vomiting and weight loss. Jaundice may be intermittent or persistent. Diagnosis is made by duodenal endoscopy and biopsy of the tumour. Ampullary carcinoma must be differentiated from carcinoma of the head of the pancreas and a cholangiocarcinoma because both these conditions have a worse prognosis.

Curative surgical treatment can be undertaken by pancreaticoduodenectomy or a segmental resection and the five-year survival may be as high as 50%. When this is impossible a palliative bypass or intubation is performed.

BENIGN GALLBLADDER TUMOURS

These are uncommon and usually found incidentally at operation or autopsy. Cholesterol polyps, sometimes associated with cholesterolosis, papillomas, and adenomas are the main types.

FURTHER READING

Blumgart L 1988 Surgery of the liver and biliary tract. Churchill Livingstone, Edinburgh

Bouchier I A D, Allan R N, Hodgson H J F, Keighley M R B 1984 Textbook of gastroenterology. Balliere Tindall, London

Shearman D J C, Finlayson N D C 1989 Diseases of the gastrointestinal tract and liver, 2nd Edn. Churchill Livingstone, Edinburgh

Sherlock S 1989 Diseases of the liver and biliary system, 8th Edn. Blackwell Scientific Publishing, Oxford

Sleisenger M H, Fordtran J S 1989 Gastrointestinal disease, 4th Edn. Saunders, Philadelphia

Wright R, Millward-Sadler G H, Alberti K G M M, Karran S 1985 Liver and biliary disease, 2nd Edn. Bailliere Tindall, London

12

Diseases of the Kidneys and Genito-urinary System

ANATOMY AND PHYSIOLOGY

The kidneys are each composed of approximately one million nephrons, the basic structure of one is illustrated in Fig. 12.1.

The blood supply of the kidneys is relatively large, about one-quarter of the cardiac output at rest, i.e. 1300 ml per minute, and subject to considerable physiological variation. The afferent arterioles which give rise to the glomerular capillaries arise from branches of the renal artery. Emerging from the glomeruli the capillaries unite to form the efferent arterioles which supply blood to proximal and distal convoluted tubules in the cortex. The medulla is supplied by arterioles arising from glomeruli in the deeper regions of the cortex.

For a short distance the afferent arterioles, and distal convoluted tubules are in contact (Fig. 12.1). At this point the tubular cells become tall and columnar, forming the macula densa and the wall of the arteriole is thickened by myoepithelial cells which contain large secretory granules of renin. These structures, together with the agranular lacis cells which lie between the glomerular hilum and the macula densa constitute the juxtaglomerular apparatus (JGA) (Fig. 12.2) which is intimately concerned in the regulation of the volume of the extracellular fluid, the blood pressure and potassium balance.

Glomerular filtration is the process whereby water and solutes pass across the glomerular membrane by bulk flow or diffusion. The mean filtration pressure, about 10 mmHg, results in production of filtrate similar in its composition with plasma except that it normally contains no fat and very little protein. Factors influencing the rate are listed in the information box (p. 549). The filtrate thus formed passes through the tubule and is modified according to the needs of the body by selective reabsorption of its constituents and by tubular secretion. The glomerular filtration rate (GFR) remains remarkably constant over a range of values of the renal perfusion and renal blood flow. This depends mainly on alterations in the relative tone of afferent and efferent arterioles brought about, in part, by release of renin from the JGA in response to changes in the delivery of solute to the macula densa.

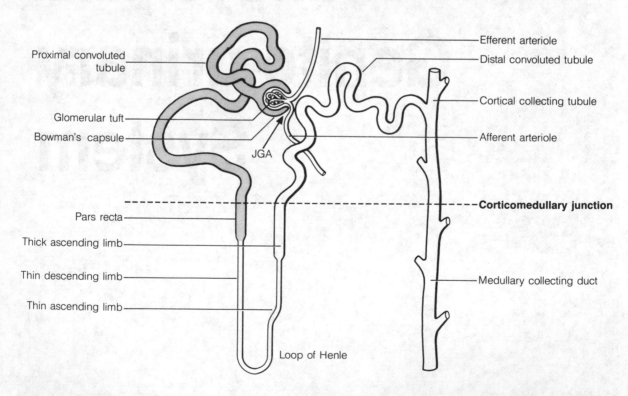

Fig. 12.1 Nephron with long loop of Henle (deep nephron). The afferent arteriole enters the glomerulus and divides into capillary loops and leaves at the efferent arteriole. From the glomerulus the proximal convoluted tubule descends to the corticomedullary junction where it becomes the loop of Henle with a thin descending limb and an ascending limb the upper third of which is thick. The nephron then progresses on to the distal convoluted tubule and then to the collecting tubule which passes through the medulla to open at the tip of the papilla.

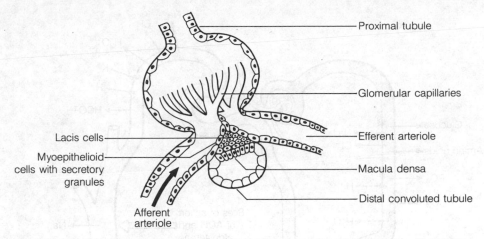

Fig. 12.2   Juxtaglomerular apparatus. The juxtaglomerular apparatus consists of (a) special myoepithelial cells which arise from the afferent arteriole and (b) lacis cells together with (c) the macula densa which consists of columnar cells of the distal convoluted tubule.

FACTORS INFLUENCING GLOMERULAR FILTRATION RATE

- Permeability of glomerular membrane
- Surface area of glomerular membrane
- Blood flow through glomerular capillaries
- Mean filtration pressure

Mean filtration pressure = mCHP − mPCOP − mTHP + TCOP

Where   mCHP = mean capillary hydrostatic pressure
         mPCOP = mean plasma colloid osmotic pressure
         mTHP = mean tubular hydrostatic pressure
         TCOP = tubular colloid osmotic pressure

FUNCTIONS OF THE KIDNEYS

In health the volume and composition of the body fluids vary within narrow limits and the kidneys are largely responsible for maintaining this state. The various renal functions are conveniently considered under the following headings and sites where some of them occur are shown in Fig. 12.3.

Regulation of the water content of the body and tonicity of body fluids

About two-thirds of the filtered water is reabsorbed with an equivalent amount of sodium in the proximal tubules. The remainder passes through the distal nephron where its reabsorption is regulated by vasopressin (Fig. 12.3). In the presence of vasopressin the collecting system becomes permeable to water which is then passively reabsorbed in response to the high concentration of sodium, chloride and urea in the medullary interstitium. The urine thus becomes concentrated. In the absence of vasopressin the distal nephron is almost impermeable to water. In these circumstances tubular reabsorption of sodium chloride without water in the thick ascending limb of the loop of Henle results in formation of a dilute urine.

Regulation of the electrolyte content of the body

This depends upon selective reabsorption and secretion of ions by the renal tubules. In the proximal convoluted tubule and pars recta about 65% of filtered sodium is reabsorbed by a complex combination of active and passive transport. In the early proximal tubule reabsorption of sodium is coupled to that of glucose and amino acids because their uptake by the cells requires sodium. About 90% of filtered bicarbonate is reabsorbed, with sodium in the proximal tubule (p. 551) and most filtered chloride is reabsorbed by a passive mechanism linked to primary active transport of sodium. About two-thirds of the filtered water is reabsorbed passively in association with the electrolytes, its movement being determined by a small transepithelial osmotic gradient.

Control of proximal tubular reabsorption of sodium and water is poorly understood. It is linked to GFR so that the fraction reabsorbed is normally constant. An increase in the extracellular fluid compartment (ECF) volume is associated with reduced reabsorption of sodium and water at this site. Among the mechanisms proposed are release of atrial natriuretic peptide, changes in physical forces operating across peritubular capillary walls, increased local release of dopamine and production of other unidentified natriuretic factors.

Most of the remaining sodium and chloride is

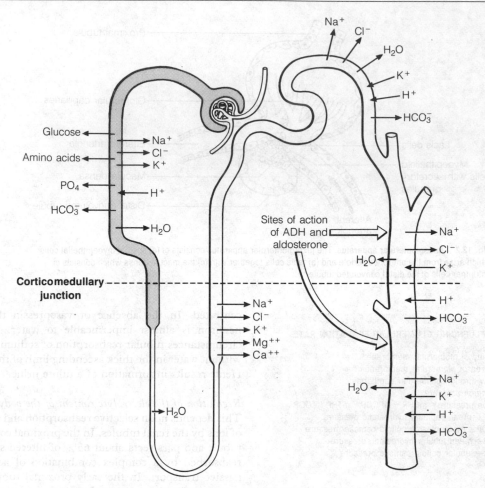

Fig. 12.3 Excretion of water and electrolytes. In the proximal tubule approximately two-thirds of filtered water is reabsorbed together with glucose, amino acids, phosphate and bicarbonate. In the thick ascending limb of the loop of Henle sodium, potassium, calcium, magnesium and chloride are reabsorbed whilst in the distal tubule sodium is reabsorbed under the influence of aldosterone with associated excretion of potassium and hydrogen ions. Water is reabsorbed from the distal nephron under the influence of ADH and the hypertonic medulla.

reabsorbed without water in the thick ascending limb of the loop of Henle. Sodium, chloride and potassium are taken up from the lumen into cells by a co-transport system. Sodium is then transported across the peritubular membrane by Na^+/K^+ ATPase. Potassium and chloride leave the cell by a KCl co-transporter which depends on the gradient for potassium across the peritubular membrane. The diuretic drug frusemide competes with chloride for the luminal co-transport exchanger thus inhibiting absorption of sodium, potassium and chloride. As in the proximal tubule reabsorption of sodium in the ascending limb is flow dependant; the amount reabsorbed depends on the proportion of filtrate delivered to the site. Unabsorbed

sodium passes into the distal tubule, a transition zone between cells having transport characteristics of the thick ascending limb and those with the characteristics of the collecting system, and thence into the collecting tubule and collecting duct. Here the cell membrane is relatively impermeable to chloride and much of the sodium is reabsorbed 'in exchange' for potassium and hydrogen ions which diffuse from cell to lumen down a lumen negative electrochemical gradient created by active sodium transport. The cells lining this part of the nephron can sustain a large concentration gradient for sodium between tubular and peritubular fluids. Thus in a sodium depleted individual the concentration of sodium in the urine can be reduced to almost zero. At this site sodium transport is stimulated by aldosterone and influenced by other hormones including prostaglandins and kinins.

More than 90% of filtered potassium is reabsorbed in the proximal tubule, where the precise mechanism is unknown, and in the ascending limb (see above). Urinary potassium is largely derived from cells in the distal nephron where active absorption of sodium in an area relatively impermeable to chloride creates a lumen negative potential difference. An electrochemical gradient is created by active transport of potassium from the peritubular fluid into the cells, a process stimulated by aldosterone, while the intraluminal potential negative with respect to the peritubular fluid favours diffusion of potassium from cells to lumen. Factors influencing the rate of potassium excretion are listed on page 216 (see Chapter 6).

The dual actions of the adrenocortical and antidiuretic hormones on the renal tubules play an important role in determining the total sodium, potassium and water content of the body. While the rate of secretion of vasopressin is determined mainly by changes in osmolality of the blood it is known to increase in response to pain, stress and a reduction in ECF volume. Aldosterone secretion is influenced, inter alia, by changes in renal perfusion pressure and the composition of the fluid reaching the macula densa. These stimuli can influence the rate of secretion of renin by the JGA.

Filtered calcium (that fraction not bound to plasma proteins) is reabsorbed throughout the nephron in a fashion similar to sodium, thus the rate of excretion of calcium usually varies with that of sodium. Proximal tubular reabsorption of both ions is inhibited by parathyroid hormone (PTH) which, however, enhances distal tubular reabsorption of calcium. Vitamin D stimulates proximal tubular calcium reabsorption. Most filtered magnesium is reabsorbed under the influence of PTH in the thick ascending limb. The differing effects of diuretics on divalent cation excretion can be explained by these different reabsorption patterns.

Maintenance of the normal acid base balance of the body fluid
This depends on the ability of the kidney to vary the rate of hydrogen ion excretion and to regenerate the base bicarbonate. The fundamental process (Fig. 12.4) is secretion of hydrogen ions, formed in the cells of proximal and distal tubules, into the lumen in exchange for sodium ions; simultaneously bicarbonate ions, formed in the cells, are reabsorbed into peritubular fluid. Filtered bicarbonate ions are reabsorbed mainly

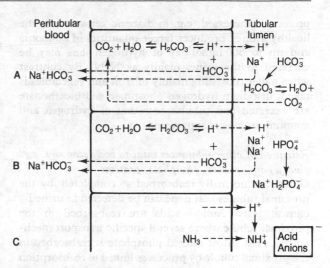

Fig. 12.4 Hydrogen ion excretion. A. Carbonic acid is generated from CO_2 and H_2O in tubular cells. Hydrogen ions (H^+) from this acid are secreted into the tubular lumen in exchange for sodium which is reabsorbed into the blood along with bicarbonate ions liberated from the carbonic acid. **B.** Some hydrogen ions are buffered by filtered disodium hydrogen phosphate in the tubular fluid forming dihydrogen sodium phosphate. **C.** Other H^+ are buffered by ammonia (NH_3) to form the weak acid NH_4^+. Anions of inorganic and organic acids are excreted largely as ammonium salts.

by this mechanism up to a threshold of a plasma concentration of 25 mmol/l. When the plasma concentration rises above this level, reabsorption is incomplete and the excess eliminated in the urine. When most filtered bicarbonate has been reabsorbed secreted hydrogen ions are taken up by other bases in the tubular fluid and the corresponding conjugate acids are formed and excreted in the urine. For each proton excreted in this way one bicarbonate ion, formed in the tubular cells, is returned to the blood so that bicarbonate reserves are regenerated. Filtered bases, of which disodium hydrogen phosphate is the most important, accept about one-third of the hydrogen ions destined for excretion (Fig. 12.4). The amount excreted in this way is limited by the magnitude of the hydrogen ion gradient between blood and tubular fluid which can be sustained by cells in the distal nephron. The urine pH cannot be reduced much below 4.5. Two-thirds of secreted protons are therefore accepted by the base ammonia (NH_3) formed within the kidney which enters the acid urine in the lumen of the distal nephron by non-ionic diffusion and accepts a proton to form the very weak acid NH_4^+. The luminal cell membrane is relatively impermeable to this charged particle and it is excreted in the urine (Fig. 12.4). A healthy person eating a mixed diet excretes 40–80 mmol of hydrogen ion in the urine daily. When the rate of production of protons is increased (e.g. in diabetic ketoacidosis) the healthy kidney produces larger quantities of ammonia and up to 500 mmol/day of hydrogen ions may be excreted in the urine, mainly as NH_4^+. By contrast when a diet consisting mainly of fruit and vegetables is taken, disodium hydrogen phosphate and bicarbonate are excreted and tubular secretion of hydrogen and ammonium ions is suppressed.

Retention of other substances vital to body economy, e.g. glucose, amino acids, phosphate, proteins
Glucose is normally reabsorbed so completely by the proximal tubules that none can be detected in urine by clinical tests. Amino acids are reabsorbed in the proximal tubule where several specific transport mechanisms exist. Most filtered phosphate is reabsorbed in the proximal tubule by processes linked to reabsorption of sodium and water, inhibited by PTH and increased by vitamin D.

In health only a small amount of protein reaches the fluid in Bowman's capsule. The volume of glomerular filtrate, however, is so great that if this small amount were not reabsorbed, more than 3 g of protein rather than the normal 50 mg would be excreted in the urine in 24 hours.

Excretion of waste metabolic products
The end-products of metabolism, especially those of protein, are excreted in the urine. Excretion of urea depends mainly on the GFR, but a certain amount is reabsorbed by diffusion down concentration gradients produced by water reabsorption, thus the proportion excreted increases during water diuresis. Creatinine is excreted mainly by filtration though a small amount is secreted. Proximal tubular reabsorption of filtered uric acid is linked to that of sodium and water and therefore increased in ECF volume depletion. In the distal nephron uric acid is both secreted and reabsorbed and certain drugs compete with it for these processes.

Hormonal and metabolic functions
The JGA secretes renin in response to a number of stimuli:

1. changes in afferent arteriolar pressure
2. changes in composition of distal tubular fluid reaching the macula densa
3. changes in sympathetic activity.

The sequence shown in Fig. 13.20 (p. 643) then takes place. Angiotensin II probably plays an important part in regulating the intrarenal circulation by constricting the glomerular efferent arteriole, stimulating aldosterone secretion by the adrenal cortex and causing systemic vasoconstriction. This may be the sequence of events whereby renal ischaemia produces hypertension.

The kidney is the main source of erythropoietin (p. 701) and hydroxylates 25 hydroxycholecalciferol to form 1:25 dihydroxycholecalciferol (p. 66). Two vasodilator prostaglandins, (PGE_2 and PGI_2) both concerned with the control of the renal circulation, are produced within the kidney which also secretes kallikrein. Kallikrein takes part in the reaction:

$$Kininogen \xrightarrow{\text{Kallikrein}} Kinin \text{ (e.g. bradykinin)}$$

The role of this system, which may influence renal blood flow and sodium and water excretion, is not yet known.

INVESTIGATION OF RENAL DISEASE

In many patients suffering from renal disease symptoms and signs are not referred to the anatomical site of the kidneys. Clinical features commonly arise from abnormalities in the chemical composition of the body or from hypertension, anaemia or metabolic bone disease and their origin may be suspected only after detection of urinary abnormalities. Thus the importance of routine examination of the urine cannot be overemphasised.

Procedures used to investigate patients with suspected renal disease are listed in Table 12.1.

EXAMINATION OF THE URINE

Urine volume
In health in temperate climates the 24-hour urine output usually varies from 800–2500 ml. The ability to concentrate urine is limited and on a normal diet a minimum volume of about 500 ml (Fig. 6.3, p. 207) is needed to excrete the urinary solutes, mainly urea and electrolytes.

Oliguria. This is the production of insufficient urine to enable solute to be excreted in adequate amounts and the *milieu interieur* to be preserved. If the renal concentrating power is seriously reduced or the solute load greatly increased, e.g. in severe infections, after trauma, a daily output of 2–3 litres of urine may be insufficient. Oliguria develops when renal blood flow and/or GFR are reduced, e.g. oligaemia, septic shock, cardiac failure, acute glomerulonephritis, acute tubular necrosis. In these circumstances urine flow occasionally ceases and *anuria* develops. Anuria more commonly indicates obstruction of the outflow from both kidneys (or from a sole functioning kidney) or

Table 12.1   Investigation of disorders of the kidneys and urinary tract

Routine examination of urine:
Volume/24 h
Dipstix (protein, blood, glucose, bile, urobilinogen)
Microscopy (r.b.c., w.b.c., casts)

Special tests performed on urine:
Quantitative culture (MSU or urine aspirated from bladder)
Urine pH. Urine acidification after administration NH_4Cl or $CaCl_2$
Urine SG or osmolality
Overnight concentration test
Water loading test
24 h output of protein
Protein/creatinine ratio
Protein selectivity

Examination of blood to assess renal function:
Blood urea, creatinine, Na^+, K^+, calcium, phosphate, uric acid, H^+, HCO_3^-, Pa_{CO_2}
Creatinine clearance, ^{51}Cr EDTA clearance, inulin clearance (measurement GFR)
24 h output Na^+, K^+, calcium, phosphate, urate, amino acids

Radiology:
Plain film abdomen (opaque calculi, calcification)
Intravenous urogram (size, shape, position of kidneys, scars, abnormalities
    outflow tract, all calculi)
Micturating cystourethrography (Pa_{CO_2} abnormalities of bladder emptying,
    examination urethra)
Cystoscopy (examination bladder)
Retrograde pyelography (examination ureter, renal pelvis)
Antegrade pyelography (obstruction urinary tract above bladder)
Renal arteriography (renal artery stenosis, AV malformation, investigation
    bleeding)

Ultrasonography:
Size, shape, position kidneys, scars, investigation renal mass, calculi,
    investigation urinary tract obstruction, demonstration retroperitoneal lesions,
    screening for invasive procedures on kidney

Computed tomography:
Investigation renal and retroperitoneal masses including aortic nodes

Radionuclide studies:
DTPA (renal perfusion, outflow obstruction, comparison function in two kidneys)
DMSA (size, shape of kidneys, cortical scars) (Fig. 12.12)

Renal Biopsy

Chemical analysis of calculi

Table 12.2   Causes of polyuria

Osmotic
Hyperglycaemia
Chronic renal failure: increased filtered solute load in surviving nephrons

Disturbance of the concentrating mechanism
A.   Lack of ADH (Diabetes insipidus)
        Inherited
        Idiopathic
        Acquired: trauma, tumours, infection
B.   Lack of response to ADH (Nephrogenic diabetes insipidus)
        Inherited
        Medullary cystic disease
        Papillary necrosis: analgesic, diabetes mellitus, sickle cell disease
        Obstructive uropathy
        Chronic interstitial (medullary) nephropathy
        Amyloidosis
        Recovery phase of acute tubular necrosis
        Potassium depletion
        Hypercalcaemia

Drugs
Osmotic diuretics (mannitol)
Diuretics
Lithium
Alcohol

Excessive water intake
Polydypsia
Psychogenic: results in inhibition of ADH secretion and reduced medullary
    osmotic gradient

---

deprivation of all functioning renal tissue of its blood supply. Anuria should be distinguished from urinary retention in which distention of the bladder will be found on examination of the abdomen and confirmed if necessary by catheterisation.

Polyuria. This is a persistent increase in urinary output and must be distinguished from frequency of micturition in which there is frequent passage of small volumes of urine without an increase in total volume.

Polyuria may be due to an increased osmotic load, disturbances of the concentrating mechanism, certain drugs or excessive water intake.

Urine concentration

This can be tested by measuring the osmolality or specific gravity (SG) of a specimen of urine obtained after water deprivation or administration of vasopressin. Urine osmolality (Uosm) is determined by the number of particles of solute per kilogram water and is essentially independent of the type of solute. Urine specific gravity depends on the number of particles, but also on their molecular weights. When urea and sodium chloride are the main solutes SG is an approximate measure of osmolality. If large amounts of high molecular weight solutes (e.g. glucose, contrast media) are present the SG is raised out of proportion to osmolality.

The ability to concentrate urine is best determined by measuring Uosm after 8 hours of water deprivation when it should reach 800 mOsm/kg (SG 1.025). Alternatively, pre-breakfast urine samples are obtained daily for a few days and if Uosm in any reaches 700 mOsm/kg (SG approx 1.021) further investigation is unnecessary. Details of a water deprivation test are given in the information box (p. 554).

The water deprivation test procedure is potentially dangerous when renal concentrating ability is impaired (e.g. diabetes insipidus) and hence patients should be weighed at the start of the test and at intervals throughout. If more than 3% of body weight is lost then the test must be stopped.

This drug should not be used in patients with cardiovascular disease.

WATER DEPRIVATION TEST

No coffee tea or smoking on test day
Free fluids until start of test
Light breakfast
No fluids for 8 hours after 08.30
Weigh patient at start and after 5 and 8 hours
Stop test if patient loses more than 3% of body weight

Time	Urine	Plasma
08.30	Empty bladder	
	Discard urine	
08.30–09.30	U_1	0900 P_1
11.30	Empty bladder	
	Discard urine	
11.30–12.30	U_2	1200 P_2
14.30	Empty bladder	
	Discard urine	
14.30–15.30	U_3	1500 P_3
15.30–16.30	U_4	1630 P_4

Osmolality measured on samples U_{1-4} and P_{1-4}. If there is a failure to concentrate urine normally then consider giving exogenous desmopression 2 μg i.m. and then collecting urine hourly for a further 4 hours. In patients with ADH deficient diabetes insipidus the urine osmolality will then increase. This does not occur in polyuria due to primary renal lesions

Urine dilution

A number of conditions interfere with urinary dilution and normal water excretion (p. 214). Occasionally, it is desirable to test these functions. Details of testing are given in the information box below.

Reaction of the urine and acid excretion

In health urinary pH ranges from about 4.3 to 8.0. A pH greater than 8 nearly always indicates urinary tract infection with an organism which forms ammonia from urea. In certain circumstances the ability to excrete hydrogen ions is depressed. This may be due to failure to form a very acid urine or inability to excrete a

TEST OF URINARY DILUTING ABILITY

The subject should drink 1000 ml water in 20 minutes
Urine collected at hourly intervals for 4 hours
Result:
● At least 750 ml of urine should be excreted in the 4 hours
● The osmolality of one sample should be less than 100 mOsm/kg (SG less than 1.003)

Note: Inadvisable in patients with adrenal insufficiency
Invalidated by pain or anxiety which stimulates release of vasopressin

sufficient quantity of ammonium ion (NH_4^+). The test for urine acidification is given in the information box below.

URINARY ACIDIFICATION TEST

● Oral ammonium chloride (0.1 g/kg) in gelatine capsules. It may be necessary to give an anti-emetic
● Collect urine hourly for 8 hours into containers holding a small quantity of liquid paraffin to prevent exposure to air
● Measure urine pH, total titratable acid, and total NH_4^+ in each sample
● During test the patient may eat normally and should drink 200 ml hourly

Failure to reduce the urine pH below 5.3 is characteristic of distal renal tubular acidosis (p. 599). In chronic renal failure the urine pH often falls below 5.3 but this disorder is characterised by a reduced rate of NH_4^+ excretion (less than 30 μmol/min after ammonium chloride)

Abnormal constituents of urine detectable by routine examination

Protein

This is detectable in the urine by dipstix or acid and is usually indicative of renal disease. Its magnitude bears little relation to overall renal function. Significant proteinuria does not occur in disease of the lower urinary tract though small amounts can be detected in severe urinary tract infection or obvious haematuria. Minor proteinuria occurs in chronic interstitial disease of the kidney, during febrile illness and in heart failure. Large amounts of protein (3 g/d or more) invariably indicate glomerular disease. The most accurate way to assess the magnitude of proteinuria is to measure the amount of protein in urine collected over a 24-hour period. When this is impractical an assessment of the total urinary protein excretion can be obtained by calculating the urine protein/creatinine ratio. As this has a diurnal variation it is best to obtain the urine sample for analysis at mid morning.

The most commonly used screening tests for detecting proteinuria are the 'stix' test and acid precipitation. The 'stix' test uses a paper strip which is impregnated with bromophenol blue dye which in the presence of protein at a suitable pH (pH3) will change colour to blue. As the strip has a yellow background this colour change is observed as green, the intensity of which is approximately proportional to the concentration of protein in the urine. The change is pH dependent and a highly alkaline urine (pH > 8) will induce colour change. The test must be performed on fresh urine and the lower limit of detection is in the range 50–100 mg/l.

It is particularly sensitive for albumin, but has a low sensitivity for other proteins such as globulins and Bence-Jones protein. A more sensitive but less specific test is the precipitation of urinary proteins by sulphasalicylic acid; 8 drops of sulphasalicylic acid are added to 2 ml urine and in the presence of protein a precipitate will develop. Other acids can be used (trichloracetic acid, phosphotungstic acid). Light chains and low molecular weight proteins will be detected by this technique. False positives may occur in the presence of certain contrast agents, penicillin and p-aminosalicylic acid. If either of these screening tests is positive then laboratory examination to detect the degree and type of proteinuria should be undertaken.

The great bulk of urinary protein is albumin, larger molecular weight plasma proteins are present in only small amounts. The pattern of proteinuria can be determined and an index of selectivity assessed. In highly selective proteinuria, the larger molecular weight proteins are virtually absent, in non-selective proteinuria they are found in significant amounts. The degree of selectivity is an indication of the amount of glomerular damage and helps predict the response to corticosteroid therapy (highly selective proteinuria usually responsive).

Postural (orthostatic) proteinuria

In a number of apparently healthy persons, usually children or adolescents, small amounts of protein are excreted without demonstrable renal disease. In such patients urine formed in recumbency is free from protein so that the specimen voided immediately on rising is normal. Urine formed during day-time activities or after vigorous exercise contains protein. Tests of renal function show no abnormality and further investigations are not justified unless required to obtain employment or for insurance purposes. Follow-up studies of such patients indicate that the condition is benign.

Microalbuminuria

Microalbuminuria is a term used to indicate an increase in urinary albumin excretion which is not manifest by an increase in urinary protein detected by conventional methods and indicates an albumin excretion rate of approximately 20–200 µg/min. As urinary albumin varies with posture and exercise it is important to collect the urine under very standard conditions; short-term (2 hours) during rest, overnight (approximately 8 hours), or early morning sample. For screening purposes an early morning urine specimen is adequate and if the albumin/creatinine ratio is found to be greater than 3.5 mg/mmol then a timed overnight sample should be obtained for estimation of the albumin excretion rate. Methods are now available for the rapid detection of urinary albumin by immunoassay and these are very specific. Interpretation of results are, however, difficult as albumin excretion will increase with exercise, hypertension, cardiac failure, urinary tract infection and also after drinking large amounts of fluid. Nonetheless it is a particularly useful test for the detection of early diabetic nephropathy. Incipient diabetic nephropathy is suspected when microalbuminuria is detected in two of three samples collected over a six-month period in patients in whom other causes of an increased urinary albumin excretion have been excluded. Overt diabetic nephropathy is indicated by finding a urinary albumin excretion of greater than 200 µg/min in two of three samples collected in an interval of six months.

Bence-Jones protein

Many patients suffering from one of the monoclonal gammopathies (p. 745) excrete light chains (Bence-Jones protein) in their urine. These proteins are not detected by dipstix and can best be identified by immunoelectrophoresis of urine.

Blood

This is found in the urine in numerous clinical conditions and may indicate serious disease of the urinary tract. The appearance of the urine varies with the amount of blood; when traces are present it appears normal; with larger amounts it appears smoky, bright red or reddish brown. Microscopic examination of the urine should be performed as the presence of red cell casts indicates a glomerular lesion. Deformed or crenated red cells suggest upper tract bleeding whereas those with normal morphology tend to indicate ureteric, bladder, prostatic or urethral bleeding. Thus haematuria may indicate blood loss from anywhere in the urinary tract (Table 12.3). The conditions which may mimic haematuria are listed in the information box (p. 556).

Pus cells and bacteria

These may be found in the urinary sediment in inflammation of any part of the urinary tract. Their presence usually indicates bacterial infection, but they are found in the absence of bacteria in acute glomerulonephritis, interstitial nephritis and polycystic disease. Bacteria may be seen under the microscope, but urine must be cultured if infection is suspected. Catheterisation should be avoided and a midstream specimen (MSU) obtained from both male and female patients and cultured within 2 hours. Suprapubic aspiration of

Table 12.3 Causes of haematuria

KIDNEY

Glomerulonephritis
Primary
  Mesangial proliferative
  Endocapillary
  Mesangiocapillary
  IgA nephropathy

Other glomerular disease
Benign familial haematuria
Loin pain haematuria syndrome
Alport's syndrome
Fabry's disease

Interstitial disease
Severe acute pyelonephritis
Papillary necrosis (diabetes mellitus, analgesic nephropathy, sickle cell disease)
Neoplastic (primary, secondary)
Arteriovenous abnormalities

Cystic disease
Adult polycystic disease, medullary cystic disease
Solitary cyst

Stone disease

Trauma

URETER
Neoplasia
Stone

BLADDER
Neoplasia
Cystitis
Stone
Trauma
Schistosomiasis (p. 165)

PROSTATE
Prostatitis
Neoplasia

URETHRA
Urethritis
Trauma

DISORDERS OF HAEMOSTASIS
Secondary
Systemic lupus erythematosus
Polyarteritis
Subacute bacterial endocarditis
Cryoglobulinaemia

CONDITIONS WHICH MAY MIMIC HAEMATURIA

- Haemoglobinuria, the urine gives a positive chemical test for haemoglobin, but no red cells are detectable
- Myoglobinuria, no red cells are seen, but chemical tests for haemoglobin are positive. Myoglobin can be distinguished by spectrometry
- Acute Intermittent porphyria in which fresh urine appears normal, but on standing for some hours a dark red colour may develop
- Beetroot, senna, dyes used to colour sweets and phenolphthalein may also mimic haematuria. Chemical test for haemoglobin negative

---

the bladder is easily performed, without local anaesthetic, when the bladder is full. This is a useful technique for obtaining an uncontaminated sample of urine particularly from small children. Quantitative culture of the urine should be performed; bacterial counts of more than 10^5/ml indicate significant infection in a properly obtained MSU. The presence of any bacteria in suprapubic aspirate must be considered significant.

Casts
These are microscopic cylindrical structures found in the urinary sediment. They are formed in renal tubules by coagulation of protein. Red cells, polymorphs or epithelial cells may be impressed upon this matrix producing erythrocyte, leucocyte and epithelial casts respectively; all such casts are found in acute glomerulonephritis and in other diseases in which there is glomerular inflammation. Leucocyte casts appear dur-

ing acute urinary infections. Granular casts are formed by degeneration of the impressed cells. Epithelial and granular casts are indicative of inflammation and degeneration of the renal tubules. Hyaline casts consist of coagulated protein without cellular elements and are found in chronic glomerulonephritis and occasionally in small numbers in normal urine, especially after vigorous exercise.

CHEMICAL ANALYSIS OF THE BLOOD

Determination of the plasma creatinine gives a useful indication of the degree of renal failure (p. 588). The blood urea, which is more readily affected by dietary protein, tissue breakdown and hydration is a less reliable guide to overall renal function. Neither plasma creatinine nor blood urea rise above the accepted normal maximum until renal function is reduced by at least 50%.

The diminishing capacity to excrete hydrogen ions results in their accumulation in blood and the severity of the consequent metabolic acidosis may be estimated by measurement of arterial $[H^+]$, $[HCO_3^-]$ and Pa_{CO_2}. Estimations of plasma sodium, potassium, calcium, phosphate and protein concentrations are of value in certain circumstances. For example in chronic renal failure metabolic acidosis is frequently accompanied by hyponatraemia, hyperkalaemia, hypocalcaemia, and hyperphosphataemia.

Renal clearance
Glomerular function is best studied by measuring renal clearance where clearance C = UV/P, U and P being the urinary and plasma concentrations of any substance and V the minute volume of urine. If a substance in plasma passes freely through the glomerular filter and is neither absorbed nor excreted by the tubules, the quantity excreted in urine (UV) is identical with the

amount filtered by the glomeruli; the clearance of such a substance therefore, equals the rate of GFR.

The polysaccharide, inulin, appears to be excreted in this way and its clearance is used to estimate GFR, which for the average adult is about 120 ml/min. A similar value is obtained using the clearance of ^{51}CrEDTA and here a single injection technique is possible. In clinical practice the clearance of creatinine, which approximates to that of inulin, is usually measured by collecting a 24-hour urine sample and withdrawing a sample of blood at the end of the collection.

RADIOLOGICAL AND OTHER IMAGING INVESTIGATIONS

A plain radiograph of the abdomen detects opaque calculi or calcification within the renal tract (Fig. 12.5). When the kidneys are outlined by perirenal fat it can give an indication of their shape, size and position, but this information is best obtained by ultrasound or intravenous urography.

Intravenous urography (IVU)

This is carried out by intravenous injection of an organic iodine-containing compound, about one-third of which is excreted, largely by glomerular filtration within the first hour. It is used, often in association with tomography, to demonstrate the size, shape and position of the kidneys and study the outflow tract. Following injection, films are taken at timed intervals. There is first an increase in the radiographic density of renal substance (nephrogram) as contrast is concentrated in the tubules and this shows the size and shape of the kidneys. Within a few minutes contrast is excreted into the calyceal system, pelvis and ureters which are best demonstrated within the first 20 minutes.

In the adult, healthy kidneys usually measure 11–14 cm in length, bi-polar diameter being similar in length to that of three lumbar vertebrae. Renal cortical thickness can be assessed and any focal or generalised cortical defect seen, e.g. scars of chronic pyelonephritis. In significant unilateral renal artery stenosis, early films show a delay on the stenotic side in the nephrogram which subsequently becomes more dense and persists longer compared with the normal side. Thus, in hypertensive patients it is useful to obtain early films to detect this difference. Abnormalities of the papillae, e.g. papillary necrosis, may be seen and the appearance of the pelvi-calyceal system, ureters and bladder will show any structural abnormality or partial

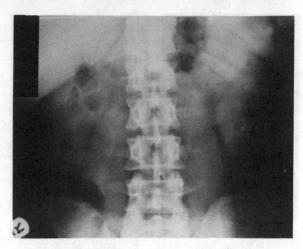

Fig. 12.5   Nephrocalcinosis.

or complete obstruction. Clubbed calyces and slow excretion are common in chronic obstruction. Severe obstruction may result in distension of the pelvis, thinning of the cortex and extravasation of contrast into extrarenal tissue. In renal tuberculosis calcification and cavitation are common. Adult polycystic disease causes bilateral renal enlargement and the calyces are stretched and spidery. Calculi may be localised.

Excretion urography is not without risk because:

1. A few patients may react to the contrast agent. In those with known atopy, diabetes mellitus or renal insufficiency and any with a history of adverse reaction to contrast agents a special low osmolar contrast medium should be used if the procedure is essential.
2. Formerly all patients were dehydrated before IVU to increase the concentration of dye in the kidneys and collecting systems. In some (diabetic patients, small children, and those with myeloma or renal failure) this resulted in significant renal impairment. Use of tomography and of modern contrast agents, which can be given in large doses, has made water deprivation unnecessary in these patients.

Micturating cystourethrography (MCU)

MCU is used to diagnose vesicoureteric reflux and to assess its severity (Fig. 12.6). Using a catheter the bladder is filled with contrast medium and while the patient voids fluoroscopic screening is carried out and films taken. MCU is used, in combination with urodynamic studies, in assessment of disordered bladder emptying and urethral abnormalities.

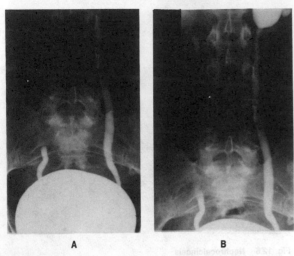

A   **B**

Fig. 12.6   Micturating cystogram. A. This demonstrates the distended bladder with free reflux to both ureters. **B.** It can be seen that the reflux extends to the pelvicalyceal system.

Cystoscopy and retrograde pyelography

These investigations are used mainly to investigate lesions of the ureter and renal pelvis and define the cause of ureteric obstruction. Cystoscopy allows direct inspection of the bladder and ureteric orifices. Contrast medium is then injected under screening control into ureteric catheters inserted during cystoscopy. Antibiotic cover is essential when the urine contains organisms.

Antegrade pyelography

This requires percutaneous insertion of a fine catheter into the pelvi-calyceal system under X-ray or ultrasound control. Injection of contrast allows detailed examination of the pelvi-calyceal system and ureters and localisation of any obstruction. The procedure can be extended to allow percutaneous drainage (nephrostomy) of an obstructed system to allow recovery of renal function, hence its value in patients shown by ultrasound to have supravesical urinary tract obstruction.

Renal arteriography

This is used to demonstrate the anatomy of the renal arterial system and is valuable when investigating renal artery stenosis, arteriovenous malformation, and persistent bleeding after trauma. It has been largely superseded by ultrasonography and computerised tomography when investigating renal masses. Following percutaneous catheterisation of the femoral artery the catheter tip is advanced and contrast injected first into the aorta and then into the renal arteries (Fig. 12.7).

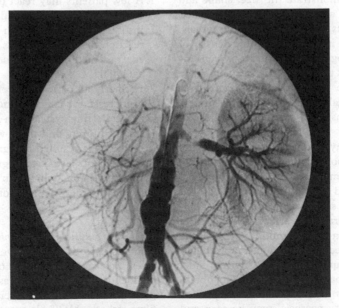

Fig. 12.7   Digital subtraction arteriogram showing renal artery stenosis. The dye has passed the stenosis and the developing nephrogram can be seen. (Courtesy of Dr D Fowler, Department of Radiology, Leeds General Infirmary.)

Arteriography can be extended:

1. to carry out balloon angioplasty to dilate the artery in patients with arterial stricture or
2. to perform arterial embolisation in patients with inoperable renal carcinoma who have haemorrhage or intractable pain.

Renal vein sampling and venography

The renal veins can be catheterised via the femoral vein and the blood taken to measure renin. This may be of value in assessing the haemodynamic significance of a renal artery stenosis. Venography will demonstrate renal vein thrombosis and invasion by tumour.

Renal ultrasound

This is the method of choice for assessing overall renal size and cortical thickness and distinguishing solid tumours from cysts. It is an excellent screening test for polycystic kidney disease. In investigation of suspected malignant renal tumours U/S can give additional information by detecting extension of tumour to renal veins, vena cava, lymph nodes or liver.

Dilatation of the pelvi-calyceal system, which may be due to obstruction (Fig. 12.8), can be demonstrated as well as perinephric abscess or haematoma. Calculi are usually detected but very small stones may be missed. Cyst puncture, renal biopsy and antegrade pyelography

A

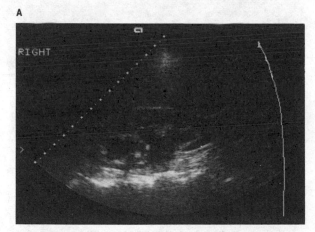

B

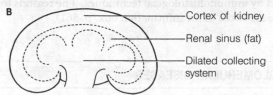

Cortex of kidney

Renal sinus (fat)

Dilated collecting system

Fig. 12.8   Ultrasound showing obstruction of the urinary tract. A. The outline of the kidney is clearly visualised with a grossly dilated pelvicalyceal system. **B.** A drawing indicating the main features.

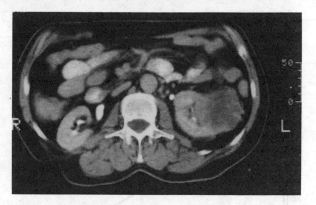

Fig. 12.9   CT of the abdomen. The left kidney contains a large tumour which is extending laterally through the capsule. Compare with the normal right kidney.

are best done under U/S screening. It is quick, inexpensive and harmless and portable equipment is available to investigate seriously ill patients.

Computed tomography (CT)

This is less widely available than ultrasound, but is particularly helpful in diagnosis of masses in the kidney and in perirenal and retroperitoneal tissues (Fig. 12.9). The information obtained can be increased by use of contrast agents. Extension of renal tumours to perirenal tissue, retroperitoneal nodes, liver and thorax can be identified. It is of value in assessing the extent of renal trauma, particular when vascular damage is suspected and in demonstrating radio-opaque stones.

Radionuclide studies (DMSA, DTPA)

These studies require the injection of gamma-ray emitting radiopharmaceuticals which are taken up and excreted by the kidney, a process which can be monitored by a computer linked gamma camera. In this way function of individual kidneys can be assessed.

Renography. Diethylenetriamine penta-acetic acid labelled with technetium (99_mTcDTPA) is excreted by glomerular filtration. Following injection of DTPA computer analysis of uptake and excretion (Fig. 12.10a) can be used to provide information about arterial perfusion of each kidney; in renal artery stenosis transit time is prolonged, peak activity delayed, and excretion reduced (Fig. 12.10b). Obstruction of the outflow tract in which persistence of nuclide in the renal artery is shown by prolongation of phase 2 and absence of phase 3 of renogram (Fig. 12.10c). Poor renal function is indicated by a curve of low amplitude. The technique can help in distinguishing poor perfusion from tubular necrosis, but it is not diagnostic.

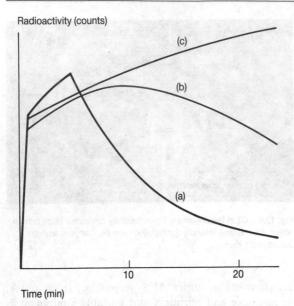

Radioactivity (counts)

Time (min)

Fig. 12.10   Isotope renogram. (a) Normal renogram showing three classical phases. (b) Renogram pattern in renal artery stenosis showing prolonged transit time, delayed peak and reduced excretion. (c) Renogram pattern in complete obstruction showing absent phase III and a fall in the slope of phase II, indicating deteriorating renal function. (Reproduced by permission from Whitworth J A, Lawrence J R (eds) 1987 Textbook of Renal Disease, 1st Edn. Churchill Livingstone, Edinburgh.)

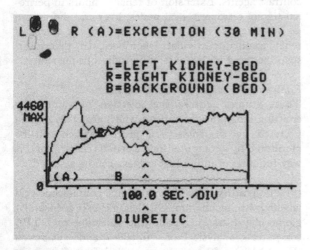

L   R (A)=EXCRETION (30 MIN)

L=LEFT KIDNEY-BGD
R=RIGHT KIDNEY-BGD
B=BACKGROUND (BGD)

4460
MAX

(A)   B

100.0 SEC./DIV

DIURETIC

Fig. 12.11   Diuretic renogram. An isotope renogram showing a normal curve from the left kidney but the tracing from the right shows an obstructive pattern with increasing isotope activity which does not diminish following the administration of a diuretic which is indicated by the arrows.

Diuretic renography. This may be used to distinguish a dilated outflow tract from urinary tract obstruction with increased pressure in the calyceal system (Fig. 12.11). The diuretic is given during the course of the renogram and if genuine obstruction is not present, activity drains away.

Renal imaging
Dimercaptosuccinic acid labelled with technetium (99_mTcDMSA) is filtered by glomeruli and partially bound to proximal tubular cells. Following intravenous injection images of the renal cortex can be obtained using a gamma camera (Fig. 12.12). These allow comparison of the two kidneys as they show the shape, size and function of each. This is a sensitive method of demonstrating early cortical scarring. It is possible to assess the relative contribution of each kidney to total function.

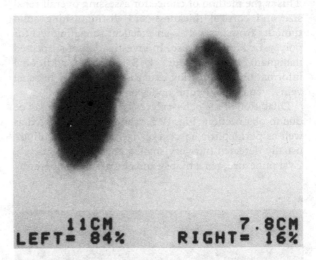

11CM
LEFT= 84%   7.8CM
RIGHT= 16%

Fig. 12.12   DMSA isotope scan showing a posterior view of a small right kidney which is contributing only 16% of renal function.

RENAL BIOPSY

This technique has greatly increased understanding of renal disease and in particular, knowledge of glomerulonephritis. To obtain the maximum information from this invasive investigation, it is important to examine the tissue obtained by light, and electronmicroscopy and by immunohistological techniques. The reasons for use are listed in the information box (p. 561).

GLOMERULAR DISEASES

The term glomerulonephritis signifies glomerular inflammation and can be considered as primary when

INDICATIONS, CONTRAINDICATIONS AND COMPLICATIONS OF RENAL BIOPSY

General indications
To determine the nature of the renal disease
To document the natural history of a disease
To establish the response to therapy

Specific indications
Adult nephrotic syndrome
Persistent proteinuria >1 g/24 hour
Adult acute nephritic syndrome
Persistent microscopic or macroscopic haematuria, (disordered haemostasis excluded)
Systemic diseases with renal involvement
Chronic renal failure with normal or near normal sized kidneys
Unexplained acute renal failure
Occasionally where documentation of specific renal disease is required for insurance or occupational purposes
Childhood nephrotic syndrome if significant haematuria present or unresponsive to corticosteroid therapy
Childhood acute nephritic syndrome if significant urinary abnormalities persist for longer than twelve months or renal functional impairment present

Contraindications to renal biopsy
Disordered coagulation
Thrombocytopenia
Uncontrolled hypertension
Solitary kidney (except in transplanted kidneys)
Small contracted kidneys i.e. less than 60% of expected bipolar length

Complications of renal biopsy
Pain — usually mild
Bleeding — usually mild but may be considerable and produce clot colic
Perirenal bleeding — may cause hypertension
Arteriovenous aneurysm — rarely clinically significant
Infection — more common where significant haematuria has developed

Table 12.4 Glomerular diseases

Primary
Minimal change glomerular disease
Proliferative glomerulonephritis
  Mesangial
  Diffuse endocapillary
  Focal
  IgA nephropathy
  Mesangiocapillary Type I (subendothelial)
                Type II (dense deposit)
  Crescentic (Goodpasture's Syndrome)
  Membranous glomerulonephritis
  Focal segmental glomerulosclerosis

Secondary

Common	Uncommon
Systemic lupus erythematosus	Pre-eclampsia,
Polyarteritis (nodosa and	Eclampsia
microscopic)	Malignancy associated
Diabetes mellitus	Paraproteinaemia
Amyloidosis	Cryoglobulinaemia
Henoch Schönlein disease	Sarcoidosis
Malarial nephropathy	Rheumatoid arthritis
(in tropical countries)	Scleroderma
	Haemolytic uraemic syndrome
	Wegener's granulomatosis
	Cytomegalovirus nephropathy
	AIDS nephropathy

niques and electron microscopy. It is now recognised that there is poor correlation between the clinical presentation and the histological appearance and only a few patients can be diagnosed accurately on clinical presentation. In addition in different types of glomerular diseases, the clinical features are present to a variable extent and not all will be present in all patients. These are listed in the information box below.

CLINICAL FEATURES OF GLOMERULONEPHRITIS

- Proteinuria
- Haematuria
- Hypertension
- Impairment of renal function

PATHOGENESIS OF GLOMERULONEPHRITIS

In the majority of patients with glomerulonephritis there is clear histological evidence of inflammation; in others such as minimal change nephropathy, there is no evidence of an inflammatory process. In some circumstances, the causative factors are known and the pathogenesis understood, in others we are ignorant of both. Experimental models of glomerular disease have been very useful in furthering the understanding of the

the major problem appears to start in the glomerulus and secondary when involvement is part of a systemic disease (Table 12.4). This distinction, while convenient, is somewhat artificial, as primary glomerulonephritis may well have systemic effects, and it is not uncommon in certain systemic diseases for the glomerular involvement to be the initial clinical feature.

The classification of glomerulonephritis was in the past confused because glomerular diseases were identified by clinical presentation. The introduction of percutaneous renal biopsy provided a detailed histological classification which has been further expanded following development of immunohistological tech-

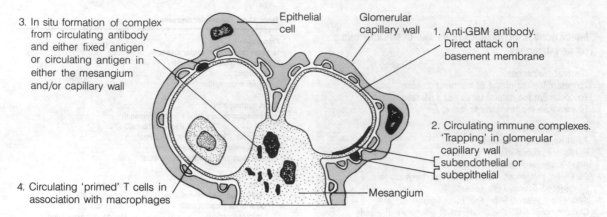

3. In situ formation of complex from circulating antibody and either fixed antigen or circulating antigen in either the mesangium and/or capillary wall

Epithelial cell

Glomerular capillary wall

1. Anti-GBM antibody. Direct attack on basement membrane

2. Circulating immune complexes. 'Trapping' in glomerular capillary wall
[subendothelial or
[subepithelial

4. Circulating 'primed' T cells in association with macrophages

Mesangium

Fig. 12.13 Pathogenesis of glomerulonephritis.

pathogenesis of glomerulonephritis (Fig. 12.13). The features of pathogenesis are listed in the information box below.

When an antigen excites antibody formation there is, normally, an excess of antibody and the complexes so formed are large, insoluble and readily removed mainly by Kupffer cells and splenic macrophages. When the complexes are relatively small and soluble, they may circulate for long periods and eventually become deposited in glomerular capillary walls. This situation usually occurs where there is a modified immune response and relative antigen excess or antigen-antibody equivalence. It is possible therefore that patients who develop immune complex glomerulonephritis suffer from some minor defect of their immune system restricting antibody production resulting in the formation of abnormal complexes. The site of deposition within the glomerulus depends on the size, solubility and electrical charge of the particles, and upon the electrical charge of the capillary basement membrane. Following interaction of antigen and antibody an inflammatory response develops.

In a number of instances of glomerulonephritis the causal antigen is known but it has become apparent that no single agent produces a uniform glomerular response. Furthermore, even in well-defined forms of glomerulonephritis the rate of progression of the disease varies greatly from patient to patient. It is possible that the glomerular response to a specific insult is genetically determined, a theory supported by the fact that a number of forms of glomerulonephritis are associated with particular HLA types, e.g. HLA BW 35 and DR4 in IgA nephropathy, HLA B12 and DRw7 in minimal change nephropathy. In addition, in some patients, the HLA type may give some indication of prognosis, e.g. HLA-B8 and DRw3 are associated with a poor prognosis in membranous glomerulonephritis. It is likely that most glomerulonephritis results from some environmental factor, such as viral or bacterial antigens, acting in a susceptible patient who is relatively immuno-incompetent due to inherited or acquired factors.

CLINICAL PRESENTATION

ACUTE GLOMERULONEPHRITIS SYNDROME ('acute nephritis')

This clinical syndrome is characterised by the sudden onset of haematuria, proteinuria, oliguria and hypertension which in some cases develops 7–20 days after a streptococcal (group A beta haemolytic streptococcus; types 1, 2, 4, 12, 18, 25, 49, 55, 57 and 60 have been implicated) or other infection (staphylococcus, pneumococcus and salmonella have been described) which may be slight or even pass unnoticed. There is no relationship between the severity of the infection and the probability of the development of acute nephritis.

PATHOGENESIS OF GLOMERULONEPHRITIS

- Binding of antibodies directed against specific glomerular basement membrane antigens (anti-GBM disease)
- 'Trapping' of circulating small soluble immune complexes in the glomerular capillary wall
- 'In situ' formation of immune complexes in the glomerular capillary wall and/or mesangium from circulating antibody and 'fixed' or planted antigen
- The action of 'primed' T-cells in association with circulating macrophages

CLINICAL FEATURES OF ACUTE GLOMERULONEPHRITIS IN CHILDREN

● History: commonly a preceding infection
● Generalised oedema: salt and water retention producing oedema most marked around the eyes
● Breathlessness: due to pulmonary oedema and in severe cases pleural effusion
● Fever
● Anorexia: sometimes associated with vomiting and upper abdominal pain
● Hypertension: rarely hypertensive encephalopathy
● Fits: febrile, hypertensive or due to sodium retention
● Urinary abnormalities: oliguria, haematuria and proteinuria

THE DIFFERENTIAL DIAGNOSIS OF THE ACUTE GLOMERULONEPHRITIS SYNDROME

● Angio-oedema: often history of atopy. Swelling of eyelids, lips and tongue frequent, urinary abnormalities absent. Deficient or defective C1 esterase inhibitor
● Acute pyelonephritis: oedema absent, loin pain and tenderness common, dysuria and frequency common urinary red cell casts absent, bacteriuria and pus cells present
● Haematuria: see Table 12.3 — red cell casts absent

CLINICAL FEATURES OF THE ACUTE GLOMERULONEPHRITIS SYNDROME IN ADULTS

● History: in many there is no history of preceding infection
● Oedema: not a marked feature
● Hypertension: variable
● Urinary abnormalities. Reduction in volume, haematuria (characteristically described as smokey), proteinuria

Clinical features

Clinical features in children and adults are listed in the information boxes above.

Characteristically the urine is slightly discoloured with a smokey appearance but occasionally it is red. Proteinuria is usually nonselective and seldom exceeds 3 g/day. Microscopic examination of the urinary deposit reveals red cells, leucocytes, epithelial cells and granular casts. Erythrocyte casts are characteristic and are formed in the tubules by binding of red blood cells with Tamm Horsfall mucoprotein. In the early stages, the urine is concentrated. The GFR is usually transiently reduced and serum creatinine and blood urea increased. During the acute phase there is evidence of complement activation by the classical pathway and acute phase proteins may be increased.

In favourable cases complete recovery occurs and this is likely in the majority of children. The acute manifestations lessen in the course of three to four days and the temperature, pulse and blood pressure return to normal. Diuresis occurs, and oedema, haematuria and the number of casts in the urine diminish. Small amounts of blood and protein may persist in the urine for weeks or months. The differential diagnosis is given in the information box (right).

Management

Patients should be advised to rest until the acute phase of the illness has resolved. Any underlying infection, particularly a streptococcal throat infection, should be treated as appropriate. Previously there was a vogue for long-term (years) antibiotic therapy but this is no longer considered necessary. If there is renal functional impairment, this should be managed by dietary and fluid control, as detailed later in this chapter; dialysis may be required transiently. Oedema requires diuretic therapy and hypertension should be controlled to maintain a blood pressure within the normal range.

NEPHROTIC SYNDROME

The nephrotic syndrome is characterised by heavy proteinuria, hypoproteinaemia and generalised oedema. Normally, only a small amount of protein crosses the glomerular capillary wall and this is reabsorbed in the proximal tubules. When the permeability of the glomerular capillary wall is increased by glomerular inflammation, change in surface charge and alteration in pore size, the amount of protein presented to the tubules exceeds their reabsorptive capacity and protein spills over into the urine. Protein reabsorbed by the tubules is catabolised and therefore the net loss of protein is always greater than can be accounted for by the measured urinary loss. If the loss exceeds the rate of hepatic synthesis hypoproteinaemia will ensue. This reduces plasma colloid osmotic pressure and as a result there will be an accumulation of fluid in the extravascular space due to a reduction in the return of extravascular ECF to the vascular space. Hypovolaemia then leads to stimulation of the renin-angiotensin-aldosterone system and other mechanisms causing increased tubular reabsorption of sodium and to an increase in ADH secretion resulting in increased water reabsorption. Not all patients have a reduced plasma volume suggesting that there may be other intrarenal mechanisms, such as redistribution of intrarenal blood flow to account for sodium and water retention. However, conservation of sodium and water by the kidney, in the presence of a low plasma colloid osmotic pressure results in further accumulation of fluid in the interstitial spaces (see Fig. 6.4, p. 210). The plasma albumin and the total plasma proteins are greatly reduced. Lipoproteins and other proteins such as fibrinogen and other coagulation factors are increased, while antithrombin 3 is lost in the urine; this may help to account for the increased incidence of atherosclerosis and thrombosis in patients with the nephrotic syndrome. Plasma cholesterol is slightly raised and the plasma may look milky due to an increase in fat and lipoproteins.

Clinical features
Patients present with gradually increasing generalised oedema which first involves subcutaneous tissues and later serous sacs. The face is characteristically pale and puffy, general health may remain good, but eventually is progressively impaired with increased liability to infection of the oedematous tissues or serous cavities. Protein malnutrition may occur.

The course and prognosis depends on the underlying renal lesion which can only be determined by renal biopsy.

Management
This is directed at relief of oedema. Patients should be advised to take a 'no-added salt diet' (100 mmol sodium). A high protein intake is now seldom advised. Increasing the plasma protein concentration will increase the amount of protein filtered by the glomerulus and therefore lost by catabolism and excretion. Moreover in patients whose renal function is already impaired, there is evidence that an increased intake of protein is associated with hyperfiltration in the remaining nephrons which may result in glomerulosclerosis and renal failure. Glomerular lesions which result in the nephrotic syndrome are listed in the information box (right). Diuretics are of great value when controlling oedema (Ch. 6, p. 211). When oedema is mild satisfactory diuresis can usually be obtained by using drugs acting on the early distal tubule, e.g. bendrofluazide 5–10 mg daily, metolazone 5–10 mg daily. They have the advantage of inducing a fairly gentle diuresis, so are particularly useful in patients who are working. In moderate oedema it is frequently necessary to start treatment with a loop diuretic, e.g. frusemide 80–120 mg daily, bumetanide 2–3 mg daily. These have the disadvantage that they induce a large diuresis rapidly and some find that this renders them house-

---

GLOMERULAR LESIONS ASSOCIATED WITH NEPHROTIC SYNDROME

Primary glomerulonephritis
Minimal change nephropathy
Membranous GN
Proliferative GN
  Mesangial proliferative, focal proliferative
  Mesangiocapillary GN

Associated with systemic disease
Systemic lupus erythematosus
Polyarteritis
Amyloidosis
Diabetes mellitus

Associated with infection
Bacterial endocarditis
Malaria
Syphilis
Hepatitis B

Associated with tumours
Carcinoma
Hodgkin's disease
Chronic lymphatic leukaemia

*Associated with drugs**
Penicillamine
Captopril
Gold, mercury
Phenindione
Heroin (contaminated)

*Many more have been reported frequently as single cases.

---

bound for up to four hours after taking the drug. In severe oedema a combination of drugs is frequently required because when there is a strong stimulus to retain sodium, it is essential to block sodium reabsorption at more than one site in the nephron. Frusemide inhibits reabsorption of sodium in the ascending limb thereby delivering more sodium to the distal nephron; when there is marked secondary aldosteronism much of this sodium will be reabsorbed in the collecting duct. Only when spironolactone 100–200 mg/day or amiloride 5–10 daily have been added will effective diuresis occur. In a few patients combined diuretic therapy with three drugs acting at different sites, frusemide, metolazone and a drug acting on the collecting ducts, is required. In patients who are profoundly oedematous, it may be necessary to give intravenous salt poor albumin (20 g in 100 ml in 1 h with frusemide 40 mg i.v.) to increase the plasma colloid osmotic pressure temporarily. When an oedema-free state has been achieved patients can frequently maintain this on a much smaller dose of diuretic.

ASYMPTOMATIC PROTEINURIA

This is defined as the chance detection of proteinuria during routine urine testing, frequently in young people who are undergoing medical examination for employment or insurance purposes. The proteinuria may be orthostatic (p. 555) or exercise induced when it is usually benign. Renal biopsy is indicated if the proteinuria exceeds 1 g daily, if there is associated hypertension, haematuria or impaired renal function, if the plasma complement is reduced or when the underlying renal disease has to be clearly defined for employment, insurance or any other purpose.

RECURRENT HAEMATURIA

Painless recurrent haematuria is most commonly confused with the acute glomerulonephritis syndrome. In recurrent haematuria, however, there is no latent period between the associated infection and appearance of macroscopic haematuria. In most patients, there are repeated episodes of frank haematuria usually appearing within 1 or 2 days of the development of a mucosal inflammatory illness. The macroscopic haematuria usually lasts for 2–3 days and between episodes microscopic haematuria can often be detected. Proteinuria rarely exceeds 2 g/day and hypertension and oliguria are uncommon. It occurs most commonly in young adults and is most frequently associated with IgA nephropathy (p. 566).

OTHER CLINICAL PRESENTATIONS

Loin pain haematuria syndrome
This consists of episodes of recurrent haematuria associated with unilateral or bilateral loin pain. It occurs most commonly in young adult women. On biopsy there is occasionally slight mesangial cell increase and complement (C_3) deposition may be seen in arterioles. The aetiology and pathogenesis are unknown. No treatment is indicated and the prognosis is good.

Hypertension
In some patients the finding of hypertension is the first indication of glomerular disease. In the absence of a typical acute glomerulonephritis syndrome this usually indicates long-standing glomerulonephritis and, not uncommonly, there is associated impairment of renal function.

Acute renal failure
This can be caused by a number of glomerular diseases, most commonly by crescentic glomerulonephritis, vasculitis and disseminated intravascular coagulation. (see pp. 569 and 574).

Chronic renal failure
Patients can present with severe renal impairment (p. 582) which has clearly developed over many months or years. These patients usually have bilateral small smooth kidneys and a presumptive diagnosis of progressive glomerulonephritis is made on the basis of significant proteinuria, haematuria and hypertension in the absence of any other obvious cause of renal failure. Renal biopsy is usually inadvisable because of the risk of bleeding, the difficulty in determining the precise histology in small contracted kidneys and the fact that treatment is unlikely to improve renal function significantly.

HISTOLOGICAL CLASSIFICATION

'PRIMARY' GLOMERULONEPHRITIS

In a number of clinical syndromes the glomerulus is primarily involved in the disease process. Renal biopsy identifies three main histological types: proliferative, membranous, and minimal change lesions. The majority of cases of glomerulonephritis belong to the proliferative group (>70%) which can be further subdivided according to certain histological appearances (Table 12.4, p. 561).

This classification is a useful working structure but many of these histological patterns may also be found in other conditions, e.g. in systemic lupus erythematosus there may be either a proliferative or membranous glomerular lesion.

Proliferative glomerulonephritis
In proliferative glomerulonephritis there is a varying degree of proliferation of mesangial, epithelial and sometimes endothelial cells associated, in the acute phase of the process, with infiltration of polymorphonuclear leucocytes and monocytes.

Aetiology
It may occur following an infection, e.g. post-streptococcal or post-viral glomerulonephritis. However, in the majority of cases it is not possible to identify the antigen which has stimulated the development of antibody and subsequently of immune complex formation. Numerous infections are associated with glomerulonephritis and although the streptococcus has been widely implicated, its incidence in Europe has declined significantly. It is still, however, common in developing countries where the site of infection is usually the skin.

Clinical features

Proliferative glomerulonephritis occurs at any age and in either sex. It presents in many different ways most commonly as acute glomerulonephritis or nephrotic syndrome. In the majority of patients unselective proteinuria is present, and may be sufficient to cause the nephrotic syndrome (i.e. greater than 3.5 g/day in adult patients). Haematuria is universal and the presence of red cell casts is diagnostic. In the majority of patients renal function is normal, but some develop significant impairment of function and a small proportion proceed to chronic renal failure. During the early or acute phase of the illness, particularly if post infective, there may be evidence of complement activation (a reduction in C_3 and C_4 indicating 'classical' pathway activation of complement). In many patients however, investigations are undertaken at a 'late' stage in the illness when complement abnormalities have frequently returned to normal. The plasma albumin will be reduced depending on the degree of proteinuria. Serum creatinine and blood urea will be increased depending on the degree of renal functional impairment.

Pathology

Histologically two main groups can be identified although these may represent a continuous spectrum rather than distinct entities:

1. severe proliferative changes (diffuse endocapillary proliferative glomerulonephritis) in which there is a marked increase of mesangial cells associated with variable infiltration with polymorphonuclear leucocytes and macrophages (Fig. 12.14);
2. mild to moderate cellular proliferation (mesangial proliferative glomerulonephritis) in which there is a less marked mesangial cell increase associated with a variable increase in mesangial matrix.

When there are severe proliferative changes on immunofluorescence microscopy, immunoglobins, complement and fibrin can usually be identified in the capillary walls and/or mesangium indicating the inflammatory nature of the condition. On electron microscopy subepithelial immune complex deposits ('humps') may be observed on the basement membrane. Frequently electron-dense deposits can be observed within the mesangium. In some patients capsular adhesions and small crescents may be seen in a few glomeruli.

When there is mild to moderate cellular proliferation on immunofluorescence microscopy, immunoglobulins may be detected within the mesangium in association with complement. There is variable inflammatory cell

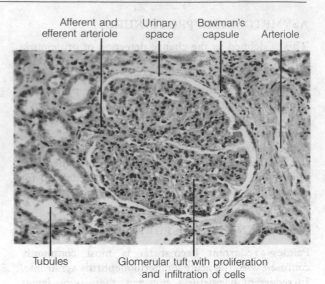

Afferent and efferent arteriole   Urinary space   Bowman's capsule   Arteriole

Tubules   Glomerular tuft with proliferation and infiltration of cells

Fig. 12.14   Proliferative glomerulonephritis. A 'solid' looking glomerular tuft in which there is an infiltration of polymorphonuclear leucocytes and a proliferation of mesangial cells with associated endothelial cell swelling and loss of capillary lumina.

infiltrate and the appearances are of a relatively benign condition.

Management

No specific therapy has yet been developed for this condition and treatment is therefore entirely symptomatic. A search should be made for any underlying infection and appropriate treatment instituted. Hypotensive therapy should be introduced as required to maintain a normal blood pressure, beta blockers (atenolol 100 mg daily), calcium channel blockers (nifedipine retard 20 mg b.d.) and ACE inhibitors (enalapril 5–10 mg daily) are particularly useful. Diuretic therapy should be introduced if peripheral oedema is manifest, loop diuretics (bumetanide, frusemide and ethacrynic acid) are frequently required initially but when oedema free maintenance therapy can frequently be maintained with metolazone (5–10 mg daily).

Prognosis

The natural history is variable and depends upon the severity of the glomerular lesion, the degree of renal impairment at the onset and the presence of hypertension. Factors indicating a poor prognosis are listed in the information box (p. 567).

IgA nephropathy

IgA nephropathy can be considered as a variant of proliferative glomerulonephritis in which the predomi-

FACTORS INDICATING A POOR PROGNOSIS IN
PROLIFERATIVE GLOMERULONEPHRITIS

- Age, older patients more frequently progress to renal failure
- Nephrotic range proteinuria
- Hypertension
- Impaired renal function at time of presentation
- Histology showing sclerosis in glomeruli or marked interstitial fibrosis

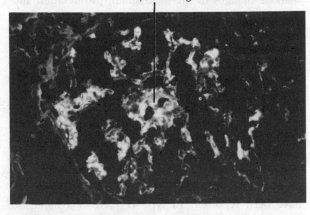

Fig. 12.15 IgA nephropathy. An immunofluorescence preparation demonstrating the deposition of IgA predominantly in the mesangium with small amounts also present in capillary walls.

nant immunoglobulin deposited, mainly in the mesangium, is IgA. It was first described more than 20 years ago by Berger and co-workers from Paris and has been subsequently reported in many countries although the incidence varies considerably. It is prevalent in Japan where it accounts for 30–40% of primary glomerulonephritis and also in southern Europe where it accounts for 20–35%. In Britain and North America it is detected in approximately 10% of renal biopsies. The geographical differences may be accounted for by different biopsy practice but in view of the known association with HLA-BW35 and DR4 it is possible that population genetics are important.

Aetiology
The pathogenesis is unknown but in view of the close association between the episodes of macroscopic haematuria and mucosal infections, it is possible that mucosal IgA plays some part. It is likely that there is mesangial deposition of IgA immune complexes or aggregates of IgA secreted by lymphocytes in mucosal tissues in response to stimulation by bacterial or viral antigens. A number of patients have chronic liver disease in which there is possibly inadequate clearing of intestinal derived IgA complexes.

Clinical features
It most commonly presents as recurrent haematuria in young adult males although it can occur at any age. In the majority of patients the episodes of macroscopic haematuria are closely associated with mucosal infections, usually of the upper respiratory tract. Between episodes of macroscopic haematuria, microscopic haematuria is common. In a small proportion of patients the haematuria is associated with loin pain. Minor proteinuria is common but approximately 20% of patients develop nephrotic syndrome. The majority of patients (80%) are normotensive but older patients most commonly present with hypertension or chronic renal failure.

Pathology
On light microscopy there is diffuse and mild mesangial proliferative glomerulonephritis or focal segmental mesangial proliferation. Commonly mesangial IgA deposition (Fig. 12.15) is associated with complement (C_3) and IgG and IgM. The diffuse increase in mesangial matrix may progress to focal glomerulonephritis.

Management
No specific therapy such as steroids or immunosuppression has been shown to affect the natural history of this condition although in patients with nephrotic syndrome or a rapidly progressing course corticosteroids may be of some value. As the episodes of macroscopic haematuria are associated with upper respiratory tract infections, long-term antibiotic therapy and/or tonsillectomy have been advocated, but have not been shown to be of value.

Prognosis
It usually follows a benign course and after an interval of 5–10 years many patients become asymptomatic. 25% of patients may develop some renal functional impairment and, in Britain, about 10% eventually require chronic dialysis. Features which indicate a poor prognosis are proteinuria in excess of 3.5 g daily, hypertension, older age onset and the appearances of focal glomerulosclerosis on biopsy. IgA nephropathy can recur in transplanted kidneys.

Mesangiocapillary glomerulonephritis
Mesangiocapillary glomerulonephritis is a variant of

proliferative glomerulonephritis in which there are marked changes in the mesangium, proliferation and expansion of matrix, associated with thickening of the glomerular capillary walls due to subendothelial deposition of the products of inflammation (type I or subendothelial type) or from the deposition of immune material within the basement membrane (type II or dense deposit type).

Aetiology

The pathogenesis is unclear. In some instances type 1 apparently follows infections or is associated with bacterial endocarditis or an infected ventriculo-atrial shunt. The activation of complement would suggest that it is immune mediated and circulating complexes have been reported. In type II there is a nephritic factor which is an IgG autoantibody which activates complement by the alternate pathway, i.e. at C_3. It is likely that the consequent low C_3 predisposes to glomerular disease. In some patients it is known that the hypocomplementaemia precedes the glomerular lesion.

Clinical features

The two types have many clinical similarities. They most commonly present between the ages of 15 and 25 years and there is slight female preponderance. The clinical presentation is usually with an acute glomerulonephritis syndrome although some may present with recurrent haematuria and a few with nephrotic syndrome. Hypertension and impaired renal function are frequently present at diagnosis. Many have hypocomplementaemia. In type I this is due to classical pathway activation whereas in type II the alternate pathway is involved due to the presence of a nephritic factor. This is an IgG autoantibody; the stimulus to production is, however, unknown.

Pathology

In mesangiocapillary glomerulonephritis (MCGN) the glomeruli show a marked enlargement of mesangial tissue due both to cellular proliferation and to a disproportionately large increase in matrix. This gives the glomeruli a lobular appearance. The capillary lumen is often diminished and may be displaced to the periphery of the lobule. Electron microscopy reveals two main subgroups. In type I large subendothelial deposits are present and the mesangial cytoplasm extends from the mesangium to the capillary wall. There is the formation of a new layer of basement membrane-like material on the luminal side giving the appearance of a double contour (Fig. 12.16). In type II the capillary wall is thickened due to the deposition of

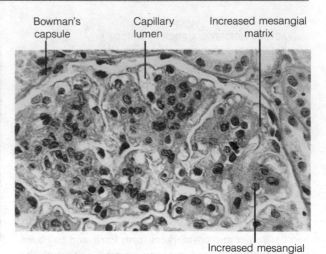

Fig. 12.16   **Mesangiocapillary glomerulonephritis type I.** Part of a glomerular tuft showing widespread proliferation of mesangial cells with increase in mesangial matrix displacing the capillary lumina to the periphery of the lobules.

electron-dense linear deposits in the lamina densa of the basement membrane (Fig. 12.17). Similar deposits can be found in Bowman's capsule and tubular membrane.

Management

There is no specific treatment for either type. A number of regimens have been suggested including corticosteroids, immunosuppressive drugs, anticoagulants and antiplatelet drugs but none has been shown to be of definite value.

Prognosis

In both types the prognosis is poor, approximately 75% of patients eventually progressing to end-stage renal failure. However, a number of patients retain stable renal function. Development of hypertension or increasing proteinuria are poor prognostic signs. Type II MCGN frequently recurs in transplanted kidneys.

Focal and segmental glomerulonephritis

This condition is characterised by proliferative and sometimes necrotic changes which occur in segments of some but not all glomeruli. 'Focal' is used to indicate that only some glomeruli are affected and 'segmental' indicates that only a segment of the glomerulus is involved.

Aetiology

It is frequently associated with systemic disease such as Henoch Schönlein purpura, microscopic polyarteritis,

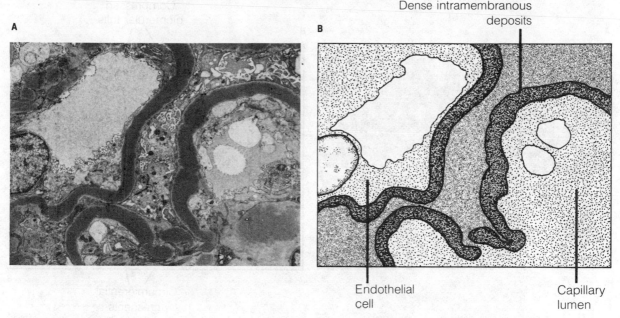

Fig. 12.17   **Mesangiocapillary glomerulonephritis type II. A.** Dense intramembranous deposits within the glomerular capillary walls. **B.** Drawing indicating main features.

Wegener's granulomatosis and bacterial endocarditis. The aetiology in cases not associated with systemic disease is unknown.

Clinical features
The most common presenting feature is haematuria or acute glomerulonephritis syndrome. It occurs most commonly in young adults and commonly there is hypertension and impairment of renal function. Complement studies are usually normal unless there is an associated systemic disease such as systemic lupus erythematosus.

Management
There is no specific treatment. A search should be made for underlying systemic disease which might be amenable to therapy.

Prognosis
The prognosis is generally good and only a small minority progress to renal impairment. In patients with an underlying systemic disease this determines the outlook.

Crescentic glomerulonephritis
In this form of proliferative glomerulonephritis the most striking feature is the presence of large cellular epithelial crescents occurring in 70% or more of glomeruli. These large crescents are associated with glomerular ischaemia and the remaining glomerular tuft usually shows no proliferation and is frequently distorted (Fig. 12.18).

Aetiology
The pathogenesis is unknown but it is likely that the initiating event is immunologically mediated and that there is rupture of the capillary basement membrane with subsequent leakage of fibrinogen into Bowman's space. This acts as a stimulus to the parietal epithelial cells to divide and thereby form crescents. Monocytes and polymorphs accumulate in Bowman's space.

There is no association with any specific agent although many patients appear to have had a preceding viral illness.

Clinical features
Clinically crescentic glomerulonephritis occurs most commonly in adults and presents as acute glomerulonephritis or acute renal failure.

Renal failure is common, hypertension usually mild and proteinuria minor. There is usually a fairly rapid clinical course with development of severe functional impairment.

Management
There is no universally successful treatment for this

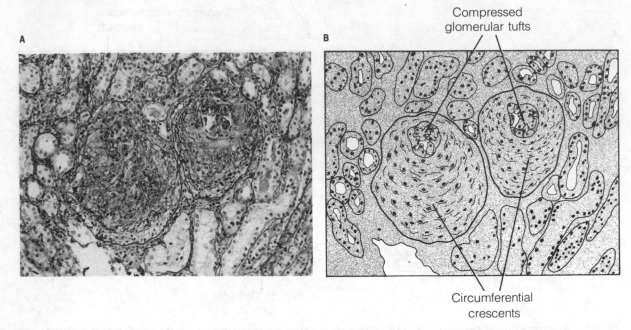

Fig. 12.18   Crescentic glomerulonephritis. A. Two glomeruli showing large circumferential crescents surrounding the compressed glomerular tufts. **B.** Drawing indicating main features.

condition although high-dose prednisolone (100 mg daily), pulse methylprednisolone (1 g i.v. daily for 3 days), cyclophosphamide (2 mg/kg/d) and plasma exchange have all been advocated. The most beneficial would appear to be pulse intravenous methylprednisolone, followed by conventional high-dose corticosteroid therapy (prednisolone 60 mg daily).

Prognosis
In the majority of patients renal function deteriorates very rapidly and haemodialysis is often required early in the illness. Although a number of patients have been shown to respond to corticosteroid therapy, the majority will develop irreversible renal failure.

Goodpasture's syndrome
This is a variety of proliferative glomerulonephritis in which there is a circulating antibody directed against antigens of the glomerular capillary basement membrane.

Aetiology
The pathogenesis is unknown but in some patients the onset appears to follow viral infection of the respiratory tract. The capillary wall is severely disrupted and fibrinogen passes through to the urinary space to stimulate formation of epithelial crescents. The result

is usually a crescentic glomerulonephritis of a type known clinically as Goodpasture's syndrome.

Clinical features
Clinically it usually presents as acute renal failure and occurs most commonly in young adult males and in spring. There is cross-reactivity between glomerular basement membrane and pulmonary basement membrane; some patients therefore have associated intrapulmonary haemorrhage and may present with haemoptysis. In such patients the chest X-ray reveals pulmonary infiltration and there may be significant impairment of lung function. In the majority of patients irreversible renal failure develops rapidly.

Pathology
On biopsy the appearances are those of crescentic glomerulonephritis and immunofluorescence microscopy reveals a linear deposition of IgG along glomerular capillary walls (Fig. 12.19).

Management
The diagnosis should be established as early as possible since plasma exchange combined with immunosuppression is highly effective in patients who still retain renal function. There is no general agreement but most would suggest pulse methylprednisolone (1 g i.v. on 3

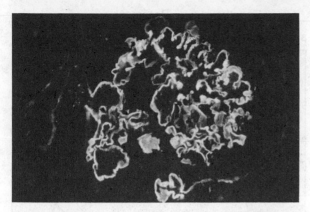

Fig. 12.19 Goodpasture's syndrome. Linear immunofluorescence to IgG from a patient with Goodpasture's syndrome.

CONDITIONS ASSOCIATED WITH MEMBRANOUS NEPHROPATHY

Infections	*Drugs*
Malaria	Gold
Syphilis	Mercury
Hepatitis B	Penicillamine
	Captopril
Malignancy	
Carcinoma	*Systemic disease*
(lung, breast, gastrointestinal)	Diabetes mellitus
Lymphoma	SLE

---

consecutive days) followed by high-dose corticosteroids (prednisolone 60 mg/d) for 4–6 weeks with a subsequent cautious and gradual reduction in dose. Many advocate the addition of either cyclophosphamide (2 mg/kg/d) or azathioprine (2 mg/kg/d) but there are no good clinical trials to support this view. After oliguria develops, plasma exchange is ineffective and should be undertaken only for life-threatening intrapulmonary haemorrhage.

Prognosis
The prognosis for renal function is poor; when oliguria develops there is not likely to be any recovery of renal function even with intensive therapy. Intrapulmonary haemorrhage carries a poor prognosis for survival and may occur in these patients in association with any intercurrent febrile illness.

Membranous glomerulonephritis
In membranous glomerulonephritis the glomerular capillary basement membrane is uniformly thickened and there is no significant proliferation of cells, although there may be a minor mesangial cell increase.

Aetiology
Membranous glomerulonephritis is found in association with a number of conditions. The pathogenesis is most likely to be in situ formation of immune complexes due to the presence of circulating antigen which is deposited in the basement membrane and subsequently reacts with a circulating low avidity antibody. Associated conditions are listed in the information box (right).

Clinical features
Most patients present with nephrotic syndrome al-

though some are detected because of asymptomatic proteinuria. Membranous glomerulonephritis is most common in middle age and in males. Proteinuria usually exceeds 3.5 g/day and is non-selective. Hypertension occurs in approximately one-third of patients and renal failure develops in approximately 50%. It is important to search for any underlying condition, particularly a malignant neoplasm.

Pathology
On light microscopy there is a diffuse regular thickening of the capillary basement membrane of all glomeruli which on electron microscopy reveals numerous small subepithelial electron-dense deposits (Fig. 12.20). On immunofluorescence microscopy these deposits contain immunoglobulins and complement and in some cases, where there is an underlying predisposing cause, relevant antigens may be detected e.g. tumour antigens.

Management
A number of therapeutic regimens have been reported to be beneficial in treatment including high-dose alternate day steroid therapy, immunosuppressive drugs, chlorambucil, antiplatelet agents and anticoagulants. As in any condition where a wide variety of different regimens is advocated it is likely that none is universally successful. Therapy should only be introduced after investigation and diagnosis in a nephrology centre. In view of the fact that only 50% of patients will progress to renal failure, it is best to reserve therapy for those with documented deterioration and to consider any such therapy experimental. Blood pressure must be controlled and oedema treated.

Prognosis
Approximately 50% of patients develop impaired renal function while 25% have complete remission. Patients who present with a severe nephrotic syndrome, chronic

A

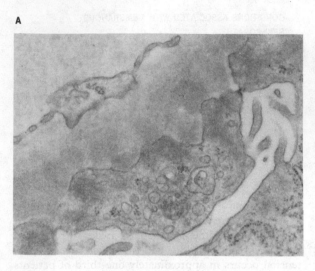

B

Endothelial cell   Basement membrane

Subepithelial deposits   Epithelial cell

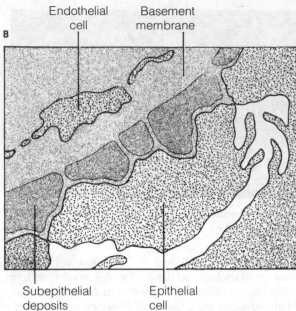

Fig. 12.20   Membranous glomerulonephritis. A. An electron micrograph from a patient with membranous glomerulonephritis showing subepithelial deposits on the outer aspect of the glomerular capillary wall basement membrane. **B.** Drawing indicating main features.

renal failure or hypertension, male patients and older patients appear to have an increased risk of developing renal failure. The presence of HLA-B8 or DRw3 is associated with a poor prognosis.

Minimal change nephropathy

Minimal change nephropathy is so-called because on light microscopy no significant abnormalities are present. It is best to use the term nephropathy instead of glomerulonephritis as in this condition there is no evidence of an underlying inflammation.

Aetiology

A number of patients are atopic. The pathogenesis is unknown, but it is thought to be immunologically related because of the universal satisfactory response to corticosteroid therapy and because relapses are frequently associated with intercurrent infections. It is likely that the condition results from many different stimuli which can induce increased suppressor T cell activity. There is an association with HLA-B12 and DRw7.

Clinical features

The lesion occurs most commonly in children between 3 and 15 years, less commonly in adults. It usually presents as a nephrotic syndrome associated with selective proteinuria (p. 555). Hypoproteinaemia is common and there is frequently a compensatory increase in beta-2 globulins and cholesterol. Haematuria and hypertension are rare. Renal function is usually normal although where there is significant hypovolaemia prerenal acute renal failure may develop.

Pathology

In minimal lesion nephropathy the morphological changes are minor and in many the renal biopsy appears normal on light microscopy. In some however, there is a very slight proliferation of mesangial cells. On electron microscopy there is usually a moderate to marked loss of epithelial pedicel structure (Fig. 12.21). This appears to be a non-specific change and may be a reflection of the heavy proteinuria.

Management

In children the diagnosis can be made without renal biopsy by finding selective proteinuria in the absence of haematuria, impaired renal function or hypertension. In adults diagnostic biopsy is required. Symptomatic treatment consists of therapy to control oedema. Diuretics may have to be combined with infusions of salt poor albumin.

Specific treatment is with corticosteroids which are most commonly given as prednisolone 60 mg/m² orally, once daily for 4 weeks or until proteinuria disappears. When the urine has been free from protein

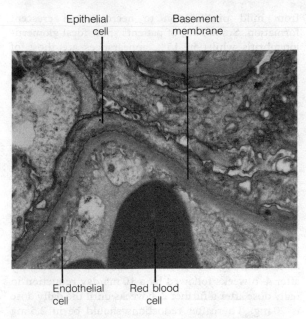

Fig. 12.21 Minimal lesion nephropathy. An electron micrograph from a patient with minimal lesion nephropathy showing smearing of the epithelial cell with loss of normal foot process structure.

for 2 weeks, prednisolone should be gradually reduced to zero over 4 weeks. Some 30% of patients will have a relapse within 3 years and for those who have frequent relapses and require repeated courses of corticosteroid the use of alternate day prednisolone therapy may reduce the incidence of steroid toxicity. For patients who have frequent relapses or develop unacceptable corticosteroid side-effects, cyclophosphamide may be of value. This is usually given in a dose of 2 mg/kg/day and continued for 2 weeks after remission or withdrawn after 6 weeks if no beneficial effect is obtained.

Prognosis
Minimal change nephropathy characteristically has a remitting and relapsing course. In time a number of patients undergo spontaneous remission but steroid therapy is indicated because of the complications of chronic hypovolaemia and the risk of infections in patients who are grossly oedematous. Relapses occurring many years later are recognised but even in the long-term there does not seem to be any deterioration of renal function.

Focal and segmental glomerulosclerosis
The term 'glomerulosclerosis' refers to partial or total replacement of a glomerulus by hyaline material, which in most cases is excess mesangial matrix. In some

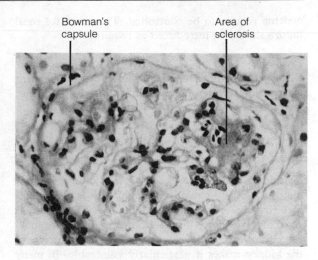

Fig. 12.22 Focal segmental glomerulosclerosis. Sclerosis is present to the right side of the glomerulus whilst in the remainder there is little abnormality apart from slight mesangial expansion.

circumstances this appears to develop in glomeruli which are chronically ischaemic whereas in other cases it seems to result from a previous focal proliferative glomerulonephritis. There is, however, a separate entity focal glomerulosclerosis, in which there is no underlying condition to account for the sclerosis which is typically focal and segmental (Fig. 12.22).

Aetiology
The aetiology is unknown.

Clinical features
In focal glomerulosclerosis the patient presents with the nephrotic syndrome and in the early stages the condition may be clinically indistinguishable from minimal change nephropathy but later haematuria, hypertension and renal failure are common. It occurs at any age, but is most common in children and young adults.

Pathology
Unlike other forms of glomerulonephritis, focal glomerulosclerosis appears initially to affect the juxtamedullary glomeruli. In these glomeruli there is an increase in mesangial matrix which gradually expands to destroy the surrounding lobule and then further until global sclerosis occurs. In time similar lesions appear in glomeruli throughout the cortex.

Management
There is no specific treatment. Hypertension and

oedema require to be controlled. Treatment for renal failure should be introduced as required.

Prognosis
Regular follow-up is mandatory in view of the frequent progression to renal failure. Unfortunately recurrence in transplanted kidneys is well recognised.

RENAL INVOLVEMENT IN SYSTEMIC DISEASES

Certain systemic diseases, e.g. systemic lupus erythematosus (SLE), vasculitis, amyloidosis and diabetes mellitus are frequently accompanied by significant renal involvement. Most of these diseases involve small blood vessels or capillaries and the vascular structure of the kidney makes it particularly vulnerable. In many patients the systemic manifestations will be apparent before any renal abnormality is found but in a small number the presenting features arise from renal involvement, the more widespread systemic manifestations becoming apparent only later. Once renal involvement is manifest, the prognosis worsens significantly.

SYSTEMIC LUPUS ERYTHEMATOSUS

Clinical renal disease is present in approximately 40% of patients at presentation and this incidence increases with time. However, even at initial presentation there is evidence of renal involvement in almost all patients subjected to renal biopsy.

Pathogenesis
The renal lesion is due to deposition of immune complexes containing DNA and anti-DNA antibodies and the subsequent inflammatory response which results.

Clinical features
SLE is a multisystem disease associated with remission and exacerbation and thus presents in a variety of ways with different clinical features. Clinically proteinuria is the most common sign of renal involvement which may be asymptomatic or sufficient to produce a nephrotic syndrome. Haematuria is also common but usually microscopic. Hypertension occurs in approximately 20% of patients and acute or chronic renal failure may develop.

Renal pathology
Most commonly there is an associated diffuse proliferative glomerulonephritis which may vary in severity from mild proliferation to necrosis and crescent formation. Some 20% of patients show focal glomerulonephritis whilst in 15% appearances are those of membranous glomerulonephritis. Wire loop lesions in the capillary walls are highly suggestive of SLE and haematoxylin bodies (disordered nuclei of cells damaged by autoantibodies) are specific to SLE.

Management
The management of SLE is fully discussed on pages 788–791. This detection of clinical renal involvement indicates a worse prognosis and requires renal biopsy and more regular clinical supervision. The mainstay of treatment has been corticosteroids but the dose required to achieve satisfactory control is very variable and can only be determined by trial and error. The initial dose should be prednisolone 60 mg/day and if disease activity is controlled, a reduction to 40 mg/day after 4–6 weeks followed by a 10 mg/day reduction in daily dose after a further 2–6 weeks until the daily dose is 20 mg. Thereafter reductions should be in 2.5 mg decrements. Patients who do not achieve satisfactory remission with corticosteroids alone should have azathioprine 2 mg/kg/day added and in very severe cases plasma exchange may be required. Disease activity can be followed by regular estimation of DNA binding and plasma complement (C_3 and C_4). Renal function must be monitored regularly.

Prognosis
The prognosis of SLE is variable and to some extent depends upon the type and severity of renal involvement. In patients whose renal biopsy reveals normal histology or only minor changes, the prognosis is good. Focal glomerulonephritis usually has a relatively benign course with a 5-year survival of approximately 65%. Patients with a membranous lesion also have a good prognosis. Those patients with diffuse proliferative changes, particularly when crescents or necrosis are present have a poor prognosis.

VASCULITIS

This is a syndrome complex due to inflammation of blood vessels, frequently associated with necrosis. It may affect arteries, capillaries or veins, alone or in combination. The inflammation usually leads to a reduction in lumen with consequent ischaemia. There is no satisfactory classification because the clinical and pathological manifestations frequently overlap and therefore the various syndromes represent a spectrum rather than distinct entities. Vasculitis may exist as a primary condition or may complicate an underlying disease due to immune stimulation or drug therapy.

Renal involvement is common in polyarteritis nodosa and Wegener's granulomatosis, it is variable in microscopic polyarteritis and Henoch-Schönlein purpura and uncommon in all other forms of vasculitis.

POLYARTERITIS

In polyarteritis nodosa (p. 794) haematuria is a feature and in some patients loin pain develops due to areas of renal infarction. Microscopic polyarteritis is a multisystem inflammation of capillaries. Renal involvement is variable consisting of either focal or segmental proliferative glomerulonephritis with or without fibrinoid necrosis or a crescentic glomerulonephritis. Hypertension is less common than in the nodosa form and the clinical presentation is usually as an acute glomerulonephritis or acute renal failure. Treatment is with corticosteroids but in both forms the prognosis is poor, renal failure being the most common cause of death.

WEGENER'S GRANULOMATOSIS

This is a variant of polyarteritis characterised by granulomatous lesions in the upper respiratory tract and lungs associated with fibrinoid necrosis of blood vessels and a focal proliferative glomerulonecrosis. Frequently patients present with nasal symptoms and renal manifestations tend to occur late. The condition responds to cyclophosphamide (2 mg/kg/day) which may have to be given on a long-term basis.

HENOCH-SCHÖNLEIN PURPURA (p. 785)

This may involve the kidneys within 4 weeks of onset and cause either symptomatic proteinuria, haematuria, acute glomerulonephritis, nephrotic syndrome or acute renal failure. Children are more commonly affected than adults and in them the prognosis is good whereas approximately 50% of adults progress to renal failure.

AMYLOIDOSIS (p. 788)

This multisystem disease may be generalised or localised and may be primary or secondary to conditions such as rheumatoid arthritis, chronic suppuration, lepromatous leprosy, and myelomatosis. When the kidney is involved the extracellular deposits of fibrils and protein damage glomerular capillaries and cause proteinuria which, in 30% of patients, will be sufficient to cause a nephrotic syndrome. Renal amyloidosis may cause proximal or distal renal tubular

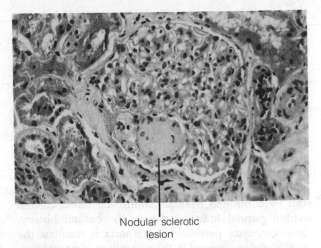

Fig. 12.23   Diabetes mellitus. Nodular diabetic glomerulosclerosis.

acidosis or nephrogenic diabetes insipidus. Renal impairment is common. There is no satisfactory treatment. Approximately 50% of patients will progress to terminal renal failure within 6 months of renal involvement becoming manifest.

DIABETIC NEPHROPATHY (p. 689)

Diabetic nephropathy occurs in both type I and type II diabetes mellitus (Fig. 12.23). The natural history of nephropathy in type I is shown in Fig. 12.24. Renal

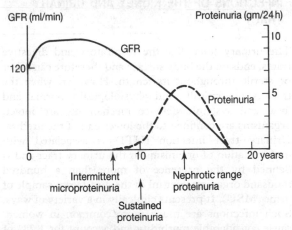

Fig. 12.24   Natural history of diabetic nephropathy. In the first few years of insulin dependant diabetes mellitus there is hyperfiltration which declines fairly steadily to return to a normal value at approximately ten years. At this time intermittent microproteinuria is noted frequently in association with exercise. After about ten years there is sustained proteinuria and by approximately 14 years it has reached the nephrotic range. Renal function continues to decline with an end stage being reached at approximately 16 years.

involvement appears more common in type I but this may be due to the long natural history and the fact that patients with type II are much older when the illness becomes clinically apparent. It is unknown why some patients develop clinically apparent renal involvement with microangiopathy while others seem to remain unaffected.

At present there is much interest in the role of diabetic control and the renal complications of diabetes mellitus. The early hyperfiltration can be abolished with very strict blood glucose control but whether this will prevent progression of the renal lesions is, as yet, not known. Once microalbuminuria appears this too can be controlled by maintaining the blood glucose within normal limits. Later in the natural history, however, once persistent proteinuria is manifest the role of glucose control in the prevention of progression is not clear. At this later stage control of blood pressure is of prime importance and there is some evidence that angiotensin converting enzymes (ACE) inhibitors, such as captopril 25–50 mg b.d. or enalapril 5–20 mg daily, may be more beneficial than other hypotensive drugs.

The renal lesions of diabetes mellitus are only one manifestation of a widespread microangiopathy and patients with renal failure frequently have clinical evidence of retinopathy, neuropathy and other system involvement. These are discussed in detail on pages 684–690.

INFECTIONS OF THE KIDNEY AND URINARY TRACT

The urinary tract, like the respiratory and digestive tracts, ends on the body surface and therefore can never be sterile throughout its length. However, when the tract is anatomically and physiologically normal and local and systemic defence mechanisms are intact, organisms are confined to the lower end of the urethra. Urinary tract infection (UTI) is associated with multiplication of organisms in the urinary tract and is defined by the presence of more than a hundred thousand organisms per ml in the midstream sample of urine (MSU). It presents clinically in a variety of ways. Such infections are much more common in women, cause considerable morbidity and account for 1.2% of all consultations in general practice. In an undetermined minority destruction of renal parenchyma and severe chronic renal failure ensues. The clinical presentations are listed in the information box (right).

Community surveys suggest that the prevalence of urinary tract infection in women is about 3% at the age

---

CLINICAL PRESENTATION OF URINARY TRACT INFECTION

Asymptomatic
Covert bacteriuria
('asymptomatic bacteriuria')

Symptomatic
Acute urethritis and cystitis
Acute prostatitis
Acute pyelonephritis
Septicaemia ± septic shock (usually Gram −ve)

---

of 20 increasing by about 1% in each subsequent decade. About 50% of women suffer symptoms of urinary tract infection sometime during their adult lives. In males such infections are uncommon except in the first year of life and in those over 60 in whom urinary tract obstruction due to prostatic hypertrophy is relatively common.

INFECTIONS OF THE LOWER URINARY TRACT

Pathogenesis

Urinary tract infections may be uncomplicated or complicated; the latter may result in permanent renal damage, the former rarely if ever does so. These infections are shown in the information box below. Uncomplicated infections are almost invariably due to a single strain of organism. In domiciliary practice *E. coli* derived from the faecal reservoir account for about 75% of infections, the remainder being due to proteus, pseudomonas species, streptococci or *Staphylococcus saprophyticus* or *epidermidis*. In hospital a higher proportion of infections are due to organisms such as klebsiella or streptococci but faecal *E. coli* still predominate. The differences between the groups are

---

INFECTIONS OF THE URINARY TRACT

Uncomplicated
Anatomically and physiologically normal urinary tract, normal renal function and no associated disorder which impairs defence mechanism

Complicated
Abnormal urinary tract, e.g. obstruction (Table 12.7), calculi, vesico-ureteric reflux, neurological abnormality, indwelling catheter, chronic prostatitis, cystic kidney, analgesic nephropathy, renal scarring
Impaired renal function
Associated disorder which impairs defence mechanisms (e.g. diabetes mellitus, immunosuppressive therapy)

mainly due to the frequency of complicated infections and the high risk of cross infection with virulent organisms in hospital patients. Certain strains of E. coli appear well adapted to invade the urinary tract, possibly because they possess surface pila or fimbriae which allow them to adhere to surface receptors on the urothelium. Haematogenous infections do occur but, particularly in women, most are ascending infections originating in the lower urinary tract. The first stage is colonisation of the periurethral zone with pathogenic faecal organisms. The urothelium of susceptible persons may have more surface receptors to which adherent strains of E. coli become attached. Colonisation is also facilitated by the tissue damage from previous UTI, by infections of the genital tract or perineal skin, by inadequate perineal hygiene and possibly by use of disinfectants, deodorants and certain toilet preparations. Ascent of organisms into the bladder is facilitated in women by the short urethra and absence of bactericidal prostatic secretions. Sexual intercourse causes minor urethral trauma and forces introital bacteria into the bladder. Instrumentation of the bladder readily introduces organisms. Urine is a good culture medium and multiplication of organisms introduced into the bladder depends on the size of the inoculum and virulence of the bacteria. Factors which limit the multiplication of organisms in the urinary tract are shown below in the information box.

FACTORS LIMITING MULTIPLICATION OF ORGANISMS

- A high rate of urine flow
- Regular complete bladder emptying
- Urinary glycoaminoglycans (Tamm–Horsfall muco protein) which may bind E. coli thus preventing their attachment to urothelium
- Mucosal defences: thin surface layer of glycoaminoglycans, secretions of IgA and IgG, mucosal phagocytosis and other unknown factors

---

Residual urine left after voiding interferes with mucosal defence mechanisms; thus patients with obstruction below the bladder, gynaecological abnormalities, pelvic floor weakness or neurological problems are susceptible to infection. In those with ureteric reflux (p. 581) urine expelled into the ureters during voiding returns to the bladder when it relaxes. Injury to the mucosa and the presence of a foreign body in the bladder also depress vesical defence mechanisms.

Clinical features

There is often an abrupt onset of frequency of micturition and dysuria. Scalding pain is felt in the urethra during micturition while cystitis may give rise to suprapubic pain during and for a few moments after voiding. After the bladder has been emptied there may be an intense desire to pass more urine due to spasm of its inflamed wall. Systemic symptoms are usually slight. Suprapubic tenderness is often present and the urine may have an unpleasant odour and appear cloudy. Gross haematuria occasionally occurs.

The diagnosis depends on:

1. the characteristic clinical features;
2. demonstration of more than 10^5/ml organisms in an MSU or any organisms in urine from suprapubic aspirations.

Pyuria is common but not invariable. Children, men and those women with recurrent infection or signs of acute pyelonephritis must be more fully investigated. Investigations are listed in the information box (p. 578).

Management

Table 12.5 shows antibiotic regimens for treatment of UTI in adults. Ideally results of urine culture should be available before starting specific therapy but if the patient is in acute discomfort an MSU should be sent for culture and treatment started while awaiting the result. Since infection is usually due to E. coli initial use of trimethoprim or amoxycillin is rational and the antibiotic can be changed if a resistant organism is identified or the response is unsatisfactory. Symptomatic relief usually occurs within 48 hours and the course need not exceed 5 days. A fluid intake of at least 2 l/day ensures regular voiding and reduces renal medullary tonicity (p. 580) oral administration of sodium bicarbonate (2 g/6 h) alkalinises the urine and may relieve dysuria. Urine culture should be repeated on the 7th day after the end of the antibiotic course. Failure to eradicate an organism or re-appearance of the same organism in the urine within a few days of stopping treatment suggests that one of the complications listed in the information box on page 576 is present and investigations should be undertaken to diagnose the underlying problem which should then be eradicated by appropriate treatment. Failing this, after completion of a further therapeutic course of antibiotics, suppressive therapy must be instituted to try to prevent recurrent symptoms, bacteraemia and further renal damage (Table 12.5). The urine is cultured at regular intervals and the drug changed as required. Reinfection with another organism or with the same organism after an interval of at least 2 weeks, is much more common than failure to eradicate the initial infection, particularly in sexually active women.

INVESTIGATION OF PATIENTS WITH ACUTE URINARY TRACT INFECTION

Investigation	Indications
Quantitative culture	All patients
MSU or urine obtained by suprapubic aspiration	
Microscopic examination	
urine for r.b.c.	
w.b.c. and casts	All patients
Examination urine for blood,	
protein, glucose (dipstix)	
Measurement 24 h urine protein excretion	When dipstix protein + + or more
Full blood count	Adults with acute pyelonephritis, prostatitis, children, infants
Blood urea, creatinine, electrolytes	Acute pyelonephritis, recurrent UTI,
Creatinine clearance	children, infants
Blood culture	Rigors, high fever, or evidence septic shock
Pelvic examination	Women with recurrent UTI
Rectal examination (to examine prostate)	Men
Intravenous urography (IVU) including	Infants, children, men after
film of bladder after voiding	single UTI
to identify physiological and	Women who
anatomical abnormalities urinary tract	(1) have acute pyelonephritis
	(2) have recurrent UTI after treatment
	(3) have had UTI or covert bacteriuria
	in pregnancy (IVU 6/52 after delivery)
Renal ultrasonography	Alternative to IVU to identify obstruction, cysts, calculi
Micturating cystourethrography (MCU)	Infants, children with abnormal IVU
to identify and quantitate vesico-	Any patient thought to have disturbance
ureteric reflux and disturbed bladder	bladder emptying
emptying	
Cystoscopy	Patients with chronic haematuria
	Patients with suspected bladder lesion

Opinions differ as to when to investigate the urinary tract; some perform intravenous urography after the second episode, others restrict investigation to patients who develop acute pyelonephritis, haematuria or bacteraemia. In women with recurrent infections the defences of the lower urinary tract may be inadequate and simple measures may prevent recurrence. If these fail, freedom from attacks may be achieved by taking a single nightly dose of a suitable antibiotic after voiding and before going to bed (Table 12.5). Prophylactic measures for women are listed in the information box (right).

Covert or asymptomatic bacteriuria
This is defined as more than 10^5/ml organisms in the MSU of apparently healthy asymptomatic patients. Surveys indicate that approximately 1% of children under the age of 1, about 1% of schoolgirls, 0.03% of school boys and men, about 3% of non-pregnant adult women and 5% of pregnant women have covert bacteriuria. There is no evidence that this condition

causes chronic interstitial nephritis (chronic pyelo-nephritis) in non-pregnant adults with normal urinary tracts. When it occurs in infants, pregnant women or in an abnormal urinary tract, investigation (information box above) and treatment (Table 12.5) are required.

PROPHYLACTIC MEASURES TO BE ADOPTED BY WOMEN WITH RECURRENT URINARY INFECTIONS

- Fluid intake of at least 2 l/day
- Regular emptying of bladder (3 h intervals by day and before retiring)
- Ensure complete emptying of bladder
  Double micturition if reflux present
  (The patient should be advised, particularly before retiring for the night, to empty the bladder and then attempt to empty the bladder a second time approximately 10–15 minutes later)
- Emptying bladder before and after intercourse
- Application of 0.5% cetrimide cream to periurethral area before intercourse

Table 12.5   Antibiotic regimens for treatment of urinary tract infections in adults[1]

Drug	Treatment of presumed urinary tract infection Dose	Duration course	Treatment of presumed pyelonephritis Dose	Duration course	Treatment of acute prostatitis Dose	Duration course	Prophylactic or suppressive therapy Dose
Trimethoprim	300 mg/d or 200 mg/12 h	5 days	200 mg/12 h	7 days	200 mg/12 h	4–6 weeks	100 mg/night
Ampicillin or Amoxycillin	250 mg/8 h	5 days	250–500 mg/8 hr oral 1 g/6 h/i.v.	7 days To start treatment in seriously ill patient	—	—	250 mg/night
Tobramycin[2]	—		2.5–3 mg/kg/i.v. 1–1.5 mg/kg/day	loading dose 7 days			
Cefuroxime	—		250 mg/12 h oral 750 mg/i.v. 6–8 h	7 days To start treatment in seriously ill patient	—	—	
Erythromycin	—				250 mg/6 h	4–6 weeks	—
Nitrofurantoin	50 mg/8 h	5 days	—		—		50 mg/night
Nalidixic acid	500 mg/8 h	5 days	—		—		

[1]Modification of dosage is necessary when renal function is impaired.
[2]As determined by plasma [creatinine] and [tobramycin]. Given in divided doses.

Any structural abnormality of the urinary tract should be corrected if possible.

Urethral syndrome

Some patients, usually female, have symptoms suggestive of urethritis and cystitis but no bacteria are cultured from the urine. Possible explanations include infection with organisms not readily cultured by ordinary methods (e.g. chlamydia, certain anaerobes), allergy to toilet preparations or disinfectants, urethral congestion related to sexual intercourse and post menopausal atrophic vaginitis. Antibiotics are not indicated, unless one of the unusual organisms is isolated.

Acute prostatitis

This is often accompanied by perineal pain and considerable systemic disturbance. The prostate is usually very tender. The diagnosis is confirmed by a positive culture from urine or from urethral discharge obtained after prostatic massage. The treatment of choice is trimethoprim or erythromycin, which penetrate prostatic secretions. A 4–6 weeks' course is required (Table 12.5).

INFECTIONS OF THE UPPER URINARY TRACT

The proportion of patients with cystitis or covert bacteriuria in whom the kidney is involved is unknown, but a figure of 50% has been suggested. Clinically, it is impossible to distinguish with certainty those with renal infection and there is no reliable test suitable for general clinical use.

Pathogenesis

Bacterial infection of the renal parenchyma is usually due to ascent of organisms by the ureter, although in a few cases it is blood borne. About 75% of infections are due to E. coli, the remainder to proteus species, klebsiella, staphylococci or streptococci. Commonly one or more complicating factors are present (information box, p. 576) but in adult women and infants infection, possibly due to a virulent organism, can occur in the absence of such factors. Stasis within the tract compromises its defences and renal cysts or medullary scars due to previous inflammation facilitate establishment of bacteria because they obstruct groups of nephrons. Very few organisms are required to infect the medulla and once established there, their eradication is difficult because low blood flow, high osmolality and high concentrations of H^+ and ammonia interfere with mobilisation of leucocytes and phagocytosis. The high osmolality probably favours conversion of bacteria to antibiotic resistant L-forms.

ACUTE PYELONEPHRITIS

Pathology
The renal pelvis is acutely inflamed and there is often co-incident cystitis. Small cortical abscesses and linear streaks of pus in the medulla are often evident. Histological examination shows focal infiltration of renal tissue by polymorphonuclear leucocytes and many polymorphs in tubular lumina.

Clinical features
There is commonly sudden onset of pain in one or both loins, radiating to the iliac fossae and suprapubic area. In some cases, particularly in children, pain is confined to the epigastrium or iliac fossae. About 30% of patients have dysuria, strangury and frequent passage of small amounts of scalding, cloudy urine due to associated cystitis. In most cases the temperature rises rapidly to 38–40°C with general manifestations of fever. Rigors and vomiting may occur and occasionally septicaemic shock supervenes. Tenderness and guarding are usually present in the renal angle and lumbar region. Characteristically there is a leucocytosis. Microscopic examination of urine reveals numerous pus cells and organisms, some red cells and epithelial cells.

Acute pyelonephritis in infants and children often presents as fever without localising symptoms. The initial feature may be a convulsion but apathy, abdominal distension and diarrhoea sometimes occur. In the febrile child the urine should always be examined for pus cells and organisms.

Acute necrotising papillitis very rarely follows a severe attack of acute pyelonephritis. Fragments of renal papillae may then be excreted in the urine and can be identified histologically. This complication, which may lead to acute renal failure, is liable to occur in patients with diabetes mellitus, paraplegia or analgesic addiction.

Differential diagnosis
Acute pyelonephritis should be distinguished from acute appendicitis, salpingitis, cholecystitis and diverticulitis in which pus and organisms are not present in the urine. Less commonly it may be mimicked by perinephric abscess due to infection by *Staphylococcus aureus*. In this condition there is marked pain and tenderness in the renal region and often bulging of the loin on the affected side. The patient is usually extremely ill, with fever, leucocytosis, and a positive blood culture. Urinary symptoms are absent and the urine contains neither pus nor organisms. An untreated perinephric abscess may eventually discharge in the loin or groin.

Management
The information box on page 578 shows the necessary investigations. Diagnosis depends on the clinical features and results of urine culture. Intravenous urography or U/S should be performed without delay if there is clinical suspicion of obstruction or septicaemia, otherwise an IVU should be done 4–6 weeks after recovery. When abnormalities of the urinary tract are found, further investigations and treatment are usually necessary.

Antibiotic regimens for adults are shown in Table 12.5. It is often necessary to start treatment without knowing the organism or its sensitivity and to change the drug, if necessary, when these become available. In most cases oral trimethoprim, ampicillin or amoxycillin, all active against *E. coli*, can be used. Severe or septicaemic cases require intravenous therapy using ampicillin, amoxycillin, an aminoglycoside such as tobramycin or a cephalosporin such as cefuroxime (Table 12.5). Urine culture should be repeated during the course and 7 and 21 days after treatment. Any abnormality of the urinary tract should, if possible, be corrected.

CHRONIC PYELONEPHRITIS

This is a form of chronic interstitial nephritis resulting from recurrent urinary tract infections. The morphological changes in the kidney are not entirely diagnostic, but the most important feature is the presence of coarse scars, each of which is associated with contraction of the related papilla and dilatation of the corresponding calyx. These features can be identified by IVU or radionuclide scanning or on examination of the kidney at operation or autopsy. Histological features are not significantly different from those of chronic ischaemia or non-infective chronic tubulointerstitial nephritis.

The incidence of chronic pyelonephritis is not known. About 20% of patients in Europe requiring treatment for end-stage renal disease are said to have chronic pyelonephritis but the precise diagnostic criteria used are not known so there is doubt about the accuracy of the figures.

Pathogenesis

In the absence of urinary tract abnormalities acute pyelonephritis in patients over the age of five rarely leads to serious chronic renal disease. Possibly the most important predisposing factor is the presence of severe vesico-ureteric reflux (VUR) in children.

Reflux of urine from the bladder into the ureter during voiding is normally prevented because the ureter passes through the vesical wall obliquely and is therefore occluded during contraction of the bladder. Abnormalities of the intramural ureter allow reflux to occur and organisms from the bladder may then reach the kidney. VUR may be unilateral or bilateral, and its severity varies. In mild cases small amounts of urine pass a short distance up the ureter during voiding returning to the bladder after cessation of micturition to form residual urine. In severe cases reflux occurs up the entire length of the ureter (Fig. 12.6); this results in a rise in intrapelvic pressure, the orifices of the compound renal papillae are forced open and urine refluxes into the renal parenchyma as far as the cortex. It is thought that the scars of chronic infective pyelonephritis are due to intraparenchymal reflux, particularly if the urine is infected. VUR is commonly congenital, but can be due to obstructive lesions at the bladder neck. It is thought that it usually occurs in utero, and that the scars of chronic infective pyelo-nephritis form during the first year of life. In young children with recurrent UTI the scars are found in 8–13%, and VUR is usually demonstrable on the side of the scarred kidney. Reflux diminishes as the child grows and usually disappears; it is rarely demonstrable in an adult with a scarred kidney due to infection in childhood. Intrarenal reflux in young children interferes with renal growth.

When UTI occurs in the presence of obstruction or stasis, whatever the cause, permanent damage may result in any age group. In pregnant women permanent damage may result from UTI. The hormonal changes in pregnancy cause reduced ureteric motility and enhanced ureteric dilatation and may also facilitate establishment of infection in the renal parenchyma. About 5% of pregnant women have covert bacteriuria and if no antibiotics are given acute pyelonephritis occurs in up to 40% of such cases; hence the importance of treating asymptomatic bacteriuria in pregnancy.

When scarring has occurred, destruction of renal tissue usually continues despite the absence of recurrent infections. Why this happens is not known. Possible explanations include damage to remaining functioning glomeruli by progressive ischaemia resulting from lesions of blood vessels sustained during acute infections or survival of bacterial variants in the hypertonic medullary tissue.

Pathology

The changes which are not diagnostic may be unilateral or bilateral and of any grade of severity. The fully developed case usually shows gross scarring of the kidneys, which may be much reduced in size with narrowing of the cortex and medulla. Renal scars are juxtaposed to dilated calyces. Histologically there is patchy fibrosis with chronic inflammatory cell infiltration, tubular atrophy, periglomerular fibrosis and eventual disappearance of nephrons. The arteries and arterioles may show sclerosis and narrowing.

Clinical features

In many cases no symptoms arise directly from the renal lesions, and the patient consults the doctor because of lassitude, vague ill-health or symptoms of uraemia or hypertension. Discovery of hypertension or proteinuria on routine examination may be the first indication of the disease. Symptoms arising from the urinary tract may also be present and include frequency of micturition, dysuria and aching lumbar pain. Occasionally weakness and fainting result from salt loss in the urine. Pyuria and a small amount of proteinuria are common, but not invariable.

Investigation

The IVU shows the diagnostic features. The kidneys are reduced in size and there is localised contraction of the renal substance associated with clubbing of the adjacent calyces (Fig. 12.25). Culture of the urine is

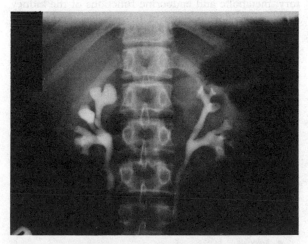

Fig. 12.25   Chronic pyelonephritis. Intravenous urogram revealing clubbing of the calyces particularly marked in the right upper pole. The appearances on the left are virtually normal.

mandatory. When infection is present *E. coli* is the most common organism. Other agents include proteus, *Pseudomonas aeruginosa* and staphylococci. Investigations such as rectal and vaginal examination, cystoscopy and urography are performed to identify any abnormality causing obstruction to the flow of urine. A micturating cystourethrogram will disclose vesico-ureteric reflux. Renal function should be assessed by estimation of the blood urea and creatinine, plasma electrolytes and creatinine clearance. It may be necessary to assess urinary acidification or renal sodium conservation.

Management

Chronic infection is difficult to eradicate. Attempts should be made to correct abnormalities of the urinary tract, including malformations, and to remove calculi. An antibiotic to which the organism is sensitive should be given for seven days. If the infection is not eradicated, suppressive therapy may be required for months (Table 12.5, p. 579) the antibiotic being changed in response to the changing pattern and sensitivity of the organisms. Simple measures outlined in the information box on page 578 should be adopted. Control of hypertension is essential and may delay the onset of uraemia.

When pyonephrosis develops or renal infection is unilateral nephrectomy may be indicated; rarely hypertension is cured by the removal of the diseased kidney. The role of surgery in correction of VUR is limited because childhood reflux tends to disappear spontaneously.

Patients who lose excessive amounts of sodium in the urine develop extracellular fluid depletion which exacerbates their uraemia. These patients benefit from taking 5–10 g/day (85–170 mmol/d) of sodium chloride by mouth. It is usual to start with 3–4 g/day and increase the dose as required. The limit for additional salt is set by development of systemic or pulmonary oedema, or aggravation of hypertension. Sodium bicarbonate may be substituted in part for sodium chloride when acidosis is severe (p. 224).

Severe renal impairment is treated as indicated on page 585.

Course and prognosis

The course is usually long and punctuated by acute exacerbations. Infection is difficult to eradicate even when underlying abnormalities are relieved and in elderly, diabetic or paraplegic patients a fulminating infection may be the terminal event.

Pyonephrosis may occur, especially in the presence of renal calculi. It is characterised by persistent lumbar pain, intermittent pyrexia, rigors, emaciation, pyuria, and, if both kidneys are involved, uraemia; one or both kidneys may become palpable. Some cases of chronic pyelonepthritis progress to chronic renal failure.

RENAL TUBERCULOSIS

Tuberculosis of the kidney is invariably secondary to tuberculosis elsewhere and occurs as a result of blood-borne infection. The initial lesion develops in the renal cortex and if untreated may ulcerate into the pelvis with consequent involvement of the bladder, epididymes, seminal vesicles and prostate. The disease tends to occur in young people and may manifest itself with recurrent haematuria and dysuria due to secondary involvement of the bladder. In addition the general features of tuberculosis, i.e. malaise, fever, lassitude and weight loss, may be present. Chronic renal failure may result from destruction of kidney tissue or be due to obstruction of the urinary tract when lesions heal by fibrosis.

Culture of the urine by ordinary methods may be sterile in spite of pyuria and indeed sterile pyuria is an indication to perform special cultures for tubercle bacilli. The extent of the infection should be ascertained by cystoscopic examination and pyelography. For treatment of TB see Chapter 9, page 367.

CHRONIC RENAL FAILURE

Chronic renal failure is irreversible deterioration in renal function. The ensuing impairment of the excretory, metabolic and endocrine functions of the kidney leads to the development of the clinical syndrome of uraemia. In general it can be assumed that in uraemia metabolic functions are adversely affected. The clinical features are listed in the information box below.

The social and economic consequences of chronic renal failure are considerable. In Britain approximately 55 new patients per million of the adult population are

---

CLINICAL FEATURES OF URAEMIA

- Anaemia
- Metabolic bone disease (renal osteodystrophy)
- Neuropathy
- Myopathy
- Endocrine abnormalities
- Hypertension and atherosclerosis
- Acidosis
- Susceptibility to infection

Table 12.6 Aetiology of chronic renal failure

Congenital and inherited diseases Polycystic kidney disease (infantile or adult) Alport's syndrome Fabry's disease	*Interstitial disease* Chronic infective interstitial nephritis (chronic pyelonephritis) Vesico-ureteric reflux Tuberculosis
Vascular disease Arteriosclerosis Vasculitis (PAN, SLE, scleroderma)	Analgesic nephropathy Nephrocalcinosis Schistosomiasis Unknown origin
Glomerular disease Proliferative GN Crescentic GN Membranous GN Mesangiocapillary GN Glomerulosclerosis Secondary GN (PAN, SLE, amyloidosis, diabetic glomerulosclerosis)	*Obstructive uropathy* Calculus Retroperitoneal fibrosis Prostatic hypertrophy Pelvic tumours Other causes (see Table 12.7)

accepted for long-term dialysis treatment each year. Introduction of dialysis and transplantation has transformed the outlook for such patients and these techniques must be regarded as amongst the most significant medical advances of this century.

Aetiology

Chronic renal failure may be caused by any condition which destroys the normal structure and function of the kidney (Table 12.6). In many patients the condition progresses insidiously over a number of years and frequently it is impossible to determine the underlying renal disease.

Pathogenesis of uraemia

Disturbances in water, electrolytes and acid-base balance undoubtedly contribute to the clinical picture in patients with chronic renal failure but the exact pathogenesis of the clinical syndrome of uraemia is unknown. Almost any substance present in abnormal concentration in the plasma has been suspected of being a 'uraemic toxin'. It is most likely that the syndrome is caused by accumulation in body fluids of a number of substances among which must be included phosphate, parathyroid hormone, urea, creatinine, guanidine, phenols, and indols. There is no satisfactory way of assessing the biological toxicity of different substances but it must be assumed that the uraemic toxins are substances eliminated by the normal kidney and retained in renal failure.

Clinical features

In the early stages of the disease, the patient may be asymptomatic and the existence of renal insufficiency may be revealed by discovery of proteinuria, anaemia, hypertension or a raised blood urea during routine examination. When renal function deteriorates slowly

it is not uncommon for patients to remain asymptomatic until the GFR is 15 ml/min or less. Subsequently, because of the widespread effects of progressive renal failure, symptoms and signs are referable to almost every system and many patients present with complaints which at first sight may not suggest their renal origin. These manifestations are listed in the information box below. None of these symptoms alone is indicative of underlying renal disease but the occurrence of more than one should suggest the possibility of renal failure.

The rate of progression to end-stage renal failure is very variable but inevitably as the disease advances, renal function deteriorates and uraemia increases, the patient looks more ill and the anaemia becomes more severe. With the exception of those who develop cardiac failure and those in whom the chronic stage of glomerular disease follows rapidly upon the initial oedematous stage, the patients are not only free from oedema but may exhibit signs of water and sodium depletion. The skin and tongue are dry and the blood pressure may fall from its previous high value. Acidosis

---

SIGNS AND SYMPTOMS OF URAEMIA

- Vague ill-health
- Generalised weakness and lack of energy
- Breathlessness on exertion
- Anorexia
- Nausea and vomiting, particularly in mornings
- Disordered intestinal motility
- Headaches
- Visual disturbances
- Pruritus
- Pallor
- Pigmentation
- Loss of libido

contributes to the dyspnoea and respirations are deep (Kussmaul's respiration). Later, hiccoughs, pruritus, muscular twitchings, fits, drowsiness and coma ensue.

Anaemia. This is common and to some extent reflects the severity of uraemia. Several factors contribute, including:

1. reduced dietary intake of iron and other haematinics due to anorexia and dietary restrictions;
2. impaired intestinal absorption of iron;
3. diminished erythropoiesis due to toxic effects of uraemia on marrow precursor cells;
4. reduced red cell survival and
5. increased blood loss due to capillary fragility and poor platelet function.

Plasma erythropoietin is usually within the normal range and thus inappropriately low for the degree of anaemia. In patients with polycystic kidneys, anaemia is less severe — possibly because the large kidneys produce more erythropoietin. Treatment is limited to correction of any iron and vitamin deficiency. Human recombinant erythropoietin has been shown to be effective in correcting anaemia but, as yet, this is very expensive and clinical trials are still in progress.

Renal osteodystrophy. This metabolic bone disease which accompanies uraemia, consists of a mixture of osteomalacia, hyperparathyroid bone disease (osteitis fibrosa) (Fig. 12.26), osteoporosis and osteosclerosis. Osteomalacia results from failure of the kidney to convert cholecalciferol to its active metabolite 1,25 dihydroxycholecalciferol. A deficiency of the latter leads to diminished intestinal absorption of calcium, hypocalcaemia and reduction in the calcification of osteoid. Osteitis fibrosa results from secondary hyperparathyroidism, the parathyroid glands being stimulated by the low plasma calcium and possibly also by hyperphosphataemia. In some patients tertiary or autonomous hyperparathyroidism develops. Osteoporosis occurs in many patients possibly related to mild malnutrition. Osteosclerosis is seen mainly in the sacral

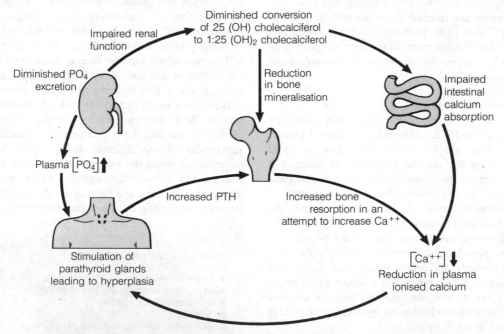

Fig. 12.26 Pathogenesis of renal osteodystrophy. A decreased hydroxylation of cholecalciferol results in a diminution in plasma, 1,25 dihydroxycholecalciferol. The effect of this is to reduce intestinal absorption of calcium resulting in a reduction in the plasma calcium with a consequent stimulation of the parathyroid glands to increase PTH secretion. The increased PTH has an effect on bone by causing increased osteoclastic activity with consequent bone resorption. In addition, the diminished 1,25 dihydroxycholecalciferol results in impaired mineralisation of bone. The nett result is a bone which exhibits increased osteoclastic activity and increased osteoid as a consequence of decreased mineralisation.

area, at the base of the skull and in the vertebrae; the cause of this unusual reaction is not known.

Generalised myopathy. This is due to a combination of poor nutrition, hyperparathyroidism, vitamin D deficiency and disorders of electrolyte metabolism.

Neuropathy. There is a demyelination of medullated fibres, the longer fibres being involved earlier. Sensory neuropathy may cause paraesthesiae and motor neuropathy may present as foot drop. Development of uraemic autonomic neuropathy may in part explain development of disorders of gastrointestinal motility and the onset of postural hypotension in the absence of sodium and water depletion. Clinical manifestations of neuropathy appear very late in the course of chronic renal failure. They improve and may, indeed, resolve when dialysis is started.

Endocrine functions. A number of hormonal abnormalities may be present. In the female, amenorrhoea is common and in both sexes there is loss of libido presumably due to the associated hyperprolactinaemia. Thyroid function is diminished although clinical hypothyroidism is uncommon. Uraemia is frequently mistaken for hypothyroidism.

Cardiovascular disorders. Hypertension develops in approximately 80% of patients with chronic renal failure and must be controlled as it causes further vascular damage thus increasing renal failure. *Atherosclerosis* is common due to abnormalities of lipid and carbohydrate metabolism and may be accelerated by hypertension. Vascular calcification may develop and be sufficiently severe to cause inadequate perfusion of the limbs. *Pericarditis* is very common in untreated end-stage renal failure.

Acidosis. Declining renal function is associated with metabolic acidosis (p. 223) which is commonly asymptomatic. Nevertheless, wherever possible, the plasma bicarbonate should be maintained at or above 18 mmol/l by giving sodium bicarbonate supplements. The dose can only be determined by clinical trial but it is appropriate to commence with 1 g t.d.s. and increase as required up to a total of 12–15 g daily. The dose may be limited by the adverse effect of the sodium which may induce hypertension and/or oedema. In such patients it is worth considering calcium carbonate (up to 9 g daily) as an alternative. Sustained acidosis results in protons being buffered in bone thereby aggravating the uraemic osteodystrophy.

Infections. Both cellular and humoral immunity are impaired and thus increased susceptibility to infection is the rule. Urinary tract infections are very common and must be treated promptly as they may lead to further destruction of functioning renal tissue.

Management

The management of chronic renal failure falls into three distinct parts:

1. Investigations to determine the nature of the underlying renal disease and to detect any reversible factors which are exacerbating the uraemic state.
2. Measures designed to limit adverse effects of loss of renal function and, when possible, to prevent further renal damage.
3. In patients with progressive destruction of renal tissue, there comes a point when supportive measures in the form of either dialysis or transplantation are required.

When the patient first presents a detailed history and physical examination are required with particular attention being paid to the cardiovascular and genitourinary systems. It is important to consider all possible underlying causes and both family history and drug history are important. Wherever possible, the nature of the underlying disease should be determined by undertaking appropriate biochemical, radiological and biopsy investigations (Table 12.1). The degree of functional impairment should be assessed and the extent of any systemic complications documented.

In every case a search must be made for reversible factors correction of which will result in improved renal function. The reversible factors are listed in the information box below.

In patients with established irreversible renal failure a number of measures can be undertaken which will

---

REVERSIBLE FACTORS IN URAEMIA

- Hypertension
- Urinary tract infection
- Urinary tract obstruction
- Reduced renal perfusion
  Sodium and water depletion
  Haemorrhage
  Cardiogenic shock
  Septic shock
- Infections which increase urea production
- Nephrotoxic medications

reduce symptoms and may slow the progression to terminal renal failure.

Hypertension and cardiac failure

Hypertension must be controlled but over-zealous treatment must be avoided and the blood pressure reduced gradually. In the majority of patients, the best results are obtained by maintaining the diastolic pressure in the region of 90 mmHg. Cardiac failure should be treated along the usual lines, great care being taken to modify the dose of any drugs used (p. 601).

Diet

When the plasma creatinine consistently exceeds 300 µmol/l, dietary protein should be restricted in the adult to approximately 40 g daily with an adequate intake of carbohydrate (250 g) and fat (60 g) to provide an energy value of at least 1700 kcal. It is not advisable to reduce the dietary protein intake further except in those patients who are unsuitable for long-term dialysis who should receive 20 g/day.

Fluid

The daily intake will depend on the nature of the underlying disease. Because of the impaired concentrating power, a large volume of urine, about 2.5 l/day, is needed to excrete end-products of metabolism and a fluid intake of 3 l/day is desirable. Fluid restriction is necessary only when the GFR is less than 5 ml/min or cardiac failure is present. Patients with cystic disease, obstructive uropathy or rare tubular lesions who have marked polyuria will require additional fluid.

Electrolytes

In the absence of oedema, cardiac failure or hypertension, sodium restriction is contraindicated. Excessive loss of sodium in the urine (salt-losing nephropathy) occurs in some forms of renal failure but not in chronic glomerular disease. Patients with salt-losing nephropathy readily become depleted of sodium and water, particularly if vomiting and when this occurs fluid and electrolytes must be given intravenously. The volume and nature of the fluid required depends on the severity of the sodium and water depletion (p. 207) and the degree of acidosis (p. 224). Thereafter oral supplements of sodium chloride and sodium bicarbonate are usually required (p. 582).

Generally in patients with glomerular diseases, and/or hypertension, a diet containing about 100 mmol of sodium per day ('no added salt' diet) should be prescribed. When the creatinine clearance has fallen below 10 ml/min, potassium restriction is often required and is achieved by advising the patient to avoid high potassium foods (e.g. bananas, coffee, tomatoes etc.).

Osteodystrophy

The plasma calcium and phosphate concentrations should be kept as near to normal as possible. Hypocalcaemia can be corrected by giving 0.25–1 µg/day of alfacalcidol, a synthetic analogue of vitamin D. The plasma calcium must be monitored regularly and the dose adjusted to avoid hypercalcaemia. Hyperphosphataemia is common and the plasma phosphate can be reduced by the dietary restriction of foods with a high phosphate content (milk, cheese, eggs) and the use of phosphate binding drugs such as aluminium hydroxide (aluminium hydroxide gel 30–60 ml or as capsules 300–600 mg after each meal). Calcium carbonate also has a mild phosphate binding effect. To prevent aluminium toxicity, the dose of aluminium hydroxide should be kept to a minimum and should only be administered immediately before meals.

Hyperparathyroid bone disease responds well to such measures but in severe osteitis fibrosa parathyroidectomy is usually indicated. Osteomalacia is frequently resistant, presumably because of some other inhibitory factors acting on the bone calcification site. The osteoporotic and osteosclerotic components of renal osteodystrophy have no satisfactory treatment.

Replacement of renal function

The excretory function of the kidney can be partially replaced by dialysis. This technique, however, does not replace the endocrine and metabolic functions and this can only be achieved by successful renal transplantation. It is beyond the scope of this text to detail the advantages and disadvantages of these therapeutic options and the reader should refer to specialised texts. The best results are obtained by an integrated approach to management by using the most appropriate form of therapy, haemodialysis, continuous ambulatory peritoneal dialysis or transplantation for the patient depending on the clinical circumstances present.

Haemodialysis. The introduction of regular intermittent haemodialysis has prolonged the lives of many patients with chronic renal failure. Haemodialysis should be started when, despite adequate medical treatment, the symptoms of uraemia have become troublesome, preferably before the patient has developed serious consequences of uraemia. An arteriovenous fistula should be formed, usually in the forearm, when the plasma creatinine is consistently in excess of 600 µmol/l so that there will be time for this to develop before it is required. Due to the increased blood pressure in the veins from the fistula there is distention and thickening of the wall, so called arterialisation, which allows for the repetitive insertion of needles for vascular access for haemodialysis. Once the patient is symptomatic, usually with a creatinine in the region of 1000 µmol/l, regular haemodialysis is started.

Haemodialysis is usually carried out for 4–6 hours 3 times weekly and many patients are trained to carry out their treatment at home. Most patients notice a gradual reduction of their uraemic symptoms during the first 6 weeks of treatment. Plasma creatinine and blood urea, however, do not return to normal, anaemia, although improved, persists, and osteodystrophy may progress. Nevertheless, many patients lead relatively normal and active lives and prolonged survival in excess of 20 years is now regularly reported.

Continuous ambulatory peritoneal dialysis (CAPD). This is a form of long-term dialysis involving insertion of a permanent intraperitoneal catheter into the abdominal cavity. Normally 2 litres of sterile isotonic dialysis fluid are introduced and left for a period of approximately 6 hours. The fluid is then drained and fresh dialysis fluid introduced. This cycle is repeated 4 times daily during which time the patient is fully mobile and able to undertake normal daily tasks. It is particularly useful in young children, in elderly patients with cardiovascular instability and in patients with diabetes mellitus. Its long-term use may be limited by episodes of peritonitis but many patients have now been treated very satisfactorily for periods in excess of 5 years without serious complications.

Renal transplantation. This offers the possibility of restoring normal kidney function and thereby correcting the many metabolic abnormalities of uraemia. The graft is usually taken from a cadaver donor or from a sibling or a parent. ABO compatibility is essential and it is customary to select donor kidneys on the basis of HLA compatibility. Results of transplantation have improved significantly in the past few years. The 3-year graft survival is now in the region of 70–80% while 3-year patient survival is approximately 90%. Long-term immunosuppressive therapy, however, is required. Many therapeutic regimens have been used but the most common involves a combination of prednisone and azathioprine. The prednisone is commenced at a dose of 60 mg daily reducing over 10 days to 30 mg daily and eventually after approximately 3–4 months to 10–15 mg daily. Azathioprine is usually given in a dose of 2 mg/kg/day but this may require reduction if there is any evidence of marrow suppres-

sion. Recently, cyclosporin has been introduced and this is of particular value in the first 3 months following transplantation; immediately post-transplant cyclosporin is commenced at a dose of 10–15 mg/kg/day in 2 divided doses 12 hours apart. The dose is gradually reduced in the following 3 months to 3–6 mg/kg/day. There is concern about the long-term nephrotoxicity of cyclosporin and many centres routinely convert patients to conventional therapy with prednisone and azathioprine 6 months post-transplant.

Immunosuppression is associated with an increased incidence of infections, particularly opportunistic infections, and a greatly increased incidence of malignant neoplasm, especially of skin; approximately 50% of patients will have some skin malignancy by 15 years post transplant. Nonetheless, transplantation does offer the best hope of complete rehabilitation and is the most cost effective of all the options.

Prognosis

Unless some form of supportive therapy such as dialysis or transplantation is available chronic renal failure is eventually fatal. When the plasma creatinine persistently exceeds 300 µmol/l there is usually progressive deterioration in renal function, irrespective of aetiology. The rate of deterioration is very variable from patient to patient, in part related to the aetiology and to development of hypertension, but it is relatively constant for any particular patient. A plot of the logarithm of the plasma creatinine concentration against time allows the physician to determine when the plasma creatinine will reach a value in the region of 1000 µmol/l and dialysis will be required. Such a plot will also detect any unexpected worsening of the renal failure (Fig. 12.27).

Information about the long-term prognosis for patients on dialysis or following transplantation is limited because these techniques have been available only for the past 30 years and technology is changing rapidly. CAPD has been available for less than 10 years and so no long-term information is available. Nevertheless, dialysis and transplantation can be considered as highly effective forms of treatment with a 5-year survival of approximately 80% for home haemodialysis, 65% for a transplanted kidney, 55% for hospital haemodialysis and 45% for CAPD. These figures are not directly comparable because of patient selection and the fact that many older patients and those with systemic disease (e.g. diabetes mellitus) are treated by CAPD. However, they can be used as a guide and clearly indicate how the outlook of end-stage renal disease is very much better than in many other potentially fatal diseases such as carcinoma.

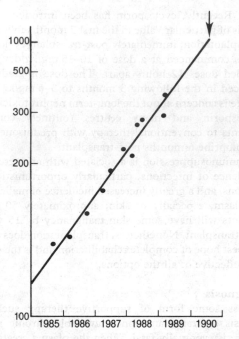

Fig. 12.27 Plot of logarithm of serum creatinine (µmol/l) against time in progressive renal failure. Serial serum creatinine estimations plotted on a reciprocal graph demonstrating a steady deterioration in renal function over a four-year period and projecting forward to indicate that a serum creatinine of 1000 µmol/l is likely to be achieved in mid 1990.

ACUTE RENAL FAILURE

Acute renal failure (ARF) is characterised by an acute and usually reversible deterioration of renal function which develops over a period of days, or, rarely, weeks and results in uraemia. A marked reduction in urine volume is usual but not invariable. The clinical features are determined by the underlying condition and by the rapidly developing uraemia and patients may present complex problems of diagnosis and management. Many of the disorders giving rise to acute renal failure carry a high mortality but, if the patient survives, renal function usually returns to normal or near normal. The classification is given in the information box (left). Prompt identification of the cause of prerenal or postrenal ARF and institution of appropriate treatment will often restore renal function. The longer the period of inadequate perfusion or obstruction the more likely it is that actual damage to kidney tissue will occur.

ACUTE RENAL FAILURE DUE TO PRERENAL DISORDER

Pathogenesis
The kidneys receive approximately 25% of the cardiac output at rest and if cardiac output falls, regional vasoconstriction occurs limiting the blood flow to organs other than the heart and brain. Initially skin blood flow is diminished and this is followed by reduction in perfusion of the gastrointestinal tract and muscles. When the renal blood supply is restricted glomerular filtration is reduced by selective cortical vasoconstriction and oliguria results. The causes of prerenal ARF are listed in the information box below.

CLASSIFICATION OF ACUTE RENAL FAILURE

- In prerenal ARF the kidneys are inadequately perfused and the GFR greatly diminished. This may be due to cardiac failure, vascular disease limiting renal blood flow, or underfilling of the vascular bed due to haemorrhage, severe fluid depletion or vasodilatation resulting from sepsis
- Renal causes of ARF include diseases of the renal arterioles, the rapidly progressing types of glomerulonephritis, injury to tubular cells (acute tubular necrosis) by toxins or ischaemia, intraluminal obstruction of nephrons from precipitation of crystals or protein and acute interstitial nephritis due to infections or drug reactions
- Postrenal ARF is caused by obstruction of the urinary tract at any point in its course

---

THE MOST IMPORTANT CAUSES OF PRERENAL ARF

Reduced circulating blood volume
Haemorrhage from any cause including complications of pregnancy, trauma and gastrointestinal bleeding
Loss of plasma as in burns and crushing injuries
Sodium and water depletion (p. 206)
  From the gastrointestinal tract in severe vomiting, diarrhoea, acute intestinal obstruction, paralytic ileus, pancreatitis, fistulae, etc.
  In urine due to excessive treatment with diuretics, diabetic ketoacidosis, etc.
  From the skin due to sweating
  Into soft tissues or body cavities

Reduction of cardiac output
Myocardial failure (cardiogenic shock) or increase in the size of the vascular bed (septic shock)

Intravascular haemolysis or rhabdomyolysis
Breakdown of skeletal muscle (due to the toxic effects on the kidney of released globins)

Diseases of the major renal vessels which result in renal underperfusion
e.g. thrombosis of the arteries, occlusive embolus of the aorta or of renal arteries, aortic aneurysm

Clinical features

Patients often present with low blood pressure and poor peripheral perfusion. However, renal vasoconstriction and prerenal ARF may occur without systemic hypotension. The cause is usually obvious but concealed blood loss can occur into the gut, following trauma (particularly with fractures of the pelvis or femur) and into the uterus. It is also difficult to assess the loss of intravascular fluid into tissues after crushing injuries or in severe inflammatory dermatoses. The diagnostic features are given in the information box below.

THE DIAGNOSIS OF PRERENAL ACUTE RENAL FAILURE

- A compatible history
- The clinical findings
- A progressive increase in blood urea and plasma creatinine
- Urine osmolality >600 mOsm/kg, urine sodium <20 mmol/l, urine/plasma urea ratio of >10:1

The urinary findings depend on the kidney's ability to respond to inadequate perfusion by intense conservation of sodium and water. They will therefore not be found in patients with pre-existing renal impairment.

Management

The cause of the disorder must be established and corrected. When hypovolaemia or septic shock is present the circulation must be restored as rapidly as possible by replacing blood, plasma or sodium and water as indicated and by judicious use of inotropic drugs. It is often necessary to monitor central venous or pulmonary wedge pressure to determine the rate of administration of fluid and/or inotropes. Occasionally more sophisticated monitoring is necessary to enable the cardiac output and systemic vascular resistance to be calculated.

Prognosis

Provided treatment is instituted early, restitution of renal blood flow is usually accompanied by a return of renal function. If oliguria persists in spite of restoration of the circulation to normal then the reversible structural changes of acute tubular necrosis are likely to have developed. In a few cases, particularly those complicated by disseminated intravascular coagulation (DIC) (p. 757), irreversible cortical necrosis may occur.

ACUTE RENAL FAILURE DUE TO INTRINSIC RENAL DISEASE

The most common cause of this condition is acute tubular necrosis due to acute ischaemia or to the effects of toxic agents such as drugs (p. 600) or bacterial endotoxins. In addition, ARF sometimes develops in conditions which affect the intrarenal arteries and arterioles such as hypersensitivity vasculitis, accelerated hypertension and DIC. A number of glomerular diseases such as crescentic nephritis or focal necrotising proliferative glomerulonephritis also produce acute deterioration in renal function and there is now good evidence that acute tubulo-interstitial nephritis (p. 592), causes ARF.

ACUTE TUBULAR NECROSIS

There are two varieties of acute tubular necrosis, the more common ischaemic type and one caused by bacterial or chemical toxins. Although the aetiology of acute ischaemic tubular necrosis varies, the common factor is a diminution in the supply of oxygen and nutrients to the metabolically active tubular cells. This results in eventual cessation of cell function and patchy necrosis. Fortunately, tubular cells can regenerate and reform the basement membrane. Thus, providing the patient can be kept alive during the regeneration phase, kidney function usually returns to near normal values.

Pathogenesis

The initial insult causes disruption of the cell membrane leading to intracellular anoxia and consequently to a rapid influx of calcium ions. This disturbs mitochondrial respiration, leading to anaerobic glycolysis and intracellular acidosis. If this process continues it causes denaturation of intracellular protein, lysozomal disruption and cell death. Small focal breaks in the tubular basement membrane then develop, and tubular contents escape into the interstitial tissue.

During shock, renal blood flow is greatly reduced. Measurements made during the established phase of acute renal failure (oliguric phase) indicate that when the circulation is restored in shocked patients, renal blood flow remains about 20% of normal until the onset of recovery. During the oliguric phase there is also significant selective reduction in cortical blood flow due in part to interstitial oedema and in part to swelling of the endothelial cells of glomeruli and peritubular capillaries, resulting in an increase in vascular resistance. Cortical blood flow may be further reduced by local and systemic vasoconstrictors such as thromboxane, vasopressin, noradrenaline and angio-

---

FACTORS CONTRIBUTING TO PERSISTENT OLIGURIA IN ACUTE RENAL FAILURE

- Reduced glomerular perfusion and glomerular permeability limit the rate of filtrate formation
- Tubular lumina may be obstructed by casts composed of necrotic tubular cells and Tamm Horsfall protein and by external compression due to raised intrarenal pressure from interstitial oedema
- Disruption of the tubular basement membrane allows back diffusion of tubular fluid into the interstitial space
- Glomerular coagulation with micro-thrombi

---

tensin II. The effects of some of these are probably counterbalanced by the action of intrarenal vasodilator prostaglandins. Factors that contribute to oliguria are listed in the information box above.

It is likely that all these mechanisms have some part to play in the pathogenesis of the oliguric phase although their relative importance may vary depending on the nature of the primary insult.

After a period of about 10–20 days, renal function returns. There is often a transient diuretic phase during which the urine output increases rapidly and remains excessive for several days before returning to normal. This is due in part to dissipation of the normal medullary concentration gradient during the period of oliguria. Maintenance of the medullary gradient depends not only on tubular transport but also on the continued delivery of filtrate to the ascending limb of the loop. Both factors are disturbed during the acute phase of ARF; the medullary concentration gradient is gradually 'washed out' and is not re-established until glomerular filtration and tubular function are are least partly restored. Not all patients exhibit the diuretic phase which is to some extent dependent on the severity of the renal damage and the rate of recovery.

Pathology
The appearances depend on the stage of the illness. In established cases, the kidneys may be enlarged and the cortex paler than normal. Histologically the glomeruli appear relatively normal, although on electron microscopy there may be endothelial cell swelling and some fibrin deposition. The most obvious abnormality is the presence of scattered breaks in tubular basement membranes, sometimes associated with visible necrosis of associated tubular cells. Actual tubular cell necrosis is surprisingly insignificant but many tubules are lined by swollen vacuolated cells. Late in the disorder the tubular epithelial cells appear flattened, and during the regenerative phase there may be evidence of mitotic activity. There is frequently interstitial oedema and infiltration with macrophages, plasma cells and a few polymorphs. In cases where the condition has been caused by drugs, the interstitial inflammatory appearances are more marked, and constitute an acute tubulointerstitial nephritis (p. 592).

Clinical features
These are those of the causal condition together with those of rapidly developing uraemia. In many patients, there is an obvious underlying cause such as trauma or septicaemia. In the majority of patients the urine volume is reduced to between 50 and 500 ml daily; anuria (urine volume less than 50 ml daily) is rare and usually indicates acute urinary tract obstruction. In about 20% of cases the urine volume is normal or increased but the quality is very poor due to a low GFR and a gross reduction of tubular function. Thus excretion is inadequate despite an apparently good urine output, the blood urea and plasma creatinine rise and the clinical picture of uraemia develops. The rate at which the blood urea and creatinine rise is determined by the rate of tissue breakdown. In patients who are suffering from severe infections or who have undergone major surgery or trauma the daily increment in blood urea usually exceeds 5 mmol/l. Disturbances of water, electrolyte and acid-base balance arise as a consequence of loss of kidney function. Hyperkalaemia is common particularly when there is massive tissue breakdown, haemolysis or metabolic acidosis and since it predisposes to ventricular arrhythmias must be promptly controlled. Patients may present with dilutional hyponatraemia, having received inappropriate amounts of intravenous fluid or having continued to drink freely despite oliguria. Hypocalcaemia, due to reduced renal production of 1,25 dihydroxycholecalciferol is common. Metabolic acidosis develops unless there has been excessive vomiting or aspiration of gastric contents.

At first the patient may feel well but after some days if treatment is inadequate, features of uraemia appear. Initially these are anorexia, nausea and vomiting. Apathy is followed by mental confusion and later muscular twitching, fits, drowsiness, coma and bleeding episodes occur. The respiratory rate is often increased due to acidosis, pulmonary oedema or respiratory infection. Pulmonary oedema may result from administration of excessive amounts of fluids. However, there is evidence that the pulmonary capillary permeability is increased in uraemia. Moreover damage to pulmonary capillaries which occurs during shock also predisposes to development of pulmonary oedema (adult respiratory distress syndrome, p. 353). Anaemia, which is common, may be due to excessive blood loss, haemolysis or decreased erythropoiesis.

Many patients have an increased bleeding tendency due to disordered platelet function and disturbances of the coagulation cascade. Gastrointestinal haemorrhage may occur, often late in the illness, from mucosal erosions throughout the length of the gastrointestinal tract. Severe infections often complicate the course of ARF because humoral and cellular immune mechanisms are depressed by uraemia.

Management
The principles are listed below:

Emergency resuscitative measures
Hyperkalaemia ($K^+ > 6$ mmol/l) must be corrected to prevent life-threatening cardiac arrhythmias (p. 219). Rapid reduction can be achieved by intravenous glucose (50 ml 50% dextrose); it is not essential to add insulin unless the patient is known to have diabetes mellitus. Correction of acidosis with intravenous sodium bicarbonate will also reduce the plasma potassium. Calcium chloride can be given intravenously for its membrane stabilising effect if cardiac arrhythmias are anticipated. Exchange resins (calcium resonium 50 g) can be given orally or rectally, their action is somewhat delayed and they are thus of use only as prophylaxis. The circulating blood volume must be corrected by prompt transfusion with appropriate fluids and this often requires monitoring of central venous or pulmonary wedge pressure. Patients who present with severe pulmonary oedema usually require haemodialysis or peritoneal dialysis to remove sodium and water.

Determination of the cause of ARF
In many cases the underlying cause is obvious. When this is not the case a wide range of investigations, including renal biopsy, may be needed to establish the diagnosis.

General management of the oliguric phase
In established acute renal failure, the main aims are to control fluid and electrolyte balance, maintain nutrition, control the disordered chemistry and protect the patient from infection. Patients with severe acute renal failure are seriously ill and require skilled nursing, preferably in single rooms designed to prevent cross-infection. Particular attention must be paid to the care of the skin and the mouth, and to prevention of infection of in-dwelling intravascular lines. Plasma urea, creatinine and electrolytes should be estimated and cultures of blood, urine and wounds carried out daily. Great care must be exercised in the use of drugs. In all but the mildest cases some form of dialysis will be required.

Fluid and electrolyte balance
Following initial resuscitation, the patient should be maintained on a daily fluid intake equal to the volume of the urine output plus 400 ml to balance (insensible loss–water of oxidation). Febrile patients require an increased allowance. As no electrolytes are lost the intake of these substances should be minimal but should abnormal losses of fluid occur, as in diarrhoea, additional fluid and electrolytes will be required. If possible the patient should be weighed daily. Large changes in body weight, or development of oedema, or, alternatively, of signs of water or electrolyte depletion, indicate the need for a reappraisal of water and electrolyte intake.

Protein and energy
In patients in whom it is hoped to avoid dialysis, dietary protein is restricted to about 40 g/day and attempts made to suppress endogenous protein catabolism to a minimum by giving as much energy as possible in the form of fat and carbohydrate. For this purpose a diet restricted in protein and electrolyte content may be supplemented by preparations containing glucose polymers. In the event of severe anorexia or vomiting, oral intake should be stopped and parenteral nutrition given (p. 74). Patients treated by dialysis may have a more liberal intake of nitrogen. In hypercatabolic patients it is often necessary to resort to parenteral nutrition in order to maintain a suitable intake of energy and nitrogen. This usually involves giving a greater volume of fluid than would be required to maintain water balance and consequently more frequent dialysis or haemofiltration may be necessary.

Dialysis
It is generally agreed that the blood urea should be kept below 30 mmol/l during an episode of ARF; when this cannot be achieved by dietary measures some form of dialysis is essential. In patients in whom the blood urea is rising rapidly early haemodialysis is required.

Haemodialysis is effective in correcting the metabolic abnormalities but requires vascular access, cardiovascular stability and adequate blood pressure. The frequency with which haemodialysis is undertaken depends upon the rate of increase of blood urea. Haemofiltration is a technique similar to haemodialysis which is better tolerated particularly by patients with cardiovascular instability. A new technique of continuous spontaneous arteriovenous haemofiltration has been introduced where a highly permeable membrane filter is employed to remove an ultrafiltrate of plasma which is replaced by reinfusing an appropriate volume of modified Ringer lactate solution. This technique is employed on a 24-hour basis and is of particular value in those patients who require long-term parenteral nutrition.

Peritoneal dialysis also is an effective means of correcting fluid balance and the metabolic disturbances in all but the most severe cases. It is particularly useful in small children and patients with cardiovascular disturbances.

Recovery phase

After approximately 10–20 days, renal function returns. In a number of patients there is the rapid onset of a diuretic phase when the urine output is frequently 3–5 litres daily. This diuretic phase persists for 3–4 days and during this time the concentration of blood urea tends to remain constant whereas the creatinine may fall slowly. Sufficient fluid must be given to replace the loss of water in the urine and frequently intravenous fluids are required. Supplements of sodium chloride and sodium bicarbonate are usually needed during the diuretic phase to compensate for increased urinary loss; potassium salts may also be required. After a few days the urine volume returns to normal as the concentrating mechanism is restored. This is associated with a gradual return of the ability to conserve sodium and potassium and regenerate bicarbonate. The blood urea and plasma creatinine return to normal and the patient can start on a normal diet.

Prognosis

The high mortality rate from acute ischaemic renal failure has been greatly reduced by the measures described above. Prognosis depends on the speed and efficiency with which these are put into operation, on the prompt recognition and effective treatment of complicating infection and on the nature and severity of the causal disorder. In cases of uncomplicated acute renal failure such as those due to simple haemorrhage, the mortality should now be negligible even when haemodialysis is required. In severe renal failure, complicated by serious infection or multiple injuries, it is still about 70%, the outcome being determined by the severity of the underlying disorder and by any complications rather than by the renal failure itself. Infection or gastrointestinal haemorrhage increase the mortality significantly.

OTHER CAUSES OF ARF

When acute renal failure arises as a result of renal disease other than acute tubular necrosis the clinical picture is that of the underlying condition complicated by the features of acute uraemia. Frequently the

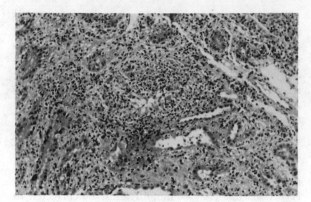

Fig. 12.28   Interstitial nephritis. Widespread interstitial infiltrate of inflammatory cells producing considerable destruction of normal architecture.

diagnosis is not immediately obvious and renal biopsy must be performed to define the nature of the pathology. Management is along the lines already discussed, but in addition specific treatment of the underlying renal disease may be required. Thus steroids, immunosuppressive drugs and rarely plasma exchange may be of value in acute renal failure due to hypersensitivity vasculitis (p. 575) and crescentic glomerulonephritis (p. 570). Control of blood pressure is critical when acute renal failure is due to accelerated hypertension.

Acute tubulo-interstitial nephritis

This is a well recognised cause of acute renal failure. It results most commonly from hypersensitivity to drugs such as penicillin, ampicillin, sulphonamides or rifampicin and other manifestations of hypersensitivity such as fever, arthralgia, rashes, marrow depression, eosinophilia and disturbance of liver function may be present. Renal biopsy usually shows an acute tubulo-interstitial nephritis associated with inflammatory cells, including eosinophils (Fig. 12.28).

POSTRENAL ACUTE RENAL FAILURE

Acute renal failure may result from obstruction (p. 593) at any point in the urinary tract. In the presence of two functioning kidneys, ureteric obstruction causes uraemia only when it is bilateral. The diagnosis may be suggested by a history of previous urinary symptoms such as loin pain, haematuria, renal colic, nocturia or difficulty in micturition. Often, however, the onset is clinically silent and the cause of obstruction discovered only after appropriate investigation. In contrast to the oliguria associated with tubular necrosis, anuria is common and is always suggestive of an obstructive cause. In patients with anuria U/S examination of both kidneys and ureters should be done as soon as possible. When pelvic or ureteric dilatation is found, percutaneous nephrostomy can be undertaken to decompress the urinary system (p. 594). Dialysis can, thereby, usually be avoided. Antegrade pyelography may reveal the cause of the obstruction. Alternatively cystoscopy and retrograde pyelography can be done. In a number of instances obstruction is caused by a malignant pelvic neoplasm such as carcinoma of the cervix or of the recto-sigmoid junction which may be palpable on rectal or vaginal examination. Unfortunately the disease is often so advanced that active intervention is seldom advisable.

When the obstruction has been relieved and the blood chemistry has returned to near normal the underlying cause must be defined and treated (p. 594).

OBSTRUCTION OF THE URINARY TRACT

Obstruction to the flow of urine from the kidney is a common disorder; it causes stasis and an increase in pressure above the obstruction which in turn predispose to infection, stone formation and renal failure. Obstruction may occur at any level but is most common at the pelvi-ureteric junction, at the bladder neck or in the urethra (Fig. 12.29). Obstruction at the pelvi-ureteric junction causes hydronephrosis; obstruction of the ureter hydroureter and subsequently hydronephrosis. Obstruction of the bladder neck or urethra distends the bladder, causes hypertrophy of its muscle, seen on cystoscopic examination as trabeculation, and subsequently leads to hydroureter and

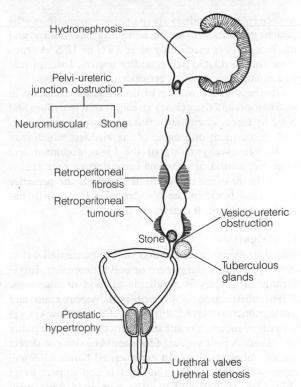

Fig. 12.29   Obstruction of the urinary tract. Obstruction to the urinary tract can arise at the pelviureteric junction, in the ureter, at the vesicoureteric junction, at bladder outflow and also in the urethra.

hydronephrosis. If obstruction is unrelieved, slow progressive destruction of renal tissue occurs. Superimposed infection often results in rapid deterioration of renal function.

Aetiology
Obstruction may be due to an organic lesion or to a congenital neuromuscular defect which prevents the contraction wave and thus the flow of urine (Table 12.7).

Clinical features
These vary with the cause and site of the lesion. When the obstruction is supravesical renal colic may occur, especially if the onset is sudden. More commonly the obstruction is gradual and aching pain in the loins, sometimes aggravated by drinking, develops. Superimposed infection causes malaise, fever, dysuria and sometimes septicaemia. Haematuria is common. In partial obstruction transmission of the increased hydrostatic pressure to the kidney interferes with the counter-current concentrating mechanism and, paradoxically, may result in polyuria. Occasionally a

Table 12.7   Important causes of urinary tract obstruction

Organic	
Lumen	Stone, blood clot, caseous or necrotic debris
	Sloughed papilla
Wall	Tumour
	Fibrosis following trauma, stone, instrumentation, surgery or infection (TB, schistosomiasis, gonorrhoea)
	Congenital bladder neck obstruction
	Urethral valves
External	Aberrant renal artery crossing upper ureter
	Retroperitoneal tumour
	Retroperitoneal fibrosis (idiopathic, leaking aortic aneurysm, drug induced, neoplastic)
	Prostatic enlargement
	Phimosis
	Accidental ligation of ureter at operation
Functional	Congenital neuromuscular defects (pelvi-ureteric junction, ureter, bladder neck)

hydronephrotic kidney is palpable. Sometimes the patient presents with anuria and acute renal failure, and the diagnosis is made only after IVU or U/S examination reveals dilated pelves and/or ureters. Intermittent anuria suggests stone or retroperitoneal fibrosis.

Obstruction below the bladder causes difficulty in micturition and the urinary stream is thin in calibre and poor in force. Complete urinary retention may occur with consequent distension of the bladder, which may be visible as a swelling of the lower abdomen and palpable; anuria or overflow incontinence may ensue. In the latter event catheterisation reveals the presence of residual urine in the bladder after the patient has voided. Infection is extremely common.

Investigation

Rectal or vaginal examination should be carried out to detect prostatic enlargement or pelvic neoplasm. Intravenous urography is a reliable method of diagnosis. When obstruction is present both nephrogram and pyelogram are delayed; dilatation of the outflow system is easily seen, and the site of obstruction usually readily identified. A post voiding film should be done to detect bladder abnormalities. In experienced hands U/S will detect dilatation of the renal pelvis and upper ureter (Fig. 12.8, p. 559) and may be combined with antegrade pyelography to identify the site of the lesion. It is particularly valuable when acute renal failure is present (p. 593) or IVU is contraindicated. Neither U/S nor IVU can distinguish a distended tract in which there is no resistance to flow (e.g. after pregnancy) from genuine urinary tract obstruction but this may often be achieved by diuretic renogram (Fig. 12.11, p. 560).

Cystoscopy, retrograde pyelography, urethrography and cystometry may be required to define lesions in the bladder, urethra or lower ureter or for removal of stones or debris from the ureter or bladder.

Culture of urine and, where appropriate, of the blood should be carried out. Assessment of overall renal function is essential and in some cases, special tests of tubular function are indicated to assess the ability to acidify the urine (p. 554) or conserve sodium or potassium.

Management

The ultimate objective is to remove the source of obstruction but in order to preserve renal function, relieve symptoms and treat infection temporary drainage of the urinary tract may be required. Intravesical obstruction should be relieved using a urethral or, rarely, a suprapubic catheter. Recent complete obstruction of the upper tract is to be treated by insertion of a catheter into the renal pelvis under U/S control. In a few cases relief of obstruction is followed by massive diuresis due to impaired tubular function and to the osmotic effect of retained solute and water, and electrolyte losses must be replaced intravenously. When obstruction is incomplete or due to stones or debris likely to be passed spontaneously, temporary drainage is rarely necessary unless infection supervenes. Antibiotics are required to treat severe infection or to cover surgical procedures. Dialysis may be necessary before surgery.

Once the underlying lesion has been identified and renal function assessed definitive treatment is often possible, e.g. removal of stone, transurethral resection of the prostate. When obstruction is irremediable the ureters may be anastomosed to an isolated loop of ileum opening on to the abdominal wall or stents left in the ureters. Patients who have undergone treatment for urinary tract obstruction should thereafter have periodic assessment of renal function. Irremediable damage to one kidney is an indication for nephrectomy. When both kidneys are permanently damaged treatment for chronic renal failure is required (p. 585).

RENAL AND VESICAL CALCULI AND NEPHROCALCINOSIS

Aetiology

Renal calculi consist of aggregates of crystals and small amounts of proteins and glycoprotein but their genesis is poorly understood. In Britain, stones in which the crystalline component consists of calcium oxalate are the most common and accounted for 39% of 1000 calculi analysed in a London series. In this series 14% of stones contained both calcium oxalate and calcium phosphate, 13% calcium phosphate alone and 15.4% magnesium ammonium phosphate. Small numbers of cystine stones and uric acid stones were found. Different types of stone occur in different parts of the world and dietary factors probably play a part in determining the varying patterns. In developing countries bladder stones are common particularly in children whereas in industrialised developed countries the incidence of childhood bladder stone is low and renal stones in adults more common. A recent Scottish survey found that 4% of the population has stones in the urinary tract but prevalence varies in different areas. It is surprising that stones and nephrocalcinosis are not more common since some of the constituents are present in urine in concentrations which exceed their maximum solubility in water. However, urine contains glycoaminoglycans, pyrophosphate and citrate

CONDITIONS ASSOCIATED WITH STONE FORMATION

Obstruction of urinary tract	Formation of calcium phosphate stones
Infection of urinary tract	Formation of magnesium ammonium phosphate stones
Climate or occupation giving rise to excessive sweating	Formation of stones due to high concentration of salts in reduced volume of urine resulting in precipitation
Hypercalciuria	Formation of calcium phosphate and calcium oxalate stones
Hyperoxaluria	Formation of calcium oxalate stones
Inherited disorders	
Cystinuria	Formation of cystine stones
Xanthinuria	Formation of xanthine stones
Gout, myeloproliferative disorders	Formation of uric acid stones
Medullary sponge kidney	Formation of stones – usually calcium phosphate

which, by forming complexes, may keep otherwise insoluble salts in solution. Certain conditions are frequently associated with stone formation and these are listed in the information box above.

The pH of urine influences the formation of stones. An alkaline urine tends to increase precipitation of calcium phosphate and may be responsible for calcium phosphate stones in patients with renal tubular acidosis whereas solubility of uric acid and cystine is reduced in acid urine. Today, in prosperous countries most calculi occur in healthy young men in whom investigations reveal no clear cause for stone formation. Multiple aetiological factors are probably present in such cases, and an alteration in the relative proportions of crystalloids and glycoaminoglycans in the urine may be of particular importance.

Pathology

Urinary concretions vary greatly in size. There may be particles like sand anywhere in the urinary tract or large round stones in the bladder. Staghorn calculi fill the whole renal pelvis and branch into the calyces (Fig. 12.30); they are usually associated with pyelone-

phritis. Deposits of calcium may be present throughout the renal parenchyma, giving rise to nephrocalcinosis (Fig. 12.5). This is especially liable to occur in chronic pyelonephritis, renal tubular acidosis, hyperparathyroidism, vitamin D intoxication and healed renal tuberculosis.

Clinical features

These vary according to the size, shape and position of the stone, and the nature of any underlying condition. Renal calculi or nephrocalcinosis may be present for years without giving rise to symptoms and may be discovered during radiological examination for another disorder. More commonly patients present with pain, recurrent urinary infection or clinical features of urinary tract obstruction. The most common complaint arising from renal calculi is intermittent dull pain in the loin or back, increased by movement. From time to time protein, red cells or leucocytes appear in the urine.

When a stone becomes impacted in the ureter an attack of renal colic develops. The patient is suddenly aware of pain in the loin, which soon radiates round the flank to the groin and often into the testis or labium in

CONDITIONS ASSOCIATED WITH HYPERCALCIURIA AND HYPEROXALURIA

Hypercalciuria
High dietary intake calcium (dairy produce)
Hyperparathyroidism
Vitamin D poisoning
Sarcoidosis
Cushing's syndrome
Myelomatosis
Renal tubular acidosis
Prolonged immobilisation
'Idiopathic' hypercalciuria
a) excessive absorption of calcium from gut
b) reduced renal tubular absorption of filtered calcium

Hyperoxaluria
High dietary intake (fruit and vegetables)
Increased absorption of oxalate from gut
a) ileal disease
b) low calcium diet

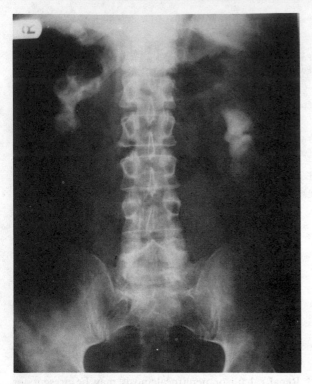

Fig. 12.30   Bilateral staghorn calculi.

the sensory distribution of the first lumbar nerve. The pain steadily increases in intensity to reach a maximum in a few minutes. The patient is restless, and generally tries unsuccessfully to obtain relief by changing position and by pacing the room. There is pallor, sweating and often vomiting, and the patient may groan in agony. Frequency, dysuria and haematuria may occur.

The intense pain usually subsides within 2 hours but may continue unabated for hours or days. The pain is usually constant during attacks, though slight fluctuations in severity may occur. Contrary to general belief, attacks rarely consist of intermittent severe pains coming and going every few minutes.

Investigation

The diagnosis of renal colic is usually easily made from the history and by finding red cells in the urine. Any patient suspected of having stones should have X-rays of the urinary tract. If there is doubt about the cause of pain an IVU during an attack may help. When the pain is due to a stone in the ureter, the radiograph shows a dense renal shadow and appearance of dye in the renal pelvis is delayed. Subsequently the site of obstruction may be visible. Appropriate investigations (Table 12.8) should be undertaken to discover any underlying disorder.

Management

The immediate treatment of loin pain or renal colic is bed-rest, application of warmth to the site of pain, and administration of analgesics, e.g. pethidine (100 mg), morphine (15–30 mg) and antispasmodic drugs, e.g. atropine sulphate (0.8 or 1.2 mg). These are given intramuscularly and may be repeated once after 2 hours. Diclofenac suppositories (100 mg) may be given as an alternative. If possible the patient should drink 2 l/day of fluid.

Small stones, less than 0.5 cm in diameter, are usually passed naturally, larger stones may require active intervention. Immediate action is required if anuria, infection or hydronephrosis develops. Indications for intervention are given in the information box below. Attempts to dissolve calculi have failed, but in a few centres a lithotripter is available, and using this apparatus, many calculi can be fragmented, in vivo, by shock waves, generated under water, focused on the stone, and applied to the body surface. The fragments are then passed in the urine. This technique requires free drainage of the tract below the stones. Stones in the renal pelvis can be removed by open operation, removed endoscopically via percutaneous nephrostomy or fragmented using the lithotripter. Ureteric stones can be removed endoscopically via the bladder or a percutaneous nephrostomy, or can be pushed up into the renal pelvis and removed through a nephrostomy or disintegrated by lithotripsy. Bladder stones are removed or fragmented during cystoscopy; rarely cystotomy is needed to remove large stones. Antibiotic cover should be given for stone removal.

A daily urine output of at least 3 l is advisable in all patients with stone disease hence the fluid intake should be about 4 l/day – more if the climate or the patient's occupation causes much sweating.

Suitable measures should be instituted to correct any known cause of stone formation. Preparations contain-

---

INDICATIONS FOR INTERVENTION IN RENAL CALCULI

- The patient is anuric*
- The ureter or pelvi-ureteric junction is obstructed, totally* or partially, by a stone unlikely to pass spontaneously or one which has not moved for several weeks
- Infection is present*
- The patient has intolerable or recurrent pain

*Indications for urgent intervention

Table 12.8 Investigation of patients with renal calculi

Investigation of urinary tract	Examination urine for protein r.b.c, w.b.c.	Indicates abnormality of urinary tract
	Quantitative culture MSU	Urinary infection
	Plain film abdomen	Shows opaque calculi, nephrocalcinosis
	IVU	Shows all calculi obstruction, abnormalities urinary tract, e.g. medullary sponge kidney
Investigation of renal function	Blood urea, plasma creatinine	
	Creatinine clearance	
Investigation to determine underlying cause	Chemical analysis calculus	Provides information as to what investigations to pursue
	Plasma calcium, phosphate	Hypercalcaemia
	Plasma PTH	If hypercalcaemia present to investigate possible hyperparathyroidism
	24 h urine calcium ($\times$ 2)	Hypercalciuria
	Plasma urate	In patients with urate stones or calcium stones
	24 h urine urate ($\times$ 2)	
	24 h urine cystine ($\times$ 2)	In patients with cystine stones
	24 h urine oxalate ($\times$ 2)	Hyperoxaluria
	Acidification of urine (p. 554)	Distal renal tubular acidosis

ing vitamin D must be avoided. In idiopathic hypercalciuria due to excessive absorption of calcium the intake of high calcium foods (milk & cheese) and of oxalate should be reduced. In this condition, bendrofluazide 5 mg/day reduces urinary calcium excretion by about 30%. An alternative is to use sodium cellulose phosphate (5 g sachet with meals). Each 5 g dose will bind approximately 350 mg of calcium. In recurrent oxalate stones foods rich in oxalate, e.g. rhubarb, spinach should be avoided. Persons who have passed several uric acid or urate stones, benefit from allopurinol in a dose of 100–300 mg/day, depending on renal function. Allopurinol also has a place in treating calcium oxalate stone disease to which urates may contribute. Phosphatic calculi are formed only in alkaline urine, hence acidifying the urine by giving ammonium chloride daily may be effective. In contrast, cystine and urate stones may be prevented or sometimes dissolved by giving sufficient sodium bicarbonate to make the urine persistently alkaline and ensuring a high urine output of 2–4 litres daily. When these measures fail or are unacceptable to the patient treatment with penicillamine, a chelating agent, in a dose of 1–1.5 g/day may be tried. This drug can cause membranous glomerulonephritis or Goodpasture's syndrome, both of which eventually recover when penicillamine is stopped, and a number of other unpleasant side-effects including fever, disturbances of taste, and blood dyscrasias.

CONGENITAL ABNORMALITIES OF THE KIDNEYS

Anomalies of the urinary tract affect more than 10% of infants and, if not immediately lethal, may lead to complications in later life. About 1 in 500 infants is born with only one kidney which, although usually compatible with normal life, is often associated with other abnormalities.

POLYCYSTIC DISEASE

This genetically determined abnormality of renal structure may be associated with other congenital abnormalities, e.g. cystic liver (p. 538). Infantile polycystic kidney disease is very rare, inherited as an autosomal recessive and usually fatal in the first year of life. Adult Polycystic Kidney Disease (APKD) affects approximately 80/100 000 of the general population and is inherited as an autosomal dominant trait, males and females being equally affected. Data obtained using recombinant DNA techniques and genetic linkage analysis indicate that the APKD gene is located on the distal short arm of chromosome 16 and genetic linkage has been shown between this gene and a) the enzyme phosphoglycolate phosphatase and b) two flanking DNA markers close to the alpha globin locus (3'HVR and 24.1).

Pathology

Small cysts, present in infancy, subsequently enlarge at a variable rate. In fully developed APKD the kidneys are asymmetrically enlarged and contain numerous cysts. These vary in size and are surrounded by a variable amount of parenchyma which often shows extensive fibrosis and arteriolosclerosis.

Clinical features

Affected subjects may be asymptomatic until late in life. After the age of 20 there is often an insidious onset of hypertension which may or may not be associated with deterioration of renal function. Common clinical features are shown in the information box below. Often one or both kidneys can be palpated and the surface may be nodular. In addition to polycystic disease, other diseases in which the kidneys may be palpable are hydro- or pyonephrosis, solitary cyst, renal carcinoma and other tumours. It should be remembered, however, that in some normal people all of the right kidney and occasionally the lower pole of the left kidney may be felt on clinical examination. This is particularly true in slim women. On the other hand, pathologically enlarged kidneys are not always palpable particularly in obese people.

About one-third of patients have hepatic cysts, but disturbance of liver function is rare. Berry aneurysms of cerebral vessels occur and about 10% of patients have a subarachnoid haemorrhage. The outlook is better than is generally appreciated; although there is a gradual reduction in renal function almost 50% of patients never require chronic dialysis.

Investigation and diagnosis

The diagnosis is made on the basis of clinical findings, family history and U/S which is a sensitive method for demonstrating cysts.

Management

Control of blood pressure is vital since uncontrolled hypertension accelerates the development of renal failure and urinary infections must be treated promptly (p. 577). Salt wasters require supplements of sodium chloride and sodium bicarbonate. When renal function is severely compromised the regimen for management of chronic renal failure must be instituted (p. 585).

Screening and counselling

Screening by U/S or occasionally by DNA analysis can be used to detect asymptomatic cases of APKD amongst patients' relatives. Screening and counselling should be offered to those over 18 years. Ultrasound is much less reliable in the 10–20 age group who, in any case, have difficulty understanding the implications of a positive diagnosis. A diagnosis made in early adult life allows regular monitoring of blood pressure and renal function and permits genetic counselling to be given before most patients start their family. It does however, have implications for life insurance, mortgages and employment and not everybody offered screening will accept it.

MEDULLARY CYSTIC DISEASE

Medullary cysts are found in two widely different conditions. In medullary sponge kidney the cysts are confined to the papillary collecting ducts. Affected patients, usually adults, present with pain, haematuria, stone, or urinary infection. The diagnosis is made by IVU. Contrast medium is seen to fill dilated or cystic tubules, which are sometimes calcified (Fig. 12.5, p. 557). The prognosis is generally good.

In uraemic medullary cystic disease small cortical cysts are also present and these lead to progressive destruction of the nephron; this condition, characterised by thirst and polyuria, occurs in younger patients and there is often a family history. Sometimes affected patients are salt wasters which aggravates the degree of renal failure but, even when treated appropriately, serious renal failure is usual.

DEFECTS OF TUBULAR FUNCTION

Renal glycosuria is a benign defect of tubular reabsorption of glucose, usually inherited as an autosomal recessive trait. Glucose appears in the urine in the presence of a normal blood glucose concentration.

Cystinuria

This is a rare condition in which reabsorption of filtered cystine, ornithine, arginine and lysine is defective. The high concentration of cystine in urine leads to cystine stone formation (p. 595). Other uncommon tubular disorders include vitamin D resistant

---

CLINICAL FEATURES WHICH MAY OCCUR IN ADULT POLYCYSTIC KIDNEY DISEASE

- Vague discomfort in loin or abdomen due to increasing mass of renal tissue
- Acute loin pain or renal colic due to haemorrhage into a cyst
- Hypertension
- Uraemia

Table 12.9 Causes of renal tubular acidosis

Distal RTA (type 1)	Proximal RTA (type 2)
Primary	
Familial autosomal dominant	Sporadic familial
Secondary	
Renal diseases	
Pyelonephritis	Nephrotic syndrome
Medullary sponge kidney	Transplanted kidney
Hydronephrosis	
Sickle cell disease	
Transplanted kidney	
Drugs	
Lithium	Tetracycline (outdated)
Amphotericin	Carbonic anhydrase inhibitors
Dysproteinaemias	
Amyloidosis	Amyloidosis
Hyperglobulinaemia	
Cryoglobulinaemia	
Disordered calcium metabolism	
Vitamin D intoxication	Cystinosis
Hyperparathyroidism	Tyrosinosis
Immunologically mediated	*Heavy metals*
Chronic active hepatitis	Cadmium
Primary biliary cirrhosis	Lead
Sjöngren's syndrome	Copper
SLE	Mercury

CLINICAL FEATURES OF DISTAL (TYPE 1) RENAL TUBULAR ACIDOSIS

- Anorexia, fatigue
- Osteomalacia, associated with buffering of retained H^+ in bone
- Muscle weakness
- Hypercalciuria, hyperphosphaturia, recurrent renal calculi, nephrocalcinosis
- Loss of excessive amounts of sodium in urine (diminished Na^+/H^+ exchange in collecting ducts)
- ECF depletion
- Loss of excessive amounts of potassium in urine (activation renin–angiotensin–aldosterone axis as a result of Na^+ and water depletion)

Young children present with failure to thrive, polyuria, thirst, constipation

rickets in which reabsorption of filtered phosphate is reduced, nephrogenic diabetes insipidus in which the tubules are resistant to the effects of vasopressin and the Fanconi syndrome.

Renal tubular acidosis (RTA) (Table 12.9)

This results from a failure of either reabsorption of bicarbonate in the proximal tubule or acidification of the urine in the distal tubule. There may be little or no overall reduction in renal function.

Distal renal tubular acidosis (classical or type 1). The ability to form a very acid urine is lost and the urine pH cannot be reduced below 5.4 even in the presence of severe systemic acidosis. This defect is demonstrated by the ammonium chloride test (p. 554) and is due to failure of the collecting ducts either to secrete hydrogen ion or to sustain the gradient for hydrogen ion between the luminal fluid and the tubular cell. Two forms have been described. In complete RTA there is persistent hyperchloraemic acidosis; in the incomplete form, the plasma bicarbonate is normal, but the urine pH exceeds 5.3 after ammonium chloride. The clinical features are listed in the information box (right).

Management

This consists of determining and dealing with the underlying cause where possible (Table 12.9). Bicarbonate supplements should be given in a dose sufficient to keep the plasma bicarbonate in excess of 18 mmol/l. Large doses may be required, starting with a dose of 1 g of sodium bicarbonate 3 times daily and increasing the dose until the desired plasma bicarbonate is achieved, and there are no signs of sodium depletion (p. 205). When hypokalaemia is present a mixture of sodium and potassium bicarbonate should be given. Initially about half of the total bicarbonate supplement is given as the potassium salt. The proportion of potassium bicarbonate is determined by regular monitoring of plasma potassium. Patients with severe osteomalacia may require alfacalcidol. The starting dose is 0.5 µg daily for adults. The plasma calcium must be checked regularly and the dose adjusted appropriately.

Proximal renal tubular acidosis (type 2). May occur as an isolated defect (primary proximal RTA). More commonly, there are multiple defects in proximal tubular function and patients have, in addition, glycosuria, aminoaciduria, phosphaturia and uricosuria (Fanconi syndrome). Proximal tubular sodium/hydrogen exchange is impaired resulting in decreased bicarbonate reabsorption, large losses of bicarbonate in the urine, and a marked reduction in plasma bicarbonate. Once the plasma bicarbonate has fallen to about 10–12 mmol/l the reduced filtered load can be reabsorbed by the proximal tubular cells, and the amount of bicarbonate reaching the distal tubular is negligible. In these circumstances it is possible to show that the collecting duct cells can secrete hydrogen ions against a gradient so that the urine pH falls below 5.3. There is

Table 12.10 Drug induced renal disease

Pathological lesion	Clinical presentation	Drugs which give rise to the lesion

Drug induced (toxic) tubular necrosis	Proteinuria
	Abnormalities of urinary sediment
	Varying degrees of renal impairment
	   including acute renal failure
	   and oliguria
		Aminoglycosides[1]
		Cephalosporins
		Iodine contrast media
		Paracetamol overdose
		Amphotericin
		Cisplatin

Acute ischaemic tubular necrosis	Hypotension
	Reduced renal perfusion
	Pre-renal failure
	Acute renal failure $\pm$ oliguria
		1. Antihypertensive drugs, opiates
		2. Drugs inducing volume depletion (diuretics, drugs
		   causing severe diarrhoea/vomiting)
		3. NSAIDs by reducing intrarenal vasodilator
		   prostaglandins

Acute tubulo-interstitial nephritis	Proteinuria, microscopic haematuria
	Varying degrees of renal
	   impairment including acute renal
	   failure and oliguria
	Arthralgia
	Rash
	Fever
	Eosinophilia
	Marrow suppression
		Penicillins
		Sulphonamides
		Cephalothin
		Rifampicin[2]
		Allopurinol
		Phenylbutazone
		Azathioprine
		Cimetidine
		NSAIDs[3]
		Frusemide

Hypersensitivity vasculitis	Proteinuria
	Micro- or macroscopic
	   haematuria
	Varying degrees of renal
	   impairment including acute renal
	   failure and oliguria
	Other manifestations of vasculitis, e.g. rash, fever,
	   eosinophilia, arthralgia
		Sulphonamides
		Penicillins
		Rifampicin
		Isoniazid
		Procainamide

Intravascular coagulation	Acute or subacute renal failure
	Manifestations of DIC, e.g.
	   coagulation disturbances, vascular lesions in other
	   organs, thrombocytopenia, fragmentation of r.b.c.
		Oral contraceptives
		Oestrogens

Glomerulonephritis	Proteinuria Nephrotic syndrome Acute renal failure Chronic renal failure	Penicillamine[4] Gold Captopril Troxidone

Disturbance of tubular function	Failure of concentration
	
	Failure to excrete water
	Renal tubular acidosis
	   Distal
	   Proximal
	
	Potassium loss
	
	Magnesium loss
		Lithium
		Demeclocycline
		Methoxyfluorane
		
		(See pp. 214–215)
		Amphotericin B, lithium
		Outdated tetracyclines
		Streptozotocin
		Amphotericin B
		Carbenicillin (large dose)
		Gentamicin
		Cisplatin

Obstruction, retroperitoneal fibrosis	Intermittent urinary tract obstruction Impaired renal function Acute renal failure Chronic renal failure	Methysergide Practolol
crystals	acute oliguric renal failure	(uric acid crystals), high-dose methotrexate therapy (crystals of drug)

Papillary necrosis and chronic interstitial nephritis	'Analgesic nephropathy
	   syndrome'
		Compound analgesics (e.g. aspirin/phenacetin/
		   codeine, aspirin/paracetamol, etc.)
		Aspirin, phenacetin, indomethacin, naproxen, possibly
		   other NSAID

[1]Combination of aminoglycosides with cephalosporin or frusemide particularly likely to induce lesion.
[2]Particularly likely if given intermittently.
[3]This lesion often associated with heavy proteinuria, suggestive of accompanying glomerular lesion.
[4]May cause Goodpasture's syndrome.

frequently associated hyperchloraemia, potassium depletion and hypocalcaemia. Distinction of proximal and distal RTA requires special tests not considered here.

Management

Any underlying cause should be treated (Table 12.9). The plasma bicarbonate should be maintained greater than 18 mmol/l with appropriate supplements of sodium bicarbonate. Very large amounts of bicarbonate are needed and it is recommended that the starting dose should be 10 mmol/kg/day. In those patients with hypokalaemia a proportion of the dose, determined by monitoring plasma potassium, is given as potassium bicarbonate. Where necessary, calcium supplements and alfacalcidol are given.

DRUGS AND THE KIDNEY

DRUG-INDUCED RENAL DISEASE

The susceptibility of the kidney to damage by drugs stems from the fact that it is the route of excretion of many water soluble compounds including drugs and their metabolites. These are delivered in large amounts to the kidney which receives 25% of the cardiac output. Drugs such as cephalosporins may reach high concentrations in the renal cortex as a result of proximal tubular transport mechanisms while others, such as aspirin, are concentrated in the medulla by the operation of the counter-current system. Renal damage can arise during treatment with a large number of drugs and a variety of lesions may result. An accurate drug history is therefore essential in all patients particularly those with unexplained impairment of renal function.

Table 12.10 gives some indication of the range of lesions, the drugs known to cause them and the ways in which patients may present. Drug induced renal failure is usually reversible but a few patients fail to recover full renal function.

ANALGESIC NEPHROPATHY

Renal papillary necrosis and chronic interstitial nepthritis due to long continued ingestion of analgesic drugs accounts for between 5 and 17% of end-stage renal disease in European countries. In animals lesions can be induced with almost any nonsteroidal antiinflammatory drug. In man mixtures containing aspirin and phenacetin were historically important, but probably all NSAID can induce the lesion if taken regularly,

even in small doses, over a long period. Dehydration, which reduces medullary blood flow and results in concentration of the drugs in the renal medulla, is an important contributory factor.

Pathogenesis

Animal experiments using aspirin and phenacetin suggest that the initial lesion is usually papillary necrosis and that the sequence of events shown in the information box below occurs.

POSSIBLE SEQUENCE OF EVENTS IN THE PATHOGENESIS OF ANALGESIC NEPHROPATHY

Data derived from animal experiments in which aspirin and phenacetin were given
- In hydropenia aspirin and phenacetin are concentrated in renal medullary cells and in the medullary interstitium
- Aspirin is also concentrated in the renal cortex
- Both drugs are transformed to cytotoxic metabolites by a P450 dependent mono-oxygenase
- These metabolites bind to cell proteins causing:
  Glutathione depletion (aspirin, phenacetin)
  Inhibition of prostaglandin synthesis (aspirin)
  Uncoupling of oxidative phosphorylation in cortical cells (aspirin)
  Inhibition of incorporation of amino acids into cell proteins (aspirin)
- Reduction in synthesis of vasodilator prostaglandins results in reversible ischaemia of medullary tissue
- Cytotoxic effects of the drugs include:
  Necrosis of cells of loop of Henle
  Lesions in the walls of vasa rectae leading to irreversible ischaemia of medullary tissue and papillary necrosis
- Toxic effect of aspirin on cortical tissue } Result in chronic interstitial nephritis in cortex
  Atrophy of nephrons involved in necrotic papillae

Pathology

Diffuse interstitial fibrosis and tubular atrophy develop particularly around the cortico-medullary junction. A variable interstitial infiltration of round cells and eosinophils is present. Ultimately there is loss of tubules in the cortex and medulla. Acute papillary necrosis is common and is probably the initial lesion in most cases. A recognised complication is development of carcinoma of the renal pelvis.

Clinical features

Most patients are women who suffer from anxiety or who have personality problems. Commonly they are apprehensive and smoke or drink alcohol to excess. Other patients have taken analgesic preparations for many years for headaches, rheumatoid arthritis or osteoarthrosis.

Asymptomatic disease may be disclosed when abnormalities of blood or urine are found during medical examination. Patients with moderate renal impairment present with malaise, thirst and polyuria due to impaired urinary concentration or recurrent urinary infection. About two-thirds are hypertensive. Renal damage is predominantly tubular and failure to conserve sodium and renal tubular acidosis are common. Renal colic or ureteric obstruction and acute renal failure may be caused by passage of fragments of necrotic papillae which can be recognised by microscopic examination of the urine. Acute renal failure may also follow urinary infection or a sudden increase in the intake of analgesics. Many present with established chronic renal failure. Analgesic nephropathy is part of a widespread syndrome associated with analgesic abuse which includes peptic ulceration, anaemia, skin pigmentation and premature ageing.

Investigations
Apart from the history of drug ingestion the diagnosis can sometimes be made on the basis of radiological findings and biochemical evidence of tubular dysfunction.

The appearance of the papillae on IVU or retrograde pyelography is often characteristic. The contrast medium appears as a small tract within the papillary substance; later the papillae may separate giving a ring shadow. Urine usually contains red cells and sterile pyuria is common. Proteinuria rarely exceeds 1 g/24 hour.

Management
Provided that analgesic preparations are withdrawn sufficiently early, there is a reasonable prospect of some recovery of function; otherwise irreversible renal failure develops. Treatment consists of withdrawing the drug, maintaining the fluid intake of 2–3 litres per day, treating hypertension and when necessary providing supplements of sodium chloride and sodium bicarbonate to restore ECF volume and correct metabolic acidosis. Regular follow-up is essential. When renal function is severely impaired the regimen for management of chronic renal failure should be instituted (p. 585).

USE OF DRUGS IN PATIENTS WITH IMPAIRED RENAL FUNCTIONS

Adverse reactions to drugs are significantly more common when renal function is impaired because urinary excretion of many drugs and their active water soluble metabolites is reduced. Moreover uraemia is associated with alterations in distribution of drugs throughout body fluids, reduced binding of drugs by plasma albumin and changes in their metabolism.

The dose of many commonly used drugs must therefore be reduced in renal failure, e.g. cephalosporins, co-trimoxazole, aminoglycosides, ranitidine, digoxin, opiates. The principles listed in the information box below should be observed when treating patients with impaired renal function.

USE OF DRUGS WITH IMPAIRED RENAL FUNCTION

- No drug should be given unless specifically indicated
- The least toxic alternative must be chosen
- The British National Formulary or other reference should be consulted to determine:
  Recommended dose for degree of renal impairment (use creatinine clearance as indication of degree of impairment)
  Adverse effects of drug
- The patient must be observed regularly for signs of adverse effects and the drug stopped or the dose reduced if these develop
- Measurement of plasma drug concentration may be helpful in monitoring dosing schedule

---

TUMOURS OF THE KIDNEY AND GENITO-URINARY TRACT

RENAL CARCINOMA

Between 1 and 2% of malignant tumours arise in the kidney. Renal adenocarcinoma, the most common, occurs most frequently in adult men. Occasionally the affected kidney contains multiple tumours or both kidneys are involved.

Pathology
The tumour, which is composed of large cells with clear cytoplasm, arises from proximal tubular epithelium. The cut surface appears yellow and large tumours contain haemorrhagic or cystic areas. Local spread is by penetration of the renal capsule and invasion of renal veins. Spread to the opposite kidney occurs via the veins. The tumour is vascular and metastases to regional lymph nodes, bone, lung, and liver.

Clinical presentation
Haematuria is the most common presenting symptom. About 20% of patients present late with haematuria, pain in the loin or renal colic and a palpable mass in the

Table 12.11   Tumour-associated syndromes

Findings	Per cent of renal tumour patients with this finding	Explanation
Raised ESR	55	Changes in serum proteins associated with many tumours
Hypertension	37	Secretion of renin by tumour
Anaemia	36	Depression of erythropoiesis plus or minus haematuria
Weight loss	34	Tumour products depress appetite
Pyrexia	17	Circulating pyrogens
Abnormal liver function	14	This may disappear after nephrectomy
Raised alkaline phosphatase	10.1	Secreted by tumour?
Hypercalcaemia	4.9	Parathyroid hormone-like peptide secretion by tumour
Polycythaemia	3.5	Erythropoietin secretion
Neuromyopathy	3.2	Tumour-associated antibodies to nerve tissue
Amyloidosis	2	Possibly associated with immunological reactions to the tumour

(Adapted by permission from Boulton Jones et al. 1982 Diagnosis and Management of Renal and Urinary Diseases. Blackwell Scientific Publications, Oxford.)

flank. In 30% changes due to systemic effects of tumour products are the first indication of disease (Table 12.11). These symptoms resolve after nephrectomy and must not be attributed to metastases. About 30% of patients present with established metastases.

Investigation

Investigations are designed:

1. to demonstrate the presence of a solid tumour
2. to determine the extent of spread of the tumour: a) local b) to nodes and c) haematogenous.

IVU with nephrotomography usually shows a renal mass with splaying and distortion of the collecting system and in the great majority of patients U/S will distinguish tumour from a simple cyst. If doubt remains cyst fluid can be aspirated under U/S control and examined histologically. The size of the tumour can be assessed from the IVU and U/S. CT scanning is of value in determining spread through the renal capsule (Fig. 12.9, p. 559). Invasion of the renal vein and vena cava can usually be shown by U/S although occasionally preoperative venography is required. Spread to lymph nodes can be assessed by CT scanning and haematogenous metastases detected by chest X-ray, CT scanning and radionuclide bone scanning.

Management

Early surgery affords the only real prospect of cure. The treatment of choice is removal of the affected kidney and the adrenal gland, en bloc, within the perinephric fascia, and simultaneous removal of regional lymph nodes. The five-year survival for tumours confined to the kidney is 60–75%. For all grades of tumour it is approximately 30%. Partial nephrectomy may be performed for carcinoma of a solitary kidney or tumour involving both kidneys. If all renal tissue must be removed chronic dialysis is instituted. Treatment of advanced disease is unsatisfactory. Nephrectomy or arterial embolisation of the kidney may be necessary for loin pain or haematuria. Radiotherapy often relieves pain due to metastases and progesterone-like hormones may slow the advance of metastatic disease but neither radiotherapy, chemotherapy, hormonal therapy nor immunotherapy has been shown to alter its course significantly.

NEPHROBLASTOMA (WILM'S TUMOUR)

This is the second most common malignant tumour of the kidney, and presents in the first decade and often in the first year of life, most commonly as an abdominal mass. Haematuria tends to occur late in the disease. The tumour is radiosensitive and responds to chemotherapy (p. 239). The best hope of cure is early diagnosis.

TUMOURS OF THE RENAL PELVIS, URETER AND BLADDER

These are histologically similar and usually transitional cell carcinomas. They spread locally by direct invasion but also by implantation to other parts of the urinary tract. While some are benign, e.g. papillomas, all urinary tract tumours are liable to recur even after apparently adequate treatment. The bladder is by far the most common site and epidemiological studies have shown that males are more often affected and that this tumour is particularly likely to develop in patients who work in industry such as dyeing and printing, where there may be exposure to aniline, in areas endemic for urinary schistosomiasis (p. 166) and as a complication of analgesic nephropathy.

Clinical features

Painless haematuria is commonly the sole presenting symptom. Unexplained frequency, dysuria or symptoms due to urinary tract obstruction also occur. The features of urinary infection may be superimposed.

Investigations

Patients with haematuria should have an IVU. Renal pelvic carcinoma appears as an abnormality on the urogram. If the IVU is normal cystoscopy is performed unless the patient is young and the haematuria is obviously associated with a urinary infection. In such a case the patient should be followed up and if haematuria persists cystoscopy should be done. Biopsy of suspicious lesions is carried out during cystoscopy. Urinary cytology may be helpful.

Local spread from tumours of the renal pelvis is apparent on CT scanning. Local spread of bladder tumours is assessed by bimanual examination under anaesthesia, from the appearances at cystoscopy and from the histology. Spread to lymph nodes is assessed at CT scanning and metastases by chest X-ray, bone scan and liver function tests.

Management

Pelvic and ureteric tumours are treated by nephroureterectomy. Radiotherapy and chemotherapy are of little value. Patients may later develop bladder tumours and therefore require regular follow-up cystoscopy. Localised well-differentiated bladder tumours (approximately 60% of such tumours) are treated by diathermy. Cystoscopy and IVU should be performed at yearly intervals thereafter to detect recurrence.

Treatment of histologically malignant tumours or those which have spread beyond the bladder mucosa is unsatisfactory. Extensive superficial tumour can be treated by intravesical chemotherapy with Epodyl or thiotepa and locally invasive lesions with radiotherapy. If this fails or if the patient has severe bladder symptoms total cystectomy and transplantation of the ureters into an ileal conduit may be required.

Systemic methotrexate and cisplatinum have been used to treat metastases but results are poor. Analgesics and palliative radiotherapy are used to relieve pain. The five-year survival of patients with superficial well-differentiated lesions is 90% whilst in those with invasive, poorly differentiated tumours it is 30%.

PROSTATIC CARCINOMA

Adenocarcinoma of the prostate accounts for 70% of all cancers in men and causes 19 deaths/100 000 males in the UK, mostly in men over 50. Autopsy reports indicate that many men over 80 have latent foci of prostatic cancer.

Clinical features

The lesion may be found incidentally on examination of tissue removed during transurethral resection for supposedly benign prostatic hypertrophy or it may present with symptoms of urethral obstruction similar to those of the benign condition. Local spread causes pain, incontinence and sometimes acute renal failure due to involvement of the lower ends of both ureters. Patients may present with bone pain due to metastases. On examination per rectum the prostate is hard and the median furrow often obliterated. Spread of tumour is often associated with increased serum acid phosphatase which acts as a tumour marker.

Investigations

The diagnosis depends on the clinical findings and examination of biopsy material. Local invasion is assessed by bimanual examination under anaesthesia and by U/S. Screening for metastases includes measurement of serum acid phosphatase, bone scan, X-rays of bones and chest and liver function tests.

Management

When asymptomatic disease is discovered incidentally it may be best, particularly in older men, to defer treatment until symptoms develop. Nevertheless radical prostatectomy, pelvic radiotherapy and hormonal treatment designed to deprive the tumour of androgens have however all been advocated for these cases. When symptoms or evidence of local spread are present, radiotherapy or androgen deprivation is indicated. The latter can be achieved by administration of oestrogens or gonadotrophin analogues or by orchidectomy. Stilboestrol has a useful palliative action. The dose should be restricted to 1–3 mg/day by mouth as larger doses, in addition to their feminising effects, are associated with increased risk of cardiovascular complications. Alternatively a gonadotrophin-releasing hormone analogue such as buserelin can be given by s.c. injection. The initial course is 500 µg/8-hourly for 7 days. Thereafter 100 µg doses delivered by a metered nasal spray are instilled into the nostrils 6 times a day. During the early days of therapy tumour growth may increase. Cyproterone acetate which blocks the effect of androgens on target tissue, can be used as a second-line drug; 100 mg orally t.d.s. after food. Transurethral resection may be required to relieve obstruction. Metastatic disease can be treated by androgen deprivation or palliative radiotherapy, or if these measures fail, hypophysectomy. Trials of chemotherapy are in progress.

BENIGN PROSTATIC HYPERTROPHY

This is most commonly found in men over 60 and may be associated with diminished androgen secretion. Histologically the inner zone of the gland undergoes hyperplasia and hypertrophy and there is an increase in fibromuscular stroma. The enlarged prostate obstructs the outflow of urine by compressing, displacing, distorting and elongating the prostatic urethra with the effects on bladder and renal function referred to on page 593.

Clinical features

These are those of progressive obstruction to urinary flow. Acute urinary retention may arise if the gland suddenly increases in size because of superimposed infection or congestion, or if cardiac failure develops in the elderly. Then the patient has a sudden desire to micturate but is unable to do so, and the bladder becomes tense and tender. Chronic retention may pass unnoticed for some time but there is a gradual increase in the volume of urine which remains in the bladder after micturition. Haematuria and urethral bleeding may also occur and may be the presenting symptom. On rectal examination the prostate may feel large, elastic and uniform in consistency. When the median lobe alone is affected the prostate feels normal and the condition can be recognised only by cystoscopy. Transurethral resection of prostatic tissues is the treatment of choice to relieve the outflow obstruction.

TESTICULAR TUMOURS

These are the most common form of malignant disease in men aged 25–34 years. The lesion may be a seminoma arising from spermatogonia, a teratoma from toti-potential germ cells or a combined tumour. These tumours occur in fit young men and should nowadays be regarded as curable. Early diagnosis and appropriate specialist treatment is essential.

Clinical features

A seminoma presents as a painless, often uniform, rapid enlargement of the testis. A teratoma causes more nodular changes and may secrete chorionic gonadotrophin producing gynaecomastia. The tumour may be overlooked if obscured by a hydrocele or if the examination is inadequate. Some cases present with metastases.

Investigations

Spread to glands can be demonstrated by CT scanning. Screening for metastases should include chest X-ray and liver function tests.

Management

The testis should be removed using the inguinal approach. Histology gives some idea of prognosis. A seminoma confined to the testicle or with metastases below the diaphragm is treated by radiotherapy to which it is very sensitive. More widespread seminoma requires chemotherapy and this is the treatment of choice for teratoma. The usual agents are cisplatinum and bleomycin. The treatment is a considerable ordeal and should be carried out in a specialised department. Circulating tumour markers, (alpha fetoprotein, human chorionic gonadotrophin and lactic dehydrogenase) are of help in assessing response to treatment and for monitoring patients in remission.

ACKNOWLEDGEMENTS

The authors are grateful to Professor J.J.K. Best and Dr P.L. Allan of the Department of Radiology, University of Edinburgh and Dr D. Thomson, Department of Pathology, University of Edinburgh for providing several of the X-rays and photographs used in this chapter.

FURTHER READING

Avery G S 1980 Drug Treatment. Adis Press. For information about drugs and renal disease (ch 21 Wright N, Robson J S).

Brenner B M, Rector F L 1985 The Kidney, 3rd Edn. vols 1 & 2. Saunders, Philadelphia. A reference book with a physiological background.

Brenner B M, Lazarus J M 1983 Acute Renal Failure. Saunders, Philadelphia. A comprehensive reference book.

Cameron J S et al. 1911 Oxford Textbook of Clinical
  Nephrology. Blackwell Scientific Publications, Oxford. A
  comprehensive textbook.
Forrester J M et al. 1986 Companion to Medical Studies,
  3rd Edn. vol 1. Blackwell Scientific Publications, Oxford.
  For information about anatomy and physiology of the
  kidney.
Kidney International. The journal of the International
  Society of Nephrology covers a wide range of clinical and
experimental topics and contains good reviews.
Munro J, Edwards C 1990 Macleod's Clinical Examination,
  8th Edn. Churchill Livingstone, Edinburgh. For further
  information about examination of the kidneys and the
  urine.
Nephrology, Dialysis, Transplantation. The journal of the
  European Society of Nephrology also covers a wide range
  of topics but is more clinically orientated than Kidney
  International.

13

Endocrine and Metabolic Diseases

Endocrinology is the biological science concerned with *the synthesis, secretion and action of hormones*. These are defined as *chemical messengers which co-ordinate the activities of different cells in multi-cellular organisms*. The body thus has two major control systems which allow specialised tissues to function in an integrated way – the nervous system and the endocrine system.

Classically the nervous system depends on electro-chemical signals passing via specific nervous pathways and the endocrine system on hormones being released into the circulation and acting at a site distant from that of secretion ((ορμαω) to stir up). However, it is becoming increasingly obvious that the situation is much more complex. Thus many hormones are now known to be neurotransmitters. In addition it is clear that the hormones may act on adjacent cells (paracrine system) or even back on the cell of origin (autocrine system) and that many have an inhibitory rather than stimulatory role. It is not surprising that this sophisticated system is associated with a large number of congenital and acquired abnormalities. Most of these endocrine diseases can be classified on the basis of being associated either with hormonal excess or deficiency (Table 13.1). The classification of endocrine disease is shown in the information box (right).

The commonest endocrine diseases are those involving the thyroid gland and that resulting from either an absolute or relative lack of insulin (diabetes mellitus). The prevalence of these conditions varies greatly in different parts of the world (Table 13.2).

CLASSIFICATION OF ENDOCRINE DISEASE ON FUNCTIONAL BASIS

	Example
Hormonal excess	
Primary gland overproduction	Adrenal tumour → cortisol → Cushing's syndrome
Secondary to excess production of trophic substance	Thyroid stimulating antibody → thyroxine → thyrotoxicosis
Hormonal deficiency	
Primary gland failure	Adrenal antibodies → adrenal failure → Addison's disease
Secondary to lack of stimulation by a trophic hormone	Pituitary disease → loss of ACTH secretion → cortisol deficiency
Target organ resistance	Defective aldosterone receptor → pseudohypoaldosteronism

---

Table 13.2 Prevalence of the commonest endocrine diseases

Disease	Area	% of population
Thyroid dysfunction (Goitre)	Endemic goitre area (e.g. Himalayas)	>10%
	Non-endemic goitre area (e.g. U.K.)	4% of women aged 20–30
Diabetes mellitus	Industrialised countries	1.5–2%
	North American Indians Australian Aborigines	>15%

Table 13.1   Diseases of the endocrine system

	Hormonal excess	Hormonal deficiency	Hormonal resistance
Hypothalamus	? Cushing's disease	Isolated releasing hormone deficiencies for LH, TSH, GH	
Pituitary	Acromegaly	Hypopituitarism	Nephrogenic Diabetes insipidus
	Cushing's disease	Diabetes insipidus	
	Prolactinoma		Laron dwarfism
Gonad	Tumours	Klinefelter's syndrome	Androgen resistance syndromes
		Turner's syndrome	
		Menopause	testicular feminisation
Thyroid	Hyperthyroidism	Hypothyroidism	Thyroid hormone resistance
Adrenal	Cushing's syndrome	Addison's disease	Glucocorticoid resistance
Parathyroids	Hyperparathyroidism	Hypoparathyroidism	Pseudo-hypopara-thyroidism
Pancreas	Insulinoma	Diabetes mellitus	Insulin resistance syndromes
	Glucagonoma		

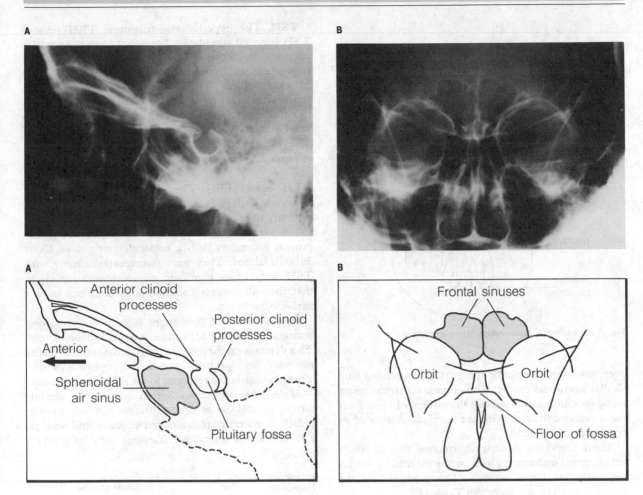

Fig. 13.1   Plain skull X-rays and diagrams showing anatomy of normal pituitary fossa. A. Lateral view. B. Postero-anterior view.

The World Health Organisation statistics indicate that endocrine diseases are a relatively rare cause of death (1–5%). However, they are an important cause of morbidity. Modern methods have resulted in earlier diagnosis and more effective therapy. The treatment of some conditions such as hypothyroidism is very satisfactory and results in return of normal function. For others, such as diabetes mellitus, however, the therapy is far from optimal.

THE HYPOTHALAMUS AND THE PITUITARY GLAND

ANATOMY AND PHYSIOLOGY

The pituitary gland is enclosed in the sella turcica, bridged over by the diphragma sellae, with the sphenoidal air sinuses below, and the optic chiasma above (Fig. 13.1). The cavernous sinuses are lateral to the pituitary fossa and contain the 3rd, 4th and 6th cranial nerves. The gland is composed of two lobes, anterior and posterior and is connected to the hypothalamus by the infundibular stalk which has portal vessels (Fig. 13.2) carrying blood from the median eminence of the hypothalamus to the anterior lobe and nerve fibres to the posterior lobe.

THE ANTERIOR LOBE

This consists of three main types of cell as identified by conventional staining: chromophobe, acidophil and basophil. Classical descriptions of pituitary tumours suggest that acidophil tumours are associated with growth hormone or prolactin excess and basophil with adrenocorticotrophic hormone hypersecretion. How-

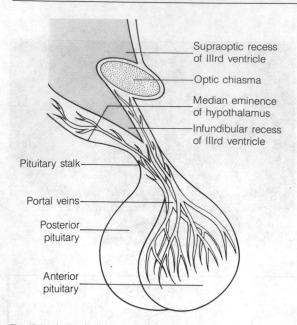

Fig. 13.2 Anatomical relationships of human pituitary.

ever, many chromophobe tumours are associated with similar hormonal excess. Thus immunohistochemistry using specific antisera against the pituitary hormones is more valuable in identifying the hormone(s) secreted by specific pituitary cells.

There are seven pituitary hormones, four of which act on target endocrine glands while the other three act primarily on target tissues. The functions of the anterior pituitary are shown in Table 13.3.

Each of these hormones is controlled by a substance produced in the hypothalamus and released into the portal blood. These hormones or factors may either stimulate or inhibit anterior pituitary hormone secretion (Fig. 13.3). Hypothalamic function is in turn dependent on a wide variety of stimuli of nervous, metabolic, physical or hormonal origin, in particular feedback control by hormones produced by the target glands (thyroid, adrenal cortex and gonads).

Table 13.3 Functions of anterior pituitary hormones

Function	Hormone	Abbreviation
Growth	Growth hormone	GH
Thyroid activity	Thyroid stimulating hormone	TSH
Sexual activity	Luteinising hormone	LH
	Follicle stimulating hormone	FSH
Lactation	Prolactin	PRL
Adrenal Glucocorticoid production	Adrenocorticotrophic hormone	ACTH
Skin pigmentation	Adrenocorticotrophic hormone + β-lipotrophin	ACTH β-LPH

TSH. The hypothalamic tripeptide TRH releases TSH (thyroid stimulating hormone) from the anterior pituitary. In its turn TSH stimulates the thyroid gland to produce the thyroid hormones, thyroxine (T_4) and triiodothyronine (T_3). These then exert a negative feedback control on TRH and TSH secretion. Even though T_4 is a prohormone which is then converted to the biologically active T_3, the pituitary secretion of TSH is more affected by circulating T_4. This is because of rapid deiodination of T_4 to T_3 by the pituitary.

LH and FSH. The gonadotrophin releasing hormone GnRH is a decapeptide and acts on the pituitary to release both luteinising hormone (LH) and follicle stimulating hormone (FSH). These are glycoprotein hormones with a molecular weight of about 30 000 Daltons. They have structural similarity with TSH and human chorionic gonadotrophin (hCG) in that they all share a common α subunit but have a variable β subunit.

Despite the fact that there is only one releasing hormone, LH and FSH can be secreted independently. This depends on the feedback of gonadal steroids on the pituitary (and probably also a polypeptide inhibin). These modulate the response to the releasing hormone.

Male: FSH stimulates Sertoli cells in the seminiferous tubules to secrete androgen binding protein (ABP), transferrin, plasminogen activator and inhibin. LH stimulates interstitial (Leydig) cells to produce

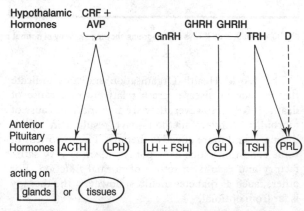

Hypothalamic hormones stimulating anterior pituitary ($\longrightarrow$)
Hypothalamic hormone inhibiting anterior pituitary ($----\rightarrow$)

Fig. 13.3 The principal direct relationships between the hypothalamus and the anterior pituitary. Hypothalamic hormones: CRF Corticotrophin releasing factor; AVP Arginine vasopressin; GnRH Gonadotrophin releasing hormone; GHRH Growth hormone releasing hormone; GHRIH Growth hormone release inhibitory hormone (somatostatin); TRH Thyrotrophin releasing hormone; D Dopamine (prolactin release inhibitory factor).

testosterone. Some oestradiol is also produced. Both FSH and LH are necessary for spermatogenesis. hCG will also stimulate interstitial cells and is used to test the ability of the testis to produce testosterone.

Female: FSH produces growth and development of ovarian follicles during the first 14 days of the menstrual cycle (the follicular phase). This leads to a gradual increase in oestradiol (E2) production. This increasing E2 level initially suppresses FSH secretion (negative feedback) but then results in increased LH secretion (positive feedback). This is due to an increase in both the frequency and amplitude of GnRH pulses. The mid-cycle peak of LH (the LH surge) induces ovulation. After release of the ovum the follicle differentiates into a corpus luteum which secretes progesterone. The second half of the cycle is known as the luteal phase.

GnRH pulsatility. GnRH is secreted in a pulsatile manner in both males and females leading to pulses of gonadotrophin secretion. This pattern of secretion is critical. Continuous administration of GnRH down regulates receptors on the pituitary gonadotrophs and therefore paradoxically inhibits gonadotrophin secretion. Thus long-acting analogues of GnRH are being used in the treatment of hormone dependent prostate and breast cancer and may have a role as contraceptives. Conversely pulsatile administration of GnRH via a portable pump is proving to be an important way of treating certain types of hypogonadotrophic hypogonadism.

In addition to steroid feedback endogenous opiates also appear to play a role in determining LH pulse frequency. Thus the opiate antagonist naloxone increases the frequency in patients with hypothalamic amenorrhoea such as that associated with excessive exercise.

Inhibin. This is a glycoprotein hormone secreted by the ovary and testis. Its major role is thought to be to act on the pituitary to suppress FSH release. It consists of an α and β subunit. Two forms of the β subunit have been isolated (β-A and β-B). Inhibin A is a heterodimer of α and β-A. Inhibin B consists of α and β-B. Recently the homodimer of the β-subunit (i.e. 2 β-A subunits) (Activin) has been isolated. Interestingly this stimulates FSH release. It is clear that the control of LH and FSH secretion is much more complex than previously thought.

GH (Growth hormone). GH is controlled by a dual system, namely growth hormone releasing hormone (GHRH) and an inhibitory hormone (GHRIH or somatostatin). GHRH was first identified from a pancreatic tumour in a patient with acromegaly and has been shown to be the same as that present in the hypothalamus. It circulates in both a 40 and an N-terminally extended 44 amino acid form. The pulsatile release of growth hormone appears to be due to stimulation by GHRH and loss of inhibition by somatostatin. This is a tetradecapeptide which has many other actions, apart from its effect on growth hormone. These are shown in the information box below.

SOMATOSTATIN

Somatostatin inhibits release of:
- GH
- Gastrin
- TSH
- Glucagon
- Gastric acid
- Insulin
- Pancreatic enzymes

Sites of production:
- Hypothalamus
- Gastrointestinal tract
- Delta cells of pancreas

The major effects of GH are mediated via an insulin-like growth factor (IGF-I) (original name somatomedin C). This polypeptide circulates in the blood bound to a specific carrier protein. The liver is a major source of IGF-I production.

PRL (prolactin). PRL secretion differs from that of other anterior pituitary hormones in that it is under predominantly inhibitory control. The inhibitory factor is dopamine which is secreted by the hypothalamus into the portal system. Thus cutting the pituitary stalk leads to an elevation of prolactin secretion but inhibits the secretion of all the other anterior pituitary hormones. Administration of TRH stimulates prolactin as well as TSH release but there is little evidence that TRH normally controls prolactin release. Vasoactive intestinal polypeptide (VIP) will also release prolactin but like TRH its physiological role is unknown.

ACTH (corticotrophin). The secretion of adrenocorticotrophic hormone (ACTH) is under the control of corticotrophin releasing factor (CRF), a 41 amino acid peptide identified in 1981. In addition the hypothalamus produces arginine vasopressin (AVP) and both CRF and AVP act synergistically to release ACTH.

ACTH is secreted as part of the large precursor molecule, pro-opiocortin, and is cleaved from the N- and C-terminal parts prior to release from the pituitary

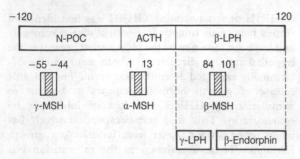

Fig. 13.4   ACTH/LPH precursor, pro-opiocortin (POC). The hatched areas represent the common core MSH sequence within different molecules. β-LPH is further broken down to γ-LPH and β-endorphin.

corticotroph (Fig. 13.4). The control of ACTH secretion is shown in the information box (right).

LPH. β-melanocyte stimulating hormone (β-MSH) is now known to be an artefact created by extracting the pituitary under harsh conditions. The β-MSH amino acid sequence is contained within β-lipotrophin (LPH) which is the C-terminal part of the ACTH precursor molecule, pro-opiocortin. This core sequence is also present within ACTH (α-MSH) and in the N-terminal part of pro-opiocortin (γ-MSH) (Fig. 13.4). Thus there are several molecules derived from pro-opiocortin which may function as melanocyte stimulating hormones and cause pigmentation of the skin and mucous membranes by increasing melanin synthesis in the melanocytes. However, the pigmenting activity of LPH is low and ACTH is probably the most important pigmenting hormone.

The C-terminal part of β-LPH (61-91) is β-endorphin, one of the endogenous substances with morphine-like actions. The first five amino acids of β-endorphin are the same as those of the pentapeptide opioid, metenkephalin. Current evidence suggests, however that metenkephalin is not derived from β-endorphin but from another precursor molecule.

THE POSTERIOR LOBE

The posterior lobe (neurohypophysis) contains neural fibres which emanate from the supraoptic and para-ventricular nuclei of the hypothalamus.

Hormones of the posterior lobe
The neurohypophysis secretes two hormones, arginine vasopressin (AVP) – here referred to as vasopressin – and oxytocin together with their specific binding proteins (neurophysins). The principal action of vaso-pressin is to increase the reabsorption of water by the

CONTROL OF ACTH SECRETION

ACTH release is affected by:
● Circadian rhythm – highest level on waking in morning, lowest level on going to bed at night
● Stress – dominant control e.g. trauma, pain, fever, hypoglycaemia
● Negative feedback – lowering cortisol levels e.g. with enzyme inhibitor metyrapone or in primary adrenal failure stimulates CRF and hence ACTH

renal tubules, and because of this action it is also known as the antidiuretic hormone (ADH). The secretion of vasopressin is controlled by three main mechanisms. A rise in plasma osmolality stimulates vasopressin release which in turn results in water retention to preserve homeostasis. A fall of about 15% in plasma volume without any change in osmolality can also stimulate vasopressin secretion by activating volume receptors in the thorax. In addition the central nervous system also can play a role. Pain, for example, produces an anti-diuresis.

The role of oxytocin in the male is unknown. In the female it has traditionally been thought to be important in parturition and the expression of milk from the breast but its role in parturition has been questioned.

INVESTIGATION OF PITUITARY FUNCTION

All the protein and peptide hormones of the pituitary gland can be measured in body fluids by radio-immunoassay and access to a laboratory with a full range of these assays is critical for the proper evaluation of pituitary function. Approximate adult reference values for hormone concentrations in the plasma are given on p. 991. In addition the hypothalamic hormones, TRH, GnRH, CRF and GHRH have been synthesised and can be used clinically to stimulate the release of the appropriate pituitary hormones. In most tests the pituitary hormone itself is measured (e.g. GH, prolactin) but in the case of ACTH it is cheaper and easier to measure cortisol as a marker of ACTH secretion. The exception is when primary adrenal disease is suspected when both ACTH and cortisol should be measured.

One of the fundamental principles of the investigation of endocrine disorders is that if high levels of a hormone are suspected then an appropriate suppression test should be used. Conversely if there is hormone deficiency a stimulation test is normally required. Thus in assessing the increased production of growth hormone in acromegaly a *glucose tolerance test* is

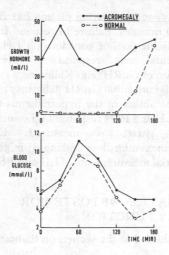

Fig. 13.5 Oral glucose tolerance tests in a normal subject and a patient with acromegaly with measurement of blood glucose and plasma growth hormone.

performed with measurement of growth hormone at half-hourly intervals for 2 hours along with measurement of blood glucose. Under physiological conditions growth hormone secretion is promptly suppressed by a rise in the blood glucose while there is either absent suppression or a paradoxical rise in patients with pituitary tumours secreting growth hormone (Fig. 13.5).

Basal function of anterior pituitary
Assessment of this should include measuring plasma:

08.00 h	cortisol
	prolactin
	thyroxine
In the male	testosterone
In the female	oestradiol
In the post-menopausal female	LH/FSH

Assessment of GH secretion
In normal subjects sampled during the day growth hormone levels are commonly undetectable. In

TESTS OF GROWTH HORMONE SECRETION

- Post-exercise
- 1 hour after going to sleep   } Physiological
- Frequent sampling during sleep

- Insulin-induced hypoglycaemia
- Clonidine
- Arginine   } Pharmacological
- Glucagon

suspected hypopituitarism, therefore, some form of dynamic function test is necessary to distinguish normal from abnormal growth hormone secretion (see the information box (left)).

Of these the insulin tolerance test remains the gold standard. It has the additional advantage that it stimulates the secretion of ACTH and hence cortisol. Prolactin is also released. It is a safe test providing it is not used when hypoglycaemia could be dangerous (i.e. in patients with):

1. ischaemic heart disease
2. epilepsy
3. severe hypopituitarism (08.00 h plasma cortisol < 180 nmol/l).

The standard dose of insulin is 0.15 u/kg body weight. It is important to achieve adequate hypoglycaemia (signs of neuroglycopaenia, tachycardia, sweating and blood glucose less than 2.2 mmol/l (40 mg/100 ml)). Blood samples are taken at 0, 30, 45, 60, 90 and 120 minutes after insulin for the measurement of blood glucose, plasma cortisol and growth hormone. In normal subjects GH levels rise to above 20 mU/l. In severe GH deficiency levels are less than 7 mU/l, whilst partial GH deficiency produces intermediate values.

GH response to GHRH is of value in distinguishing patients who lack the releasing hormone (the usual cause of isolated GH deficiency).

ACTH
If the basal plasma cortisol is normal (> 180 nmol/l) then this indicates that basal ACTH secretion is normal. However, it does not mean that the patient can respond normally to stress (e.g. surgery). To determine whether or not the stress response is normal further dynamic function testing is usually necessary (the exception is a patient with 08.00 h plasma cortisol > 550 nmol/l).

The best simple, safe screening test is that giving synacthen (β-24 tetracosactrin, ACTH) (250 μg i.m.). If after 30 minutes the plasma cortisol is > 550 nmol/l then this indicates a normal stress response. If it is less than this then an insulin hypoglycaemia test should be carried out as some patients will respond normally to insulin (and stress) and yet have a subnormal response to synacthen. In patients in whom hypoglycaemia is contraindicated (see above) then other tests such as that giving glucagon can be performed. However, this is a less reliable index of the ability of the hypothalamic-pituitary-adrenal axis to respond to stress.

ACTH/cortisol response to CRF is of little value in determing stess responsiveness but is helpful in distinguishing pituitary-dependent Cushing's disease (exaggerated ACTH/cortisol response) from the ectopic ACTH syndrome (no response) (p. 645).

TSH, prolactin

The ability of the pituitary to secrete TSH and prolactin can be tested by giving TRH 200 μg intravenously and measuring the serum TSH and prolactin before and at 20 and 60 minutes after. It should be stressed that the value of this test is limited. In secondary hypothyroidism (i.e. due to hypothalamic or pituitary disease) a normal TSH response may be found and the diagnosis is made on the thyroxine level and not the TSH response to TRH. In primary hypothyroidism there will be an exaggerated TSH response to TRH but the diagnosis can be made on the basis of the elevated basal TSH.

The prolactin response to TRH may be absent in post-partum pituitary necrosis (Sheehan's syndrome). It is blunted in patients with prolactinomas. However, the overlap with other causes of hyperprolactinaemia is such that the prolactin response to TRH has little discriminatory value in the individual patient. The basal prolactin level is much more valuable.

LH and FSH

The pulsatile release of LH and FSH makes it difficult to assess the results of single blood samples with the exception of those from the post-menopausal patient. Here, one would expect the values of LH and FSH to be high reflecting ovarian failure. If, however, they are not then this suggests hypothalamic or pituitary disease.

The ability of the pituitary to synthesise and release LH and FSH can be tested by giving GnRH (100 μg intravenously) and measuring plasma LH and FSH at 0, 20 and 60 minutes. Failure to respond indicates no readily releasable pool of gonadotroph LH and FSH. Such patients may respond to the pulsatile administration of GnRH (e.g. Kallmann's syndrome in which there is congenital GnRH deficiency).

To test the ability of the hypothalamus to produce GnRH the LH and FSH response to the anti-oestrogen clomiphene citrate is measured. Clomiphene (3 mg/kg/d, maximum dose 150 mg/d) is given for 10 days with serial measurements of LH and FSH.

INVESTIGATION OF POSTERIOR PITUITARY FUNCTION

This is considered in the section on diabetes insipidus (p. 621).

SYNDROMES DUE TO ANTERIOR PITUITARY HYPOSECRETION

HYPOPITUITARISM

Aetiology

The causes of hypopituitarism are best classified on the basis of whether the lesion is in the hypothalamus or pituitary.

Clinical features

These depend on the underlying lesion. In the congenital defects of the hypothalamus where there is an isolated failure of production of a releasing hormone (e.g. GnRH) then apart from the failure of LH and FSH production and hence of gonadal steroids, the rest of hypothalamic-pituitary function is normal. There is, however, in this case an important associated abnormality, anosmia, which often points to the diagnosis.

With progressive lesions of the pituitary such as a gradually expanding non-functioning pituitary tumour there is a characteristic sequence of loss of pituitary hormone secretion. GH secretion is often the earliest to be lost but this produces no obvious symptoms in the adult. Next LH secretion becomes impaired with, in the male, loss of libido and impotence and, in the female, oligomenorrhoea or amenorrhoea. Later in the male there may be gynaecomastia and decreased frequency of shaving. In both sexes axillary and pubic hair eventually becomes sparse or even absent. The skin becomes characteristically finer and more wrinkled. FSH secretion tends to be lost later than LH.

The next hormone to be lost is usually ACTH and thus cortisol resulting in symptoms of adrenal in-

Table 13.4 Hypopituitarism

	Lesion/hormone deficiency	Clinical features
Hypothalamus		
Congenital	GnRH (Kallmann's syndrome)	Delayed puberty
	TRH	Hypothyroidism
	GHRH	Short stature
	CRF	Adrenal insufficiency
Acquired	Craniopharyngioma	See text
	Sarcoidosis	See text
	Tuberculosis	See text
	Histiocytosis-X	See text
	Head injury	See text
	Surgery	See text
	Tumour – primary or secondary	See text
	Radiotherapy	See text
Pituitary	Tumour – primary or secondary	See text
	Surgery	See text
	Radiotherapy	See text
	Post-partum necrosis (Sheehan's)	See text
	Haemorrhage (apoplexy)	See text
	Head injury	See text
	Autoimmune	See text

Table 13.5   Coma in patient with hypopituitarism

Possible cause	Measure	Aetiology
Hypoglycaemia	Blood glucose (low)	lack of GH → ↑ sensitivity to insulin
Water intoxication	Electrolytes (Na decrease, K decrease, urea decrease)	Cortisol required for excretion of water load
Hypothermia	Rectal temperature (may be <32°C)	Hypothyroidism

sufficiency. In contrast to primary adrenal insufficiency zona glomerulosa function is not lost and hence angiotensin II-induced aldosterone secretion maintains normal plasma electrolytes. In some patients, however, there may be a dilutional hyponatraemia. Cortisol is required for normal water handling by the kidney. In contrast to the pigmentation of Addison's disease a striking degree of pallor is usually present principally because of lack of melanin in the skin.

Finally TSH secretion is lost with consequent secondary hypothyroidism. This further contributes to the apathy and cold intolerance. In contrast to primary hypothyroidism frank myxoedema is not seen.

Untreated severe hypopituitarism eventually results in *coma*. This may follow some mild infection or injury. Several factors may contribute to this (Table 13.5). Investigation is detailed on p. 613.

Management

The aim should be to provide adequate substitution therapy according to the deficiencies demonstrated.

Cortisol replacement. This should be started if there is ACTH deficiency. In someone who is not critically ill cortisol should be given by mouth, 20 mg on waking and 10 mg at 18.00 h. The precise dose may need to be adjusted for the individual patient. Excess weight gain usually indicates over-replacement whilst persistent lethargy may be due to an inadequate dose. Measurement of plasma cortisol levels during the day – a cortisol day curve (Fig. 13.6) – may be helpful in assessing the requisite dose. As indicated above mineralocorticoid replacement is not required.

Thyroid replacement. If this is required then thyroxine 0.1–0.15 mg once daily should be given. It is

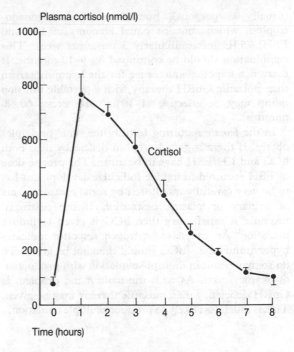

Fig. 13.6   Plasma cortisol levels following the oral administration of hydrocortisone 20 mg in 12 patients with adrenal insufficiency.

dangerous to give thyroid replacement to patients with adrenal insufficiency without first giving glucocorticoid therapy.

Sex hormone replacement therapy. This is indicated if there is gonadotrophin deficiency to restore normal sexual function and to prevent osteoporosis. Male sex hormone replacement in shown in Table 13.6.

In *pre-menopausal females* the treatment is cyclical oestrogen therapy (e.g. ethinyloestradiol 20–30 μg for 3 weeks) with a progestogen such as medroxy-progesterone acetate (5 mg daily) for days 14–21.

Patients requiring *fertility* will usually need to be given gonadotrophin therapy. In the *post-pubertal male* it is usual to give human chorionic gonadotrophin (hCG) (3000 IU intramuscularly weekly) to stimulate testosterone production by the interstitial cells for the first 6 months and then hCG weekly together with FSH

Table 13.6   Sex hormone replacement therapy in males

Preparation	Dose	Route of administration	Frequency	Comment
Depot testosterone esters (Sustanon)	250–500 mg	Intramuscular injection	Every 2–4 weeks	Monitor on basis of symptoms + packed cell vol (every 6–12 months)
Testosterone undecanoate	80–120 mg	Oral	Twice daily	May produce variable blood levels
Testosterone implant	600–800 mg	Subcutaneous	3–6 months	Probably best method for obtaining normal blood levels

(usually as pergonal, human menopausal gonado-trophin, which contains equal amounts of LH and FSH) 75 IU intramuscularly 3 times per week. This combination should be continued for 9–12 months. If there is a hypothalamic cause for the hypopituitarism then pulsatile GnRH therapy with a portable infusion pump may be effective (1–10 μg/pulse every 60–90 minutes).

In the *female* requiring fertility the same principles obtain. If there is gonadotrophin deficiency then both hCG and LH/FSH have to be given. The precise dose of FSH required to induce follicular development has to be very carefully monitored by serial measurements of urinary or plasma oestradiol. If the oestrogen response is satisfactory then hCG is given to induce ovulation. An excessive oestrogen response indicates hyperstimulation – hCG should then not be given. To do so may result in multiple ovulation with production of ovarian cysts. As with the male if the problem is GnRH deficiency then pulsatile therapy may be given. This is much less likely to produce multiple ovulation.

GROWTH HORMONE DEFICIENCY

In children hyposecretion of GH causes short stature. This is usually due to an inability to secrete GHRH rather than a primary pituitary abnormality. The next most common cause would be a craniopharyngioma.

In children with short stature it is essential that accurate records of height and weight are kept and entered on a percentile chart. Single measurements are of less value than serial estimates. With the latter the growth velocity can be plotted. If a child is below the 3rd centile or has measurements which cross the centile lines then careful serial measurements are necessary. If growth velocity is below the 25th centile or above the 75th centile then the child should be referred to a specialist growth clinic. The parental heights should be noted. There is a clear relationship between the mid-parental height and the expected height of the child – 95% of normal children will be within 8.5 cm of the mid-parental height.

Differential diagnosis of short stature
Short stature may be due to a large number of different reasons – both endocrine and non-endocrine. The presenting growth velocity may be normal or impaired as shown in the information box (right).

Diagnosis of GH deficiency
The tests used to assess GH secretion are detailed on page 613.

DIFFERENTIAL DIAGNOSIS OF SHORT STATURE

Impaired growth velocity
- Endocrine
  Isolated GH deficiency
  Panhypopituitarism
  Primary hypothyroidism
  Cushing's syndrome
  Pseudohypoparathyroidism
- Abnormal body proportions
  Short limbs for spine (e.g. achondroplasia)
  Short limbs and very short spine (e.g. mucopolysaccharidoses)
- Other conditions
  Chromosome abnormalities (e.g. Turner's)
  Malabsorption (coeliac, Crohn's, colitis)
  Systemic illness (asthma, heart, renal disease)
  Malnutrition
  Psychosocial deprivation

Normal growth velocity on presentation
- Prior problem affecting growth but no longer active
  Intra-uterine growth retardation
  Congenital heart disease
- Constitutional short stature
  Normal bone age
- Physiological growth delay
  Retarded bone age

Management of GH deficiency
In children with documented GH deficiency and impaired growth GH therapy is indicated (biosynthetic GH 24 units/m²/week divided into daily bedtime subcutaneous injections). Patients with other causes of short stature such as Turner's syndrome may benefit from GH therapy. In the case of a normal short child the role of GH treatment is not yet clear and is being examined in a series of clinical trials.

TUMOURS OF THE PITUITARY GLAND

The pathology of tumours is shown in the information box (p. 617).

GH hypersecretion is usually due to an acidophil (or a mixed acidophil and chromophobe) macroadenoma. Very rarely it may result from ectopic production of GHRH (e.g. by pancreatic tumour).

Excess secretion of ACTH and of β-lipotrophin is usually associated with a microadenoma (75% cases) of basophil (or mixed basophil and chromophobe) cells (Cushing's disease). There is usually little or no enlargement of the pituitary fossa. If, however, the Cushing's is treated by bilateral adrenalectomy with no definitive treatment for the pituitary then Nelson's syndrome may develop (hyperpigmentation associated with aggressive pituitary tumour).

PATHOLOGY OF TUMOURS OF THE PITUITARY GLAND

Pituitary tumours may be:
- Macroadenomas > 10 mm diameter
- Microadenomas < 10 mm diameter

The large tumours may:
- Produce hypofunction by pressure on surrounding normal pituitary tissue (see p. 614).
- Involve adjacent structures
  - Dura – headache
  - Optic chiasma, nerve or tract – visual field loss
  - Cavernous sinus – IIIrd, IVth, or VIth nerve palsy
- Prevent prolactin inhibitory factor, dopamine, from reaching pituitary lactotroph – disconnection hyperprolactinaemia

Both micro- and macroadenomas may be functional or non-functional. The functional tumours may secrete:
- GH – Acromegaly/gigantism
- prolactin – Galactorrhea/menstrual dysfunction/impotence
- ACTH – Cushing's syndrome
- TSH – Hyperthyroidism

There may also be mixed tumours secreting more than one hormone e.g. GH and prolactin.

Prolactin-secreting tumours are the most common of the pituitary adenomas. They may be acidophil (densely granulated) or more commonly chromophobe (sparsely granulated). It is important to understand that the conventional classification of pituitary tumours based on the staining characteristics of the cells may be misleading. Thus many tumours with hormone secretion have little stored hormone and hence are chromophobe. For this reason the increased sensitivity of immunohistochemistry is useful in characterising these tumours. Specific antibodies against the pituitary hormones can then be used to localise hormones.

Craniopharyngiomas are tumours, usually cystic, developing in cell rests of Rathke's pouch, and may be located within the sella turcica, or commonly in the suprasellar space, where they frequently calcify. In either situation their clinical presentation is likely to be due to pressure on adjacent structures, e.g. the visual pathways.

Primary carcinoma of the pituitary gland is rare, but a metastatic tumour from a primary in the breast, lung, kidney or elsewhere may occur in the hypothalamus and reduce pituitary function. Other tumours, for example pinealoma, ependymoma or meningioma, may occasionally be associated with some disturbance of the pituitary or hypothalamus. Conditions such as sarcoidosis or syphilis may mimic pituitary tumours.

Clinical features

These vary, depending on the type of lesion in the pituitary gland and the effect of that lesion on sur-rounding structures. Enlarging tumours of the gland may present with signs attributable to increased output of hormones or to failure of secretion. Some tumours secreting hormones compress the remaining pituitary tissue, so that there may be failure of some functions of the gland in the presence of an excess of others. Headache is the most constant but least specific symptom.

Involvement of an optic nerve, the optic chiasma, or an optic tract leads to impaired visual fields. Bitemporal hemianopia is the most characteristic finding associated with pressure upon the chiasma. Optic atrophy may be apparent on ophthalmoscopy. Diplopia and strabismus may follow pressure on the third, fourth or sixth cranial nerves.

Some tumours expand sufficiently to interfere with ADH secretion and so cause diabetes insipidus. Damage to the posterior pituitary per se will not normally produce diabetes insipidus as vasopressin secretion by the hypothalamus continues. Thus if there is diabetes insipidus it usually indicates that the tumour has a suprasellar extension. Tumours which expand upwards to impinge on the hypothalamus may cause obesity and disturbance of sleep, thirst, temperature control and appetite.

Investigation

Anatomy: radiological investigation

Plain X-rays. X-rays of the pituitary fossa may demonstrate enlargement of the sella turcica (Fig. 13.7)

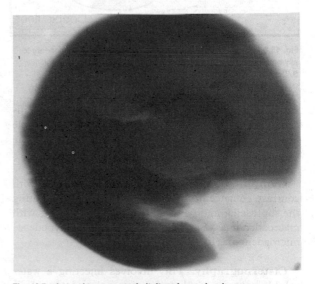

Fig. 13.7   Lateral tomogram of pituitary fossa showing gross enlargement by pituitary tumour.

A

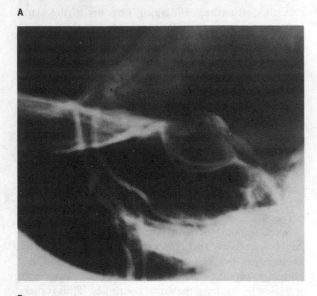

B

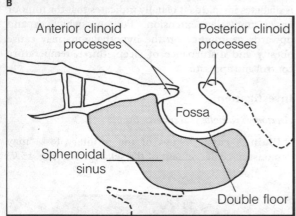

Fig. 13.8   X-ray of pituitary fossa showing double floor secondary to asymmetrical expansion of fossa by pituitary tumour. A. Lateral view. **B.** Diagram of the same view.

and erosion of the clinoid processes. Suprasellar calcification may be seen in a craniopharyngioma. A 'double floor' of the sella (Fig. 13.8) may be present if the tumour enlarges the fossa asymmetrically.

Computed tomography (CT). This (usually with contrast enhancement) is essential for demonstrating the suprasellar and parasellar anatomy in patients with macroadenomas (Fig. 13.9) and may show a hypodense microadenoma (Fig. 13.21).

Cisternography. This involves injecting a water soluble contrast medium by cisternal puncture. It is usually done in conjunction with CT scanning to

A

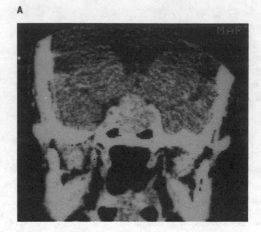

B

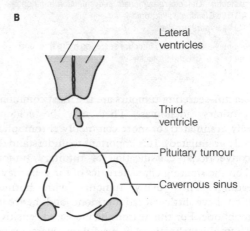

Fig. 13.9   CT scan of pituitary. A. Coronal view showing suprasellar extension of pituitary tumour. **B.** Diagram of the same view.

demonstrate an empty sella, the superior aspect of a pituitary tumour or a hypothalamic lesion.

Nuclear magnetic resonance scanning (NMR). This is another very valuable imaging technique for pituitary lesions but is only available in relatively few centres.

Visual fields. Both central and peripheral visual fields should be plotted (i.e. not just perimetry). Classically pressure on the optic chiasma produces a bitemporal hemianopia. However, it is important to recognise that *any type of visual field defect* may result from suprasellar extension of a pituitary tumour as the growth may involve the optic nerve to produce unilateral loss of acuity or a scotoma, the optic chiasma or the optic tract (homonymous hemianopia).

Function

Both anterior (p. 612) and posterior (p. 621) pituitary function need to be assessed. The latter cannot be done until the anterior pituitary function has been tested and, if there is ACTH or TSH insufficiency, the patient started on replacement therapy (cortisol and thyroxine necessary for normal water handling by the kidney).

If the clinical features suggest hormonal hypersecretion then this must be assessed as detailed below.

Management

If there is evidence of pressure on the visual pathways then urgent treatment is required. The type of treatment depends on the nature of the pituitary tumour. If this is a prolactinoma then bromocriptine should be given (p. 620) as this will shrink about 80% of these tumours and surgery can be avoided. If, however, bromocriptine is stopped then the tumour can rapidly (i.e. over a few days) re-enlarge and thus many patients are given definitive treatment with external radiotherapy (3500 rads in 33 fractions is often used).

If there is a non-functioning tumour with visual field defect then surgery is required. Almost all tumours can be decompressed by a trans-sphenoidal approach rather than the trans-frontal which has a higher morbidity and mortality. Following decompression external radiotherapy is necessary to prevent recurrence.

When there is hyperfunction of the pituitary sufficiently severe to affect the patient's welfare and prognosis, then treatment aimed at either destroying the tumour, or affecting its capacity to grow or secrete should be considered. In Cushing's disease (pituitary dependent Cushing's syndrome), prolactinomas and acromegaly it may be possible by trans-sphenoidal surgery to selectively remove an adenoma and leave sufficient pituitary tissue to maintain normal function. Alternatively, suppression of tumour growth and, to a less predictable extent, of secretory capacity may be achieved by external radiotherapy usually with a linear accelerator. The implantation of yttrium in the pituitary fossa is an alternative form of irradiation used only in certain specialist centres. The same is true for proton beam therapy.

SYNDROMES OF ANTERIOR PITUITARY HYPERSECRETION

GIGANTISM AND ACROMEGALY

Clinical features

If growth hormone hypersecretion occurs before epiphyses have fused then gigantism will result. More commonly GH excess occurs in adult life after epiphyseal closure and acromegaly ensues. If hypersecretion starts in adolescence and persists into adult life then the two conditions may be combined. The clinical features are listed in the information box (below).

CLINICAL FEATURES OF ACROMEGALY

Soft tissue changes
Skin thickening
Increased sweating
Increased sebum production
Enlargement of lips, nose and tongue
Increased heel pad thickness
Arthropathy
Myopathy
Carpal tunnel syndrome
Visceromegaly (e.g. thyroid, heart, liver)

Acral enlargement
Large hands (difficult to remove rings)
Large feet (↑ shoe size, ↑ width)

Other bone changes
Growth of lower jaw – prognathism
Skull growth – prominent supraorbital ridges with large frontal sinuses
Kyphosis

Metabolic effects
Glucose intolerance (25%)
Clinical diabetes mellitus (10%)
Hypertension (25% associated increase in total exchangeable sodium)

In addition the pituitary tumour, almost invariably the source of GH, may produce headaches, visual field defect or cranial nerve palsies (p. 617). The tumour may also affect other anterior pituitary hormone secretion (p. 614). In about 30% of patients prolactin levels are elevated.

Investigation

These patients should be investigated in the same way as the patients with non-functioning pituitary tumours (p. 612). The clinical diagnosis must be confirmed by measuring GH levels during an oral glucose tolerance test (Fig. 13.5). In normal subjects GH suppresses to below 2 mU/litre. In acromegaly it does not suppress and in about 50% of patients there is a paradoxical rise. In 70% of acromegalics there is a GH rise after TRH administration. This is not found in normal subjects. The tissue effects of raised GH result in high circulating insulin-like growth factor, IGF-1.

Management

Medical. Bromocriptine, a long-acting dopamine agonist, will lower GH in about 75% of patients but only a small number of patients get levels below 10 mU/litre. The usual dose is 20–30 mg/day in divided doses with food. This must be started at low dose, 1.25–2.5 mg/day, and then gradually increased. It may initially cause nausea, vomiting and postural hypotension especially if too large a dose is given. On maintenance therapy constipation may occur. More recently a long-acting analogue of somatostatin (octreotide) has been used with considerable success. It has to be given by subcutaneous injection usually 3 times daily.

Surgical. Trans-sphenoidal surgery may enable selective removal of an adenoma with cure. However, with large tumours surgical cure of GH excess is much more difficult. Surgery may, however, be required if there is a visual field defect. After decompression external radiotherapy should be given.

Radiotherapy. Conventional external radiotherapy given using a linear accelerator is an effective treatment of acromegaly in that it stops tumour growth and lower GH levels. The problem is that GH levels fall slowly and hypopituitarism occurs in about 35% of patients. In a few centres interstitial irradiation is given by implanting rods of yttrium into the pituitary via a transnasal stereotaxic operation.

CUSHING'S DISEASE

This is dealt with in the section on Cushing's syndrome (p. 643).

HYPERPROLACTINAEMIA

Elevation of plasma prolactin levels is a common endocrine finding and may arise from a variety of causes. Even though the list is long it is usually possible by taking a careful history, especially with regard to drug therapy, to rapidly reach a presumptive diagnosis. The causes are listed in the information box (right).

Clinical features

Hyperprolactinaemia may be associated with galactorrhoea and therefore the breasts in both sexes must be examined. Hippocrates was one of the first to observe that milk secretion was associated with decreased gonadal function. Thus in women amenorrhoea, oligomenorrhoea, deficient luteal phase progesterone production or menorrhagia may all be associated with hyperprolactinaemia. It is important to measure prolactin in cases of unexplained infertility.

In men hyperprolactinaemia usually presents with

CAUSES OF ELEVATED PLASMA PROLACTIN

Physiological
Stress
    Pregnancy
    Lactation

Drugs
Dopamine antagonists
    Phenothiazines e.g. chlorpromazine
    Butyrophenones e.g. haloperidol
    Metoclopramide
Dopamine depleting
    Reserpine
    Methyldopa
Oestrogens
TRH

Pathological
Hypothalamic disease
    Dopamine depletion
Stalk section ⎫
Non-functioning   Disconnection
pituitary tumours ⎭   hyperprolactinaemia
Prolactinomas
Mixed pituitary tumours
    e.g. GH + prolactin
Primary hypothyroidism
    30% cases
Chest wall reflex
    e.g. nipple stimulation, post herpes zoster
Renal failure
Ectopic source

---

loss of libido or impotence. Unfortunately at this stage many have a macroadenoma often with associated visual field defects.

Investigation

Plasma prolactin levels greater than 4000 mU/litre almost invariably indicate a diagnosis of prolactinoma (upper limit of normal for many assays is 360 mU/l). Because of variation with stress of venepuncture it is useful to have more than one basal prolactin level. The value of dynamic function tests of prolactin secretion and the assessment of pituitary anatomy and function are detailed on p. 612.

Management

Medical. In almost all cases of hyperprolactinaemia dopamine agonist therapy with bromocriptine will lower prolactin levels, often to below normal, with return of gonadal function (regular periods with fertility in women, return of libido and potency in males). The usual dose is 2.5 mg orally 3 times daily with meals. As with acromegaly the drug must be started at a low dose, 1.25 mg daily, and gradually increased. If gonadal function does not return despite effective lowering of prolactin then there may be associated gonadotrophin deficiency or, in the female, the onset of a premature or natural menopause.

Surgical. As discussed on p. 619 bromocriptine not only lowers prolactin levels but shrinks the majority of prolactin-secreting macroadenomas. Thus surgical decompression of these large tumours is not usually necessary unless they are cystic. However, microadenomas can be removed selectively by transsphenoidal surgery with a cure rate of about 80%.

Radiotherapy. External irradiation may be required as definitive treatment for some macroadenomas to prevent regrowth if bromocriptine is stopped.

Pregnancy. Prolactinomas may enlarge rapidly during pregnancy and thus these patients need careful assessment prior to becoming pregnant and supervision with assessment of prolactin levels and visual fields during pregnancy.

DIABETES INSIPIDUS (DI)

This uncommon disease is characterised by the persistent excretion of excessive quantities of dilute urine, and by constant thirst. Diabetes insipidus can be divided into:

Cranial – deficient production of anti-diuretic hormone (ADH), arginine vasopressin (AVP)

Nephrogenic DI – renal tubules unresponsive to vasopressin

Aetiology

The aetiology of cranial and nephrogenic diabetes insipidus are shown in the information boxes below and right.

CAUSES OF CRANIAL DIABETES INSIPIDUS

Genetic defect
Dominant
Recessive (DIDMOAD syndrome – association of DI with diabetes mellitus, optic atrophy, deafness)

Hypothalamic or high stalk lesion
e.g. histiocytosis-X, sarcoidosis, craniopharyngioma, pituitary tumour with suprasellar extension, basal meningitis, head injury, surgery, encephalitis

Idiopathic

CAUSES OF NEPHROGENIC DIABETES INSIPIDUS

This may be due to:
- Genetic defect
  Sex-linked recessive
  Cystinosis
- Metabolic abnormality
  Hypokalaemia
  Hypercalcaemia
- Drug therapy
  Lithium
  Demethylchlortetracycline
- Poisoning
  Heavy metals

If there is associated cortisol deficiency then diabetes insipidus may not be manifest until glucocortoid replacement therapy is given.

Clinical features

The most marked symptoms are polyuria and polydipsia. The patient may pass 5–20 or more litres of urine in 24 hours. This is of very low specific gravity and osmolality (less than plasma usually). In the unconscious patient or one with damage to the hypothalamic thirst centre DI is potentially lethal unless the condition is recognised and appropriate therapy given.

Investigation

The key test is that involving water deprivation to distinguish between DI and psychogenic polydipsia. If DI is suspected then the test is followed by vasopressin administration to demonstrate whether the kidney can (cranial) or cannot (nephrogenic) respond. The details of this test are given on page 554.

In cranial DI the pre-testing plasma osmolality is usually high and with fluid deprivation often exceeds 300 mOsm/kg. The urine osmolality of the DI patients is usually less than that of the plasma at the end of the test but rises when vasopressin is given whereas in normal subjects urine osmolality after 8 hours fluid deprivation is about 800 mOsm/kg and does not increase when vasopressin is given.

In psychogenic polydipsia the initial plasma osmolality is usually below normal and the urine osmolality fails to rise normally with water deprivation. The renal response to exogenous vasopressin is also impaired because of the effect of long-term overhydration on the kidney.

In nephrogenic DI appropriate tests include electrolytes, plasma calcium and investigation of the renal tract.

The suprasellar anatomy in patients with cranial DI needs to be assessed as indicated on p. 618.

Management

This is usually with the long-acting analogue of vasopressin, desmopressin (DDAVP). The amount of vasopressin required to keep the patient in water balance must be determined by measuring the fluid output. Desmopressin is given intranasally; $10-20\,\mu g$ once or twice daily elicits a response as effectively as vasopressin given by injection.

A variety of other drugs have been used. Chlorpropamide ($125-250\,mg/d$), the oral hypoglycaemic agent, enhances the renal responsiveness to vasopressin. As might be anticipated hypoglycaemia can be a problem. An alternative drug with a similar action is carbamazepine ($100-200\,mg/d$). Thiazide diuretics (e.g. bendrofluazide $5-10\,mg/d$) remain the only effective drug therapy for nephrogenic DI and reduce urine volume in this condition by about 50%. Plasma potassium levels need to be carefully monitored.

THE THYROID GLAND

PHYSIOLOGY

The thyroid secretes predominantly thyroxine (T_4), and only a small amount of triiodothyronine (T_3); approximately 85% of T_3 is produced by mono-deiodination of T_4 in other tissues such as liver, muscle and kidney. T_4 is probably not metabolically active until converted to T_3 and may be regarded as a pro-hormone. T_3 and T_4 circulate in plasma almost entirely bound ($> 99.9\%$) to transport proteins, mainly thyroxine binding globulin (TBG). It is the minute fraction of unbound or free hormone which diffuses into tissues and exerts its metabolic action. It is possible to measure the concentration in plasma of total or free T_3 and T_4, but the advantage of the free hormone measurements is that they are not influenced by changes in concentration of binding proteins, e.g. in pregnancy TBG levels are increased and total T_3 and T_4 may be raised but free thyroid hormone levels are normal.

Production of T_3 and T_4 in the thyroid is stimulated by thyrotrophin (thyroid-stimulating hormone, TSH), a glycoprotein released from the thyrotroph cells of the anterior pituitary in response to the hypothalamic tri-peptide, thyrotrophin-releasing hormone (TRH) (see p. 610). A circadian rhythm of TSH secretion can be demonstrated with a peak at 01.00 hours and trough at 11.00 hours, but the variation is small and does not influence the timing of blood sampling for assessment of thyroid function.

There is a negative feedback of thyroid hormones on the thyrotrophs such that in hyperthyroidism when plasma concentrations of T_3 and T_4 are raised, TSH secretion is suppressed, and in hypothyroidism due to disease of the thyroid gland, low T_3 and T_4 are associated with high circulating TSH levels. The anterior pituitary is very sensitive to minor changes in thyroid hormone levels within the normal range. Although the reference range for total T_4 is $60-150\,nmol/l$, a rise or fall of $20\,nmol/l$ in an individual in whom the level is usually $100\,nmol/l$ would on the one hand be associated with undetectable TSH and on the other hand with a raised TSH. The combination of 'normal' T_3 and T_4 and suppressed or raised TSH is known as subclinical hyperthyroidism (p. 629) or subclinical hypothyroidism (p. 634) respectively.

Non-thyroidial illness

In ill patients, e.g. myocardial infarction or pneumonia, not only is there a decreased peripheral conversion of T_4 to T_3, but also there are alterations in the concentrations of binding proteins and in their affinity for thyroid hormones. In addition TSH levels may be sub-normal, or may even rise into the hypothyroid range during convalescence. It follows that the biochemical assessment of thyroid function may be difficult in such patients and should not be undertaken unless there is strong clinical evidence of thyroid disease requiring urgent treatment.

HYPERTHYROIDISM

Hyperthyroidism is the clinical syndrome which results from exposure of the body tissues to excess circulating levels of free thyroid hormones. It is a common disorder with a prevalence of about $20/1000$ females; males are affected five times less frequently.

Causes

It is important to identify the cause of hyperthyroidism (Table 13.7) in order to prescribe appropriate treatment. In over 90% of patients the hyperthyroidism is due to Graves' disease, multinodular goitre or an autonomously functioning solitary thyroid nodule (toxic adenoma). Excess pituitary secretion of TSH which may or may not originate from a tumour, intrinsic thyroid stimulating activity of human chorionic gonadotrophin in hydatidiform mole and choriocarcinoma, ovarian teratoma containing thyroid tissue (struma ovarii) and metastatic differentiated carcinoma of the thyroid are extremely rare causes.

Table 13.7 Causes of hyperthyroidism and their relative frequencies in a series of 2087 patients presenting to the Royal Infirmary, Edinburgh in the 10-year period 1979–1988

Cause	Frequency (%)
Graves' disease	76
Multinodular goitre	14
Autonomously functioning solitary thyroid nodule	5
Thyroiditis	
Subacute (de Quervain's)*	3
Postpartum*	0.5
Iodide-induced	
Drugs*, e.g. amiodarone	1
Radiographic contrast media*	—
Iodine-prophylaxis programmes*	—
Extra-thyroidal source of thyroid hormone excess	
Factitious hyperthyroidism*	0.2
Struma ovarii*	—
TSH-induced	
Inappropriate TSH secretion by pituitary	0.2
Choriocarcinoma and hydatidiform mole	—
Follicular carcinoma ± metastases	0.1

* These causes of hyperthyroidism are characterised by a negligible radioiodine uptake test result.

Clinical features

Hyperthyroidism usually develops insidiously and most patients have had symptoms for at least six months before presentation. Almost every system is affected and the clinical features are listed in the information box (right). There is great individual variation in the dominant features; for example the initial presentation may be to a cardiologist on account of palpitations, to a dermatologist because of pruritus or to a gastro-intestinal clinic with diarrhoea. Weight loss in older patients may be associated with anorexia raising the possibility of carcinoma. Atrial fibrillation which is seldom seen in young patients unless there is severe long-standing disease, occurs in up to 50% of patients over 60 years of age and characteristically the ventricular rate is uninfluenced by digoxin. In children medical attention may be sought because of behaviour disorders, deteriorating academic performance or a premature growth spurt.

GRAVES' DISEASE

Graves' disease is distinguished clinically from other forms of hyperthyroidism by the presence of diffuse thyroid enlargement, ophthalmopathy and rarely pre-tibial myxoedema. It can occur at any age but is unusual before puberty and most commonly affects the 30–50-year age group.

Pathogenesis

Graves' disease is the major immunologically-mediated form of hyperthyroidism, the other being postpartum thyroiditis (p. 628). The hyperthyroidism results from

---

CLINICAL FEATURES OF HYPERTHYROIDISM

Goitre
Diffuse ± bruit[1]
Nodular

Gastrointestinal
Weight loss despite normal or increased appetite[2]
Hyperdefaecation[2]
Diarrhoea and steatorrhoea
Anorexia[3]
Vomiting

Cardiorespiratory
Palpitations[2], sinus tachycardia, atrial fibrillation[3]
Increased pulse pressure
Ankle oedema in absence of cardiac failure
Angina, cardiomyopathy and cardiac failure[3]
Dyspnoea on exertion[2]
Exacerbation of asthma

Neuromuscular
Nervousness, irritability, emotional lability[2], psychosis
Tremor
Hyper-reflexia, ill-sustained clonus
Muscle weakness, proximal myopathy, bulbar myopathy[3]
Periodic paralysis (predominantly Chinese)

Dermatological
Increased sweating[2], pruritus
Palmar erythema, spider naevi
Onycholysis
Alopecia
Pigmentation, vitiligo[1]
Finger clubbing[1]
Pretibial myxoedema[1]

Reproductive
Amenorrhoea/oligomenorrhoea
Infertility, spontaneous abortion
Loss of libido, impotence

Ocular
Lid retraction, lid lag[1]
Grittiness[1], excessive lacrimation[1]
Chemosis[1]
Exophthalmos[1], corneal ulceration[1]
Ophthalmoplegia[1], diplopia[1]
Papilloedema[1], loss of visual acuity[1]

Other
Heat intolerance[2]
Fatigue[2], apathy[3]
Gynaecomastia
Lymphadenopathy[1]
Thirst

[1]Features of Graves' disease only.
[2]The most common symptoms of hyperthyroidism, irrespective of its cause.
[3]Features found particularly in elderly patients.

---

the production of IgG antibodies directed against the TSH-receptors on the thyroid follicular cell which stimulate thyroid hormone production and, in the majority, goitre formation. These antibodies are termed thyroid stimulating immunoglobulins or TSH-receptor antibodies (TRAb) and can be detected in the serum of most patients with Graves' disease. Why these antibodies are produced is not clear but there are important genetic and environmental considerations.

In Caucasians there is an association of Graves' disease with HLAB8, DR3 and DR2, and with inability to secrete the water soluble glycoprotein form of the ABO blood group antigens coded for on chromosomes 6 and 19 respectively. Family studies show that 50% of monozygotic twins are concordant for hyperthyroidism as opposed to 5% of dizygotic twins. The trigger for the development of hyperthyroidism in genetically susceptible individuals may be infection with viruses or bacteria. Certain strains of the gut organisms *Escherichia coli* and *Yersinia enterocolitica* possess cell-membrane TSH receptors. The production of antibodies to these microbial antigens which might cross-react with the TSH receptor on the host thyroid follicular cell could result in the development of hyperthyroidism. Stress is usually dismissed as aetiologically unimportant but many experienced endocrinologists are impressed from time to time by the temporal relationship between the onset of hyperthyroidism and a major life event such as the death of a close relative.

The concentration of TRAb in the serum is presumed to fluctuate because of the natural history of Graves' disease (Fig. 13.10). The ultimate thyroid failure in some patients is thought to result from the presence of yet another immunoglobulin, a blocking antibody against the TSH receptor, and from tissue destruction by cytotoxic antibodies and cell-mediated immunity.

The pathogenesis of the ophthalmopathy and dermopathy is less well understood. Both are immunologically mediated but TRAb is not implicated. Within the orbit there is proliferation of fibroblasts which secrete hydrophilic glycosaminoglycans. The resulting increased interstitial fluid content combined with a chronic inflammatory cell infiltrate causes marked swelling of the extra-ocular muscles (Fig. 13.11) and a rise in retrobulbar pressure. The eye is displaced forwards (proptosis, exophthalmos) and in more severe cases there is optic nerve compression.

Clinical features

Goitre. The diffusely enlarged gland is usually 2–3 times the normal volume and increased blood flow may be manifest by a thrill or bruit. In some patients, particularly the elderly, no thyroid enlargement is palpable or the gland may be nodular. The largest goitres tend to occur in young men.

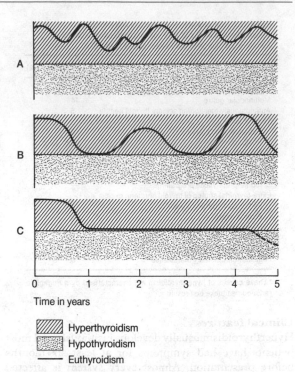

Fig. 13.10   Natural history of the hyperthyroidism of Graves' disease. The majority (60%) of patients have either prolonged periods of hyperthyroidism of fluctuating severity (**A**), or periods of alternating relapse and remission (**B**). It is the minority who experience a single short-lived episode followed by prolonged remission and in some cases by the eventual onset of hypothyroidism (**C**). [Cross-hatched areas represent hyperthyroidism, stippled areas hypothyroidism and the horizontal lines between, euthyroidism].

Ophthalmopathy. This is only present in 50% of patients when first seen but may also develop after successful treatment of the hyperthyroidism of Graves' disease, or precede its development by many years (exophthalmic Graves' disease). The most frequent presenting symptoms are related to increased exposure of the cornea resulting from proptosis and lid retraction. There may be excessive lacrimation made worse by wind and bright light, and pain may be due to conjunctivitis or corneal ulceration. In addition there may be loss of visual acuity and/or visual field resulting from corneal oedema or optic nerve compression. If the extraocular muscles are involved and do not act in concert, diplopia will result.

Pretibial myxoedema. This infiltrative dermopathy takes the form of raised pink coloured or purplish plaques on the anterior aspect of the leg extending on to the dorsum of the foot. The lesions may be itchy and the skin may have a *peau d'orange* appearance with growth

A

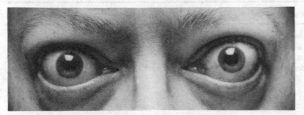

B

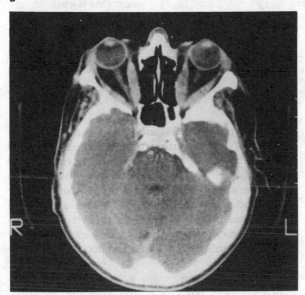

Fig. 13.11   A. Bilateral ophthalmopathy of Graves' disease in a 42-year-old man developing two years after successful treatment of hyperthyroidism with [131]**I.** The main symptoms were those of diplopia in all directions of gaze and reduced visual acuity in the left eye. The periorbital swelling is due to retrobulbar fat prolapsing into the eye lids, and increased interstitial fluid as a result of raised intra-orbital pressure. **B. Transverse CT scan of the orbits of the same patient as in A showing the extraocular muscles enlarged to three times their normal bulk.** This is most obvious at the apex of the left orbit, causing compression of the optic nerve and reduced visual acuity.

of coarse hair; less commonly the face and arms may be affected.

Investigation

A clinical diagnosis can usually be made, but in view of the likely need for prolonged medical treatment or destructive therapy, it is essential to confirm the diagnosis biochemically by more than one test of thyroid function. Serum T_3 and T_4 concentrations are elevated in the majority, but T_4 is in the upper part of the normal range and T_3 raised (T_3-thyrotoxicosis) in 5% of patients, particularly those with recurrent hyper-

thyroidism following surgery or a course of antithyroid drugs. TSH is undetectable if a sensitive assay capable of recording values of 0.1 mU/l or less is used. If this is not available it will be necessary to demonstrate an absent serum TSH response following the intravenous administration of 200 µg TRH. Measurement of ^{131}I uptake by the thyroid and TRAb may be of value in diagnosing Graves' disease if exophthalmos, goitre and pretibial myxoedema are not present. Other non-specific abnormalities are given in the information box below.

NON-SPECIFIC BIOCHEMICAL ABNORMALITIES IN HYPERTHYROIDISM

Hepatic dysfunction
Slightly raised concentrations of bilirubin, alanine aminotransferase and gamma-glutamyl transferase; elevated alkaline phosphatase derived from bone and liver

Mild hypercalcaemia (5%)

Glycosuria
Associated diabetes mellitus
'Lag storage' (p. 667)

Management of hyperthyroidism of Graves' disease

Table 13.8 compares the different treatments. If it were possible to predict with confidence the natural history of the hyperthyroidism in an individual patient at presentation it would be appropriate to give an antithyroid drug for 12–18 months to those in whom a single episode was anticipated and to advise destructive therapy with ^{131}I or surgery for those likely to experience recurrent disease. With the exception of young men with large goitres and those with severe hyperthyroidism such a prediction is not possible. For patients under 40 years of age many centres adopt the empirical approach of prescribing a course of carbimazole and recommending surgery if relapse occurs. Although there is no evidence that thyroid carcinoma or leukaemia is induced by ^{131}I, or that its use results in an increased frequency of congenital malformation among subsequent offspring, radioactive iodine treatment is usually reserved in the UK for patients over the age of 40.

Antithyroid drugs

The most commonly used are carbimazole and its active metabolite, methimazole (not available in the UK). Propylthiouracil is equally effective but the dose is 10 times that of carbimazole. These drugs reduce the synthesis of new thyroid hormones by inhibiting the iodination of

Table 13.8 Comparison of the different treatments for the hyperthyroidism of Graves' disease

Treatment	Indications	Contraindications	Disadvantages/complications
Antithyroid drugs, e.g. carbimazole	1st episode in patients <40 years	Hypersensitivity Breast feeding – (propylthiouracil suitable)	>50% relapse rate usually within 2 years of stopping drug
Subtotal thyroidectomy	1 Recurrent hyperthyroidism after course of antithyroid drugs in patients <40 yrs	Previous thyroid surgery Dependence upon voice, e.g. opera singer, lecturer	Transient hypocalcaemia (10%) Hypoparathyroidism (1%) Recurrent laryngeal nerve palsy[2] (1%)
	2 Initial treatment in males with large goitres and in those with severe hyperthyroidism i.e. total T_3 > 9.0 nmol/l		
	3 Poor drug compliance		
Radioiodine	1 Patients >40 yrs[1]	Pregnancy or planned pregnancy within 6 months of treatment	Hypothyroidism, approx. 40% in 1st year, 80% after 15 years
	2 Recurrence following surgery irrespective of age		
	3 Other serious illness, e.g. multiple sclerosis irrespective of age		

[1] In certain parts of the world, ^{131}I is used more liberally and prescribed for young women in the 20–40 age group. It is likely that with recent more restrictive regulations governing the use of isotopes in the U.K. that ^{131}I will become less popular as a form of therapy.
[2] It is not only vocal cord palsy which alters the voice following thyroid surgery; the superior laryngeal nerves are frequently transected and result in minor changes in voice quality.

tyrosine. Carbimazole also has an immunosuppressive action, leading to a reduction in serum TRAb concentrations, but this is not enough to influence the natural history of the hyperthyroidism significantly. The dosage is given in the information box below.

CARBIMAZOLE

Dosage
0–3 weeks: 15 mg t.d.s.
4–8 weeks: 10 mg t.d.s.
Maintenance: 5–20 mg daily

Adverse effects
rash 2%
agranulocytosis 0.2%

Duration of treatment
18–24 months

There is subjective improvement within 10–14 days of starting carbimazole and the patient is usually clinically and biochemically euthyroid at 3–4 weeks. The maintenance dose is determined by measurement of T_4 and TSH, attempting to keep both hormones within their respective reference ranges. In most patients it can be taken as a single dose and is continued for 18–24 months in the hope that during this period permanent remission will occur. Unfortunately, hyperthyroidism recurs in at least 50%, usually within 2 years of stopping treatment. Rarely, despite good drug compliance, T_4 and TSH levels fluctuate between those of hyperthyroidism and hypothyroidism at successive review appointments, presumably due to rapidly changing concentrations of TRAb. In such patients satisfactory control can be achieved by blocking thyroid hormone synthesis with carbimazole 10 mg t.d.s. and adding T_4 150 μg daily as replacement therapy.

The adverse effects of the antithyroid drugs develop within 7–21 days of starting treatment. Agranulocytosis cannot be predicted by routine measurement of white blood cell count, and is fortunately reversible. Patients should be warned to stop the drug and contact their medical attendant immediately should a severe sore throat develop. Cross sensitivity between the antithyroid drugs is unusual and another member of the group can be substituted with good effect.

Subtotal thyroidectomy
Patients must be rendered euthyroid before operation. The antithyroid drug is stopped 2 weeks before surgery and replaced by potassium iodide 60 mg t.d.s. orally. This maintains euthyroidism in the short term by inhibiting thyroid hormone release and reduces the size and vascularity of the gland making surgery technically easier. Complications of surgery are rare (Table 13.8). One year after surgery 80% of patients are euthyroid, 15% permanently hypothyroid and 5% remain thyrotoxic. Thyroid failure within 6 months of operation may be temporary. Long-term follow-up of patients treated surgically is necessary, as the late development of hypothyroidism and recurrence of thyrotoxicosis are well-recognised.

Radioactive iodine
^{131}I acts either by destroying functioning thyroid cells or by inhibiting their ability to replicate. The variable radiosensitivity of the gland means that the choice of dose is empirical. In most centres 185–370 MBq (5–10 mCi) is given orally depending upon clinical assessment of goitre size. This regimen is effective in 75% of patients within 4–12 weeks. During the lag

period symptoms can be controlled by propranolol 160 mg per day or, in more severe cases, by carbimazole 15 mg t.d.s. for 4–6 weeks starting 48 hours after radio-iodine therapy. If hyperthyroidism persists at 12 weeks a further dose of ^{131}I should be employed. The disadvantage of ^{131}I treatment is that the majority of patients eventually develop hypothyroidism and long-term follow-up is therefore necessary.

Beta-adrenoceptor antagonists

A non-selective member of this group, such as propranolol, will alleviate but not abolish symptoms of hyperthyroidism within 24–48 hours. The usual dose is 160 mg daily. β-adrenoceptor antagonists cannot be recommended for long-term treatment, but they are extremely useful in the short-term, e.g. patients awaiting hospital consultation or following ^{131}I therapy. Propranolol alone or in combination with potassium iodide has been used in the preparation of patients for subtotal thyroidectomy, but this treatment cannot be recommended as standard practice.

Management of ophthalmopathy

The majority of patients require no treatment other than reassurance. Lid retraction will resolve when the patient becomes euthyroid and exophthalamos usually lessens gradually over a period of 2–3 years. For those with symptomatic ophthalmopathy, methylcellulose eyedrops will counter the gritty discomfort of dry eyes and tinted glasses or side shields attached to spectacle frames will reduce the excessive lacrimation triggered by sun or wind. Corneal ulceration is an indication for lateral tarsorrhaphy. Persistent diplopia can be corrected by extraocular muscle surgery but this should be delayed until the degree of diplopia is stable.

Papilloedema, loss of visual acuity or visual field defect require urgent treatment with prednisolone 60 mg daily if blindness is to be prevented. Close co-operation between endocrinologist and ophthalmologist is necessary and if significant improvement is not evident within 7–10 days, orbital decompression is indicated.

Treatment of dermopathy

The pretibial myxoedema of Graves' disease rarely requires to be treated. Local injections of triamcinolone or the application of betamethasone ointment under occlusive dressings may be effective.

TOXIC MULTINODULAR GOITRE

Like Graves' disease, this form of hyperthyroidism is more common in women. The mean age of presentation is 60 years. Thyroid hormone levels are usually only slightly elevated, but as an older age group is affected, cardiovascular features such as atrial fibrillation or cardiac failure tend to predominate. Treatment is usually with a large dose of ^{131}I (555–1850 MBq, 15–50 mCi) as the gland is relatively resistant to radiation. Hypothyroidism is less common than after treatment of Graves' disease. If there is significant tracheal compression or retrosternal extension of the goitre, partial thyroidectomy is indicated. Long-term treatment with anti-thyroid drugs is not appropriate as relapse is invariable after drug withdrawal.

TOXIC ADENOMA

The presence of a toxic solitary nodule is the cause of less than 5% of all cases of hyperthyroidism. The nodule is a follicular adenoma which autonomously secretes excess thyroid hormones and inhibits endogenous TSH secretion with subsequent atrophy of the rest of the thyroid gland. The adenoma is usually greater than 3 cm in diameter. In some cases spontaneous resolution of hyperthyroidism has occurred as a result of infarction of the adenoma.

Most patients are female and over 40 years of age. Although most nodules are palpable, the diagnosis can be made with certainty only by isotope scanning. The hyperthyroidism is usually mild and in almost 50% of patients the plasma T_3 alone is elevated (T_3 thyrotoxicosis). Treatment is by hemithyroidectomy or by ^{131}I, 555–1110 MBq (15–30 mCi). Permanent hypothyroidism does not occur following surgery and is unusual after treatment with ^{131}I, since the atrophic cells surrounding the nodule will have received little or no irradiation.

HYPERTHYROIDISM ASSOCIATED WITH A LOW IODINE UPTAKE

In patients with hyperthyroidism, the thyroid uptake of ^{131}I is usually high but a low or negligible uptake of iodine occurs in some rarer causes. If the radioactive iodine uptake test is not routinely performed in patients with thyrotoxicosis who do not have obvious Graves' disease or nodular goitre, the correct diagnosis may not be made and inappropriate treatment given.

Subacute (de Quervain's) thyroiditis

This form of hyperthyroidism is characterised by pain in the region of the thyroid gland which may radiate to the angle of jaw and the ears and is made worse by swallowing, coughing and movement of the neck. The thyroid is usually palpably enlarged and tender. Systemic upset is common. Affected patients are usually females aged 20–40 years.

Subacute thyroiditis is a virus-induced (Coxsackie, mumps, adenovirus) inflammation of the thyroid gland which results in release of colloid and its constituents into the circulation. Thyroid hormone levels are raised for 4–6 weeks until the preformed colloid is depleted. The iodine uptake is low because the damaged follicular cells are unable to trap iodine and because endogenous TSH secretion is suppressed. Low titre thyroid auto-antibodies appear transiently in the serum, and the erythrocyte sedimentation rate (ESR) is usually raised. The hyperthyroidism is followed by a period of hypo-thyroidism which is usually asymptomatic, and finally by full recovery of thyroid function within 4–6 months. The pain and systemic upset usually respond to simple measures such as aspirin or other non-steroidal anti-inflammatory drugs. Occasionally, however, it may be necessary to prescribe prednisolone 40 mg daily for 3–4 weeks. The hyperthyroidism is mild and treatment with propranolol, 160 mg per day, is usually adequate. Anti-thyroid drugs are of no benefit.

Postpartum thyroiditis

The maternal immune response which is modified during pregnancy to allow survival of the fetal homo-graft is enhanced after delivery and may unmask previously unrecognised subclinical autoimmune thyroid disease. Surveys have shown that transient bio-chemical disturbances of thyroid function, i.e. hyper-thyroidism, hypothyroidism and hyperthyroidism followed by hypothyroidism, lasting a few weeks, occur in 5–10% of women within 6 months of delivery. Those affected are likely to possess antithyroid microsomal antibodies in the serum in early pregnancy. Thyroid biopsy shows a lymphocytic thyroiditis. Symptoms of thyroid dysfunction are rare and there is no association between post-natal depression and abnormal thyroid function tests. However symptomatic hyperthyroidism presenting for the first time within 6 months of child-birth is unlikely to be due to Graves' disease, and the diagnosis of postpartum thyroiditis can be confirmed by a negligible radioiodine uptake.

If treatment of the hyperthyroid phase is necessary, a β-adrenoceptor antagonist should be prescribed and not an antithyroid drug. Postpartum thyroiditis tends to recur after subsequent pregnancies and eventually patients progress over a period of years to permanent hypothyroidism.

A similar painless form of thyroiditis, unrelated to pregnancy, has been increasingly recognised in North America and Japan, and accounts in these countries for up to 20% of all cases of hyperthyroidism.

Iodine-induced hyperthyroidism

The administration of iodine either in prophylactic iodinisation programmes, radiographic contrast media or drugs such as the anti-arrhythmic agent amiodarone, may result in the development of hyperthyroidism which is usually mild and self-limiting. Affected individuals are thought to have underlying thyroid autonomy or Graves' disease in remission. If it is not possible to discontinue amiodarone or substitute another drug, hyperthyroidism can be controlled with carbimazole.

Factitious hyperthyroidism

This uncommon condition occurs when an emotionally disturbed person, usually a nurse, has been taking excessive amounts of a thyroid hormone preparation, most often thyroxine. The exogenous T_4 suppresses pituitary TSH secretion and hence iodine uptake, serum thyroglobulin and release of endogenous thyroid hormones. As a result the $T_4:T_3$ ratio (approximately 30:1 in conventional hyperthyroidism) is increased to approximately 70:1 because circulating T_3 in factitious thyrotoxicosis is derived exclusively from the peripheral monodeiodination of T_4. The combination of negligible iodine uptake high $T_4:T_3$ ratio and a low or undetectable thyroglobulin is diagnostic and has made what was often a difficult diagnosis much simpler.

SPECIAL SITUATIONS

Hyperthyroidism in pregnancy

The coexistence of pregnancy and hyperthyroidism is unusual as anovulatory cycles are common in thyrotoxic patients and autoimmune disease tends to remit during pregnancy. The hyperthyroidism is almost always caused by Graves' disease.

The hyperthyroidism is treated with carbimazole which crosses the placenta and also treats the fetus whose thyroid gland is exposed to the action of maternal TRAb. It is important to use the smallest dose of carbimazole (optimally less than 15 mg per day) which will maintain maternal (and presumably fetal) free hormones and TSH within their respective normal ranges in order to avoid fetal hypothyroidism and goitre.

The patient should therefore be reviewed every 4 weeks and it is a wise precaution to discontinue carbimazole 4 weeks before the expected date of delivery to avoid any possibility of fetal hypothyroidism at the time of maximum brain development. If the assay is available measurement of TRAb in the maternal serum at this stage is valuable; a high titre identifies those fetuses at particular risk of developing neonatal hyperthyroidism.

If maternal hyperthyroidism occurs after delivery, and the patient wishes to continue breast feeding, propylthiouracil (p. 625) is the drug of choice as it is excreted in the milk to a much lesser extent than carbimazole.

If subtotal thyroidectomy is necessary because of poor drug compliance or hypersensitivity, it is most safely performed in the middle trimester. Radioactive iodine is absolutely contraindicated as it invariably induces fetal hypothyroidism.

Hyperthyroidism in childhood
Graves' disease is almost invariably the form of thyrotoxicosis in childhood and usually presents in the second decade. Treatment should be with carbimazole until the patient is about 18 years of age in an attempt to guarantee the important stages in the physical and educational development of the child.

Hyperthyroid crisis
This is a rare and life-threatening increase in the severity of the clinical features of hyperthyroidism. The most prominent signs are fever, agitation, confusion, tachycardia or atrial fibrillation and, in the older patient, cardiac failure. It is a medical emergency and, despite early recognition and treatment, the mortality rate is 10%. Thyrotoxic crisis is most commonly precipitated by infection in a patient with previously unrecognised or inadequately treated hyperthyroidism. It may also develop shortly after subtotal thyroidectomy in an ill-prepared patient or within a few days of ^{131}I therapy when acute irradiation damage may lead to a transient rise in serum thyroid hormone levels.

Management
Patients should be rehydrated and given a broad spectrum antibiotic. Propranolol is rapidly effective orally (80 mg q.d.s.) or intravenously (1–5 mg q.d.s.). Sodium iopodate 500 mg per day orally will restore serum T_3 levels to normal in 48–72 hours. It is a radiographic contrast medium which not only inhibits the release of thyroid hormones, but also reduces the conversion of T_4 to T_3 and is therefore more effective than potassium iodide or Lugol's solution. Carbimazole 15 mg t.d.s. orally inhibits the synthesis of new thyroid hormone. If the patient is unconscious or unco-operative carbimazole can be administered rectally with good effect, but no preparation is available for parenteral use.

Sodium iopodate and propranolol can be withdrawn after 10–14 days and the patient maintained on carbimazole.

Subclinical hyperthyroidism
This term is used to describe clinically euthyroid patients in whom serum thyroid hormone concentrations are normal, but usually in the upper part of the reference range, and TSH undetectable in the absence of non-thyroidal illness. Subclinical hyperthyroidism occurs most often in patients with exophthalmic Graves' disease (50%), multinodular goitre (25%) and in a variable proportion following therapy of hyperthyroidism. Although there is evidence from studies of hepatic, renal and cardiac function that such patients are probably mildly hyperthyroid, treatment is not usually instituted. There is a significant risk of overt hyperthyroidism developing and follow-up is indicated.

PRIMARY HYPOTHYROIDISM

In primary hypothyroidism there is an intrinsic disorder of the thyroid gland e.g. following ^{131}I therapy for Graves' disease, in which low levels of thyroid hormones are associated with raised TSH. The classification is shown in the information box below.

A CLASSIFICATION OF PRIMARY HYPOTHYROIDISM
- Spontaneous atrophic
- Goitrous
  Hashimoto's thyroiditis
  Drug-induced
  Iodine deficiency
  Dyshormonogenesis
- Post-ablative
- Transient
- Subclinical
- Congenital

Spontaneous atrophic hypothyroidism, thyroid failure following ^{131}I or surgical treatment of hyperthyroidism and the hypothyroidism of Hashimoto's thyroiditis account for over 90% of cases in those parts of the world which are not iodine deficient. The prevalence of primary hypothyroidism is 10/1000 but increases to 50/1000 if patients with subclinical hypothyroidism (normal T_4, raised TSH) are included. The female: male ratio is approximately 6:1.

SPONTANEOUS ATROPHIC HYPOTHYROIDISM

This form of primary hypothyroidism increases in incidence with age and, like Graves' disease and Hashimoto's thyroiditis, is an organ-specific auto-immune disorder. There is destructive lymphoid infiltration of the thyroid, ultimately leading to fibrosis and atrophy. There is also evidence for the presence of TSH-receptor antibodies which block the effects of endogenous TSH. In some patients there is a history of Graves' disease treated with antithyroid drugs 10–20 years earlier and, very occasionally, patients with this form of hypothyroidism develop Graves' disease. As with any of the immunologically-mediated thyroid disorders, patients are at risk of developing other organ-specific autoimmune conditions such as type I diabetes mellitus, pernicious anaemia and Addison's disease, and autoimmune disease is not uncommon in their first and second degree relatives.

Clinical features

These depend on the duration and severity of the hypothyroidism. In the patient in whom complete thyroid failure has developed insidiously over months or even years many of the clinical features listed in the information box (right) are likely to be present. A consequence of prolonged hypothyroidism is the infiltration of many body tissues by the mucopolysaccharides, hyaluronic acid and chrondroitin sulphate, resulting in a low-pitched voice, poor hearing, slurred speech due to a large tongue and compression of the median nerve at the wrist. Infiltration of the dermis gives rise to non-pitting oedema or myxoedema which is most marked in the skin of the hands, feet and eyelids. The resultant periorbital puffiness is often striking and when combined with facial pallor due to vasoconstriction and anaemia, or a lemon-yellow tint to the skin due to carotinaemia, purplish lips and malar flush the clinical diagnosis is simple. Most cases of hypothyroidism are not so obvious, however, and unless the diagnosis is positively entertained in a middle-aged woman complaining of symptoms such as tiredness, weight gain, or depression, or with the carpal tunnel syndrome an opportunity for early treatment will be missed. On the other hand many patients are asymptomatic and thyroid failure is detected by screening during hospital admission or by routine testing of thyroid function in patients known to be at risk of developing hypothyroidism, e.g. following ^{131}I therapy of Graves' disease. It is in this group of patients that there is often little or no subjective benefit from thyroxine replacement therapy.

CLINICAL FEATURES OF HYPOTHYROIDISM

General
Tiredness, somnolence
Weight gain
Cold intolerance
Hoarseness
Goitre

Cardiorespiratory
Bradycardia, hypertension, angina, cardiac failure*
Xanthelasma
Pericardial and pleural effusion*

Neuromuscular
Aches and pains, muscle stiffness
Delayed relaxation of tendon reflexes
Carpal tunnel syndrome, deafness
Depression, psychosis*
Cerebellar ataxia*
Myotonia*

Haematological
Macrocytosis
Anaemia
    Iron deficiency (pre-menopausal women)
    Normochromic
    Pernicious

Dermatological
Dry flaky skin and hair, alopecia
Purplish lips and malar flush, carotenaemia
Vitiligo
Erythema ab igne (Granny's tartan)
Myxoedema

Reproductive
Menorrhagia
Infertility
Galactorrhoea*, impotence*

Gastrointestinal
Constipation
Ileus*
Ascites*

* Rare but well-recognised features.

Investigations

Serum T_4 is low and TSH raised, usually in excess of 20 mU/l. T_3 concentrations do not discriminate reliably between euthyroid and hypothyroid patients and should not be measured. Other non-specific abnormalities include elevation of the enzymes lactate dehydrogenase and creatine kinase, raised cholesterol and triglyceride levels and low serum sodium. In severe prolonged hypothyroidism the electrocardiogram (ECG) classically demonstrates sinus bradycardia with low voltage complexes and ST-T wave abnormalities.

Management

Hypothyroidism should be treated with thyroxine

which is available as 25, 50 and 100 µg tablets. It is customary to start slowly and a dose of 50 µg per day should be given for 3 weeks increasing thereafter to 100 µg per day for a further 3 weeks and finally to 150 µg per day. In the elderly and in patients with ischaemic heart disease the initial dose should be 25 µg per day. Thyroxine should always be taken as a single daily dose as it has a plasma half-life of approximately 7 days. The correct dose of thyroxine is that which restores serum TSH to normal. There is some evidence that the finding of an undetectable TSH concentration indicates over treatment even in the presence of a normal T_4, although in certain circumstances, e.g. Hashimoto's thyroiditis and differentiated thyroid carcinoma, the aim is to suppress TSH without inducing overt hyperthyroidism.

Patients feel better within 2–3 weeks. Reduction in weight and periorbital puffiness occurs quickly, but the restoration of skin and hair texture and resolution of any effusions may take 3–6 months.

Special problems

Ischaemic heart disease. Untreated primary hypothyroidism is associated with hyperlipidaemia but there is doubt whether, in the absence of hypertension, it leads to increased coronary atheroma. However, 5% of patients with long-standing hypothyroidism complain of angina at presentation or develop it during treatment with thyroxine. Although angina may remain unchanged in severity, or paradoxically, disappear with restoration of metabolic rate, exacerbation of myocardial ischaemia, infarction and sudden death are well-recognised complications, even using doses of thyroxine as low as 25 µg per day. Approximately 40% of patients with angina cannot tolerate full replacement therapy despite the use of β-adrenoceptor antagonists and vasodilators. Although there is still reluctance to operate on patients with untreated or partially treated hypothyroidism, coronary artery surgery and balloon angioplasty can safely be performed in such patients and, if successful, allow full replacement dosage of thyroxine in the majority.

Myxoedema coma. This is a rare presentation of hypothyroidism in which there is a depressed level of consciousness, usually in an elderly patient who appears myxoedematous. Body temperature may be as low as 25°C, convulsions are not uncommon and cerebrospinal fluid (CSF) pressure and protein content are raised. Mortality rate is 50% and survival depends upon early recognition and treatment of hypothyroidism and other factors contributing to the altered conscious level, e.g.

drugs such as phenothiazines, cardiac failure, chest infection, dilutional hyponatraemia, and hypoxia and hypercapnia due to hypoventilation.

Myxoedema coma is a medical emergency and treatment must begin before biochemical confirmation of the diagnosis. Thyroxine is not usually available for parenteral use and triiodothyronine is given as an intravenous bolus of 20 µg followed by 20 µg every 8 hours until there is sustained clinical improvement. In survivors there is a rise in body temperature within 24 hours and, after 48–72 hours, it is usually possible to substitute oral thyroxine in a dose of 50 µg per day. Unless it is apparent that the patient has primary hypothyroidism, e.g. thyroidectomy scar or goitre, the thyroid failure should be assumed to be secondary to hypothalamic or pituitary disease and treatment given with hydrocortisone sodium succinate 100 mg intramuscularly 8-hourly, pending the results of T_4, TSH and cortisol concentrations. Other measures include slow rewarming by wrapping the patient in a space blanket, cautious use of intravenous fluids, broad spectrum antibiotics and high-flow oxygen. Occasionally, if hypoxia, hypercapnia and respiratory acidosis persist assisted ventilation may be necessary.

Ensuring compliance. Patients often do not take long-term medication in the recommended dose and thyroxine is no exception (Fig. 13.12). It is, therefore, important to measure thyroid function tests every 1–2 years once the dose of thyroxine is stabilised and at each visit to reinforce the need for regular medication. In some patients in whom tablet taking is erratic, thyroxine is taken diligently or even in excess for the few days prior to a clinic visit, resulting in the seemingly anomalous combination of a high serum T_4 and high TSH.

Inappropriate thyroxine therapy. In some patients treatment with thyroxine may have been started in the past without biochemical confirmation of the diagnosis for a variety of complaints such as obesity, tiredness or alopecia and may have been given for many years to patients in whom thyroid failure could have been short-lived, e.g. post-partum thyroiditis. Thyroxine should be stopped and serum T_4 and TSH concentrations measured 4–6 weeks later. This period allows for any thyroxine-induced suppression of pituitary thyrotrophs to recover and a biochemical distinction to be made between primary and secondary hypothyroidism. If the patient is truly hypothyroid, lack of thyroxine for 4–6 weeks will be relatively easily tolerated.

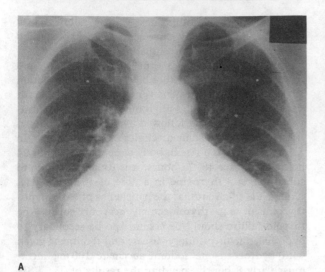

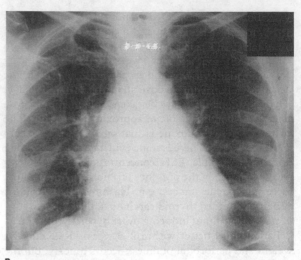

A

B

C

Fig. 13.12   Sequential chest X-rays in a patient with severe long-standing hypothyroidism. A. Before treatment. Cardiomegaly is due to a combination of dilatation and pericardial effusion. **B. After treatment with thyroxine for 9 months. C. After patient had defaulted from follow-up and had discontinued thyroid replacement therapy 2–3 years earlier**. Note the redevelopment of cardiomegaly.

GOITROUS HYPOTHYROIDISM

The following conditions are not always associated with hypothyroidism and should therefore be included in the differential diagnosis of a euthyroid patient with goitre.

Hashimoto's thyroiditis

This is the most common cause of goitrous hypo-thyroidism. It typically affects 20–60-year-old women who present with a small or moderately sized diffuse goitre which is characteristically firm or rubbery in consistency. The goitre may be soft, however, and impossible to differentiate from simple goitre by palpation alone. Thyroid status depends upon the relative degrees of lymphocytic infiltration, fibrosis and follicular cell hyperplasia within the gland but 25% of patients are hypothyroid at presentation. In the remainder serum T_4 is normal and TSH normal or raised but these patients are at risk of developing overt hypothyroidism in future years. In 90% of patients with Hashimoto's thyroiditis thyroid microsomal antibodies are present in the serum. In those under the age of 20 years the ANF may be positive.

Thyroxine therapy is indicated not only for hypothyroidism but also for goitre shrinkage. In this context the dose of thyroxine should be sufficient to suppress serum TSH to undetectable levels without inducing hyperthyroidism (usually 150 µg daily but in some patients 200 µg daily).

Drug-induced hypothyroidism

Lithium carbonate. This is widely used for the treatment of manic-depressive illness. Like iodide, lithium inhibits the release of thyroid hormones. Although the most common evidence of thyroid dysfunction is a raised serum TSH, some patients, usually those with underlying autoimmune thyroiditis, develop goitre and hypothyroidism.

Iodine. When taken for prolonged periods iodine may cause goitrous hypothyroidism. This is usually seen in patients with chronic respiratory diseases given expectorants containing potassium iodide, or in patients receiving the antidysrhythmic drug, amiodarone, which contains a significant amount of iodine.

Iodine deficiency

In certain parts of the world, such as the Andes, Himalayas and central Africa, where there is dietary iodine deficiency, thyroid enlargement is common (more than 10% of the population) and is known as endemic goitre. Most patients are euthyroid and have normal or raised TSH levels. In general the more severe the iodine deficiency, the greater the incidence of hypothyroidism.

Dyshormonogenesis

Dyshormonogenesis is an unusual genetically determined defect in thyroid hormone synthesis. The mode of inheritance is autosomal recessive. Although several forms have been described, the most common results from deficiency of the intrathyroidal peroxidase enzyme. Homozygous individuals present with congenital hypothyroidism; heterozygotes present in the first two decades of life with goitre, normal thyroid hormone levels and a raised TSH. The combination of dyshormonogenetic goitre and nerve deafness is known as Pendred's syndrome.

TRANSIENT HYPOTHYROIDISM

This is often observed during the first 6 months after subtotal thyroidectomy or ^{131}I treatment of Graves'

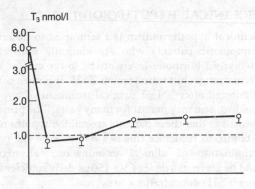
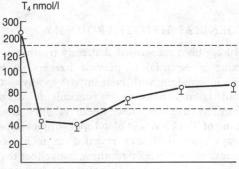
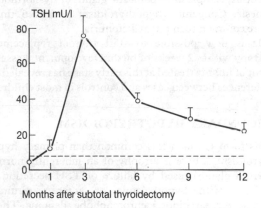

Months after subtotal thyroidectomy

Fig. 13.13   Total T_3, T_4 and TSH levels before and after subtotal thyroidectomy in a series of patients with temporary hypothyroidism. The normal ranges are indicated by the broken lines. (Adapted from Toft et al 1978 New England Journal of Medicine, 298, 643.)

disease, in the post-thyrotoxic phase of subacute thyroiditis and in post-partum thyroiditis (Fig. 13.13). In these conditions thyroxine treatment should not be necessary as the patient is usually asymptomatic during the short period of thyroid failure. In some neonates transplacental passage of TSH-receptor blocking antibodies from a mother with autoimmune thyroid disease is a cause of hypothyroidism which, like neonatal thyrotoxicosis is temporary.

SUBCLINICAL HYPOTHYROIDISM

Subclinical hypothyroidism is a term used to describe asymptomatic patients who are clinically euthyroid with thyroid hormone levels at the lower end of the reference range, but raised serum TSH. It is most often encountered after ^{131}I or surgical treatment of hyperthyroidism and may persist for many years. The present consensus is that these patients are mildly hypothyroid and failure to recognise this is a reflection of the poor discrimination of clinical examination. Thyroxine should be given in a dose of 50–150 µg daily sufficient to restore TSH concentrations to normal.

CONGENITAL HYPOTHYROIDISM

It has long been recognised that early treatment with thyroxine is essential to prevent irreversible brain damage in children with congenital hypothyroidism. Thyroid failure, however, is difficult to diagnose clinically in the first few weeks of life. Routine screening of TSH levels in blood spot samples obtained 5–7 days after birth has revealed an incidence of approximately one in 3000 resulting from either thyroid agenesis, ectopic or hypoplastic glands or dyshormonogenesis. Congenital hypothyroidism is thus 6 times more common than phenylketonuria.

It is now possible to start thyroid replacement therapy within 2 weeks of birth. Developmental assessment of infants treated at this early stage has revealed no differences between cases and controls in most children.

SECONDARY HYPOTHYROIDISM

This form is much less common than primary hypothyroidism. There is atrophy of an inherently normal thyroid gland caused by failure of TSH secretion in patients with hypothalamic or anterior pituitary disease, e.g. sarcoidosis, chromophobe adenoma. There is usually deficiency of other anterior pituitary hormones and clinical evidence of hypopituitarism or, in the case of hypothalamic dysfunction, diabetes insipidus may be present. Recently there have been reports that pituitary hypothyroidism may result from an autoimmune lymphoid hypophysitis.

SIMPLE GOITRE

This is the term used to describe diffuse or multinodular enlargement of the thyroid which occurs sporadically and is of unknown aetiology. It is likely, however, that suboptimal dietary iodine intake, minor degrees of dyshormonogenesis and stimuli such as epidermal growth factor and growth stimulating immunoglobulins are important in the development of simple goitre. Affected patients are euthyroid, usually female and often have a family history of goitre.

SIMPLE DIFFUSE GOITRE

This form of goitre usually presents between the ages of 15–25 years, often during pregnancy, and tends to be noticed not by the patient but by friends and relatives. Occasionally, there is a tight sensation in the neck, particularly when swallowing. The goitre is soft, symmetrical and enlarged 2–3 times normal. There is no tenderness, lymphadenopathy or overlying bruit. Concentrations of T_3, T_4 and TSH are normal and no thyroid autoantibodies are detected in the serum. No treatment is necessary and in most cases the goitre regresses. In some, however, the unknown stimulus to thyroid enlargement persists and as a result of recurrent episodes of hyperplasia and involution during the following 10–20 years the gland becomes multinodular with areas of autonomous function (simple multinodular goitre, Fig. 13.14).

SIMPLE MULTINODULAR GOITRE

Presentation is rare before middle age. The patient may have been aware of goitre for many years, perhaps slowly increasing in size. Rarely, medical advice may have been sought because of painful swelling lasting a few days caused by haemorrhage into a nodule or cyst. The goitre is nodular or lobulated on palpation and may

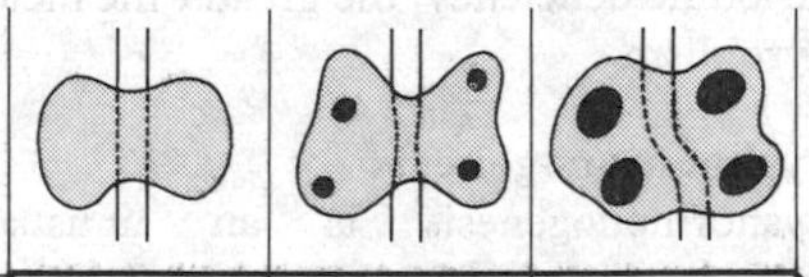

Age (year)	15-25	35-55	>55
Goitre	Diffuse	Nodular	Nodular
Tracheal compression/ deviation	No	Minimal	Yes
T_3, T_4	Normal	Normal	Raised
TSH	Normal	Normal or undetectable	Undetectable

Fig. 13.14 Natural history of simple goitre.

extend retrosternally. Very large goitres may cause mediastinal compression with stridor, dysphagia and obstruction of superior vena cava. Hoarseness due to recurrent laryngeal nerve palsy can occur but is strongly suggestive of thyroid carcinoma. Serum T_3 and T_4 are normal and in the majority are associated with normal TSH. In approximately 25% thyroid hormone levels are in the upper part of their respective normal ranges and TSH is undetectable (subclinical hyperthyroidism). Radiographs of the thoracic inlet may show tracheal displacement or compression, intrathyroidal calcification and the extent of retrosternal extension.

If the goitre is small no treatment is necessary other than annual review as the natural history is progression to a toxic multinodular goitre. Partial thyroidectomy is indicated for large goitres which cause mediastinal compression or which are cosmetically unattractive. Unfortunately recurrence 10–20 years later is not uncommon and cannot be prevented by the long-established custom of treatment with thyroxine which may serve to aggravate any associated hyperthyroidism.

SOLITARY THYROID NODULE

Palpable thyroid nodules occur in approximately 5% of females and are even more commonly found at post-mortem examination. Whereas multinodular goitre is benign, solitary nodules may be malignant. In those who seek medical attention it is important therefore to determine whether the nodule is benign, e.g. cyst, colloid nodule, or malignant. With the exception of haemorrhage into a cyst when thyroid enlargement is of rapid onset and painful, or the presence of cervical lymphadenopathy which is highly suggestive of carcinoma, it is rarely possible to make this distinction on clinical grounds alone. However, a solitary nodule presenting in childhood or adolescence, particularly if there is a past history of head and neck irradiation, or presenting in the elderly, should raise the suspicion of malignancy. Very occasionally a secondary deposit from a renal, breast or lung carcinoma presents as a painful, rapidly growing solitary thyroid nodule.

Investigations
The most useful is fine-needle aspiration of the nodule. This is performed in the outpatient clinic without local anaesthetic, using a standard 21 gauge venepuncture needle and a 20 ml syringe. Aspiration may be therapeutic in the small proportion of patients in whom the swelling is a pure cyst, although recurrence on more than one occasion is an indication for surgery. Usually 2–3 aspirates are taken from the nodule. Cytological examination will differentiate benign (80%) from suspicious or definitely malignant nodules (20%) of which half are confirmed as cancer at surgery. The advantage of fine-needle aspiration over long-established tests such as isotope and ultrasound scanning is that a much higher proportion of patients avoid surgery. The limitation of the method is that it cannot differentiate between follicular adenoma and carcinoma.

It is important to measure serum T_3, T_4 and TSH in all patients with a solitary thyroid nodule. The finding of undetectable TSH is very suggestive of an autonomously functioning thyroid adenoma which can only be confirmed by thyroid scanning, is for practical purposes always benign, and is treated with ^{131}I or surgery.

MALIGNANT TUMOURS

Primary thyroid malignancy is rare, accounting for less than 1% of all carcinomas and has a prevalence of 25 per million. As shown in Table 13.9 it can be classified according to the cell-type of origin. With the exception of medullary carcinoma, thyroid cancer is always more common in females.

Table 13.9 Malignant thyroid tumours

Origin of tumour	Type of tumour	Frequency (%)	Usual age of presentation (years)	Approximate 10-year survival (%)
Follicular cells	Differentiated carcinoma			
	Papillary	70	20–30	95
	Follicular	10	30–40	80
	Undifferentiated carcinoma			
	Anaplastic	5	>60	<1
Parafollicular C-cells	Medullary carcinoma	5–10	>40*	50
Lymphocytes	Lymphoma	5–10	>60	10

* Patients with medullary carcinoma as part of multiple endocrine neoplasia syndromes usually present in childhood.

DIFFERENTIATED CARCINOMA

In most patients presentation is with a palpable solitary nodule.

Papillary carcinoma. This is the commonest of the malignant thyroid tumours and accounts for 90% of irradiation-induced thyroid cancer. It may be multi-focal, and spread is to regional cervical lymph nodes. Some patients present with cervical lymphadenopathy and no apparent thyroid enlargement and the primary lesion may be less than 10 mm in diameter.

Follicular carcinoma. This is always a single encapsulated lesion. Spread to cervical lymph nodes is rare. Metastases are blood-borne and are most often found in bone, lungs and brain.

Management
This is usually by total thyroidectomy followed by a large dose of ^{131}I (3000 MBq) in order to ablate any remaining thyroid tissue, normal or malignant. There-after long-term treatment with thyroxine in a dose sufficient to suppress TSH (usually 150–200 µg daily) is important as there is some evidence that differentiated thyroid carcinoma may be TSH-dependent. Follow-up is by measurement of serum thyroglobulin which should be low or undetectable in patients taking a suppressive dose of thyroxine. A level in excess of 15 µg/l is strongly suggestive of tumour recurrence or metastases which may be detected by whole body scanning with ^{131}I and which may respond to further radioiodine therapy.

Prognosis
Most patients have an excellent prognosis when treated appropriately. Patients under 50 years of age with papillary carcinoma can anticipate a near normal life expectancy if the tumour is less than 2 cm in diameter, confined to the thyroid and cervical nodes and of low-grade malignancy histologically. Even for patients with distant metastases at presentation the 10-year survival is approximately 40%.

ANAPLASTIC CARCINOMA AND LYMPHOMA

These two conditions are difficult to distinguish clinically but not by cytological examination of fine-needle aspiration biopsy. Patients are usually elderly women in whom there is rapid thyroid enlargement over 2–3 months. The goitre is hard and symmetrical. There is usually stridor due to tracheal compression and hoarseness due to recurrent laryngeal nerve palsy.

There is no effective treatment of anaplastic carcinoma although radiotherapy may afford temporary relief of mediastinal compression. The prognosis for lymphoma which may arise from pre-exisiting Hashimoto's thyroiditis, is better. External irradiation often produces dramatic goitre shrinkage and when combined with chemotherapy may result in survival for 5 years or more.

MEDULLARY CARCINOMA

This tumour arises from the parafollicular C-cells of the thyroid. In addition to calcitonin, the tumour may secrete serotonin, ACTH and prostaglandins. As a consequence carcinoid syndrome and Cushing's syndrome have been described in association with medullary carcinoma.

Patients usually present in middle age with a firm thyroid mass. Cervical lymphadenopathy is common, but distant metastases are rare initially. Diarrhoea may be profuse but is unexplained. Serum calcitonin levels are raised and are useful in monitoring response to treatment. Despite the very high levels of calcitonin found in some patients, hypocalcaemia is extremely rare.

Treatment is by total thyroidectomy with removal of affected cervical nodes. Since the C-cells do not concentrate iodine there is no role for ^{131}I therapy. Prognosis is very variable, some patients surviving 20 years or more and others less than one year.

Medullary carcinoma of thyroid as a component of multiple endocrine neoplasia (MEN) syndrome
Whereas medullary carcinoma usually occurs sporadically and in isolation it may present, usually in childhood, as part of two complex syndromes.

MEN IIa. This is inherited as an autosomal dominant and is characterised by medullary carcinoma, phaeochromocytoma which is usually bilateral and parathyroid hyperplasia. The gene responsible has been mapped to chromosome 10. Only 50% of gene carriers present with symptoms by the age of 55 years because clinical penetrance is incomplete. It follows that the family history of an affected individual may be mis-leading. Before a diagnosis of sporadic or isolated medullary carcinoma is made, not only should patients be screened for the presence of phaeochromocytoma, but also their first degree relatives should be examined for goitre and serum calcitonin measured.

MEN IIb. This is much less common. In addition to the features of MEN IIa, there are mucosal neuromas, a marfanoid habitus with poor muscle development and skeletal abnormalities such as kyphosis, pectus excavatum, pes cavus and high arch palate. The facial appearance is characteristic with thick lips (Fig. 13.26), broad based nose, everted eye lids and grossly abnormal dental enamel. MEN IIb is likely to be inherited as an autosomal dominant, but the medullary carcinoma is aggressive and few patients survive into adulthood.

RIEDEL'S THYROIDITIS

This is not a form of thyroid cancer but the presentation is similar and the differentiation can usually only be made by thyroid biopsy. It is an exceptionally rare condition of unknown aetiology in which there is extensive infiltration of the thyroid and surrounding structures with fibrous tissue. There may be associated mediastinal and retroperitoneal fibrosis. Presentation is with a slow growing goitre which is irregular and stony-hard. There is usually tracheal and oesophageal compression necessitating partial thyroidectomy. Other recognised complications include recurrent laryngeal nerve palsy, hypoparathyroidism and eventually hypothyroidism.

THE PARATHYROID GLANDS

PHYSIOLOGY

Parathyroid hormone (PTH) is a single chain polypeptide of 84 amino acids which is synthesised by the chief cells of the parathyroid glands. The important actions of PTH are on renal function, vitamin D metabolism and bone.

Renal function
PTH stimulates tubular reabsorption of calcium, but decreases reabsorption of phosphate and bicarbonate.

Vitamin D metabolism
Vitamin D_3 (cholecalciferol) is the major dietary form of vitamin D and is the form synthesised in skin exposed to ultraviolet light. Cholecalciferol is hydroxylated in the liver to give 25-hydroxycholecalciferol (25-HCC) which is the predominant circulating form of the vitamin. Further hydroxylation occurs in the kidney to give 1 alpha, 25-dihydroxycholecalciferol (1,25-DHCC) which is the most potent form of the vitamin known. It is this second hydroxylation which is stimulated by PTH. The major actions of 1,25-DHCC are to increase intestinal absorption of calcium and phosphate, and in combination with PTH, to mobilise calcium from bone.

Bone
Bone represents 99% of the total body calcium and is in dynamic equilibrium with the extracellular fluid by processes of bone resorption and deposition. The initial effect of PTH on bone is to stimulate osteolysis returning calcium from bone to extracellular fluid. Prolonged exposure of bone to PTH is associated with increased osteoclastic activity, extensive bone remodelling and osteoblastic repair.

Role of PTH in calcium homeostasis
This is summarised in Figure 13.15. The normal response to a fall in serum ionised calcium is an increase in circulating levels of PTH. The actions of PTH on renal handling of calcium, on vitamin D metabolism and on bone resorption combine to return serum ionised calcium to normal. Conversely, an elevation in serum ionised calcium is normally corrected by suppression of PTH secretion. Calcitonin, a peptide secreted by the parafollicular C-cells of the thyroid, may have a role in reducing serum ionised calcium in response to an acute increase by opposing the action of PTH on renal tubular reabsorption of calcium and phosphate and on bone resorption. Parathyroid disease results in failure of calcium homeostasis, the clinical features being a consequence of tissue exposure to abnormal concentrations of ionised calcium and PTH.

HYPERPARATHYROIDISM

It is customary to distinguish three categories of hyperparathyroidism. In primary hyperparathyroidism there is usually autonomous secretion of PTH by a single parathyroid adenoma varying in size from a few millimetres to several centimetres in diameter. The categories are shown in the information box below. Secondary hyperparathyroidism is present when there is hyperplasia with increased PTH secretion in an

---

HYPERPARATHYROIDISM

Primary
Single adenoma (90%)
Multiple adenomata (4%)   serum calcium
Nodular hyperplasia (5%)   and PTH raised
Carcinoma (1%)

Secondary
Chronic renal failure
Malabsorption   serum calcium
Osteomalacia and rickets   low, PTH raised

Tertiary   serum calcium
                             and PTH raised

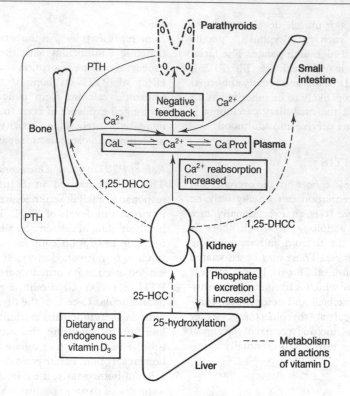

Fig. 13.15 Outline of calcium homeostasis showing response to decreased serum ionised calcium level. Calcium in serum exists as 50% ionised (Ca^{2+}), 10% non-ionised or complexed with organic ions such as citrate and phosphate (CaL) and 40% protein-bound, mainly to albumin (Ca prot). It is the ionised calcium concentration which regulates PTH and 1,25 DHCC production.

attempt to compensate for prolonged hypocalcaemia. Its effect is to restore serum calcium levels at the expense of the skeleton.

In a very small proportion of cases of secondary hyperparathyroidism continuous stimulation of the parathyroids may result in adenoma formation and autonomous PTH secretion. This is known as tertiary hyperparathyroidism.

PRIMARY HYPERPARATHYROIDISM

This is the commonest of the parathyroid disorders with a prevalence of about 1 in 800. The current detection rate is 20–30 per 100 000 annually and reflects the increasing number of asymptomatic cases discovered as a result of biochemical profile investigations performed in the hospital population. It is 2–3 times more common in women than men and 90% of patients are over 50 years of age.

Clinical features

About 50% of patients with biochemical evidence of primary hyperparathyroidism are asymptomatic. Many others have non-specific symptoms. These include anorexia, nausea, vomiting, constipation and weight loss; polyuria and polydipsia; weakness, tiredness and lassitude; drowsiness, poor concentration, memory loss and depression. Such vague symptoms may progress to acute hypercalcaemic crisis.

Calculus disease is a common renal manifestation, and 5% of first stone formers and 15% of recurrent stone formers have hyperparathyroidism. Nephrocalcinosis may also occur and is due to deposition of calcium salts in the renal parenchyma, particularly the medullary region and the collecting ducts. Renal function may be adversely affected as evidenced by uraemia, hypokalaemia, hyperuricaemia, hyperchloraemic acidosis and poor urine concentrating ability.

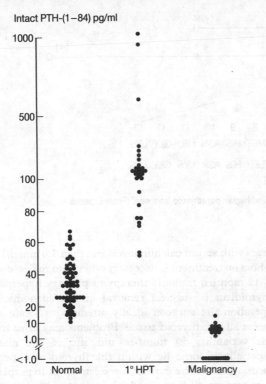

Intact PTH-(1–84) pg/ml

Fig. 13.16 Intact PTH 1–84 measurements by immunoradiometric assay in sera from normal individuals, patients with surgically proven primary hyperparathyroidism and patients with malignancy associated hypercalcaemia. (From Nussbaum et al. Clinical Chemistry, 33, 1987.)

Osteitis fibrosa, in which there is increased bone resorption by osteoclasts with fibrous replacement in the lacunae is the characteristic skeletal disorder. Cystic expansion may accompany the osteitis fibrosa. These changes may present clinically as bone pain and tenderness, fracture and deformity. Rarely, primary hyperparathyroidism may present as a local swelling, usually of the mandible, due to an isolated cyst. Chondrocalcinosis is due to deposition of calcium pyrophosphate crystals within articular cartilage. This typically affects the menisci at the knees and can result in secondary degenerative arthritis or predispose to attacks of acute pseudogout, especially following parathyroidectomy.

Other features of primary hyperparathyroidism include corneal calcification best seen by slit-lamp examination, ectopic calcification in arterial walls and soft tissues of hands, peptic ulceration, hypertension, myopathy and pruritus.

Investigations

Biochemical. The diagnosis of primary hyperparathyroidism depends upon the finding of a raised serum calcium and raised PTH (Fig. 13.16). It is preferable to avoid artefactual increases in serum calcium by collecting blood under standardised conditions with the patient supine and avoiding the use of a tourniquet while withdrawing the sample. Although changes in serum calcium in response to dietary intake are small, specimens should be collected with the patient fasting. If serum albumin is low the value for calcium should be adjusted upward by 0.1 mmol/l for each 6 g/l that the albumin is below the laboratory mean. Serum phosphate is usually low in hyperparathyroidism and chloride elevated. Serum alkaline phosphatase, an index of osteoblastic activity, may be raised depending on the degree of involvement of bone.

The most common other cause of hypercalcaemia is malignancy. Those malignancies most frequently causing hypercalcaemia are breast, kidney, lung, thyroid, ovary and colon. The primary is usually obvious and in 90% of cases there are radiologically evident metastases in bone. The hypercalcaemia of multiple myeloma is also caused by bone destruction. In the absence of metastases, the hypercalcaemia of malignancy is due to the production by the tumour of a PTH-like peptide the structure of which shows considerable homology with the biologically critical NH_2 terminal region of PTH (Fig. 13.17). This is not detected by the newer PTH assays (Fig. 13.16) and, as in all other causes of hypercalcaemia, e.g. vitamin D intoxication, milk-alkali syndrome, hyperthyroidism, sarcoidosis, untreated Addison's disease and long periods of immobilisation in patients with Paget's disease, PTH will be low or undetectable.

Radiological. In the early stages there may be demineralisation and subperiosteal erosions may be noted in the phalanges (Fig. 13.18). These are most marked on the radial side of the middle phalanx. There may also be resorption of the terminal phalanges. A 'pepper-pot' appearance may be seen on lateral radiographs of the skull. Cystic changes are rare. In nephrocalcinosis scattered opacities may be visible within the renal outline. There may be soft tissue calcification elsewhere.

Localisation of parathyroid tumour. In over 90% of patients an experienced surgeon will locate the adenoma without difficulty and routine preoperative localisation is not usually performed. If surgical exploration has been unsuccessful, however, ultrasonography, selective neck vein catheterisation with PTH measurements, CT scanning and subtraction imaging may prove useful. In this last technique the neck is imaged during the successive injections of two short-

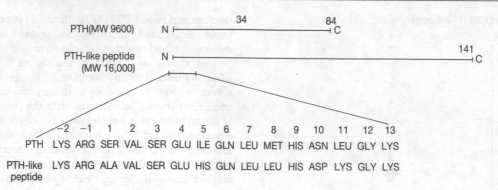

Fig. 13.17   Structures of the parathyroid hormone-like peptide and human parathyroid hormone. (From Broadus et al New England Journal of Medicine, 319, 1988.)

lived isotopes, thallium-201 (taken up by thyroid and parathyroid), followed by technetium-99m (taken up by thyroid only). Computer subtraction of the two images leaves a parathyroid image if an adenoma is present. Recent improvements in ultrasound technology are likely to make ultrasound one of the most useful methods of localising parathyroid tumours.

Management

Apart from asymptomatic patients over the age of 65

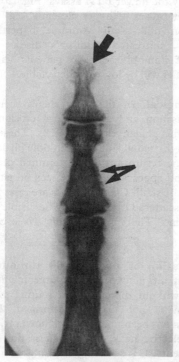

Fig. 13.18   X-ray of subperiosteal erosions in a phalanx with terminal resorption in a patient with primary hyperparathyroidism.

years with serum calcium levels less than 3.0 mmol/l for whom no treatment is necessary other than review every 6–12 months, the only therapy of primary hyperparathyroidism is surgical removal of the adenoma. At operation the surgeon ideally attempts to locate and assess all parathyroid tissue. Problems may arise from the variability in number and site of the glands especially if some lie within the thyroid or superior mediastinum. The current management of hyperplasia is to remove all four glands and to transplant some of the excised tissue to the forearm. If hypercalcaemia returns part of the transplant can be removed under local anaesthetic.

Postoperative hypocalcaemia is not uncommon during the first two weeks while residual suppressed parathyroid tissue recovers. It is usually mild or asymptomatic and can be controlled with oral calcium supplements, e.g. 80 mmol daily. It is recognised that patients with particularly high preoperative serum calcium levels and obvious bone or renal damage are especially likely to develop prolonged symptomatic hypocalcaemia after operation as there is a major net shift of calcium into healing bone. This hypocalcaemia can be minimised by giving 1 alphahydroxycholecalciferol 2 µg daily for 48 hours before surgery and continuing for 1–2 weeks after operation. Intravenous calcium gluconate as 10 ml of 10% solution which can be given every 3–4 hours and oral calcium supplements may also be necessary.

Hypercalcaemic crisis. In recent years this condition has been increasingly recognised as a mode of presentation of primary hyperparathyroidism, especially in the elderly. The clinical features are those of dehydration and hypotension, associated with abdominal pain, vomiting, pyrexia and altered conscious level. Treatment is a medical emergency and is aimed at replacing fluid deficit, correcting electrolyte imbalance and lowering serum calcium levels which are usually in excess of 4.0 mmol/l. The ultimate treatment is surgery and this should be performed as soon as possible after the patient has been rehydrated and an adequate fall in serum calcium achieved.

In the first 24 hours it is usually necessary to replace 4–6 litres of 0.9% saline (145 mmol/l). Any associated hypokalaemia and hypomagnesaemia should also be corrected by intravenous supplements. In most cases intravenous fluids alone will reduce serum calcium to approximately 3.0 mmol/l, allowing safer surgery. However it may be necessary to use additional methods to lower calcium and these include:

1. salmon calcitonin (Calsynar) in a dose of 200–400 i.u. 8-hourly subcutaneously suppresses bone turnover and will reduce serum calcium by up to 0.7 mmol/l;
2. mithramycin, a cytotoxic drug, in a dose of 25 μg/kg intravenously;
3. 500 ml 0.1 M neutral phosphate intravenously over 6–8 hours is effective in lowering serum calcium but at the expense of causing the precipitation of calcium phosphate in non-articular tissues.

Neither treatment with mithramycin nor phosphates should be given on more than one occasion, but should allow time for emergency surgery or rapid investigation of the possibility that the diagnosis is not primary hyperparathyroidism but malignancy-related hypercalcaemia.

Familial hypocalciuric hypercalcaemia

This is a poorly understood syndrome, inherited as an autosomal dominant in which there is increased renal tubular reabsorption of calcium with resultant low urinary calcium in the presence of hypercalcaemia. Serum PTH levels are normal or marginally elevated. Patients have few if any symptoms and it is difficult to make the distinction from primary hyperparathyroidism. Surgery of the parathyroid glands which are hyperplastic fails to correct the hypercalcaemia. In this circumstance a search for hypercalcaemia should be made in other members of the family. Surgery is not indicated in those identified as the course of the condition should be uneventful.

Association of primary hyperparathyroidism with other endocrine disorders

Hyperparathyroidism may occur, usually in the form of hyperplasia, with pancreatic islet cell tumours secreting insulin or gastrin and pituitary tumours (MEN I) or in association with medullary carcinoma of the thyroid and phaeochromocytomas (MEN II, p. 636).

HYPOPARATHYROIDISM

This unusual condition may arise from a variety of causes, but with each the clinical feature in common is tetany (see p. 642). Biochemically, a depressed concentration of calcium and a raised concentration of phosphate in serum are characteristic.

Postoperative hypoparathyroidism. The commonest cause of hypoparathyroidism is damage to the parathyroid glands or their blood supply during thyroid surgery, although this complication occurs in only 1% of thyroidectomies. Transient hypocalcaemia develops in 10% of patients 12–36 hours following subtotal thyroidectomy for Graves' disease.

Infantile hypoparathyroidism. This may be transient and associated with maternal hyperparathyroidism or calcium deficiency. It persists in thymic aplasia (Di George syndrome).

Idiopathic hypoparathyroidism. This may develop at any age, and is sometimes associated with autoimmune disease of the adrenal, thyroid or ovary especially in young people. In addition to tetany other features of prolonged hypocalcaemia include grand mal epilepsy, psychosis, cataracts, calcification of basal ganglia and papilloedema. In addition there is an association with mucocutaneous candidiasis particularly affecting finger nails, mouth and oesophagus.

Pseudohypoparathyroidism. This is the term applied to a congenital variety in which there is tissue resistance to the effects of parathyroid hormone. The PTH receptor is normal but there is a defective post-receptor mechanism. Pseudohypoparathyroidism also presents with the biochemical and clinical features of hypoparathyroidism. Unlike patients with idiopathic hypoparathyroidism there is no associated mucocutaneous candidiasis, but patients may have mental retardation and characteristically there are skeletal abnormalities such as small stature and short 4th and 5th metacarpals and metatarsals (Fig. 13.19). These patients have elevated levels of serum PTH.

The term pseudo-pseudohypoparathyroidism is given to patients exhibiting the above skeletal abnormalities but in whom serum calcium concentration is normal.

Management

Commercial preparations of parathyroid hormone are unsatisfactory for the treatment of parathyroid insufficiency because they have to be given by frequent

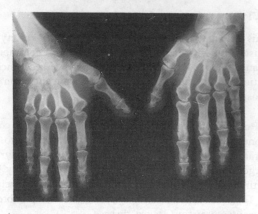

Fig. 13.19   X-ray of hand in a patient with pseudohypoparathyroidism showing short fourth and fifth metacarpals.

injections, and soon become ineffective because of antibody formation. In the acute phase, calcium is given intravenously as for tetany, substitution therapy for persistent hypoparathyroidism and for pseudohypoparathyroidism is provided by 1 α-hydroxycholecalciferol (alfacalcidol) or 1,25 dihydroxycholecalciferol (calcitriol) to which it is hydroxylated in the liver. The dose of these preparations is 1–3 μg daily. It is important to monitor the serum calcium level every 3–6 months once the dose has been stabilised.

TETANY

Aetiology

There is an increased excitability of peripheral nerves due either to a low serum calcium or to alkalosis in which the proportion of the serum calcium in the ionised form is decreased, although the total calcium concentration remains unaltered. Magnesium depletion should also be considered as a possible contributing factor, particularly in malabsorption. The most common cause of hypocalcaemia is a low serum concentration of albumin which does not result in tetany. The causes are listed in the information box (left).

Clinical features

In *children* a characteristic triad of carpopedal spasm, stridor and convulsions occurs, though one or more of these may be found independently of the others. The hands in carpal spasm adopt a characteristic position. The metacarpophalangeal joints are flexed, the interphalangeal joints of the fingers and thumb are extended and there is opposition of the thumb (*main d'accoucheur*). Pedal spasm is much less frequent. Stridor is caused by spasm of the glottis.

Adults complain of tingling in the hands, feet and around the mouth. Less often there is painful carpopedal spasm while stridor and fits are rare.

Latent tetany may be present when signs of overt tetany are lacking. It is best recognised by eliciting *Trousseau's sign*. Inflation of the sphygmomanometer cuff on the upper arm to more than the systolic blood pressure is followed by carpal spasm within 3 minutes. A less specific sign of hypocalcaemia is that described by *Chvostek* in which tapping over the brances of the facial nerve as they emerge from the parotid gland produces twitching of the facial muscles.

Management

Control of tetany

Injection of 20 ml of a 10% solution of calcium gluconate slowly into a vein will raise the serum calcium concentration immediately. An intramuscular injection of 10 ml may also be given to obtain a more prolonged effect. In severe cases of alkalotic tetany, intravenous calcium gluconate often relieves the spasm, while specific treatment of the alkalosis, which will vary with the cause, is being applied. If tetany is not relieved by giving calcium the administration of magnesium may be required.

Correction of alkalosis

In persistent vomiting, intravenous isotonic saline is the most effective treatment.

When alkalis have been given to excess their withdrawal may suffice to stop the tetany, but if not, ammonium chloride 2 g should be given 4-hourly by mouth until relief has been obtained.

The inhalation of 5% carbon dioxide in oxygen may be prescribed for the correction of the alkalosis of hyperventilation, or more simply, the patient should be made to rebreathe expired air from a suitable bag. The hysterical patient should also have appropriate psychotherapy.

CAUSES OF TETANY

Due to hypocalcaemia	*Due to alkalosis*
Malabsorption	Repeated vomiting of gastric juice
Osteomalacia	
Hypoparathyroidism	Excessive intake of oral alkalis
Acute pancreatitis	
Chronic renal failure*	Hyperventilation
	Primary hyperaldosteronism

* Coincident acidosis usually prevents tetany.

THE ADRENAL GLANDS

ANATOMY AND PHYSIOLOGY OF THE ADRENAL CORTEX

Each adrenal consists of an inner medulla and an outer cortex. This is divided into three zones:

zona glomerulosa → aldosterone (mineralocorticoid)
zona fasciculata → cortisol (glucocorticoid)
zona reticularis → androgens

ZONA GLOMERULOSA

Aldosterone, the body's most important sodium retaining hormone (*mineralocorticoid*), is produced by the outermost zone of the adrenal and is principally under the control of angiotensin II (AII). ACTH and hyperkalaemia are less important stimuli. Low salt intake stimulates aldosterone secretion by activating the renin-angiotensin system. It also enhances the response of the zona glomerulosa to AII. High salt intake has the opposite effect. Standing levels of plasma renin activity are about double those when lying down. Factors controlling the increase of renin are thus key to understanding aldosterone secretion.

Angiotensin-converting enzyme (ACE) is present in the lung, in the circulation and in the blood vessel walls. The introduction of ACE inhibitors such as captopril or enalapril has been of major importance in the treatment of hypertension and congestive heart failure (see pp. 290 and 321).

Aldosterone acts on the distal nephron to produce sodium retention and urinary potassium loss. Thus hypokalaemia is an important clue to the possibility of hyperaldosteronism.

ZONA FASCICULATA

Cortisol is the major product of this zone. Under most circumstances this acts as a *glucocorticoid* hormone.

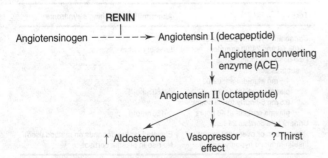

Fig. 13.20   Renin-angiotensin-aldosterone system.

Such steroids have anti-insulin effects and raise blood sugar by converting amino acids from protein breakdown to glucose (gluconeogenesis). Glucocorticoids are very important anti-inflammatory agents. This effect is probably mediated via production of lipocortin which then inhibits the synthesis of prostaglandins and leukotrienes. Cortisol is converted by 11β-hydroxysteroid dehydrogenase (11β-OHSD) into inactive cortisone. This conversion is used by the kidney to protect the non-specific mineralocorticoid receptor from exposure to cortisol. Loss of this protection by inhibition of 11β-OHSD by liquorice results in cortisol acting as a potent sodium-retaining steroid.

ZONA RETICULARIS

The innermost zone of the adrenal cortex produces androgens such as dehydroepiandrosterone sulphate, dehydroepiandrosterone and androstenedione. These are increased during the adrenarche which results in initial pubic hair development. The control of adrenal androgen production is unclear. Certainly ACTH plays a role. However, there may possibly be a separate androgen stimulating hormone (ASH).

HYPERFUNCTION OF THE ADRENAL GLAND

GLUCOCORTICOID EXCESS

Cushing's syndrome is defined as the symptoms and signs associated with prolonged inappropriate elevation of free corticosteroid levels.

Patients with Cushing's syndrome can be classified into two groups on the basis of whether the condition is ACTH-dependent or independent (Table 13.10).

Table 13.10   Classification of Cushing's syndrome

ACTH-dependent	Non-ACTH dependent
Iatrogenic (ACTH therapy)	Iatrogenic (e.g. prednisolone)
Pituitary-dependent bilateral adrenal hyperplasia (Cushing's disease)	Adrenal adenoma
Ectopic ACTH syndrome (benign or malignant non-endocrine tumour)	Adrenal carcinoma

Epidemiology

Cushing's syndrome of pituitary origin or associated with an adrenal tumour is four times more common in women than men. In contrast the ectopic ACTH syndrome (often due to a small cell carcinoma of the bronchus) is more common in men. When the iatrogenic and ectopic groups are excluded pituitary-

Table 13.11   Clinical features of Cushing's syndrome (after Ross & Linch 1982)

Symptoms	Patients presenting (%)	Signs	Patients presenting (%)
Weight gain	91	Obesity	97
Menstrual irregularity	84	Plethora	94
Hirsutism	81	Moonface	88
Psychiatric	62	Hypertension	74
Backache	43	Bruising	62
Muscle weakness	29	Striae	56
		Muscle weakness	56

dependent Cushing's disease is the commonest cause of Cushing's syndrome, acounting for about 80% of adult cases.

Clinical features

The features common to all causes of glucocorticoid excess are indicated in Table 13.11. Weight gain is the commonest symptom and obesity the most frequent sign. The distribution of fat is classically described as centripetal (like a lemon on toothpicks) but generalised obesity may be just as common. Because of this it is useful to compare the prevalence of the symptoms and signs in patients with Cushing's syndrome with those in patients with simple obesity. Using this approach bruising, myopathy and hypertension are the best discriminants and thus the features to look for in an obese patient in whom Cushing's syndrome is suspected.

Glucocorticoid excess leads to collagen breakdown which results in thinning of the skin and blood vessels with resultant bruising, striae (livid stretch marks especially over the abdomen, buttocks and thighs) and a plethoric appearance. The loss of protein in muscle leads to a proximal myopathy (difficult or impossible to get up from a squatting position) and the changes in bone to osteoporosis. The latter may present with back pain from vertebral compression fractures. Other fractures such as in the ribs are more common and tend to heal with exuberant callus formation.

Increased gluconeogenesis may lead to impaired glucose tolerance. This is much more common in the ectopic ACTH syndrome secondary to a small cell carcinoma of the bronchus in which plasma cortisol levels tend to be very high. These patients also usually have a severe hypokalaemic alkalosis. This hypokalaemia may inhibit insulin secretion and, if severe, produce muscular weakness or paralysis.

Increased adrenal androgen secretion (especially with adrenal carcinomas) can contribute to the hirsutism but this occurs with glucocorticoid therapy alone.

Skin pigmentation may be a feature especially of the ectopic ACTH syndrome. This relates to the α-melanocyte stimulating hormone (α-MSH) sequence which is part of the ACTH molecule. In addition the rest of the ACTH precursor molecule (pro-opiocortin) contains two other MSH sequences (β-MSH in β-lipotrophin and γ-MSH in the N-terminal part (p. 612)). In patients with pituitary-dependent Cushing's disease treatment by bilateral adrenalectomy may lead to the development of a locally invasive pituitary tumour with very high levels of ACTH and hyperpigmentation (Nelson's syndrome). This tumour contrasts with the microadenoma (less than 10 mm in diameter) which is found in the pituitary of about 75% of patients with Cushing's disease. Hence local symptoms related to the pituitary tumour (e.g. visual field defect) are rare in untreated Cushing's disease.

Skin infections especially with fungi such as *Tinea versicolor* are common. Minor trauma produces gaping skin wounds which heal poorly.

Hypertension is common. Glucocorticoids increase plasma volume. This appears not to relate to sodium retention. Cortisol also enhances vascular responsiveness to noradrenaline.

Gonadal function is frequently abnormal with oligomenorrhoea or amenorrhoea in women and impotence in men.

Growth retardation is almost invariable in children. Adults frequently present with psychiatric problems (especially depression).

Investigation

In a patient suspected of having Cushing's syndrome the investigations should be divided into two stages to answer these questions:

1. Diagnosis: Does the patient have Cushing's syndrome (Table 13.12).
2. Differential diagnosis: What is the cause of the adrenocortical hyperfunction (Table 13.13).

Only if the answer to Question 1 is 'yes' should any further tests be performed.

Table 13.12   Does the patient have Cushing's syndrome?

Test	Abnormality in Cushing's syndrome
Circadian rhythm of plasma cortisol (08:00 and 24:00 samples)	Loss of rhythm
Low dose dexamethasone suppression	
1.5 mg at midnight: 09:00 plasma cortisol next day*	>180 nmol/l
0.5 mg 6-hourly for 48 hours: plasma cortisol at 48 hours	>180 nmol/l
Urinary free cortisol 24-hour excretion or overnight excretion*	Elevated (value depends on method used)
Insulin-induced hypoglycaemia	No rise in plasma cortisol

* Useful outpatient screening tests.

Table 13.13   What is the cause of Cushing's syndrome

Test	Pituitary dependent	Ectopic ACTH	Adrenal tumour
Plasma ACTH 08:00	N or ↑	↑ or ↑↑	Undetectable
Metyrapone 750 mg 4-hourly × 6 doses: measure 11-deoxycortisol at 24:00	↑↑	↑	→↑
High dose dexamethasone 2 mg 6-hourly for 48 hours: plasma cortisol 48 hours	↓	→	→
Plasma K⁺	N	<3.5 mmol/l	N
Corticotrophin-releasing factor 1µg/kg body weight plasma ACTH and cortisol over 3 hours	↑	→	→

N = normal; ↑ = increased; → = no change; ↑↑ = markedly increased; ↓ = suppressed.

In Cushing's syndrome there is a characteristic loss of the circadian rhythm of plasma cortisol (i.e. instead of cortisol levels being lowest at midnight they are about the same throughout the 24 hours). This may also be lost by stress caused from hospital admission, depression or heart failure. Negative feedback control is abnormal and cortisol levels are not suppressed by low doses of dexamethasone. This synthetic glucocorticoid is not measured by the cortisol radioimmunoassay (this test may be invalid in patients on enzyme-inducing drugs such as phenytoin which markedly reduce dexamethasone half-life).

Urinary-free cortisol is a reflection of the free (i.e. non-protein bound) cortisol in plasma and is a very useful index of increased cortisol secretion.

Insulin-induced hypoglycaemia stimulates a rise in plasma cortisol in normal and depressed subjects but not in patients with Cushing's syndrome.

Measurement of plasma ACTH is the key to establishing the differential diagnosis (Table 13.13). Very high levels (above 300 ng/l) suggest the ectopic ACTH syndrome and are typical of patients with small cell carcinoma of bronchus. Levels within the normal range for 0800 h plasma ACTH (10–80 ng/l) usually indicate a pituitary source. Values between 80 and 300 ng/l may relate to either pituitary-dependent disease or the ectopic ACTH syndrome (usually from a benign tumour such as bronchial carcinoid). Techniques such as venous catheterisation with measurement of inferior petrosal sinus ACTH (i.e. draining directly from the pituitary) may be necessary to distinguish these. Other tests include giving the enzyme inhibitor metyrapone. This blocks the last step in cortisol biosynthesis (11-deoxycortisol to cortisol) and thus activates negative feedback control (Table 13.13). In addition, high-dose dexamethasone suppression, measurement of plasma potassium and the ACTH/cortisol response to corticotrophin-releasing factor are helpful in distinguishing the different causes of Cushing's syndrome.

Radiological and other investigations
Plain skull X-rays are usually normal in patients with pituitary-dependent Cushing's disease. High resolution CT scanning may be of value (Fig. 13.21A) but false positive and false negative results are not uncommon. Plain X-ray of the chest may show a bronchogenic carcinoma. If this is normal and an ectopic source of ACTH is suspected then CT scans of the anterior mediastinum and upper abdomen to include the pancreas should be done. If ACTH is undetectable, suggesting an adrenal tumour, then an adrenal scan using selenium-75-labelled cholesterol is useful in locating an adrenal adenoma. Carcinomas do not usually take up the isotope.

Management
This is essential as untreated Cushing's syndrome has a 50% five-year mortality. Treatment of choice depends on the cause.

Adrenal tumours
Adrenal adenomas should be surgically removed via a loin approach. It may take several months for the contralateral adrenal and the hypothalamus and pituitary to recover. During this time suboptimal replacement therapy is required (0.5 mg dexamethasone mane). Adrenal carcinomas should also be resected if possible, the tumour bed irradiated and the patient given the adrenolytic drug o,p'DDD (usually 6–9 g/d). This may produce nausea and ataxia. Cortisol overproduction can be reduced by metyrapone (start with 250 mg 8-hourly) or the more toxic aminoglutethimide (250 mg 6–8-hourly).

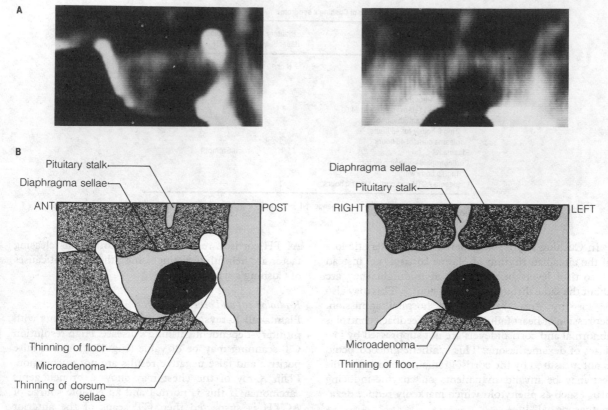

A

B

Pituitary stalk

Diaphragma sellae

ANT

POST

Thinning of floor

Microadenoma

Thinning of dorsum sellae

Diaphragma sellae

Pituitary stalk

RIGHT

LEFT

Microadenoma

Thinning of floor

Fig. 13.21 CT scan of pituitary in patient with Cushing's disease (5 mm tumour subsequently removed by trans-sphenoidal surgery). **A**. Lateral and coronal views. **B**. Diagrams of the same views.

Cushing's disease

Trans-sphenoidal surgery with selective removal of the adenoma (found in 75% of cases) is the treatment of choice and results in cure in about 80% of patients. Recurrence is rare. If no tumour is found and the diagnosis is definitely pituitary-dependent Cushing's then a radical hypophysectomy may be required. If the diagnosis is not certain then bilateral adrenalectomy with pituitary irradiation to prevent the development of Nelson's syndrome may be the correct treatment. External pituitary irradiation alone is of little value in adults but is surprisingly effective in children with Cushing's disease. The implantation of yttrium-90 (interstitial irradiation) produces good results in both adults and children. Medical treatment with drugs such as metyrapone is usually only of value in preparing patients for surgery.

Following successful selective adenomectomy plasma cortisol should be undetectable as the ACTH-producing cells around the adenoma are suppressed. The patient should be given dexamethasone 0.5 mg mane and plasma cortisol measured at 08.00 hours (before dexamethasone) at 2-weekly intervals. When the level is above 180 nmol/l dexamethasone can be stopped. An insulin hypoglycaemia test should then be performed to demonstrate if the response to stress is normal. The rest of the pituitary function will also need to be assessed.

Nelson's syndrome. This should not occur if pituitary irradiation is given to patients who have had bilateral adrenalectomy. If it does happen then surgery, radiotherapy and drugs such as the γ-aminobutyric acid inhibitor, sodium valproate, may all be necessary but are often ineffective.

Ectopic ACTH syndrome

Benign tumours causing this syndrome (e.g. bronchial carcinoid) should be removed. Malignancies such as small cell carcinoma of bronchus may initially respond to radiotherapy and chemotherapy. When they recur then lowering cortisol levels with metyrapone or amino-glutethimide may help to control severe hypokalaemia and hyperglycaemia.

MINERALOCORTICOID EXCESS

Overproduction of aldosterone (hyperaldosteronism), the major salt-retaining hormone, may be due to a primary abnormality in the zona glomerulosa or secondary to stimulation of aldosterone secretion by angiotensin II following activation of the renin-angiotensin system (p. 643).

Primary hyperaldosteronism (Conn's syndrome)

In this syndrome overproduction of aldosterone by either an adenoma (about 60% of cases) or bilateral zona glomerulosa hyperplasia is associated with hypertension and hypokalaemia (Fig. 13.22). This is a rare cause of hypertension (about 1%) but is more common in Negroid than in Caucasian subjects. The hypokalaemia may result in muscle weakness, occasionally tetany because of the metabolic alkalosis with low ionised calcium, and polyuria with polydipsia secondary to renal tubular damage (nephrogenic diabetes insipidus). If the patient is on a low salt intake plasma potassium may be normal. Conversely diuretic therapy (especially with thiazides) may produce marked hypokalaemia.

Investigations

Diagnosis

1. Several measurements of plasma potassium should be made off diuretics and when the hypertension has been controlled. Blood samples should be taken without occlusion or muscular exercise of the arm and the samples separated soon after being drawn with care to avoid haemolysis. The patient should be on a normal salt intake (i.e. not low).
2. If hypokalaemia persists then measure plasma and/ or urinary aldosterone and plasma renin activity (PRA). In Conn's syndrome aldosterone levels will be elevated and PRA suppressed (Fig. 13.22).

If possible antihypertensive drugs should be stopped for at least two weeks beforehand as many of these affect the renin-angiotensin system (e.g. β-adrenoceptor blocking drugs inhibit whilst thiazide diuretics stimulate renin secretion). If this is not possible then change to the adrenergic neurone-blocking drug bethanidine 10 mg t.i.d. which has minimal effect on the renin-angiotensin system.

Differential diagnosis

If aldosterone levels are high and renin suppressed then further investigation is necessary to differentiate between an adenoma and hyperplasia (may be either idiopathic or ACTH-dependent and is often referred to

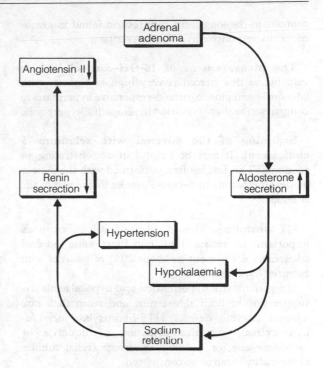

Fig. 13.22   Primary hyperaldosteronism.

as glucocorticoid-responsive or dexamethasone-suppressible). These tests are:

Aldosterone response to posture and time. This depends upon the fact that in normal subjects standing elevates plasma renin activity and hence aldosterone. In idiopathic hyperplasia the zona glomerulosa is very sensitive to angiotensin II and the small rise with standing increases aldosterone. In contrast Conn's adenoma is very responsive to ACTH as is the adrenal in glucocorticoid-responsive hyper-aldosteronism. During the course of the morning ACTH levels normally fall and hence aldosterone decreases.

Adrenal vein catheterisation. A difficult investigation to perform but necessary in some cases where other tests are equivocal. Adrenal venous cortisol levels should be measured in addition to aldosterone to demonstrate that the catheter is correctly positioned. In patients with an adenoma there is unilateral hypersecretion of aldosterone in comparison to bilateral elevation in those with hyperplasia.

Dexamethasone. This lowers plasma aldosterone transiently in Conn's adenoma patients (24–48 h) in contrast to the long-term suppression found in gluco-corticoid-responsive hyperaldosteronism.

The measurement of 18-OH-cortisol. This is valuable as this steroid is very high in patients with adenomas and glucocorticoid-responsive hyperplasia in comparison to slight elevation in idiopathic hyperplasia.

Scanning of the adrenal with selenium-75 cholesterol. It may be helpful in demonstrating an adenoma. This test is often performed with the patient on dexamethasone to decrease uptake by the rest of the adrenal.

CT scanning. This is also of value but it is important to realise that non-functioning adrenal adenomata are present in about 20% of patients with essential hypertension.

If a patient with hypertension and hypokalaemia has suppression of both aldosterone and renin then rare adrenal enzyme defects (11β-hydroxylase or 17α-hydroxylase), excessive ingestion of liquorice or carbonoxolone, or Liddle's syndrome (renal tubular abnormality) need to be considered.

Management
The aldosterone antagonist spironolactone is valuable in treating hypokalaemia and hypertension. High doses (up to 400 mg/d) may be required. The blood pressure response to spironolactone correlates well with the results of removal of an adenoma by unilateral adrenalectomy (60% normotensive, 20% improved). Idiopathic hyperplasia may respond to spironolactone but often requires additional therapy for the hypertension. Surprisingly, ACE inhibitors are often of value. Up to 20% of males develop gynaecomastia on spironolactone. Amiloride (10–40 mg/d) can then be substituted.

Secondary hyperaldosteronism
This is a very common clinical problem resulting from excessive activity of the renin-angiotensin system (Fig. 13.23). The reasons for this can be divided into physiological and pathological.

Physiological
Salt depletion either by inadequate intake or by excessive loss from the kidney or gastrointestinal tract activates the renin-angiotensin-aldosterone axis by reducing the intravascular and extracellular fluid volume which leads to renin release and also by increasing the sensitivity of the zona glomerulosa to angiotensin II. In pregnancy the natriuretic steroid

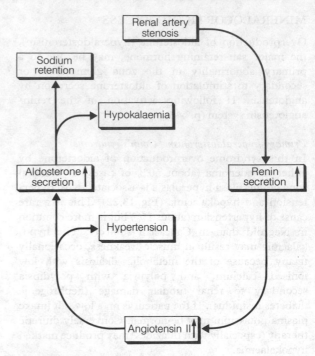

Fig. 13.23   Secondary hyperaldosteronism.

progesterone is produced and higher levels of aldo-sterone are necessary to maintain salt balance.

Pathological
In conditions such as the nephrotic system, cirrhosis with ascites and congestive heart failure, there is a reduced effective intravascular volume which leads to decreased renal perfusion and hence increased renin release. Bartter's syndrome usually presents with short stature. Investigations show hypokalaemia, gross elevation of renin with less marked hyperaldosteronism, hyperplasia of the juxtaglomerular apparatus and increased urinary prostaglandin excretion.

Whereas secondary hyperaldosteronism is common in accelerated or malignant phase hypertension it is unusual in renovascular disease unless there is a severe renal artery stenosis. Renin-secreting tumours (haemangiopericytomas) are very rare. Diuretic therapy, especially when excessive, is by far the commonest cause of secondary hyperaldosteronism.

Investigations

Diagnosis

1. The plasma electrolytes reveal hypokalaemia often associated with plasma sodium levels which are in the lower part of the reference range or subnormal.

2. Plasma aldosterone and plasma renin activity are both elevated.

Management

This depends on the underlying cause. If this is salt depletion then intravenous saline may be required. In congestive heart failure, treatment with either spirono-lactone or an angiotensin-converting enzyme (ACE) inhibitor (e.g. captopril 25–50 mg b.d.) may produce considerable haemodynamic and electrolyte improvement. In Bartter's syndrome spironolactone often with indomethacin to inhibit prostaglandin synthesis is indicated.

With effective antihypertensive therapy plasma potassium usually returns to normal in patients with accelerated or malignant phase hypertension. Reno-vascular disease can be effectively treated by an ACE inhibitor but definitive therapy such as transluminal angioplasty of a stenosed renal artery needs to be considered. If diuretic therapy (e.g. with a thiazide) produces problems with hypokalaemia then a potassium-sparing drug such as amiloride, triamterene or spironolactone can be given.

ADRENOCORTICAL INSUFFICIENCY

This can be divided into primary and secondary causes as shown in the information box below.

CAUSES OF ADRENOCORTICAL INSUFFICIENCY

Primary
Addison's disease   → ACTH ↑
Congenital or acquired enzyme defects   → ACTH ↑

Secondary
Hypothalamic or pituitary disease   → ACTH ↓
Glucocorticoid therapy   → ACTH ↓

PRIMARY – ADDISON'S DISEASE

Aetiology

Addison's classic description *Diseases of the suprarenal capsules* published in 1855 included detailed drawings of caseating adrenal tuberculosis. However, in one case in which the patient had gross vitiligo (a marker of autoimmune disease) he was unable to get an autopsy. Most likely this patient had autoimmune adrenalitis, now the commonest cause of primary adrenal failure. As with other autoimmune diseases this is more common in females than males (2:1). The causes are listed in the information box (right).

CAUSES OF ADDISON'S DISEASE

- Autoimmune adrenalitis
- Tuberculosis
- Bilateral adrenalectomy
- Bilateral adrenal haemorrhage or infarction
- Metastases (esp. small cell carcinoma of bronchus)
- Haemochromatosis
- Amyloidosis

Clinical features

These result from glucocorticoid usually together with mineralocorticoid insufficiency, loss of adrenal androgen production and increased ACTH secretion. The clinical features are listed in the information box below.

CLINICAL FEATURES OF ADDISON'S DISEASE

Glucocorticoid insufficiency
Weight loss
Malaise
Weakness
Anorexia
Nausea
Vomiting
Gastrointestinal – diarrhoea or constipation
Postural hypotension
Hypoglycaemia

Mineralocorticoid insufficiency
Hypotension

Increased ACTH secretion
Pigmentation
    Sun exposed areas
    Pressure areas, e.g. elbows, knees
    Palmar creases, knuckles
    Mucous membranes
    Conjunctivae
    Recent scars

Loss of adrenal androgen
Decreased body hair esp. in female

The patient may present with an acute, chronic or acute on chronic illness. The initial symptoms are often misdiagnosed and it is the pigmentation that commonly raises the suspicion of the diagnosis.

The blood pressure may be normal with the patient lying down. Hence, the pressure should also be measured after standing for 1 minute. Postural hypotension is almost invariably present.

The cause of the pigmentation is probably the high circulating level of ACTH stimulating melanin production rather than the associated pro-opiocortin peptides (β-LPH and N-POC), even though both of these have common core MSH sequences (Fig. 13.4).

Vitiligo is present in about 10–20% (Fig. 13.24). Other autoimmune diseases which may be present are listed in the information box (p. 650).

Surgery or other stress may precipitate an acute adrenal crisis. Alternatively such patients may take much longer than normal to recover from an illness or operation.

AUTOIMMUNE DISEASES PRESENT IN ADDISON'S DISEASE

- Hashimoto's thyroiditis
- Primary atrophic hypothyroidism
- Pernicious anaemia
- Type I diabetes mellitus
- Primary ovarian failure
- Hypoparathyroidism

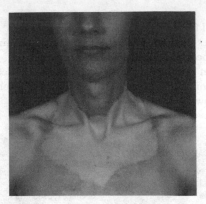

Fig. 13.24   Vitiligo in a patient with Addison' disease.

Investigation

Biochemical tests are essential to confirm the diagnosis of Addison's disease. The key investigations are:

ACTH stimulation test

In Addison's disease there is almost always a failure of the plasma cortisol to rise following administration of ACTH. The basal 08.00 h plasma cortisol is usually low but may be normal; in this context 'normal' is difficult to define as the level may be within the normal reference range but actually inappropriately low for a seriously ill patient.

The usual ACTH test involves giving β1-24 ACTH (i.e. the biologically active 24 out of the total 39 amino acids in the natural molecule). This is tetracosactrin (synacthen); 0.25 mg is given either intramuscularly or intravenously. Blood samples for the measurement of plasma cortisol should be taken at 0, 30 and 60 minutes. In normal subjects in response to ACTH the plasma cortisol should exceed 550 nmol/litre.

Patients with secondary adrenocortical insufficiency may also get a subnormal cortisol rise. They can be distinguished from primary adrenal failure either by measurement of ACTH (see below) or by giving depot tetracosactrin (1 mg i.m. daily for 3 days). In secondary insufficiency there is a progressive increase in plasma cortisol whereas in primary it is less than 700 nmol/l at 8 hours after the last injection.

If glucocorticoids have to be given prior to testing the adrenal response to ACTH then the corticosteroid should be changed to a steroid such as dexamethasone (0.75 mg/d) which does not cross-react in the plasma cortisol radioimmunoassay.

Measurement of plasma ACTH

The simultaneous measurement of 08.00 h plasma cortisol and ACTH is the most sensitive test of primary adrenal failure. Thus even if the plasma cortisol is normal the ACTH value will be elevated (> 80 ng/l).

Plasma electrolytes

The plasma sodium is usually low, the potassium high normal or frankly elevated and the plasma urea raised.

Blood glucose

This may be low especially in severe adrenal insufficiency.

Plasma renin activity (PRA) and aldosterone. PRA values are nearly always high with plasma aldosterone being either low or normal.

After the diagnosis has been made the specific cause must be identified. A chest X-ray should be taken to look for evidence of TB. Such patients may have adrenal calcification which may be visible on a plain abdominal radiograph or CT scan. Blood should be sent for adrenal and other organ-specific antibodies. Associated thyroid disease, pernicious anaemia and diabetes should be excluded.

Management

Patients with Addison's disease always need glucocorticoid replacement therapy and usually mineralocorticoid. *Cortisol (hydrocortisone)* is the drug of choice. In the past cortisone acetate was given but this has to be converted to cortisol by the liver and in some patients this may be impaired. Hydrocortisone 20 mg is given orally on getting up in the morning and 10 mg at 18:00 h (see p. 615 for assessment of dose). Cortisone acetate 25 mg in the morning and 12.5 mg in the evening.

Fludrocortisone is the mineralocorticoid used to replace aldosterone. The usual dose is 0.05–0.1 mg daily. Adequacy of replacement can be assessed by measurement of blood pressure, plasma electrolytes and plasma renin activity.

If the Addison's disease results from tuberculosis then this will need to be appropriately treated (p. 367).

Advice to patients is given in the information box (p. 651).

ADVICE TO PATIENTS WITH ADDISON'S DISEASE

Intercurrent stress
E.g. febrile illness – double dose of hydrocortisone

Surgery
Minor operation – hydrocortisone 100 mg by intramuscular injection with premedication
Major operation – hydrocortisone 100 mg 6-hourly for 24 hours → 50 mg i.m. 6-hourly

Gastroenteritis
Must have parenteral hydrocortisone if unable to take by mouth

Steroid card
Patient should carry this at all times. Should give information regarding diagnosis, steroid, dose and doctor

Bracelet
Patients should be encouraged to buy one of these engraved with the diagnosis and reference number

ADRENAL CRISIS

This requires intravenous hydrocortisone hemi-succinate 100 mg and intravenous fluid (normal saline and 5% dextrose if hypoglycaemia). Parenteral hydrocortisone should be continued (100 mg i.m. 6-hourly) until the gastrointestinal symptoms abate before starting oral therapy. The precipitating cause should be sought. This is often an infection.

PRIMARY – CONGENITAL ENZYME DEFECTS

Defects in the cortisol biosynthetic pathway result in activation of ACTH secretion via negative feedback control. ACTH then stimulates the production of steroids up to the enzyme block. This produces adrenal hyperplasia. The commonest enzyme defect is that of the 21-hydroxylase enzyme (Fig. 13.25). In about one-third of cases this defect affects both mineralocorticoid (aldosterone) and glucocorticoid (cortisol) production. This results in severe salt wasting which may be fatal in the first few weeks of life if untreated. In the other two-thirds mineralocorticoid secretion is not affected.

The increased ACTH drive results in high levels of 17-OH-progesterone and androgens. The latter produce clitoromegaly, accelerated growth and premature fusion of the epiphyses. In boys there may be enlargement of the penis and pubic hair development but without testicular enlargement (precocious pseudo-puberty).

Defects of all the other enzymes have been described but are much rarer. 17-hydroxylase and 11β-hydroxylase deficiency may produce hypertension due to excess mineralocorticoid production.

Investigation

High levels of plasma 17-OH-progesterone are found in 21-hydroxylase deficiency. These can be measured in

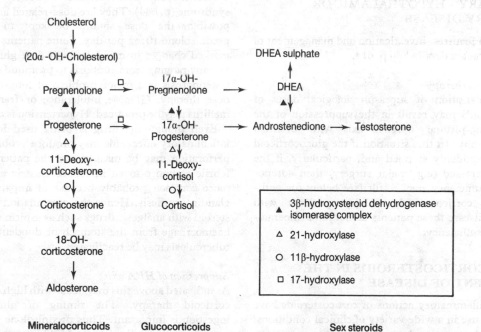

Fig. 13.25   The major pathways of synthesis of adrenal corticosteroids. (DHEA Dehydroepiandrosterone.)

blood spot samples taken in the first week of life from heel pricks for phenylketonuria testing. In the past the metabolite of 17-OH-progesterone, pregnanetriol, was measured in the urine. Specific antenatal diagnosis can now be made. Plasma electrolytes, renin activity and aldosterone should be measured. Bone age should be carefully followed.

Management
The aim is to suppress ACTH and hence adrenal androgen production by glucocorticoid therapy. Treatment of the female can be started in utero if the diagnosis is made and hence clitoromegaly prevented. Under-replacement with glucocorticoid will fail to control the initially increased growth velocity. However, excess glucocorticoid will suppress growth. It is usual to give reverse replacement therapy, i.e. larger dose of glucocorticoid just before going to bed to suppress nocturnal ACTH rise and smaller dose in the morning.

PRIMARY – ACQUIRED ENZYME DEFECTS

Certain drugs can inhibit cortisol biosynthesis by enzyme inhibition. The most commonly used is metyrapone which blocks 11β-hydroxylase (Fig. 13.25) (see p. 651).

SECONDARY – HYPOTHALAMIC OR PITUITARY DISEASE

The clinical features, investigation and management of this condition are detailed on p. 614.

Glucocorticoid therapy
The administration of supra-physiological doses of glucocorticoids may result in the suppression of the hypothalamic-pituitary-adrenal axis with eventual adrenal atrophy. In this situation if the glucocorticoid therapy is suddenly stopped and, particularly, if the patient is stressed (e.g. major surgery) then adreno-cortical insufficiency may result (see below for withdrawal of corticosteroids). Unlike patients with Addison's disease these patients do not have mineralo-corticoid insufficiency.

USE OF CORTICOSTEROIDS IN THE TREATMENT OF DISEASE

The anti-inflammatory actions of corticosteroids have led to their use in a wide variety of clinical conditions. The first glucocorticoid used was cortisone acetate. When given in high dose this had significant sodium retaining effects (the active metabolite cortisol can bind to type I mineralocorticoid and type 2 glucocorticoid receptors). This led to the synthesis of a large number of other steroids with more selective binding to the type 2 receptor (e.g. prednisolone and especially beta-methasone and dexamethasone). Doses are listed in the information box below.

EQUIVALENT DOSES OF GLUCOCORTICOIDS (ANTI-INFLAMMATORY POTENCY)

● Hydrocortisone	20 mg
● Cortisone acetate	25 mg
● Prednisolone	5 mg
● Betamethasone	0.75 mg
● Dexamethasone	0.75 mg

SIDE-EFFECTS OF CORTICOSTEROID THERAPY

These can be divided into:

Metabolic effects
Suppression of the hypothalamic-pituitary-adrenal axis

Metabolic effects
These are identical to those found in Cushing's syndrome (p. 644). They are dose-related and hence, if possible, the dose should be kept to less than prednisolone 10 mg per day. Some patients experience marked changes in mood on high-dose glucocorticoid therapy ranging from euphoria to profound depression. Osteoporosis is a major problem of long-term, high-dose therapy. Glucose intolerance or frank diabetes mellitus may be produced. Hypertension is common.

Even though the drug is being used for its anti-inflammatory effect this may produce problems. Thus perforation may be masked and the patient show no febrile response to an infection. Gastric erosions are more common probably because of impaired prosta-glandin synthesis. Hence the combination of corticosteroid with analgesic drugs such as aspirin may lead to haemorrhage from the stomach or duodenum. Latent tuberculosis may be reactivated.

Suppression of HPA axis
As indicated above this may occur with high dose glucocorticoid therapy. The timing of glucocorticoid ingestion is important. Thus prednisolone 5 mg orally on going to bed will suppress ACTH secretion whereas 5 mg in the morning will have little or no effect on the

HPA axis. Thus if the condition being treated permits the glucocorticoid should be taken as a single morning dose.

Withdrawal of corticosteroid therapy

If possible corticosteroids should be withdrawn slowly unless they have only previously been given for a short period. As indicated the dose should be given in the morning as this will enhance recovery of the HPA axis. Giving ACTH to stimulate adrenal recovery is of no value as the hypothalamus remains suppressed. In a patient with a completely suppressed axis it may take months or years to recover. If the gluco-corticoid-requiring condition allows then giving dexamethasone 0.5 mg in the morning instead of the gluco-corticoid will usually result in gradual recovery. This can be monitored by measuring 08.00 h plasma cortisol just before the dexamethasone dose.

When the plasma cortisol exceeds 180 nmol/l then dexamethasone can be stopped and a short synacthen test performed (p. 613). A rise of plasma cortisol to > 550 nmol/l indicates that the patient will respond normally to stress and thus does not require cortico-steroid cover for surgery etc.

PHAEOCHROMOCYTOMA

This is a rare tumour of chromaffin tissue which secretes catecholamines and is responsible for less than 0.1% of cases of hypertension. The tumours are usually benign (10% malignant) and may arise from any part of the sympathetic chain. However, in over 90% of cases the tumour is found in the adrenal medulla. In multiple endocrine neoplasia (MEN) type IIa phaeochromo-cytoma (almost invariably involving both adrenals) is associated with medullary carcinoma of thyroid and hyperparathyroidism (usually hyperplasia). In MEN IIb the same abnormalities are associated with

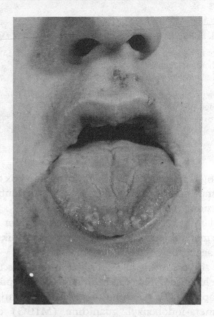

Fig. 13.26   Bumpy lips and tongue neuromas in patient with multiple endocrine neoplasia type IIb who presented with vomiting and paroxysmal hypertension, bilateral phaeochromocytomas and medullary carcinoma of thyroid.

Marfanoid body habitus, bumpy lips, mucosal neuromas of tongue, eyelids and cornea (Fig. 13.26). Both these conditions may arise spontaneously or be inherited as an autosomal dominant.

Clinical features

These depend on the catecholamine secretion. The clinical features are listed in the information box (left).

Some patients may present with a complication of the hypertension e.g. stroke, myocardial infarction, left ventricular failure. Occasionally the patients may be hypotensive (especially dopamine secreting tumours). Neurofibromatosis is associated with an increased incidence of phaeochromocytomas.

Investigation

The diagnosis is made on the basis of biochemical testing. Provocative tests of catecholamines release should not be used. The enzyme that synthesises adrenaline from noradrenaline is phenylethanolamine-N-methyl transferase (PNMT). This is induced by high glucocorticoid levels. Hence small adreno-medullary tumours bathed in cortisol by the centripetal blood flow of the adrenal produce the highest levels of adrenaline. Large adrenal tumours which have out-grown the normal cortical supply or extra-adrenal tumours produce almost entirely noradrenaline.

CLINICAL FEATURES OF PHAEOCHROMOCYTOMA

- Hypertension (usually paroyxsmal) (often postural drop of BP)
- Attacks with:
    - Pallor (sometimes flushing)
    - Palpitations
    - Sweating
    - Headache
    - Anxiety (fear of death – angor animi)
- Abdominal pain, vomiting
- Constipation
- Weight loss
- Glucose intolerance

USUAL SCREENING TESTS FOR PHAEOCHROMOCYTOMAS

24-hour urine for 3-methoxy-4-hydroxymandelic acid (VMA)
or 24-hour metanephrines
or 24-hour free urinary catecholamines

Plasma noradrenaline and adrenaline should be measured in:
Established or borderline cases
Paroxysmal hypertension
Renal failure

Screening tests are given in the information box above.

In some patients the diagnosis remains in doubt and a suppression test may be useful (e.g. plasma catecholamines 10 minutes after pentolinium 2.5 mg i.v.: normal subjects' levels will suppress unlike those with phaeochromocytoma).

Once the diagnosis has been made then the tumour must be localised. This can be done using computerised tomography (CT) scanning (Fig. 13.27). Scintigraphy using meta-iodobenzyl guanidine (MIBG) can be useful: MIBG labelled with radioactive iodine is taken up by both benign and malignant phaeochromocytomas. If the tumour cannot be localised then selective venous sampling with measurement of plasma noradrenaline may be required.

Management

This requires excision of the tumour or, failing this, long-term treatment with alpha (and usually beta) adrenoceptor blockade. Prior to surgery it is essential to give alpha blocking drugs such as phenoxybenzamine 10–20 mg orally 3–4 times daily preferably for a minimum of 6 weeks to allow restoration of normal plasma volume. If alpha-blockade produces a marked

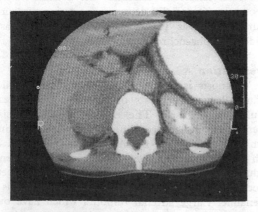

Fig. 13.27   CT scan of abdomen showing large right phaeochromocytoma.

tachycardia then a β-blocking drug such as propranolol (10–20 mg 3 times daily) should be added. On no account should the β-blocker be given before the α-blocker as vasoconstriction due to unopposed α-adrenoceptor activity may occur with a further increase in blood pressure. During surgery sodium nitroprusside and the short acting α-blocker phentolamine are very useful in controlling hypertensive episodes which may result from anaesthetic induction or tumour mobilisation. Postoperative hypotension may occur and require volume expansion and very occasionally noradrenaline. This is uncommon if the patient has been prepared with phenoxybenzamine for at least 6 weeks.

SEXUAL DISORDERS IN THE MALE

These can be classified on the basis of hypogonadism and precocious puberty. Hypogonadism is classified in the information box below.

CLASSIFICATION OF HYPOGONADISM

Secondary hypogonadism
Hypothalamic-pituitary disease
    Hypogonadotrophic ($\downarrow$ LH $\downarrow$ FSH) (see p. 614)
Primary testicular failure
    Hypergonadotrophic ($\uparrow$ LH $\uparrow$ FSH or $\uparrow$ FSH alone)
        Anorchia
        Klinefelter's syndrome (p. 655)
        Mumps orchitis – bilateral
        Tuberculosis
        Testicular tumours
        Idiopathic
        Chemotherapy/irradiation

Clinical features

These will depend on the underlying pathology. Thus in Kallmann's syndrome with isolated GnRH deficiency there is associated anosmia (p. 614). Pituitary tumours may present with symptoms of the tumour such as a visual field defect. The age of presentation is also important. If the defect is present prior to the normal onset of puberty then this will be delayed. Such a delay may be constitutional (often positive family history and short stature) or due to a variety of other conditions other than hypothalamic-pituitary-gonadal disease. These conditions are listed in the information box (p. 655).

Failure to go into puberty results in failure of normal fusion of the epiphyses of long bones with consequent

CLINICAL FEATURES OF HYPOGONADISM IN PRE-PUBERTY

- Systemic disease
  (e.g. malnutrition, cystic fibrosis, renal failure, heart disease, malabsorption)
- Androgen receptor defect
  (testicular feminisation or partial defects)
- 5α-reductase deficiency
- Anorexia nervosa
- Emotional deprivation
- Excessive exercise

excessive height (long arms and long legs in comparison to trunk height – eunuchoid proportions). The typical eunuch is tall with a hairless face, high-pitched voice, small external genitalia and rather immature personality. Some pubic hair is usually present as the result of adrenal androgen production – adrenarche.

If the hypogonadism develops *post pubertally* then the clinical features are usually those relating to loss of testosterone secretion. These are listed in the information box below.

CLINICAL FEATURES OF HYPOGONADISM IN POST PUBERTY

- Impotence ⎫
- Loss of libido ⎬ Early symptoms
- Tiredness ⎭

- Decreased shaving ⎫
- Decreased body hair ⎬ Late symptoms
- Decreased muscle power ⎭

Sudden loss of testosterone as with surgical castration may produce hot flushes and profuse sweating unless replacement therapy is given.

The loss of testosterone allows unopposed effects of oestrogen. The latter is increased when there is increased LH drive to the interstitial cells as in Klinefelter's syndrome. This leads to breast enlargement (gynaecomastia). Oestrogen secreting tumours may arise from interstitial cells and present with impotence and gynaecomastia. The tumour is often very small.

Males with hyperprolactinaemia frequently present with impotence, and occasionally with galactorrhoea. Thus the breasts should be carefully examined.

In cases of delayed puberty the extent of development should be classified using the 5 stages described by Marshall and Tanner. In GI the patient is

prepubertal: in G2 there is testicular enlargement to 4 ml (measured using a Prader orchidometer with a series of ellipsoids of known volumes); in G3 there is further scrotal and testicular enlargement (8–10 ml) with increased length of penis: G4-length and breadth of penis increases with development of glans, testicular volume 12 ml: G5-genitalia adult in size and shape with testes > 15 ml.

Pubic hair is associated in a similar manner (see the information box below).

CLASSIFICATION OF PUBIC HAIR

- PH 1 – no pubic hair
- PH 2 – sparse growth of straight lightly pigmented hair
- PH 3 – hair spreads over pubes, darker, coarser, curlier
- PH 4 – adult in character but smaller area
- PH 5 – hair extends onto inner aspects of thighs and up towards umbilicus

In complete androgen resistance (testicular feminisation) the phenotype is female and the condition due to defective androgen receptors in target tissues. The testes may be found in the groins. Pubic hair is absent. Breasts develop normally and the patient may present with primary amenorrhoea.

In 5alpha-reductase deficiency there is failure of conversion of testosterone to dihydrotestosterone. The latter is required for the development of the external genitalia. Thus these patients are usually brought up as females but have growth of the phallus at puberty. They then often change sexual orientation to that of a male.

The loss of FSH secretion leads to failure of spermatogenesis. This is also affected by LH deficiency as testosterone is required for spermatogenesis. If there is damage to testicular germ cells (e.g. by chemotherapy for malignant disease) then this can be detected by finding elevated FSH with normal LH.

Investigation

The tests for hypothalamic-pituitary dysfunction are detailed on p. 612.

In primary gonadal disease plasma testosterone, LH and FSH should be measured. If there is gynaecomastia then oestradiol should also be estimated. If elevated then the source must be determined (?exogenous, ?adrenal or testicular tumour). If indicated a karyotype should be performed. Bone age should be assessed in boys with delayed puberty.

Management

This depends on the cause. The androgen deficiency

should be replaced using one of the drugs and routes indicated on p. 615.

With delayed puberty there are various possibilities including intramuscular testosterone oenanthate 50–100 mg at 6-weekly intervals, hCG injections (1500 IU i.m. weekly) or pulsatile GnRH therapy (see p. 616).

The treatment of infertility in secondary hypogonadism is given on p. 616. There is no effective therapy for infertility resulting from primary gonadal failure. However, it is important to exclude causes such as sulphasalazine therapy when the effects are reversible.

CRYPTORCHIDISM

Cryptorchidism (undescended testis) usually occurs in otherwise normal boys but may be the presenting feature of hypogonadotrophic hypogonadism. Highly retractile testes, particularly in an obese boy, may be mistaken for cryptorchidism. If the testes remain in the inguinal canal they are more liable to trauma than if situated in the scrotum. The seminiferous tubules will fail to develop in an undescended gland, and if the condition is bilateral, sterility will follow. Even in testes which remain undescended into adult life the interstitial cells function normally, so that the secondary sex characteristics develop in the usual way. A course of chorionic gonadotrophin should be given at about 6 years of age. Alternatively GnRH can be given intranasally for 1–4 weeks. With inguinal testes the success rate for descent is about 40% which is similar to that with gonadotrophin. If medical treatment is unsuccessful the testis or testes should be placed in the scrotum surgically.

In maldescent the testis takes an abnormal route and is liable to develop malignancy. Such testes should either be brought down into the scrotum or, if discovered in the adult, removed.

IMPOTENCE

Erectile dysfunction or failure (impotence) was thought to be due to psychological causes in the majority of cases. However, the incidence of this condition increases with age; vascular disease involving the internal pudendal artery or its branches is common in these patients. This alone may be the cause of the impotence or a trigger for psychological dysfunction. Impotence may also be an early symptom in diabetes mellitus, multiple sclerosis and tabes dorsalis. Endocrine causes of impotence are uncommon and there is usually an associated loss of libido.

PRECOCIOUS PUBERTY

True precocious puberty results from the premature activation of the hypothalamic-pituitary-gonadal axis and needs to be distinguished from precocious pseudo-puberty associated with gonadal or adrenal tumours or congenital adrenal hyperplasia (p. 651). True precocious puberty is usually idiopathic in girls and there is frequently a positive family history. In boys it is more commonly indicative of central nervous system disease. Long-acting analogues of gonadotrophin releasing hormone are now being used to treat precocious puberty and thus improve the adult height prognosis and avoid the physical and psychological problems.

SEXUAL DISORDERS IN THE FEMALE

As with the male these can be classified into those arising from either hypothalamic-pituitary or primary gonadal defects. The presentation is often with menstrual abnormalities such as primary or secondary amenorrhoea.

PRIMARY AMENORRHOEA

This may be due to a chromosomal abnormality, e.g. Turner's syndrome (p. 13). These patients are usually short and have features such as a webbed neck and increased carrying angle. However, some cases have none of these phenotypic features.

Unrecognised or ineffectively treated congenital adrenal hyperplasia (p. 651) may present with primary amenorrhoea. The testicular feminisation syndrome due to defective androgen receptors is usually obvious because of the lack of pubic hair and good breast development (p. 655).

Any hypothalamic (e.g. craniopharyngioma) or pituitary (i.e. prolactinoma) lesion may be first manifest with failure to start menstruation. Primary autoimmune ovarian failure is a rare cause.

Structural abnormalities of the genital tract need to be excluded. It is important to recognise that any chronic systemic disease may delay the onset of menstruation.

SECONDARY AMENORRHOEA

This is a relatively common problem. The differential diagnosis is included in the information box (p. 657).

SECONDARY AMENORRHOEA

Hypothalamic dysfunction (see p. 614) +
Anorexia Nervosa, excessive exercise, psychogenic

Pituitary disease (see p. 614)
Especially hyperprolactinaemia

Ovarian dysfunction
Polycystic ovary syndrome
Androgen secreting tumours
Autoimmune (premature menopause)
Turner mosaic
Menopause (see below)

Adrenal disease
Cushing's syndrome, congenital adrenal hyperplasia, androgen secreting tumours

Thyroid disease
Hypo and hyperthyroidism

Other conditions
Severe systemic disease, e.g. renal failure, endometrial TB

Clinical features

These will depend on the condition. If there is weight loss then this may be primary as in anorexia nervosa or secondary to an underlying disease such as TB, malignancy or hyperthyroidism. Weight gain may suggest Cushing's syndrome, hypothyroidism or, very rarely, a hypothalamic lesion. Hirsutism may indicate androgen excess. A very common cause of this is the polycystic ovary syndrome. Androgen secreting tumours are much rarer. They may produce virilisation, e.g. clitoromegaly, deepening of the voice, temporal recession, breast atrophy. The breasts need to be carefully examined for milk (p. 620). The presence of other autoimmune disease should raise the possibility of autoimmune ovarian failure.

Investigation

High levels of LH and FSH suggest primary ovarian failure. This may be premature as with autoimmune ovarian failure. Elevated LH is common in the polycystic ovary syndrome together with slightly increased plasma testosterone with low levels of sex hormone binding globulin. High levels of plasma testosterone may be due to an androgen secreting tumour. If prolactin levels are elevated then this requires detailed investigation (p. 612). Low levels of gonadotrophins and oestradiol suggest hypothalamic or pituitary disease (p. 614).

Management

This depends on the cause. Androgen excess as in the polycystic ovary syndrome is a common problem. The hirsutism is usually of more concern to the patient than the menstrual abnormality. In about 75% of cases this improves with cyproterone acetate (anti-androgen). In pre-menopausal patients this is usually given as cyproterone acetate 50 mg b.d. on days 1–10 with ethinyl oestradiol 30 μg daily on days 1–21. This allows regular menstruation. In primary ovarian failure, especially if premature, oestrogen replacement will normally be required (see below).

THE MENOPAUSE

The cessation of menstruation in Western women occurs at a median age of 50.8 years. In the 5 years before there is a gradual increase in the number of anovulatory cycles. This period is referred to as the climacteric. Oestrogen secretion falls and negative feedback results in increased pituitary secretion of LH and FSH.

Clinical features

Irregular periods commonly precede the menopause and hence the exact timing of it can only be recognised in retrospect (e.g. 6 months after last period). The symptoms relate to oestrogen deficiency. In some patients they are relatively minor but in others a major problem. The symptoms are given in the information box below.

MENOPAUSAL SYMPTOMS

- Vasomotor effects
    Hot flushes
    Sweating
- Psychological
    Anxiety
    Emotional lability
    Irritability
- Genitourinary
    Dyspareunia ('senile vaginitis')
    Vaginal infections ↑
    Urgency of micturition

The flushes may start when the patient still has regular periods. In most patients the vasomotor symptoms gradually improve but in about one quarter they go on for more than 5 years. They are almost invariably relieved by oestrogen therapy. Their precise cause remains unknown. They are associated with an LH pulse. The fall in oestrogen secretion is associated with increased bone resorption. There is an initial rapid loss of bone mass which is most marked in the axial skeleton (1–3% per annum for 4 years and then 0.5% per annum). This eventually results in osteoporosis with an increased incidence of vertebral compression fracture, fractured neck of femur and distal radius in comparison to the male. This is a major and apparently increasing problem with significant morbidity, mortality (17% per 30 000 women per annum in the UK with hip fractures) and enormous cost. It is not at present possible to predict with accuracy a population at risk. This depends on bone density at the time of menopause and the rate of bone loss. However, those women who smoke cigarettes appear to be at particular risk. The earlier the menopause the greater the problem. Excessive alcohol and lack of exercise seem to be additional risk factors. Oestrogen started at the time of menopause has been shown to prevent the normal post-menopausal bone loss.

Management

Many women seek explanation and reassurance rather than treatment. In some the vasomotor symptoms may be the main problem. These may be helped by clonidine 50 μg b.d. but in many patients oestrogen therapy is required. This has the advantage of not only improving symptoms but also having beneficial effects on bone and soft tissues. Giving oestrogen is referred to as hormone replacement therapy (HRT). It can be given in a variety of different ways. These are included in the information box below.

OESTROGEN REPLACEMENT THERAPY

Oral oestrogens
e.g. cyclical ethinyl oestradiol 0.01–0.02 mg/day for 21 days with medroxyprogesterone acetate 5 mg daily for last 10 days

Percutaneous
Patches with reservoir of oestradiol giving oestradiol 25–50 μg/day. Change every 3–4 days. Add oral progestogen for 10 days per month

Topical oestradiol
e.g. for atrophic vaginitis 0.01% dienoestrol cream

Percutaneous oestrogen is a relatively new form of treatment. It has the advantage of not having the same effect on liver production of coagulation factors as oral oestrogen. Patients should not be given long-term unopposed oestrogen as this increases the risk of endometrial cancer (× 5). Nausea and breast tenderness may be a problem. The blood pressure should be measured before and at 6-monthly intervals on treatment. The duration of treatment is debatable. For symptoms such as hot flushes a year may be reasonable with gradual withdrawal. For prevention of osteoporosis much longer treatment is necessary. For patients with a premature menopause oestrogen should be given until at least aged 50. A cervical smear should be taken and the breasts and pelvis examined before giving oestrogen.

DIABETES MELLITUS

Diabetes Mellitus is a clinical syndrome characterised by hyperglycaemia due to absolute or relative deficiency of insulin. This can arise in many different ways (Table 13.14). Lack of insulin, whether absolute or relative, affects the metabolism of carbohydrate, protein, fat, water and electrolytes. Death may result from acute metabolic decompensation while long-standing metabolic derangement is frequently associated with permanent and irreversible functional and structural changes in the cells of the body, those of the vascular system being particularly susceptible. These changes lead in turn to the development of well-defined clinical entities, the so called 'complications of diabetes' which most characteristically affect the eye, the kidney and the nervous system.

EPIDEMIOLOGY

Epidemiological study of whole populations has shown that the distribution of blood glucose concentration is unimodal with no clear division between normal and abnormal values. Diagnostic criteria are therefore arbitrary. Population studies involving Pima Indians in Arizona and civil servants in Whitehall have shown that hyperglycaemia represents an independent risk factor for the development of disease of small and large blood vessels respectively. Current diagnostic criteria for diabetes (Table 13.15) have been selected on the basis of identifying those who have a degree of hyperglycaemia which has been shown to be associated with a significantly increased risk of disability and death from vascular disease, irrespective of the basic cause of the hyperglycaemia.

Diabetes is by far the most common of the endocrine disorders. It is world-wide in distribution and the incidence of both types of primary diabetes, that is Insulin Dependent Diabetes Mellitus (IDDM) and Non-Insulin Dependent Diabetes (NIDDM) is rising throughout the world. However the prevalence of both varies considerably in different parts of the world. This seems to be due to differences in both genetic and environmental factors. The prevalence in Britain is between 1 and 2% but almost 50% of cases of NIDDM remain undetected. The great majority of cases seen world-wide have primary diabetes and in Europe and

Table 13.14 Classification of diabetes mellitus

	Examples
A *Primary*	
Type 1 Insulin-dependent diabetes mellitus (IDDM)	
Type 2 Non-insulin-dependent diabetes mellitus (NIDDM)	
B *Secondary to other pathology*	
1 Pancreatic pathology	Pancreatitis
	Haemochromatosis
	Neoplastic disease
	Pancreatectomy
	Cystic fibrosis
2 Excess endogenous production of hormonal antagonists	
to insulin	Growth hormone (acromegaly)
	Glucocorticoids (Cushing's syndrome)
	Thyroid hormones (hyperthyroidism)
	Catecholamines (phaeochromocytoma)
	HPL (pregnancy)
	Glucagon (glucagonoma)
	Severe burns (glucagon, cortisol, catecholamines)
3 Medication with	Corticosteroids
	Thiazide diuretics
	Phenytoin
4 Liver disease	
C *Associated with genetic syndromes*	DIDMOAD (i.e. diabetes insipidus, diabetes mellitus, optic atrophy, nerve deafness)
	Lipoatrophy
	Muscular dystrophies
	Friedreich's ataxia
	Down's syndrome
	Klinefelter's syndrome
	Turner's syndrome

North America the ratio of NIDDM:IDDM is approximately 7:3.

AETIOLOGY

Although the precise aetiology is still uncertain in both main types of diabetes environmental factors interact with a genetic susceptibility to determine which of those with the genetic predisposition actually develop the clinical syndrome and the timing of its onset. However both the pattern of inheritance and the environmental factors differ in IDDM and NIDDM.

IDDM

The inheritance of human IDDM is polygenic. It has

Table 13.15 Diagnostic criteria for diabetes mellitus using an oral glucose (75 g) tolerance test (WHO 1985)

	Venous plasma (whole blood) glucose concentration mmol/l	
	Normal	Diabetic
Fasting	<6.1 (5.6)	≥7.8 (6.7)
2 hours after glucose	<8.9 (6.7)	≥11.1 (10.0)

Note:
1. These figures refer to the concentration of glucose estimated by a specific enzymatic assay.
2. Most hospital laboratories measure the concentration of glucose in plasma samples.

been estimated that over 50% of the heritability is contributed by the HLA class II genes (that is the D loci on the short arm of chromosome 6) which determine immune responsiveness. Associations with alleles at other loci occur because of linkage disequilibrium. About 95% of patients with IDDM are either HLA DR3 and/or 4 (Table 13.16) but since 50%

Table 13.16 Relative risk of developing IDDM conferred by HLA-DR antigens

HLA-DR	Relative risk
DR2	0.12
DR3	7.39
DR4	9.25
DR7	0.12
DR3, DR4	14.26
DR3. DR	0.80
DR4, DR	0.95
DR, DR	0.04

of the general population are also DR3/4 the search for IDDM specific HLA genes has continued. Recently analysis of DNA sequences from diabetic patients has been performed. Although so far no unique class II sequences have been found it has been shown that susceptibility to IDDM is directly related to the amino acid at position 57 of the N-terminal B-1 domain of the HLA-DQ beta chain. Thus maximum, in fact almost complete HLA-linked resistance to the development of IDDM is conferred by inheritance of two alleles with aspartic acid at position 57 (Asp 57-positive homozygosity), while maximum susceptibility is associated with Asp 57-negative homozygosity (that is alanine, valine or serine substituted for aspartate), and Asp 57 heterozygosity carries a much lower risk of developing IDDM (10% of IDDM patients). It has been suggested that DQ beta polymorphisms determine the specificity and extent of an autoimmune response against pancreatic islet insulin secreting cells and are necessary, but not in themselves sufficient, for the development of IDDM. This implies either the existence of another/other specific IDDM related gene(s) or involvement of more than one HLA-D gene controlling the intensity of the beta cell destructive process (which appears to be mediated by cytokines), or an important role for environmental factors in clinical expression of the disease in genetically susceptible persons. The latter hypothesis is supported by the fact that about 50% of pairs of monozygotic twins are discordant for IDDM.

Environmental factors

Viruses

The evidence that viral infection might cause some forms of human IDDM is derived from epidemiological studies and isolated case reports. Studies in mice have shown that viruses can induce diabetes by two distinct pathogenic mechanisms: destruction of the pancreatic beta cells by direct cytolysis results from infection with the D variant of the EMC virus, Mengo virus 2T and Coxsackie B4 virus, while induction of an autoimmune destructive process results from infection with reo virus type 1 and rubella virus. The ability of viruses to induce diabetes in mice is dependent on the genetic background of the host as well as on the genetic makeup of the virus. The induction of diabetes by infection with EMC, Mengo or Coxsackie B4 viruses can be prevented by administration of live attenuated vaccine while reo virus induced diabetes can be prevented by immunosuppression.

Diet

Dietary factors have been invoked as a possible explanation for the rising incidence of IDDM in Northern Europe and North America. There are no direct data relating diet after weaning to the development of IDDM in genetically susceptible children however two reports have provided circumstantial evidence supporting the proposition that dietary factors may at least in certain circumstances influence the development of human IDDM. Thus an unusually high incidence of IDDM in boys born in the month of October in Iceland has been linked to the high nitrosamine content of a smoked mutton traditionally consumed at Christmas. Subsequent experiments in mice suggested that this effect was mediated via the parental germ cells rather than by a direct effect on the pancreatic beta cells of the fetus. In the second report anti-gliadin antibodies were reported in 54% of children (none of whom had coeliac disease) at diagnosis of IDDM under two years of age. In addition studies using the spontaneously diabetic, insulin dependent BB rat suggest that certain components of the diet may be essential for the expression of clinical diabetes in diabetes-prone animals. Wheat and milk protein have been shown to have the strongest diabetogenic effect and are evidently capable of triggering the string of events which results ultimately in destruction of pancreatic islet insulin-secreting cells.

Immunological factors

The information box below summarises the evidence that IDDM is a slow autoimmune disease. Detailed family studies have produced evidence that contrary to clinical impression destruction of the insulin-secreting cells in the pancreas is a slow process occurring over many years. Hyperglycaemia accompanied by the classical symptoms of diabetes occurs only when 90% of insulin-secreting cells are already destroyed. It is clear also that in both man and animals with spontaneous insulin-dependent diabetes the immune system retains the capacity to recognise and destroy transplanted insulin-secreting cells indefinitely.

EVIDENCE THAT IDDM IS A SLOW AUTOIMMUNE DISEASE

- HLA-LINKED genetic predisposition
- Association with other autoimmune disorders
- Circulating islet cell cytoplasmic and surface and insulin-autoantibodies in new cases
- Mononuclear cell infiltration of pancreatic islets resulting in selective destruction of insulin-secreting cells.
- Recurrence of insulitis and selective destruction of insulin-secreting cells in pancreatic grafts

---

Pancreatic pathology

Three outstanding features characterise the pathological picture in the pre-diabetic pancreas in IDDM. Firstly, 'insulitis', that is infiltration of the islets with mononuclear cells. Secondly, the initial patchiness of this lesion, with, until a very late stage, lobules containing heavily infiltrated islets commonly

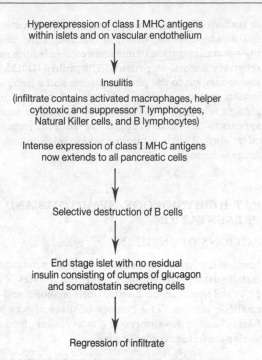

Hyperexpression of class I MHC antigens
within islets and on vascular endothelium

↓

Insulitis

(infiltrate contains activated macrophages, helper
cytotoxic and suppressor T lymphocytes,
Natural Killer cells, and B lymphocytes)

Intense expression of class I MHC antigens
now extends to all pancreatic cells

↓

Selective destruction of B cells

↓

End stage islet with no residual
insulin consisting of clumps of glucagon
and somatostatin secreting cells

↓

Regression of infiltrate

Fig. 13.28   Sequence of pancreatic events in the development of IDDM.

seen immediately adjacent to unaffected lobules. Thirdly, the striking beta cell specificity of the destructive process within infiltrated islets where the glucagon and other hormone secreting cells invariably remain intact. Figure 13.28 shows the sequence of pancreatic events in the development of IDDM.

NIDDM

Genetic factors

NIDDM is not HLA linked and there is no evidence that autoimmunity or viruses have anything to do with its development. Studies of monozygotic twins have shown that genetic factors are more important in the development of this type of diabetes than in IDDM, with concordance for NIDDM approaching 100%, but there is little information about what is inherited.

Environmental factors

Lifestyle

Epidemiological studies of NIDDM provide evidence that over-eating, especially when combined with obesity and underactivity, is associated with the development of NIDDM. Other more direct studies have shown that middle-aged diabetic patients eat significantly more and are fatter and less active than their non-diabetic siblings. The majority of middle-aged diabetic patients are obese but only a few obese people develop diabetes. Obesity probably acts as a diabetogenic factor (through increasing resistance to the action of insulin) in those genetically predisposed to develop NIDDM.

Age

In Britain over 70% of all cases of diabetes occur after the age of 50 years. In contrast to IDDM which mainly affects younger people, NIDDM is principally a disease of the middle aged and elderly. Thus ageing is an important risk factor for NIDDM.

Pregnancy

There are rather more young male diabetics than female but in middle age more females are affected. During normal pregnancy the level of plasma insulin is raised by the action of placental hormones, thus placing a burden on the insulin-secreting cells of the pancreatic islets. The pancreas may be unable to meet these demands in women genetically predisposed to develop both types of diabetes. The term 'gestational diabetes' refers to hyperglycaemia occurring for the first time during pregnancy. This may or may not disappear following delivery. Repeated pregnancy may increase the likelihood of developing permanent diabetes, particularly in obese women. Long-term studies show that some 80% of women with gestational diabetes ultimately develop permanent clinical diabetes requiring treatment.

Pancreatic pathology

In contrast to IDDM where at diagnosis the insulin-secreting cells have largely disappeared from the pancreas so that plasma immunoreactive insulin is either very low or undetectable, in NIDDM there is only moderate reduction in the total mass of islet tissue consistent with a measurable, though reduced, concentration of insulin in plasma. There are however some pathological changes which are typical of NIDDM and demonstrable in most, although not all cases. The most consistent of these changes is probably deposition of amyloid which is accompanied by atrophy of the normal tissue, particularly islet epithelial cells. In more advanced lesions, the islet is more or less converted to amyloid and the reduction in the number of insulin-secreting cells is more pronounced than that of glucagon-secreting cells. Islet amyloid is not a qualitative marker of NIDDM but rather a quantitative one. Heavy deposition of amyloid in islets is rare without diabetes. Small quantities of islet amyloid are very common in elderly non-diabetic patients. Deposition of amyloid is probably not a cause of diabetes but rather reflects a pathological process which is increased in NIDDM.

Simple deficiency of insulin cannot entirely account for the diabetic syndrome in NIDDM. Increased hepatic production of glucose and resistance to the action of insulin are characteristic features of this disorder. Insulin resistance is also seen in obesity which so often accompanies NIDDM. However many non-obese patients with NIDDM are also insulin resistant.

Insulin resistance may be due to any one of three general causes: an abnormal insulin molecule, an excessive amount of circulating antagonists, and target tissue defects. The last is the common cause of insulin resistance in NIDDM. The specific mechanisms underlying this insulin resistant state are heterogeneous. In patients with relatively mild impairment of glucose tolerance the defect in insulin action is associated with a decreased number of cellular insulin receptors. Patients with more severe hyperglycaemia usually combine a reduced number of receptors with a post-receptor defect in the action of insulin and the latter seems to be the predominant abnormality.

Increased hepatic production of glucose and/or decreased peripheral utilisation of glucose cannot lead to sustained hyperglycaemia unless the pancreatic islets fail to adapt to the situation. Although the absolute plasma concentration of immunoreactive insulin may be relatively normal in patients with mild NIDDM it is low in relation to the plasma glucose and a delay in the insulin response to glucose is commonly seen during a glucose tolerance test. This defect in insulin secretion appears to be selective for glucose since the response to other stimuli such as amino acids and sulphonylurea drugs is normal.

PATHOPHYSIOLOGY, SYMPTOMS AND PRESENTATION

ACTIONS OF INSULIN

Insulin has profound effects on the metabolism of carbohydrate, fat, protein and electrolytes (Table 13.17). These can be divided into anabolic and anti-catabolic actions. The balance of these effects in the fasting and post-absorptive states, after food, and during exercise is controlled by:

1. variation in the relative circulating concentration of insulin (the only anabolic hormone) and several catabolic hormones namely glucagon, growth

Table 13.17   Actions of insulin

	Increase (anabolic effects)	Decrease (anticatabolic effects)
Carbohydrate metabolism	Glucose transport (muscle, adipose tissue) Glucose phosphorylation Glycogenesis Glycolysis Pyruvate dehydrogenase activity Pentose phosphate shunt	Gluconeogenesis Glycogenolysis
Lipid metabolism	Triglyceride synthesis Fatty acid synthesis (liver) Lipoprotein lipase (adipose tissue) activity	Lipolysis Lipoprotein lipase (muscle) Ketogenesis Fatty acid oxidation (liver)
Protein metabolism	Amino acid transport Protein synthesis	Protein degradation
Electrolytes	Cellular potassium uptake	

Table 13.18   Probable actions of hormones countering the effect of insulin in man

	Insulin release	Muscle glucose uptake	Hepatic glucogenesis	Ketogenesis	Lipolysis	Proteolysis
Catecholamines	↓	↓	↑	↑	↑	↑
Glucagon	—	—	↑	↑	—	—
Growth hormone	—	↓	—	↑	↑	—
Glucocorticoids	—	—	↑	↑	↑	↑
Thyroid hormones	—	—	↑	↑	↑	↑

↑ = increase; ↓ = decrease; — = no significant primary effect.

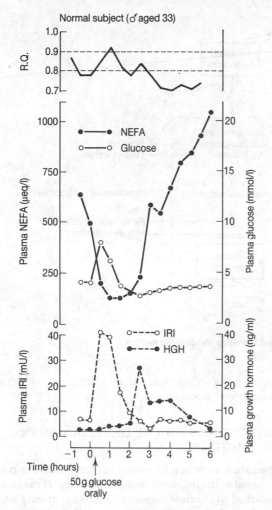

Fig. 13.29 **Changes in respiratory quotient and plasma concentration of** glucose, non-esterified fatty acids, immunoreactive insulin and human growth hormone following ingestion of 50 g glucose by a normal, thin young man.

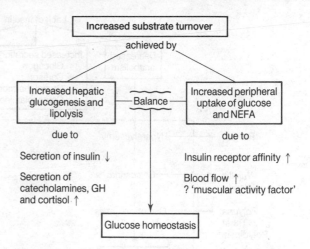

Fig. 13.30 **Main features of the metabolic adaptation to moderate exercise.**

hormone, cortisol, catecholamines and thyroid hormones (Table 13.18);

2. the fact that insulin exerts its anticatabolic effects at a lower concentration than that required for its anabolic actions.

During an oral glucose tolerance test (Fig. 13.29) or a mixed meal the first one and half hours are dominated by increased secretion of insulin and both growth hormone and glucagon secretion are inhibited. Cortisol and adrenaline levels do not change significantly.

Exercise represents a special stress with a rapid increase in the demand for metabolic fuel. At rest 90% of the energy requirements of muscle come from fatty

acids and ketone bodies. In the initial stages of strenuous exercise energy comes from oxidation of stored glycogen but if the demand for oxygen outstrips supply anaerobic glycolysis becomes all important. Glycogen supplies are rapidly depleted and glucose is extracted from the circulation independent of insulin. Blood glucose levels fall and secretion of insulin also decreases. Catecholamine and cortisol levels rise stimulating lipolysis and gluconeogenesis. The increase in hepatic glucose production matches the increased extra hepatic utilisation so that glucose levels do not change markedly (Fig. 13.30). As anaerobic glycolysis continues blood lactate concentration rises and this is recycled by the liver as new glucose.

PATHOPHYSIOLOGY

Whatever the aetiology, in all cases the hyperglycaemia of diabetes develops because of an absolute (IDDM) or relative (NIDDM) deficiency of insulin which leads to:

1. a reduced rate of removal of glucose from the blood by peripheral tissues;
2. an increased rate of release of glucose from the liver into the circulation.

When the concentration of glucose in the plasma exceeds the renal threshold (that is the capacity of renal tubules to reabsorb glucose from the glomerular filtrate), glycosuria occurs. The renal threshold is approximately 10 mmol/l but there is wide individual variation.

Figure 13.31 relates the pathophysiology of diabetes to its symptoms. Note that the severity of the classical

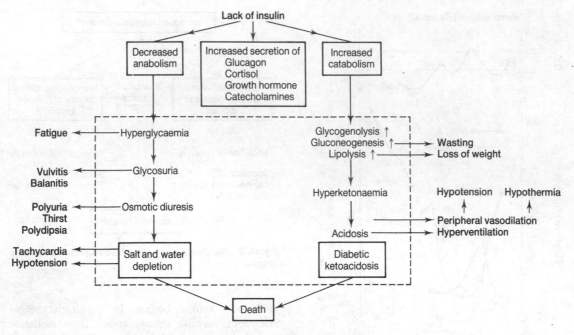

Fig. 13.31 Pathophysiological basis of the symptoms and signs of untreated or uncontrolled diabetes mellitus.

symptoms of diabetes, namely polyuria and polydipsia, is related directly to the degree of glycosuria. If hyperglycaemia develops slowly over many months or even years, as in NIDDM, the renal threshold for glucose rises and both glycosuria and the symptoms of diabetes are then correspondingly slight. This is one reason for the large number of undetected cases of NIDDM. Such individuals may have significant but symptomless hyperglycaemia for many years before glycosuria is noted on routine urine testing. Sometimes they eventually present with symptoms due to one or more of the complications of long-term diabetes: paraesthesiae, pain, and muscle atrophy in the legs, or impotence due to neuropathy; deterioration of vision due to retinopathy; or ulceration of the feet due to a combination of neuropathy, peripheral vascular disease and infection. Uncontrolled diabetes is associated with an increased susceptibility to infection and patients may present with skin sepsis, intractable and recurrent urinary tract infections, pulmonary tuberculosis or poor healing of a wound following surgery.

A minority of cases of diabetes may first present as severe ketoacidosis, either associated with an acute infection or other illness or even without evidence of a precipitating cause. In such cases abdominal pain and vomiting may be the presenting complaints. This is more likely to occur in IDDM. Diabetic ketoacidosis must therefore be considered in the differential diagnosis of a patient who complains of acute abdominal symptoms.

MECHANISMS OF THE DEVELOPMENT OF KETOACIDOSIS

The extent to which increased lipolysis occurs is proportional to the degree of insulin deficiency. If the latter is marked the normal response to feeding, namely suppression of lipolysis, may be lost and the plasma concentration of non-esterified fatty acids may remain constantly elevated. Fatty acids are taken up by the liver and degraded through eight steps within the mitochondria of the liver cells. Each stage yields one molecule of acetyl-co-enzyme A. Normally most of these molecules enter the citric acid cycle by condensing with oxaloacetic acid, but in the absence of insulin more is formed than can enter the citric acid cycle and acetyl-co-enzyme A is converted to aceto acetic acid. Most of this is then reduced to beta hydroxy-butyric acid, while some is decarboxylated to acetone. These ketone bodies, when formed in small amounts, are oxidised and utilised as metabolic fuel. However, the rate of utilisation of ketone bodies is limited. When the rate of production by the liver exceeds that of removal by the peripheral tissues then hyperketonaemia results.

Ketone bodies increase the osmolality of plasma and

so also lead to withdrawal of water from cells. They are acids which dissociate almost completely at physiological pH, releasing hydrogen ions into the body fluids. The fall in pH is countered by the buffers of the blood, the most important being bicarbonate. The dissociation of carbonic acid is reduced, the ratio of bicarbonate ions to carbonic ions falls, and measurement of plasma bicarbonate will show a lower value than normal. The rise in hydrogen ion concentration in the arterial blood stimulates pulmonary ventilation so that clinically hyperpnoea or 'air hunger' is observed.

The extent to which the clinical features of dehydration and ketoacidosis are seen in the individual case will depend on such factors as the speed at which the condition develops and the extent to which the patient increases the intake of fluid as well as on the degree of insulin deficiency present. Thus when insulin deficiency is partial, as in patients with NIDDM, the anticatabolic effect of insulin may be relatively well preserved while its anabolic action is more seriously defective. In these circumstances lipolysis is not markedly accelerated and the concentration of ketone bodies in the blood remains relatively normal despite severe hyperglycaemia. This state has been designated 'hyperosmolar diabetic coma'.

CLINICAL FEATURES

In Table 13.19 the classical clinical features of the two main types of diabetes are compared. While the distinction between IDDM and NIDDM is broadly true in relation to the features listed, overlap occurs in relation particularly to age at onset of diabetes, duration of symptoms and family history. Thus some young people have a form of NIDDM designated Maturity Onset Diabetes in Young people (designated the MODY Syndrome) while some middle-aged and elderly patients present with typical autoimmune Type I IDDM.

Patients with IDDM usually show no physical signs attributable to diabetes. In the fulminating case the

Table 13.19 Clinical features of IDDM and NIDDM

	IDDM	NIDDM
Age at onset	<40 years	>50 years
Duration of symptoms	Weeks	Months–years
Body weight	Normal or low	Obese
Ketonuria	Yes	No
Rapid death without treatment with insulin	Yes	No
Autoantibodies	Yes	No
Diabetic complications at diagnosis	No	10–20%
Family history of diabetes	No	Yes
Other autoimmune disease	Yes	No

Table 13.20 Approximate empirical risk of development IDDM up to the age of 25 years

First degree relative with IDDM	Risk of IDDM (%)
Father	2.5
Mother	1.5
Both parents	15–20
Mother and sibling	13
Sibling	3
Monozygotic twin	40

most striking features are those of salt and water depletion, that is a loose dry skin which lifts in folds, a dry furred tongue and cracked lips, tachycardia, hypotension and reduced intraocular pressure. Breathing may be deep and sighing due to acidosis, the breath is usually fetid and the sickly sweet smell of acetone may be apparent. Mental apathy, confusion or coma may also be present.

The physical signs present in patients with NIDDM at diagnosis depend on the mode of presentation. Pruritus vulvae or balanitis is a common presenting symptom since the external genitalia are especially prone to infection by fungi (candida) which flourish on skin and mucous membranes contaminated by glucose. Ophthalmoscopy may show the typical appearances of diabetic retinopathy. Depression or loss of the tendon reflexes at the ankles and impaired perception of vibration sensation distally in the legs indicate neuropathy. Other abnormalities of neurological examination are less common. The presence of diabetic nephropathy may be indicated by proteinuria in addition to glycosuria. Signs of atherosclerosis are common and may include hypertension, diminished or impalpable pulses in the feet, bruits over the carotid or femoral arteries, and gangrene of the feet. Signs of water and salt depletion with associated mental changes may be seen in cases with severe hyperglycaemia with or without ketoacidosis.

Apart from patients with established clinical diabetes two other categories are recognised – potential and latent diabetes.

Potential diabetics are persons with a normal glucose tolerance test who have an increased risk of developing diabetes for genetic reasons, for example the children of two diabetic parents, the sibling of a diabetic, the non diabetic member of a pair of monozygotic twins where the other is diabetic. Table 13.20 shows the approximate empirical risk of an individual developing IDDM up to the age of 25 years when various first degree relatives already have IDDM, while Table 13.21 shows the risk of developing NIDDM up to the age of 80 years for siblings of probands with NIDDM subdivided according to age at onset.

Table 13.21 Risk of developing NIDDM up to the age of 80 years for siblings of probands with NIDDM

Age at onset of NIDDM in Proband	Age corrected risk of NIDDM for siblings (%)
25–44	52.9
45–54	36.5
55–64	38.4
65–80	30.7
Overall 25–80	37.9

Latent diabetics are persons in whom the glucose tolerance test is normal but who are known to have given an abnormal result under conditions imposing a burden on the pancreatic cells, for example during pregnancy, infection or other severe stress, mental or physical, during treatment with corticosteroids, thiazide diuretics or other diabetogenic drugs, or when over-weight.

Potential and latent diabetic patients usually complain of no symptoms and show no abnormality on examination. However, certain features are recognised as being characteristic of such states without necessarily implying that such individuals will progress to clinical diabetes. For example, they are predisposed to coronary and peripheral arterial disease, may show abnormal lipid patterns in response to oral contraceptives, and have an increased incidence of still-born, abnormally large and heavy babies and babies with congenital defects.

DIAGNOSIS

When the symptoms suggest diabetes the diagnosis may be confirmed by finding glycosuria, with or without ketonuria, and a random blood glucose concentration greater than 14 mmol/l. This is shown in the information box below.

DIAGNOSIS OF DIABETES

Patient complains of symptoms suggesting diabetes
● Test urine for glucose and ketones
● Measure random blood glucose, plasma electrolytes, HbA,
Diagnosis confirmed by random plasma glucose
> 14 mmol/l ± HbA, > 9.0%

Indications for glucose tolerance test
● Glycosuria ± ketonuria found on routine urine test
● Patient has minimal or no symptoms
● Random plasma glucose – 6.0–13.0 mmol/l ± HbA, 8–9%

The severity of the classical symptoms of diabetes, namely polyuria and polydipsia, is directly related to the degree of glycosuria. Some individuals may have significant but symptomless hyperglycaemia for many years before glycosuria is noted on routine urine testing in the course of a medical examination being conducted for various reasons.

Urine testing

Testing the urine for glucose is the most usual procedure for detecting diabetes, both in the consulting room and in population screening surveys. Sensitive and glucose-specific dipstick methods are available. A positive response gives a rough indication that the urinary glucose concentration exceeds 0.55–1.11 mmol/l. If possible, the test for urinary glucose should be performed on urine passed $1\frac{1}{2}$–2 hours after a main meal since this will detect more of the milder cases of diabetes than a fasting urine specimen.

The most serious disadvantage of using urinary glucose as a diagnostic or screening procedure is the individual variation in renal threshold. On the one hand some undoubtedly diabetic individuals will have a negative urine test and on the other hand non-diabetic individuals with a low renal threshold for glucose will give a positive result. Estimation of the blood glucose concentration (either in a random sample of blood or following a 75 g oral glucose load), using an accurate laboratory method rather than a side room technique, is therefore essential in making the diagnosis (see information box left)).

Clinically important amounts of ketone bodies can be recognised by the nitroprusside reaction which is conveniently carried out using tablets or test papers. Ketonuria may be found in normal people who have been fasting or exercising strenuously for long periods, who have been vomiting repeatedly or who have been eating a diet very high in fats and low in carbohydrate. Ketonuria is therefore not pathognomonic of diabetes, but if both ketonuria and glycosuria are found, the diagnosis of diabetes is practically certain.

Gestational diabetes

The term 'gestational diabetes' is used to refer to hyperglycaemia occurring for the first time during pregnancy in individuals who have an inherited predisposition to develop diabetes. Both IDDM and NIDDM are involved. The hyperglycaemia may or may not disappear following delivery. Normal pregnancy is characterised by hyperinsulinaemia in response to the production of hormonal insulin antagonists such as human placental lactogen and progesterone. A suboptimal endocrine pancreas may be unable to meet this demand. Since even minimal hyperglycaemia in

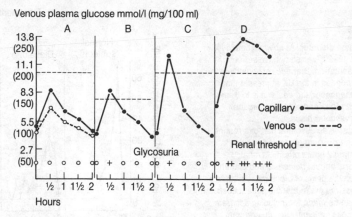

Venous plasma glucose mmol/l (mg/100 ml)

Fig. 13.32   The glucose tolerance test: blood glucose curves after 75 g glucose by mouth, showing (A) normal curve, (B) renal glycosuria, (C) alimentary (lag storage) glycosuria and (D) diabetes mellitus of moderate severity.

pregnancy is associated with increased perinatal mortality and morbidity it is important to detect and treat these cases effectively. Detection may present problems. Glycosuria is common in normal pregnancy (due to a fall in the renal threshold for glucose secondary to an increase in the glomerular filtration rate) and in late pregnancy through lactose appearing in the urine. The finding of reducing substances in the urine of a pregnant women should however never be lightly dismissed and in all cases the blood glucose concentration should be carefully measured, using an accurate laboratory assay specific for glucose, in the fasting state, and then at accurately timed intervals after a 75 g glucose load, and during a glucose profile in the course of a normal day.

The oral glucose tolerance test

The patient, who should have been taking an unrestricted carbohydrate diet for at least three days or more prior to the test, fasts overnight. Ideally out-patients should rest for at least half an hour before starting the test, and should remain seated and refrain from smoking during the test. A sample of blood is taken to measure the fasting plasma glucose level and 75 g glucose dissolved in 300 ml of water is then given by mouth. Thereafter samples of blood are collected at half-hourly intervals for at least two hours and their glucose content is estimated. The diagnostic criteria for diabetes mellitus and normality recommended by WHO in 1985 are shown in Table 13.15. Intermediate readings are classified as Impaired Glucose Tolerance and indicate the need for further evaluation of the

patient including the history. It may be necessary to keep the patient under observation and to repeat the test at a later date. The diagnostic criteria for diabetes in pregnancy are more stringent than those recommended for non-pregnant subjects and pregnant women with impaired glucose tolerance should be treated as diabetic.

Renal glycosuria

Apart from diabetes the commonest cause of glycosuria is a low renal threshold for glucose (Fig. 13.32) which commonly occurs temporarily in pregnancy and is a much more frequent cause of glycosuria than diabetes in young people. Renal glycosuria is a benign condition unrelated to diabetes and is not accompanied by the classical symptoms associated with glycosuria due to diabetes.

Alimentary (lag storage) glycosuria

In some individuals an unusually rapid but transitory rise of blood glucose follows a meal and the concentration exceeds the normal renal threshold; during this time glucose will be present in the urine. This response to a meal or to a dose of glucose is traditionally known as a 'lag storage' blood glucose curve although alimentary glycosuria is a better term (Fig. 13.32). It may occur in otherwise normal people or after gastric surgery when it is due to rapid gastric emptying leading to an increased rate of absorption into the blood stream. It is not uncommonly seen in patients with hyperthyroidism or hepatic disease. This type of blood glucose curve is usually regarded as benign and unrelated to diabetes:

SUMMARY OF DIAGNOSIS

- Diabetes is a very common disorder. At any one time 50% of cases are undiagnosed. 10–20% already have serious vascular disease at presentation. Diabetic retinopathy is the commonest cause of blindness in the UK at present time
- The earlier diabetes is diagnosed the easier it is to treat effectively and the greater the chance of avoiding the development of serious vascular disease.
- Testing the urine for sugar is an essential part of a routine clinical examination. The urine sample tested should preferably be passed within 2 hours of a main meal.
- All patients with glycosuria should be considered diabetic until proved otherwise on the basis of blood measurements.
- A negative urine test does not mean that the patient does not have diabetes. A case can be made for including *accurate* measurement of the glucose concentration in a random plasma sample as an essential component of a routine clinical examination.
- Wherever practicable, estimation of the blood glucose concentration 2 hours after 75 g glucose orally should be used as the screening test for detecting diabetes.
- HbA₁ alone is not sensitive enough to detect early, relatively mild cases of diabetes.
- Particular attention should be paid to high-risk groups such as the first-degree relatives of known diabetics, the obese, and pregnant women.

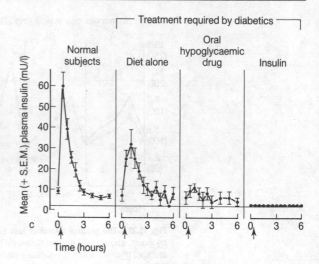

Fig. 13.33   Mean (±SEM) plasma concentration of immunoreactive insulin in the fasting state and at half-hourly intervals after 50 g glucose orally (indicated by ↑) in normal subjects and in newly diagnosed untreated diabetic patients grouped on the basis of the treatment they were subsequently found to require on clinical grounds. The solid line at the foot of the section relating to insulin secretion indicates the lower limit of sensitivity of the assay.

although the peak blood glucose concentration is abnormally high the value two hours after oral glucose is normal.

Diagnosis of diabetes

This is given in the information box above.

MANAGEMENT

Three methods of treatment are available: diet alone, diet and an oral hypoglycaemic drug, and diet and insulin. Approximately 50% of new cases of diabetes can be controlled adequately by diet alone, 20–30% will need an oral hypoglycaemic drug, and 20–30% will require insulin. Regardless of aetiology the type of treatment required is determined by the circulating plasma immunoreactive insulin concentration (Fig. 13.33). At a clinical level the age and weight of the patient at diagnosis are closely correlated with the plasma insulin concentration and indicate with a high degree of probability the type of treatment likely to be required (Fig. 13.34) but the regimen eventually adopted in each individual case is ultimately chosen by therapeutic trial.

DIETARY MANAGEMENT

General principles

Dietary measures are required in the treatment of all diabetic patients to achieve the overall therapeutic goal: normal metabolism. The specific aims of treatment are to prevent the development of diabetic microangiopathy (p. 683) by avoiding sustained hyperglycaemia and to reduce the incidence of atherosclerosis by lowering blood lipids, maintaining an ideal body weight, and avoiding hyperinsulinaemia.

The first step in preparing any dietary regimen is to decide what the individual patient's daily energy requirement is. This must be estimated after considering such factors as age, sex, actual weight in relation to desirable weight, activity and occupation. An

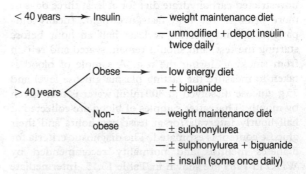

Fig. 13.34   The long-term type of treatment probably required by any individual patient can be determined by considering their age and weight at diagnosis of diabetes.

Table 13.22   Proportion of energy derived from carbohydrate, protein, fat

	UK national diet	Recommended diet
Carbohydrate	46%	50–60%
Protein	12%	10–15%
Fat	46%	30–35%

METHODS OF SLOWING THE RATE OF CARBOHYDRATE ABSORPTION

- Nibbling rather than gorging
- Use of soluble fibre supplements and soluble fibre foods
- Use of foods with Low Glycaemic Index
- Alpha-glucosidase inhibition

approximate range for the various groups of patients might be: an obese middle-aged or elderly person, 1000–1600 kcal daily; an elderly person not overweight, 1400–1800 kcal daily; a young active person 1800–3000 kcal daily. The body weight should be maintained at or slightly below the ideal for the patient's height. Thus these suggested ranges for energy intake for the various groups of patients may have to be extended after considering this. For example young overweight patients may have to have their daily intake reduced to below 1800 kcal while elderly thin patients may require more than 1800 kcal to maintain weight.

Next the proportion of energy derived from carbohydrate, protein and fat must be allocated. Table 13.22 shows the approximate ratio in the British National diet. The intake of fat is high and a large proportion of this consists of saturated fat. This type of diet is generally considered to be atherogenic and it is recommended that the percentage of calories derived from carbohydrate should be increased and that from fat reduced. Diabetic patients are peculiarly prone to develop atherosclerosis and it is therefore particularly important that the general guidelines issued to the public by nutritional organisations concerned with heart disease should be followed by diabetic patients. It is important to realise, and to explain to the individual diabetic patient, that the 'diabetic diet' is simply that which is now recommended for the population in general.

Carbohydrate and fibre
All the carbohydrate prescribed should be taken in the form of starches and other complex sugars. Rapidly absorbed simple sugars such as glucose and sucrose should generally be avoided because they result in a sudden rise in the blood glucose concentration. The intake of carbohydrate ranges from 100 g (the minimum sufficient to prevent ketonuria) to a maximum of 300 g. In the latter case each of three main meals can provide 60 g carbohydrate, each of three snacks 30 g, and 30 g comes in 0.5 l milk taken in the course of the day.

Slowing the rate of carbohydrate absorption may be usefully exploited in the treatment of diabetes. The information box (right) lists methods by which this has been achieved.

Spreading the nutrient load throughout the day as three main meals and three snacks ('nibbling' as opposed to 'gorging') not only results in lower blood lipid as well as reduced blood glucose and insulin concentrations in all diabetic patients but also in the case of those taking insulin or an oral hypoglycaemic agent safeguards against the development of hypoglycaemia. Consumption of both soluble fibre supplements (for example guar, pectin, locust bean gum) and fibre-rich foods (for example barley, oats, legumes, beans, peas, and lentils) has been associated with improved blood glucose control and lower blood lipids in both normal, diabetic and hyperlipidaemic persons. Long-term compliance is better with fibre-rich foods than with soluble fibre supplements. Classification of foods according to their acute effect on the blood glucose concentration ('Glycaemic Index') has been suggested as a useful means of determining the optimal carbohydrate foods for diabetic patients but is not in general use. This applies also to the use of enzyme inhibitors (anti-amylase, sucrase and maltase activity). Although their use has been shown to reduce postprandial glucose, insulin and triglyceride concentrations the side-effects are troublesome in some patients and the long-term effects are uncertain.

Protein
Consumption of protein is determined largely by social and economic considerations and will usually be 60–110 g daily. In patients with NIDDM consumption of protein along with carbohydrate will lower the blood glucose concentration due to amino-acid stimulation of insulin secretion which helps to compensate for the defect in glucose mediated insulin secretion seen in so many of these patients. Protein also promotes satiety and helps both types of diabetic patient to adhere to the carbohydrate allowance.

Fat
The total intake of fat should be reduced and the proportion of unsaturated fat increased if possible. Plasma lipids should be checked regularly and if significantly elevated the diet may be further modified (p. 696). The most important determinant of the fat content of the

diet is the type of food eaten but the way it is cooked is also important. Fried food is a traditional way of cooking for many people and they need to be made aware of other methods of cooking such as grilling, baking, poaching and steaming. Fish is particularly rich in long-chain polyunsaturated fatty acids.

Alcohol

In general, diabetic individuals should take the same precautions regarding alcohol intake as the general population. However account must be taken of:

1. the energy and sometimes the carbohydrate content of alcoholic drinks;
2. the fact that alcohol may potentiate the hypoglycaemic action of oral hypoglycaemic drugs and of insulin;
3. the tendency of alcohol to predispose towards the development of lactic acidosis in patients taking biguanides (p. 673);
4. the fact that alcohol can induce a disulfiram type of reaction (p. 672) in patients taking sulphonylurea drugs.

Abstinence should be encouraged if obesity, hypertension or hypertriglyceridaemia is present.

Salt

Diabetic patients should follow the advice given to the general population, namely to reduce sodium intake to no more than 6 g daily. Further restriction of sodium intake (to less than 3 g daily) is important in the management of hypertensive diabetic patients.

Diabetic foods and sweeteners

Low calorie and sugar-free drinks are useful for patients on low calorie diets. These drinks usually contain nonnutritive sweeteners. Many 'diabetic foods' contain sorbitol or fructose which may have gastrointestinal side-effects, are relatively high in energy, may be expensive and are therefore not particularly recommended as part of the diabetic diet.

Non-nutritive sweeteners: saccharin, aspartame, sucramate and acesulphame K are the most widely used non-nutritive sweeteners and provide means for reducing energy intake without loss of palatability.

Nutritive sweeteners, sorbitol and fructose are particularly useful in baking. They contain as many calories as sucrose and their total intake should not therefore exceed 50 g daily. Gastrointestinal side-effects do not usually occur at these quantities provided the intake is spread over the day.

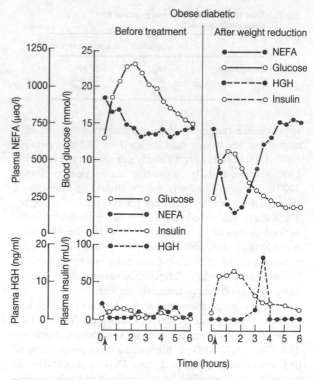

Fig. 13.35 Changes in the concentration of blood glucose and plasma non-esterified fatty acids, immunoreactive insulin, and human growth hormone following ingestion of 50 g glucose (↑) in an obese patient with NIDDM at diagnosis and after reduction in weight. Note the marked rise in plasma IRI and the restoration of the normal postabsorptive surge of HGH following treatment with a low energy diet.

Types of diabetic diets

Two basic types of diet are used in the treatment of diabetes: low energy, weight reducing diets and weight maintenance diets. The benefits of a reduction in body weight on the metabolism of the obese patient with NIDDM are striking (Fig. 13.35). Even where the initial blood glucose concentration is high and the plasma immunoreactive insulin low, additional treatment with insulin or an oral hypoglycaemic agent can often be avoided. The benefit of weight reduction on the mortality rate of obese non-diabetic persons is well known and applies even more strikingly to obese diabetics. Treatment of obese people (both diabetic and non-diabetic) with a diet low in refined and high in unrefined carbohydrate and restricted in total energy content, results in increased insulin sensitivity which is associated with a rapid fall in the blood glucose concentration in diabetic, obese patients. The precise mechanism of this effect is uncertain. Reduction in body weight increases this effect and, in the long run the plasma insulin concentration rises in many patients as shown in Figure 13.35.

Low energy, weight-reducing diet

Diabetics who are obese should be treated with a strict low calorie diet. The method of achieving reduction in weight is the same for obese diabetic patients as for those with simple obesity. The diet on page 986 will meet the needs of many. The portions in this diet can be weighed with scales but more usually are dispensed using household measures as described in this diet. It should be explained that such a strict diet is to be followed only temporarily until the standard weight is reached; thereafter the diet may be increased, and if the patient is sufficiently intelligent, advice can then be given on how to avoid monotony by using a list of exchanges for diabetic diets (p. 987). The administration of a sulphonylurea or insulin should be avoided if at all possible in these patients since both increase appetite and weight and intensify the total disability. Metformin has a place in the treatment of obese, non-insulin dependent patients who remain hyperglycaemic either after losing weight or because they fail to lose weight.

Weight maintenance diet

Dietary measures are an essential part of the treatment of diabetic patients who require treatment with a sulphonylurea drug or insulin. The purpose of the diet is to keep the intake of food constant in content and pattern of distribution from day to day. The dose of insulin or hypoglycaemic agent is then adjusted to match this. If a fixed daily intake is to be achieved and monotony avoided an exchange system is necessary. The 'exchanges' or portions employed as units are arbitrary and decided mainly on the basis of the food habits of each particular country. In most parts of the world the carbohydrate unit recommended is 10 g. In Britain the staple carbohydrate food is bread and the basic carbohydrate exchange for the purposes of calculating an individual diet is 20 g bread which contains 10 g carbohydrate along with 1.5 g protein and

Table 13.23   Basic food units used in diabetic diets

	Food	Carbohydrate (g)	Protein (g)	Fat (g)	Energy (kcal)
Carbohydrate	20 g bread	10	1.5	0.3	50
Protein	30 g meat	—	7	5	70
Fat	15 g butter	—	—	15	110
Milk	585 ml	30	18	24	400

Using Atwater calorie conversion factors of 4, 4 and 9 kcal/g for carbohydrate, protein and fat respectively to calculate the energy content.

Table 13.24   Method of constructing a diabetic weight-maintenance diet

Exchanges	Carbohydrate (g)	Energy (kcal)
21 carbohydrate	210	1050
2/3 pint milk	20	260
4 protein	—	280
2 fat	—	220
Total	230	1810

1. The diet contains approximately 1800 kcal (7560 kJ) with 230 g carbohydrate, 72 g protein, 66 g fat providing 51%, 16% and 33% of calories respectively.
2. The 23 carbohydrate and 4 protein exchanges are distributed throughout the day according to the eating habits and daily routine of the patient.

0.3 g fat. Table 13.23 shows the basic food units used in diabetic diets in the UK. Table 13.24 shows how a diabetic weight maintenance diet is constructed. When this has been done the figures must be translated into practical instructions in the form of a diet book individually prepared for each patient and which includes a comprehensive list of carbohydrate exchanges. The information box below lists examples of useful carbohydrate exchanges.

USEFUL CARBOHYDRATE EXCHANGES

Each item on this list =
1 carbohydrate exchange =
10 g carbohydrate
- $\frac{1}{2}$ slice bread from a large loaf
- 1 large digestive biscuit
- 2 cream crackers
- $\frac{2}{3}$ teacup natural unsweetened orange or grapefruit juice
- 1 medium-sized eating apple or orange

- 10 grapes
- 1 small banana
- $\frac{1}{3}$ pint (200 ml) milk
- 1 teacup cooked porridge
- 1 teacup cream or tinned soup
- $\frac{2}{3}$ teacup cornflakes
- 1 small packet crisps
- 1 small potato

Unmeasured diets

If insulin or an oral hypoglycaemic agent is not required, marked obesity is not present, or hyperglycaemia is relatively mild it may not be necessary for the patient to follow such accurate diets as described above. Sometimes, for various reasons, it may be impracticable to do so. In such cases an unmeasured diet of the type listed in the information box (p. 672) may be adequate.

ORAL HYPOGLYCAEMIC DRUGS

A number of compounds are effective in reducing hyperglycaemia in patients with NIDDM who are not

UNMEASURED DIABETIC DIET

Foods to be avoided altogether
Sucrose, glucose and foods high in sucrose/glucose

Carbohydrate foods to be eaten in moderation
Breads of all kinds, rolls, scones, biscuits, crispbreads;
breakfast cereals and porridge; potatoes, peas, baked beans;
all fresh and dried fruit; pasta, custard, thick soups; 'diabetic
foods'; milk; meat, fish, eggs, cheese

Foods which can be eaten as desired
Green vegetables; clear soups, meat extracts, tomato or lemon
juice; tea and coffee

adequately controlled by dietary measures alone and who would otherwise require treatment with insulin. These drugs fall into two categories: the sulphonylureas and the biguanides. Although their mechanism of action is different, the effect of both groups of drugs depends upon a supply of endogenous insulin and they therefore have no hypoglycaemic effect in patients with IDDM.

Sulphonylureas

Mechanism of action
The initial effect of sulphonylurea compounds in lowering the blood glucose concentration is due to stimulation of the release of insulin from the pancreatic beta cell. The long-term hypoglycaemic action however seems to be due to extra pancreatic effects, particularly in reducing the hepatic release of glucose and diminishing insulin resistance.

Sulphonylureas are valuable in the treatment of non-obese patients with NIDDM who fail to respond to dietary measures alone.

Although sulphonylureas will lower the blood glucose concentration of obese patients with NIDDM such patients should be treated energetically by individually prescribed and carefully designed dietary measures only in the first instance since treatment with sulphonylureas is associated with an increase in weight which in the long run will intensify the total disability and increase insulin resistance which commonly leads to secondary failure to respond to the drugs, so that ultimately treatment with insulin may be required. The diabetic dietary prescription often involves a major change in lifestyle and its effective implementation requires the skill of an experienced dietitian. Only if it is clear that dietary measures alone are insufficient should patients be started on an oral hypoglycaemic drug.

Table 13.25 lists the sulphonylureas in common use. The main differences between the individual compounds is in their potency, length of action and cost.

Tolbutamide is the mildest and probably also the safest of the sulphonylureas. It is very well tolerated and toxic reactions are rare. Its duration of action is relatively short so that it has to be given 2 or 3 times daily. The usual maintenance dose is 250–500 mg 2 or 3 times daily. Tolbutamide is a useful drug in the elderly where the risk and the consequences of inducing hypoglycaemia are increased.

Chlorpropamide has a biological half-life of about 36 hours and an effective concentration can be maintained in the blood by a single dose at breakfast. The usual maintenance dose is between 100 and 350 mg daily; larger doses should not be used on a long-term basis since above this level there is an increased risk of toxic effects such as cholestatic jaundice, skin rashes and blood dyscrasia. Facial flushing and other features of a disulfiram-like reaction occur in some patients after taking alcohol. Occasionally chlorpropamide can induce the syndrome of inappropriate antidiuretic hormone secretion (SIADH). Chlorpropamide may cause severe and prolonged (due to its long biological half-life) hypoglycaemia. Care must be taken to avoid

Table 13.25 Sulphonylureas – comparative features

Approved name	Daily dose range (mg)	Potency	Approximate biological half life (hours)	Special points
First generation drugs				
Acetohexamide	500–1500	Medium	5	
Chlorpropamide	100–500	Strong	36	Risk of serious hypoglycaemia particularly in the elderly Disulfiram-like reaction with alcohol Occasionally cholestatic jaundice, SIADH, exfoliative dermatitis
Tolbutamide	500–3000	Relatively weak	4	
Tolazamide	100–750	Strong	7	
Second generation drugs				
Glibenclamide	2.5–20	Strong	12	Particularly prone to induce severe hypoglycaemia, especially in the elderly
Gliclazide	40–320	Medium	10–12	
Glipizide	2.5–30	Strong	3.5	

this, particularly in elderly patients, and in this group once glycosuria has been abolished and symptoms relieved the daily dose should be reduced to a minimum. Many patients requiring 250–330 mg daily initially can be maintained on a long-term basis on 50–100 mg per day.

Second generation sulphonylureas are more expensive and usually offer little advantage over tolbutamide and chlorpropamide but may be useful in individual patients. Glibenclamide is particularly prone to induce severe hypoglycaemia in the elderly and should be avoided in those over 70 years of age.

Patients with NIDDM who fail to achieve initial control with sulphonylureas are considered 'primary treatment failures'. The incidence of primary treatment failure depends mainly on the criteria for initial selection and patient compliance with diet. With continuing follow-up 'secondary failure' affects 3–10% of patients each year. These patients are not a homogeneous group, they include some with Type I IDDM who have an absolute deficiency of insulin and others with significant circulating insulin levels who are commonly obese and have failed to lose weight while supposedly taking a low energy diet. Failure to comply with the diet is the commonest cause of secondary treatment failure.

Biguanides

The biguanides are less widely used than the sulphonylureas because of a high incidence of side-effects, particularly gastrointestinal symptoms, and because there has been a significant number of deaths from lactic acidosis in patients taking these drugs.

Mechanism of action

The mechanism of action of these compounds has not been precisely defined. They have no hypoglycaemic effect in normal people but, in the diabetic, insulin sensitivity and peripheral glucose uptake are increased. There is some evidence that they also impair glucose absorption and reduce hepatic gluconeogenesis. Although secretion of some endogenous insulin is mandatory for their hypoglycaemic action these compounds do not increase insulin secretion and hypoglycaemia does not occur in patients being treated with these drugs.

Indications for use

Some of the biguanides are associated with the development of lactic acidosis and are no longer in clinical use. However metformin is less associated with this development and may be useful in two difficult clinical situations. Firstly, its administration is not associated with a rise in body weight and it may therefore be preferred when an obese patient with NIDDM must be treated because hyperglycaemia persists despite efforts to adhere to a diet and reduce weight. Secondly, as the hypoglycaemic effect of metformin is synergistic with that of the sulphonylurea drugs there is a place for combining the two when sulphonylureas alone have proved inadequate in both primary and secondary treatment failure. Such combined therapy should be used however only when there are clear contraindications to treatment with insulin since, despite euglycaemia, the plasma concentration of intermediary metabolites (including lactate, pyruvate, alanine, glycerol and ketone bodies) is abnormal in patients treated in this way.

Metformin is given with food 2 or 3 times daily. The usual starting dose is 500 mg twice daily with a gradual increase as required to a maximum of 1 g 3 times daily. Its use is contraindicated in patients with impaired renal or hepatic function and in those who take alcohol in excess because the risk of lactic acidosis is significantly increased in such patients. Its administration should be discontinued, at least temporarily, if any other serious medical condition develops. In such circumstances treatment with insulin should be substituted.

Lactic acidosis

The increased blood lactate levels seen in patients taking biguanides seem to result from an increased flow of glucose through glycolysis combined with reduced lactate removal due, partly at least, to inhibition of gluconeogenesis. Lactic acidosis has a high mortality – at least 50% even in specialist centres. It is further discussed on page 682.

INSULIN

Two main types of insulin preparations are used clinically: unmodified, rapid onset, short acting; and modified or 'depot', delayed onset, long-acting (Table 13.26).

Unmodified insulins are clear solutions which, when injected subcutaneously, produce an effect in about 30 minutes which lasts for approximately 6 hours. Unmodified insulin is essential in new cases of diabetes with dehydration and/or ketoacidosis, in acute metabolic decompensation in established cases of diabetes (both IDDM and NIDDM) from whatever cause, in combination with depot insulins for the day-to-day management of nearly all patients with IDDM, and in any situation where intravenous insulin is required, for example in infusion pumps.

Table 13.26 Insulin preparations in common use

Type	Proprietary preparations*	Species	Approximate duration (hours)
Unmodified			
Clear solutions	Actrapid (Novo-Nordisk)	Human	
Rapid onset	Velosulin (Novo-Nordisk)	Human	
Short action		Porcine	6
	Humulin S (Lilly)	Human	
	Hypurin Neutral (CP Pharm)	Bovine	
Modified (depot)			
Cloudy solutions	Monotard (Novo-Nordisk)	Human	
Delayed onset	Insulatard (Novo-Nordisk)	Human	
Prolonged action		Porcine	12
	Humulin I (Lilly)	Human	
	Hypurin Isophane (CP Pharm)	Bovine	
	Ultratard (NOVO)	Human	
	Humulin Zn (Lilly)	Human	24
	Hypurin Protamine (CP Pharm)	Bovine	

* In Britain and the U.S.A. all these insulin preparations are available only in 100 i.u./ml strength for routine clinical use. In other parts of the world insulins are also available in 40 and 80 i.u./ml strength.
Pre-mixed insulin preparations, containing a wide range of fixed ratios of unmodified and intermediate depot, are also available.

LA

Depot insulin preparations are cloudy solutions. Their delayed and prolonged action is achieved in two main ways. In isophane preparations insulin is adsorbed on to a foreign protein, namely fish protamine, in exactly equivalent amounts, from which it is gradually released in the tissues. Although a foreign protein, protamine is virtually non immunogenic. As with all the complexed insulins isophane preparations may only be used by subcutaneous injection. Unmodified insulin mixed with isophane retains it characteristic action. Insulin zinc suspensions do not contain foreign protein. The duration of their action depends on the size and form of the insulin crystals as well as on the rate at which these crystals are dissolved and absorbed. The former is achieved by carefully controlling the conditions of precipitation; the latter is delayed by buffering with acetate and adding zinc. These insulin zinc suspensions must contain excess free zinc in solution and when mixed with unmodified insulin the zinc will blunt the onset of its action.

For many years insulin was regarded as non antigenic. It is now known that even homologous pancreatic insulin can, in some circumstances, act as a weak antigen. The factors determining the immunogenicity of therapeutic preparations of insulin are listed in the information box (right).

The older preparations of insulin were strongly antigenic because they consisted usually of bovine insulin, were commonly prepared at low pH, frequently contained added protein to delay their action, and always contained trace amounts of pro-insulin and

FACTORS DETERMINING THE IMMUNOGENICITY OF THERAPEUTIC PREPARATIONS OF INSULIN

Species
Bovine > Porcine > Human

Addition of protein
To delay and prolong action increases immunogenicity

Purity
Older preparations contain trace amounts of pro-insulin and other islet hormones which stimulate the formation of antibodies cross-reacting with insulin

pH
Acidity increases immunogenicity: new preparations neutral

other pancreatic hormones. Care must be taken to avoid hypoglycaemia when transferring patients from the older to the newer preparations.

Most patients with IDDM do best by taking unmodified insulin along with one of the intermediate depot-insulins before breakfast and repeating this combination before the evening meal. However various combinations of the numerous preparations of insulin available can be tried and the time at which they are administered altered on the basis of the results of blood glucose estimations at different times of the day until good metabolic control is achieved over 24 hours. It is impossible to forecast the response of a patient to insulin and the daily dose required to establish satisfactory control varies widely and is established by clinical trial.

Factors determining the type and amount of insulin required in an individual case include the patient's sensitivity to the action of insulin (thin subjects are generally more sensitive than the obese) and way of life, (for example meal pattern, occupation and hours of work, and the amount and timing of exercise). More insulin will be needed to cover main meals and periods of inactivity, and vice versa. Figure 13.36 shows an example of a patient poorly controlled by one insulin regime but well controlled by another. The aim is to achieve preprandial blood glucose readings within the

Table 13.27 Adjusting the dose of insulin

Blood glucose reading:	Before Breakfast ↑	Before Lunch	Before Evening ↑ Meal	At Bedtime
Gives information about:	Evening cloudy insulin	Morning clear insulin	Morning cloudy insulin	Evening clear insulin

↑ Indicates times at which insulin combination (unmodified, clear + depot cloudy) taken.

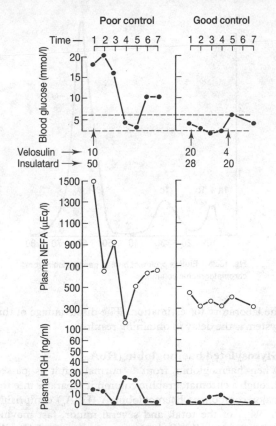

Poor control | Good control

Fig. 13.36 Blood glucose and plasma non-esterified fatty acids (1) fasting, (2) 1½ hours after breakfast, (3) and (4) before and 1½ hours after the midday meal, (5) and (6) before and 1½ hours after the evening meal, and (7) before going to bed, in a non-obese, 14-year-old girl with IDDM, undertaking normal activity in the course of the day. Diabetes had been diagnosed 11 years previously and she was following a diet of 9.2 MJ distributed in three main meals and three snacks taken at mid-morning, mid-afternoon and bedtime. Her diabetes was poorly controlled by 60 units of insulin taken in a single daily dose before breakfast. Greatly improved control was achieved by a slight increase in the total daily amount of insulin given and by administering this in two doses. The broken lines in the upper panel indicate the physiological range for the blood glucose concentration.

range 4–7 mmol/l. Each of the four insulins is adjusted individually on the basis of the appropriate blood glucose measurement (Table 13.27).

METHODS OF ASSESSING BLOOD GLUCOSE CONTROL

Urinary glucose
Preprandial tests
24-hour collection

Blood glucose
Single, random clinic measurements
Day profile:
    Inpatients
    Day patients
Capillary blood spot profiles: home-based patients
Patient home monitoring
    Test-strips (visual)
    Test-strips (meters)

Glycosylated proteins
Haemoglobin
Albumin
Total serum proteins (fructosamine)

ASSESSMENT OF METABOLIC CONTROL

The aim of treatment is to achieve as near normal metabolism as is practicable. It is clear that the nearer the body weight approaches the ideal level and the closer the blood glucose concentration is kept to normal the more normal is the body's total metabolic profile. The various methods of assessing blood glucose control are listed in the information box above.

Semi-quantitative preprandial urine testing is the time honoured method of assessing blood glucose control. However its limitations in this role have become increasingly apparent, not only in patients with IDDM (Fig. 13.37) but also in NIDDM patients where a raised renal threshold for glucose (which is very common in these patients) may mask persistent hyperglycaemia. In addition, negative urine tests also fail to distinguish between normal and low blood glucose levels which is a particular disadvantage since hypoglycaemia is a major cause of iatrogenic morbidity and mortality in both types of diabetes. Thus wherever possible all patients should be taught to perform blood glucose measurements at home using blood glucose test strips read either visually or with a reflectance meter (Table 13.28). The great advantage of self-monitoring

Table 13.28 Blood glucose testing strips and meters

Meter	BG range (mmol/l)	BM test 1–44	Dextrostix	Exactech	Glucostix	Hypoguard GA
Exactech (Baxter)	2.2–25			✓		
Glucochek 90 (Medistron)	0.6–27.8	✓			✓	✓
Hypocount (Hypoguard, UK)	2.0–22.0	✓	✓			✓
Reflolux 11 M (BCL)	0.5–27.7	✓				
Glucometer 11	1.3–22.2	✓			✓	

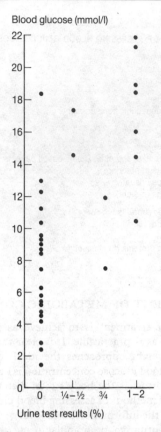

Fig. 13.37   Simultaneous urinary and blood glucose estimations performed over a two-week period in a 14-year-old girl taking twice daily injections of insulin for one year. Note that when the urinary test records 0 the blood glucose concentration ranges from 1.5–18 mmol/l even when the bladder has been emptied $\frac{1}{2}$–1 hour before passing the urine to be tested.

of capillary blood glucose concentration by patients is that information is immediately available and permits those well informed and motivated to make appropriate adjustments in insulin, oral hypoglycaemic agent and/or diet on a day-to-day basis. Thus the development of serious ketoacidosis can be avoided and a normal or near normal metabolism achieved without frequent and disabling hypoglycaemia. Single random blood glucose estimations obtained at routine clinic visits are of limited value. The main disadvantage of day profiles obtained in hospital or in day patients is that they are obtained in a highly artificial situation. The advantage of the capillary blood spot profile is that tests are performed in the real-life situation while at the same time the estimations are accurate. In this technique patients collect serial capillary blood samples by finger prick on to filter paper strips previously soaked in boric acid. When the series is complete the strips are posted to

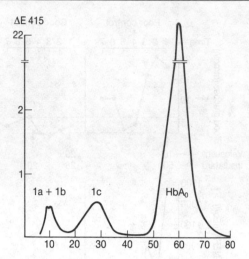

Fig. 13.38   Elution profile of human haemoglobin from chromatographic column.

the laboratory for estimation. The disadvantage of this system is the delay in obtaining results

Glycosylated haemoglobin (HbA$_1$)

When haemoglobin from a normal adult is passed through a chromatographic column it separates into the major component haemoglobin A (HbA$_0$) comprising 92–94% of the total, and several minor, fast moving components collectively known as haemoglobin A$_1$ (HbA$_1$) comprising 6–8% of the total (Fig. 13.38). The latter are structurally identical to HbA$_0$ except for the addition of a glucose group to the terminal amino acid of the B chain of the haemoglobin molecule. This is a post-synthetic, non-enzymatic reaction and the rate of synthesis of HbA$_1$ is therefore a function of the exposure to the red cell to glucose. Since the glucose linkage to haemoglobin is relatively stable, HbA$_1$ accumulates throughout the life-span of the erythrocyte and its concentration reflects the mean blood glucose concentration over the previous few months. Measurement of HbA$_1$ can therefore be used as a supplement to blood glucose estimations to monitor the overall degree of diabetic control achieved. Figure 13.39 shows the close relationship between HbA$_1$ and the mean blood glucose concentration in 40 patients with IDDM over a 3-month period. The very close correlation obtained between HbA$_1$ and mean blood glucose concentration supports the expectation that such measurements taken during a normal working day are more representative of the usual prevailing blood glucose levels than those obtained in hospital or in day patients.

Glycosylation of haemoglobin is just one example of the many glycosylation reactions which occur in the

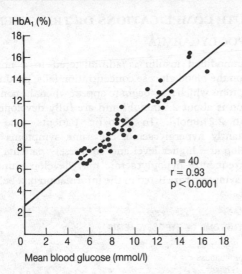

Fig. 13.39 The relationship between %HbA₁ and mean blood glucose levels in the previous three months. Each dot represents the mean blood glucose concentration for a single patient. Each patient collected capillary blood samples before and two hours after each main meal for 24 hours every two weeks for three months. Glycosylated haemoglobin is expressed here as HbA₁ (that is $HbA_{1a} + {}_{1b} + {}_{1c}$). HbA_{1c} (the largest fraction) is sometimes reported alone in which case the normal range is significantly lower than that for HbA₁.

body. Glycosylated serum proteins can also be measured and, because of their shorter half-life, give an indication of glycaemic control over the preceding few weeks rather than months.

Blood lipids

Concentration of serum lipids is another important index of overall metabolic control in diabetic patients and should be monitored regularly. Ideally the concentration of total cholesterol, triglyceride, and HDL cholesterol should be measured in blood samples obtained from patients who have fasted overnight.

GOALS OF TREATMENT

The ideal treatment for diabetes would allow the patient to lead a completely normal life, to remain not only symptom-free but in good health, to achieve a normal metabolic state, and to escape the micro and macroangiopathy associated with long-term diabetes. Nowadays diabetic patients rarely die in ketoacidosis but the major problem which has emerged is the serious morbidity and disability suffered by many of those whose duration of life has been extended by treatment. In addition, even today expectation of life is reduced by 30% in diabetic patients. The factors which have been shown to be associated with increased mortality and

> **FACTORS ASSOCIATED WITH INCREASED MORTALITY AND MORBIDITY IN DIABETIC PATIENTS**
>
> - Duration of diabetes
> - Early age at onset of disease
> - High HbA₁
> - Raised BP
> - Proteinuria
> - Obesity
> - Hyperlipidaemia

morbidity in diabetic patients are listed in the information box above.

Although the relationship between the degree of control and the development of micro and macroangiopathy is not a simple one, it appears that the vascular abnormalities are secondary to the metabolic disturbance seen in diabetes since they are found in both primary and secondary diabetes and can be produced experimentally in animals rendered diabetic by various methods. Moreover data from several clinical epidemiological studies involving thousands of patients followed for over two decades show that serious morbidity and disability due to diabetic retinopathy, nephropathy and neuropathy can be largely avoided if the mean blood glucose concentrations set out in the information box below are achieved on a long-term basis. This represents a mean overall blood glucose of approximately 9 mmol/l corresponding to an HbA₁ of 9–9.5% (Fig. 13.39). Such figures can be used as practical treatment goals in terms of blood glucose concentration.

> **CRITERIA OF 'GOOD' DIABETIC CONTROL (PIRART 1978)**
>
> Mean blood glucose concentration (mmol/l)
> Fasting   < 6.7
> 2 hour post-prandial < 11.1

INITIATING TREATMENT AND EDUCATING PATIENTS

It is essential that the diabetic patient learns to manage all aspects of their treatment as quickly as possible and this can best be done on an outpatient basis while leading a relatively normal existence at home and work. However, patients requiring insulin have to be seen daily at first and if this is not practicable, admission to hospital will be necessary. Hospital admission will also be required for patients presenting with ketoacidosis.

Every patient who is capable of learning must be taught how to perform capillary blood glucose estimations and tests of urinary ketones, to keep a record of the results and to understand their significance.

Those requiring insulin need to learn how to measure their dose of insulin accurately with an insulin syringe, to give their own injections and to adjust the dose themselves on the basis of blood glucose estimations and other factors such as illness, unusual exercise and hypoglycaemic episodes. They must be familiar with the symptoms associated with hypoglycaemia (right). They must therefore have a working knowledge of diabetes and must also have ready access to medical advice when the need arises. Such education is time consuming but only in this way can patients safely undertake normal activities while maintaining good control.

It is a wise precaution for diabetic patients who are taking insulin or an oral hypoglycaemic drug to carry a card with them at all times stating their name and address, the fact that they are diabetic, the nature and dose of any insulin or other drugs they may be taking, and giving the name, address and telephone number of their family doctor and any specialist diabetic clinic they may be attending.

Supervision

Diabetic patients should be seen at regular intervals for the remainder of their lives either at a specialist diabetic clinic or by their general practitioner if he has a particular interest and training in diabetes. A check list for follow-up visits is detailed in the information box below. The frequency of visits is very variable ranging from weekly during pregnancy to annually in the case of patients with well-controlled mild NIDDM.

CHECK LIST FOR FOLLOW-UP VISITS OF PATIENTS WITH DIABETES MELLITUS

- Body weight
- Urinalysis of fasting specimen for glucose, ketones, albumin (both macro and micro albuminuria)
- Glycaemic control
  HbA$_1$
  Inspection of home blood glucose monitoring record
- Hypoglycaemic episodes
  Number of serious (requiring assistance in treatment) and mild episodes
  Time when 'hypos' experienced
- BP (supine and erect)
- Visual acuity
  Ophthalmoscopy
- Lower limbs
  Peripheral pulses
  Tendon reflexes
  Perception of vibration sensation
  Feet: ulceration, callus skin indicating pressure areas, nails, need for chiropody

---

ACUTE COMPLICATIONS OF TREATMENT

HYPOGLYCAEMIA

If unmodified insulin is administered to a normal person the blood glucose concentration falls, producing symptoms which may begin to appear when the concentration is about 2.5 mmol/l and are fully developed at about 2.2 mmol/l. In diabetic patients who are constantly hyperglycaemic the same symptoms may develop at a higher level and conversely patients who are frequently hypoglycaemic may develop blunting. The symptoms are listed in the information box below.

SYMPTOMS OF HYPOGLYCAEMIA

- Weakness
- Emptiness
- Hunger
- Diplopia
- Blurring of vision
- Mental confusion
- Abnormal behaviour (e.g. aggression, poor co-ordination)
- Lassitude
- Somnolence } Particularly in children
- Muscular twitchings
- Vomiting
- Coma (sometimes with convulsions may follow)

Hypoglycaemia induces secretion of 'counter-regulatory' hormones namely catecholamines (which raise the blood glucose concentration by increasing glycogenolysis and are responsible for inducing some of the classical clinical features of hypoglycaemia such as pallor, palpitations, tachycardia and tremor), glucagon (which increases both hepatic glycogenolysis and gluconeogenesis), glucocorticoids, and growth hormone. This mechanism partly explains why patients rarely die of hypoglycaemia from too much unmodified insulin. In contrast, coma is likely to be more severe and dangerous when it occurs as a result of an overdose of depot-insulin or a long-acting sulphonylurea. Permanent brain damage may result from prolonged hypoglycaemia.

Hypoglycaemia due to over-dosage with unmodified insulin is liable to occur at the time when the insulin has its maximum effect. On the standard twice daily insulin regime this is likely to be in the late morning or early evening. Classical symptoms are usually elicited and response to oral glucose is generally rapid. Hypoglycaemia from excessive depot-insulin given before breakfast usually occurs in the late afternoon, while depot-insulin given before the evening meal is commonly responsible for hypoglycaemia developing through the night and in the early hours of the morning. In this case the fall in blood glucose concentration may be more gradual and elicit little catecholamine response, become persistent and profound and respond more slowly to treatment. The predominant warning symptoms, which are very variable, include headache, night sweats, nausea leading sometimes to troublesome vomiting, mental confusion and drowsiness, especially before breakfast.

The incidence of nocturnal hypoglycaemia in patients with IDDM treated conventionally with twice daily doses of insulin is difficult to establish. It is certainly common. The basic cause is the physiological diurnal variation in the amount of insulin required to achieve homeostasis (Table 13.29) which is probably related to the diurnal rhythm in secretion of counter regulatory hormones such as glucocorticoids and growth hormone which act as insulin antagonists. Thus there is a tendency for hypoglycaemia to occur between midnight and 03.00 hours and this may be combined with hyperglycaemia at 08.00 hours. This problem is compounded by the quicker, shorter action of human depot-insulins so that intermediate preparations are likely to exert their maximum action at 03.00 hours when the insulin requirement is lowest and vice versa. This problem can be dealt with effectively by splitting the evening dose of insulin, with unmodified insulin only taken before the evening meal and the evening depot-insulin taken at 23.00 hours.

Table 13.29   Nocturnal hypoglycaemia in IDDM

Incidence	Uncertain
Cause	Variation in overnight requirement for insulin: 24:00–04:00 h = 8 mIU/kg/h 04:00–08:00 h = 16 mIU/kg/h Quicker, shorter action of human depot insulins compared with older insulins with greater immunogenicity
Diagnosis	Accurate blood glucose estimations at 03:00 and 08:00 h
Treatment	Split evening dose of insulin: Take unmodified insulin only before the evening meal and depot insulin at 23:00 h

Exercise

Figure 13.40 shows that the effect of exercise in treated IDDM depends on the prevailing metabolic state. On the one hand, well-controlled patients are invariably hyperinsulinaemic so that during exercise the increased peripheral glucose uptake is not compensated for in the normal way by an increase in the hepatic release of glucose so that hypoglycaemia occurs; on the other hand poorly controlled patients are relatively hypoinsulinaemic and exercise may aggravate hyperglycaemia and ketonaemia.

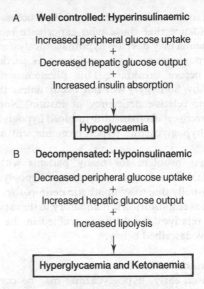

A   Well controlled: Hyperinsulinaemic

Increased peripheral glucose uptake
+
Decreased hepatic glucose output
+
Increased insulin absorption
↓
| Hypoglycaemia |

B   Decompensated: Hypoinsulinaemic

Decreased peripheral glucose uptake
+
Increased hepatic glucose output
+
Increased lipolysis
↓
| Hyperglycaemia and Ketonaemia |

Fig. 13.40   The effect of exercise in diabetic patients being treated with insulin. A. Well controlled: Hyperinsulinaemic patients. **B.** Decompensated: Hypoinsulinaemic patients.

Cause and prevention

The most common causes of hypoglycaemia in patients taking insulin or a sulphonylurea drug are unpunctual meals and unaccustomed exercise. Both are avoidable. The preceding dose of insulin should be reduced appropriately if unusual activity is anticipated, and extra carbohydrate may also be required. Diabetic patients should experience hypoglycaemia under supervision so that they can learn to recognise the early symptoms. They should also carry some tablets of glucose for use in an emergency.

Patients with long-standing IDDM may have particular problems associated with insulin-induced hypoglycaemia (Table 13.30). In many such patients the increased secretion of counter-regulatory hormones which corrects insulin induced hypoglycaemia in normal people is defective. In particular, sympathetic neuropathy (p. 687) may result in the loss of both glucagon and catecholamine responses to hypo-

Table 13.30   Particular problems associated with insulin-induced hypoglycaemia

Impaired recovery from insulin-induced hypoglycaemia due to:
1 glucagon response   ↓
2 catecholamine response   ↓
3 plasma free insulin   ↑
Post-hypoglycaemic hyperglycaemia due to:
1 sympatho-adrenal activation
    +
2 insulin deficiency
Loss of symptoms of hypoglycaemia

glycaemia so that glucose recovery fails to occur. There is also evidence that those who experience recurrent hypoglycaemia may develop hypothalamic dysfunction.

Post-hypoglycaemic hyperglycaemia is particularly common before breakfast. This phenomenon (first described by Somogyi) will not occur unless there is absolute or relative deficiency of insulin. Note that impaired recovery from insulin-induced hypoglycaemia and post-hypoglycaemic hyperglycaemia will not co-exist.

A further problem for many patients with long standing IDDM is loss of symptoms of hypoglycaemia which is usually due to sympathetic neuropathy. Home blood glucose monitoring is mandatory in these patients and their relatives should be instructed in the use of glucagon as described below.

Management

If recognised early, hypoglycaemia may be corrected easily by ingestion of carbohydrate, preferably in an easily absorbable form.

If patients are so stuporose that they cannot swallow, a subcutaneous or intramuscular injection of 1 mg glucagon may be given, repeated if necessary after 10 minutes. The hyperglycaemic effect is due to stimulation of hepatic glycogenolysis and is transitory so that carbohydrate must be ingested as soon as the patient recovers consciousness. Glucagon may not be effective in severe and prolonged hypoglycaemia due to depot-insulins and in this case intravenous glucose (40–50 ml, 50% dextrose) may be required. Note that in addition to increasing hepatic glycogenolysis, glucagon stimulates the secretion of insulin and therefore should not be used to treat hypoglycaemia induced by an oral hypoglycaemic drug.

As soon as the patient is able to swallow glucose should be given orally. Full recovery may not occur immediately. Further, when hypoglycaemia has occurred in a diabetic using a depot-insulin or a sulphonylurea, particularly chlorpropamide, the possibility of relapse within a day or more should be anticipated.

Repeated episodes of hypoglycaemia may lead to permanent intellectual deterioration. Unless the reason for a hypoglycaemic episode is clear and will not recur the patient should reduce the next and subsequent dose of insulin by 20% and seek medical advice about further adjustments in dose.

DIABETIC KETOACIDOSIS

Prior to the discovery of insulin more than 50% of diabetic patients died in ketoacidosis. Today this complication should account for less than 2% of deaths among diabetics. However both the incidence and the mortality rate are still regrettably high. Failure of the patient to understand the disease and to appreciate the significance of symptoms of poor control are the most common causes. Its prevention is largely a matter of education of both patients and doctors. A significant number of new patients still present in diabetic keto-acidosis and in established diabetics a common course of events is that patients develop an intercurrent infection, lose their appetite, and either stop or drastically reduce their dose of insulin (on either their own initiative or their doctor's advice) in the mistaken belief that under these circumstances less insulin is required. Any form of stress particularly that produced by infection, may precipitate severe ketoacidosis in even the mildest case of diabetes.

A clear understanding of the biochemical basis and pathophysiology of this problem (p. 663) is essential for its efficient treatment. Hyperglycaemia and ketoacidosis are not always necessarily closely correlated. Even moderate hyperglcaemia may be associated with life threatening acidosis, particularly in young patients with IDDM, while coma can occur, usually in elderly patients, with extreme hyperglycaemia and dehydration but no ketoacidosis. This metabolic state is known as *hyperosmolar diabetic coma*.

Table 13.31   Average loss of fluid and electrolytes in an adult with diabetic ketoacidosis of moderate severity

Water:	6 litres
Sodium:	500 mmol
Chloride:	400 mmol
Potassium:	350+ mmol

Table 13.31 shows the average loss of fluid and electrolytes in moderately severe diabetic ketoacidosis in an adult. About half the deficit of total body water is derived from the intracellular compartment and occurs comparatively early in the development of acidosis with relatively few clinical features; the remainder represents loss of extracellular fluid sustained largely in the latter stages. It is at this time that marked contraction of the size of the extracellular space occurs, with haemo-concentration, a decreased blood volume, and finally a fall in blood pressure with associated renal ischaemia and oliguria.

Every patient in diabetic ketoacidosis is potassium depleted, but the plasma concentration of potassium and sodium give very little indication of the total body deficit. They may even be raised initially due to disproportionate loss of water and catabolism of protein and glycogen. However soon after treatment with

Table 13.32 . Differences in coma due to hypoglycaemia and ketoacidosis in IDDM

	Hypoglycaemic coma	Coma with ketosis
History	No food; too much insulin; unaccustomed exercise	Too little or no insulin; an infection; digestive disturbance
Onset	In good previous health; related to last insulin injection	Ill-health for several days
Symptoms	Hypoglycaemia; occasional vomiting from depot insulins	Of glycosuria and dehydration; abdominal pain and vomiting
Signs	Moist skin and tongue	Dry skin and tongue
	Full pulse	Weak pulse
	Normal or raised BP	Low blood pressure
	Shallow or normal breathing	Air hunger
	Brisk reflexes	Diminished reflexes
Urine	No ketonuria	Ketonuria
	No glycosuria, if bladder recently emptied	Glycosuria
Blood	Hypoglycaemia	Hyperglycaemia
	Normal plasma bicarbonate	Reduced plasma bicarbonate

insulin is started there is likely to be a precipitous fall in the plasma potassium due to dilution of extracellular potassium by administration of intravenous fluids, the movement of potassium into cells as a result of treatment with insulin, and the continuing renal loss of potassium.

The severity of ketoacidosis can be assessed rapidly by measuring the plasma bicarbonate: less than 12 mmol/l indicates severe acidosis. The hydrogen ion concentration in the blood gives an even more precise measure but may not be so readily available. There is no simple and accurate quantitative method for determination of ketones in plasma although a test strip (ketostix) can be used as a semi-quantitative guide to the plasma concentration of acetoacetate and acetone.

Clinical features

The clinical features of coma due to ketoacidosis are listed in Table 13.32 where they are compared with those of hypoglycaemia. It should be remembered however that the state of consciousness is very variable in patients with diabetic ketoacidosis and a patient with dangerous ketoacidosis requiring urgent treatment may walk into the consulting room. For this reason the term diabetic ketoacidosis is to be preferred to 'diabetic coma' which suggests that there is no urgency until unconsciousness occurs. In fact it is imperative that energetic treatment is started at the earliest possible stage.

Management

Diabetic ketoacidosis is a medical emergency which should be treated in hospital. Intravenous fluid replacement is required since even when the patient is able to swallow fluids given by mouth may be poorly absorbed. Treatment must be checked against the plasma concentration of glucose, potassium and bicarbonate estimated at intervals of 1–2 hours initially. The components of treatment are:

1. the administration of unmodified insulin by intramuscular or intravenous injection
2. fluid replacement
3. potassium replacement
4. the administration of antibiotics if infection is present.

Note that although leucocytosis is invariably seen this represents a stress response and does not necessarily indicate infection, also that pyrexia may not be present initially because of vasodilatation secondary to acidosis. Guidelines for the management of ketoacidosis are shown in Table 13.33.

Insulin

A loading dose of 10–20 units unmodified insulin is given by intramuscular injection immediately followed by 4–6 units hourly thereafter either by intramuscular injection or intravenous infusion, preferably using a constant rate pump. The blood glucose concentration should fall by 3–6 mmol/l per hour. If there is no fall in the blood glucose concentration by 2 hours after treatment, then the dose of insulin should be doubled until a satisfactory response is obtained. Ketosis, dehydration, acidaemia, and stress combine to produce severe insulin resistance in some cases but most will respond to a low dose insulin regime. When the blood glucose concentration has fallen to 10.0 mmol/l the dose of insulin should be reduced to 1–4 units hourly.

Fluid replacement

The deficit of extracellular fluid should be made good by infusing isotonic saline (0.9% NaCl). Early rapid rehydration is essential otherwise the administered insulin will not reach the poorly perfused tissues. In cases which are severely acidotic (pH < 7.0), 500 ml of isotonic sodium bicarbonate (1.4%) may be given in place of the same volume of isotonic saline. Correction of the total bicarbonate deficit should not be attempted

Table 13.33 Management of diabetic ketoacidosis*.

Time (hours)	Insulin units (U) (unmodified preparation)		IV fluid	IV potassium (rate of infusion: mmol/hour)
	Intramuscular	Intravenous (rate of infusion: units/hour)		
0	10–20 U		Isotonic (0.9%) saline 1.0 litre in 30 minutes	Check urinary output Obtain results for plasma electrolytes
	6 U	6 U/hour	0.5 litre in 30 minutes	If plasma concentration (mmol/l) is:
				>6 6–4.5 4.5–3 <3
				↓ ↓ ↓ ↓
	If plasma Na$^+$ > 155 mmol/l give 0.45% saline		Give mmol K$^+$/hour	0 13 26 39
1	6 U	6 U/hour	0.5 litre in 30 minutes	
			0.5 litre/hour	Monitor plasma concentration every 1–2 hours and change infusion rate accordingly
2	6 U	6 U/hour	0.5 litre/hour	
	If fall in blood glucose <3 mmol/l/h switch to IV	If fall in blood glucose <3 mmol/l/h double rate		
3	6 U every hour, continue until blood glucose concentration 1–4 U hourly	6 U/hour <10 mmol/l, then give 1–4 U/hour	0.25 litre/hour 5% glucose: 0.25 litre/hour	

NB: Average fluid deficit = 6 litres ⟨ 3.0 litres from Extra-cellular compartment replaced by NaCl
3.0 litres from Intra-cellular compartment replaced by glucose

Procedures:
Intravenous line; catheterise after 3 hours if no urine passed; nasogastric tube to keep stomach empty. Central venous pressure line if cardiovascular system compromised so that volume of IV fluid can be adjusted.
Monitor:
Blood glucose and electrolytes hourly for 3 hours and then 2–4 hourly; temperature, pulse, respiration, BP hourly; urinary output; urinary ketones; ECG, blood osmolality, arterial pH, in some cases.
* These guidelines for a typical, 'average' case should be modified appropriately in the individual patient after considering the blood biochemistry and clinical features.

however since there is some evidence that rapid correction of acidosis may aggravate tissue hypoxia and also reduce the level of consciousness by causing a paradoxical acidosis of the cerebrospinal fluid (CSF). The combined administration of bicarbonate and insulin will also increase the risk of hypokalaemia and potassium should be given along with bicarbonate.

The intracellular deficit of water must be replaced by using 5 or 10% dextrose and not by more saline. It is best given when the blood glucose concentration approaches normal.

Potassium

As the plasma potassium is often high at presentation treatment with intravenous potassium chloride should be started cautiously (Table 13.33) and carefully monitored by frequent estimations. Sufficient should be given to maintain a normal plasma concentration and large amounts may be required (10–300 mmol in the first 24 hours).

Antibiotics

Infections must be carefully sought and vigorously treated since it may not be possible to abolish ketosis until they are controlled.

Non-ketotic hyperosmolar diabetic coma

The aetiology of this condition is discussed on page 665. Its treatment differs from that of ketoacidosis in two main respects. Firstly, these patients are usually relatively sensitive to insulin and approximately half the dose of insulin recommended for the treatment of keto-acidosis should usually be employed at least initially. Secondly, the plasma osmolality should be measured or, less accurately, calculated (using the formula 2 × plasma sodium + 2 × plasma potassium + plasma glucose + plasma urea mmol/l = 280–300 mOsm/l normally) and if it is high (> 360 mOsm/l) 0.45% saline should be given until the osmolality approaches normal, when 0.9% should be substituted. The rate of fluid replacement should be regulated on the basis of the central venous pressure, and plasma sodium concentration checked frequently. Too rapid a fall in osmolality may be associated with the development of cerebral oedema.

Lactic acidosis

In coma due to lactic acidosis the patient is likely to be a diabetic taking a biguanide who is very ill and over-breathing but not so profoundly dehydrated as is usual in coma due to ketoacidosis, whose breath does not smell of acetone, with mild or even absent ketonuria yet whose plasma bicarbonate and pH are markedly reduced (pH < 7.2). The diagnosis is confirmed by a high (usually > 5.0 mmol/l) concentration of lactic acid in the blood. Treatment is with intravenous bicarbonate sufficient to raise the plasma pH to above 7.2 along with insulin and glucose. Despite energetic treatment the mortality in this condition is > 50%.

Acute circulatory failure

Acute circulatory failure occurring in any of these types of acute metabolic decompensation should be treated as described on page 681.

LONG-TERM RESULTS OF MANAGEMENT

The long-term results of treatment of diabetes are disappointing in many patients. Table 13.34 shows that

Table 13.34   Mortality ratios for diabetics and matched controls

		Significance of increased ratio seen in diabetics
Overall	2.6	P < 0.001
Coronary heart disease		
Cerebrovascular disease	2.8	P < 0.001
Peripheral vascular disease		
All other causes including renal failure	2.7	P < 0.05

treated diabetic patients incur an overall mortality $2\frac{1}{2}$ times greater than that for a comparable non-diabetic population. Large blood-vessel disease accounts for about 70% of all deaths (Table 13.35). Atherosclerosis occurs commonly and extensively in diabetic patients with pathological changes similar to those seen in non-diabetics but occurring earlier and being more widespread.

Disease of small blood vessels is specific to diabetes and is termed *diabetic microangiopathy*. It contributes to the mortality, particularly that incurred by younger people, by causing renal failure due to *diabetic nephropathy*.

Diabetic patients also incur substantial morbidity and disability due to both types of vascular disease. Diabetic retinopathy can cause severely impaired vision

Table 13.35   Approximate figures for causes of deaths in treated diabetic patients

Atherosclerosis	70%
Renal failure	10%
Cancer	10%
Infections	6%
Diabetic ketoacidosis	1%
Other	3%

and blindness (it is now the commonest cause of blindness in the 35–65 age group in most developed countries); diabetic neuropathy can cause difficulty in walking, chronic ulceration of the feet, and bowel and bladder dysfunction; while atherosclerosis results in angina, cardiac failure, intermittent claudication and gangrene.

AETIOLOGY OF THE LONG-TERM COMPLICATIONS OF DIABETES

The development of vascular disease in both large and small blood vessels of treated diabetic patients appears to be secondary to metabolic abnormalities present in these patients since it occurs in cases of both primary and secondary diabetes being treated in various ways and can be produced experimentally in animals rendered diabetic by various methods. Moreover data from numerous clinical studies published within the last ten years show that the incidence of the clinical syndromes arising from the vascular disease is mainly related to duration of diabetes and the degree of metabolic control (indicated by the mean blood glucose concentration) achieved. Although it is unlikely that hyperglycaemia per se is the only, or even the main factor involved in the aetiology of diabetic complications and numerous functional abnormalities have been identified in diabetic patients being treated conventionally, it is clear that the more normal the blood glucose concentration the fewer and less severe the functional abnormalities seen (Table 13.36).

The hallmark of diabetic microangiopathy at the

Table 13.36   Functional abnormalities with a possible pathogenic role in diabetic vascular and neuropathic disease

Microangiopathy and neuropathy
Protein glycosylation ↑
Capillary basement membrane ↑
Sorbitol synthesis ↑
Myo-inositol metabolism ↓

Capillary permeability ↑
Blood flow ↑

Red cell deformability ↓
Red cell aggregation ↑
Blood viscosity ↑
Platelet aggregation and adhesiveness ↑
Fibrinolysis ↓

Hypertension

Macroangiopathy
Hyperlipidaemia
Hyperinsulinaemia
Hypertension
Arterial endothelial permeability ↑

ultrastructural level is thickening of the capillary basement membrane with associated increased vascular permeability throughout the body. A considerable body of evidence indicates that increased metabolism of glucose to sorbitol is of central importance in the pathogenesis of diabetic microangiopathy, neuropathy and macroangiopathy. Haemodynamic, vascular permeability and structural changes in capillaries are prevented in diabetic animals by a variety of structurally different aldose reductase inhibitors. The development of the characteristic clinical syndromes of diabetic retinopathy, nephropathy, neuropathy, and atherosclerosis are thought to result from the imposition of organ and tissue specific factors (anatomical, haemodynamic and metabolic) on generalised vascular injury. Thus increased permeability of arterial endothelium, particularly when combined with hyperinsulinaemia (stimulating the uptake of lipid in large arteries) and hypertension, would increase the deposition of atherogenic lipoproteins into the vessel wall.

Reversibility of diabetic complications

The possibility of reversing early vascular disease by improved metabolic control has been examined in three prospective, randomised, controlled clinical trials involving patients with background retinopathy and minimal proteinuria. None of these independently conducted studies produced any evidence of reversal of either retinopathy or nephropathy, and indeed retinopathy worsened abruptly in some cases when control was improved. Thus the 'point of no return' seems to be past by the time retinopathy and nephropathy are clinically detectable. This has had two effects. Firstly, it has stimulated a search for markers of early, reversible, retinal, renal, and neural dysfunction. Micro-albuminuria is now validated as a marker for the subsequent development not only of diabetic nephropathy but also of hypertension and ultimately of lethal large blood vessel disease. Secondly, the whole emphasis in the management of diabetes has shifted to primary prevention of complications.

It must be stressed that there is nothing mild about NIDDM in relation to the development of severe complications. These will develop with increasing frequency as the mean overall blood glucose concentration rises independently of the type of diabetes.

DIABETIC RETINOPATHY

Diabetic retinopathy is the most common cause of blindness in adults between 30 and 65 years of age in developed countries. This fact is all the more depressing when one realises that although the precise mechanism underlying the development of diabetic retinopathy is still not clear, retinal photocoagulation is an effective treatment provided it is given at an early stage when the patient is usually symptomless. This means that regular ophthalmoscopy, with the pupils fully dilated, is mandatory in all diabetic patients.

Clinical features

The clinical features characteristic of diabetic retinopathy are listed in the information box below. These occur in varying combinations in different patients. Abnormalities of the capillary bed, which are not clinically visible are the earliest lesions. They include capillary dilatation and closure.

THE CLINICAL FEATURES CHARACTERISTIC OF DIABETIC RETINOPATHY

- Microaneurysms
- Retinal haemorrhages
- Hard exudates
- Soft exudates
- Venous changes
- Neovascularisation
- Preretinal haemorrhage
- Vitreous haemorrhage
- Fibrous proliferation

Microaneurysms. In most cases these are the earliest clinical abnormality detected. They appear as minute, discrete, circular, dark red spots near to but apparently separate from the retinal vessels. They look like tiny haemorrhages but photographs of injected preparations of retina shows that they are in fact minute aneurysms arising mainly from the venous end of capillaries near areas of capillary closure.

Haemorrhages. These most characteristically occur in the deeper layers of the retina and hence are round and regular in shape and described as 'blot' haemorrhages. The smaller ones may be difficult to differentiate from microaneurysms and the two are often grouped together as 'dots and blots'. Superficial flame shaped haemorrhages may also occur, particularly if the patient is hypertensive

Hard exudates. These are characteristic of diabetic retinopathy. They vary in size from tiny specks to large confluent patches and tend to occur particularly in the perimacular area. They result from leakage of plasma from abnormal retinal capillaries and overlie areas of neuronal degeneration.

Soft exudates. Sometimes referred to as 'cotton wool spots' these are similar to those seen in hypertension, and also occur, particularly within five disc diameters of the optic disc. They represent arteriolar occlusions and are most often seen in rapidly advancing retinopathy or in association with uncontrolled hypertension.

Neovascularisation. This may arise from mature vessels on the optic disc or the retina. The earliest appearance is that of fine tufts of delicate vessels forming arcades on the surface of the retina. As they grow they may extend forwards towards the vitreous. They are fragile and leaky and are liable to rupture causing haemorrhage which may be intra-retinal, pre-retinal ('sub-hyaloid') or into the vitreous. Serous products leaking from these new vessel systems stimulate a connective tissue reaction, *retinitis proliferans*. This first appears as a white, cloudy haze among the network of new vessels. As it extends, the new vessels may be obliterated and the surrounding retina covered by a dense white sheet. At this stage bleeding is less common but retinal detachment can occur due to contraction of adhesions between the vitreous and the retina.

Venous changes. These include venous dilatation, 'beading' (that is sausage-like changes in calibre) and increased tortuosity including 'oxbow lakes' or loops. These changes often indicate widespread capillary non-perfusion.

CLASSIFICATION OF DIABETIC RETINOPATHY BASED ON PROGNOSIS FOR VISION

Background retinopathy without maculopathy[1]: observe carefully
Peripheral
   Microaneurysms
   Small blot retinal haemorrhages
   Small hard exudates

Pre-malignant retinopathy: refer for specialist opinion
Macular oedema with reduced visual acuity
Perimacular exudates ± retinal haemorrhages
Multiple soft exudates
Sheets/clusters/large retinal haemorrhages
Venous loops and beading

Malignant retinopathy: urgent treatment mandatory[2]
Exudative maculopathy
Pre-retinal haemorrhage
Neovascularisation
Fibrous proliferation

[1]Good five-year prognosis.
[2]If untreated 50% are blind within five years.

Classification

A classification of diabetic retinopathy based on prognosis for vision is shown in the information box (left).

Microaneurysms, abnormalities of the veins, and small blot haemorrhages and hard exudates situated in the periphery will not interfere with vision unless they are associated with macular oedema in the perimacular or macular area. This is not easy to detect by ophthalmoscopy but should be suspected particularly if there is marked impairment of visual acuity in association with mild peripheral background retinopathy and no other obvious pathology.

New vessels may be *completely symptomless* until sudden visual loss occurs from a haemorrhage into the vitreous. Although these frequently clear, the risk of recurrence is high and the more frequent the haemorrhage the slower and less complete the recovery. Fibrous tissue may seriously interfere with vision by obscuring the retina and/or causing retinal haemorrhage or detachment.

Prevention and management

Since there is mounting evidence that good metabolic control, particularly in the early years following the development of diabetes, reduces the chance of developing retinopathy every effort should be made to achieve a metabolic state as near normal as is practicable in all diabetic patients from the time of presentation. As previously mentioned it is a common error to suppose that NIDDM is a 'mild' condition carrying little risk of complications. This is not so. Whatever the type of diabetes duration of the disorder and sustained hyperglycaemia are the main factors associated with the development of retinopathy. Early diagnosis followed by effective treatment is particularly important for those with NIDDM 15–20% of whom present with the complications already established. In some cases retinopathy is untreatable at diagnosis of diabetes while in others untreatable retinopathy is diagnosed only when the patient is referred for a specialist opinion after years of ineffective treatment of NIDDM.

No specific treatment is required for simple background retinopathy. Control should be assessed by reviewing the HbA_1 result, control of diabetes and hypertension should be maximised and patients should be urged to stop smoking and limit their intake of alcohol. Rapid lowering of the blood sugar may result in abrupt worsening of the retinopathy in some cases with the appearance of soft exudates and an increased number of retinal haemorrhages. Such patients may require laser treatment and should be referred for a specialist opinion. Despite this initial deterioration (which is thought to be due to a reduction in retinal blood flow) long-term follow-up studies show that the rate of progression of retinopathy is significantly less in these intensively treated patients than in matched control subjects. All patients with background retinopathy should have their eyes examined at least annually and more frequently if risk factors are present. These include early onset of diabetes, long duration of diabetes, hypertension, poor glycaemic control, pregnancy, use of the oral contraceptive pill, heavy smoking, abuse of alcohol, and evidence of microangiopathy elsewhere particularly patients with neuropathy and persistent proteinuria.

Pre-malignant and malignant retinopathy can be treated with retinal photocoagulation. Photocoagulation is used:

1. to destroy areas of retinal ischaemia (since it is thought that this plays a major role in the development of neovascularisation)
2. to seal leaking microaneurysms and exudates
3. to obliterate new vessels directly.

Two types of photocoagulation are available: xenon-arc (white light) and laser beam (monochromatic blue/green light). The latter is less uncomfortable for the patient and the smaller size of beam allows greater accuracy in delivering shots. This procedure can be done under local anaesthesia and in skilled hands is a simple procedure which carries little risk and can be very effective. New vessels can be eliminated and vision maintained in up to 90% of patients with new vessels on the retina and/or disc. Successfully treated patients must be reviewed regularly to check for further development of new vessels.

Vitrectomy may be used in selected cases with advanced diabetic eye disease causing permanent visual loss due to vitreous haemorrahge or retinal detachment resulting from retinitis proliferans. The more severe types of retinopathy may be accompanied by the development of new vessels on the anterior surface of the iris: 'rubeosis iridis'. These vessels may obstruct the anterior angle of the eye and the outflow of aqueous fluid causing glaucoma. Various techniques for the treatment of rubeosis are now available but the main method of management is the prevention of extension of the rubeosis by early retinal photocoagulation.

Cataract

Very rarely a type of cataract specific to diabetes occurs in young patients with poorly controlled diabetes. Senile cataract also occurs commonly in elderly diabetics but is probably no more common than in non-diabetic people in this age group. The indications for cataract extraction are similar to the general population and depend on the degree of visual impairment caused by the cataract. An additional indication in the diabetic is when adequate assessment of the fundus is precluded or laser treatment to the retina is prevented. The extracapsular method of extraction is preferable in diabetics and there is no contraindication to an intraocular lens.

DIABETIC NEUROPATHY

This is a relatively early and common complication in diabetic patients. Although it can cause severe disability in a few, it is symptomless in the majority. Like retinopathy it occurs secondary to the metabolic disturbance and the prevalence is related to the duration of diabetes and the degree of metabolic control. Although there is evidence that the central nervous system is affected in long-term diabetes the clinical impact of diabetes is mainly on the peripheral nervous system. The main pathological features are listed in information box below.

DIABETIC NEUROPATHY: HISTOPATHOLOGY

- Axonal degeneration of both myelinated and unmyelinated fibres
  Early: axon shrinkage
  Late: axonal fragmentation; regeneration
- Thickening of Schwann cell basal lamina
- Patchy, segmental demyelination
- Abnormalities of intraneural capillaries; thickening of basement membrane and microthrombi

---

They can occur in motor, sensory and autonomic nerves. Various classifications of diabetic neuropathy have been proposed. One is shown in the information box (p. 687). None of the proposed classifications is entirely satisfactory since motor, sensory and autonomic nerves may be involved in varying combinations so that clinically mixed syndromes usually occur.

Clinical features

Symmetrical sensory polyneuropathy

This is frequently asymptomatic. The most common signs found on physical examination are loss of tendon reflexes in the lower limbs, diminished perception of vibration sensation distally, and 'glove-and-stocking' impairment of all other modalities of sensation. Symptoms include paraesthesiae in the feet and sometimes in the hands, pain in the lower limbs (dull, aching and/or lancinating, worse at night, and mainly felt on the anterior aspect of the legs), burning sensations in the soles of the feet, cutaneous hyper-

CLASSIFICATION OF DIABETIC NEUROPATHY

Somatic
Polyneuropathy
 Symmetrical, mainly sensory and distal
 Asymmetrical, mainly motor and proximal
Mononeuropathy (including mononeuropathy multiplex)

Visceral (autonomic)
Cardiovascular
Gastrointestinal
Genitourinary
Sudomotor
Vasomotor
Pupillary
Loss of awareness of hypoglycaemia

aesthesia and an abnormal gait (commonly wide-based) often associated with a sense of numbness in the feet. There may be perforating, relatively or completely painless, ulcers on the feet and painless distal arthropathy characterised by disorganisation of the joint (Charcot joints). There may also be some motor involvement causing muscle weakness and wasting. The toes may be 'clawed up' due to wasting of the interosseous muscles which results in increased pressure on the plantar aspects of the metatarsal heads with the development of callous skin at these sites. Callous skin may also develop at other pressure points. On investigation both motor and sensory conduction velocity is reduced and CSF protein may be raised.

Asymmetrical motor diabetic neuropathy
Sometimes called diabetic amyotrophy. This presents as severe and progressive weakness and wasting of the proximal muscles of the lower (and occasionally also the upper) limbs and is commonly accompanied by severe pain mainly felt on the anterior aspect of the leg. Sometimes there may also be marked loss of weight ('neuropathic cachexia'). Hyperaesthesia and paraesthesiae are also common. The patient may look extremely ill and may be unable to get out of bed. Tendon reflexes may be absent on the affected side(s). Sometimes there are extensor plantar responses and again the CSF protein is commonly raised. This condition is now known to involve the lower motor neurones of the lumbosacral plexus. Other lesions involving this plexus such as lower abdominal neoplasms and lumbar disc disease must be excluded.

Mononeuropathy
Either motor or sensory function can be affected within a single peripheral or cranial nerve. The nerves most commonly affected are the third and sixth cranial nerves resulting in diplopia due to impaired ocular movement; the ulnar and median nerves leading to the clinical picture of carpal tunnel compression syndrome; and the femoral, sciatic and lateral popliteal nerves leading to foot drop. Rarely involvement of other single nerves results in bizarre paresis and paraesthesiae in the thorax and trunk.

Autonomic neuropathy
This is not necessarily associated with peripheral somatic neuropathy. Either parasympathetic or sympathetic nerves may be predominantly affected in any one or more system(s). Although autonomic neuropathy can affect virtually all bodily systems in any one patient system involvement is patchy. The information box below lists the symptoms and signs arising from autonomic neuropathy affecting the various systems. The development of autonomic neuropathy is less clearly

FEATURES, SYMPTOMS, AND SIGNS OF AUTONOMIC NEUROPATHY

Cardiovascular
Postural hypotension
Resting tachycardia
Fixed heart rate
Sudden cardiorespiratory arrest

Gastrointestinal
Dysphagia, due to oesophageal atony
Abdominal fullness, nausea and vomiting, unstable diabetes, due to delayed gastric emptying ('gastroparesis')
Nocturnal diarrhoea ± faecal incontinence
Constipation, due to colonic atony

Genitourinary
Difficulty in micturition urinary incontinence, recurrent infection, due to atonic bladder
Impotence and retrograde ejaculation

Sudomotor
Gustatory sweating
Nocturnal sweats without hypoglycaemia
Anhidrosis-fissures in the feet

Vasomotor
Feet feel constantly cold, due to loss of skin vasomotor responses
Dependent oedema, due to loss of vasomotor tone and increased vascular permeability
Bullous formation

Pupillary
Decreased pupil size
Resistance to mydriatics
Delayed or absent response to light

Loss of awareness of hypoglycaemia
Due to parasympathetic/sympathetic denervation and hypothalamic dysfunction – impaired responses of counter-regulatory hormone responses

related to poor metabolic control than somatic neuro-pathy, and improved control rarely results in amelioration of symptoms. Five years after developing symptoms of autonomic neuropathy 50% of patients are dead – many from sudden cardiorespiratory arrest, the cause of which is unknown.

Management

Symptomatic relief and a degree of functional improvement can often be achieved in somatic neuropathy by maintaining a near normal blood glucose concentration ($HbA_1 < 9\%$) on a long-term basis. However rapid improvement of glycaemic control in patients with symptomless somatic neuropathy may sometimes precipitate the development of severe symptomatic neuropathy in the short-term. Continuing treatment of these cases also gives good results in the long-term. This is true for proximal motor neuropathy as well as for the more common mainly sensory distal type. Intensive insulin treatment may be required not only to achieve an adequate degree of control but also to improve the general nutritional state. With intensive insulin treatment the prognosis is good for most patients with diabetic amyotrophy who recover over a period of months, up to two years.

The pain of diabetic neuropathy can be extremely distressing and unremitting particularly since it is commonly worse through the night, preventing sleep. It does not respond well to conventional analgesics but the tricyclic antidepressants amitriptyline or imipramine are often rapidly effective long before their anti-depressant effect is apparent. Side-effects include a dry mouth and postural hypotension which may be particu-larly important if the patient also has autonomic neuropathy with associated postural hypotension.

Aldose reductase inhibitors are now available. These have been shown to reverse or prevent most of the acute changes seen in animal models of diabetic neuropathy but their place in the treatment of patients with neuropathy is still being assessed.

Postural hypotension may be improved by support stockings and fludrocortisone. When the latter is used patients require careful monitoring in relation to the possible development of hypertension or oedema.

The dopamine antagonists metoclopramide and domperidone are used in the treatment of gastroparesis but have several disadvantages including the fact that they tend to lose their effectiveness as time goes on, sometimes produce extra-pyramidal reactions and may worsen impotence. Cisapride is a new pro-kinetic agent chemically related to metoclopramide which facilitates or restores motility throughout the gastrointestinal tract. It is thought to act mainly by indirectly enhancing

acetyl choline release from the neurones of the myenteric plexus thereby increasing motor activity in gastrointestinal smooth muscle.

Diabetic diarrhoea is difficult to treat but a few patients respond to tetracycline.

Problems arising from a neurogenic bladder are also difficult to treat effectively. In a few cases stimulation of the detrusor muscle by a sympathomimetic drug such as carbachol or bladder-neck resection are effective but many end up with an in-dwelling catheter.

Again there is no really satisfactory treatment for diabetic impotence which affects at least 25% of diabetic males. A variety of penile prostheses have been used; one of the simplest consists of a semi-rigid silicone rod implanted into the corpus cavernosa. Alter-natively the patient may be taught how to inject the corpus cavernosa with papaverine before intercourse. However priapism may be a troublesome side-effect which occasionally requires surgical decompression. It should be remembered that several antihypertensive drugs including betablockers and methyldopa can affect sexual functional and that although neuropathy is usually the cause of impotence in diabetic men a few will have an endocrine cause and all should be screened for this.

Anti-cholinergic drugs such as propantheline may relieve gustatory sweating and nocturnal drenching sweats (which are not associated with hypoglycaemia) but have the disadvantage that gastric atony and urinary retention may worsen.

THE DIABETIC FOOT

Tissue necrosis in the feet is a common reason for hospital admission in diabetic patients. Such admissions tend to be prolonged (weeks or months rather than days) and not unusually end with amputation at various levels. Three main factors lead to tissue necrosis in the feet of diabetic patients: neuro-pathy, infection and ischaemia. In most cases all three are involved but sometimes neuropathy or ischaemia may predominate (Table 13.37). There is evidence that shunting of blood via peripheral arterio-venous anastomoses occurs in neuropathic feet thereby reducing blood flow in the smallest vessels. Thus there is probably reduced blood supply to most peripheral tissues even when the circulation is apparently good. The most common cause of ulceration is a plaque of callous skin beneath which tissue necrosis occurs. This eventually breaks through to the surface. If there is cellulitis the patient should be admitted to hospital immediately for bed rest, intravenous antibiotics, and surgical debridement and drainage of pus. Neuro-

Table 13.37   Clinical features of the diabetic foot

Primarily neuropathic	Primarily ischaemic
Warm	Cold
Bounding pulses	Absent pulses
Diminished sensation	Sensation intact
Pink skin	Skin blanches on elevation
Anhidrosis	
Callous formation	
Cracks and fissures	
Painless ulceration	Painful ulceration
Digital gangrene	Digital gangrene
Charcot's joints	
Wasting of interosseous muscles	
Clawed toes	
Neuropathic oedema	Oedema associated with cardiac decompensation

pathic oedema can be treated with ephedrine 300 mg t.d.s. which reduces peripheral blood flow and increases sodium excretion.

In the ischaemic foot ulceration usually results from localised pressure necrosis which is often complicated by secondary infection. Peripheral oedema is commonly secondary to cardiac failure associated with extensive and severe atherosclerosis. Medical management includes bed rest, eradication of infection, diuretics if there is oedema, and analgesics. Amputation is indicated for uncontrolled infection, osteomyelitis, extensive tissue destruction or intractable pain at rest in a limb in which vascular reconstruction has failed or more commonly is impossible due to extensive large blood-vessel disease.

Prevention is clearly the most effective way of dealing with this problem. A specialist chiropodist is an integral part of the diabetes team not only to ensure regular and effective chiropody but also to educate patients in foot care.

DIABETIC NEPHROPATHY

Diabetic nephropathy accounts for approximately 14% of all deaths in diabetic patients and some 25% of those developing diabetes under the age of 30 die from renal failure due to diabetic nephropathy.

Histopathology

Figure 13.41 relates the renal histopathology to the development of diabetic nephropathy. The earliest functional renal change detected is glomerular hyperperfusion. This is followed by renal hypertrophy. At this stage there may be microalbuminuria (albumin excretion $> 30\,\mu g/min$) which is reversible by strict control of the blood glucose concentration and of hypertension, if present. Its importance is that it predicts the development of irreversible renal damage indicated by the development of proteinuria detectable by dipstix ($> 150\,mg/l$).

Management

Once proteinuria is established glomerular filtration declines steadily with time in a linear fashion. The rate of progression of the disease can be reduced by energetic treatment of hypertension and a low protein (40–60 g daily) diet. Since many patients are relatively young a diastolic blood pressure $> 95\,mmHg$ usually indicates the need for treatment of hypertension. Standard hypotensive drugs are used but there are particular problems in their use in diabetic patients. For example thiazide diuretics, by inhibiting the secretion of insulin, raise the blood glucose concentration in patients with NIDDM, while non-cardioselective beta-blockers, by inhibiting muscle glycogenolysis, may not only lead to the development of symptomless hypoglycaemia in some patients taking a sulphonylurea or

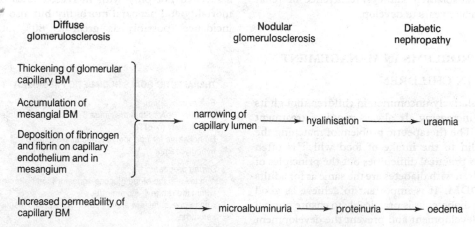

Fig. 13.41   Renal histopathology and development of diabetic nephropathy. (BM = basement membrane.)

insulin but also aggravate impotence and peripheral vascular disease both of which are common problems in these patients. Calcium antagonists and angiotensin converting enzyme inhibitors are commonly used with a loop diuretic.

The management of patients with renal failure (serum creatinine > 200 μmol/l) is essentially the same as in other forms of chronic renal disease. Diabetes often becomes unstable and the dose of insulin required may have to be adjusted daily on the basis of capillary blood glucose monitoring. Increased sensitivity to the action of exogenous insulin is often seen resulting in an overall decrease in the dose of insulin required. Treatment with metformin should never be used since the risk of lactic acidosis increases with impaired renal function and long acting sulphonylureas should be avoided and replaced by those which are metabolised rather than excreted such as tolbutamide or glipizide.

When the serum creatinine level exceeds 450 μmol/l most patients are unwell and should be considered for renal support treatment. Unfortunately some will not qualify for active intervention because of another major disability arising from severe large blood-vessel disease, neuropathy or retinopathy. The results of haemodialysis are less good than in non-diabetics and most diabetic patients start treatment with continuous ambulatory peritoneal dialysis (CAPD). The results of renal transplantation in carefully selected cases can be almost as good as in non-diabetics and the use of cyclosporin has improved results in diabetic as in non-diabetic patients.

Large blood-vessel disease causing cardiac failure and ischaemic gangrene, and retinopathy and neuropathy show continued progression even after successful transplantation and need constant attention. Although characteristic glomerular and arterial changes develop in transplanted kidneys recurrence of renal failure takes many years to develop.

SPECIAL PROBLEMS IN MANAGEMENT

DIABETES IN CHILDREN

Diabetes is relatively uncommon in children though its incidence is increasing. It always requires treatment with insulin. The therapeutic problem of matching the dose of insulin to the intake of food which is often variable raises practical difficulties but the principles of treating children with diabetes are the same as for adults who have IDDM. It is important to achieve as good control of the diabetes as is practicable to ensure normal growth and development and prevent the development of long-term complications of diabetes. Thus children

and their parents need to be educated in the management of diabetes to the limit of their ability. They need to have sufficient knowledge to make daily alterations in the dose of insulin on the basis of the results of pre-prandial capillary blood glucose measurements and consideration of such factors such as exercise and illness. Families with a diabetic child require much support and open access to specialist advice by means of a 'hot line' telephone is an important component of this. The greater the integration of the medical paediatric and adult diabetes services the less the trauma for diabetic children and their families as they grow up.

PREGNANCY AND DIABETES

Pregnancy in diabetic women is associated with an increased perinatal mortality rate (that is still-births and neonatal deaths within the first week of life). The main causes of this are intra-uterine death in the third trimester of pregnancy, prematurity (due to a high incidence of spontaneous premature labour and of elective premature delivery in an attempt to avoid late intra-uterine death), low birth weight and congenital malformation. Birth trauma is also more common due to a high incidence of excessively large, macrosomic babies. All these problems are directly related to poor metabolic control and largely disappear if near normoglycaemia is maintained before and at conception and during pregnancy and delivery. The therapeutic goals are listed in the information box below. The components of a successful diabetic pregnancy are listed in the information box (p. 691).

Gestational diabetes
Gestational diabetes, defined as diabetes diagnosed for the first time in pregnancy, is a common problem. It is associated not only with increased rates of perinatal mortality and neonatal morbidity but also with a high incidence (possibly as great as 80% at 25 years

---

THERAPEUTIC GOALS IN DIABETIC PREGNANCY

Before conception
Establish HbA, within the range 8–9% by use of 3 injections of insulin daily (p. 677)
Do not strive for normoglycaemia at the expense of hypoglycaemia

During pregnancy
Aim to keep the blood glucose concentration before meals within the range 4–5.5 mmol/l
Aim to give sufficient dietary carbohydrate and insulin to avoid ketonuria

COMPONENTS OF SUCCESSFUL DIABETIC PREGNANCY

- Pregnancy planned
- Maintain blood glucose/HbA, goals before and at conception and during pregnancy and delivery
- Delivery not before 38 weeks' gestation
- Supervision by experienced medical/obstetric/paediatric team at specialist centre throughout pregnancy

1. too insensitive
2. changes too slowly
3. is affected by things other than changes in the blood glucose concentration, such as the influx of new young red cells into the circulation
4. since it reflects the overall integrated mean blood glucose concentration, it gives no information about fluctuations in the blood glucose level and may therefore be misleading.

postpartum) of subsequent clinical diabetes (both insulin dependent and non-insulin dependent) in the mother. Normalisation of the metabolism whether by treatment with dietary measures alone or with additional treatment usually in the form of insulin undoubtedly reduces the fetal risk but its effect on diminishing the maternal risk of subsequent diabetes is less certain.

A screening procedure for gestational diabetes involving the measurement of true venous plasma glucose concentration 1 hour after a 50 g oral glucose load followed by a formal 3-hour 100 g oral glucose tolerance test in suspicious cases has been validated but is complicated and an accurate laboratory measurement of the basal (that is the fasting or more than 2 hours post meal) prevailing venous true plasma glucose concentration can be recommended for the following reasons:

1. It is a simple test which avoids the need for special preparation and can be incorporated readily as part of routine antenatal care thus encouraging assessment two or three times during pregnancy in all pregnant women.
2. It is more physiological and relevant to the clinical problem, since the prevailing maternal blood glucose concentration is the important thing as far as the fetus is concerned.

Thus this measurement selects those in need of treatment. Table 13.38 indicates the basal plasma glucose concentrations which indicate the need to consider instituting treatment.

Although measurements of glycosylated plasma albumin or total proteins may be more useful than glycosylated haemoglobin in pregnancy (since their rate of turnover is of the order of 1 compared with 3 months) they can only complement and not substitute for measurement of the blood glucose concentration which is the cornerstone of management in diabetic pregnancy.

Management of diabetes at delivery

Because of the risk of sudden intra-uterine death in the third trimester diabetic women have traditionally been delivered at 36–38 weeks' gestation either by caesarian section or by vaginal delivery following induction. Today improved metabolic control makes later delivery possible and most are now delivered between 38 and 39 weeks' gestation after induction of labour or if necessary, by caesarian section, while an increasing number are allowed to proceed to spontaneous vaginal delivery at term.

On the morning of delivery the usual breakfast and insulin should be replaced by an intravenous infusion of 10% dextrose with 10 units of unmodified insulin added to each 500 ml. This should be given at a rate of 100 ml hourly. The blood glucose concentration should be monitored at intervals of 1–2 hours and the concentration of insulin adjusted to keep the blood glucose concentration within the range 5–6 mmol/l. An alternative method is to give the insulin separately from the glucose infusion by means of a constant rate infusion pump at a rate of 1–2 units hourly. Whatever method is used administration of insulin should be stopped immediately on delivery and subcutaneous insulin resumed according to need as determined by capillary blood glucose estimations. Little or no insulin may be required for 12 hours after delivery. Thereafter the pre-pregnancy dose of subcutaneously administered insulin can be gradually resumed.

Table 13.38 Screening for gestational diabetes

Gestation	Basal true venous plasma glucose concentration – mmol/l
Up to 20 weeks	>5.5
20–40 weeks	>6.5

Note:
Assess further and consider need for treatment.

HbA$_1$ is unreliable as a screening test for gestational diabetes and for assessing diabetic control during pregnancy because it is:

SURGERY AND DIABETES

Surgery, whether performed electively or in an emergency, represents stress and invariably elicits secretion of the catabolic hormones cortisol, catecholamines, glucagon, and growth hormone in both normal and diabetic subjects. This results in increased glycogenolysis, gluconeogenesis, lipolysis, proteolysis, and insulin resistance, while the release of insulin is suppressed. In the non-diabetic person these metabolic effects lead to a secondary increase in the secretion of insulin which exerts a restraining and controlling influence. In diabetic patients there is either absolute deficiency of insulin (IDDM) or insulin secretion is delayed and impaired (NIDDM) so that in untreated or poorly controlled diabetes the uptake of metabolic substrate is significantly reduced, catabolism is increased, and ultimately metabolic decompensation in the form of diabetic ketoacidosis may develop in both types of diabetic patients. Starvation will exacerbate this process. In addition hyperglycaemia impairs phagocytic function (leading to reduced resistance to infection) and wound healing. Thus surgery must be carefully planned and managed in the diabetic patient with particular emphasis on good metabolic control along with avoidance of hypoglycaemia which is obviously particularly dangerous in the unconscious or semiconscious patient.

Preoperative assessment
Careful preoperative assessment is mandatory and is summarised in the information box below. Much of this can be done on an outpatient basis but if cardiovascular or renal function is impaired, there are signs of neuropathy (particular autonomic), diabetic control is poor, and alterations need to be made in the patient's usual treatment then admission to hospital some days before operation will be required.

PREOPERATIVE ASSESSMENT IN DIABETIC PATIENTS

- Assess cardiovascular and renal function
- Check for signs of neuropathy, particularly autonomic
- Assess diabetic control
    Measure HbA,
    Monitor preprandial blood glucose 4 times daily
- Review treatment of diabetes
    Replace long-acting with intermediate insulin
    Stop metformin and long-acting sulphonylureas: replace with insulin if necessary

---

Perioperative management
The management of diabetic patients undergoing surgery requiring general anaesthesia is summarised in Figure 13.42. Postoperatively the glucose/insulin/potassium infusion should be continued until the patient's intake of food is adequate when the normal insulin or tablet regimen can be resumed. If the intravenous infusion has to be continued for more than 24 hours plasma electrolytes and urea should be measured and urinary ketones checked daily. If the infusion is prolonged the concentration of potassium may require adjustment and if dilutional hyponatraemia occurs a parellel saline infusion may be necessary. If fluids need to be restricted, for example in patients with cardiovascular or renal disease, the volume of the glucose infusion can be halved by using a 20% dextrose solution and doubling the concentration of insulin and potassium. The infusion rate should then be 50 ml/hour. The insulin requirement is likely to be higher than that indicated in Figure 13.42 in patient's with hepatic disease, obesity, or sepsis and in those being treated with corticosteroids or undergoing cardiopulmonary bypass surgery.

Surgical emergencies
If the patient is significantly hyperglycaemic and/or ketoacidotic this should be corrected first with an intravenous infusion of saline and/or glucose plus insulin 6 units per hour plus potassium as required on the basis of repeated plasma potassium levels. Subsequently treatment as described in Figure 13.42 can be used during and after the operation.

Emergency surgery in a patient with well-controlled insulin-dependent diabetes depends on when the last subcutaneous injection of insulin was given. If this was recent an infusion of glucose only may be sufficient but frequent monitoring is essential.

PROSPECTS IN DIABETES MELLITUS

Management
The scale of the clinical problem presented by diabetic patients with severe vascular disease, the suggestion that good control of the blood glucose may prevent or retard the development of diabetic microangiopathy, the introduction of better methods of assessing diabetic control, the realisation that at present good control is achieved in only a minority of diabetic patients, and increased understanding of the deficiencies of con-

---

NEW SYSTEMS FOR DELIVERING INSULIN

- 'Open loop': pumps
- 'Closed loop': artificial pancreas
- Organ transplantation
    Whole pancreas
    Isolated islets

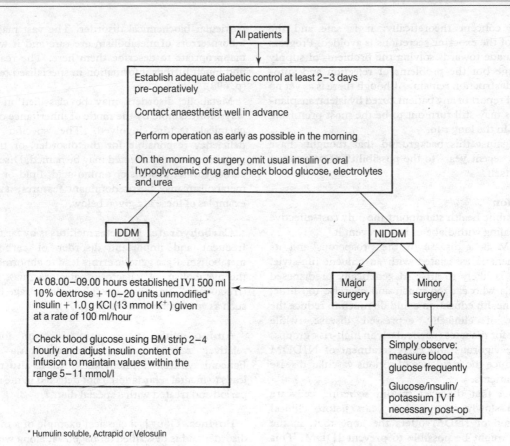

All patients

Establish adequate diabetic control at least 2–3 days pre-operatively

Contact anaesthetist well in advance

Perform operation as early as possible in the morning

On the morning of surgery omit usual insulin or oral hypoglycaemic drug and check blood glucose, electrolytes and urea

IDDM

At 08.00–09.00 hours established IVI 500 ml 10% dextrose + 10–20 units unmodified* insulin + 1.0 g KCl (13 mmol K$^+$) given at a rate of 100 ml/hour

Check blood glucose using BM strip 2–4 hourly and adjust insulin content of infusion to maintain values within the range 5–11 mmol/l

NIDDM

Major surgery

Minor surgery

Simply observe: measure blood glucose frequently

Glucose/insulin/ potassium IV if necessary post-op

* Humulin soluble, Actrapid or Velosulin

Fig. 13.42 Management of diabetic patients undergoing surgery and general anaesthesia. (IVI = intravenous infusion.)

ventional treatment with insulin has led to a search for better methods of treating IDDM and these are listed in the information box (p. 692).

'Open-loop' systems are battery powered portable pumps providing continuous subcutaneous, intra-muscular or intravenous infusion of insulin, delivered at fixed rates (a low basal rate and one or more higher rates before main meals) without reference to the blood glucose concentration. In practice the 'loop' is closed by the patient performing blood glucose estimations and the use of these devices requires a high degree of patient motivation and has the particular disadvantage that if the pump fails the onset of ketosis tends to be more rapid than with conventional treatment because there is no subcutaneous depot of insulin. These systems will not be suitable for general therapeutic use until they incorporate an automatic failure alarm and a miniaturised glucose sensor. Unfortunately the latter is not yet available.

'Closed loop', sometimes referred to as 'artificial pancreas' systems consist of three basic components: a

glucose sensor, an insulin delivery pump, and a computer control which regulates the administration of insulin on the basis of the blood glucose concentration. Ideally such a device should be small enough for implantation, deliver insulin intra-portally, and measure the blood glucose concentration rapidly without consuming blood. Existing systems deliver insulin peripherally, use blood, and are large, extra-corporeal, relatively slow and unreliable, and very expensive. However technology is advancing rapidly, particularly in relation to miniaturisation and glucose sensor devices.

Pancreatic transplantation is an alternative approach but there are particular problems relating to the exocrine pancreatic secretions and long-term immuno-suppression is of course necessary. While results are steadily improving they remain significantly less good than for renal transplantation and it is questionable if it will ever be considered justifiable to transplant young diabetics before vascular disease is clinically apparent.

Transplantation of isolated pancreatic islets is an

attractive concept theoretically: it is safe and the problem of the exocrine secretions is avoided. Progress is being made towards solving the problems of supply and storage but the problems of rejection and auto-immune destruction remain. Although there is as yet no published report of any patient cured by islet transplantation this may still turn out to be the most promising approach in the long run.

It is against this background that thoughts have turned in recent years to the possibility of preventing diabetes itself.

Prevention

From a public health standpoint the only cost-effective way of dealing with diabetes is to prevent it.

NIDDM is a disease of the prosperous and its development is associated with an affluent life-style. NIDDM is likely to arise in genetically predisposed individuals who eat too much and exercise too little. Effective health education could do much to reduce the incidence of clinically expressed disease, while screening for diabetes (particularly in high-risk groups) and more vigorous and early treatment of NIDDM would reduce the incidence of serious vascular disease in these patients.

The fact that the islet insulin secreting cells are destroyed slowly over several years before clinical presentation of IDDM offers the hope that, in the future, it might be possible to prevent IDDM. This depends on:

1. the availability of accurate, predictive markers for the development of clinical diabetes in genetically predisposed individual subjects
2. an understanding of the precise sequence of events leading to pancreatic beta cell destruction
3. the development of methods of intervention based on specifically targetted immunomodulation which could be applied early in the pre-diabetic period before most of the insulin secreting cells have been destroyed.

OTHER METABOLIC DISEASES

Metabolism is as fundamental as life itself; in medicine the term is usually restricted to disorders which can best be described in biochemical terms.

Many metabolic disorders are acquired. Others are congenital. The genetic aetiology of numerous inborn errors of metabolism has been identified with abnormalities of the structure or function of DNA and the pattern of their inheritance mapped by the study of a particular biochemical disorder. The vast majority of inborn errors of metabolism are rare and it would be inappropriate to describe them here. The reader will find much further information in specialised textbooks (p. 698).

Metabolic disorders may be classified in various ways, for example by the mode of inheritance or by the chemical factors involved. The specific enzyme deficiency responsible for the disorder, or the body system principally affected may be named. Disorders of carbohydrate, protein or amino acid, lipid or mineral metabolism may be predominant features, and a few examples of these are given below.

Carbohydrate. Diabetes mellitus is by far the most frequent and important disorder of carbohydrate metabolism. Rare genetic errors lead to abnormalities in the metabolism of galactose (galactosaemia), fructose (fructosuria), and glycogen (glycogen storage diseases, such as von Gierke's disease, p. 795).

Amino acids. Inborn errors account for many relatively rare diseases such as cystinuria and the Fanconi syndrome. Phenylketonuria is also rare but leads to mental retardation if not detected in the neonatal period and treated with a special diet.

Purines. Gout is a classical example of a metabolic disorder and is described on page 794, along with other causes of arthritis.

Lipids are complex substances among which cholesterol and triglyceride are the most useful indices for the detection and monitoring of hyperlipidaemia. Lipids circulate as lipoproteins (chylomicrons, low and high density lipoproteins), while free fatty acids are bound to albumin (p. 489). Analysis of fasting serum lipids and particularly of lipoproteins provides a useful classification of the hyperlipidaemias as devised by WHO, and based particularly on the work of Fredrickson (Table 13.39). In this classification there are five major types (I–V) of hyperlipidaemia due either to genetic defects in lipid metabolism or to environmental factors such as diet, alcohol and drugs, including oestrogens and corticosteroids. Measurement of lipoproteins is usually not necessary for management which can generally be determined by clinical observation along with measurement of fasting serum cholesterol and triglyceride. Family screening and specific diagnostic tests based on ultracentrifigation, apolipoprotein analysis, enzyme measurements and receptor studies which are available in specialist centres may be indicated in a few cases. Newer techniques in genetics

Table 13.39 Classification of primary hyperlipidaemia

Primary hyperlipidaemia	CHD risk	Risk of pancreatitis	Plasma cholesterol	Plasma triglyceride	Lipoprotein phenotype*	Treatment group
Common, polygenic hypercholesterolaemia	+	—	↑ (7–10)	—	IIa (LDL↑)	A
Familial combined hyperlipidaemia	++	—	↑ (7–10)	↑ (3–6)	IIb (LDL↑) (VLDL↑)	B
Familial hypercholesterolaemia (autosomal dominant)	+++	—	↑ (8–16) (heterozygotes) ↑ (16–32) (homozygotes)	— —	IIa (LDL↑) due to impaired function of LDL receptors	A
Remnant hyperlipidaemia	+++	?	↑ (8–15)	(5–15)	III (VLDL↑) (LDL↑) associated with abnormal apo-protein E	B
Familial hypertrigylceridaemia (autosomal dominant)	?	++	↑ (5–8)	(4–40)	IV (VDDL↑) cause unknown	B
Chylomicronaemia (autosomal recessive)	—	+++	↑ (8–12)	(20–80)	I due to deficiency of extra hepatic lipoprotein lipase or of apo-protein C-II V cause unknown	C

* Based on WHO/Fredrickson lipoprotein typing system.
LDL = low density lipoproteins.
VLDL = very low density lipoproteins.

are likely to facilitate more precise diagnosis in the next few years.

HYPERLIPIDAEMIA

PRIMARY HYPERLIPIDAEMIA

Such patients can for most clinical purposes be placed into one of three treatment groups two of which are metabolically heterogeneous (Table 13.40).

Clinical features

Group A
This group consists of those with hyper-cholesterolaemia and normal triglycerides. The serum is clear.

Common polygenic hypercholesterolaemia is by far the most frequent cause of the serum cholesterol exceeding 5.2 mmol/l (the recommended cut-off point for intervention). It reflects an interaction between multiple genes and dietary and other environmental factors and has more than one metabolic basis. Variation in its prevalence is the main reason for differences in cholesterol levels between countries and in the prevalence of coronary heart disease. The diagnosis is made by exclusion of other causes of hyperlipidaemia. Most patients have mild to moderate hypercholesterolaemia and no physical signs but early arcus

Table 13.40 Treatment of hyperlipidaemia

Treatment group	Type of hyperlipidaemia	Diet	Drugs
A	*Hypercholesterolaemia (IIa)*	Low energy if obese Low fat → <35% energy Increased proportion of polyunsaturated fat → PUS/S fat ratio >1 : 1 Restricted cholesterol	
	Common polygenic	Usually diet only	± Bile acid sequestrant or reductase inhibitor
	Rare dominant	Diet	+ Bile acid sequestrant + reductase inhibitor
B	*Hypertriglyceridaemia*	Diet as above *plus* Omit sucrose and alcohol	(see Table 13.41)
	Common familial combined hyperlipidaemia (IIb)	Usually diet only	± Nicotinic acid or fibrate
	Relatively uncommon familial Hypertriglyceridaemia (IV) Rare remnant hyperlipidaemia (III)	Diet	1 Nicotinic acid ± 2 Fibrate 3 1+2
C	*Chylomicronaemia (I, V)*	Restrict fat to <25 g daily	—

senilis or xanthelasma may be present. Those with such stigmata, particularly if combined with a positive family history of coronary heart disease and obesity are more likely to have a higher plasma cholesterol level than those without these characteristics.

About 5% of patients with hypercholesterolaemia have a more sharply defined disorder transmitted as an autosomal dominant and due to impaired function of LDL receptors. This is a serious disease which affects 1 person in 500. Heart disease may be present in the fourth or even the third decade of life. The condition is present in 1 out of 25 patients presenting with myocardial infarction before the age of 60. Serum cholesterol levels range from 8–16 mmol/l in heterozygotes and from 16–32 mmol/ in the rare homozygotes. The diagnosis of familial hyper-cholesterolaemia can be made at birth in the infant of an affected parent by measuring LDL cholesterol in cord blood. Tendon xanthomas, polyarthritis affecting the large joints, arcus senilis and xanthelasma are common. An aortic systolic murmur may be present due to supra-vulvar aortic stenosis. In homozygotes these manifestations appear in childhood or adolescence and untreated the expectation of life is about 20 years.

Group B

This group comprises those with predominant hyper-triglyceridaemia. The serum is cloudy. Cholesterol may be normal or if increased the rise is usually less pronounced than that of triglyceride.

Familial combined hyperlipidaemia is probably the commonest genetic disorder of lipoprotein metabolism associated with coronary heart disease. In both affected families and individuals the pattern of hyperlipidaemia (namely raised cholesterol, triglyceride or both) may vary at different times. The majority however have elevated plasma levels of apoprotein B, the structural protein of VLDL and LDL. At present the diagnosis depends on a family history: the condition should be suspected when moderate hyperlipidaemia is accompanied by a strong family history of coronary heart disease. Xanthomas do not occur.

Remnant hyperlipidaemia is another rare cause of early onset coronary heart disease and of peripheral vascular disease affecting the lower limbs and carotid arteries. Typically both cholesterol and triglyceride levels are markedly raised. The disorder can appear in childhood but is usually not diagnosed until adult life when typically skin xanthomas are seen in the palmar creases and/or on the elbow, although these are not invariable. The diagnosis can be confirmed by demonstrating an abnormal apoprotein E and/or raised VLDL cholesterol.

Familial hypertriglyceridaemia may be pronounced or relatively mild and in the more severe forms there is usually also chylomicronaemia. Most of the triglyceride in plasma is of endogenous rather than dietary origin. The metabolic defect is unknown. It is uncertain whether there is an excess risk of coronary heart disease. Recurrent pancreatitis is a common manifestation when the hypertriglyceridaemia is marked. There is also increased risk of thrombosis. Diabetes mellitus may be present. This may simply represent the coexistence of two diseases, alternatively diabetes might result from pancreatic damage secondary to recurrent sub-clinical pancreatitis. Family studies show autosomal dominant transmission with considerable variation in severity of the hyperlipidaemia. Unlike the chylomicronaemia syndrome familial hypertriglyceridaemia is not ameliorated, and may even be exacerbated, by a fat deprivation test. Lipoprotein lipase activity is usually either normal or slightly subnormal.

Group C

Chylomicronaemia is a rare cause of severe hypertri-glyceridaemia presenting in childhood or adult life. It is caused by deficiency of the enzyme lipoprotein lipase or of the protein which activates this enzyme, apo-protein C2. Transmission is by autosomal recessive inheritance, hence hyperlipidaemia is not usually found in family members. Recurrent pancreatitis (or sometimes a history of attacks of undiagnosed abdominal pain dating from childhood or infancy), crops of eruptive xanthomas on extensor surfaces, retinal-lipaemia, and hepatosplenomegaly are all characteristic. Since the hypertriglyceridaemia is due to accumulation in the plasma of fat of dietary origin the diagnosis can be confirmed by a fat deprivation test in which a fat free diet (that is containing less than 5% of energy derived from fat) is given for 3 days. In a positive test there is a steep fall in plasma triglyceride concentration to near normal values and disappearance of chylomicrons. A definitive diagnosis can be confirmed by assaying the lipoprotein lipase in a plasma sample collected 10 minutes after injecting heparin 40 units/kg body weight intravenously. Some patients have normal or high levels of this enzyme but lack its activator the apo-protein C2. This can be measured either by electrophoresis or by using a specific antibody.

SECONDARY HYPERLIPIDAEMIA

Common causes of secondary hyperlipidaemia include diabetes mellitus, alcohol abuse, hypothyroidism, chronic renal failure, nephrotic syndrome, cholestasis, and bulimia.

Rarer causes include severe liver dysfunction, anorexia nervosa, myelomatosis, and glycogen storage disease.

Commonly used drugs that can cause, usually moderate, hyperlipidaemia, include thiazide and other diuretics, oral contraceptives, retinoids, and corticosteroids. Their effect is exaggerated in patients with primary hyperlipidaemia. Anabolic steroids and progestogens may elevate LDL cholesterol. Oestrogen, phenytoin, phenobarbitone, cimetidine, rifampicin, and alcohol increase HDL cholesterol.

Cardiovascular disease is a frequent complication of diabetes mellitus and of chronic renal failure being treated with dialysis or renal transplantation. This is probably related in part to hyperlipidaemia.

Management

Primary hyperlipidaemia
The treatment of primary hyperlipidaemia is shown in Table 13.40.

Control of primary hyperlipidaemia always requires dietary measures. Obesity must be corrected in every

Table 13.41 Lipid lowering drugs

Class of drugs	Effect	Problems
Bile acid sequestrant resins		
Cholestyramine	Cholesterol↓ 20–30%	Inconvenient: long-term compliance poor
Colestipol	HDL↑	Dyspepsia Constipation Absorption of other medications
Fibrates		
Bezafibrate	Triglyceride↓ 25–60%	Creatine kinase↑ ± myopathy
Ciprofibrate		Impotence
Clofibrate	Cholesterol↓	AST↑
Fenofibrate	10–25%	Gallstones↑
Gemfibrozil	HDL↑	Warfarin potentiated Contraindicated when renal function impaired ? excess mortality
HMG CoA reductase inhibitors		
Simvastin	Cholesterol↓ 30–40%	Creatine kinase↑ ± myopathy
Lovastin		AST↑
Pravastin	HDL↑	Lens opacities ↑ Potentiates Warfarin Rhabdomyolysis
Miscellaneous		
Nicotinic acid	Triglyceride↓ 40–60% Cholesterol↓ 10–25% HDL↑	Flushing Hyperuricaemia ± gout
Probucol	Cholesterol↓ 5–15% HDL↓	Prolongs QT complex Contraindicated when ventricular arrhythmia or prolonged QTc
Fish oils	Triglyceride↓	Not yet adequately evaluated

case. The low energy diet on page 986 can be appropriately modified in relation to the fat content. An abnormal sensitivity to sucrose and/or alcohol is responsible for inducing hyperlipidaemia in some of those in Group B who should be advised to restrict their consumption of these dietary components even if they are not obese.

Patients in Group C improve dramatically with restriction of fat intake to about 25 g daily.

If dietary measures alone are insufficient lipid lowering drugs (Table 13.41) should be considered. All have some disadvantages and the balance between the benefits and the risks and side-effects of drug therapy must be carefully reviewed. In all cases every effort should be made to ensure effective dieting and dietary treatment alone should be continued for a sufficiently long period (9–12 months) so that its maximum effect can be seen. When lipid lowering drugs are used this should always be in conjunction with continuing careful attention to diet.

Bile acid sequestrant resins are well tried and widely used but many patients find their preparation and consumption inconvenient. Nicotinic acid is a potent lipid lowering agent but it has side-effects. Indications for the use of clofibrate came under scrutiny when two extensive clinical trials of this drug for the primary prevention of ischaemic heart disease revealed an increased mortality among treated individuals from ischaemic heart disease, cerebrovascular disorders and neoplasms, particularly of the respiratory and gastrointestinal tracts. This excess mortality is unexplained and it is uncertain if the use of other members of this group of drugs has similar disadvantages. For this reason use of the fibrates should be strictly confined to the few cases of severe hyperlipidaemia which have failed to respond to other measures and where the clinical benefit seems likely to be greater than the risk associated with medication. Those in this category are likely to include patients with the relatively uncommon familial hypertriglyceridaemia, rare remnant hyperlipidaemia, and some cases of chylomicronaemia where there is a risk of acute relapsing pancreatitis when the plasma triglyceride concentration remains elevated above 6–7 mmol/l despite dietary measures and other drugs. HMG CoA reductase inhibitors are the most promising of recently developed cholesterol lowering drugs. They are very potent and fully effective when given once daily after the evening meal. However large-scale, long-term evaluation is not yet available and careful monitoring for undesirable effects is essential particularly in relation to a possible increase in the incidence of lens opacities, hepatotoxicity, and rhabdomyolysis. The cholesterol lowering effect of probucol is limited and the fall in HDL cholesterol undesirable.

Epidemiologically there is an inverse relation between consumption of fish and coronary heart disease but the safety and the ability of fish oil preparations to protect against coronary heart disease have not been established in man. Highly unsaturated fatty acids are prone to lipid peroxidation, the products being toxic. To prevent this an antioxidant must be added. Long-term evaluation is desirable before widespread use of marine oil preparations can be recommended.

A single drug in combination with diet not infrequently fails to achieve adequate reduction of lipids in patients with severe hyperlipidaemia. Bile acid sequestrant drugs are often used in combination with CoA reductase inhibitors, nicotinic acid, fibrates, and probucol. However such combination therapy is associated with an increased incidence of side-effects and the cost can become very high.

Secondary hyperlipidaemia
This condition usually responds to treatment of the underlying condition when this is possible. If it is not possible treatment should be along the same lines as for primary hyperlipidaemia.

FURTHER READING

Endocrinology:
Edwards C R W 1986 Integrated clinical science: endocrinology. Heinemann, London. This book provides the undergraduate with both the basic science and clinical aspects of endocrinology including diabetes mellitus
Hall R, Besser M 1989 Fundamentals of clinical endocrinology, 4th Edn. Pitman Medical, London. A very good general textbook
Williams D H 1985 Textbook of endocrinology. Saunders, Philadelphia. A large comprehensive source of reference of particular value to the postgraduate student
Belchetz P E 1984 Management of pituitary disease. Chapman and Hall, London. A useful book covering all aspects of the physiology and pathophysiology of the pituitary

Specialist texts for further reference
Ingbar S H, Braverman L E (eds) 1986 The Thyroid, 5th Ed. Lippincott, Philadelphia
Lazarus J H, Hall R (eds) 1988 Hypothyroidism and goitre. Clinical Endocrinology and Metabolism. Bailière Tindall, London

Toft A D (ed) 1985 Hyperthyroidism. Clinics in Endocrinology and Metabolism. Saunders, London
Wilson J D, Foster D W 1985 William's Textbook of Endocrinology, 7th Ed. Saunders, Philadelphia

Diabetes mellitus:
Alberti K G M M, Krall L P (1985, 1986, 1987) The Diabetes Annual, 1, 2, 3. Elsevier, Amsterdam
Keen H, Jarrett R J (1982) Complications of diabetes, 2nd Ed. Arnold, Sevenoaks
Nattrass M, Santiago J V (1983) Recent Advances in Diabetes 1. Churchill Livingstone, Edinburgh
Nattrass M (1986) Recent Advances in Diabetes 2. Churchill Livingstone, Edinburgh
Creutzfeldt W, Lefebvre P (1988) Diabetes Mellitus: Pathophysiology and Therapy. Springer-Verlag, Heidelberg and Berlin
Krall L P, Alberti K G M M, Turtle J R (1988). World Book of Diabetes in Practice, Volume 3, Elsevier.

14

Diseases of the Blood

BLOOD CELL FORMATION

Blood cells are formed both in liver and spleen up to the fifth month of fetal life. Thereafter normal production is found increasingly in the medullary cavity of bones and from birth onwards is restricted to these sites.

At birth the whole marrow cavity is utilised for haemopoiesis. During childhood there is a progressive diminution in the amount of red haemopoietic marrow so that in the young adult it is confined to the heads of the femur and humerus, to flat bones such as the sternum, ribs and ilia and to the vertebrae. The rest of the marrow cavity is occupied by fat. Red marrow reappears in the shafts of the long bones, replacing the fat, when there is increased demand for blood formation.

All blood cells are derived from a totipotent haemopo-

ietic stem cell (THSC). Cells which will mature into lymphocytes appear to arise from this cell at a very early stage of differentiation, pre-B and pre-T stem cells are formed which mature to become B and T lymphocytes respectively (Fig. 14.1). Cells destined to become the 'myeloid' elements appear at a slightly later stage (Fig. 14.1). Pluripotent myeloid stem cells (PMSC) are formed and, in turn, give rise to cells committed to either erythroid, granulocyte/monocyte or megakaryocyte cell maturing pathways.

Certain disease states which involve the totipotent stem cell affect all the haemopoietic cell lines while other disorders may affect only one or other of the lines. The latter are, in some instances, easier to treat since there is the possibility of regenerating normal marrow from the normal totipotent stem cells.

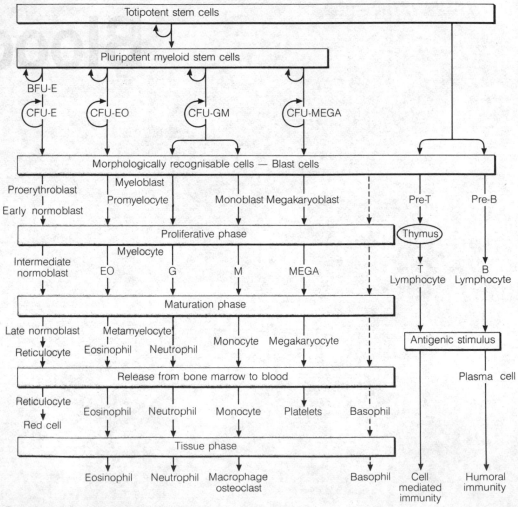

Fig. 14.1 Origin and development of blood cells.

Of the three types of cell found in the blood, erythrocytes and platelets are true blood cells. They differ from most other cells in the body in that they have no nuclei. Leucocytes are cells which use the blood to migrate from the marrow or other production sites to the tissues where they function. Thus leucocytes in the circulation form only a very small fraction of the total leucocyte mass in the body.

ERYTHROCYTES

The earliest identifiable erythrocyte precursor in the marrow is the pro-erythroblast, a large cell with a nucleolated nucleus and deeply basophilic cytoplasm. This cell undergoes a series of divisions rapidly so that the daughter cells do not have time to regrow between divisions and become progressively smaller. At the same time maturation proceeds with the formation of haemoglobin in the cytoplasm. Early, intermediate and late normoblasts can be identified.

Proliferation ceases at the intermediate normoblast stage and maturation is then completed with condensation of the nuclear chromatin and eventual ejection of the nuclear remnant. At this stage the cell still has the capacity to synthesise haemoglobin, due to the presence of ribosomes in the cytoplasm. This ribosomal material (RNA) gives the cell a faintly bluish colour with Romanowsky stains. Supravital staining with new methylene blue causes condensation of the ribosomes to form reticular material which makes the cells easy to identify. They are called reticulocytes and are easily counted. The reticulocyte matures into an adult red cell in about 3 days and is released to the circulation about half way through this period. Normally between $10-100 \times 10^9$ l reticulocytes are found in the circulating blood of healthy adults.

Under stress, reticulocytes can be released sooner from the marrow, raising the reticulocyte count without an increase in erythropoiesis. These 'marrow' reticulocytes can be recognised as they have a much more dense central aggregate of reticulum when stained with supravital stains. However an absolute increase in the number of reticulocytes usually reflects increased erythropoiesis.

After the first few days of life there are, in health, no nucleated red cells in the peripheral blood. The presence of normoblasts indicates excessive or abnormal blood formation or irritation of the bone marrow by invasion with foreign elements.

The mature erythrocyte is a circular biconcave disc with a mean diameter of 7.2 μm (Fig. 14.2). There is an excess of membrane which is partly responsible for the biconcave shape but the maintenance of this shape

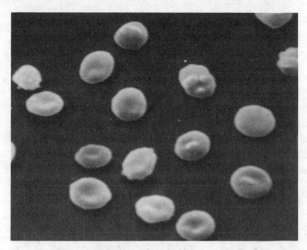

Fig. 14.2 Scanning electron microphotograph of human erythrocytes. The bioconcave disc shape is easily seen (magnification × 5000).

requires energy supplied by glycolysis. This unusual morphology gives the erythrocyte considerable plasticity enabling it to pass through capillaries and other structures of small diameter. In some disorders erythrocytes may lose membrane becoming progressively more spherical and rigid. As a result they are more susceptible to destruction particularly in the spleen, which is uniquely adapted to filtering out such cells. The spleen also removes inclusion bodies such as Howell Jolly bodies and Pappenheimer bodies (p. 706) from erythrocytes without destroying the cells.

The red cell membrane has a lipid bilayer structure in which the membrane proteins are found and is a complex dynamic structure, one function of which is to maintain high levels of potassium and low levels of sodium in the cell by means of ionic pumps. The surface of the membrane also carries antigenic determinants for the various blood groups.

Erythropoietin

Erythropoiesis is controlled by a hormone, erythropoietin, produced mainly in the kidneys. There, cells which are probably located in the tubules, monitor the provision of oxygen to the tissues and respond to hypoxia by the production of erythropoietin. Erythropoietin acts on the erythropoietic stem cells stimulating increased proliferation and reducing ineffective erythropoiesis (Fig. 14.3).

HAEMOGLOBIN

Haemoglobin in the erythrocyte provides the oxygen transport mechanism of the blood. Erythrocytes also carry carbon dioxide from the tissues to the lungs

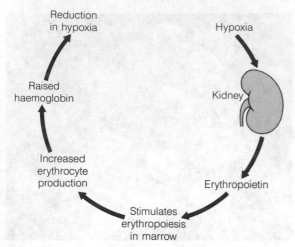

Fig. 14.3 Erythropoietin and erythropoiesis.

buffering the carbonic acid formed in the red cell (p. 221). Haemoglobin is a complex globular protein molecule, a conjugate of a red pigment (haem) with protein (globin). Haem is formed under the control of the enzyme ALA synthetase by the condensation of glycine and succinyl coenzyme A to form amino-levulinic acid. There follows a series of synthetic steps which build the porphyrin ring, at the end of which the enzyme haem-synthetase (ferrochelatase) inserts iron into the ring and haem is formed. Each step in this synthetic pathway requires its own enzyme; deficiencies of these enzymes give rise to the various forms of porphyria.

The globin fraction of normal human haemoglobin consists of four polypeptide chains, two alpha chains of 141 amino acids and two other chains of 146 amino acids. The chains are the product of four structural genes, all on autosomal chromosomes. The genes and their polypeptide chains are designated alpha, gamma, beta and delta and are responsible for the production of the three main haemoglobins seen after birth, namely haemoglobins F, A and A2 (Table 14.1). The α genes are on chromosome 16 and the β, γ and δ genes on chromosome 11.

Table 14.1 Polypeptide chain construction of normal haemoglobins

	Schematic	Written
Hb F	$\alpha\gamma$ $\gamma\alpha$	$\alpha_2\gamma_2$
Hb A	$\alpha\beta$ $\beta\alpha$	$\alpha_2\beta_2$
Hb A2	$\alpha\delta$ $\delta\alpha$	$\alpha_2\delta_2$

One molecule of oxygen is carried by each haem fraction of the haemoglobin molecule which is therefore capable of carrying four molecules of oxygen. Beta, gamma and delta chains are incapable of accepting oxygen until the alpha chains have taken up oxygen. When this occurs a configurational change in the haemoglobin molecule prises open the haem pockets of the other chains, allowing them to accept oxygen. Thus the more oxygen the haemoglobin molecule has, the more easily it acquires further oxygen until saturated. In the tissues the reverse occurs, easy loss becoming more difficult as haemoglobin becomes desaturated.

This function can be influenced further by a by-product of glucose metabolism, 2–3-diphosphoglycerate (2–3-DPG). The concentration of 2–3-DPG in the erythrocyte affects the avidity of the haemoglobin molecule for oxygen by reversible combination with deoxygenated haemoglobin. Increased levels of 2–3-DPG decrease haemoglobin's oxygen affinity and improve release to the tissues. Under hypoxic conditions, 2–3-DPG levels in the erythrocytes increase as a compensatory mechanism. This is the first step in acclimatisation at high altitude and occurs within 24–48 hours, long before increased erythropoietin production stimulates an increase in erythrocyte numbers.

Iron metabolism

Iron is essential for the synthesis of the haem fraction of haemoglobin. It is also present in myoglobin and enzymes such as the cytochromes. Iron in food (p. 56) is absorbed from the upper small intestine, mainly in the ferrous form bound to amino acids and sugars, but is also absorbed in haem from red meat. Iron readily takes the inabsorbable ferric form but the low pH of the stomach contents helps to preserve it in the ferrous form (Fig. 14.4).

Each cell obtains iron from the iron transport system (transferrin) in the blood by transfer across its membrane. The intestinal mucosal cell is no exception but it also receives iron by absorption from the gut lumen. When body stores of iron are adequate the intestinal mucosal cell is well supplied and absorption from the gut is discouraged. Iron is lost when the mucosal cells are sloughed into the gut. Thus excessive iron absorption is prevented.

When demand for iron increases, or the body stores are low, the mucosal cell becomes iron depleted and therefore avid for iron. Absorption from the gut increases and the iron is passed rapidly to the iron transport system in the blood. Little is lost when the cell is sloughed.

Iron for erythropoiesis comes mainly from transfer-

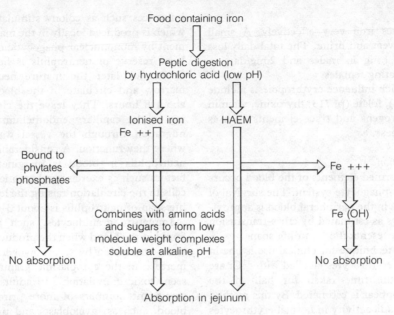

Fig. 14.4   Iron absorption.

rin and almost all iron absorbed from the gut goes preferentially to the bone marrow to be used by the developing red cells. Increased erythropoiesis associated with a variety of disorders may promote iron absorption by using this iron even when iron stores are increased. Thus some forms of prolonged anaemia, not due to blood loss or iron deficiency, can be associated with excessive iron stores. Haem absorbed by the mucosal cell is split in the cell and iron liberated. The iron is then treated in the same way as that absorbed by other means. This is a very useful additional means of iron absorption provided mainly by red meat. Iron obtained from the catabolism of haemoglobin from destroyed red cells is recycled either to the bone marrow, or, if there is excess, to the iron stores. Iron is stored in cells in two forms (Fig. 14.5) and these are listed in the information box below.

FORMS IN WHICH IRON IS STORED

- Ferritin from which iron is fairly readily available
- Haemosiderin which is a more stable form and constitutes the bulk of the iron stores. Haemosiderin is probably formed by the degradation of ferritin and can be stained by the Prussian blue reaction. This stain is used to provide a crude measurement of iron stores in the marrow

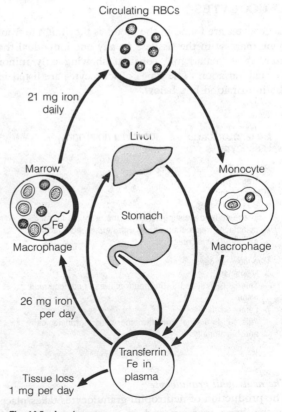

Fig. 14.5   Iron turnover.

Iron loss

The body conserves iron very effectively. A small amount is lost in sweat and urine. The total daily loss amounts to about 1 mg in males and 2 mg/day on average in menstruating females.

Other factors which influence erythropoiesis include vitamin B_{12} (p. 711), folate (p. 713) thyroxine, vitamin C, vitamin E, androgens and trace elements such as copper and manganese.

Erythrocyte destruction

Destruction of all formed elements of the blood occurs in the mononuclear-phagocyte system. The survival of mature erythrocytes in the peripheral blood is approximately 110–120 days as estimated by cross-transfusion experiments and represents the mean life span.

A more practical technique for clinical use is one in which the patient's erythrocytes labelled with ^{51}Cr are retransfused and the time taken for half of the radioactivity to disappear is estimated. By this method the half-life of the radioactivity in normal erythrocytes is 25–35 days and is shorter than the true half life because of the elution of chromium from the cells.

LEUCOCYTES

Leucocytes are found in the blood as they migrate from bone marrow to the tissues. In any one individual the number is remarkably constant showing only minor diurnal variation. The types of leucocytes are listed in the information box below.

MORPHOLOGICALLY DISTINCT TYPES OF BLOOD LEUCOCYTE

Polymorphonuclear granulocytes
- Neutrophil
- Eosinophil
- Basophil
  These cells are distinguished by the granules in the cytoplasm which stain either with neutral, acid (eosin) or alkaline (basic) reactions.

Mononuclear cells
- Monocyte
  This cell is related to the neutrophil and finds common origin.
- Lymphocyte
  This cell is distinct from the other cells morphologically and functionally.

The neutrophil granulocyte

The production of neutrophil granulocytes takes place in the bone marrow and is regulated by humoral influences such as colony stimulating factor some of which is produced locally in the marrow microenvironment by mononuclear phagocytic cells and fat cells. A large reserve of neutrophils is held in the marrow. Sooner or later the mature neutrophils leave the marrow and circulate in the blood, on average, for about 8 hours. They leave the circulation by adhering to the capillary endothelium (margination) and migration through the vessel wall into the tissues where they function. A considerable proportion of the neutrophils in blood is marginated. Certain stress factors such as exercise and emotion may return these cells to the circulation raising the leucocyte count. The life span of neutrophils is about 3–4 days.

Immature granulocytes, such as myelocytes, are found in the blood when the production of leucocytes is being stimulated by severe pyogenic infection and an increase in the cytoplasmic granulation may also be seen (toxic granulation). In adults the appearance of significant numbers of more primitive forms in the blood, such as myeloblasts and promyelocytes, indicates a serious disturbance of marrow function such as invasion by metastases or neoplastic change as in leukaemia.

Neutrophil granulocytes are phagocytic cells which ingest bacteria and fungi. Neutrophils are attracted to bacteria by chemotaxis and phagocytosis is enhanced by opsonisation. Having engulfed a bacterium the neutrophils kill it:

1. by the production of hydrogen peroxide (oxygen dependent)
2. release of myeloperoxidase into the phagosome (oxygen dependent)
3. release of lysozyme, lactoferrin and pH reduction in the phagosome (oxygen independent).

The products of autodigestion of cells killed by organisms (pus cells) are potent stimulants of fresh neutrophil formation by the marrow. Pyrogens are also released. Neutrophils also ingest uric acid crystals and may disintegrate in the process, liberating tissue damaging substances causing local inflammation.

Apart from responding to infection, neutrophils also produce a vitamin B_{12} binding protein, transcobalamin III which explains the high levels of vitamin B_{12} in the serum in conditions in which there is a greatly increased number of neutrophils, e.g. chronic myeloid leukaemia.

The degree of segmentation of neutrophils varies from unsegmented to five segments. The number of segments appears to have no functional importance. A failure to segment with the formation of 'band' cells, occurs in toxic conditions and under such circumstances the degree of segmentation tends to diminish. This is commonly called a 'shift to the left'. A 'shift to the right' in which there is increased segmentation, occurs in disorders such as vitamin B_{12} and folate deficiency and also iron deficiency.

Eosinophil granulocytes

These are also produced in the marrow. The absolute count in blood is normally less than $0.4 \times 10^9/l$. Factors influencing production are poorly understood but T lymphocytes appear to exert some control. Eosinophils are also phagocytic but less actively so than neutrophils. They are associated with allergic reactions, ingest antigen-antibody complexes and are concerned in processes involving foreign proteins, such as hypersensitivity reactions and have a role in the containment of parasitic infections (see p. 30). Their numbers are severely reduced by corticosteroid therapy.

Basophil granulocytes

These are poorly phagocytic and possess the Fc portion of the IgE molecule on specific binding sites on the surface membrane. Activation of this by antigens results in degranulation of the cell with release of histamine. Thus basophils participate in hypersensitivity reactions in the same way as mast cells (tissue basophils) as described on page 30. Basophils also contain heparin which may be released to participate in lipid metabolism.

Monocytes

These derive from the same precursors (CFU-GM) as the granulocyte. The monocyte is a cell with an irregularly shaped nucleus in a cloudy blue cytoplasm containing numerous minute red granules. Monocytes are motile and phagocytic and migrate into the tissues where they develop further into various types of macrophages such as tissue macrophages, Kupffer cells and osteoclasts. There they constitute the mononuclear phagocyte system (previously but wrongly known as the reticuloendothelial system) which removes debris as well as microorganisms by phagocytosis and collects and presents antigenic material to lymphocytes. Lysis of tumour cells is another important function. Their production of platelet derived growth factor is important in promoting healing and tissue remodelling. They also produce interleukin-I and tumour necrosis factor; mediators of the acute phase response. Production of tissue thromboplastin in response to bacterial endotoxin may activate the extrinsic coagulation mechanism and promote intravascular coagulation. Macrophages may survive for months.

Lymphocytes

These originate from committed stem cells in the bone marrow. Some migrate to the thymus where they become T (thymic) lymphocytes. Others become B (bursa) lymphocytes and a few become cytotoxic killer cells. About 75% of circulating lymphocytes are T cells. The rest are B cells and a few are 'null' cells showing neither T nor B characteristics. Both B cells and T cells respond to antigenic stimuli by transformation, in the case of B lymphocytes to plasma cells producing immunoglobulin. T cells mediate cellular immunity. They are divided into 'helper' and 'suppressor' types. Their functions are described on page 27. The life span of lymphocytes may vary from as short as a few days to many years. The latter may re-enter the circulation at intervals.

THE PLATELETS (THROMBOCYTES)

These are described on page 748.

NORMAL HAEMATOLOGICAL VALUES

These are given in Table 20.9 (p. 992).

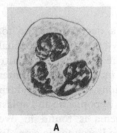 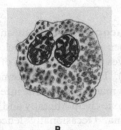 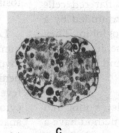 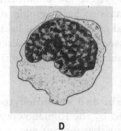

Fig. 14.6 The types of blood leucocyte. A. The neutrophil granulocyte. **B.** The eosinophil granulocyte. **C.** The basophil granulocyte. **D.** The monocyte. **E.** The lymphocyte.

TERMS DESCRIBING ABNORMAL BLOOD FILM APPEARANCES AND THEIR MEANING

Microcytosis. This means that the average size of the red cells is reduced. It is commonly found in iron deficiency anaemia and other disorders of haemoglobin synthesis.

Macrocytosis. This means that the average size of red cells is greater than normal. It is seen, for instance, in megaloblastic anaemias but its occurrence does not necessarily mean megaloblastic change in the marrow. A common cause is excessive alcohol consumption.

Hypochromia. This exists when the red cells contain less than the normal amount of haemoglobin. They stain less deeply and show greater than normal central pallor. Hypochromia is commonly associated with microcytosis and is a characteristic feature of disorders of haemoglobin synthesis, most commonly iron deficiency.

Anisocytosis. This means inequality in the size of the red cells. It is found in many forms of anaemia but is very prominent in megaloblastic anaemia.

Poikilocytosis. This means marked irregularity in the shape of the red cells. It is never present without anisocytosis and usually reflects dyserythropoiesis.

Elliptocytosis. This means elliptical red cells; ovalocytosis refers to a less marked abnormality. Such cells are found in small numbers in a variety of disorders such as megaloblastic and hypochromic anaemias. When the majority of cells are oval or elliptical it indicates a hereditary disorder of dominant type which is usually clinically benign; in less than 10% of cases a haemolytic state exists and may cause anaemia.

Target cells. These are abnormally flat red cells with a central mass of haemoglobin surrounded by a ring of pallor and an outer ring of haemoglobin. They are commonly associated with liver disease, impaired or absent splenic function (hyposplenism) and haemoglobinopathies.

Polychromasia and reticulocytosis. Young red cells when stained by the Romanowsky method have a faint bluish colour (basophilia) due to residual ribosomal material. A blood film in which such cells are present in increased numbers along with those of normal orange colour is said to show polychromasia. This, like reticulocytosis (p. 701), indicates increased production of new red cells by the bone marrow.

Punctate basophilia. Pathologically damaged young red cells may show scattered deep blue dots in the cytoplasm with Romanowsky staining. Such punctate basophilia may be found in any severe anaemia, but the presence of many of these cells is most commonly seen in β thalassaemia and chronic lead poisoning where it may occur when the anaemia is slight.

Howell Jolly bodies. These are remnants of nuclear material left in the erythrocyte after the nucleus is extruded. They are normally removed by the spleen and their presence usually indicates a nonfunctioning or absent spleen. Their numbers are greatly increased in certain erythropoietic disorders, e.g. megaloblastic anaemia.

Pappenheimer bodies. These are iron-protein complexes (siderotic granules) found in red cells in certain iron overload states and are increased when the spleen is nonfunctioning or absent.

Nucleated red cells. These are usually normoblasts and are found in the blood when erythropoiesis is very vigorous or when there is irritation of the bone marrow, as in leukaemia, or infiltration by secondary tumour.

Leucocytosis. This means an increase in the total number of white blood cells (over $11.0 \times 10^9/l$ in adults). This may take the form of a polymorphonuclear leucocytosis in which the increase is due to the outpouring of many young neutrophil granulocytes, as occurs in the presence of pyogenic infections. Alternatively it may take the form of a lymphocytosis, as is frequently found in whooping cough. Infants commonly respond to infections by producing a lymphocytosis.

Leucopenia. This means a decrease in the total number of white cells below $4.0 \times 10^9/l$ and usually involves a reduction only of the granulocytes (neutropenia). Leucopenia is found in tuberculosis, enteric fever, many acute viral infections, brucellosis, during cytotoxic chemotherapy and in hypoplastic and aplastic anaemia. Occasionally leucopenia is found in overwhelming infections and is a bad prognostic sign. In a small number of patients it may be constitutional and represent no threat to health. In others it may have an immune aetiology or be early evidence of developing acute leukaemia.

Eosinophilia. This is the term used when the number of eosinophil granulocytes exceeds $0.4 \times 10^9/l$. Eosinophilia is found most commonly in infections with worms, in allergic diseases, Hodgkin's lymphoma and polyarteritis nodosa. Rarely it may be familial or idiopathic.

Monocytosis. This refers to a monocyte count exceeding $0.8 \times 10^9/l$ and is found in advanced tuberculosis, malaria, in some neutropenic states, reactive leucocytosis and in leukaemic disorders.

Thrombocytopenia. This means a diminution in the number of blood platelets and is clinically significant only below a figure of $100 \times 10^9/l$. Capillary bleeding tends to occur when the platelet count falls below $40 \times 10^9/l$ but there is a variable correlation between the platelet count and bleeding tendency.

Leucoerythroblastic. This is used to describe a blood picture in which primitive granulocytes and erythroblasts are simultaneously present in the peripheral blood. It is usually but not necessarily associated with anaemia and reflects bone marrow irritation, as in malignant infiltration of the marrow, or disordered haemopoiesis, as in myclofibrosis.

Extramedullary haemopoiesis. This means that production of blood cells takes place outside the normal sites. It occurs not uncommonly in the first year of life when the available bone marrow space is insufficient to allow for an increased demand for blood formation.

DISEASES OF THE ERYTHROCYTES

THE ANAEMIAS

Anaemia may be defined as a state in which the blood haemoglobin level is below the normal range for the patient's age and sex.

At birth the haemoglobin is high (200 g/l) because fetal haemoglobin has a higher oxygen affinity than adult haemoglobin. In the first 3 months of life lower affinity haemoglobin A replaces haemoglobin F. The haemoglobin level rapidly drops, partly by removal of effete red cells but also by reduced production, reaching about half the birth level when the baby is 3 months of age.

Thereafter the average level rises gradually until the child reaches puberty when a further rise occurs which is more marked in males than females.

Adult males have haemoglobin levels on average 20 g/l higher than adult females. This reflects the stimulus of androgens on erythropoiesis. A haemoglobin level of 120 g/l is regarded as anaemic in an adult male, but normal in an adult female. In practice, most adults who are otherwise in reasonably good health function satisfactorily if the haemoglobin is above 100 g/l, provided this lower level has not appeared quickly.

The presence of symptoms related to anaemia depends partly on its severity but also on how rapidly the anaemia develops. Thus a patient who has a reduction of haemoglobin from 130 g/l to 80 g/l in 1 week may have severe symptoms, while another patient whose anaemia has developed slowly to a similar level over months may be asymptomatic.

Aetiology

The causes of anaemia are summarised in the information box below.

CLASSIFICATION OF ANAEMIA

- Blood loss, which may be either acute or chronic (haemorrhage)
- Inadequate production of normal red cells by the bone marrow (hypoplasia; aplasia)
- Excessive destruction of red blood cells (haemolysis)

This classification of the anaemias helps to guide the clinician in planning investigation as it reflects what is happening. Most anaemias are multifactorial in their aetiology and many causes are relatively rare. The vast majority of anaemias are due to inadequate erythrocyte production caused by failure of haemoglobin synthesis due to iron deficiency, the commonest reason for which is blood loss.

Alternatively, anaemias can be classified on the basis of the morphology of the red cell as:

1. normocytic
2. microcytic and
3. macrocytic.

Clinical features of anaemia reflect the diminished oxygen carrying capacity of the blood. Their severity depends on the degree of anaemia and the rapidity of its development, but are independent of its type.

The symptoms and signs of anaemia are listed in Table 14.2.

Table 14.2   Symptoms and signs of anaemia

Symptoms	Signs
Lassitude	Pallor of
Fatigue	Skin
Breathlessness	Mucous membranes
on exertion	Palms of hands
Palpitations	Conjunctivae
Throbbing in head	Tachycardia
and ears	Cardiac dilatation
Dizziness	Systolic flow murmurs
Tinnitus	Oedema
Headache	
Dimness of vision	
Insomnia	
Paraesthesia in fingers and toes	
Angina	

ANAEMIAS DUE TO BLOOD LOSS

Classification

1. Acute (large volume over short period)
2. Chronic (small volume over long period)

Acute blood loss
A healthy adult can lose about half a litre of blood without ill effect. When more is lost, compensatory mechanisms come into play which reduce the blood flow to peripheral tissues such as skin and muscle, and conserve the supply for central organs. The pulse rate rises and blood pressure is maintained. The patient is pale, cold and sweaty and has to lie flat in order to maintain the cerebral circulation; hypovolaemic shock may ensue. At this stage the haemoglobin level and haematocrit of the blood is unchanged and in some cases it may be higher than before the acute blood loss. If no further bleeding occurs, plasma production

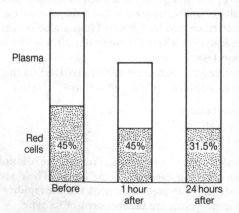

Fig. 14.7   Effect of acute blood loss of 30% of total blood volume on the haematocrit.

replenishes the volume, diluting the remaining red cells, and anaemia appears in about 24–36 hours (Fig. 14.7). If blood loss is very severe, compensatory mechanisms fail and irreversible hypovolaemic shock supervenes, progressing to death. Anaemia may not have had time to appear.

The primary problem in acute blood loss is lack of blood volume which must be replaced by transfusion of whole blood, red cell concentrate, plasma or plasma substitutes. The anaemia which appears later, if red cells are not given or if plasma or plasma substitutes are used, will be corrected in the ensuing few weeks by increased red cell production unless the body iron stores are depleted. When acute blood loss is associated with other diseases, which themselves impair erythropoiesis, recovery of the haemoglobin level may be slow and the anaemia may become chronic. Immediately after acute blood loss there may be a transient leucoerythroblastic blood picture. A few days later a reticulocytosis develops, subsiding gradually as the haemoglobin level recovers. A transient rise in platelet count may also occur.

Chronic blood loss
This does not give rise to reduction in blood volume or immediately to anaemia because the body has time to compensate by increased plasma and red cell production. Eventually, however, the continued loss of red cells depletes the iron stores, red cell production is impaired, and anaemia due to iron deficiency appears.

ANAEMIAS DUE TO INADEQUATE PRODUCTION OF RED CELLS

The causes of inadequate production of red blood cells are listed in the information box (p. 709).

IRON DEFICIENCY ANAEMIA

Iron deficiency is by far the commonest cause of anaemia in most parts of the world.

Aetiology
Iron deficiency usually results from either loss of iron due to bleeding, an inadequate diet (p. 56) or malabsorption (p. 446). Occasionally iron may be lost in the urine in the form of haemosiderin. Of these causes, loss due to bleeding in greater amounts than can be balanced in absorption is by far the most common.

There are periods in life when iron deficiency may be regarded as almost physiological. At birth the normal infant has a store in the form of a very high haemoglobin level and in addition some iron is

CAUSES OF INADEQUATE PRODUCTION OF ERYTHROCYTES

Deficiency of essential factors
Iron, vitamin B_{12} or folate

Toxic factors
Inflammatory disease
Hepatic and renal failure
Drugs

Endocrine deficiencies
Hypothyroidism
Hypoadrenalism
Hypopituitarism
Hypogonadism
Reduced production of erythropoietin

Invasion of bone marrow
Leukaemia, secondary carcinoma, fibrosis

Disorders of developing red cells
Sideroblastic anaemia
Neoplastic disorders of erythropoiesis
Other idiopathic refractory anaemias
Hereditary disorders of haemoglobin synthesis (thalassaemia)

Failure of stem cells
Hypoplastic and aplastic anaemia

available in the liver. This is adequate for erythropoietic requirements in the first few months of life. Thereafter a mild degree of deficiency appears because milk is a very poor source of iron. If weaning is delayed for 1 or 2 years, as is the custom in certain parts of the world, deficiency may become marked. The deficiency is fairly quickly corrected if the child is weaned to a good diet. When prematurity and haemorrhage from the cord at birth deprive the infant of the normal store of iron, deficiency may appear sooner and be more severe.

In adolescents, in whom a marked growth spurt occurs, iron requirements may outstrip absorption. Food fads are not uncommon at this age and may contribute.

Menstruation causes an average loss of 30 mg of iron per month requiring increased absorption of approximately 1 mg daily. Although this loss disappears during pregnancy, the mother requires additional iron for the fetus, the placenta, her own increased red cell mass and blood loss at parturition. The daily requirements will be about 2.5 mg plus her own basic requirement of 1 mg a day, a total of 3.5 mg. This increased demand for iron rises as pregnancy progresses and is therefore greatest in the second half of pregnancy. Because of these factors iron deficiency is more common in females than males during the reproductive years.

In post-menopausal women and adult men the commonest cause of iron deficiency is gastrointestinal bleeding, for example from erosions associated with anti-inflammatory drugs, neoplastic disease and peptic ulcers. Infestation with hookworm and schistosomiasis is very common and is the main cause of iron deficiency in many parts of the world.

At all ages, a diet containing inadequate iron (p. 56) can cause or contribute to iron deficiency anaemia. Elderly people, particularly men, living alone, are susceptible.

Clinical features

There are often no symptoms and the deficiency may be discovered incidentally. Vague symptoms of tiredness are insufficient to make some patients seek medical help. The symptomatology of iron deficiency is mainly that of anaemia (Table 14.2). However, there are some characteristic features. Angular stomatitis, glossitis and brittle finger nails are relatively common. Evidence of nail cracking is common but flattening or concavity of the nails, (koilonychia), is rare. Dysphagia is very rare but when present should raise the possibility of a post-cricoid web (Plummer-Vinson Syndrome). Pica, the eating of strange items, such as coal, earth, or foods in great excess, such as tomatoes or greens is more common than generally realised and may be uncovered only if the patient is specifically asked. Splenomegaly is uncommon unless the anaemia is severe and may reflect other disease such as portal hypertension, of which the iron deficiency is also symptomatic.

Investigations

The first abnormality to appear is microcytosis. Later, hypochromia occurs due to a reduced amount of haemoglobin in the red cells. Elliptical cells and later poikilocytes are also seen. Some target cells may be found but often indicate other disorders (p. 706). The haematological findings are a reduced haemoglobin with normal or slightly reduced red cell count and a low mean cell volume (MCV) of less than 76 fl. The white cell and differential counts are usually normal, although hypersegmentation of the neutrophils commonly occurs. The erythrocyte sedimentation rate (ESR) is usually lower than would be expected for the degree of anaemia or associated disease. A raised platelet count may suggest that bleeding is the cause of the deficiency (Table 14.3). Bone marrow iron stores are found to be empty when stained by the Prussian blue technique.

The iron transport protein transferrin is normally about one-third saturated with iron. Saturation below

Table 14.3 Diagnostic features of iron deficiency

Haemoglobin (Hb)	Variably reduced
Mean cell volume (MCV)	Reduced – microcytosis
Erythrocyte count	Normal or reduced less than Hb level would suggest
Blood film	Hypochromia, microcytosis, oval and elliptical cells, poikilocytes in more severe cases
Leucocyte count and differential	Normal Normal
Platelet count	Normal or raised
ESR	Less elevated than degree of anaemia might suggest
Bone marrow iron stores	Empty
Plasma transferrin	Raised
Plasma iron	Reduced
Serum ferritin	Reduced

15% indicates iron deficiency and above 50%, iron overload or failure to utilise available iron as in pernicious anaemia. Serum ferritin is present in minute quantities and is measurable only by radio-immunometric means. The range is wide in both sexes, mean values being higher in males. The levels, which generally correlate well with body iron stores, are very low in iron deficiency and raised in iron overload.

Diagnosis of the cause of iron deficiency
The direction of the investigations will obviously be influenced by the age and sex of the patient, the history and the findings on examination. Excessive menstrual loss and repeated pregnancy are common causes. In the absence of any clear lead, evidence of gastrointestinal blood loss should first be sought with faecal occult blood tests, barium meal, enema and endoscopy. Negative barium studies or occult blood tests should not be accepted as evidence of the absence of lesions. ^{51}Cr-labelled red cells may be used to measure blood loss into the gut. The patient's erythrocytes are labelled and reinfused. The level of radioactivity in the stool provides an accurate measurement of the amount of blood lost.

In tropical countries the stools and urine should be examined for hookworm infestation and schistosomiasis. Patients in whom there is a known cause of intravascular red cell destruction, such as a prosthetic heart valve, should have the urine tested for haemosiderin.

Management
Most patients can be treated orally and the cheapest preparation is dried ferrous sulphate given as a tablet containing 200 mg of the salt (60 mg elemental iron) 3 times daily. A small proportion of patients develop dyspepsia, constipation or diarrhoea. If this occurs more expensive proprietary preparations may be tried. Delayed release preparations are to be avoided as they release little iron in the upper jejunum where absorption is best. Proprietary liquid preparations may be used.

A response to oral medication usually appears in under 2 weeks. If no response is seen, it may be that the patient is not taking the tablets. A check may be made by examining the stool which will be grey or black if the patient is taking iron.

The reticulocyte response to iron therapy is usually modest and seldom above 10%. Iron should be continued for at least 6 months after the haemoglobin level has returned to normal, and in some patients for a year in order to replenish iron stores. In patients with malabsorption, or chronic loss as in haemosiderinuria, continuous oral therapy may be required or the iron may be given parenterally.

Parenteral iron therapy
This is suitable for the very few patients who are genuinely unable to take iron by mouth because of pain, vomiting or diarrhoea, who are unable to absorb iron because of some disorder of the gastrointestinal tract or who are unreliable in taking oral preparations. Iron given by injection has also been used for the treatment of the anaemia of rheumatoid arthritis, for the correction of severe anaemia in the late stages of pregnancy and following major operations.

The recommended single dose of iron-sorbitol is 1.5 mg of iron per kg of body weight given daily. It is assumed that about 250 mg of iron are required to increase the haemoglobin level by 10 g/l but the total dosage of iron should not exceed 2.5 g. *Iron-sorbitol should be given by intramuscular injection, never intravenously.*

Iron-dextran is seldom given intramuscularly because of local irritation and reports of sarcomatous change in experimental animals. It can be given intravenously by what is known as the 'total dose infusion method' in a suitable diluent. Alarming systemic anaphylactic reactions can occur.

Hypochromic anaemia of chronic disease
A blood film appearance similar to that of iron deficiency anaemia may be seen in chronic inflammatory or neoplastic diseases despite the presence of abundant stores of iron in the marrow. There is inhibition of mobilisation of storage iron for haemo-

globin formation. The microcytic, hypochromic blood picture is associated with a low serum iron but also normal or low levels of transferrin; the saturation of the transferrin is usually less reduced than in iron deficiency anaemia with a similar level of serum iron. Saturation of the transferrin below 15% almost always means iron deficiency. Although iron can be observed in the storage cells in the marrow virtually no sideroblasts are seen. Serum ferritin levels are normal reflecting the true state of the body iron stores.

THE MEGALOBLASTIC ANAEMIAS

Haemopoietic tissue is one of a number of rapidly proliferating tissues in which DNA synthesis is intense. Both vitamin B_{12} and folate are essential for DNA synthesis and deficiency of either or both causes a failure of DNA synthesis and disordered cell proliferation. Haemopoiesis is particularly susceptible and division of cells is delayed and eventually halted. Morphological changes appear in the marrow cells. In the erythrocyte series these changes are described as megaloblastic because the cells appear abnormally large. Changes also occur in the granulocyte precursors (giant metamyelocytes) and megakaryocytes and disordered morphology can be seen in other rapidly dividing cells such as those of the gastrointestinal tract.

Cell division occurs rapidly in normal erythrocyte production. Between divisions the cells do not have time to regrow to their full size and a progressive size reduction occurs. When DNA synthesis is impaired, the time between divisions increases, more cell growth occurs and the cells become larger. The cells also undergo less divisions probably because the synthesis of haemoglobin is unimpaired. Haemoglobin production appears to be one of the factors limiting proliferation. Once a certain haemoglobin level has been reached, division stops. Thus in megaloblastic disorders not only do the erythrocyte precursors have time to grow to a larger size between division, they also undergo less divisions, both factors contributing to the macrocytosis. The end products are abnormally large and misshapen red cells which are well haemoglobinised. As dysplasia becomes advanced erythrocyte fragments appear and the MCV may drop. Despite anaemia the reticulocyte count is low. There is usually leucopenia and thrombocytopenia.

The massive destruction of marrow cells from dyserythropoiesis liberates large amounts of enzyme including lactate dehydrogenase (LDH) which rises to very high levels in the blood. Eventually, in the absence of treatment, cell production fails.

Excessive doses of anti-metabolites such as those used in the treatment of cancer which interfere with DNA synthesis (p. 239) have similar effects and may induce severe dysplasia and morphological changes in the marrow and blood very similar to those produced by vitamin B_{12} and folate deficiency.

The findings on investigation of a megaloblastic anaemia whatever the cause are given in Table 14.4.

Table 14.4   Diagnostic features of a megaloblastic anaemia

Investigation	Result
Haemoglobin	Often reduced, may be very low
Mean cell volume (MCV)	Usually raised, commonly > 120 fl
Erythrocyte count	Low for degree of anaemia
Reticulocyte count	Low for degree of anaemia
Leucocyte count	Low normal or reduced
Platelet count	Low normal or reduced
Blood film	Oval macrocytosis, poikilocytosis, red cell fragmentation, neutrophil hypersegmentation
Bone marrow	Increased cellularity, megaloblastic change in erythroid series, giant metamyelocytes, dysplastic megakaryocytes, increased iron in stores, pathological non-ring sideroblasts
Serum iron	Elevated
Iron binding capacity	Increased saturation
Serum ferritin	Elevated
Plasma LDH	Elevated, often markedly

Most patients with megaloblastic anaemia suffer from deficiency of either vitamin B_{12} or folate which is demonstrated by deficiency blood levels of these vitamins.

Vitamin B_{12}. This is a cobalt-containing porphyrin, cobalamin. The absorption of vitamin B_{12} from the lower ileum is facilitated by gastric intrinsic factor, a glycoprotein synthesised by gastric parietal cells, which complexes with ingested vitamin B_{12} in the stomach. The complex is taken up at special binding sites in the ileum where the vitamin B_{12} is released to the ileal cells. Intrinsic factor is not absorbed. After absorption vitamin B_{12} is bound to a carrier protein in the plasma, transcobalamin II, transported to the tissues and taken up by cells as required. Vitamin B_{12} is stored in the liver where there may be up to 3 years supply.

Deficiency of vitamin B_{12}. This vitamin is obtained mainly from animal foodstuffs. Vegetables alone are an inadequate source. Normal requirements of vitamin B_{12} are 1–2 µg daily. Deficiency takes at least 3

CAUSES OF VITAMIN B₁₂ DEFICIENCY

- Inadequate diet (true vegans)
- Intrinsic factor deficiency due to:
  Gastric atrophy as in pernicious anaemia
  Gastrectomy
  Congenital deficiency without gastric atrophy (rare)
- Disease of the terminal ileum reducing or eliminating the absorption site
  e.g. Crohn's disease
- Vitamin B₁₂ may be removed from the gut either by:
  Bacterial proliferation in blind loops
  Parasites such as the fish tapeworm
  (Table 5.36, p. 171)

---

years to appear and occurs because of the factors listed in the information box above.

Prevalence. The majority of patients with vitamin B_{12} deficiency have pernicious anaemia. Addisonian pernicious anaemia appears to be relatively uncommon in tropical countries and in some areas quite rare.

ADDISONIAN PERNICIOUS ANAEMIA

The term Addisonian pernicious anaemia should be limited to megaloblastic anaemia due to a failure of secretion of intrinsic factor by the stomach other than from total gastrectomy. It is an autoimmune disease and in about 50% of patients antibodies to intrinsic factor can be demonstrated. The disease is rare before the age of 30, occurs mainly between 45–65 years and affects females more than males.

Pathology

There is evidence of increased blood destruction – including unconjugated hyperbilirubinaemia and increased deposition of iron (haemosiderin) in the liver, spleen, kidneys and bone marrow. The gastric mucosa is thin and atrophic.

Clinical features

The onset is insidious and the degree of anaemia is often great before the patient consults the doctor. In addition to the general symptoms of anaemia there may be intermittent soreness of the tongue and periodic diarrhoea.

The patient generally appears well nourished despite the fact that weight loss is a common feature. The skin and mucous membranes are pale and in severely anaemic cases the skin and conjunctivae may show a lemon yellow tint. The surface of the tongue is usually smooth and atrophic, but sometimes it is red and

inflamed. The spleen may be palpable. In many patients paraesthesiae occur in the fingers and toes and occasionally there are signs of subacute combined degeneration (p. 903), which can appear before the anaemia. Dementia may also occur. In young females there may be infertility.

Investigations

Helpful findings in the diagnosis of Addisonian pernicious anaemia are given in the information box below.

DIAGNOSTIC FEATURES OF ADDISONIAN PERNICIOUS ANAEMIA

Diagnostic findings
Very low serum vitamin B₁₂ often less than 50 ng/l
Anti-intrinsic factor antibodies in serum (present in 50%)

Corroborative findings
Macrocytic, dysplastic blood picture
Megablastic marrow
Abnormal vitamin B₁₂ absorption test corrected by addition of intrinsic factor (Schilling Test)
Pentagastrin fast achlorhydria

OTHER CAUSES OF MEGALOBLASTIC ANAEMIA DUE TO VITAMIN B₁₂ DEFICIENCY

Dietary insufficiency. This is rare unless meat and other animal foodstuffs are not eaten. The deficiency is readily corrected by the parenteral administration of vitamin B_{12}. Thereafter the vitamin should be given by mouth.

Gastrectomy. Total resection of the stomach results in a complete loss of intrinsic factor production and failure to absorb vitamin B_{12}. The patient requires life-long vitamin B_{12} injections. Partial gastrectomy reduces vitamin B_{12} absorption, in some cases to the point that deficiency occurs. Gastritis may, in part, be responsible. The Schilling test often demonstrates reduced absorption. One annual injection of 1000 µg of hydroxocobalamin is adequate prophylaxis for a patient who has had a partial gastrectomy.

Disease of the terminal ileum. This should be suspected if the Schilling test is not corrected by the addition of adequate amounts of intrinsic factor.

Bacterial colonisation of the small intestine (p. 450). This results in an abnormal Schilling test, both without and with intrinsic factor; this is corrected by the administration of tetracycline.

Folic acid and interaction with vitamin B$_{12}$
Folic acid (pteroylglutamic acid) and related compounds are known as folates. Folic acid as such is available only as a medicinal compound. The body obtains folates by the breakdown of food polyglutamates to monoglutamates in the small intestine or mucosal cell. In the plasma, folate appears as methyl tetrahydrofolate which is changed to tetrahydrofolate (THF) by a pathway for which vitamin B$_{12}$ is essential (Fig. 14.8). Without this, active folate coenzymes are poorly formed. 5, 10 methylene THF is the form essential for the synthesis of DNA. Dihydrofolate from this step is reconverted to THF by dihydrofolate

reductase, an enzyme inhibited by the folate antagonist, methotrexate. Formyl THF (folinic acid) will bypass both the metabolic blocks created by vitamin B$_{12}$ deficiency or methotrexate and acts as an antidote to this drug. Clinically folinic acid or folic acid must not be used to treat vitamin B$_{12}$ deficiency or severe neurological damage may result (p. 903) although the anaemia may be corrected. Daily requirement of folate for a normal healthy adult is 100 μg.

MEGALOBLASTIC ANAEMIAS DUE TO FOLATE DEFICIENCY

Folate occurs mainly in the form of polyglutamates in both vegetable and animal foodstuffs. Much is destroyed by cooking. Body stores are relatively small, lasting only a few weeks. It is absorbed mainly in the jejunum. Its metabolism thereafter is shown in Fig. 14.8. The causes of folate deficiency are shown in the information box below.

Prevalence
Approximately 60% of all megaloblastic anaemias in

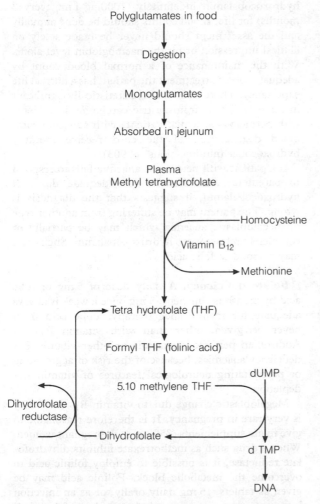

Fig. 14.8 **Metabolic pathway showing interaction of vitamin B$_{12}$ and folate in the synthesis of DNA.**

CAUSES OF FOLATE DEFICIENCY

Inadequate intake
Diets which totally lack fresh vegetables and meat or which consist of overcooked food, may not provide enough folate.

Disease of upper small bowel
As in coeliac disease or sprue; very rarely extensive resection of the small bowel has a similar effect.

The body's demands exceeding intake
● When there is very active cell proliferation, e.g. haemolytic anaemia, leukaemias and other neoplastic disease, during periods of acute or chronic infection and in extensive psoriasis.

● Pregnancy, when the demands of the fetus and placental growth require large amounts of folate. In this situation folate is taken by the fetus in amounts adequate for its needs, even when the mother is folate deficient. There is no evidence that the fetus is ever affected by folate deficiency in the mother.

Interference with the dihydrofolate reductase system
This enzyme system may be blocked by certain drugs, particularly, methotrexate. In theory trimethoprim may also do this but a real danger appears to exist only in patients deficient in folate from another cause.

An unexplained mechanism
Alcoholism and the anti-epileptic drugs phenytoin and primidone may cause folate depletion by an unknown mechanism not related to interference with the dihydrofolate reductase system.

Britain are due to folate deficiency. In tropical countries most megaloblastic disease is due to folate deficiency associated with malnutrition, infection and pregnancy.

Clinical features

These are those of anaemia and of the underlying cause. Glossitis is less common than in vitamin B_{12} deficiency. Neurological problems are very rare.

Investigations

Diagnostic features of a folic acid deficiency anaemia are given in the information box below.

DIAGNOSTIC FEATURES OF FOLIC ACID DEFICIENCY

Diagnostic findings
Low serum folate levels (fasting blood sample)
Red cell folate levels low (but may be normal if folate deficiency is of very recent onset)

Corroborative findings
Macrocytic dysplastic blood picture
Megaloblastic marrow
Normal or only marginally reduced serum vitamin B_{12} levels

---

Management

General

The decision to give a blood transfusion in a patient with a megaloblastic anaemia is based on general principles concerning the clinical state of the patient. It should be seriously considered when the haemoglobin level is so low as to endanger life, e.g. under 40 g/l. In all types of chronic anaemia of sufficient severity to require transfusion the blood should be given very slowly, preferably as red cell concentrate, because of the danger of producing cardiac failure. A diuretic is given simultaneously (frusemide, 40–80 mg).

Specific

Vitamin B_{12} deficiency. Hydroxocobalamin is given parenterally in a dosage of 1000 μg twice during the first week, then 1000 μg weekly for a further 6 doses. Within 48 hours of the first injection the bone marrow shows a striking change from a megaloblastic to a normoblastic state. The serum iron drops precipitously and hypokalaemia may be a problem sufficient to require replacement therapy. Within 2–3 days the reticulocyte count begins to rise, reaching a maximum between the fifth and tenth days. The response may be delayed if there is coexisting inflammatory disease or if the patient has been transfused. There is a brief peak of erythrocyte output due to the maturation of the large number of cells held in maturation arrest by the vitamin B_{12} deficiency. Depending on the initial erythrocyte count the proportion of reticulocytes may rise above 50% but soon falls to below 10% as more normal production is resumed.

In some patients the rapid regeneration of the blood depletes the iron reserves of the body and recovery is halted. To prevent this, ferrous sulphate 200 mg t.i.d. should be given soon after the commencement of treatment. A combined deficiency of vitamin B_{12} and iron is recognised by the presence of macrocytosis and hypochromia – a dimorphic blood picture.

Maintenance treatment

The patient must be given regular parenteral doses of hydroxocobalamin indefinitely (1000 μg i.m. every 3 months) for life. Blood counts should be done annually and the assessment should never be made solely on clinical impression or on the haemoglobin level alone. With the maintenance of a normal blood count by adequate specific treatment the patient has a normal life expectancy. There is, however, a statistically significant increase in deaths from gastric carcinoma in patients with pernicious anaemia. Patients with subacute combined degeneration of the cord receive monthly hydroxocobalamin injections (p. 903).

If a patient with pernicious anaemia fails to respond to parenteral administration of adequate doses of hydroxocobalamin, it suggests that the diagnosis is wrong. The patient may be suffering from another type of megaloblastic anaemia which may be partially or completely refractory to hydroxocobalamin. Such cases may respond to folic acid.

Folate deficiency. A daily dose of 5 mg of folic acid by mouth is sufficient; 5 mg once a week is always adequate for maintenance therapy. Folic acid must never be given, other than with vitamin B_{12}, in Addisonian pernicious anaemia or other vitamin B_{12} deficiency anaemias, because of the risk of aggravating or precipitating neurological features of vitamin B_{12} depletion.

Megaloblastic change due to vitamin B_{12} deficiency is very rare in pregnancy. It is therefore reasonable to give folate supplements (350 μg/d) to pregnant women. When a drug such as methotrexate inhibits dihydrofolate reductase, it is possible to employ folinic acid to overcome the metabolic block. Folinic acid may be given as tablets, 15 mg daily orally, or as an injection intravenously or intramuscularly at a dose of 3 mg/ml. Folinic acid mouthwashes are used to counteract the oral side-effects of folate antagonist drugs. Megaloblastic disorder caused by other cytotoxic drugs which inhibit DNA synthesis is not reversed by either vitamin B_{12} or folate administration.

PRIMARY IDIOPATHIC ACQUIRED APLASTIC ANAEMIA

This is a rare but grave disease of the stem cells which fail to a varying degree, producing serious hypoplasia of the marrow elements. An autoimmune mechanism may be responsible.

Clinical features
The disorder may occur at any age, the peak incidence being around 30 years. The onset is insidious and the clinical problems are due to the reduction or virtual absence of production of erythrocytes, granulocytes and platelets. Infections and haemorrhage are the most troublesome complications and may prove lethal. Bleeding occurs in the skin and mucous membranes. Haematuria and epistaxis are common. Intracranial bleeding is always a risk. Necrotic mouth and throat ulcers and monilial infections reflect the neutropenia.

Investigations
Known causes of hypoplastic and aplastic anaemia must first be excluded. A careful inquiry into exposure to drugs, chemicals and radiation should be made. A history of viral illness, particularly hepatitis may be important. A full blood count demonstrates a pancytopenia. Neutropenia is the most marked aspect of the leucopenia, although leucopenia may not be the first development. The anaemia is normocytic, normochromic and often marked. Platelet production is often the most severely affected and the last to recover.

The bone marrow should be examined by aspiration and trephine. The latter provides a better assessment of cellularity; an aspirate may be difficult to obtain (dry tap). Studies with ^{59}Fe show poor clearance of the isotope from the blood, poor uptake and utilisation by the marrow and no extramedullary haemopoiesis.

Management
Bone marrow transplantation (p. 733) should be considered urgently in children and adults up to 50 years. No blood products from relatives should be given until compatibility testing has been completed in order to avoid the risk of immunisation against potential donor antigens. Bone marrow transplantation now offers the best prognosis for patients under 20 years (p. 733).

There are two aspects to the management of patients unable to have bone marrow transplantation.

1. Support for the patient with replacement therapy. This consists of maintaining a reasonable haemoglobin level with red cell concentrate and platelet transfusion for bleeding. Vigorous antibiotic therapy for infection is required as outlined in the management of acute myeloblastic leukaemia (p. 730). Corticosteroids may be used to reduce bleeding but carry the risk of promoting infection.
2. Treatment to stimulate haemopoiesis and promote recovery. Androgenic steroids with low virilising activity and corticosteroids are employed, oxymetholone, 2 mg/k daily orally for 3–6 months plus prednisolone, 60 mg daily orally for 6 weeks, thereafter weaning down to lower doses. High doses (2 g daily) of methyl prednisolone may also be used.

Erythrocyte production and to a lesser extent granulocyte production benefit most from these drugs which unfortunately have undesirable and troublesome side-effects when used over long periods. This is particularly so in children in whom secondary sexual characteristics may be stimulated and premature fusion of epiphyses may occur if the treatment is not suitably curtailed. Androgens may also cause cholestasis; fluid retention and prostatic enlargement with obstruction in older men.

Intravenous antilymphocyte or antithymocyte globulin may be given where an autoimmune process is thought to be an aetiological factor. Risks include anaphylaxis and serum sickness.

Prognosis
The course tends to be prolonged. Spontaneous improvement and recovery may occur and is one reason why treatment should be vigorous and prolonged. Androgens may be ineffective in the early phase of the disease but become effective later and should not be abandoned because of initial failure. The prognosis is poor and more than 50% of patients die usually within the first year. Patients who survive longer than 1 year have a better chance of remission. In a few leukaemia supervenes and it is probable that these are patients with leukaemia presenting with an aplastic or hypoplastic phase.

Secondary pancytopenia
The causes of this condition are listed in the information box (p. 716).

In some instances the cytopenia is more selective and affects only one cell line, most often the neutrophils. Frequently this is an incidental finding unassociated

CAUSES OF SECONDARY PANCYTOPENIA

- Idiosyncrasy to certain drugs such as chloramphenicol, antithyroid drugs, indomethacin, sulpha-methoxypyridazine and tolbutamide, sulphonamides, gold compounds, anticonvulsants, antimalarials, certain industrial chemicals and insecticides chiefly benzene and its derivatives such as trinitrophenol, trinitrotoluene and gamma-benzene hexachloride
- The majority of drugs used in the chemotherapy of malignant disease
- Exposure to radiation
- Replacement of the bone marrow by abnormal cells such as tumour or fibrous tissue
- Viral infections, particularly viral hepatitis
- Deficiency states such as severe lack of vitamin B_{12} or folate

with ill health. It probably has an immune basis but this is difficult to prove.

The clinical features and methods of diagnosis are the same as for primary idiopathic aplastic anaemia. The noxious agent if identified should be removed but otherwise treatment is as for the idiopathic form. Bone marrow transplantation may be required in young patients who have HLA matched sibling donors.

DISORDERS DUE TO EXCESSIVE RED CELL DESTRUCTION

HAEMOLYTIC DISORDERS

Various abnormalities either in the erythrocyte may shorten the normal life span of 120 days. Anaemia develops when marrow output no longer compensates. The increased output of new erythrocytes is reflected in a raised reticulocyte count which gives an indication of the severity of the process. Normoblasts may be released under extreme stress.

The catabolic pathways for haemoglobin degradation are overloaded and there is a modest increase in unconjugated bilirubin in the blood and increased reabsorption of urobilinogen from the gut, which is then excreted in the urine in increased amounts. Bile does not appear in the urine. Jaundice is mild (p. 502).

Intravascular haemolysis. Haemoglobin is liberated into the plasma where it is bound mainly by the α-2 globulin, haptoglobin, to form a complex too large to be lost in the urine. It is taken up by the liver and degraded. Some haemoglobin is partially degraded and bound to albumin to form methaemalbumin. This is the basis of the *Schumm's test* for haemoglobin in the plasma.

If all the haptoglobin has been consumed, free haemoglobin may be lost in the urine. In small amounts this is reabsorbed by the renal tubules where the haemoglobin is degraded and the iron stored as haemosiderin. Sloughing of the renal tubular cells gives rise to haemosiderinuria which, if found, always indicates intravascular haemolysis. When greater amounts of haemoglobin are lost haemoglobinuria occurs, giving the urine a black appearance (black water).

Extravascular haemolysis. This occurs in the phagocytic cells of the spleen, liver, bone marrow and other organs and there may be little or no depletion of haptoglobin. Estimation of the haptoglobin level in the blood is not always easily interpreted. Inflammatory disease and steroid therapy both increase haptoglobin levels. Ahaptoglobinaemia may occur as an inherited disorder. Nevertheless absence of haptoglobin is usually a strong indicator of haemolytic disease. Its presence does not exclude haemolysis.

Blood and marrow findings

The peripheral blood shows a moderate macrocytosis and polychromasia due to reticulocytosis while specific red cell abnormalities may give a clue to the type of haemolytic disease (see information box (p. 717)). There may be a polymorphonuclear leucocytosis. The marrow shows erythroid hyperplasia. If megaloblastic change occurs it usually reflects depletion of folate reserves.

Increased erythropoietic turnover in the marrow is associated with increased levels of lactic dehydrogenase in the blood, which, in the absence of folate deficiency, closely follows the severity of the haemolytic disorder. Red cell survival can be measured crudely using radioactive chromium (^{51}Cr). Surface counting done at the same time over liver and spleen may give an indication of the site of haemolysis. If transfusion has been given the patient's blood contains a mixed cell population which is not suitable for ^{51}Cr studies. In these circumstances cross-matched donor cells should be used for labelling.

The causes of haemolytic anaemias are listed in the information box (p. 717).

HAEMOLYTIC ANAEMIA DUE TO INTRAERYTHROCYTIC CAUSES

The principal disorders are hereditary spherocytosis, glucose-6-phosphate dehydrogense (G6PD) deficiency, haemoglobinopathies (e.g. sickle-cell disease and thalassaemia). G6PD deficiency and haemoglobinopathies are

---

THE CAUSES OF HAEMOLYTIC ANAEMIA

Intra-erythrocytic defects
Hereditary
    Spherocytosis
    Disorders of glycolysis (enzyme deficiencies)
    Haemoglobinopathies (abnormal haemoglobins and
    thalassaemias)
Acquired
    Red cells produced by dyserythropoietic states, e.g.
    vitamin B_{12} and folate deficiency

Extra-erythrocytic abnormalities
    Antibodies (autoimmune and isoimmune)
    Physical trauma (prosthetic heart valve, burns)
    Chemical trauma (drugs, e.g. dapsone)
    Infections (malaria)
    Toxic factors associated with inflammatory or neoplastic
    disease and metabolic failure

---

most common in African Blacks and thalassaemia in the Mediterranean area. There has been a rise in the incidence of these disorders in other countries including Britain because of immigration.

HEREDITARY SPHEROCYTOSIS

This is an autosomal dominant disorder in which the principal abnormality appears to be a deficiency of spectrin, a red cell membrane protein. The erythrocyte envelope is abnormally permeable and the sodium pumps are overworked. The erythrocytes lose their biconcave shape, become spherical and are more susceptible to osmotic lysis. These spherocytes are destroyed almost exclusively by the spleen. The severity of the disorder is very variable even within an affected family. Haemolysis is mainly extravascular.

Clinical features

Symptoms vary from none to those of severe anaemia. Episodic jaundice may be noted. The spleen is often but not always palpably enlarged. The severity of the disorder tends to vary in any one patient with episodes of increased haemolysis (haemolytic crises) at times. The transient hypoplasia of red cell production, which can occur in normal persons in association with parvovirus infections, presents as aplastic crises in these patients because of the greatly increased red cell turnover. There is a liability to form pigment gallstones and cholecystitis may be the presenting event. Leg ulcers sometimes occur.

Investigations

The diagnosis is made by demonstrating a haemolytic state (see p. 716) together with spherocytes in the blood film, increased osmotic fragility due to the spherocytes and the demonstration of the same disorder in other members of the family. The Coomb's test is negative. There is an increased loss of urobilinogen in the urine. Red cell survival studies with ^{51}Cr show destruction of red cells almost exclusively in the spleen. The differential diagnosis is from other causes of spherocytosis, particularly the various forms of immune haemolysis (p. 723).

Management

Splenectomy results in striking and usually permanent improvement both in the symptoms and in the anaemia and should be advised when:

1. the anaemia causes persistent impairment of health;
2. when severe haemolytic or aplastic crises have occurred;
3. when other members of the family have died from the disease;
4. where evidence of cholecystitis and cholelithiasis is present.

Opinion differs as to the desirability of operation for patients with no disability. The operation should be performed during a period of remission, and in young children should be deferred until they are as old as possible and should be preceded by vaccination against pneumococcal infection. Following splenectomy, resistance to some infections may be impaired and daily penicillin V, 250 mg b.d., is prescribed for at least 5 years.

Severe haemolytic crises require treatment by blood transfusion. Blood must be matched very carefully and administered very slowly, as gross haemolytic transfusion reactions are common in this disease. Folic acid, 5 mg daily orally, is prescribed to support the increased erythropoiesis. Iron is of no value unless a genuine deficiency is demonstrated. Treatment with corticosteroids is not indicated.

GLUCOSE-6-PHOSPHATE DEHYDROGENASE DEFICIENCY

Glucose-6-phosphate dehydrogenase (G6PD) is the first enzyme in the hexose monophosphate shunt of the Embden Myerhof glycolytic pathway from which red cells derive most of their metabolic energy. The function of this shunt is to service the enzyme glutathione reductase and glutathione peroxidase which protect the red cells against damage due to oxidation. In the absence of G6PD this protective mechanism is crippled and certain drugs in sufficient concentration can seriously injure the erythrocyte.

The deficiency is inherited as a X-linked disorder with a high frequency among African Blacks among whom there is an electrophoretic enzyme polymorphism with A and B type enzymes. The enzyme is A type (A−) in deficient African Blacks. In Caucasians only the normal B type enzyme is found and the deficient type is also B (B−). In West and East Africa about 20% of male (hemizygotes) and about 4% of females (homozygous for the abnormal gene) are affected and the enzyme activity is about 15% of normal. Heterozygous females have two populations of red cells, one deficient and the other normal. 100 million persons are affected by this disorder worldwide.

The deficiency in Caucasian and Oriental populations is more severe, enzyme activity being less than 1% of normal. Favism (haemolytic anaemia from the ingestion of the broad bean, Vicia faba) is due to deficiency of G6PD of the severe variety (B−). Some cases of haemolytic disease of the newborn are caused by this deficiency. Other rare types of G6PD, biochemically different from the above may be associated with congenital nonspherocytic haemolytic disease and occur sporadically in all races.

Many drugs in common clinical use, e.g. some antimalarials and sulphonamides, are capable of precipitating haemolysis in individuals with G6PD deficiency. Infections may also potentiate the haemolytic action of drugs such as aspirin, chloramphenicol, and chloroquine.

Clinical features

Persons with G6PD deficiency normally enjoy good health but are liable to haemolysis if any of the incriminated drugs or foods are ingested. However the haemolytic effect is dose related and will not be clinically detectable if the amount does not exceed a critical level. It is often possible to employ doses which are not toxic. The anaemia, when it occurs, may be rapid in onset, becoming obvious between 2 and 10 days after exposure to the precipitating agent and may be sufficiently severe to cause haemoglobinuria as well as the other classical signs of haemolysis. In the relatively mild type of deficiency prevalent in Blacks only older cells which have lost enzyme activity are involved so that the haemolysis is to some extent self-limiting even when the offending agent is continued. Young red cells have some G6PD activity and remain viable until their enzyme complement decays. The enzyme deficiency is much more severe in the B-variety, and destruction tends to be greater. Anuria is an infrequent but serious complication.

Investigation

The diagnosis can be confirmed by estimating the G6PD activity of the red cell but this may not be entirely accurate if there is a considerable reticulocytosis. A number of screening tests are also available. The characteristics of intravascular haemolysis are usually present: haemoglobinaemia, methaemalbuminaemia, haemoglobinuria, ahaptoglobinaemia and later haemosiderinuria.

Management

This is by removal of the toxic agent. Recovery is usually rapid but if the anaemia is severe, transfusion of red cells with a normal enzyme complement may be required. Thereafter the patient should be advised to avoid drugs which may precipitate the disorder. Splenectomy is valueless.

THE HAEMOGLOBINOPATHIES

The haemoglobinopathies can be classified into two subgroups:

1. Where there is an alteration in the amino acid structure of the polypeptide chains of the globin fraction of haemoglobin, commonly called the abnormal haemoglobins. The best known example is haemoglobin S found in sickle-cell anaemia. Some 'abnormal' haemoglobins function as normal variants.
2. Where the amino-acid sequence is normal but polypeptide chain production is impaired or absent for a variety of reasons; these are the thalassaemias.

Abnormal haemoglobins are caused by amino acid substitutions in their polypeptide chains. These in turn reflect mutations in the structural genes controlling the production of these chains. There are several hundred haemoglobin variants known, some functionally normal, most not. Originally they were designated by letters of the alphabet, e.g. S, C, E and so on. Now this does not suffice and for some years new variants have been given names, often of the towns or districts in which they were discovered. Sickle-cell haemoglobin or haemoglobin S is the most important but haemoglobin C, D and E are also significant in some parts of the world, particularly when inherited along with haemoglobin S or with beta thalassaemia (p. 722).

Modern nomenclature includes a statement of the site of the amino acid substitution. Thus sickle haemoglobin may be defined as:

$$\text{Hb S}^{6\text{GLU−VAL}} \qquad \text{Hb S}^{\text{A3GLU−VAL}}$$

The second method is more accurate since it defines the helix or bend in which the substitution occurs.

Control of haemoglobin synthesis is inherited from both parents. Thus a normal adult can be depicted as having the haemoglobin genotype AA, sickle-cell trait by AS and sickle-cell anaemia or homozygous S disease by SS. The inheritance when both parents have sickle-cell trait can be shown thus:

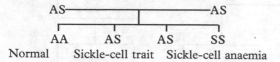

Normal   Sickle-cell trait   Sickle-cell anaemia

There is a 1:4 chance with each pregnancy that the offspring will have sickle-cell anaemia.

SICKLE-CELL ANAEMIA (HOMOZYGOUS Hb S DISEASE)

Epidemiology

The patient with sickle-cell trait is relatively resistant to the lethal effects of falciparum malaria in early childhood. The high incidence of this deleterious gene in equatorial Africa is thus explained by the selective advantage for survival it confers in an environment of endemic falciparum malaria. Patients with sickle-cell anaemia do not have correspondingly greater resistance to falciparum malaria.

Pathogenesis

When haemoglobin S is deoxygenated, the molecules of haemoglobin polymerise to form pseudo-crystalline structures known as 'tactoids'. These distort the red cell membrane and produce characteristic sickle-shaped cells. The polymerisation is reversible when reoxygenation occurs. The distortion of the red cell membrane, however, may become permanent and the red cell 'irreversibly sickled'. The greater the concentration of sickle-cell haemoglobin in the individual cell, the more easily are tactoids formed, but this process may be enhanced or retarded by the presence of other haemoglobins. Thus haemoglobin C participates in the polymerisation more readily than haemoglobin A, whereas haemoglobin F strongly inhibits polymerisation.

In sickle-cell anaemia most of the red cells contain haemoglobin S and little else and are very prone to sickle even in vivo under normal conditions. This happens particularly in those parts of the microvasculature which are sinusoidal and where the flow is sluggish. Sickled cells increase blood viscosity, traverse capillaries poorly and tend to obstruct flow, thereby increasing the sickling of other cells and eventually

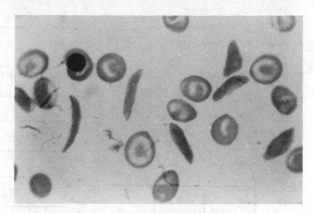

Fig. 14.9   Blood film from a patient with sickle cell anaemia. It shows characteristic sickled cells, target cells and a normoblast.

stopping the flow. Thrombosis follows and an area of tissue infarction results causing severe pain, swelling and tenderness (infarction crisis). In addition these cells are phagocytosed in large numbers by the mononuclear-phagocyte system, reducing their life span considerably and giving rise to haemolysis.

Clinical features

The two major problems are chronic anaemia due to reduced erythrocyte survival and episodes of tissue infarction (Fig. 14.10).

Anaemia

Problems do not arise until about the fourth month of life when haemoglobin F containing cells give way to haemoglobin S containing cells. The anaemia is haemolytic in type and severe, the haemoglobin seldom rising above 100 g/l and averaging approximately 80 g/l. Secondary folate deficiency is common and exacerbates the anaemia. When folate deficiency is chronic, growth may be retarded and puberty delayed. Episodes of increased sequestration and destruction of red cells (haemolytic crises) occur, sometimes for no apparent reason and may lead to a swift fall in haemoglobin with rapidly enlarging spleen and liver. Aplastic crises occur in association with parvovirus infections as in hereditary spherocytosis (p. 717) but the effect of the temporary cessation of erythropoiesis may be more dramatic as the haemolysis is severe.

The chronic anaemia is responsible for fatigue, reduced exercise tolerance, increased susceptibility to infection, cardiomegaly, leg ulcers and cholelithiasis. Hyperplasia of the marrow in the first year of life expands the marrow cavity producing bossing of the skull, prominent malar bones and protuberant teeth.

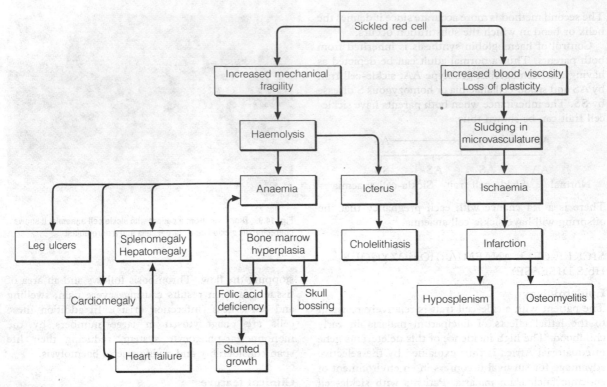

Fig. 14.10   Clinical effects of sickled red cells.

Infarction crises

These are characterised by episodes of severe pain and these punctuate the patients' lives. They occur commonly in bones and spleen but no tissue is exempt. In the infant they classically affect the fingers and toes, producing large fusiform swellings (dactylitis). Metacarpal and tarsal bones may be affected and shortened digits due to epiphyseal involvement may occur. Mesenteric infarction may produce an acute abdominal emergency at any age. The renal papilla is another site of damage and infarction may give rise to painless haematuria. In adults aseptic necrosis of the head of the femur is a disabling complication. An acute chest syndrome can occur resembling pneumonia but is probably due to pulmonary infarction.

Precipitating factors include dehydration, chilling and infection, but sometimes the attacks occur spontaneously. The onset is usually rapid and the pain excruciatingly severe (pain crisis) in the first 24 hours, thereafter abating over the next few days. Fever, increasing jaundice and malaise are frequent and, if persistent, may suggest the establishment of infection in the infarcted site. Salmonella osteomyelitis is common.

Pregnancy is hazardous unless careful antenatal care is provided and as full-term approaches, infarctive crises in the bones may liberate large amounts of fat and bone marrow emboli which cause diffuse microembolism of the lungs with pulmonary infarction, cor pulmonale and even death. A pseudo-toxaemia syndrome may develop. These complications may also be seen in the less severe haemoglobin SC disease.

Sickle-cell anaemia should always be suspected in a patient who has had symptoms of anaemia and 'rheumatism' since infancy and who belongs to a race which is often affected. In areas where sickle-cell anaemia is common, it should be considered in the differential diagnosis of many disorders. Patients must be adequately screened before major surgery and bloodless field surgery should never be employed because infarction of the entire limb below the tourniquet may occur.

Investigations

Diagnosis is based on the patient's race, history, clinical findings and investigations which demonstrate the presence of Hb S and no other major haemoglobin in the blood. These include solubility screening tests and haemoglobin electrophoresis. A family study should reveal that both parents carry the abnormal gene for Hb S. In this way true sickle-cell anaemia can be differentiated from other diseases in which haemoglobin S is combined with thalassaemia or some other abnormal haemoglobin such as C or D.

Antenatal diagnosis is discussed on page 22.

Management
There is no method of changing the genetic constitution of an individual and therefore no means of curing this disease other than by bone marrow transplantation. Management is aimed at alleviation of the symptomatology and the promotion of a way of life that will minimise the ill effects of the disorder. Regular folic acid supplements (5 mg daily) are prescribed to support the greatly increased erythropoietic activity.

Exacerbation of the chronic haemolytic anaemia is commonly associated with infections and these should be treated promptly and prevented, e.g. life-long antimalarials taken where appropriate. Young patients with hyposplenism should be given phenoxymethylpenicillin, one 250 mg tablet daily, and pneumococcal vaccine. Patients should avoid becoming chilled, dehydrated or exposed to hypoxia, e.g. at high altitudes.

An acute exacerbation of the anaemia may have no obvious precipitating cause. The spleen and liver may enlarge rapidly and the haemoglobin drops, sometimes with alarming speed (sequestration crisis). Transfusion with red cell concentrate is urgently required.

In less severe illness the patient should be adequately hydrated but transfusion with red cell concentrate is used only if essential because of the risk of allo-antibody formation and subsequent reactions. Most patients are habituated to a haemoglobin level of about 80 g/l and should be transfused only when the haemoglobin drops below 50 g/l. Transfusion is used before planned surgery in order to raise the haemoglobin and reduce susceptibility to sickling. In acute cases, exchange transfusion is desirable to reduce haemoglobin S levels.

In *pain crises*, powerful, potentially addictive, analgesics may be necessary in the early stages; after 24–48 hours they should be replaced by milder non-addictive preparations. The prompt correction of dehydration often helps to relieve pain. Antibiotics will be necessary if there are infective complications such as osteomyelitis. At the end of pregnancy these episodes may precipitate a pseudo-toxaemia syndrome that requires heparin therapy and no sedation.

Many other lines of therapy to prevent in vivo sickling have been tried but even those with a theoretical hope of success have proved disappointing.

Prognosis
It is probable that in Africa, without medical attention, few children with sickle-cell anaemia survive to adult life. With full medical facilities and improved social and economic circumstances many patients survive and, although subject to recurrent ill health, lead a fairly normal life but are unlikely to reach old age.

OTHER SICKLE-CELL DISEASES

Sickle-cell trait
Most patients who are carriers of the sickle gene lead healthy lives. However, under certain circumstances they may be liable to sickling. These include bloodless field surgery and flying at altitudes over 15 000 feet (4575 m) if pressurisation is inadequate. In addition these patients are liable to attacks of painless haematuria due to infarction of the renal papillae.

Haemoglobin SC disease
This disorder behaves like a mild variety of sickle-cell anaemia. Episodes of infarction are less frequent and anaemia is either absent or less severe. Aseptic necrosis of the femoral head, retinal vein thrombosis and painless haematuria are not uncommon complications.

Pregnancy is the main hazard because the same complications occur as in sickle-cell anaemia, particularly fat and bone marrow embolisation of the lungs and pseudo-toxaemia.

Haemoglobin C disease
This is a benign haemoglobinopathy which, in its homozygous form, is not associated with much morbidity. It may cause megaloblastic anaemia in pregnancy and considerable splenomegaly in adult life. No specific treatment is required other than folic acid supplements in pregnancy.

THE THALASSAEMIAS

Thalassaemia is an inherited impairment of haemoglobin production, in which there is partial or complete failure to synthesise a specific type of globin chain. The exact nature of the defect varies and it is probable that a number of different faults occur along the pathway which translates the genetic information into a polypeptide chain. The gene itself may be deleted and usually is in α thalassaemia. When the abnormality is heterozygous, synthesis of haemoglobin is only mildly affected and little disability occurs. Synthesis is grossly impaired when the patient is homozygous, and there is an imbalance in polypeptide chain production. The chains produced in excess precipitate in the cell forming Heinz bodies.

Beta-thalassaemia

Failure to synthesise beta chains (β-thalassaemia) is the most common type and is seen in highest frequency in the Mediterranean area. Heterozygotes have thalassaemia minor, a condition in which there is usually mild anaemia and little or no clinical disability. Homozygotes (thalassaemia major) are either unable to synthesise haemoglobin A or at best produce very little and, after the first 4 months of life, develop a profound hypochromic anaemia. The diagnostic features are listed in the information box below.

DIAGNOSTIC FEATURES OF β-THALASSAEMIA

Major
- Profound hypochromic anaemia
- Evidence of severe red cell dysplasia
- Erythroblastosis
- The absence or gross reduction of the amount of haemoglobin A
- Raised levels of haemoglobin F
- Evidence that both parents have thalassaemia minor

Minor
- Mild anaemia
- Microcytic hypochromic erythrocytes (not iron deficient)
- Some target cells
- Punctate basophilia
- Raised resistance of erythrocytes to osmotic lysis
- Raised haemoglobin A2 fraction
- Evidence that one or other parent has thalassaemia minor

Clinical features of β-thalassaemia major

The anaemia is crippling and the probability of survival for more than a few years without transfusion is low. Bone marrow hyperplasia early in life may produce head bossing and prominent malar eminences. The skull radiograph shows a 'hair on end' appearance and general widening of the medullary spaces which may interfere with the development of the paranasal sinuses. Development and growth are retarded and folate deficiency may occur. Splenomegaly is an early and prominent feature. Hepatomegaly is slower to develop but may become massive especially if splenectomy is undertaken. Transfusion therapy inevitably gives rise to haemosiderosis. Cardiac enlargement is common and cardiac failure, in which haemosiderosis may play a part, is a frequent terminal event.

β-thalassaemia minor is often detected only when iron therapy for a mild hypochromic anaemia fails. The diagnostic features are summarised in the information box (left). Symptoms are absent or minimal. Intermediate grades of clinical severity occur.

Management

The treatment of β-thalassaemia major is given in Table 14.5.

Table 14.5   Treatment of β-thalassaemia major

Problem	Management
Erythropoietic failure	Allogeneic bone marrow transplantation from HLA compatible sibling Hypertransfusion to maintain Hb 1000 g/l Folic acid 5 mg daily
Iron overload	Iron therapy forbidden Desferrioxamine therapy
Splenomegaly causing mechanical problems excessive transfusion required	Splenectomy performed as late as possible

Prevention

It is possible to identify a fetus with homozygous β-thalassaemia by obtaining chorionic villus material for DNA analysis sufficiently early in pregnancy to allow termination of pregnancy. This examination is appropriate if both parents are known to be carriers (β-thalassaemia minor) and will accept a termination.

Alpha thalassaemia

The reduction or absence of alpha chain synthesis is

ALPHA THALASSAEMIA

Cause
Failure of production of haemoglobin chain due to gene deletion

Age and sex
Both sexes from birth onward

Genetics
Four chains genes (2 loci)

Presentation
Hydrops fetalis. All genes deleted
Haemoglobin H. 3 genes deleted
Mild hypochromic microcytic anaemia 2 genes deleted

Treatment
Hydrops fetalis – none
Haemoglobin H as for thalassaemia intermedia
Avoid iron therapy. Folic acid if necessary

---

common in South East Asia. There are two alpha gene loci on chromosome 16 and therefore four alpha genes. If one is deleted there is no clinical effect. If two are deleted there may be a mild hypochromic anaemia. If three are deleted the patient has haemoglobin H disease and if all four are deleted the baby is stillborn (hydrops fetalis). Haemoglobin H is a β chain tetramer formed from the excess of chains. It is functionally useless. Treatment of haemoglobin H disease is similar to that of β thalassaemia of intermediate severity. In some patients the disorder is due to a combination of α thalassaemia genes with genes which produce a functionally useless globin chain, Hb Constant Spring. The combinations are shown in the information box (p. 722).

HAEMOLYTIC DISEASE DUE TO EXTRAERYTHROCYTIC CAUSES

Autoimmune haemolytic disease

In this disorder antibodies are formed against red cell antigens and cause inappropriate destruction of the cells (p. 39). There are two main types categorised on the basis of the thermal characteristics of the antibody.

'Warm' antibodies. These have a thermal optimum of 37°C, this being characteristic of most acquired antibodies. The majority are IgG. Warm type autoimmune haemolytic anaemia has antibodies of this type and can almost always be shown to have Rhesus specificity.

'Cold' antibodies. These have a thermal optimum of 4°C, but sometimes a thermal range of up to 37°C. Naturally occurring antibodies tend to be of this type, most are IgM and bind complement strongly. About 50% of 'warm' type antibodies are also seen to bind complement but less strongly.

Warm type autoimmune haemolytic anaemia

Many cases are idiopathic but some occur in association with chronic lymphatic leukaemia, lymphoma, systemic lupus erythematosus or certain drugs (e.g. methyldopa).

Clinical features

Patients of all ages are affected. Symptoms vary with the severity of the disease and its cause and are mainly those of anaemia. In addition, in severe cases there may be fever, vomiting and prostration. Splenomegaly and sometimes hepatomegaly is present.

Investigations

The diagnosis is established by demonstrating evidence of antibody on the red cells by the direct antiglobulin test (Coomb's test). This test detects the presence of antibodies on the surface of erythrocytes using an anti-human globulin antiserum (AHG). Antibodies being human globulin are recognised by the AHG which attacks them and causes agglutination of the erythrocytes. This is the 'direct' test. When antibodies are present in serum they must first be attached to red cells with the appropriate antigen before their presence can be detected as described above. This is known as the 'indirect' test. Elution of antibody from the red cells allows investigation of specificity against a panel of cells. The majority of these antibodies can be shown to have anti-Rhesus specificity. Of these, anti-e is the commonest. If possible, identification of specificity is useful as blood for transfusion which does not carry the specific antigen can be chosen. The blood film almost always shows polychromasia, spherocytosis and nucleated red cells.

Management

This is with prednisolone 60 mg daily for 3–4 weeks, the dose thereafter being slowly reduced. Response to treatment can be monitored with reticulocyte counts and haemoglobin estimations. The dosage should be raised if relapse occurs, and maintained for a further 3 weeks, when reduction may be tried again. If treatment fails from the beginning or, if after 6 months of steroid therapy the patient still has active haemolytic disease, splenectomy should be considered.

If splenectomy fails, immune suppression with drugs such as azathioprine, 100 mg daily, may be tried. However, disease which behaves in this way usually turns out to be chronic. Blood transfusion should be avoided unless an antibody specificity has clearly been identified and antigen-free blood is available. In life-threatening situations, the least incompatible blood available can be given, covered by high doses of prednisolone.

Cold agglutinin disease

Idiopathic cold agglutinin disease. This occurs mainly in the elderly. Symptoms reflect a tendency of the red cells to agglutinate and sludge in the microvasculature of the extremities where the blood is cooled. Raynaud's phenomenon is usually present and also acrocyanosis. A low-grade chronic haemolytic anaemia occurs. All these problems are worse in cold weather. Investigations demonstrate an increased erythrocyte turnover and a 'cold' antibody in enormously high titres with anti I or i specificity. The antiglobulin test is almost always positive and demonstrates complement binding.

Treatment consists of keeping the extremities warm. Transfusion should be avoided if possible. Steroids and splenectomy are of little value but immunosuppressive therapy may decrease antibody levels in severe cases.

Cold agglutinin disease secondary to other disorders. Paroxysmal cold haemoglobinuria may be associated with syphilis or be idiopathic. The Donath Landsteiner IgG antibody may be found which has anti P specificity. Cold antibody-type disease may also occur in association with Mycoplasma pneumoniae infection and infectious mononucleosis when the haemolysis is usually self limiting. If found in lymphoma the haemolysis tends to be more chronic.

ISOIMMUNE HAEMOLYTIC DISEASE

The term isoimmune is used to indicate that the antigen and the antibody come from different persons, although of the same species. This distinguishes it from autoimmune disease in which the antigen and the antibody are from the same individual.

Haemolytic disease of the newborn (HDN)

This disorder, previously called erythroblastosis fetalis, occurs in either sex and is due to attack in the fetal erythrocytes by maternal antibodies of IgG type which can pass the placental barrier. Causes are listed in the information box below.

CAUSES OF HAEMOLYTIC DISEASE OF THE NEWBORN

ABO incompatibility
This form is the commonest and is usually mild and can affect first pregnancies. It occurs in Group O mothers carrying A or B infants and is due to immune anti A or anti B

Rhesus incompatibility
This form occurs in Rhesus negative mothers carrying rhesus positive babies. The first pregnancy is seldom affected unless the mother has been previously sensitised

Other blood group system incompatibilities
e.g. anti-Kell. These are rare

The various degrees of severity of HDN are listed in the information box right.

Rhesus HDN

In about 1 pregnancy in 10 the mother is Rh-negative and the fetus Rh-positive. However haemolytic disease of the newborn is very rare in first pregnancies provided the mother has not previously been sensitised

---

TYPES OF HAEMOLYTIC DISEASE OF THE NEWBORN

- Haemolytic disease of the newborn is the mildest
- Icterus gravis neonatorum is more severe and carries the risk of severe brain damage unless treated urgently but is compatible with survival
- Hydrops fetalis is the most severe and causes death in utero

---

by transfusion (see below). Furthermore, sensitisation does not occur as often as might be anticipated and the risk of an Rh-negative woman having a baby with haemolytic disease of the newborn in any pregnancy other than the first is about 1 in 22.

If a mother is Rh-negative and the father Rh-positive, the maternal serum must be tested for antibodies between the 32nd and 36th week of each pregnancy. If found, delivery should be undertaken in hospital. If no antibodies are detected the infant will probably escape the disease, but nevertheless the cord blood should be tested for antibodies. If present, preventive treatment can be instituted.

Clinical features

These are of severe haemolytic anaemia with oedema and enlargement of the liver and spleen. Clinical jaundice may be absent for 24 hours after birth. Thereafter deep unconjugated hyperbilirubinaemia leading to kernicterus may occur. The severity of the jaundice is largely due to the immaturity of the fetal liver which is unable to conjugate the large amounts of bilirubin. The haemoglobin level, which should normally be about 180 g/l at birth, falls rapidly. Enormous numbers of nucleated red cells and a reticulocytosis of 10–50% are seen in the blood film (erythroblastosis). The direct Coombs test is positive.

Management

Exchange transfusion should be given to all severely affected infants (Hb. < 140 g/l, cord serum bilirubin > 60 mmol/l, infant's serum bilirubin > 300 mmol/l), as this is the only treatment which will overcome heart failure in a very anaemic infant and prevent deep jaundice and kernicterus. Early diagnosis is essential. Antenatal prediction from tests for antibodies in the maternal serum gives the infant the best chance. In mild cases simple transfusion and phototherapy will be sufficient, and in some instances no treatment is required.

Prevention

It is now believed that the most common cause of

primary Rh immunisation is transplacental haemorrhage during the third stage of labour. The likelihood of an Rh-negative woman developing anti-Rh antibodies is related to the number of Rh-positive red cells present in her circulation immediately after delivery. These can be stained and quantified. If found the mother should receive an injection of gammaglobulin containing a high titre of anti-D immunoglobulin within 72 hours of delivery. This will destroy the infant cells that have leaked into the mother's circulation and will prevent the development of antibodies in the mother and haemolytic disease in subsequent offspring.

HAEMOLYTIC ANAEMIA DUE TO OTHER ABNORMALITIES

Physical trauma to red cells. This is seen in:

1. prosthetic heart valves;
2. bacteraemia with certain organisms e.g. *C. Welchi*;
3. intravascular fibrin formation (disseminated intravascular coagulation). Fragmented cells may be seen in the blood film.

Drugs. Such as:

1. sulphasalazine or dapsone stress the erythrocyte metabolism;
2. antigen-antibody reactions (drugs acting as haptens).

Malaria. Haemolysis always accompanies malaria and in severe or prolonged attacks very considerable anaemia may ensue (p. 153). The destruction of erythrocytes is always greater than can be explained by parasitisation and may be due to an immune mechanism.

Inflammatory and neoplastic disease. This shortens the life span of the erythrocyte. The mechanisms are complex and not completely understood. Excessive erythrophagocytosis by macrophages occurs. Erythrocytes are damaged as they pass through affected tissue and drugs used in treatment may also harm them.

Paroxysmal nocturnal haemoglobinuria. This is a very rare disease in which a clone of erythrocytes with an acquired defect is abnormally sensitive to lysis by complement in the blood causing intermittent haemolytic anaemia, haemoglobinuria and thrombotic episodes.

Transfusion with incompatible blood. The reasons are given in the information box (right).

TRANSFUSION WITH INCOMPATIBLE BLOOD

- Clerical or checking errors, usually at the bed side, leading to the wrong blood being given
- Infused red cells are of the wrong main blood group due to careless typing of the blood
- The blood of the recipient and donor are of compatible main groups but contain incompatible subgroups. Direct cross-matching of recipient's serum against donor cells greatly reduces this risk
- From the transfusion of Rh-positive blood to a sensitised Rh-negative recipient

---

Clinical features

Symptoms usually begin after only a few millilitres of blood have been given, and if the transfusion is immediately stopped there may be no serious consequences. In severe reactions the patient complains of shivering and restlessness, nausea and vomiting, precordial and lumbar pain. Pulse and respiration rates increase. The blood pressure falls and the patient passes into a state of shock.

Jaundice appears after a few hours. There is haemoglobinaemia, and possibly even haemoglobinuria; oliguria may occur with renal failure due to acute tubular necrosis. In severe cases anuria persists and uraemia develops, from which the patient may die. In others diuresis occurs even after several days and the patient recovers. In the majority the acute features subside in 24–48 hours. Problems may arise later from immune complexes causing renal damage.

Management

Treatment of the established reaction involves:

1. giving hydrocortisone (100 mg i.v.)
2. inducing a diuresis with mannitol
3. treating the patient for shock. If acute tubular necrosis occurs the measures recommended on page 591 must be instituted at once.

ERYTHROCYTOSIS AND POLYCYTHAEMIA

A raised haemoglobin level usually, but not always, indicates an absolute increase in the number of circulating erythrocytes. In some patients it may be a spurious finding, the apparently high haemoglobin level being due to a reduction in plasma volume. This may occur because of dehydration or because of unknown mechanisms often associated with stress (Fig. 14.11).

A genuine increase in erythrocyte numbers (erythrocytosis) occurs for a number of reasons which are shown in the information box (p. 726).

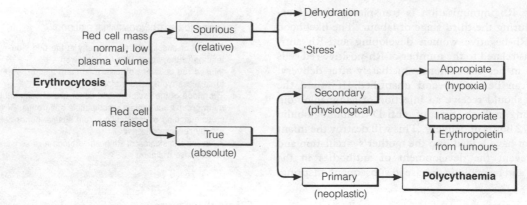

Fig. 14.11 Erythrocytosis and polycythaemia.

ERYTHROCYTOSIS/POLYCYTHAEMIA

Causes of erythrocytosis ·
When there is a physiological response to a pathological stimulus, as in hypoxia (p. 702) in which the production of erythropoietin is increased. Hypoxia may be due to:
  Altitude
  Pulmonary disease or congenital heart disease with cyanosis
  Abnormal haemoglobins with a high oxygen affinity. The white cells and platelets are unaffected and there is no splenomegaly
When there is a physiological response to a pathological stimulus. In this group the red cells are increased secondary to the production of abnormal amounts of substances with erythropoietin activity; this is occasionally found with certain benign and malignant tumours, e.g. of the kidney, liver, bronchus, uterus and cerebellum (haemangioblastoma) and with renal cysts. As in the first group the white cells and platelets are usually normal and there is no splenomegaly. However, the blood counts may be affected by the underlying disease

Causes of polycythaemia
When there is a pathological (neoplastic) proliferation of red cells without erythropoietin stimulus. This is primary proliferative polycythaemia (Fig. 14.11)

Stress or spurious erythrocytosis
Some patients with a high haemoglobin are found to have a red cell mass which is normal or even subnormal. The cause is a reduced plasma volume. This latter disorder tends to occur in middle-aged males who carry heavy responsibility or who are under stress for other reasons. It is often associated with hypertension and vascular disease. A reduction in stress or the use of tranquillisers or beta-blocking drugs sometimes has a beneficial effect with recovery of normal blood values.

PRIMARY PROLIFERATIVE POLYCYTHAEMIA

Polycythaemia is one of a group of disorders of the pluripotential stem cells called 'myeloproliferative disorders' (p. 727) which have features in common and may progress from one form to another.

Clinical features
Polycythaemia occurs mainly in patients over the age of 40 years and is more common in males than females. There may be no symptoms and the disorder is diagnosed incidentally. Common symptoms are lassitude, loss of concentration, headaches, dizziness, blackouts, pruritus, epistaxis and 'indigestion'. Some present with manifestations of peripheral vascular disease or a cerebrovascular accident.

The patients often have a high colour, suffused conjunctivae, deep red palate and dusky red hands; retinal vein engorgement may be found. The spleen is palpable in 75% of patients at diagnosis. Thrombotic complications may occur and peptic ulceration is common, sometimes complicated by bleeding.

Investigations
Diagnosis is established along the lines indicated in the information box (p. 727).

In some patients the results listed in the information box may be marginal and the diagnosis uncertain. However, the presence of a raised red cell mass together with splenomegaly is virtually diagnostic.

Management
Venesection is the simplest therapeutic measure and the best to use if the diagnosis is in doubt; 500 ml of blood (less if the patient is elderly) may be removed and

THE DIAGNOSIS OF PRIMARY PROLIFERATIVE POLYCYTHAEMIA

- The haemoglobin level is usually greater than 180 g/l in males and 160 g/l in females
- An associated elevation of white cell and platelet counts occurs in many patients
- The bone marrow is hypercellular with erythroid hyperplasia, very active granulopoiesis and increased numbers of megakaryocytes
- Depletion of marrow iron stores is usual
- The red cell mass is greatly increased and the plasma volume is often normal
- The neutrophil alkaline phosphatase score is normal or elevated and urate levels are often high
- Whole blood viscosity is increased

this venesection repeated within a day or two if necessary until the haematocrit reading is reduced to 45%. Clinical improvement occurs rapidly with the reduction of blood viscosity. Iron deficiency appears, if not already present, but iron therapy is withheld until the disease has been controlled by other methods of treatment.

Venesection should be used with caution when the platelet count is very high because of the risk of thrombosis.

Radioactive phosphorus (5 mCi of ^{32}P i.v.) is an excellent form of treatment for older patients when the diagnosis is certain. The full effect will not appear for 3 months but the white cell count and platelets respond more quickly. Further doses will be required, usually 6–18 months later, and may be repeated until the disease becomes refractory.

Chemotherapy with busulphan (2–4 mg/d), melphalan (2–4 mg/d) or hydroxyurea (2 g daily) until the disease is brought under control is equally effective but requires more supervision and more frequent blood counts than with radioactive phosphorus. Chemotherapy is preferred for patients under 50 years. Busulphan carries a slightly greater risk of severe marrow depression. Pyrimethamine may be used if no other treatment is available but can be associated with drug-induced ill health. Chlorambucil is contraindicated as it is associated with an increased incidence of secondary acute leukaemia.

Prognosis
The median life span after diagnosis in treated patients exceeds 10 years. Some survive more than 20 years. Progress to a refractory state with anaemia, myelofibrosis or acute leukaemia eventually occurs if the patient does not succumb to intercurrent disease.

OTHER MYELOPROLIFERATIVE DISORDERS

There are a number of other myeloproliferative conditions in addition to primary proliferative polycythaemia which are closely related and are either malignant or pre-malignant. These include myelofibrosis (p. 736) and essential thrombocythaemia (p. 753). There is a tendency for these disorders to terminate in an acute leukaemic phase.

DISORDERS OF THE WHITE BLOOD CELLS AND THE MONONUCLEAR-PHAGOCYTE SYSTEM

The term 'mononuclear-phagocyte' system is now replacing the widely used 'reticulo-endothelial' system as the latter has little meaning and is inaccurate in the light of current knowledge.

NEUTROPENIA AND AGRANULOCYTOSIS

A reduction in the number of circulating neutrophil leucocytes (neutropenia) or their absence (agranulocytosis) is a potentially serious disorder.

Aetiology
In some cases the cause is an idiosyncrasy or sensitisation to, or poisoning by, one of a variety of drugs. These are listed in the information box below.

NONCYTOTOXIC DRUG CAUSES OF NEUTROPENIA AND AGRANULOCYTOSIS

Antibiotics
Chloramphenicol
Penicillin
Sulphonamides including co-trimoxazole

Anticonvulsants
Phenytoin

Antithyroid
Propylthiouracil

Hypoglycaemics
Chlorpropamide

Phenothiazines
Chlorpromazine

Antimalarials
Maloprim

Almost every drug in use has been occasionally implicated. Exposure to insecticides or other industrial poisons should also be considered.

Neutropenia or agranulocytosis may follow excessive irradiation or the use of cytotoxic drugs or antimetabolites and is also found as an integral part of the pancytopenia of aplastic anaemia, leukaemia and some cases of hypersplenism. Rarely the disorder is inherited. In a few patients there is no discoverable cause – idiopathic agranulocytosis.

Pathology

In many patients the bone marrow shows a virtual disappearance of the granular cells and their precursors. In some the marrow contains early myelocytes, with few mature forms – an arrest of maturation, but such appearances may indicate early recovery. In others the appearances are those of an underlying blood disease.

Clinical features

There may be a history of exposure to one of the agents mentioned above. The onset may be either sudden or gradual. In acute and severe cases the condition begins with sore throat, fever and often rigors. There is rapidly advancing necrotic ulceration in the throat and mouth, with little evidence of pus formation. In fulminating cases the patient may die in a few days from toxaemia and septicaemia. In less acute cases there may be a preliminary period of malaise and weakness.

A chronic type has been described in which there is a persistence of neutropenia. Rarely the neutropenia occurs in cycles of 3–4 weeks (cyclic neutropenia.) In such cases the symptoms are chiefly recurrent malaise, low-grade fever and sore throat.

Investigation

The outstanding and sometimes only abnormality is the reduction in absolute numbers of neutrophils which may be absent in the most severe disease. Where the cause is another disorder such as leukaemia, evidence of this may be found and a reduction in haemoglobin and platelet count observed.

Management

The most important measure is removal of the offending agent if it can be identified. The patient is at risk from septicaemia. Blood cultures should be taken and the patient managed in the same way as those with the neutropenia and agranulocytosis following ablative chemotherapy used for acute myeloblastic leukaemia (p. 732). If the patient survives the acute phase, the outlook is fairly good, with recovery in many cases. In more chronic cases and where there is only neutropenia, infections should be dealt with if they arise.

Prevention

All the drugs mentioned at the beginning of this section should be regarded as potentially dangerous and must be employed carefully. Patients taking them should be warned to report unusual symptoms, fever or a sore throat.

THE LEUKAEMIAS

Leukaemias are a group of malignant disorders of the haemopoietic tissues characteristically associated with increased numbers of leucocytes in the blood. They are progressive and fatal conditions resulting in death most often from haemorrhage or infection. The course may vary from a few days or weeks to many years depending on the type.

Epidemiology

The incidence of leukaemia of all types in the population is approximately 10 per 100 000 per annum, of which just under half are acute leukaemias. Males are affected more frequently than females, in acute leukaemia the ratio being about 3:2, in chronic lymphocytic leukaemia 2:1 and in chronic myeloid leukaemia 1.3:1. Geographic variation in incidence does occur, the most striking being the rarity of chronic lymphocytic leukaemia in the Chinese and related races.

Age incidence

Acute leukaemia occurs at all ages. Acute lymphoblastic leukaemia shows a peak of incidence in the 1–5 age group. All forms of acute leukaemia have their lowest incidence in young adult life and there is a striking rise over the age of 50. Chronic leukaemias occur mainly in middle and old age.

Aetiology

In the majority of patients the cause of the leukaemia is unknown. Several factors, however, are associated with the development of leukaemia and these are listed in the information box (p. 729).

Terminology and classification

The terms 'acute' and 'chronic', when applied to leukaemias, refer to the clinical behaviour of the disease. In acute leukaemia the history is usually brief and life expectancy, without treatment, short. In chronic leukaemias the patients have usually been unwell for years, and survival is measured in years.

Not all leukaemias are associated with an increased leucocyte count or even the appearance of abnormal cells in the blood. The term 'subleukaemic' is used when the leucocyte count is within or below normal limits but abnormal cells are seen in the blood. 'Aleukaemic' is used when there are no abnormal cells to be seen and the leucocyte count is normal or subnormal. Almost all patients who present with subleukaemic or aleukaemic disease have acute leukaemias. The diagnosis is made from the marrow.

FACTORS ASSOCIATED WITH THE DEVELOPMENT OF LEUKAEMIA

Ionising radiation
A significant increase in myeloid leukaemia followed the atomic bombing of Japanese cities. An increase in leukaemia was observed after the use of radiotherapy for ankylosing spondylitis and diagnostic X-rays of the fetus in pregnancy

Cytotoxic drugs
These, particularly alkylating agents, may induce myeloid leukaemia, usually after a latent period of several years

Exposure to benzene in industry

Retroviruses
One rare form of T cell leukaemia lymphoma appears to be associated with a retrovirus similar to the viruses causing leukaemia in cats and cattle

Genetic
There is a greatly increased incidence of leukaemia in the identical twin of patients with leukaemia. Increased incidence occurs in Down's syndrome and other genetic disorders

Immunological
Immune deficiency states are associated with an increase in haematological malignancy

Occasionally acute leukaemia presents as an aplastic anaemia.

The classification of leukaemia is given in Tables 14.6 and 14.7.

Table 14.6   A classification of leukaemia

Acute	Chronic
Lymphoid (Lymphoblastic)	Lymphoid (Lymphocytic)
Myeloid (Myeloblastic)	Myeloid (Myelocytic)

Erythaemic myelosis. This is a disorder of erythropoiesis analogous to acute or subacute leukaemia. It is closely related to and overlaps the M6 variety of acute myeloid leukaemia.

Although leukaemias are divided into lymphoid or myeloid varieties, recent advances have shown that this division may be artificial since in acute leukaemias both types may coexist in the same patient. Nevertheless there is a value in maintaining the distinction since the drug therapy of the two main types is substantially different.

The subclassification of the lymphoblastic varieties is possibly of greater value since the subtype dictates greater variation in treatment. The 'common' type

Table 14.7   Subclassifications of leukaemia

1. Acute lymphoblastic	Acute myeloblastic
Common type (pre B)	FAB* classification
T cell	M1, undifferentiated
B cell	M2, differentiated
Undifferentiated	M3, promyelocytic
	M4, myelomonocytic
	M5, monocytic
	M6, erythrocytic
	M7, megakaryocytic
2. Chronic lymphocytic	Chronic myeloid leukaemia
Common B cell	Ph.ˣ positive
Rare T cell	Ph.ˣ negative, BCRˣˣ positive
Hairy cell	Ph.ˣ negative, BCRˣˣ negative
Prolymphocytic	Eosinophilic leukaemia

* FAB = French, American, British
x = Philadelphia chromosome   xx = Breakpoint Cluster Region

which constitutes 70% of all patients responds well to treatment and carries the best chance of long-term remission. The classification of acute myeloblastic leukaemia into seven varieties reflects the variable degree of maturation of the granulocyte series, the common involvement of the monocyte series with the granulocyte series and also the involvement of erythrocytic and megakaryocytic elements.

ACUTE LEUKAEMIAS

There is a failure of cell maturation in acute leukaemias. Proliferation of cells which do not mature leads to an increasing accumulation of useless cells which take up more and more marrow space at the expense of the normal haemopoietic elements. Eventually this proliferation spills into the blood. The evolution of acute leukaemia is illustrated schematically in Fig. 14.12.

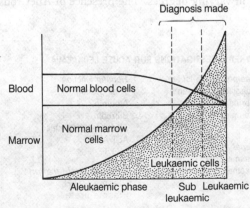

Fig. 14.12   Development of leukaemia.

Acute myeloblastic leukaemia is about eight times more common than acute lymphoblastic leukaemia in adults. In young children the lymphoblastic variety is more common.

Clinical features

The patient usually presents with non specific 'flu-like' symptoms or vague malaise and tiredness. Often the diagnosis of acute leukaemia is not obvious from the symptomatology and is uncovered by laboratory investigation. Where there are bleeding manifestations such as purpura, epistaxis and gum bleeding, it may be suspected but similar signs are found in thrombocytopenic purpura. Mouth ulcers, herpes labialis and sore throats are common to many disorders.

On examination the spleen and liver are often enlarged, particularly when the disease is advanced. There may be cervical lymphadenopathy secondary to pharyngeal sepsis but enlarged lymph nodes due to the disease is a common feature of the lymphoblastic form.

Investigations

Blood examination usually shows a profound anaemia of normochromic type. The MCV is either normal or raised. The leucocyte count may vary from as low as $1 \times 10^9/l$ to as high as $500 \times 10^9/l$ or more. In the majority the count is below $100 \times 10^9/l$. The blood film appearance of blast cells and other primitive cells are usually diagnostic. Sometimes in aleukaemic forms a bone marrow is necessary to establish the diagnosis. Severe thrombocytopenia is usual but not invariable.

The bone marrow is the most valuable diagnostic investigation and will provide material for cytology, cytogenetics and immunological phenotyping. If no marrow is obtained (dry tap) a trephine biopsy should be taken. The marrow is usually hypercellular with replacement of normal elements by leukaemic blast cells in varying degrees. The presence of Auer rods in

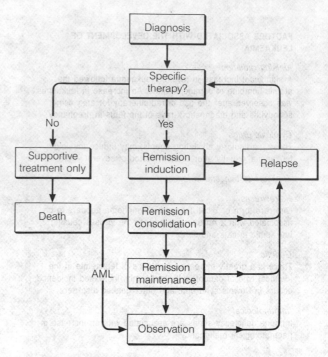

Fig. 14.13   Treatment strategy in acute leukaemia.

the cytoplasm of blast cells indicates a myeloblastic type of leukaemia.

Other basic investigations required at diagnosis are given in the information box (left).

Management

The general strategy for acute leukaemia is given in Fig. 14.13. The first decision must be whether or not to give specific treatment. Since specific treatment is of necessity aggressive and unpleasant, it may not be appropriate for the following groups of patients:

1. the very elderly (over 80 years of age)
2. patients with other serious disorders
3. patients who decline specific therapy
4. patients with types of leukaemia known to be very unresponsive to specific treatment.

In these patients supportive treatment only should be given and can result in considerable improvement in well-being. These decisions must, if possible, be made with the understanding and co-operation of the patient and his or her relatives.

Specific therapy

If a decision to embark on specific therapy has been taken, the patient should be prepared in the ways listed in the information box (p. 731).

OTHER INVESTIGATIONS FOR ACUTE LEUKAEMIA	
Haemostatic function	**Hepatic function**
Coagulation screen	Total protein
Fibrinogen	Albumin
d-dimers	Bilirubin
	Alkaline phosphatase
	AST/ALT
Renal function	γ-G.T.
Plasma urea	
Plasma creatinine	**Cellular proliferation**
	Plasma L.D.H.
	Plasma urate

PREPARATIONS FOR SPECIFIC THERAPY

- Existing infection should be identified and treated (e.g. urinary tract infection, oral candidiasis, dental, gingival and skin infections)
- Anaemia corrected with red cell concentrate infusion
- Thrombocytopenic bleeding controlled with platelet transfusion
- If possible, insertion of sylastic catheter into the neck veins for venous access
- Careful explanation of the therapeutic regimen to the patient

It is unwise to attempt aggressive management of acute leukaemia unless adequate services are available for the provision of the various forms of supportive therapy outlined later.

The aim of treatment is to destroy the leukaemic clone of cells without destroying the residual normal stem cell compartment from which repopulation of the haemopoietic tissues will occur. There are three phases.

Remission induction. In this phase the bulk of the tumour is destroyed by combination chemotherapy. The patient often goes through repeated periods of severe bone marrow failure requiring intensive support and in-patient care from specially trained medical and nursing staff.

Remission consolidation. If remission has been achieved by induction therapy, residual disease is attacked by therapy during the consolidation phase. This includes intrathecal drug therapy to deal with disease which may have survived in the sanctuary of the nervous tissues where it is not easily reached by systemic chemotherapy. Cranial irradiation is also given for the same purpose, particularly in acute lymphoblastic leukaemia. Much of the treatment in this phase can be given on an outpatient basis.

Remission maintenance. If the patient is still in remission after the consolidation phase, a period of maintenance therapy is given consisting of a repeating cycle of drug administration. This may extend for up to two years if relapse does not occur and is usually given on an outpatient basis. Thereafter specific therapy is discontinued and the patient observed. This phase is often omitted in patients with acute myeloblastic leukaemia who have been brought into complete remission by induction and consolidation therapy. The detail of the treatment schedules for these treatments is

Table 14.8   Drugs commonly used in the treatment of acute leukaemia

Lymphoblastic	Myeloblastic
Induction	
Vincristine (i.v.)	Daunorubicin (i.v.)
Prednisolone (oral)	Cytosine arabinoside (i.v.)
L-asparaginase (i.v.)	Etoposide (i.v. and oral)
Daunorubicin (i.v.)	Thioguanine (oral)
Methotrexate (intrathecal)	
Etoposide (i.v. and oral)	
Cytosine arabinoside (i.v.)	
Consolidation	
Mercaptopurine (oral)	Cytosine arabinoside (i.v.)
Methotrexate (intrathecal)	Amsacrine (i.v.)
	Etoposide (i.v. and oral)
	Mitozantrone (i.v.)
Maintenance	
Prednisolone (oral)	Mercaptopurine (oral)
Vincristine (i.v.)	Cytosine arabinoside (i.v. or s.c.)
Mercaptopurine (oral)	OR
Methotrexate (oral)	**No drugs.** This phase is often omitted

beyond the scope of this chapter. In any event no agreed treatment schedules exist but there is broad similarity between the experimental regimens currently used. The drugs most commonly employed for the two main varieties of acute leukaemia are given in Table 14.8. If a patient fails to go into remission with induction treatment, alternative drug combinations may be tried but generally the outlook is poor. Alternatively a decision may be taken not to give any further specific therapy and the patient is given supportive treatment only.

Disease which relapses during treatment or soon after the end of treatment carries a poor prognosis and is difficult to treat. The longer after the end of treatment relapse occurs, the more likely it is that further treatment will be effective.

Bone marrow transplantation
This is a therapeutic option for young patients (under the age of 40) who have histocompatible sibling donors. It is generally offered to patients with acute myeloblastic leukaemia in first remission and those with acute lymphoblastic leukaemia in first, second or subsequent remission (p. 733). Autologous bone marrow transplantation may also be used as a form of therapy intensification.

Supportive therapy
Aggressive and potentially curative therapy which involves periods of severe bone marrow failure would not be possible without adequate and skilled supportive care. The following problems commonly arise.

Anaemia. This is treated with red cell concentrate infusion to maintain a haemoglobin above 100 g/l.

Thrombocytopenic bleeding. This requires platelet transfusions unless the bleeding is trivial. Freshly harvested platelets from five donors are pooled and provided as a pack. One or two packs daily may be required if bleeding is severe.

Infection. Unexplained fever (greater than 38°C) lasting over 6 hours in a neutropenic patient (absolute neutrophil count less than $0.5 \times 10^9/l$) indicates probable septicaemia. Parenteral antibiotic therapy is required. When the organism is unknown, as is usually the case, an aminoglycoside (e.g. gentamicin) is given with an acylureido penicillin (e.g. azlocillin). This combination is synergistic and bacteriocidal and should be continued for at least 9 days unless a specific organism is isolated when therapy can be suitably adjusted. The organisms most commonly associated with severe neutropenia are Gram-negative bacteria such as *Escherichia coli*, *pseudomonas* and *Klebsiella* and Gram-positive bacteria such as *Staphylococcus aureus*. *Staphylococcus epidermis* is troublesome if there is an indwelling silastic catheter.

Patients with lymphoblastic leukaemia are susceptible to infection with the protozoon sp. *Pneumocystis carinii* which causes a severe pneumonia. Diagnosis may be difficult and is obtained either from bronchial washings or open lung biopsy. Treatment is with high dose Co-trimoxazole (20 mg Trimethoprim and 100 mg sulphamethoxazole per kg per day in two divided doses for a period of 3 weeks) initially intravenously with change to oral treatment as soon as possible.

Fungal infections. Oral and pharyngeal monilial infection is common. Prophylaxis with oral nystatin is standard practice: 1 ml of suspension (100 000 units) held in the mouth for as long as possible 4 times per day. Lozenges are less effective. For established infection nystatin suspension or amphotericin suspension, 1 ml (100 mg per ml) 4 times per day or amphotericin lozenges, 10 mg dissolved slowly in the mouth 4 times per day, should be given. Topical gentian violet paint may be effective for severe infection.

For systemic fungal infection with candida or pulmonary aspergillosis intravenous amphotericin is required: 0.5–1 mg/kg/day until response, then 1.2 mg/kg on alternate days for at least three weeks. The addition of flucytosine, 100–200 mg/kg daily given intravenously or orally in 4 divided doses may enhance the therapeutic effect of amphotericin. However, flucytosine is myelotoxic and may delay recovery from bone marrow failure. Amphotericin is nephrotoxic and hepatotoxic. Renal and hepatic function should be monitored closely particularly if the patient is receiving antibiotics which are also nephrotoxic.

Viral infections. Herpes simplex infection occurs frequently round the lips and nose during ablative therapy for acute leukaemia. Acyclovir applied to the lesions as a cream 5 times per day may control minor lesions but generally acyclovir tablets, 200 mg 5 times per day for 5–10 days will be required. The intravenous dose is 5 mg/kg over 1 hour repeated every 8 hours. Herpes zoster can also be treated in the early stage with acyclovir at a dose of 10 mg/kg/8-hourly intravenously for 5 days.

Protected environments. The value of these such as laminar flow rooms is debatable but may contribute to the awareness of staff for careful barrier nursing practice. The isolation is often psychologically stressful for the patient.

Supportive observation. Continuous monitoring of renal, hepatic and haemostatic function is necessary together with fluid balance measurements. Patients are often severely anorexic and may find drinking difficult. The necessary fluids and electrolytes often have to be given intravenously for as long as necessary. Renal toxicity occurs with some antibiotics (e.g. aminoglycosides) and anti-fungal agents (amphotericin).

Psychological support. Psychological support of the patient is very important. The patient should be continuously kept informed, questions answered and fears allayed as far as possible. An optimistic attitude from the staff is vital. Delusions, hallucinations and paranoia are not uncommon during periods of severe bone marrow failure and septicaemic episodes and should be met with patience and understanding.

Alternative chemotherapy. Gentle chemotherapy not designed to achieve remission may be used to curb excessive leucocyte proliferation. Drugs used for this purpose include hydroxyurea up to 4 g daily and mercaptopurine up to 150 mg daily. The effect is to reduce the leucocyte count without inducing bone marrow failure.

Prognosis

Without treatment the median survival of patients with acute leukaemia is about 5 weeks. This may be extended to about 10 weeks with supportive treatment. Patients who achieve remission with specific therapy have a better outlook. About 79% of adult patients with acute lymphoblastic leukaemia and 60% with acute myeloblastic leukaemia achieve remission. Median survival for acute lymphoblastic leukaemia patients is about 30 months and for acute myeloblastic leukaemia patients about 13 months if remission is achieved. Bad prognostic factors for survival are given in the information box below.

POOR PROGNOSTIC FEATURES IN ACUTE LEUKAEMIA

- Increasing age
- Male sex
- High leucocyte levels at diagnosis
- Cytogenic abnormalities
- CNS involvement at diagnosis

ALLOGENEIC BONE MARROW TRANSPLANTATION (BMT)

This is the only therapeutic measure which holds out the hope of 'cure' for persons with a variety of haematological and other disorders, particularly those listed in the information box below.

GENERAL INDICATIONS FOR USE OF ALLOGENEIC BONE MARROW TRANSPLANTATION

- Neoplastic disorders affecting the totipotent or pluripotent stem cell compartment (e.g. leukaemias)
- Those with a failure of haemopoiesis (e.g. aplastic anaemia)
- A major inherited blood defect in blood cell production (e.g. thalassaemia, immunodeficiency diseases)
- Inborn errors of metabolism with missing enzymes or cell lines

---

Healthy marrow from a donor is injected intravenously into a recipient who has been suitably 'conditioned' with chemotherapy and radiotherapy. Conditioning ablates the recipient's haemopoietic and immunological tissues. The injected cells 'home' to the marrow and produce enough erythrocytes, granulocytes and platelets for the patient's needs in about 3–4 weeks. It takes up to 3 or more years to regain good lymphocyte function and immunological stability. During this period, particularly in the first year, the patient is at great risk from opportunistic infections.

The preferred donors are histocompatible siblings

and the best results are obtained in patients aged under 20. Older patients can be transplanted, but results become progressively worse with age. The patient must be sufficiently stable psychologically to contend with a period of grave illness during the transplantation process. The patient should be free of other disorders which might seriously limit life span.

Bone marrow transplantation is not a particularly difficult or complicated procedure but requires highly specialised supervision and supportive facilities and fully trained staff. It is best performed in units established for the care of acute leukaemias under the primary care of haematologists, with the co-operation of immunologists, microbiologists, radiotherapist and full laboratory services.

Haematological indications. Transplantation may be syngeneic (identical twin donor) or allogeneic (non identical donor). Disorders for which allogeneic transplantation is currently offered are shown in the information box below.

HAEMATOLOGICAL INDICATIONS FOR ALLOGENEIC BONE MARROW TRANSPLANTATION

- Acute myeloblastic leukaemia in first remission
- Chronic myeloid leukaemia in chronic phase
- T and B cell lymphoblastic leukaemia in first remission
- Acute lymphoblastic leukaemia (common pre-B type) in second remission
- Severe aplastic anaemia
- Acute myelofibrosis
- Severe immunodeficiency syndromes

Transplantation is also a possibility for resistant acute leukaemia and selected patients with lymphoma.

Graft-versus-host disease (GVHD). Problems of GVHD and interstitial pneumonitis may cause serious morbidity and death if the graft is successful. Even low-grade GVHD, which is probably advantageous in terms of survival, can reduce the quality of life. GVHD is due to the cytotoxic activity of donor T lymphocytes which become sensitised to their new host which they regard as foreign. This may cause either an acute or chronic form of GVHD. The *acute GVHD* usually appears 14–21 days after the graft, although it may appear earlier or up to 70 days later. It causes diarrhoea, hepatitis, cholestasis and exfoliative dermatitis. All these features may vary from being mild to lethally severe. It appears to be associated with infection, although the relationship is not fully understood. Methotrexate, cyclosporin, antithymocyte glob-

Table 14.9   Infection during recovery from bone marrow transplant

Infection	Period after BMT	Treatment
Herpes simplex	0	Acyclovir
Bacterial Fungal	0–4 weeks	As for acute leukaemia (See p. 732)
Cytomegalovirus	7–21 weeks	If patient CMV negative, use CMV negative blood products. Hyperimmune sera for infected patient
Varicella zoster	After 13 weeks	Prophylaxis Hyperimmune globulin Acyclovir, 10mg/kg/day for 1–2 weeks i.v.
Pneumocystis carinii	8–26 weeks	Co-trimoxazole 20 mg trimethoprim 100 mg sulphamethoxazole/kg daily in 2 divided doses for 3 weeks
Non infective Interstitial pneumonitis of unknown aetiology	6–18 weeks	No specific therapy. Prednisolone, 60 mg daily orally may be tried

ulin, high dose corticosteroids and T cell depletion of the donor marrow have all been used to treat the disorder. The more severe forms prove very difficult to control.

Chronic GVHD. This may follow acute GVHD or arise independently; it occurs later than acute GVHD. It often resembles a connective tissue disorder, although in mild cases a rash may be the only manifestation. Chronic GVHD is usually treated with azathioprine and corticosteroids. It may be useful in preventing disease relapse in some patients.

Infection. This is the other major problem during recovery from BMT. Details are given in Table 14.9.

Autografting or autologous bone marrow transplantation. In this the patient's own marrow is harvested to be given back again after intensive therapy. It may be used for disorders which do not primarily involve the haemopoietic tissues or in patients in whom very good remissions have been achieved in conditions such as acute leukaemias and high-grade lymphomas. For chronic myeloid leukaemia, autografting with the patients own chronic phase cells harvested and stored at the time of presentation has been used to treat the disease when it enters the acute phase.

CHRONIC LEUKAEMIAS

CHRONIC MYELOID LEUKAEMIA

Chronic myeloid leukaemia is a disorder of proliferation which is unrestrained and excessive. Maturation proceeds fairly normally.

Epidemiology

The disease occurs chiefly between the ages of 30 and 80 years with a peak at 55 years. The ratio of males to females is 1.3:1. The disease is found in all races. The aetiology is unknown.

Cytogenetic and molecular aspects

Ninety per cent of patients with chronic myeloid leukaemia have a chromosome abnormality known as the Philadelphia (Ph.) chromosome. This is a shortened number 22 chromosome and is the result of a reciprocal translocation of material with chromosome 9. The break on the number 22 chromosome occurs in the BCR (breakpoint cluster region). The fragment from chromosome 9 that joins the BCR carries the Abelson (ABL) oncogene which forms a chimeric gene with the remains of the BCR. This chimeric gene codes for 210 kDa protein with tyrosine kinase activity which may play a causative role in the disease. Some Ph negative patients also have evidence of the same molecular abnormality.

Natural history

The disease has three phases:

1. a chronic phase in which the disease is responsive to treatment, is easily controlled and is essentially a benign neoplasm;
2. an accelerated phase (not always seen) in which disease control becomes more difficult;
3. a blast crisis phase in which the disease transforms into an acute leukaemia, either myeloblastic (70%) or lymphoblastic (30%) which is relatively refractory to treatment. Blast crisis occurs

Table 14.10 Symptoms at presentation of chronic myeloid leukaemia

Symptoms	Percentages
● Tiredness	37
● Weight loss	26
● Breathlessness	21
● Abdominal pain and discomfort	21
● Lethargy	13
● Anorexia	12
● Sweating	11
● Abdominal fullness	10
● Bruising	7
● Vague ill health	7

randomly and is the cause of death in the majority of patients. Patient survival is therefore dictated by the timing of the blast crisis which cannot be predicted.

Clinical features

The frequency of the more common symptoms at presentation are given in Table 14.10. About 11% of patients are asymptomatic at diagnosis. About 2% of males present with an attack of priapism. On examination the principal clinical finding is usually splenomegaly which is present in 90% of patients. In about 10% the enlargement is massive extending to over 20 cm below the coastal margin. The spleen is usually firm, smooth and painless but occasionally infarction may occur, giving rise to exquisite tenderness. A friction rub may be heard over it. Hepatomegaly occurs in about 50% of patients. Lymphadenopathy is unusual.

Investigations

Examination of the blood usually shows a normocytic normochromic anaemia. The mean haemoglobin is 100.5 gm/l with a range from 70–150 g/l. The mean leucocyte count is $220 \times 10^9/l$ with a range of 9.5–600. The mean platelet count is $445 \times 10^9/l$ with a range of 162–2000.

In the blood film the full range of granulocyte precursors from myeloblasts to mature neutrophils is seen with peaks at the myelocyte and mature granulo-

cyte stage of maturation. Myeloblasts are usually less than 10%. There is often an absolute increase in eosinophils and basophils and nucleated red cells are common.

If the disease progresses through an *accelerated phase* the percentage of the more primitive cells increases. There is a dramatic increase in the number of circulating myeloblasts as the disease enters blast transformation. In about a third of patients very high platelet counts are seen during treatment, both in chronic and accelerated phase, but usually drop dramatically at blast transformation. Basophilia tends to increase as the disease progresses.

The peripheral blood is the most useful diagnostically but bone marrow material should be obtained for chromosome analysis to demonstrate the presence of the Philadelphia chromosome. Increasingly DNA analysis is being undertaken to demonstrate the presence of the chimeric Abelson-BCR gene.

Other characteristic findings on investigation include a very low neutrophil alkaline phosphatase score and very high vitamin B_{12} levels in the plasma. Lactate dehydrogenase levels are also substantially elevated.

Management

No specific therapy may be required if the patient is asymptomatic and the leucocyte count not greatly elevated. In the majority of patients however treatment is necessary.

Chemotherapy

The two most widely used drugs both given orally are busulphan and hydroxyurea although melphalan is as satisfactory as busulphan. Control of the leucocyte count is smoother with busulphan than hydroxyurea but carries greater risk of serious marrow suppression and, rarely, of serious interstitial pulmonary fibrosis (busulphan lung). The dosage used to induce control of disease and thereafter maintenance is given in Table 14.11. Busulphan may be given either as low dose continuous or high dose intermittent therapy.

The induction doses shown in Table 14.11 other than high dose busulphan are given until the leucocyte count drops to around $20 \times 10^9/l$ when the drug is tempor-

Table 14.11 Drugs used in the treatment of chronic myeloid leukaemia

Drugs	Induction	Maintenance
Busulphan (low dose)	4 mg daily	2–4 mg daily 1–7 days per week
Busulphan (high dose)	50–150 mg stat.	50 mg stat. not more often than 4-weekly
Hydroxyurea	0.5–2 gm daily	0.5–2 g daily 1–7 days per week
Melphalan	4–12 mg daily	2–4 mg daily 1–7 days per week

arily stopped in order to avoid excessive marrow suppression. This is least likely to occur with hydroxyurea. The drug is reintroduced as soon as the leucocyte count plateaus and starts to rise again. Usually dose adjustments are required at this stage and the aim is to give a dose which will maintain the leucocyte count within the normal range $(4-11 \times 10^9/l)$.

After some months of satisfactory maintenance treatment the drug may be stopped, sometimes for as long as a year or more and reintroduced when the leucocyte count rises above $20 \times 10^9/l$. However, it is seldom possible to stop hydroxyurea for long periods as the leucocyte count tends to rise quickly. None of these treatments affect the onset of blast cell transformation and therefore do little to prolong life, but they do substantially improve the quality of life.

Alpha interferon. This is given i.m. or s.c., 3–9 mega units daily. It can induce control and maintain control of this disease in chronic phase in about 70% of patients. Reduction in the percentage of Ph positive cells is seen in about 20% and apparent elimination of the Ph chromosome in about 5%. It is hoped that this may prolong survival, in responsive patients. Interferon therapy causes 'flu-like' symptoms initially, tiredness, somnolence, weight loss, dizziness, nausea, vomiting, loss of taste, diarrhoea and headache. Some of these side-effects may be controlled with paracetamol; others such as severe bone pain and severe weight loss are reasons for discontinuation. The majority of patients tolerate the therapy well, particularly if the dose can be reduced to 3 mega units 3 times per week. It is probably unwise to use interferon therapy in patients over 75 years of age because of neurotoxicity. During treatment the aim should be to maintain the leucocyte count at low levels between 2 and $5 \times 10^9/l$.

Splenectomy. Splenectomy does not prolong survival and is indicated only to relieve symptoms of discomfort and pain such as may occur because of size or repeated infarctions.

Thrombocythaemia. Very high platelet counts are not uncommon but generally give rise to few problems and can usually be ignored. Interferon therapy is probably the most effective in reducing the platelet count.

Treatment of the accelerated phase of the disease is more difficult. Hydroxyurea is the most effective single agent. When blast transformation occurs, the type of blast cells should be ascertained by cytochemical and immunological techniques. If lymphoblastic, the response to appropriate treatment (p. 731) is better than

if myeloblastic. Response to treatment for the latter is very poor. There is a strong case for supportive therapy only, particularly in older patients.

Bone marrow transplantation. Allogeneic or syngeneic bone marrow transplant from a matched sibling donor provides the only means of obtaining long-term remission in this disease. It is available to those under the age of 40 years who have a suitable donor. The best results are obtained in patients in early chronic phase when about 50% can expect prolongation of survival and possible cure. The results of transplantation in accelerated and blast transformation phases are poor. Autografting as a means of prolonging chronic phase has not been very successful.

Prognosis

Patients treated conventionally have a 15% chance of death in the first 12 months and thereafter an annual risk of 20–25%. Median survival is about 3 years. A few patients survive over 10 years.

Philadelphia chromosome negative chronic myeloid leukaemia

About half of these patients have the classical molecular abnormality (BCR positive) without a demonstrable Philadelphia chromosome and behave as Philadelphia chromosome positive patients. They should be managed in the same way. The remainder (BCR negative) tend to be older, mostly males, have lower platelet counts, higher absolute monocyte counts and respond poorly to treatment. Median survival is less than one year.

Eosinophilic leukaemia

This is a rare variant of chronic myeloid leukaemia and shows features of the hypereosinophilic syndrome in which cardiomyopathies and endomyocardial fibrosis occur, leading to severe cardiac failure. Treatment is difficult.

MYELOID METAPLASIA AND MYELOFIBROSIS

Myeloid metaplasia is the appearance of precursors of red cells, granulocytes and platelets in abnormal sites such as the liver and spleen, and is usually associated with a leucoerythroblastic blood picture (p. 707). This is not a phenomenon compensating for loss of marrow activity but is evidence of disordered behaviour by the precursor cell lines.

Myelofibrosis

Myeloid metaplasia is seen in myelofibrosis. Early in

myelofibrosis the marrow may have little fibrous tissue and be hypercellular with an excess of all cell lines particularly megakaryocytes. As the disease progresses fibrous tissue increases and may eventually fill most of the marrow space. The fibrosis is a reactive response to the disease process not part of the neoplastic disorder.

Clinical features

These are very variable. Most patients with myelofibrosis suffer lassitude, weight loss, night sweats and some intolerance of heat. The spleen may be greatly enlarged and splenic infarcts may occur. Rarely splenomegaly is absent.

Investigations

Anaemia, sometimes macrocytic, is common. The leucocyte count varies, with an increase in granulocytes and usually a leucoerythroblastic blood picture. The erythrocytes show very characteristic tear drop poikilocytes. The platelet count may be very high, normal or low and giant forms are seen in the blood film. The neutrophil alkaline phosphatase score is frequently raised as are urate levels. The marrow is often difficult to aspirate and a trephine biopsy shows an excess of megakaryocytes and increased reticulin and fibrous tissue replacement. Folate deficiency is very common.

Management

Treatment is largely supportive with blood transfusion, folic acid (5 mg daily), and non-virilising androgen therapy (oxymetholone 50 mg daily if tolerated). Corticosteroids (prednisolone) may be helpful in some patients. Cytotoxic therapy with drugs such as hydroxyurea up to 2 g daily (p. 735) should be used very cautiously, starting at a smaller dose. Splenectomy may be required if the grossly enlarged spleen is causing distress or because transfusion requirements are excessive but the outcome is unpredictable. Prognosis is variable and survival may exceed 10 years. The disease is progressive with steady deterioration. Bone marrow transplantation should be considered for young patients.

Myelodysplastic syndrome

This syndrome consists of a group of disorders which represent steps in the progression to the development of leukaemic malignancy and are characterised by variable cytopenia, hypogranular neutrophils with nuclear hyper- or hyposegmentation and hypercellular marrow with dysplastic changes in all three cell lines. Included in the syndrome are:

1. refractory anaemia
2. refractory anaemia with ring sideroblasts
3. chronic myelomonocytic leukaemia
4. refractory anaemia with excess of blasts (RAEB)
5. refractory anaemia with excess of blasts in transformation (RAEB).

The first two are relatively chronic disorders while the latter three show a more aggressive course with a tendency to terminate as acute myeloid leukaemia. They occur mainly in the elderly.

Treatment is difficult. Transfusional support is often required. Pyridoxine 300 mg daily may produce some response in sideroblastic anaemia and folate deficiency should be excluded. Some response has been obtained using low dose cytosine arabinoside therapy (20 mg b.d., s.c. for 3 weeks) in RAEB and REB.

Essential thrombocythaemia

This is a rare myeloproliferative disorder and most patients are elderly. Clinical features and treatment are described on page 753.

CHRONIC LYMPHOCYTIC LEUKAEMIA

This is the commonest variety of leukaemia. The male:female ratio is 2:1 and the majority of patients are over the age of 45 with a peak at 65. The disease is very rare in the Chinese and related races.

Pathology

There is moderate enlargement of lymph nodes and other lymphoid tissues throughout the body, the normal structure being replaced by sheets of lymphocytes. The histology is that of diffuse well-differentiated lymphocytic disease, nodular histology being rare. The spleen and liver are moderately enlarged and show lymphocytic infiltration. The bone marrow becomes progressively infiltrated with lymphocytes which eventually replace the haemopoietic tissue.

In this disease B lymphocytes which would normally respond to antigens by transformation and antibody formation, fail to do so. An ever increasing mass of immuno-incompetent cells accumulate to the detriment of immune function and normal bone marrow haemopoiesis. The receptor profile of the lymphocytes almost always demonstrates a B cell type of disease. T cell disease occurs rarely (1.5%). The light chains of immunoglobulins produced by these B cells tend to be either kappa or lambda in type (p. 30) indicating in the majority of cases, a monoclonal expansion of cells. The disease is closely related to and indeed overlaps with well-differentiated lymphocytic lymphoma (p. 743).

Clinical features

The onset is very insidious. Tiredness and vague ill-health are common although about 25% of patients are symptom free and the disorder is found incidentally. The development of anaemia tends to be slower than in chronic myeloid leukaemia and the presenting feature is usually the finding of firm rubbery, discrete and painless lymph nodes in the cervical, axillary and inguinal regions. The spleen is usually palpable but smaller than in chronic myeloid leukaemia. The liver may also be enlarged. As a result of immunosuppression there is an increasing tendency to recurrent infections.

Investigations

Peripheral blood examination usually shows a mild but gradually increasing anaemia. Haemolytic anaemia may occur and is usually autoimmune in type. In the majority of patients the leucocyte count is between 50 and $200 \times 10^9/l$ although it may occasionally be greatly increased up to $1000 \times 10^9/l$. Of these cells about 95% or more are lymphocytes which are predominantly of the small variety. Lymphoblasts are rare but undifferentiated lymphocytes may increase in number in the terminal stages. The platelet count is either low normal or only mildly reduced.

Examination both by aspiration and trephine is required to assess the degree of marrow involvement. Folate deficiency may occur. Estimations of total proteins and immunoglobulin levels should be undertaken to establish the degree of immunosuppression which is common and progressive. In some patients immunoglobulin levels may be raised and there may be a monoclonal band. Urate levels are seldom raised because cell turnover is low.

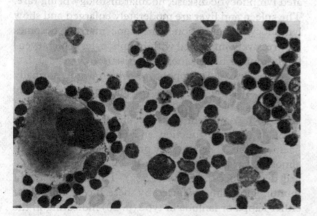

Fig. 14.14   Marrow aspirate in chronic lymphocytic leukaemia. It shows marked infiltration with mature lymphocytes. The large cell is a megakaryocyte.

Staging

The disease may be staged according to the criteria of the International Classification. These are given in the information box below.

> **STAGING OF CHRONIC LYMPHOCYTIC LEUKAEMIA**
>
> *Clinical Stage A*
> No anaemia or thrombocytopenia and less than three areas of lymphoid enlargement
>
> *Clinical stage B*
> No anaemia or thrombocytopenia, with three or more involved areas
>
> *Clinical stage C*
> Anaemia and/or thrombocytopenia regardless of the number of areas of lymphoid enlargement

Management

The treatment depends upon the stage of the disease.

Clinical Stage A. No specific treatment required. In older patients life expectancy is normal. The patient should be reassured.

Clinical Stage B. If asymptomatic no treatment may be required. Chemotherapy with chlorambucil may be initiated in symptomatic patients. Local radiotherapy to troublesome lymph nodes may be given.

Clinical Stage C. Anaemia may require transfusion with red cell concentrate. Bone marrow failure, if present, is treated initially with prednisolone, 40 mg daily, for 3–6 weeks supplemented by oxymetholone, 50 mg on alternate days, to stimulate erythropoiesis. A degree of bone marrow recovery is usually achieved.

Cytotoxic therapy. Chlorambucil, 5 mg orally daily, over long periods with dose adjustment according to blood counts will reduce the abnormal lymphocyte mass and produce symptomatic improvement in most patients. Alternatively chlorambucil may be given as intermittent high dose therapy, 0.4 mg/kg every 2 weeks incrementing by 0.1 mg/kg until the maximum tolerated dose is reached. This is continued until the desired therapeutic effect is obtained.

Radiotherapy. Total body irradiation employing very small doses spread over 5 weeks in 10 fractions is also effective and well tolerated, especially by the elderly. Local radiotherapy may be used to reduce spleen size or treat local problems due to the disease.

Combination chemotherapy. This may induce more rapid disease control but is more toxic; there is no evidence that it improves survival. It may be reserved for the later stages of the disease. A combination of cyclophosphamide, doxorubicin, vincristine and prednisolone (CHOP) is often used and a total of 6 or more pulses given.

Infections. These must be vigorously treated with antibiotics as appropriate. Recurrent viral or non-specific infections (often respiratory) sometimes respond to immunoglobulin replacement therapy. Acyclovir is indicated for herpetic infections.

Splenectomy. This may be required to treat auto-immune haemolytic anaemia or because of gross splenic enlargement.

Prognosis
The overall median survival is about 6 years. Clinical Stage A patients have a median survival over 12 years and Stage C patients between 2 and 3 years. Fifty per cent of patients die of infection and 30% of causes unrelated to chronic lymphocytic leukaemia. Unlike chronic myeloid leukaemia, chronic lymphocytic leukaemia rarely transforms to an acute phase.

Hairy cell leukaemia
This is a variant of chronic lymphocytic leukaemia.

Clinical features
The male female ratio is 6:1 and the median age is 50. Presenting symptoms are generally those of ill health and recurrent infections. Splenomegaly occurs in 90% but lymph node enlargement is unusual.

Investigations
Severe neutropenia, monocytopenia and the characteristic hairy cells in blood and bone marrow are typical. These cells usually type as B lymphocytes. The diagnostic test is to show that the acid phosphatase staining reaction in the cells is resistant to the action of tartrate. The neutrophil alkaline phosphatase score is almost always very high.

Management
Alpha interferon, 3 mega units daily, reducing eventually to 3 times a week subcutaneously, should be given until the disease is brought under control. Splenectomy

may also be valuable. Corticosteroids are of limited value and cytotoxic therapy is seldom rewarding.

Prolymphocytic leukaemia
This is another variant of chronic lymphatic leukaemia found mainly in males over the age of 60; 25% are of the T cell variety. There is massive splenomegaly with little lymphadenopathy and a very high leucocyte count, often in excess of $400 \times 10^9/l$. The characteristic cell is a large lymphocyte with a prominent nucleolus. Treatment is generally unsuccessful and the prognosis very poor. Leucapheresis for very high white counts, splenectomy and chemotherapy may be tried.

THE LYMPHOMAS

This group of malignant neoplasms is divided into two main types: Hodgkin's lymphoma and non-Hodgkin lymphoma.

HODGKIN'S LYMPHOMA

This disease is characterised by progressive, painless enlargement of lymphoid tissues throughout the body. It occurs in both sexes but more commonly in men, with two peaks of incidence, one in adolescence and early adult life, and a second in the 45–75 age group. The pathogenesis is unknown. The condition is usually regarded as a form of malignant disease related to other neoplastic processes of haemopoietic tissue. It is distinguished from non-Hodgkin lymphoma by the presence of Reed-Sternberg (R.S.) cells, now thought to be the malignant cells.

Pathology
This neoplasm is unusual in that the malignant cells form only a small proportion of the cell mass of the tumour. In addition to R.S. cells there are cells known as Hodgkin cells which are mononuclear whereas R.S. cells are binuclear or multinuclear (Fig. 14.15). The remainder of the cell mass is made up of lymphocytes, granulocytes, plasma cells, histiocytes and fibrous tissue. The numbers of well-differentiated lymphocytes vary from many to few and the degree of lymphocyte depletion forms the basis for the main pathological classification of the disease. In some cases the fibrous stroma is increased. Caseation and necrosis are most unusual. Infiltration with areas of Hodgkin's tissue causes enlargement of the spleen and liver. The bone marrow, lungs, kidneys and alimentary tract may also be involved but deposits in the nervous system are rare. The disease can be divided pathologically into four types which are shown in the information box (p. 740).

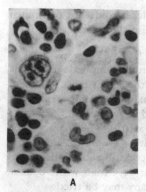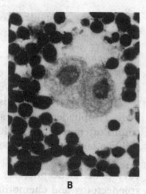

A   B

Fig. 14.15   Hodgkin's disease: Reed Sternberg cells. **A.** Histological preparation. **B.** Cytological preparation. Binucleate mirror image nuclei with large nucleoli.

PATHOLOGICAL CLASSIFICATION OF HODGKIN'S LYMPHOMA

- Lymphocyte predominant
- Nodular sclerosing
- Mixed cellularity in which neutrophils, eosinophils and plasma cells are common
- Lymphocyte depleted

The nodular sclerosing variety is the most commonly encountered, particularly in young women, with the mixed cellularity type, commoner in older men, coming second. Lymphocyte predominant is third and lymphocyte depleted the least often seen. The last is sometimes difficult to distinguish from a high grade non-Hodgkin lymphoma.

Clinical features

The onset is insidious, usually with enlargement of one group of superficial nodes which may fluctuate in size. While the cervical nodes are often the first to be involved, the disease may also appear to start in the mediastinal and axillary nodes and more rarely in abdominal, pelvic and inguinal areas. Involved lymph nodes are usually painless, discrete and rubbery, though tenderness does occur in some cases, particularly when the nodes have enlarged rapidly. The overlying skin is freely mobile. Extension of the disease from the lymph nodes to adjacent tissues may occur, and is found particularly in the mediastinum. Pressure by node masses on neighbouring structures may cause a variety of problems, such as dysphagia, dyspnoea, venous obstruction, jaundice and paraplegia. Splenomegaly is uncommon at the onset and even when present does not always signify organ involvement; but absence of splenomegaly does not exclude involvement.

General features may include progressive weakness, loss of weight and drenching night sweats. Fever may be present. In some there is a low-grade pyrexia and in others swinging fevers. The classical Pel-Ebstein intermittent fever is seldom seen now because the disease is modified by treatment. Pruritus is troublesome in about 10% of patients. Some patients experience discomfort at the site of disease infiltration shortly after an alcoholic drink.

Staging

Hodgkin's disease is thought to arise in one area and spread to others. It is important to establish the extent of the disease at the time of diagnosis because staging largely determines the therapeutic approach. For clinical staging investigations required include chest radiographs, bipedal lymphangiography, abdominal ultrasound, computed tomography, marrow trephine and aspirate. Magnetic resonance imaging may also contribute, but is not yet widely available. A laparotomy for splenectomy, liver and lymph nodes biopsies is rarely carried out as a means of establishing the extent of intra-abdominal disease but when performed enables pathological staging to be made. There are four clinical stages based primarily on the extent of the disease (Ann Arbor Classification, Table 14.12).

Table 14.12   Clinical stages of Hodgkin's disease

Stage	Definition
I	Involvement of a single lymph node region (I) or extralymphatic site (IE)
II	Involvement of two or more lymph nodes regions (II) or an extra-lymphatic site and lymph node regions on the same side (above or below) the diaphragm (IIE)
III	Involvement of lymph nodes regions on both sides of the diaphragm with (IIIE) or without (III) localised extra-lymphatic involvement or involvement of the spleen (IIIS) or both (IIISE)
IV	Diffuse involvement of one or more extra-lymphatic tissues, e.g. liver or bone marrow. The lymphatic structures are defined as the lymph nodes, spleen, thymus, Waldeyer's ring, appendix and Peyer's patches

Each stage is sub-divided into 'A' or 'B' categories, according to whether they have systemic symptoms or not. The symptoms that place a patient in the 'B' category are:

1. unexplained weight loss of more than 10% of the body weight in the previous 6 months
2. unexplained fever above 38°C
3. heavy night sweats.

Investigations

Anaemia is common and progressive. It is usually

normochromic and normocytic but occasionally has an immune haemolytic component. There is no diagnostic change in the white cells although a modest eosinophilia occurs in about 10–15% of patients. The total white cell count may be normal but is sometimes considerably raised and there is a neutrophil leucocytosis.

Lymphopenia, when it occurs, has a bad prognosis and an indicator of lympyhocyte depletion. In the terminal phase there may be leucopenia and thrombocytopenia which may be as much a reflection of treatment as of the disease. Bone marrow involvement is very uncommon at the outset but may be found later in the disease. The diagnosis can be established with certainty only by tissue biopsy, usually of a lymph node. Liver biopsy may provide the diagnosis in patients with hepatic enlargement.

Management

There are two main modalities of treatment, radiotherapy and chemotherapy (p. 239). Megavoltage radiotherapy can eliminate the disease in a high proportion of patients provided the disease is localised. Chemotherapy alone or combined with radiography is employed when there is any suspicion that the disease is more widespread. The indications for radiotherapy and chemotherapy are given in the information box below.

THERAPEUTIC GUIDELINES FOR HODGKIN'S LYMPHOMA

Indications for radiotherapy
- Stage I disease
- Stage II A disease with 3 or less areas of involvement
- After chemotherapy to sites where there was originally bulk disease
- To lesions causing serious pressure problems

Indications for chemotherapy
All patients with 'B' symptoms
Stage II disease with more than three areas of involvement
Stage III and Stage IV disease

Radiotherapy. Megavoltage radiotherapy to a dose of 3500–4000 cGy is given over a period of 4 weeks, 5 days each week, to involved areas and a slightly lower dose to adjacent areas. Extensive radiotherapy, however, prejudices future chemotherapy by destroying too much of the bone marrow reserves. The tendency is therefore to opt for chemotherapy if the disease is extensive followed by radiotherapy if necessary.

Chemotherapy. Combination chemotherapy has been shown to be highly effective in obtaining lasting remissions in this disease. The most widely used regimen is given in Table 14.13 and is a variation of the MOPP/MVPP regimens which employ mustine hydrochloride as the alkylating agent. In this regimen chlorambucil replaces mustine.

Table 14.13 The CHLVPP regimen

Drug	Dose		
Chlorambucil	6 mg/m	(up to 10 mg total)	Days 1–14 orally
Vinblastine	6 mg/m	(up to 10 mg total)	Days 1 and 8 i.v.
Procarbazine	100 mg/m		Days 1–14 orally
Prednisolone	40 mg		Days 1–14 orally

These drugs are given on a 28-day cycle for a minimum of 6 pulses and up to 9 if necessary. The chlorambucil-based regimen is better tolerated causing less vomiting and epilation than that based on mustine hydrochloride. The regimen using vinblastine (MVPP) is less neurotoxic than that employing vincristine (MOPP). Chlorambucil can be given orally. All regimens are myelotoxic and bone marrow tolerance is monitored with repeated blood counts. Dose modification or delay may be required if leucocyte and platelet counts do not recover adequately by the time the next pulse of chemotherapy is due. There is a small (5%) risk that patients treated with chemotherapy, particularly if combined with radiotherapy, will develop acute leukaemia, usually 7–10 years later. Attempts have been made to compile regimens that do not carry this risk. One such regimen employs doxorubicin, bleomycin, vinblastine and decarbazine (ABVD) although the last drug is now often replaced by VP16–213. This may be used as an alternating regimen with chlorambucil VPP or as salvage therapy.

Combined modality treatment. This is employed usually where there is bulk disease. The chemotherapy is given first and radiotherapy subsequently to the original sites of bulk disease which have been shrunk by the chemotherapy.

Relapse. Patients who relapse while on therapy have a poor prognosis. If relapse occurs more than one year after the cessation of chemotherapy, the same drugs may be used again. Otherwise salvage chemotherapy or radiotherapy is required. Autologous bone marrow transplantation may be employed for patients whose marrow is not involved who have relapsed or for bad prognosis type of disease.

Chemotherapy carries a fairly high risk of inducing sterility in males and this may be permanent. It is less of a risk in females, in whom evidence of premature menopause may also appear. Because many of these patients are young, the males in particular may require counselling about the effect of chemotherapy and should be offered the possibility of sperm storage. In women if premature menopause occurs replacement therapy may be required to preserve the skeleton.

Prognosis

If the patient is untreated the disease is fatal. With stage IA disease, the 5-year survival rate in patients treated with radiotherapy exceeds 90%, and in stage IIA disease is greater than 70%. In more advanced disease the results of chemotherapy are very satisfactory and more than 50% of patients remain disease free after 5 years. Just how effective combination chemotherapy is, remains to be seen because many patients who were treated in this way are still alive. The prognosis so far as histological type is concerned seems to matter less when chemotherapy is used. Chronic relapsing disease occurs in some patients who may survive with repeated treatment for over 20 years.

NON-HODGKIN'S LYMPHOMA

In this group of disorders there is a malignant monoclonal proliferation of lymphoid cells, the majority of cases identifiable as B cell and a minority as T cell. Non-Hodgkin's lymphomas merge with lymphoblastic and lymphocytic leukaemias with which they have many features in common.

Pathology and classification

In the past the most widely use classification was that of Rappaport which had the merit of simplicity. It drew attention to the division between lymphomas which retained a nodular structure (nodular or follicular) and those in which the architecture was lost (diffuse) (Fig. 14.16). Another classification, the Kiel, has also been widely adopted. More recently a 'Working Formulation' has been drawn up from these two classifications in which cases are allotted to one of three grades:

1. low
2. intermediate
3. high.

The criteria by which patients are allotted are complex but this grading provides a practical guide for the clinician and can be easily understood. For treatment purposes intermediate and high-grade lymphomas are often taken as one group. The size of the lymphoid cells is also a guide to prognosis. Small cell disease (mature

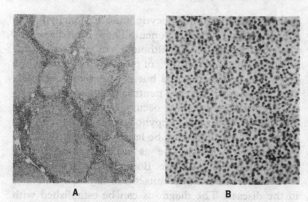

Fig. 14.16 Non-Hodgkin's lymphoma. A. Follicular or nodular pattern. **B.** Diffuse pattern of histology.

lymphocytes) is associated with low-grade and large-cell disease (immature lymphoid cells) with high-grade disease. Most nodular lymphomas are low grade and most diffuse lymphomas high grade. Low-grade lymphomas carry the best prognosis and high grade the worst. However, high-grade lymphomas may respond better to treatment and patients can achieve long-term remission if treated properly.

Staging

The Ann Arbor classification outlined in the section on Hodgkin's disease is used. Unlike Hodgkin's lymphoma the disease in non-Hodgkin lymphoma is frequently widespread at diagnosis (Stage III or IV), often involving not only lymph nodes, but also bone marrow, spleen and other tissues. Early involvement of bone marrow is typical of nodular lymphoma. Extra-lymphatic tissue involvement at the time of presentation is more common and almost every organ or tissue in the body may be the site of initial disease. In gastrointestinal lymphomas the stomach is most frequently and the rectum least frequently involved. Thryoid lymphomas tend to be associated with gastro-intestinal involvement. Some skin lymphomas are T cell in type, e.g. mycosis fungoides. Most lymphomas originating in extra-lymphatic tissues are of the diffuse variety and therefore have a rather poor prognosis unless well localised.

Epidemiology

These lymphomas occur at all ages, are rare under 2 years and become more frequent with increasing age. Males are more frequently affected than females. Nodular lymphomas occur mainly in adults between the ages 30 and 60.

Clinical features

Lymph node enlargement is the most common presenting finding, and is usually painless unless it has developed very quickly. The nodes are discrete and firm. The patient usually complains of tiredness, lassitude, loss of weight and occasionally fever and sweating. However, the patient may be symptom free. When the presentation is extra-lymphatic the symptoms will reflect the tissues involved. Frequently the diagnosis of lymphoma comes as a surprise at laparotomy or during other investigative procedures.

Weakness of the legs progressing to paraplegia may be due to an extradural lymphoma compressing the cord. Pressure effects in other areas may cause dysphagia, breathlessness, vomiting, intestinal obstruction or ascites and limb oedema. Pain is the main symptom of bone involvement which may present with a pathological fracture.

Physical examination often reveals more widespread node involvement than the patient has noticed. Unexplained lymphadenopathy which fails to resolve spontaneously within a few weeks should always be suspect. Moreover lymphomatous nodes may wax and wane in size and the shrinkage of nodes does not exclude a diagnosis of lymphoma. Splenomegaly usually indicates that the spleen is involved.

Investigations

Laparotomy may be required for diagnostic purposes when only retroperitoneal nodes are involved. Bone marrow aspiration and trephine biopsy should be done early in the investigation since marrow involvement is common and indicates stage IV disease. Blood counts usually show normal values unless there is splenomegaly with hypersplenism or a complicating autoimmune haemolytic anaemia when a reduced haemoglobin level, reticulocytosis and positive direct antiglobulin test (Coombs' test) will be found (p. 723). In some patients a slight excess of lymphocytes may be present. Thrombocytopenia is uncommon. Moderate degrees of anaemia may be present if there is considerable bone marrow involvement.

FACTORS DETERMINING MANAGEMENT STRATEGY IN NON-HODGKIN LYMPHOMA

- The age of the patient
- The degree of ill health (concomitant disease)
- The type of lymphoma
- The staging of the disease
- The patient's wishes

Immunophenotyping of blood, lymph node and marrow lymphoid cells provides invaluable information on cell lineage (B or T or other), the degree of cell differentiation and cell clonality. It may also identify patients who are non-lymphomatous or demonstrate lymphoma in cases thought not to be. An assessment of immune competence is also important and immunoglobulin levels should be measured. In some cases a monoclonal band may be found.

Management

Treatment stategy in lymphoma is determined by factors listed in the information box left.

There are two principal modalities of treatment, radiotherapy and chemotherapy.

Radiotherapy. If used, this is usually given as 'involved field' treatment. No benefit is gained in survival terms from more extensive treatment. Total nodal irradiation (TNI) unfortunately causes much marrow damage and makes future chemotherapy difficult to give. Total body irradiation (TBI) is a different technique in which the body is bathed in very small doses of irradiation twice each week for 5 weeks to a total dose of 150 cGy. It is used mainly for low-grade disease.

Chemotherapy. This may be given as simple single agent treatment or as combination therapy with multiple drug regimens designed to optimise tumour toxicity and minimise damage to the normal tissues particularly the haemopoietic tissues.

Disease relapsing during chemotherapy generally carries a poor prognosis unless alternative therapy is available. If relapse occurs years after cessation of therapy response to the same chemotherapy as was originally used may be good.

Management of low-grade lymphoma

No specific therapy may be required if the disease is not advanced. Some patients can be observed for years before active measures are indicated. Where treatment is required, either radiotherapy or chemotherapy may be used. The indications are:

Stage I and IIA	Involved field radiotherapy
Stage IIB, III and IV	Chemotherapy, single agent or combination Whole body irradiation

Treatment with radiotherapy should be given for very localised disease as there is the possibility of cure. No combination chemotherapy regimen has been shown to give longer survival than single agent chlorambucil therapy. The latter is better tolerated by the patient. Chlorambucil is administered usually at a dose of 5 mg daily although this may be adjusted upwards or downwards as dictated by blood counts until response is obtained. This may take many weeks or months. Dose reduction will be necessary if the leucocyte and platelet count fall significantly below the normal range. Once response has been achieved the patient may be off therapy sometimes for a number of years and the same treatment used again on relapse. Eventually the disease becomes more aggressive with the appearance of more primitive lymphocytes. At this stage combination chemotherapy is very often required and the palliative use of radiotherapy for local problems can be useful.

Management of high grade lymphoma

The indications for radiotherapy and chemotherapy in high grade lymphoma are:

Stage I disease (adequately staged)	Involved field radiotherapy
Stage II, III and IV disease	Intensive combination chemotherapy to the limit of patient tolerance

Over 90% of these patients require chemotherapy. Stage I disease is uncommon and difficult to prove. Intensive combination chemotherapy will give long-term remission in over 50% of patients with the most malignant varieties of high-grade lymphoma. The treatment should be pushed to the limits of tolerance and may require the services of highly specialised units capable of supporting patients with severe bone marrow failure as for the treatment of acute leukaemia (p. 730).

Lymphoblastic lymphoma

This is a highly malignant lymphoma usually of T cell phenotype found in young persons. Over 70% are males, adolescent or young adults. Presentation is with bulky mediastinal disease in about 50% and 30% have marrow involvement at diagnosis. There is a tendency to develop CNS disease. Aggressive chemotherapy as for poor prognosis acute lymphoblastic leukaemia is given together with CNS prophylaxis.

Elderly patients may not tolerate the aggressive chemotherapeutic approach. More gentle combination chemotherapy such as the CHOP regimen (cyclophosphamide, adriamycin, vincristine, prednisone) may be possible or the disease palliated with involved field radiotherapy.

Bone marrow transplantation. For patients young enough (less than 40 years) with compatible donors, allogeneic or syngeneic bone marrow transplantation is a possibility and long-term remissions have been achieved. It can be offered as salvage therapy for relapsing disease and has about a 25% success rate. Unfortunately the majority of patients with high-grade lymphoma are outside this age group.

Prognosis

This is given in Table 14.14. Low grade lymphomas are almost never cured but high-grade lymphomas have a 50% chance of long-term remission and possibly cure if treated properly.

Table 14.14   Prognosis of non-Hodgkin lymphoma

Grade	Median survival
Low	7–8 years
Intermediate	2 years
High	1 year

BURKITT'S LYMPHOMA

This form of lymphoblastic B cell non-Hodgkin's lymphoma occurs predominantly in tropical Africa and New Guinea, although it also occurs less frequently in other parts of the world. There is strong evidence that the Epstein-Barr (EB) virus plays an important aetiological role in its development. The majority of cases occur in children with a peak incidence between the ages of 4 and 8 years, although cases found outside the tropics show an older age distribution and a lower incidence of EB viral infection.

Clinical features

The disorder affects predominantly extranodal tissues with a marked predilection for the mandible and the maxillary bones. This may cause marked bone deformity, loosening of the teeth and, if the orbit is involved, extrusion of the eye with loss of sight. In the abdomen, involvement often bilaterally, of the kidneys, adrenals, ovaries or lymph nodes may give rise to abdominal tumours.

Extradural lesions of the spinal cord may cause sudden onset of paraplegia. Other sites which may be involved include long bones, the salivary glands, the thyroid, testes and the heart. Bilateral tumours of the breast may be seen in young adult women. Abdominal tumours are the most common finding in patients outside the tropics and lymph nodes and marrow are more frequently involved.

Investigations

The cytological appearance of Burkitt's lymphoma is characteristic with lymphoblast-type cells showing vacuolation in the cytoplasm and nucleus. Histologically the 'starry sky' appearance created by histiocytes scattered amongst sheets of primitive lymphoid cells is typical. Chromosome analysis shows an 8/14 translocation in a high proportion of cases and less often 2/8 or 8/22 translocation. Antibody to EB viral capsid antigen is found in most patients with the African variety.

Management

Response to chemotherapy, particularly in the African variety if the disease is localised, is very good. Cyclophosphamide is given intramuscularly, 40–60 mg/kg every 2 weeks for up to 6 doses. Prophylactic intrathecal methotrexate may also be given because meningeal involvement often occurs later in the disease. The response to treatment is often dramatic with resolution of the disease following the first dose of cyclophosphamide. The cases found randomly throughout the world in an older age group are much more difficult to treat and require exceptionally aggressive chemotherapy.

MULTIPLE MYELOMA (MYELOMATOSIS)

This is a malignant disorder of plasma cells.

Immunopathology

Normal plasma cells are derived from B lymphocytes by transformation after exposure to antigenic stimuli; individual plasma cells manufacture immunoglobulins with only one type of light chain. The finding that in myeloma, and in other related malignant disorders of B lymphocytes, all the malignant cells produce the same immunoglobulin indicates that the tumour is derived originally from one cell by cloning; the disease is therefore monoclonal.

The immunoglobulin is called a paraprotein and appears on electrophoretic strips as a clear-cut band. Each of the five normal types of immunoglobulin has light chains of either lambda or kappa variety (Fig. 2.3, p. 30). In myeloma the paraprotein produced belongs to one of these immunoglobulin types and has one or other of the two light chains. In some patients only part of the immunoglobulin molecule is produced by the tumour cells, most commonly the light chains. These appear in the urine as Bence-Jones proteinuria and if myeloma is associated only with light chains it is known as Bence-Jones myeloma.

The classification of myeloma by type of paraprotein and their relative frequency are given in Table 14.15.

Table 14.15   Classification of multiple myeloma

Type of paraprotein	Relative frequency %
IgG	55
IgA	21
Light chain only	22
Others (D, E, nonsecretory)	2

Patients with a myeloma which produces complete immunoglobulin molecules may also excrete increased amounts of light chain in their urine (Bence-Jones proteinuria). In some this appears later as a new phenomenon and usually indicates an acceleration of the disease.

Epidemiology

The disease is very uncommon under the age of 30. Thereafter it becomes increasingly frequent, with a peak incidence between 60 and 70 years. Males are affected rather more frequently than females and Black people of Central African origin two to three times more often than Caucasians.

Pathology

In the majority of patients the bone marrow is heavily infiltrated with atypical plasma cells which are usually larger and paler staining than normal plasma cells and contain nucleoli. Some cells may be multinucleated. Progressive replacement of the marrow occurs with eventual reduction of the normal cell lines, inducing anaemia, leucopenia and thrombocytopenia. Osteoclasts are stimulated and absorption of bone occurs, producing diffuse osteoporosis. Local tumour formation by the myeloma causes punched out translucencies in the bone radiograph. Rarely the disease may present as a solitary plasmacytoma either in bone or soft tissue.

Excessive production of the myeloma paraprotein is associated with progressive reduction in normal immunoglobulin levels and impairment of immune function.

Clinical features

There is a long preclinical phase, in some instances up to 25 years. The disorder may be discovered incidentally by laboratory tests during this phase and the patient may be observed for years before symptoms appear. The symptoms and their mechanism are given in Table 14.16.

Investigations

A diagnosis of myeloma requires the detection of at least two of the following abnormalities:

1. monoclonal immunoglobulin or light chains in blood or urine;

Table 14.16 The relationship between pathology, the effect of the disease process and the symptoms

Pathology	Effect	Symptoms
Marrow involvement with malignant plasma cells	Bone erosion due to stimulation of osteoclasts	Pain in weight-bearing skeleton of wandering and persistent type
	Pathological fractures	Severe local pain
	Hypercalcaemia	Lethargy and coma
	Anaemia	Tiredness, malaise
	Bone marrow failure Leucopenia Thrombocytopenia	Infections and bleeding
Excess production of paraprotein and light chains	Renal damage	None until uraemic
	Increased blood viscosity	None until severe, then blurred vision, headache, vertigo, stupor, coma
	Amyloidosis – renal damage	Azotaemia
Reduction in number of plasma cells	Impaired immune function	Susceptibility to infection, particularly respiratory

2. infiltration of the marrow with malignant plasma cells;
3. osteolytic bone lesions.

Once a diagnosis has been established investigations should be undertaken to clarify the questions listed in Table 14.17.

Table 14.17 Rationale for investigations in multiple myeloma

	Investigations
State of renal function?	Urea and electrolytes, creatinine, urate
Presence of hypercalcaemia?	Blood calcium Albumin
Presence of bone fractures?	Radiographs Blood alkaline phosphatase Bone scan
Degree of immune paresis?	Plasma immunoglobulins
Degree of bone marrow failure?	Blood counts Reticulocyte count
Disorder of haemostasis?	Bleeding time Coagulation screen
Blood viscosity?	Plasma viscosity
Disease activity?	Serum $\beta 2$ microglobulin

POINTS TO NOTE IN DIAGNOSIS OF MYELOMA

- In the absence of fractures or bone repair the plasma alkaline phosphatase and the bone scan are normal
- Serum B-microglobulin estimations may provide a useful assessment of prognosis
- The absence of immune paresis (reduction of normal immunoglobulins below normal levels) should cast doubt on the diagnosis
- Only about 5% of patients with ESRs persistently above 100 mm in the first hour have myeloma

The points listed in the information box (left) should be noted.

Management

Sometimes myeloma is diagnosed when the disease is at an early stage and not causing symptoms or any other problems. At this stage it is reasonable to observe the patient as no specific treatment may be required for several years. Treatment should be started if the patient is symptomatic or there is other evidence of disorder due to the myeloma.

All patients must take at least 3 litres of fluid each day indefinitely unless there is no evidence of renal impairment, a serum B2-microglobulin level of less than 4 mg/l and less than 0.1 unit of free light chains per gramme creatinine in the urine.

The high fluid intake is particularly important in patients with compromised renal function. In these the addition of oral sodium bicarbonate enough to make the urine neutral or alkaline may be helpful, particularly if the plasma bicarbonate falls below 20 mmol/l.

Chemotherapy

If the patient can tolerate aggressive therapy, a regimen which includes adriamycin, BCNU, cyclophosphamide and melphalan in 6-weekly pulses achieves the best results. This is unsuitable for patients over 75. A more gentle regimen consists of melphalan 7 mg/m^2 daily for 4 days every 4–6 weeks with or without prednisolone 40 mg/m^2 for 4 days. Cytopenic patients can be given cyclophosphamide i.v. 300 mg/m^2 weekly. Allopurinol 300 mg daily is given in the early stages of treatment to prevent excessive formation of uric acid. Treatment is continued until 'plateau phase' after which there is no value in continuing. Plateau phase is that stage at which the patient's paraprotein level, haemoglobin and β-

microglobulin level have become stable and the patient is well or only minimally symptomatic over a period of at least 3 months. Further chemotherapy with the same or other regimens may be given if the patient relapses and further response may be obtained. Eventually the disease becomes increasingly refractory to treatment.

Radiotherapy. Radiotherapy is uniquely useful in the treatment of local problems such as severe bone pain, pathological fractures and tumorous lesions. Hemi-body irradiation in which the lower half of the body and then 6–8 weeks later the upper half is irradiated, may be employed for disseminated skeletal pain but is moderately toxic to bone marrow and lungs.

Renal failure. In the early stages of the disease when there is the possibility of life extending chemotherapy, renal failure should be treated vigorously. Renal dialysis may be necessary.

Infections. Patients and their GP should be warned of the need to treat any infections early with referral to hospital if necessary. Patients may be given an antibiotic such as amoxicillin to be taken if an infection develops.

Hypercalcaemia. This is most commonly seen in IgA myeloma. It increases the dehydration and causes drowsiness, confusion, leading on to coma and death, if not treated. The patient should be rehydrated and given prednisolone, 30–40 mg daily for as short a period as possible, consistent with obtaining a response. Mithramycin is also highly effective at doses of up to 25 µg/kg body weight daily for 2–4 days. The drug is cytotoxic and may cause a marked drop of the platelet count and also, if high doses are used, a bleeding diathesis. It acts by inhibiting osteoclast stimulating factor thus reducing bone resorption and the liberation of calcium from the bones.

Progress
Episodes of bone pain and fracture are liable to occur despite good control of the general disease. Prophylactic irradiation of eroded vertebrae may be warranted before crush fractures occur. At all times bed-rest should be minimised to avoid further loss of calcium from the skeleton.

Hyperviscosity problems, if they arise, will require plasmapheresis. The discrete use of anabolic steroids such as oxymetholone 50 mg on alternate days may be helpful in arresting further deterioration of the skeleton. Almost inevitably the disease develops eventually to a crippling and painful phase when it may be very

difficult to maintain the morale of the patient. At this stage adequate and effective use of analgesic support is essential. Death is often associated with terminal respiratory infection.

Prognosis
Without treatment the disease progresses relentlessly to death. With treatment the outlook for the majority of patients is considerably improved and a few may survive for many years. Bad signs at the time of diagnosis are shown in the information box (p. 748).

Prognosis should be guarded in any individual until the response to treatment has been assessed; this may take 6 months or more.

Waldenström's macroglobulinaemia
This is a rare disease of the elderly, more common in males than females. There is a monoclonal IgM

Table 14.18   Cytotoxic drugs and diseases in which they may be used

Antimetabolite	
Methotrexate	All NHL intrathecal
Mercaptopurine	ALL AML CML
Thioguanine	AML CML ALL
Cytarabine	AML MDS ALL NHL CML
Asparaginase	ALL
Alkylating agent	
Mustine	HD NHL
Cyclophosphamide	HD NHL AL ALL MY PL
Chlorambucil	CLL NHL HD WM
Busulphan	CML PV ET MF
Melphalan	MY CML PV ET
Ifosamide	NHL HD
Plant alkaloid	
Vincristine sulphate	ALL AML HD NHL CLL PL MY
Vinblastine sulphate	HD NHL
Vindesine sulphate	HD NHL
Etoposide (VP-16)	HD NHL AML
Nitrosoureas	
Carmustine (BCNU)	MY HD NHL
Lomustine (CCNU)	MY HD NHL
Antibiotic	
Daunorubicin	ALL ALL
Doxorubicin	NHL HD PL
Bleomycin sulphate	NHL HD
Mitoxantrone	ALL AML NHL
Miscellaneous	
Hydroxyurea	CML MF PV ET AML
Dibromomannitol	CML
Procarbazine	HD
Deoxycoformycin	T cell leukaemia/lymphoma HCL
Interferon	HCL CML MY
Glucocorticoids	ALL NHL CLL MY MF

Note: ALL = acute lymphoblastic leukaemia; AML = acute myeloblastic leukaemia; CLL = chronic lymphocytic leukaemia; CML = chronic myeloid leukaemia; ET = essential thrombocythaemia; HCL = hairy cell leukaemia; HD = Hodgkin's disease; MDS = myelodysplastic syndrome; MF = myelofibrosis; MY = myeloma; NHL = non-Hodgkin's lymphoma; PL = prolymphocytic leukaemia; PV = polycythaemia vera; WM = Waldenstrom's macroglobulinaemia.

POOR PROGNOSTIC FEATURES AT DIAGNOSIS IN MULTIPLE MYELOMA

- A haemoglobin level of less than 70 g/l
- Severe hypoalbuminaemia
- Intractable renal failure
- Thrombocytopenia
- High β2-microglobulin levels
- Plasma cell leukaemia

paraproteinaemia and a tendency to develop a hyperviscosity syndrome. The marrow is infiltrated with neoplastic lymphocytes.

Untreated, the progress is often slow with eventual immune deficiency and susceptibility to infection. Chlorambucil on a long-term low dose basis, such as 2 mg daily, may control the lymphocyte proliferation and the advance of the disease. Some patients are unresponsive. Plasmapheresis may be required. The majority of patients survive 2–5 years and some live considerably longer.

A summary of the drug regimens of use in malignant disease of the haematopoietic system is given in Table 14.18.

HAEMOSTASIS

The prevention of bleeding depends upon maintaining the integrity of the blood vessel walls by mechanisms which ensure that any breaches are rapidly sealed by deposition of platelets and fibrin. This process can be arbitrarily divided into two stages. Firstly primary haemostasis in which the vessel constricts; activated platelets adhere to the damaged wall and subsequently aggregate to form a platelet plug which arrests haemorrhage. During secondary haemostasis the platelet plug is stabilised by deposition of a network of fibrin. The initial platelet plug formation takes place over a few minutes whilst its stabilisation by fibrin, within the aggregated platelets, takes much longer. Although haemostasis is arbitrarily divided into these two stages they are in fact closely interrelated. There are receptors on the activated platelet surface for components of the coagulation cascade ensuring that they are brought into close proximity resulting in a greatly enhanced rate of fibrin generation compared to the reactions that occur in a platelet free environment. Fibrinolysis is initiated by tissue plasminogen activator released from local endothelial cells; this converts fibrin bound plasminogen to plasmin which lyses the fibrin.

PLATELETS

Each megakaryocyte liberates several thousand individual platelets into the circulation where each has a life span of approximately 10 days. They are complex highly specialised cells capable of responding quickly to a variety of activators, e.g. ADP, thrombin and collagen, by contracting into spheres and sending out long pseudopodia which adhere to subendothelial vessel wall components and neighbouring platelets.

Within the cytoplasm are three types of storage organelles; alpha granules, containing a variety of coagulation factors, e.g. fibrinogen and von Willebrand factor; dense granules which store low molecular weight substances, e.g. ADP and serotonin; and lysosomes containing acid hydrolases. When platelets are activated the contents of these granules are discharged and promote further platelet aggregation and fibrin deposition on the platelet surface. The platelet surface contains many well-characterised glycoproteins which act as receptors for external activators and transmit stimuli into the cytoplasm. During activation arachidonic acid is liberated from membrane lipids and converted by platelet cyclo-oxygenase and thromboxane synthetase to thromboxane A_2 which is the most potent stimulator of platelet aggregation known. Aspirin, and other non-steroidal anti-inflammatory drugs, being potent inhibitors of cyclo-oxygenase, reduce platelet function resulting in a predisposition to haemorrhage.

Thrombocytopenia causes characteristic bleeding with purpura, bruising and mucosal haemorrhage of the nose, mouth, gastrointestinal and genito-urinary tracts. A severe reduction in platelet numbers may result in fundal haemorrhage and intracranial bleeding which is often fatal.

COAGULATION SYSTEM

The cascade of the coagulation mechanism consists of a series of inactive zymogens; each activates a subsequent enzyme by its protease activity. The cascade is often considered to be composed of two distinct parts, the intrinsic and extrinsic systems, which both converge to activate factor X. Although the system is often envisaged as illustrated in Fig. 14.17, and from a practical viewpoint such a scheme is very helpful in understanding deficiencies, it is a gross simplification of the many interactions. Many more reactions between different components take place than are illustrated. The plasma concentration of the components increases down the cascade; there being only trace amounts of factor XII but relatively very high levels of fibrinogen (Table 14.19). Such amplification allows for small

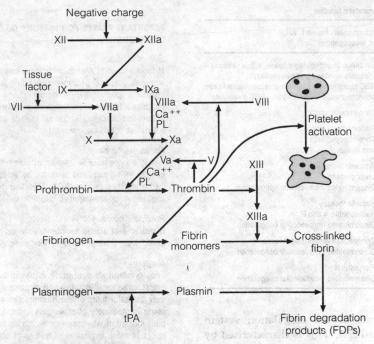

Fig. 14.17 Cascade of the coagulation mechanism. (PL = platelet, tPA = tissue plasminogen activator.)

initiating stimuli to result in the deposition of large amounts of fibrin.

The intrinsic pathway, consisting of factors XII, XI, IX and VIII is activated by negatively charged surfaces and activated platelets. It is assessed in vitro by the activated partial thromboplastin time (APTT) (Table 14.20).

The extrinsic pathway measured by the prothrombin time (PT), depends upon tissue factor, liberated from

damaged cells, activating factor VII. Both these in vitro tests of the coagulation cascade are more sensitive to deficiencies of the initial components than those in the final common pathway subsequent to factor X activation. For this reason neither the APTT nor the PT can be relied upon to reflect the concentration of fibrinogen and this is therefore measured specifically when the whole coagulation cascade is being screened.

Deficiencies, either congenital or acquired, of single

Table 14.19   Components of the haemostatic system

Factor	Synonym	Half-life	Treatment of single deficiency
I	Fibrinogen	4 days	Cryo
II	Prothrombin	3 days	Concentrate II, IX, X
V	Proaccelerin	12–15 h	FFP
VII	Proconvertin	4–6 h	Concentrate VII
VIII	Antihaemophilic factor	12–15 h	Concentrate VIII
IX	Christmas factor	20 h	Concentrate II, IX, X
X	Stuart-Prower factor	10–15 h	Concentrate II, IX, X
XI	Plasma thrombo-plastin antecedent (PTA)	3 days	Concentrate XI
XII	Hageman factor		—
XIII	Fibrin stabilising factor	12–15 days	Concentrate XIII
ATIII	Antithrombin III	2 days	Concentrate ATIII
	Platelets	3–4 days	Platelet concentrates

Cryo. = cryoprecipitate, FFP. = fresh frozen plasma

Table 14.20 Investigation of haemostatic function

Investigation	Information obtained. Value of investigations
Blood film	Evidence of underlying disease, e.g. leukaemia Platelets numbers and morphology RBC morphology, e.g. liver disease – target cells Microangiopathic haemolysis – RBC fragments
Platelet count	Thrombocytopenia
Bleeding time	Platelet dysfunction Thrombocytopenia von Willebrand's disease
Prothrombin time (extrinsic pathway)	Warfarin therapy Liver disease Disseminated intravascular coagulation
Activated partial thromboplastin time (intrinsic pathway)	Heparin therapy Haemophilia A and B Disseminated intravascular coagulation
Fibrinogen concentration	Congenital hypofibrinogenaemia Disseminated intravascular coagulation
D dimers	Fibrinolysis Disseminated intravascular coagulation

or multiple components of the coagulation system result in a bleeding diathesis. This is characterised by joint and muscle haemorrhage and prolonged bleeding after surgery or trauma, for example as in haemophilia. Occasionally autoantibodies may arise, sometimes in association with autoimmune disorders, which specifically inhibit one of the components, e.g. factor VIII, resulting in a severe bleeding disorder, e.g. acquired haemophilia. It may be very difficult to treat because when the deficient factor is transfused it is quickly neutralised by the antibody.

Once activated the coagulation proteins are inhibited by the protease inhibitors antithrombin III and protein C. A deficiency of either of these may result in a predisposition to venous thromboembolism.

ASSESSMENT OF PATIENT WITH A POSSIBLE BLEEDING DISORDER

A careful history of all bleeding episodes is essential as well as a full clinical examination prior to the laboratory investigation. A history of bleeding is often remarkably reproducible particularly after dental extraction; if a socket oozes for two days after removal of a tooth on one occasion it is likely to do so again following each subsequent extraction.

History

It is important to consider the points listed in the information box (right).

IMPORTANT POINTS FOR HISTORY OF BLEEDING DISORDERS

Site of bleeds
Muscle and joint bleeds indicate a coagulation defect, whereas purpura, prolonged bleeding from superficial cuts, epistaxis, gastrointestinal haemorrhage or menorrhagia indicate a failure of platelets or possibly the presence of von Willebrand disease. Recurrent bleeds at a single site suggest a local structural abnormality

Duration of history
It may be possible to assess whether the patient has a congenital or acquired disorder by whether the patient has had a life-long propensity to bleeding or a short history suggestive of an acquired cause

Precipitating causes
Bleeding that arises spontaneously indicates a more severe defect than if haemorrhage only arises after trauma

Surgery
Enquiry about all operations is useful but particularly dental extractions, tonsillectomy and circumcision as these are all very stressful tests of the haemostatic system. Bleeding that starts immediately after surgery indicates defective platelet plug formation whereas that which comes on after several hours is more indicative of failure of platelet plug stabilisation by fibrin due to a coagulation defect

Family history
Absence of other relatives with clinically significant bleeding does not exclude a hereditary bleeding diathesis; about one-third of cases of haemophilia arise in individuals without a family history

Systemic illnesses
Many diseases, or their treatment may occasionally be associated with bleeding but it is particularly important to consider the possibility of hepatic or renal failure, paraproteinaemia or a collagenosis

Drugs
Almost any drug can potentially produce bleeding either by depressing marrow function with consequent thrombocytopenia or by interacting with warfarin. Nonsteroidal anti-inflammatory drugs inhibit platelet function; the effect of aspirin may last for up to 10 days after a single tablet

---

Superficial examination may reveal bruises and purpura. Telangectasia of lips and tongue are diagnostic of hereditary haemorrhagic telangectasia. Joints should be carefully scrutinised for evidence of haemarthroses. A full general medical examination is important because it may give clues of systemic illness.

Investigations

Screening investigations and their interpretation are given in Table 14.20. If the patient has a referent history and all the preliminary tests give normal results it may be appropriate to perform further investigations. The clinical history may be a useful guide as to whether attention should be directed to platelet function (von Willebrand disease) or coagulation disturbance, e.g. haemophilia.

VESSEL WALL ABNORMALITIES

Abnormalities of the vessel walls both congenital and acquired, e.g. vasculitis, may result in a propensity to bleed.

HEREDITARY HAEMORRHAGIC TELANGIECTASIA

This is a dominantly inherited condition in which telangiectasia and small aneurysms are found on the fingertips, face, nasal passages, tongue and gastrointestinal tract.

Clinical features

Patients present either with recurrent bleeds particularly epistaxis or iron deficiency due to occult gastrointestinal bleeding.

Management

Treatment can be difficult because of the multiple bleeding points but regular iron therapy often allows the marrow to compensate for blood loss. Local cautery or laser therapy may prevent single lesions from bleeding. A variety of medical therapies has been tried, but none has been found to be universally effective.

Ehlers-Danlos. This is a congenital disorder of collagen synthesis in which the capillaries are poorly supported by subcutaneous collagen and ecchymoses are commonly observed.

QUALITATIVE ABNORMALITIES OF PLATELETS

Even in the presence of a normal platelet count an individual may bleed if the function of the platelets is reduced. Congenital abnormalities include disorders of the membrane glycoproteins, e.g. thrombasthenia and Bernard Soulier syndrome, or the presence of defective platelet granules, e.g. storage pool disorders. Such patients exhibit bleeding of platelet type which varies between patients, some presenting with severe recurrent bleeds whilst others are only diagnosed because of excessive post-operative haemorrhage.

Many drugs inhibit platelet function. Aspirin and other non-steroidal drugs inhibit platelet cyclo-oxygenase preventing the conversion of arachidonic acid to the potent platelet aggregator, thromboxane B2. Other drugs which inhibit platelets are listed in the information box below.

DRUG INHIBITING PLATELET FUNCTION	
Non-steroidal anti-inflammatory agents	*Antibiotics*
Aspirin	Penicillins
Indomethacin	Cephalosporins
Phenylbutazone	*Dextran*
Sulphinpyrazone	
	Heparin
	Beta-blockers

QUANTITATIVE DISORDERS OF PLATELETS

THROMBOCYTOPENIA

A reduced platelet count may arise by one of three mechanisms; failure of megakaryocyte maturation, excessive platelet consumption after their release into the circulation or platelet sequestration in an enlarged spleen. The common causes of thrombocytopenia are listed in the information box below.

CAUSES OF THROMBOCYTOPENIA
Marrow disorders
Hypoplasia
Idiopathic
Drug induced
Cytotoxic
Antimetabolites
Thiozides
Infiltration
Leukaemia
Myeloma
Carcinoma
Myelofibrosis
Osteopetrosis
B_{12}/folate deficiency
Increased consumption of platelets
Disseminated intravascular coagulation
Idiopathic thrombocytopenic purpura (ITP)
Viral infections
Epstein-Barr virus
Human immunodeficiency virus
Bacterial infections — e.g. gram negative septicaemia
Hypersplenism
Lymphomas
Liver disease

Clinical features

Spontaneous bleeding does not usually occur until the platelet count falls below about $30 \times 10^9/l$ unless their function is also compromised, for example following aspirin ingestion. Purpura and spontaneous bruising are characteristic but there may also be oral, nasal, gastrointestinal or genito-urinary bleeding. Severe thrombocytopenia results in fundal haemorrhage which may be a prelude to a rapidly fatal intracranial bleed.

Investigations

These are performed to ascertain the possible cause of thrombocytopenia and should be directed towards the conditions listed in the information box (p. 53). A blood film may give diagnostic information as in acute leukaemia. A bone marrow will reveal whether there is an infiltrate, e.g. carcinoma; a reduced number of megakaryocytes, e.g. hypoplastic anaemia; or an increased number of megakaryocytes indicating excessive peripheral destruction, e.g. idiopathic thrombocytopenic purpura.

Management

Thrombocytopenia causing clinically significant bleeding constitutes a haematological emergency which should be promptly investigated and appropriately treated. Treatment should be directed to the underlying condition. Platelet transfusions for thrombocytopenia should be given only to treat troublesome bleeding, for example persistant epistaxis, or potentially life-threatening bleeding, e.g. gastrointestinal haemorrhage. Such transfusions provide only temporary relief because the survival of the platelets is only a few days at most and in many instances may be only a matter of minutes or hours if the thrombocytopenia is due to increased platelet consumption as in ITP or disseminated intravascular coagulation.

IDIOPATHIC THROMBOCYTOPENIC PURPURA (ITP)

The presence of auto-antibodies, often directed against membrane glycoprotein IIb–IIIa, causes the premature removal of platelets by the monocyte-macrophage system. Occasionally antigen-antibody immune complexes adhere to platelets at their Fc receptor resulting in their premature removal from the circulation.

Clinical features in children

In children, ITP often presents 2–3 weeks after a viral illness with the sudden onset of purpura and sometimes oral and nasal bleeding. The peripheral blood film is normal apart from a greatly reduced platelet number whilst the bone marrow reveals an obvious increase in megakaryocytes. It is important to ascertain that the child does not have any other systemic illness and in particular disseminated intravascular coagulation.

Management

It is usual to withhold any specific treatment if the child has only mild bleeding symptoms as the condition, in the majority, is self limiting within a few weeks. The presence of moderate to severe purpura, bruising or epistaxis and a platelet count that is usually less than $10 \times 10^9/l$ is an indication for prednisolone 2 mg/kg/day. The platelet count usually rises promptly within 1–3 days. Increasingly intravenous immunoglobulin is used as primary therapy. Persistent epistaxis, gastrointestinal bleeding, fundal haemorrhages or any suggestion of intracranial bleeding should be treated immediately by a platelet transfusion. If fresh bleeding persists for more than a few days following the introduction of steroids, intravenous immunoglobulin should be given.

Clinical features in adults

In adults, ITP more commonly affects females and has a more gradual insidious onset. It is unusual for there to be a history of a preceding viral infection. Some patients at presentation may have symptoms or signs of a collagenosis or rheumatoid arthritis, whilst in others these disorders may become apparent several years later. The condition is likely to become chronic, with remissions and relapses.

Management

Treatment with prednisolone 1 mg/kg/day is less rewarding than in children; often the platelet count rises in response to therapy but falls again when the dose is reduced or stopped. Persistent or potentially life-threatening bleeding should be treated with platelet transfusion.

Relapses should be treated by increasing the dose of prednisolone. If a patient has two relapses it is customary to consider splenectomy. This should be preceded by pneumococcal vaccination; because so many adult patients with ITP require splenectomy it is prudent to vaccinate all patients at presentation (subcutaneously; if given by the customary intramuscular route it may result in a muscle haematoma) before they become immuno-suppressed with a prolonged course of steroids. Splenectomy is curative in about 70% of patients and in the remainder the aim should be to keep the patient free of symptoms rather than treat the platelet count alone. Often such patients have counts of $20–30 \times 10^9/l$ without symptoms; some require long term maintenance with prednisolone at 5 mg/day. If significant bleeding persists despite splenectomy and a small dose of steroids e.g. 5 mg/daily, vincristine, immunosuppressive therapy, e.g. cyclophosphamide, or intravenous immunoglobulin should be considered.

THROMBOCYTOSIS

An increase in platelet count may either occur as a direct result of malignant proliferation of megakaryocytes or as non-specific reactive response to chronic bleeding or inflammation. Secondary thrombocytosis is much more common than primary malignant disorders (Table 14.21). Malignant increase of megakaryocytes

Table 14.21   Causes of a raised platelet count

Reactive thrombocytosis	Malignant thrombocytosis
Chronic inflammatory disorders	Essential thrombocythaemia
Malignant disease	Primary proliferative polycythaemia
Tissue damage	Myelofibrosis
Haemolytic anaemias	Chronic myeloid leukaemia
Post-splenectomy	
Post-haemorrhage	

may occur alone resulting in essential thrombocythaemia or may be accompanied by a more fundamental defect of the bone marrow stem cell as in chronic myeloid leukaemia, polycythaemia vera or myelofibrosis.

ESSENTIAL THROMBOCYTHAEMIA

This malignant condition of megakaryocytes results in a raised level of circulating platelets which may in addition have aberrant function.

Clinical features
Patients may present with excessive bruising and bleeding or with venous or arterial thrombosis. Splenomegaly may be present but in some patients the blood film reveals changes due to splenic atrophy, e.g. Howell Jolly bodies, as a result of asymptomatic splenic infarction. In most individuals the condition is chronic with the platelet count only gradually increasing.

Management
Treatment of essential thrombocythaemia is by intravenous radioactive phosphorous (^{32}P) or alkylating reagents, e.g. busulphan. On rare occasions it rises rapidly, sometimes accompanied by blast cells in the peripheral blood when it is more correctly termed megakaryocytic leukaemia and should be treated like acute myeloid leukaemia.

COAGULATION DISORDERS

HAEMOPHILIA A

Of the various congenital disorders of coagulation factors the commonest is that causing a reduction of factor VIII resulting in haemophilia A which affects 1:10 000 individuals. Factor VIII is primarily synthesised by the liver but other organs, e.g. spleen, kidney and placenta, may also contribute to the plasma level. Plasma factor VIII has a half life of about 12 hours and is carried non-covalently bound to the von Willebrand factor. The very large 286 kilobase factor VIII gene is located on the X chromosome and consists of 26 exons. A large number of different defects in the gene have been identified, for example single base changes resulting in amino acid substitutions or nonsense codons (causing premature chain termination) or deletions. The normal factor VIII gene has been cloned and small amounts of synthetic factor VIII have been synthesised to treat a few patients. It is anticipated that within the next few years this supply will greatly increase potentially providing almost an unlimited amount of factor VIII.

Clinical features
Although haemophilia A is a congenital disorder it is unusual for excessive bleeding to be noticed until babies are about 6 months old when superficial bruising or a haemarthrosis is observed. This apparent delay in presentation is presumably due to the relative inactivity of babies in the first few months of life and it is only when they begin to move about that more trauma results in the excessive bleeding. It is not uncommon for children to be initially classified as having non-accidental injury unless all such children are appropriately investigated for the presence of a bleeding disorder.

The normal factor VIII level is 0.50–1.50 i.u./ml and is usually measured by a clotting assay. The propensity to bleeding is related to the plasma factor VIII level; those with less than 0.02 i.u./ml are classified as having severe haemophilia; 0.02–0.10 i.u./ml as moderate and those with greater than 0.10 i.u./ml as a mild form of the disorder.

Individuals with severe haemophilia experience recurrent haemarthroses in large joints (Fig. 14.18). Bleeding usually occurs spontaneously without apparent trauma and the joints most commonly affected are knees, elbows, ankles and hips. The patient is aware that bleeding has started because of an abnormal sensation in the joint. If treatment is not given at this stage bleeding continues resulting in a hot, swollen very painful joint; severe pain and swelling may last for

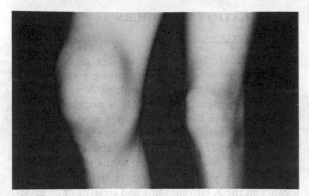

Fig. 14.18   Acute haemarthrosis of right knee.

many days before gradually subsiding. Recurrent bleeds into joints lead to synovial hypertrophy, destruction of the cartilage and secondary osteoarthrosis (Fig. 14.19). The resultant limitation of movement may greatly reduce the function of joints making walking difficult.

Muscle haematoma is the other bleeding problem faced by haemophiliacs. These occur most commonly in the calf (Fig. 14.20) and psoa muscles but almost any muscle may develop a haematoma. Although relatively less common than haemarthroses a single episode can leave severe lasting damage if not effectively treated. A large psoas bleed, for example, may extend to press on the femoral nerve with consequent parasthaesia in the thigh and weakness of the quadriceps; although some of this injury may be reversible, the patient is often left with some weakness in the leg. Furthermore if the bleed does not resolve completely recurrences may occur leading to progressive muscle and nerve damage. Calf haematomas are also serious because of the inflexible facial sheath surrounding the soleus and gastrocnaemius muscles; untreated haemorrhage causes a rise in pressure with eventual ischaemia, necrosis, fibrosis and subsequent contraction and shortening of the Achilles tendon (Fig. 14.21).

Although joint and muscle bleeds are the commonest places for haemorrhage, bleeding can occur at almost any site. Clearly it is particularly serious if it takes place in a confined anatomical space associated with vital structures. Thus intracranial haemorrhage is often fatal, unless it is treated promptly.

Individuals with moderate haemophilia usually only experience haemorrhage after minor trauma and those with the mild form of the disorder following more major trauma or surgery. Whereas severe haemophilia is usually diagnosed within the first two years of life individuals with moderate and mild forms may escape diagnosis until adulthood.

Management

Bleeding episodes should be treated early by raising the factor VIII level. This is most commonly accomplished by intravenous infusion of factor VIII concentrate prepared from blood donor plasma. Such concentrates are freeze dried and stable at 4°C and can therefore be stored in domestic refrigerators. This enables many patients to treat themselves at home and has revolutionised haemophilia care. Until recently cryoprecipitate has been used to treat patients particularly those individuals with mild haemophilia who were only rarely exposed to blood products. This was because cryoprecipitate was perceived to carry a smaller chance of transmitting hepatitis than factor VIII concentrate which is prepared from a plasma pool composed of many thousands of individual blood donations. How-

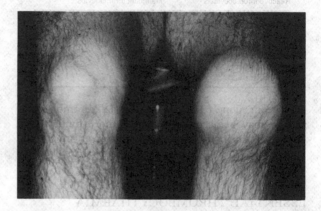

A

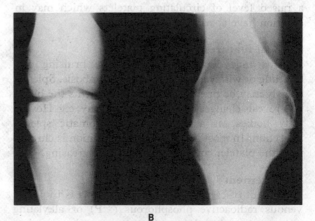

B

Fig. 14.19   Haemophilic arthropathy of left knee. A. Bony enlargement of femoral condyles and head of tibia.
B. Destruction of joint; loss of articular cartilage, cysts in bone, osteophytes and broadening of condyles.

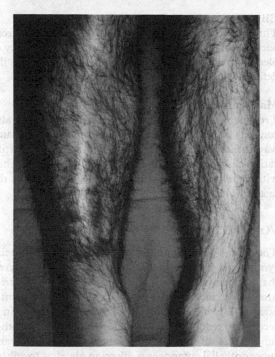

Fig. 14.20 Muscle haematoma in the calf of the leg.

ever, all factor VIII concentrates are now treated either by heat or chemicals to reduce greatly transmission of viruses and are probably safer than cryoprecipitate.

Resting of the bleeding site helps reduce bleeding and is therefore an important adjuvant to factor VIII

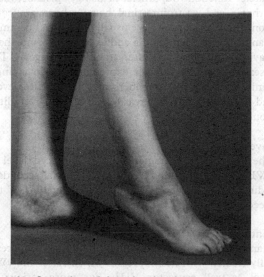

Fig. 14.21 Contraction and shortening of the Achilles tendon as a result of fibrosis following a previous haematoma in the calf.

therapy. As soon as bleeding has settled the patient should be mobilised and receive physiotherapy to restore strength to the surrounding muscles.

Factor VIII concentrates have transformed the lives of haemophiliacs by allowing many to lead near normal lives but this is at the expense of side-effects from repeated injection of concentrate particularly hepatitis and human immunodeficiency virus (HIV) infections. Most severe haemophiliacs have been exposed to hepatitis B virus and have developed immunity; a small percentage become chronic HBsAg carriers and may infect sexual partners who should therefore be offered hepatitis B vaccine. They are also at risk of delta virus infection. Virus or viruses that cause non-A non-B hepatitis (for example, hepatitis C virus) were ubiquitously transmitted by concentrates prior to 1984 resulting in virtually all recipients developing non-A non-B hepatitis. The long-term consequences of this are unknown although there is increasing evidence that many may have severe progressive liver disease.

Prior to 1985, HIV was transmitted by concentrates resulting in approximately 60% of severe haemophiliacs becoming infected. By February 1989, approximately 15% had developed AIDS but it is clear that this percentage will rise. All factor VIII concentrates are now heated or treated with virucidal chemicals. This is effective against HIV and it also reduces the infectivity of contaminating hepatitis B and non-A non-B viruses.

The other serious consequence of factor VIII infusion is the development of antifactor VIII antibodies which arise in about 10% of severe haemophiliacs. Such antibodies rapidly neutralise therapeutic factor VIII infusions making treatment relatively ineffective. Individuals may be treated with porcine factor VIII or activated factor IX concentrates.

In individuals under the age of 40 years, without evidence of cardiovascular disease and with a basal factor VIII level of 0.07 i.u./ml or greater it may be possible to raise the level approximately 3–5 fold with intravenous desmopressin (0.3 µg/kg). This is often sufficient to treat a mild bleed or cover minor surgery, e.g. dental extraction. Injections can be repeated 6–8 hourly although the response to second or subsequent infusions is not as good due to the development of tachyphylaxis. Desmopressin is an important form of therapy because it may avoid patients with moderate or mild haemophilia being exposed to blood products.

Surgery in haemophiliacs can be safely performed provided the patient does not have an inhibitor to factor VIII and receives appropriate doses of factor VIII. For simple dental extractions in an individual with severe haemophilia, a single infusion of factor

VIII is usually adequate along with a 10-day course of tranexamic acid and antibiotic. Major surgery, e.g. orthopaedic surgery, requires twice daily therapy for about 14 days or longer.

GENETICS OF HAEMOPHILIA A

The factor VIII gene is localised on the X chromosome making haemophilia A a sex-linked disorder. Thus on pedigree grounds all daughters of haemophiliacs are obligate carriers and sisters have a 50% chance of being a carrier. If a carrier has a son, he has a 50% chance of having haemophilia, and a daughter has a 50% chance of being a carrier. Haemophilia 'breeds true' within a family, as all members will have the same abnormality of the factor VIII gene, i.e. if one individual has severe haemophilia all others affected will also have a severe form of the disorder. Female carriers of haemophilia tend to have reduced factor VIII levels because of random inactivation of the X chromosome in the developing fetus (Lyonisation). An indication of carriership can be ascertained by measurement of factor VIIIC:von Willebrand factor (vWF) ratio which is reduced in carriers compared to normal individuals.

Tracing of the haemophilia gene within families can be accomplished using gene probes which detect restriction fragment length polymorphism (RFLPs). The most useful probes are those that detect an endonuclease restriction site within the gene and these are known as genomic probes. Other probes detect endonuclease sites close to, but outwith, the gene and these linked probes are less reliable because recombination, between the factor VIII gene and the endonuclear site, may occur during meiosis. Antenatal diagnosis can be undertaken in a female who has a high probability of being a carrier. This is accomplished by chorion villus sampling (CVS) at about 8–9 weeks' gestation, sexing the fetus and using informative factor VIII probes. Alternatively the fetus can be sexed at 16 weeks' gestation by amniocentesis and, if male, a fetal blood sample obtained at about 19–20 weeks. The CVS technique is preferable because it allows for the possibility of therapeutic termination at about 10–12 weeks compared to 20 weeks following fetal blood sampling.

HAEMOPHILIA B (CHRISTMAS DISEASE)

Aberrations of the factor IX gene, which is also present on the X chromosome, results in a reduction of the plasma factor IXC level giving rise to haemophilia B.

Clinical features
This disorder is clinically indistinguishable from haemophilia A but it is less common. The frequency of bleeding episodes is related to the severity of the deficiency of the plasma factor IX level.

Management
Treatment is with a factor IX concentrate (which also contains factors II and X); it is used in much the same way as factor VIII for haemophilia A. Carrier identification and antenatal diagnosis can be accomplished with gene probes although different ones than for the factor VIII gene.

VON WILLEBRAND'S DISEASE

The von Willebrand factor (vWF) is a protein, synthesised by endothelial cells and megakaryocytes, that performs two principal functions. It acts as carrier protein for factor VIII to which it is non-covalently bound. A deficiency of vWF therefore results in a secondary reduction in the factor VIII level. Its other function is to form bridges between platelets and subendothelial components allowing platelets to adhere to damaged vessel walls. A deficiency of vWF therefore also leads to prolonged primary haemorrhage after trauma.

Clinical features
As vWF participates, along with platelets, in primary haemostasis patients present with haemorrhagic manifestations which are similar to individuals with reduced platelet function. Superficial bruising, epistaxis, menorrhagia and gastrointestinal haemorrhage are common. Bleeding episodes are usually much less common than in severe haemophilia and excessive haemorrhage may only be observed after trauma or surgery. The disease is of very variable expression within a single family so that some members may have quite severe and frequent bleeds whereas others are relatively little troubled.

Investigations
The disorder is characterised by a reduced level of vWF which is often accompanied by a secondary reduction in factor VIII and a prolongation of the bleeding time.

Management
Many episodes of mild haemorrhage can be successfully treated with desmopressin which raises the vWF level as well as factor VIII. For more serious or persistent bleeds, haemostasis can be achieved with

cryoprecipitate or factor VIII concentrates, which contain a considerable quantity of vWF in addition to factor VIII.

Genetics
The gene for vWF is located in chromosome 12 and therefore the disorder is inherited as an autosomal dominant condition. Probes are available to trace the gene in a family although in most instances antenatal diagnosis is not indicated because of the relatively mild nature of the disorder.

ACQUIRED BLEEDING DISORDERS

DISSEMINATED INTRAVASCULAR COAGULATION

Disseminated intravascular coagulation (DIC) can be initiated by a variety of different mechanisms in a number of diverse, but distinct clinical situations. These are listed in the information box below.

CAUSES OF DISSEMINATED INTRAVASCULAR COAGULATION

Infections
E. coli
Neisseria meningococcus
Streptococcus pneumoniae
Malaria

Obstetric
Abruptio placentae
Retained dead fetus
Pre-eclampsia
Amniotic fluid embolism

Cancers
Lung
Pancreas
Prostate

Clinical features
Endothelial damage due to many causes, for example endotoxin produced during Gram-negative septicaemia, may activate platelets, leukocytes and factor XII leading to initiation and promotion of the coagulation cascade. The presence of thromboplastin from damaged tissues, placenta, fat embolus or following brain injury, may also activate coagulation. Intravascular coagulation takes place with consumption of platelets, factors V and VIII and fibrinogen. This results in a potential haemorrhagic state, due to the depletion of haemostatic components, which may be exacerbated by activation of the fibrinolytic systems secondary to the deposition of fibrin.

Investigations
DIC should be suspected when any of the conditions in the information box (left) are encountered. Definitive diagnosis depends on the finding of thrombocytopenia, prolongation of the prothrombin time (due to factor V deficiency) and an activated partial thromboplastin time (due to factors V and VIII deficiency), a low fibrinogen and increased levels of D dimer (evidence of fibrin lysis).

Management
Therapy should be aimed at treating the underlying condition causing the DIC. Exacerbating factors of acidosis, dehydration, renal failure and hypoxia should be corrected.

If the patient is bleeding therapy should be given with blood products to correct identified abnormalities, for example, platelets and/or cryoprecipitate (which is enriched in factor VIII and fibrinogen). Severe coagulation abnormalities should be treated in the absence of frank bleeding to prevent sudden catastrophic haemorrhage such as an intracranial bleed or massive gastrointestinal haemorrhage.

LIVER DISEASE

In severe parenchymatous liver disease bleeding may arise from many different causes. Local anatomical abnormalities are often the site of major bleeding, e.g. oesophageal varices or peptic ulcer, which may be difficult to arrest because of deficiencies in components of the haemostatic systems. These may arise because of reduced hepatic synthesis of factors II, VII, IX, X and fibrinogen, or DIC, or reduced clearance of plasminogen activator, or thrombocytopenia secondary to hypersplenism. Treatment should be reserved for acute bleeding episodes.

Cholestatic jaundice reduces vitamin K absorption and leads to a deficiency of factor II, VII, IX and X. This deficiency can be readily and effectively treated with vitamin K_1 10 mg parenterally for several days.

RENAL FAILURE

The severity of the haemorrhagic state in renal failure is proportional to the plasma urea concentration. Bleeding manifestations are of platelet type with gastrointestinal haemorrhage being particularly common. The causes are multifactorial including anaemia, mild thrombocytopenia and the accumulation of low molecular waste products that inhibit platelet function. Treatment is by dialysis and platelet concentrate infusions; red cell transfusions may raise the haemo-

Table 14.22 Predisposing factors to thromboembolism

Mainly arterial	Arterial and venous	Mainly venous
Smoking	Systemic lupus erythematosus	Malignant disease
Rheumatic heart disease	Behçet's disease	Pregnancy
Prosthetic heart valves	Homocystinaemia	Obesity
Atrial fibrillation	Oestrogens	Trauma
Hypertension	Polycythaemia vera	Surgery
Hypercholesterolaemia		
Diabetes mellitus	Myelofibrosis	
Chronic renal failure		
		Immobility/paralysis
		Heart failure
		Nephrotic syndrome
		Varicose veins
		Deficiencies of
		Antithrombin III
		Proteins C and S
		Plasminogen
		Dysfibrinogenaemias
		Paroxysmal nocturnal
		haemoglobinuria (PNH)

globin and decrease the propensity to bleed. There is some evidence that increasing the concentration of vWF either by cryoprecipitate or desmopressin may promote haemostasis.

THROMBOSIS
Both arterial and venous thrombosis may arise either because of damage to vessels, e.g. atheroma or varicose veins, or as a result of changes in the plasma or cellular elements. Predisposing conditions are listed in Table 14.22.

Clinical features
Arterial thromboembolism is usually easy to diagnose clinically becaue of the sudden onset of the local symptoms resulting from occlusion of the arterial supply. The symptoms arising from venous thrombo-embolism often lead to incorrect clinical diagnosis and investigations are therefore appropriate in most individuals in whom the diagnosis is suspected. An angiogram may be appropriate particularly if surgical thrombectomy is to be undertaken.

Antithrombin III deficiency
Antithrombin III is a protease inhibitor which inactivates factors IIa, IXa, Xa and XIa especially in the presence of heparin which greatly potentiates its antiprotease activity. Congenital deficiency of antithrombin III, which is a dominantly inherited disorder, is associated with a predisposition to venous thromboembolism. Such patients may be relatively resistant to anticoagulation with heparin because of the low level of antithrombin III which is necessary for heparin to produce its anticoagulant effect.

Protein C and S deficiencies
Protein C is a vitamin K dependant protein which when activated by traces of thrombin in the presence of protein S, inactivates factor VIII. Thus a deficiency of either protein C or S results in a prothrombotic state due to reduced inhibition of activated factor VIII.

Investigations
Venography is a reliable technique for assessing the presence and extent of thrombus and an isotope lung scan for the diagnosis of pulmonary embolism. When doubt remains a pulmonary angiogram is the definitive investigation.

Management
The use of fibrinolytic drugs, e.g. tissue plasminogen activator or streptokinase, or anticoagulants, e.g. heparin or warfarin depends upon the site, extent and age of the thrombus and whether it is arterial or venous. Prior to any antithrombotic therapy it is essential to consider whether the patient may have a significant contraindication to a anticoagulant therapy. Such contraindications include hypertension, recent central nervous system (CNS) surgery, proliferative diabetic retinopathy, peptic ulcer or other potentially haemorrhagic gastrointestinal disease such as ulcerative colitis, pre-existing bleeding disorder, hepatic or renal failure. On occasions antithrombotic therapy may have

to be given to a patient who has a contraindication to anticoagulation and in this instance the potential benefits have to be weighed against the risk of serious haemorrhage.

Heparin
Heparin produces its anticoagulant effect by potentiating the activity of antithrombin III which inhibits the procoagulant enzymic activity of factors II, IX, X and XI. For the treatment of established venous thrombosis a loading dose of 5000 units is given intravenously followed by a continuous infusion of 20 units/kg/hr initially. The level of anticoagulation is assessed daily by use of a coagulation test which is appropriately sensitive to heparin, e.g. APTT or thrombin time. The aim is for a patient time which is 2–3 × the control time of the test. Treatment should continue for 3–10 days depending upon the extent of the thrombus. It is usually appropriate to start overlapping with warfarin therapy for about 3 days until its effect becomes apparent.

Warfarin
Warfarin inhibits the vitamin K-dependent carboxyla-

tion of factors II, VII, IX and X in the liver. Carboxylation of glutamyl residues in these coagulation factors increases their negative charge and allows them to bind, via calcium bridges, to negatively charged phospholipid surfaces particularly on the platelet.

Therapy with warfarin must be initiated with a loading dose, e.g. 10 mg orally, on the first day, and subsequent daily doses depending on the prothrombin time ratio. This should be in the range 2.0–4.0; lower degrees of anticoagulation are usually adequate to prevent venous thromboembolism whereas values at the upper end of the therapeutic range are usually more appropriate when treating established venous thrombosis or to prevent arterial thromboembolism. Nearly all drugs can potentially modify the degree of warfarin therapy, e.g. non steroidal anti-inflammatory drugs, and the prothrombin ratio should be checked 2 or 3 days after stopping or starting any other medicine.

The anticoagulant effect of warfarin, may be reversed quickly if the patient bleeds, by infusing fresh frozen plasma or by giving vitamin K_1, 5 mg slowly intravenously. Its effect becomes apparent within about 6 hours although it may not fully reverse anticoagulation for 1 or 2 days.

FURTHER READING/REFERENCES

General haematology
Barnard D L, McVerry B A, Norfolk D R 1989 Clinical Haematology. Heinemann Medical Books, Oxford. A comprehensive, readable review of basic haematology.
Thompson R B, Proctor S J 1984 A Short Textbook of Haematology 6th Edn. Pitman, London. A comprehensive, readable account of haematology.

Practical haematology
Allan N C 1990 In: Munro J, Edwards C R (eds) Macleod's Clinical Examination 8th Edn. Churchill Livingstone, Edinburgh. Describes basic haematological investigations and their interpretation.
Dacie J V, Lewis S M 1984 Practical Haematology 6th Edn. Edn. Churchill Livingstone, Edinburgh. For information regarding investigative procedures.
Hirsh J, Brain E 1983 Haemostasis and thrombosis: a conceptual approach 2nd Edn. Churchill Livingstone, Edinburgh. An excellent and easily understood introduction to coagulation.
Ludlam C A 1990 Clinical Haematology. Churchill Livingstone, Edinburgh. A comprehensive textbook of haematology.

Reference volumes
Coleman R W, Hirsh J, Marder V J & Salzman E W 1987 Haemostasis and Thromboses, Basic Principles and Clinical Practice. J P Lippincott Company, Philadelphia.
Dacie J V 1988 The Haemolytic Anaemias 1 & 2 The Hereditary Haemolytic Anaemias 3rd Edn. Churchill Livingstone, Edinburgh. A very detailed review of these disorders.
Wintrobe M M 1981 Clinical Haematology 8th Edn. Kimpton, London. Probably the best comprehensive reference (9th Edn. due out in 1991).

15

Diseases of the Connective Tissues, Bones and Joints

The 'Rheumatic Diseases' are a heterogeneous group of disorders of connective tissues, joints and bones in which pain and stiffness affecting some part of the musculoskeletal system are prominent.

PREVALENCE

Rheumatic diseases affect people of both sexes, all ethnic groups and ages. Their frequency increases with age and as many as 40% of persons over the age of 65 years in the UK have had some kind of rheumatic disorder. In Britain 20 million people experience a rheumatic complaint each year. Five million suffer from osteoarthrosis, 500 000 have rheumatoid arthritis and there are 12 000 children with juvenile chronic arthritis. Rheumatic complaints account for more than 10% of all consultations in general practice (Fig. 15.1). In the UK rheumatic diseases are the commonest cause of physical impairment in the community. The lives of more than one million people are physically impaired by rheumatic disorders and one-fifth of these are severely disabled; no other group of diseases is responsible for greater loss of earnings. The cost to the United States economy attributed to the musculoskeletal disorders is more than 20 billion dollars.

CLASSIFICATION

A classification of diseases of the connective tissues, joints and bones is given in the information box (p. 763).

INFLAMMATORY JOINT DISEASE

RHEUMATOID ARTHRITIS

Rheumatoid arthritis (RA) is the commonest form of chronic inflammatory joint disease. In its typical form RA is a symmetrical, destructive and deforming polyarthritis affecting small and large peripheral joints with associated systemic disturbance, a variety of extra-articular features and the presence of circulating anti-globulin antibodies (rheumatoid factors). Characteristically the course of the disease is prolonged with exacerbations and remission but atypical, asymmetrical and incomplete forms are not uncommon.

Epidemiology
Rheumatoid arthritis occurs throughout the world and in all ethnic groups. Climate, altitude and geography do not appear to influence its prevalence but a higher

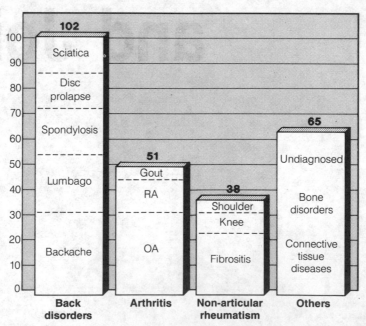

Fig. 15.1 Rheumatic complaints in an Edinburgh general practice. Annual number of patient consultations/2500 population. Total 256 = 10% of all patients registered.

		66	67			70			74	75
Haplotypes associated with RA	DR1	D	L	L	E	Q	R	R	A	A	A
	DR4DW4	D	L	L	E	Q	K	R	A	A	A
	DR4DW14	D	L	L	E	Q	R	R	A	A	A
	DR4DW15	D	L	L	E	Q	R	R	A	A	A
	DRW10	D	L	L	E	R	R	R	A	A	A
Haplotypes not associated with RA	DR4DW10	D	I	L	E	R	E	R	A	A	A
	DR4DW53	D	L	L	E	D	R	R	A	E	A
	DR7	D	I	L	E	D	A	R	G	Q	A

One letter aminoacid code

A = Ala, D = Asp, E = Glu, G = Gly, I = Ile, K = Lys, L = Leu, Q = Gln, R = Arg

Fig. 15.2   The RA susceptibility determinant: a common epitope on the third hypervariable region of HLA DR beta 1 which is shared by 85% of patients with rheumatoid arthritis.

CLASSIFICATION OF RHEUMATIC DISEASES

Inflammatory joint diseases
Rheumatoid arthritis
Ankylosing spondylitis
Reiter's disease
Psoriatic arthritis
Enteropathic arthropathy
Juvenile chronic arthritis
Behcet's disease
Whipple's disease

Infectious arthritis
Bacterial
Viral
Fungal

Connective tissue diseases
Systemic lupus erythematosus
Mixed connective tissue disease
Progressive systemic sclerosis
Polymyositis
Polyarteritis nodosa
Churg-Strauss vasculitis
Wegener's granulomatosis
Giant cell arteritis
Takayasu's disease

Crystal deposition diseases
Gout
Chondrocalcinosis

Osteoarthrosis

Soft tissue rheumatism

Miscellaneous

Disorders of bone

Aetiology

Although the cause of rheumatoid arthritis remains tantalisingly obscure, there is increasing evidence that the disease is triggered by T lymphocyte activation in genetically predisposed individuals with defined HLA Class II haplotypes. HLA-DR4 is the major susceptibility haplotype in most ethnic groups but DR1 is more important in Indians, Israelis and Yugoslavs, DW15 in Japanese and alleles of DW10, DW13 and DW14 have also been implicated.

The molecular basis for disease susceptibility resides in a shared epitope found in the third major allelic hypervariable region of HLA DR beta 1 between amino acid residues 67–74 which flank the T cell recognition site (Figs 15.2, 15.3). Whether or not one

proportion of patients in western and urban communities have more severe and disabling disease. The overall prevalence of RA in Caucasian populations is about 1% with a female to male ratio of 3:1. The disease starts most commonly between the third and fifth decades but the age of onset follows a normal distribution curve and no age group is exempted. With an annual incidence of new cases of about 0.02%, 5% of women and 2% of men over age of 55 are affected.

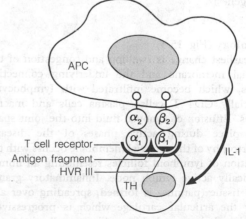

Fig. 15.3   Schematic diagram of antigen presentation by Class II molecules. APC Antigen presenting cell; TH T helper lymphocyte; HVR III 3rd hypervariable region of DR B1.

or more exogenous or auto-antigenic peptides can bind this disease susceptibility epitope to initiate or perpetuate disease is still unclear, but it is of interest that an Epstein-Barr virus glycoprotein (gp 110) contains the identical amino acid sequence. The search for other potential mechanisms for persistent antigenic stimulation and altered immune reactivity include a search for the presence of retroviral or parvoviral gene products, partially degraded bacterial cell wall peptidoglycans, cross reaction between bacterial or viral antigens and articular components, viral induction of immune complexes or viral immunosuppression. Alternatively, it has been suggested that sensitisation to self antigens could be a consequence of enzymatic or free radical damage to proteins such as immunoglobulin (IgG) or Type II collagen, the development of antiidiotypic antibodies or a defect in glycosylation of IgG.

Whatever the initiating stimulus, RA is characterised by persistent cellular activation, autoimmunity and the presence of immune complexes at sites of articular and extra-articular lesions (Table 15.1). The development of amyloidosis in some cases provides further clinical evidence for chronic immune stimulation while the striking remissions of activity that can follow lymphocyte depletion by thoracic duct drainage, lymphocytophoresis or cytotoxic drug therapy attest to the importance of lymphocytes and cellular immunity. Thus rheumatoid arthritis is both an extravascular immune complex disease and a disorder of cell mediated immunity in which the events depicted in Fig. 15.4 lead to chronic inflammation, granuloma formation and joint destruction. The severity of tissue damage is related to joint movement and physical stress as well as the activity of the inflammatory disease indicating that mechanical factors are also important in pathogenesis.

Pathology (Fig. 15.5)

The earliest change is swelling and congestion of the synovial membrane and the underlying connective tissues, which become infiltrated with lymphocytes (especially CD4 T cells), plasma cells and macrophages. Effusion of synovial fluid into the joint space takes place during active phases of the disease. Hypertrophy of the synovial membrane occurs with the formation of lymphoid follicles resembling an immunologically active lymph node. Inflammatory granulation tissue (pannus) is formed, spreading over and under the articular cartilage which is progressively eroded and destroyed. Later, fibrous adhesions may form between the layers of pannus across the joint space and fibrous or bony ankylosis may occur.

Localisation of antigen in joints
▽
Processing by antigen presenting cells
▽
Interaction with T cell receptor
▽
Release of immunopotentiating cytokines (e.g. IL-1)
▽
Endothelial cell activation
▽
Expression of adhesion molecules
▽
Homing of T lymphocytes
▽
IL-2 production and T cell proliferation
▽
Production of T cell cytokines (IL-2, IL-6, TNF alpha)
▽
B lymphocyte proliferation
▽
Local synthesis antiglobulin antibodies
▽
Formation of immune complexes
▽
Activation of complement pathway
▽
Neutrophil chemotaxis and cytolysis
▽
Lymphokine production
▽
Macrophage activation
▽
Release monokines and other monocyte mediators
▽
Immune complex phagocytosis by neutrophils and monocytes
▽
Release of mediators of acute inflammation (Vasoactive amines, proteases, polypeptides, prostaglandins, leukotrienes, oxygen radicals)
▽
Activation macrophages and chondrocytes
▽
Pannus formation
▽
Enzymatic destruction of cartilage and bone (IL-1, collagenase, neutral proteinases)
▽
Fever, acute phase response, muscle wasting

Fig. 15.4   Pathogenesis of RA: possible sequel of events.

Muscles adjacent to inflamed joints atrophy and there may be focal infiltration with lymphocytes.

Subcutaneous nodules have a characteristic histological appearance. There is a central area of fibrinoid material consisting of swollen and fragmented collagen fibres, fibrinous exudate and cellular debris, surrounded by a palisade of radially arranged proliferating

Table 15.1 Evidence for cellular activation, autoimmunity and immune complex pathology in RA

Cellular activation	Autoantibodies	Immune complex pathology
DR expression (Dendritic and synovial lining cells)	Rheumatoid factors (IgM, IgA, IgG)	IgG-IgG IgG-IgM complexes in SF
Endothelial cell expression of adhesion molecules	ANF Anticollagen antibodies	Complement activation with ↑ C3, C4, CH50
Leukocyte emigration		
CD4 lymphocytes		
B lymphocytes Plasma cells Monocytes		
Cytokine production (IL1, TNF, IL6, IL2)		
Prostaglandins Leukotrienes Metalloproteinases Acute phase proteins Heat shock proteins O₂ free radicals		

mononuclear cells. The nodules have a loose capsule of fibrous tissue. Similar granulomatous lesions may occur in the pleura, lung, pericardium and sclera. Lymph nodes are often hyperplastic showing many lymphoid follicles with large germinal centres and numerous plasma cells in the sinuses and medullary cords. Immunofluorescence shows that plasma cells in the synovium and lymph nodes synthesise rheumatoid factors.

Clinical features

Onset

The different patterns of onset are shown in Table 15.2. In the majority of patients the onset is *insidious* with joint pain, stiffness and symmetrical swelling of a number of peripheral joints. Initially pain may be experienced only on movement of joints, but rest pain and especially early morning stiffness are characteristic features of all kinds of active inflammatory arthritis.

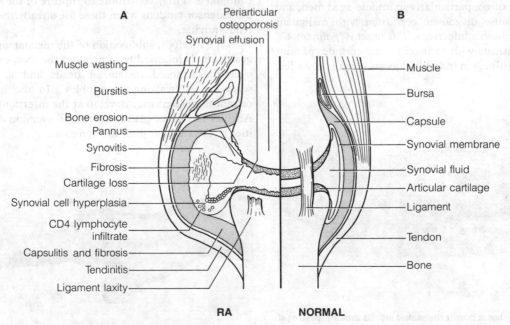

Periarticular osteoporosis
Synovial effusion

A

Muscle wasting
Bursitis
Bone erosion
Pannus
Synovitis
Fibrosis
Cartilage loss
Synovial cell hyperplasia
CD4 lymphocyte infiltrate
Capsulitis and fibrosis
Tendinitis
Ligament laxity

B

Muscle
Bursa
Capsule
Synovial membrane
Synovial fluid
Articular cartilage
Ligament
Tendon
Bone

RA   **NORMAL**

Fig. 15.5 The pathology of rheumatoid arthritis.

Table 15.2   Patterns of onset in rheumatoid arthritis

	%
Acute	15
Palindromic	5
Insidious	70
Systemic	10
Monoarticular	21
Oligoarticular	44
Polyarticular	35

In the typical case the small joints of the fingers and toes are the first to be affected. Swelling of the proximal, but not the distal, interphalangeal joints gives the fingers a 'spindled' appearance (Fig. 15.6) and swelling of the metatarsophalangeal joints results in 'broadening' of the forefoot. As the disease progresses with or without intervening remissions, there is a tendency for it to spread to involve the wrists, elbows, shoulders, knees, ankles, subtalar and midtarsal joints. The hip joints become involved only in the more severely affected but neck pain and stiffness from cervical spine disease is common. The temperomandibular, acromioclavicular, sternoclavicular and cricoarytenoid joints are sometimes involved, as indeed are all synovial joints.

In 10–15% of patients the disease starts as an *acute polyarthritis* with severe systemic symptoms. A more insidious *systemic onset* with fever, weight loss, profound fatigue and malaise without joint symptoms occurs less often, particularly in middle-aged men, and this can cause diagnostic confusion with malignant disease or chronic infections. The onset is '*palindromic*' in some patients with recurrent acute episodes of joint pain and stiffness in individual joints lasting only a few hours or days. In about a third of such cases the disease sooner or later evolves into a more typical arthritis. The onset of RA in the elderly can be indistinguishable from polymyalgia rheumatica with pain and stiffness in the region of the hip and shoulder girdles without apparent synovitis. The presence of rheumatoid factor in such patients may be a clue to the true diagnosis before typical joint changes have developed.

Progression

As the disease advances, muscle atrophy, tendon sheath and joint destruction result in limitation of joint motion, joint instability, subluxation and deformities. At first deformities are correctable, but later permanent contractures develop and the joints may become completely disorganised.

Characteristic deformities include flexion contractures of the small joints of the hands and feet, the knees, hips and elbows. Anterior subluxation of the metacarpophalangeal joints in common with ulnar deviation of the fingers. Other finger deformities lead to greater loss of joint function. These include the 'swan neck' deformity (hyperextension of the proximal interphalangeal joint with fixed flexion at the distal interphalangeal joints) (Fig. 15.7), the Boutonniere or 'button-hole' deformity (fixed flexion of the proximal interphalangeal joint and extension of the terminal interphalangeal joint) and a Z deformity of the thumb. Dorsal subluxation of the ulnar styloid at the wrist is common and may contribute to rupture of the 4th and 5th extensor tendons when these are already the site of tenosynovitis.

In the forefoot, subluxation of the metatarsophalangeal joints is followed by clawing of the toes, callosites over the exposed metatarsal heads and a painful sensation of 'walking on pebbles'. In the hindfoot calcaneal erosions may develop at the insertions of the Achilles tendon or plantar fascia and eversion deformities at the subtalar joint are common.

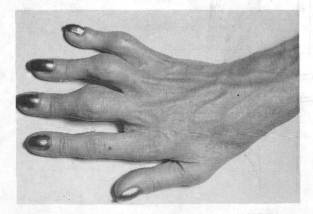

Fig. 15.6   The hands in early rheumatoid arthritis showing spindling of the fingers due to swelling of the PIP joints.

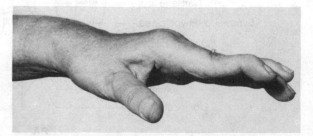

Fig. 15.7   The hand in rheumatoid arthritis: swan neck deformity.

Extra-articular features

Rheumatoid arthritis is a systemic disease. Anorexia, weight loss, lethargy and myalgia occur commonly throughout its course and may precede the onset of articular symptoms by weeks or months. The many extra-articular features of the disease are given in Table 15.3.

Table 15.3 Extra-articular manifestations of rheumatoid disease

Systemic	*Vasculitis*
Fever	Digital arteritis
Weight loss	Ulcers
Fatigue	Pyoderma gangrenosum
Susceptibility to infection	Mononeuritis multiplex
	Visceral arteritis
Musculoskeletal	
Muscle wasting	*Cardiac*
Tenosynovitis	Pericarditis
Bursitis	Myocarditis
Osteoporosis	Endocarditis
	Conduction defects
Haematological	Coronary vasculitis
Anaemia	Granulomatous aortitis
Thrombocytosis	
Eosinophilia	*Pulmonary*
	Nodules
Lymphatic	Pleural effusions
Lymphadenopathy	Fibrosing alveolitis
Splenomegaly	Bronchiolitis
Felty's syndrome	Caplan's syndrome
Nodules	*Neurological*
Sinuses	Cervical cord compression
Fistulae	Compression neuropathies
	Peripheral neuropathy
Ocular	Mononeuritis multiplex
Episcleritis	
Scleritis	*Amyloidosis*
Scleromalacia	
Keratoconjunctivitis sicca	

Raynaud's phenomenon. This may occur in the prodromal period as well as during the course of the disease.

Lymphadenopathy. This is usually found in nodes draining actively inflamed joints but more generalised lymphadenopathy can give rise to diagnostic confusion when arthritis is minimal or quiescent.

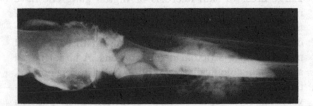

Fig. 15.8 Arthrogram of the knee following rupture of popliteal cyst into the calf.

The nodes are discrete and not tender. Histology shows a reactive hyperplasia which can be mistaken for lymphoma.

Osteoporosis, muscle weakness and wasting. These occur adjacent to inflamed joints and as part of the systemic disturbance. Although often seen early in the course of the disease they progress to become prominent features in very active or advanced cases.

Tenosynovitis and bursitis. These are frequent accompaniments of active arthritis as tendon sheaths and bursae are also lined with synovium. 'Triggering' of the fingers may be associated with nodules in the flexor tendon sheaths which can progress to permanent flexion contractures or tendon rupture if left untreated.

Popliteal cysts (Baker's cysts). These communicate with the knee, but fluid is prevented from returning to the joint by a valve-like mechanism. The high pressure generated by flexion of the knee, especially when effusions are present, can cause gradual extension or rupture of the cyst into the calf. Rupture is accompanied by calf pain, swelling, tenderness and pitting oedema. Diagnostic confusion with deep vein thrombosis can usually be avoided by careful consideration of the history but ultrasound examination, venogram or arthrogram are occasionally required to establish the correct diagnosis (Fig. 15.8).

Subcutaneous nodules. These appear at some time in the course of the disease in about 20% of patients. They are usually seen at sites of pressure or friction such as the extensor surfaces of the forearms below the elbow, the scalp, sacrum, scapula and Achilles tendon, as well as on the fingers and toes. Ulceration and secondary infection are common. Nodules are almost invariably associated with positive tests for rheumatoid factor.

Ocular manifestations

Episcleritis. This is a frequent and benign feature in patients with nodular seropositive disease. The intermittent inflammation of the superficial sclera is usually painless. It is not associated with visual disturbance and requires no specific therapy.

Scleritis. This is a rarer but more serious condition. The eye is red and painful with inflammatory changes throughout the sclera and uveal tract. The pupil may be irregular from adhesions (synechiae) which can cause secondary glaucoma and visual impairment.

Scleromalacia. Thinning of the sclera may follow episodes of scleritis and is seen as a blue discolouration of the white of the eye.

Scleromalacia perforans. This follows necrosis of a scleral rheumatoid nodule and may require grafting or enucleation of the eye.

Keratoconjunctivitis. This occurs in 10% of patients. Lack of lacrimal secretion results in grittiness, burning or itching associated with sticky mucous threads. The diagnosis can be confirmed by finding a reduction in the rate of tear secretion (Schirmer test).

Sjögren's syndrome. This is the association of xerostomia and keratoconjunctivitis sicca with a connective tissue disorder. Most often this is rheumatoid arthritis but other associations of Sjögren's syndrome are listed in the information box below.

SECONDARY SJÖGREN'S SYNDROME

- Age onset 40–60
- F > M
- HLA B$_8$ DR$_3$
- Incidence 10% RA patients
- Common clinical features
  - Mild keratoconjunctivitis sicca
  - Dry mouth
- Other associated autoimmune disorders
  - Systemic lupus erythematosus
  - Progressive systemic sclerosis
  - Primary biliary cirrhosis
  - Chronic active hepatitis
  - Myasthaenia gravis
  - Polymyositis
  - Thyroiditis
- Autoantibodies frequently detected
  - Rheumatoid factor
  - ANF
  - Salivary duct
  - Gastric parietal cell
  - Thyroid

Sicca syndrome (primary Sjögren's syndrome). This is the term used when severe keratoconjunctivitis sicca and xerostomia occur in the absence of an associated connective tissue disorder. The pathological feature which can be detected in the minor salivary glands on a simple lip biopsy is intense infiltration with lymphocytes and plasma cells. The clinical features are listed in the information box (right).

PRIMARY SJÖGREN'S (SICCA SYNDROME)

- Age onset 40–60
- F > M
- HLA B$_8$ DR$_3$
- Common clinical features
  - Keratoconjunctivitis sicca
  - Xerostomia
  - Salivary gland enlargement
- Rarer clinical features
  - Anaemia, leukopaenia, thrombocytopaenia
  - Lymphadenopathy
  - Hepatomegaly
  - Hyperglobulinaemic purpura
  - Vasculitis
  - Neuropathy
  - Myositis
  - Fibrosing alveolitis
  - Glomerulonephritis
  - Renal tubular acidosis
  - Lymphoreticular malignancy
- Autoantibodies frequently detected
  - Rheumatoid factor
  - ANF
  - SS-A (Anti-Ro)
  - SS-B (Anti-La)
  - Salivary duct
  - Gastric parietal cell
  - Thyroid

Cardiovascular manifestations

Asymptomatic pericarditis. This is a common and benign feature of seropositive rheumatoid arthritis while pericardial effusions and constrictive pericarditis occur infrequently. Rarely the formation of granulomatous lesions leads to heart block, cardiomyopathy, coronary artery occlusion or aortic regurgitation.

Vasculitis

Diffuse necrotising vasculitis is relatively common in patients with nodules and positive tests for rheumatoid factor. Clinical manifestations vary with the size and site of the vessel involved. Small vessel disease of the terminal arterioles or capillaries is often associated with no more than nail fold infarcts, leg ulcers or purpura. Large areas of skin necrosis or digital gangrene have more sinister significance and may herald the onset of 'malignant rheumatoid disease'. These patients are often febrile with severe systemic disturbance and multiple extra-articular manifestations. A larger vessel arteritis, histologically resembling polyarteritis nodosa, may result in catastrophic mesenteric, renal, cerebrovascular or coronary artery occlusion. Such patients frequently have evidence of circulating immune complexes, cryoglobulins and hypocomplementaemia.

Pulmonary manifestations

Pleurisy or pleural effusions. These occur in about 1% of men with rheumatoid arthritis. Diagnostic aspiration should be undertaken to exclude other causes.

Pulmonary nodules, Caplan's syndrome and fibrosing alveolitis. These are rarer manifestations of rheumatoid disease.

Neurological manifestations

Entrapment neuropathies. These result from compression of peripheral nerves by hypertrophied synovium. Median nerve compression in the carpal tunnel is the most common and may be an early clinical manifestation of the disease. Others include ulnar nerve compression at the elbow, peroneal nerve palsy at the knee and a posterior tibial nerve entrapment in the flexor retinaculum at the ankle (tarsal tunnel syndrome).

Peripheral neuropathy. This is usually symmetrical and limited to symptoms and signs of mild 'glove and stocking' sensory loss.

Mononeuritis multiplex. This follows occlusion of vasa nervorum in patients with arteritis.

Cervical cord compression. This may result from subluxation of the cervical spine at the atlanto-axial joint or at a subaxial level. Atlanto-axial subluxation is a common finding in long-standing rheumatoid arthritis and can be diagnosed from lateral radiographs of the cervical spine taken in full flexion (Fig. 15.9). Although usually associated with no more than neck pain radiating to the occiput, it can result in cord compression and sudden death if the neck is manipulated inadvertently under an anaesthetic. Progressive cervical myelopathy may develop more insidiously with limb weakness, difficulty in holding up the head and tetraparesis. These problems occur more often following subluxation at a subaxial level and may require operative decompression and fixation.

Haematological manifestations

These are very common in active rheumatoid disease. A normochromic normocytic anaemia of chronic disease which does not respond to oral iron may be complicated by true iron deficiency secondary to gastrointestinal blood loss from treatment with analgesic anti-inflammatory drugs. Much less frequently there may be a macrocytic anaemia associated with folate deficiency.

Felty's syndrome

This is the association of splenomegaly and neutropaenia with rheumatoid arthritis. Symptoms are listed in the information box below.

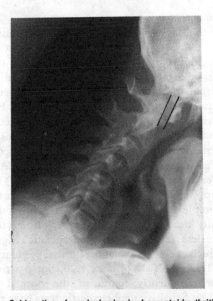

Fig. 15.9   Subluxation of cervical spine in rheumatoid arthritis. Lateral radiograph in flexion shows atlanto-axial subluxation (>4 mm gap between odontoid peg and arch of atlas).

FELTY'S SYNDROME

- Age onset 50–70
- F > M
- Caucasian > Blacks
- Incidence < 1% RA patients
    Longstanding RA
    Deforming but inactive disease
    Seropositive
- Common clinical features
    Splenomegaly
    Lymphadenopathy
    Weight loss
    Skin pigmentation
    Keratoconjunctivitis sicca
    Nodules
    Vasculitis
    Leg ulcers
    Recurrent infections
- Laboratory findings
    Anaemia
    Neutropaenia
    Thrombocytopaenia
    Impaired T and B cell immunity
    Abnormal liver function

Complications

Septic arthritis may complicate rheumatoid arthritis, particularly in patients with long-standing nodular seropositive disease. In debilitated patients, fever and leucocytosis may be absent and the signs of infection limited to malaise and slight exacerbation of inflammation in one or more joints. *Staphylococcus aureus* is commonly implicated secondary to invasion from an ulcerated nodule or infected skin lesion. *Amyloidosis* is a complication of prolonged active disease and is found in 25–30% of patients at autopsy making rheumatoid arthritis a leading cause of secondary amyloidosis.

Diagnosis

A diagnosis of rheumatoid arthritis can be established in patients with clinical features of inflammatory arthritis of six weeks' duration. The criteria for diagnosis are shown in the information box below.

CRITERIA FOR THE DIAGNOSIS OF RHEUMATOID ARTHRITIS
(American Rheumatism Association 1988 Revision)

- Morning stiffness (>1 hour)*
- Arthritis of 3 or more joint areas*
- Arthritis of hand joints*
- Symmetrical arthritis*
- Rheumatoid nodules
- Rheumatoid factor
- Radiological changes

*Duration of six weeks or more.
Diagnosis of RA made with 4 or more criteria.

Markers of active inflammatory disease are listed in the information box below. These can be used to help establish the diagnosis and follow the activity of disease in response to therapy.

MARKERS OF ACTIVE INFLAMMATORY DISEASE

- Anaemia of chronic disease
- Thrombocytosis
- ↑ Acute phase proteins (e.g. C-reactive protein)
- ↑ Plasma viscosity
- ↑ Erythrocyte sedimentation rate.

Investigations

These are listed in the information box (right).

INVESTIGATIONS IN RHEUMATOID ARTHRITIS

Establish diagnosis
Clinical criteria
Markers of inflammation
Serological tests
X-rays
Synovial analysis

Document extent of pathological changes
X-rays
Occasionally
  Arthrography
  Scintigraphy
  Ultrasound
  CT scanning
  MRI

Monitor disease activity in response to therapy
Clinical measures
ESR, plasma viscosity or
Acute phase protein (eg. CRP)
Haemoglobin

Assess progression of disease
X-rays
Functional index
Outcome assessment

Monitor for safety of drug therapy
Haematology
Urinalysis
Biochemistry
Other tests

Serological tests

Rheumatoid factors (RF) are immunoglobulins of the IgG or IgM class which react with the Fc portion of IgG. In clinical immunological practice RF of the IgM class can be detected and measured semiquantitatively by testing the ability of the patient's serum to agglutinate carrier particles coated with IgG. Polystyrene particles coated with human IgG are used in the latex slide test. Sheep or human erythrocytes coated with rabbit anti-erythrocyte antibodies are used in the Rose Waaler sheep-cell agglutination test (SCAT), the human erythrocyte agglutination test (HEAT) and the differential agglutination test (DAT). The latex fixation test is simple and sensitive but less specific so that it is frequently used as a screening test. The erythrocyte tests are less sensitive but more specific. Significant titres which exclude 95% of the normal population are: SCAT 1:32; DAT 1:16; latex 1:20; but positive tests are more frequently found in the normal elderly population. Sensitive nephelometric tests have recently been developed.

The Rose Waaler test is positive in 70% of patients

with RA but may not become so for 1–2 years. Positive tests are also found in other autoimmune diseases and chronic infections and these are listed in the information box below.

DISEASES WHICH MAY BE ASSOCIATED WITH POSITIVE RHEUMATOID FACTOR TESTS

Autoimmune and connective tissue diseases
Rheumatoid arthritis
Sjögren's syndrome
Systemic lupus erythematosus
Progressive systemic sclerosis
Polymyositis/dermatomyositis
Fibrosing alveolitis
Chronic active hepatitis
Liver cirrhosis
Sarcoidosis
Waldenström's macroglobulinaemia

Chronic infections
Infectious mononucleosis
Infectious hepatitis
Bacterial endocarditis
Tuberculosis
Syphilis
Yaws
Leprosy
Kala-azar
Schistosomiasis
Filariasis

Up to 30% of patients with rheumatoid arthritis have positive tests for antinuclear factor.

Synovial analysis
Analysis of synovial fluid is an important diagnostic procedure in patients presenting with a joint effusion and essential for the immediate diagnosis of joint infections and crystal arthropathies. Synovial fluid analysis can however also be useful in the differential diagnosis of inflammatory and degenerative arthropathies (Table 15.4).

Low levels of synovial fluid complement (CH_{50}, C_3, C_4) reflecting activation of the classical pathway of complement by immune complexes are only found in patients with classical rheumatoid arthritis. Blood contamination can follow a traumatic tap but evenly blood-stained haemarthroses are characteristically associated with haemophilia and Von Willebrand's disease, villonodular synovitis, neuropathic joints, pyrophosphate arthropathy, resolving infections, as well as traumatic arthropathies.

Synovial biopsy
This is seldom useful in distinguishing different types of inflammatory arthritis but it can be undertaken by blind needle biopsy, arthroscopy or open surgery if tuberculosis or a tumour are suspected.

Arthroscopy
This is particularly useful for excluding meninscal tears in the knee and it can also be used to establish the extent of erosive cartilage damage.

Imaging techniques
X-rays are most frequently used to follow the progression of erosive inflammatory disease of osteoarthrosis. The stages are listed in the information box below. Other imaging techniques such as arthrography, scintigraphy, ultrasound, CT scanning and NMR are occasionally used to establish the extent of local pathology in joints.

Tenography, myelography, radiculography and discography are also occasionally required for demonstrating pathology in the tendon sheaths and spine and

---

STAGES OF X-RAY PROGRESSION IN RHEUMATOID ARTHRITIS

- I   Periarticular osteoporosis
- II Loss of articular cartilage ('joint space')
- III Erosions
- IV Subluxation and Ankylosis

Table 15.4 Synovial fluid analysis

	Colour	Viscosity	Clarity	Cell count/mm³	Other tests
Normal	Colourless	Very high	Clear	0–200	—
OA	Colourless	High	Clear	200–4000	—
RA	Yellow	Low	Cloudy	2000–40 000	Low complement
Seronegative inflammatory arthritis	Yellow	Low	Cloudy	2000–40 000	Normal complement
Gout/Pseudo-gout	Variable	Low	Variable	2000–40 000	Crystals MSU/CPPD on polarising microscopy
Septic arthritis	Yellow	Low	Very turbid	>50 000	Gram stain culture and GLC

sialography and angiography are used as adjuncts to the diagnosis of Sjogren's syndrome and various forms of necrotising vasculitis.

Management

Because the aetiology of rheumatoid arthritis is unknown treatment is empirically directed towards

1. relief of symptoms;
2. suppression of active and progressive disease;
3. conservation and restoration of function in affected joints.

To a greater or lesser extent those are achieved by combining:

1. treatment of the patient — drugs, rest, physiotherapy, surgery with
2. modification of the environment — aids, appliances, housing, occupation, statutory social benefits.

In a chronic and frequently progressive disease characterised by exacerbations and remissions over many years, as well as by systemic, psychiatric and social complications, periodic assessment of disease progression (information box, p. 771), disease activity (Table 15.5) and disability (Table 15.6) are required

Table 15.5 Assessment of disease activity in rheumatoid arthritis

Clinical

Pain	Visual analogue scale
Early morning stiffness	Minutes
Joint tenderness	{ Number of inflamed joints / Articular index

Laboratory

Acute phase proteins
Erythrocyte sedimentation
  rate
Plasma viscosity

and general practitioners and hospital physicians have a special responsibility to co-ordinate a team of medical specialists, orthopaedic surgeons, occupational therapists, physiotherapists, nurses, social workers and other health professionals in an integrated programme of multidisciplinary care and rehabilitation.

Patient education, counselling and continuing medical support are usually required for successful management while physical rehabilitation, reconstructive surgery and environmental adaptation assume increasing importance when advancing joint damage and deformity are associated with functional impairment.

In a disease which is as complex and changeable as

Table 15.6 Grading of function in rheumatoid arthritis

I	Fit for all activities	No handicap
II	Moderate restriction	Independent despite handicap and limitation of joint movement
III	Marked restriction	Limited self-care. Some assistance required
IV	Confined to chair or bedbound	Largely incapacitated and dependent

rheumatoid arthritis repeated medical, functional and social assessment are required if patients are to maintain their maximum physical, psychological, social and vocational potential, and outcome should be assessed using a comprehensive health status questionnaire (Table 15.7) as well as simple process measures.

Table 15.7 Outcome measures in rheumatoid arthritis

Functional
Grip strength
Activities of daily living
Functional index

Health Status Questionnaire

Dimensions	Subdimensions	Components (e.g.)
Death		
Disability	Upper / Lower	Grip, feed, walk, / climb
Discomfort	Physical / Psychological	Pain, fatigue, / Depression, anxiety
Iatrogenic	Medical / Surgical	Dyspepsia, haemorrhage / Prosthesis infection and loosening
Economic	Direct / Indirect	Drugs, consultations, / Loss of work, social

General treatment in the active phase

Physical rest, anti-inflammatory drug therapy and maintenance exercises are the cornerstones of treatment for exacerbations of rheumatoid disease. Admission to hospital is necessary in a minority of patients when widespread active polyarthritis is associated with signs of constitutional disturbance and there has been no response to rest at home and optimal doses of nonsteroidal analgesic anti-inflammatory drugs (NSAID).

The rest from physical and emotional stress provided by 2–3 weeks in hospital is usually sufficient to induce a marked remission of symptoms without recourse to strict bed-rest. The time in hospital allows for detailed assessment by all members of the arthritis team. It ensures that the programme of medical and physical rehabilitation best suited to the individual's needs can be started under supervision and it provides an opportunity to plan the solution of outstanding functional and social problems with appropriate aids and social services.

In a few patients a period of complete bed-rest may be required to induce a remission. In these circumstances it is essential to prevent the development of 'bed deformities'. The mattress should be firm or fracture boards inserted beneath it. A back rest with the minimum number of pillows should be in position during the day and only one firm pillow used at night. Pillows behind the knees must be avoided and a bed cage with padded footrest provided. Foot and quadriceps exercises should be performed daily, along with maintenance exercises for muscle groups in unaffected limbs.

Anaemia of chronic disease responds best to induction of disease remission and oral iron is only indicated in those patients with super added true iron deficiency. Folic acid is occasionally required to treat an associated macrocytic anaemia.

Local measures in the active phase

Rest splints. These can be useful to support a particularly painful joint, such as the knee or wrist, and splints are used to prevent or correct flexion deformities.

Intra-articular corticosteroid injections. These are particularly useful for settling inflammation in isolated joints that remain painful and inflamed despite general measures. Local injection of a long-acting microcrystalline corticosteroid such as methylprednisolone acetate (20–80 mg large joints; 4–10 mg small joints) or triamcinolone hexacetonide (10–30 mg large joints; 2–6 mg small joints) can bring symptomatic relief lasting weeks or months. Repeated injections at short intervals, particularly in weight bearing joints, should be avoided. Local injection of a corticosteroid is also the treatment of choice for bursitis, tenosynovitis and carpal tunnel syndrome when rest, splints, and other general measures have not been effective.

Non-steroidal anti-inflammatory drugs

These are the mainstay of therapy for active inflammatory arthritis in optimal anti-inflammatory doses (Table 15.8). They can be very effective in relieving pain and stiffness but they do not alter the course of the disease and the margin between effective and toxic doses is often small.

Inhibition of prostaglandin synthetase is a major pharmacological action common to all these agents but simultaneous inhibition of the cytoprotective effect of prostanoids on gastric mucosa makes them all liable to cause gastrointestinal side-effects such as dyspepsia, ulceration and haemorrhage. NSAID associated upper

Table 15.8 Non-steroidal analgesic anti-inflammatory drugs (NSAID)

Drug	Usual dose
CARBOXYLIC ACIDS	
Salicylic acids	
Aspirin	600–900 mg × 6/d
Aloxiprin	1200 mg × 4/d
Benorylate	10 ml b.d.
Diflusinal	500 mg b.d.
Salsalate	1–1.5 g b.d.
Trilisate	1–1.5 g b.d.
Anthranilic acids	
Mefenamic acid	500 mg × 4/d
Propionic acids	
Fenbufen	300 mg mane
	600 mg nocte
Fenoprofen	600 mg × 4/d
Flurbiprofen	100 mg t.i.d.
Ibuprofen	400–800 mg × 4/d
Ketoprofen	100 mg t.i.d.
Naproxen	500 mg b.d.
Tiaprofenic acid	200 mg t.i.d.
Acetic acids	
Diclofenac	50 mg t.i.d.
Naphthylalkanones	
Nabumetone	1000 mg daily
Heterocyclic acetic acids	
Tolmetin	400 mg × 4/d
Indole acetic acids	
Indomethacin	25–50 mg t.i.d.
Sulindac	200 mg b.d.
Pyranocarbolxylic acids	
Etodolac	200 mg b.d.
ENOLIC ACIDS	
Pyrazolones	
Azapropazone	600 mg b.d.
Phenylbutazone	100 mg t.i.d.
(severe, active ankylosing spondylitis only)	
Oxicams	
Piroxicam	20 mg daily
Tenoxicam	20 mg daily

gastrointestinal haemorrhage is the most frequent serious adverse drug-related event to be reported to the Committee on Safety of Medicines. Elderly women are particularly susceptible and case control studies suggest that a fifth of all admissions to hospital in patients over the age of 60 with bleeding gastric or duodenal ulcers are directly attributable to taking NSAID. Treatment with these agents should be avoided in patients with peptic ulceration but it is important to realise that endoscopic evidence of ulcers is found in 20% of NSAID treated patients even in the absence of symptoms. The overall risk of an individual developing a life-threatening gastrointestinal side-effect following treatment with an NSAID is approximately 1 in 10 000. When NSAID treatment cannot be avoided peptic ulcers can be made to heal by concomitant administration of H2 antagonists (cimetidine, ranitidine) or prostaglandin E analogues (misoprostol). In high-risk patients the risk of NSAID induced gastric ulceration can be reduced by the simultaneous administration of misoprostol 100–200 μg q.i.d.

Other side-effects of NSAID include fluid retention, rashes, interstitial nephritis, occasional hepatotoxicity and rarely asthmas and anaphylaxis.

It is advisable for initial treatment to use one of the established, less expensive NSAID, with a low incidence of side-effects, in moderate dosage for a trial period of about 2–3 weeks. Another NSAID with which the clinician is familiar can be tried if the response is not satisfactory but simultaneous administration of more than one NSAID generally result in an increase in the risk of adverse events without significant therapeutic benefit.

Simple analgesics

Those without appreciable anti-inflammatory action include peripherally acting agents such as paracetamol and centrally acting narcotic analgesics such as dextropropoxyphene, dihydrocodeine and nefopam. Although centrally acting narcotic analgesics should generally be avoided in the management of rheumatic diseases, simple analgesics are frequently used as additions to therapy when pain relief is inadequate and combination drugs such as co-proxamol (paracetamol and dextropropoxyphene) can be safe and effective when used in moderate doses.

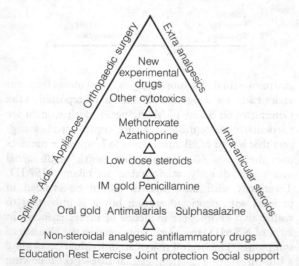

Fig. 15.10 The pyramidal approach to therapy in patients with rheumatoid arthritis.

Slow acting and anti-rheumatic drugs

The addition of a 'second-line' or 'disease-modifying' suppressive anti-rheumatic drug should be considered in all patients where symptoms and signs of active inflammatory arthritis have persisted for 3–4 months despite adequate general measures and optimal doses of an NSAID. Drugs of this type do not possess immediate anti-inflammatory effects but characteristically cause an improvement in joint pain, stiffness and swelling and a reduction in systemic symptoms, acute phase proteins, sedimentation rate and rheumatoid factor titre over a period of months. If started early they may have a marginal effect in reducing the rate of radiological progression of disease but their main benefit is in inducing a symptomatic remission for one to two years in 40–60% of patients. They are usually introduced in a pyramidal fashion starting with the safest agent (Fig. 15.10) because they are all potentially associated with serious adverse reactions.

Antimalarials. Chloroquine phosphate (250 mg/d) or hydroxychloroquine sulphate (200 mg b.d.) are often used as the initial adjunct to basic therapy. Clinical benefit is noted in about half the patients in 4–12 weeks and the drug should be discontinued if there is no effect within 6 months. Occasional side-effects include nausea, diarrhoea, rashes, haemolytic anaemia, ototoxicity and neuromyopathy and there is a small risk of ocular toxicity after more than a year of therapy. Deposits of the drug in the cornea may produce disturbances of vision which tend to disappear when the drug is withdrawn. More rarely retinopathy can result in permanent visual impairment. If the drug is effective it is advisable to check the visual acuity and ophthalmoscopic appearance of the maculae after one year and at six-monthly intervals thereafter. In order to reduce the risks of ocular toxicity antimalarials are often given for only 10 months in each year. In some the dose can be halved without exacerbation of symptoms. Although antimalarials are generally less effective than gold salts or d-penicillamine, their use is associated with fewer patient drop-outs for toxicity.

Sulphasalazine. This also has a good benefit to risk profile. Approximately 50% of patients respond in three to six months. Nausea and vomiting can be troublesome but these symptoms can usually be avoided if treatment is started with 500 mg daily and increased gradually to a maximum of 500 mg q.d.s. over a period of 4 weeks. Depression, rashes, megaloblastic anaemia and hepatitis are rarer side-effects and the full blood count and liver function tests should be monitored monthly.

Auranofin. This oral gold compound is less toxic than parenteral preparations but short and medium-term efficacy are also less. The usual dose is 6 mg daily but this can be increased to 9 mg daily if there has been no response after three to four months. Diarrhoea is a common side-effect during the early phases of treatment. Mouth ulcers, dermatitis, proteinuria and bone marrow suppression are significantly less likely than with intramuscular gold but the full blood count including platelets and routine urinalysis do need to be monitored regularly.

Penicillamine and parenteral gold. These are slow acting suppressive antirheumatic drugs which have been shown to decrease the progression of erosive changes as well as reduce the activity of the disease in 50–60% of patients. Because of a high incidence of toxic effects, treatment with these agents should only be considered as an addition to basic therapy when there are clear indications for the use of a disease modifying drug and the patient has failed to respond to antimalarials or sulphasalazine. Indications for use are listed in the information box below.

INDICATIONS FOR DISEASE MODIFYING DRUGS

- Persistent symptoms and signs of inflammatory arthritis despite optimum therapy with NSAIDs
- Evidence of progressive radiological damage
- Troublesome extra-articular manifestations
- Palindromic rheumatoid arthritis

Penicillamine. This treatment is commenced with a single evening dose of 125 or 250 mg and dosage is increased by no more than 250 mg monthly to a maximum of 1 g daily. Clinical benefit is noted several weeks after an effective dose has been achieved and reaches a maximum only after 4–6 months.

Rashes, loss of taste, nausea, vomiting and serious febrile reaction can occur early after starting treatment. Later side-effects include mouth ulcers, proteinuria and the nephrotic syndrome. Very rarely diseases resembling systemic lupus erythematosus, myasthenia gravis, pemphigus and Goodpasture's syndrome can occur. Thrombocytopaenia and pancytopaenia may occur at any time and are potentially the most serious toxic effects.

Patients should be monitored, initially at weekly intervals, by urinalysis and full blood counts, including platelets. Proteinuria and mild thrombocytopaenia are indications for cessation of therapy followed by re-introduction of the drug at a lower dose if the abnormalities disappear. It is advisable to withdraw penicillamine altogether if the side-effects recur. Febrile reactions and pancytopaenia are absolute indications for drug withdrawal.

The likelihood of side-effects with penicillamine is increased in slow sulphoxidisers.

Parenteral gold. After a test dose of 10 mg, weekly intramuscular injections of 50 mg sodium aurothiomalate are given until a response is obtained usually by 2–3 months. The intervals between injections are progressively increased provided the remission is maintained and the drug is continued indefinitely. Gold injections should be stopped if there has been no clinical benefit after 6 months.

Adverse effects include pruritic rashes, exfoliative dermatitis, mouth ulcers, enterocolitis, proteinuria and the nephrotic syndrome, thrombocytopaenia, agranulocytosis and aplastic anaemia. All are potentially serious and preclude further therapy. Patients who are HLA-DR3 positive are particularly at risk of developing a gold-induced immune complex glomerulonephritis. Monitoring should include a routine urinalysis and full blood counts with platelets, initially prior to each injection.

Pruritus may respond to antihistamines and exfoliative dermatitis, thrombocytopaenia, agranulocytosis and nephropathy to corticosteroids. Patients with agranulocytosis almost invariably recover if they can be protected from serious infection; those with aplastic anaemia have a more serious prognosis. Dimercaprol (BAL) combines with heavy metals to form a stable compound which is rapidly excreted in the urine; 3 mg/kg body weight should be administered intramuscularly 6-hourly for 3–4 days in patients with aplastic anaemia who have not responded to withdrawal of gold injections after 4–5 days.

Other disease modifying antirheumatic drugs
Dapsone is associated with slow clinical improvement and reduction of acute phase proteins but haemolytic anaemia can be a troublesome side effect, particularly in slow acetylators. Other compounds which have been shown to have slow acting antirheumatic activity include the antibacterial agent rifampicin, the antihypertensive agent captopril, the penicillamine analogues 5-thiopyridoxine, pyrithioxine and thyopronine, the pentapeptide thymosin and the cytokine gamma interferon.

Corticosteroids and corticotrophin

These have a very potent anti-inflammatory activity but doses required to maintain adequate symptomatic relief on a long-term basis are accompanied by an unacceptable level of side-effects and it remains uncertain to what extent they possess the 'disease modifying' properties of the slow acting antirheumatic agents. Indications for their use are therefore restricted and a slow acting antirheumatic agent is usually commenced simultaneously with a view to gradual withdrawal of corticosteroid therapy when remission has been obtained.

The main indications for the use of systemic corticosteroids are:

1. in exceptionally severe exacerbations which are not remitting with rest, intra-articular injections of corticosteroids and non-steroidal anti-inflammatory drugs;
2. when other measures fail to control persistently disabling symptoms in breadwinners or young mothers who have to return to work;
3. in some elderly patients when acute disease is threatening to render them bedbound;
4. in life or sight threatening visceral disease such as severe pericarditis, polyarteritis or scleritis.

Prednisolone. This is the corticosteroid of choice. It should ideally be administered as a single morning dose of no more than 7.5 mg daily to minimise suppression of the hypothalamo-pituitary-adrenal axis. An evening dose of 5 mg is sometimes more useful in overcoming intractable early morning stiffness. Enteric coated tablets or small doses of corticotrophin may be preferred in patients with a previous history of peptic ulceration. In other circumstances any possible advantages of corticotrophin seem to be outweighed by the disadvantages, namely the need for injections, the difficulty in knowing the dose of steroid being effectively administered and the high prevalence of mineralocorticoid side-effects. The potential side-effects of steroids are numerous (Table 15.9). Infection and osteoporosis are particularly troublesome in patients with RA and patients commencing systemic steroid therapy should be given oral calcium supplements.

Immunomodulation

Because rheumatoid arthritis is associated with evidence of both immune hyper-reactivity and suppression of some cell-mediated immune responses both 'immunosuppressive' and 'immunostimulant' drugs have been considered for the management of the disease. Increasing understanding of the complexity of

Table 15.9   Side-effects of systemic corticosteroids

Endocrine	*Immunological*
Moon face	Suppression delayed hypersensitivity
Truncal obesity	Reactivation TB
Hirsutism	Susceptibility to infection
Impotence	
Menstrual irregularity	*Gastrointestinal*
Suppression HPA axis	Peptic ulceration
Growth suppression	Pancreatitis
Metabolic	*Cardiovascular*
Negative Ca, K, N balance	Hypertension
Sodium and fluid retention	Congestive cardiac failure
Hyperglycaemia	
Hyperlipoproteinaemia	*Ocular*
	Glaucoma
Musculoskeletal	Posterior, subcapular, cataracts
Myopathy	
Osteoporosis	
Avascular necrosis	
	CNS
Skin	Changes in mood and
Acne, striae	personality
Skin atrophy	Psychosis
Bruising	Benign intracranial
Impaired wound healing	hypertension

regulation of the immune system and the 'immunopharmacology' of cytotoxic and immunostimulant drugs makes it clear that these agents may have variable and even paradoxical effects on the expression of immune responses depending on the dose, the timing of administration and the subpopulation of cells predominantly affected. Net immune stimulation may result from treatment with a drug which predominantly inhibits a suppressor cell sub-population of lymphocytes while functional immunosuppression can follow use of an immunostimulant which selectively activates these cells. Many immunoregulatory drugs are cell cycle specific so their action depends on the relationship of the cell cycle to target function. Receptors for growth factors and cytokines as well as the processing and release of these peptides are important targets for potential immunomodulation but nearly all the drugs currently in use were originally developed for the chemotherapy of malignant diseases. They tend therefore to be rather non-specific cytotoxic and cytostatic agents which predominantly interfere with events involved in the cellular proliferation of all cells without specificity for receptors involved in the processes of cellular differentiation.

In practice a number of cytotoxic and immunostimulant agents have been found empirically to have both symptomatic and slow acting 'disease modifying' activity in rheumatoid arthritis. The effects are mediated as much by 'anti-inflammatory' as by 'immunoregulatory' activity and their usefulness is very strictly limited by immediate and potential long-term toxicity.

Table 15.10   Mechanism of action of the immunomodulating drugs

Drug	Class	Effects
Azathioprine	Purine analogue	Inhibits purine synthesis DNA and RNA
Cyclophosphamide	Alkylating agent	Direct binding DNA, RNA and proteins
Methotrexate	Folic acid antagonist	Binds dihydrofolate reductase. Blocks de novo purine and thymidylate synthesis
Cyclosporin A	Fungal polypeptide	Inhibits IL2 transcription: CD4 and cytotoxic lymphocytes

Table 15.11   Toxic effects of immunosuppressive drugs

	Azathioprine	Methotrexate	Cyclophosphamide	Chlorambucil	Cyclosporin A
GI tract	+	+ +	+	+	+
Bone marrow	+ +	+ +	+ +	+ + +	+
Bladder	0	0	+ + +	0	0
Kidneys	0	+	0	0	+ + +
Liver	+	+ + +	0	0	+ +
Lungs	+	+ + +	+	+	+ +
Gonads	0	0	+ + +	+ + +	0
Fetus	±	+ + +	±	±	±
Neoplasia	+ + +	0	+ +	+ +	+

0–+ + + = no toxicity–severe toxicity.

The indications for use of these agents at present are limited to:

1. life threatening extra-articular manifestations which have failed to respond to corticosteroids or second-line agents;
2. severe active symptomatic and progressive joint disease that has failed to respond to all other forms of therapy;
3. patients receiving unacceptably high doses of corticosteroids in whom dose reduction has not been possible.

Mechanisms of action of commonly used agents are summarised in Table 15.10 and toxic effects in Table 15.11.

Azathioprine. This has been shown to be effective in both high (2.5 mg/kg) and low doses (1.25 mg/kg). Adverse effects include vomiting, stomatitis, diarrhoea, hepatitis and particularly bone marrow suppression and susceptibility to infection. Monitoring is with fortnightly or monthly full blood counts.

Cyclophosphamide. This has a narrow therapeutic range but is effective in a daily dose of 1–2 mg/kg. Adverse effects include alopecia, azoospermia, anovulation, cystitis, nausea and vomiting, susceptibility to infection, bone marrow suppression and teratogenesis. Monitoring is by fortnightly or monthly full blood counts and routine urinalysis. Toxicity may

be reduced by intermittent, intravenous infusion (0.5–1.5 g/m^2) every 1–3 months.

Methotrexate. This is effective in low oral pulse doses of 7.5–15 mg/week. It is very rarely associated with bone marrow suppression; liver function must be monitored regularly and interstitial lung disease can be a rare complication.

Levimasole. This is an antihelminthic which has been shown to augment T lymphocyte responses as well as polymorph and macrophage chemotaxis and phagocytosis. It can be effective in patients with rheumatoid arthritis as a single weekly dose of 150 mg. Adverse effects include febrile reactions, vomiting, urticarial and vasculitic rashes. A high risk of agranulocytosis even with weekly monitoring of blood counts precludes its use routinely.

Medical synovectomy

Synovial obliteration can be achieved with osmic acid or a variety of radiocolloids if pain, effusion and synovitis persist despite local corticosteroid injections, systemic drug therapy and physical measures. Yttrium-90 silicate is used for large joints such as the knee and erbium-159 acetate for the small joints of the hands. Joints are immobilised for 72 hours to reduce spread to regional lymph nodes. Patients under the age of 45 should not be treated in this manner.

Table 15.12   Some useful surgical procedures in rheumatoid arthritis and osteoarthrosis

Procedure	Joint(s)	Indication
Soft tissue release (decompression)	Carpal tunnel	Median nerve compression
	Tarsal tunnel	Posterior tibial nerve entrapment
	Flexor tendon sheaths hand	Relief of 'trigger fingers'
	Rerouting ulnar nerve at elbow	Ulnar nerve entrapment
Tendon repairs and transfers	Extensor tendons hands	Rupture extensor tendons
	Flexor tendons thumb and fingers	Rupture flexor tendons
Synovectomy	Wrist and extensor tendon sheaths (+ excision ulnar)	Pain relief and prevent extensor tendon rupture
Osteotomy	Keller's operation	Correct hallux valgus
	Femoral osteotomy	Pain relief. Correct deformity early OA hip
	Tibial osteotomy	Pain relief. Correct deformity unicompartmental OA knee
Excision arthroplasty	Radial head	Pain subluxation radio-ulnar joint
	Lateral end clavicle	Pain acromio-clavicular joint
	Fowler's operation (metatarsal head resection)	Forefoot pain MTP joint subluxation
Joint replacement	Hip, knee, elbow, shoulder, ankle MCP joints hands	Pain relief. Maintain, restore and improve function
Arthrodesis	Interphalangeal joint thumb or fingers	Improve hand function
	MCP joint thumb	Improve pinch grip
	Wrist	Pain relief. Improve grip
	Ankle and subtalar joints	Pain relief. Stabilise hind foot

Surgical treatment and rehabilitation

There are many circumstances in the overall management of patients with severe and progressive rheumatoid arthritis when orthopaedic surgical procedures are required to relieve pain and conserve or restore locomotor function (Table 15.12).

Surgical decompression and synovectomy of the wrist and tendon sheaths of the hands are often needed when non-steroidal anti-inflammatory drugs, local injections of corticosteroids and simple physical measures have failed to relieve a carpal tunnel syndrome or flexion contractures of the fingers resulting from fibrosis and nodule formation. Flexor and extensor tendon synovectomy, the latter often accompanied by resection of a subluxated ulnar styloid, can be important measures in preventing tendon ruptures. Synovectomy of joints will not prevent disease progression but may be indicated for pain relief when drug therapy, local rest, intra-articular injections and radiocolloids have failed to provide symptomatic relief.

At a later stage, when tendons, cartilage and bone have been eroded and the mechanics of joints disturbed, reconstructive tendon surgery, osteotomy, arthrodesis and a variety of arthroplasties with or without prostheses play a major part in the rehabilitation of the patient.

If surgical treatment is to be successful the aims and consequences of each operation should be carefully considered as part of an integrated programme of management and rehabilitation. This is often best achieved where physicians and surgeons with special experience work together in a combined rheumatology/orthopaedic clinic with other allied health professionals. Assessment of motivation, social support and environment are no less important than careful consideration of the patient's general health and detailed assessment of the extent of disease in other joints, the integrity of the cervical spine, the presence or absence of infection, arteritis or osteoporosis. In particular it must be appreciated that whereas many patients with slowly progressive disease can be maintained mobile and functionally independent by a series of major joint replacements carried out over a number of years, it is seldom possible to mobilise a patient who has been chair- or bedbound for a long period by multiple joint replacement during a single lengthy hospital admission. In these and other circumstances pain relief and functional independence are better served by provision of a suitable wheelchair, home adjustments, physical aids and social services.

When a patient cannot return to a former occupation it may be necessary to suggest a change of employment where less strain will be thrown on the damaged joints. Although disablement resettlement officers, industrial rehabilitation units and government retraining centres are sometimes helpful in such circumstances it should be emphasised that patients have the best chance of returning to active work with their former employers. It cannot be stressed too strongly that adequate treatment in the early stages and throughout the course of the disease enables most patients to return to some form of wage earning activity. Disabilities of all kinds can be reduced even in the 25% of patients running a severe progressive course.

Prognosis

The course and prognosis in rheumatoid arthritis is very variable. In those patients with disease of such severity as to require admission to hospital, review after ten years shows that: 25% will have a complete remission of symptoms and remain fit for all normal activities; 40% will have only moderate impairment of function despite exacerbations and remissions of disease; 25% will be more severely disabled; 10% will be severely crippled (this rises to 20% after 20 years). The overall prognosis is much better if the many patients in the community are considered whose symptoms are never of such severity as to require admission to hospital. A poor prognosis may be associated with:

1. high titres of rheumatoid factor
2. insidious onset of disease
3. more than a year of active disease without remission
4. early development of nodules and erosions and
5. extra-articular manifestations.

Patients with Sjögren's syndrome require scrupulous oral and ocular hygiene and the instillation of artificial tears (hypermellose eye drops). Drug hypersensitivity is sometimes a problem. Corticosteroids are used in Felty's syndrome but the outcome is unsatisfactory. Splenectomy is reserved for patients with serious or life-threatening infections and is followed by remission in 60% of patients.

THE SPONDARTHRITIDES

This is a group of diseases in which an inflammatory arthritis, characterised by persistently negative tests for IgM rheumatoid factor, is variably associated with a number of other common articular, extra-articular and genetic features. These are listed in the information box (right). The features held in common by the spondarthritides are shown in the information box (right).

Current concepts of the aetiology of these disorders are that they may arise as an abnormal response to

---

THE SPONDARTHRITIDES

- Ankylosing spondylitis
- Reiter's disease
- Reactive arthritis
- Enteropathic arthritis
  - Ulcerative colitis
  - Crohn's disease
- Behcet's syndrome
- Juvenile chronic arthritis

FEATURES COMMON TO THE SPONDARTHRITIDES

- Sacroiliitis and/or spondylitis
- Asymmetrical oligoarthritis
- Enthesitis
- Anterior uveitis
- Familial association
- High prevalence HLA-B27

---

infection in genetically predisposed persons carrying the HLA-B27 antigen. In some, an inciting organism has been identified as in Reiter's disease which can follow bacterial dysentry or chlamydial urethritis, or in the reactive arthritis following infection with *Yersina enterocolitica*. In the others the infectious agent remains obscure. It is uncertain whether possession of HLA-B27 predisposes towards disease because:

1. it is merely a marker for an immune response gene;
2. susceptibility to infection is increased as a result of cross-reactivity between an HLA-B27 determined host gene product and an antigen carried by the invading organism or
3. the inciting organism modifies HLA-B27 positive cellular receptors in such a way as to initiate an autoimmune reaction or render the cells more susceptible to cytotoxic lymphocytes.

ANKYLOSING SPONDYLITIS

In its typical form this is a chronic inflammatory arthritis with a predilection for the sacroiliac joints and spine and characterised by progressive stiffening and fusion of the axial skeleton.

Epidemiology

Typically ankylosing spondylitis is a disease with a peak onset in the second and third decades and a male to female ratio of about 4:1. More than 90% of affected persons carry the histocompatibility antigen HLA-B27. First degree relatives of patients with ankylosing spondylitis have a greatly increased incidence of psoriatic arthritis, inflammatory bowel disease and

Reiter's syndrome. Chronic prostatitis is more common than would be anticipated but it is not possible to isolate organisms from prostatic fluid. Faecal carriage of some Klebsiella species is increased in ankylosing spondylitis and this may be related to exacerbation of the disease.

Pathology

Biopsy material from peripheral joints shows changes similar to those found in rheumatoid arthritis. Bony ankylosis, however, occurs more frequently. The characteristic *enthesopathy* comprises multiple foci of inflammation with lymphocytes and plasma cells at ligamentous attachments with adjacent erosion of bone. Healing of similar lesions at the junction of the vertebral bodies and annulus fibrosus of the intervertebral discs leads to the new bone formation (syndesmophytes) which is the hallmark of the disease.

Clinical features

The onset is usually insidious with recurring episodes of low back pain and stiffness sometimes radiating to the buttocks or thighs. Characteristically the symptoms are worse in the early morning and after inactivity. Occasionally the onset may be acute, resembling a lumbar disc protrusion. A few patients present with symptoms referable to the dorsal or cervical spine but such cases usually reveal evidence of previous sacroiliitis and lumbar spine involvement.

Chest pain aggravated by breathing results from involvement of the costovertebral joints. Plantar fasciitis, Achilles tendonitis and tenderness over bony prominences such as the iliac crest, ischial tuberosity and greater trochanter are typical. 25% of patients have an attack of acute anterior uveitis during the course of the disease and this may occasionally be the presenting feature. A peripheral joint is first affected in 10% and in a further 10% symptoms begin in childhood as one variety of pauciarticular juvenile chronic arthritis.

Early signs include failure to obliterate the lumbar lordosis on forward flexion, pain on sacroiliac compression, and restriction of movements of the lumbar spine in all directions. As the disease progresses, stiffness increases throughout the spine, and chest expansion frequently becomes restricted. Severe spinal fusion and rigidity occurs in only a minority and in most of these is not associated with much deformity. A few develop kyphosis of the dorsal and cervical spine which can be incapacitating especially when associated with hip involvement.

Iritis occurs in up to 25% of patients but other extra-articular features are rare. These manifestations are listed in the information box (right).

EXTRA-ARTICULAR MANIFESTATIONS OF ANKYLOSING SPONDYLITIS

- Iritis
- Aortic regurgitation
- Conduction defects
- Apical pulmonary fibrosis
- Amyloidosis
- Osteoporosis
- Myelopathy secondary to atlanto-axial subluxation
- Corda equina syndrome

Diagnosis

The erythrocyte sedimentation rate (ESR) is usually raised but may be normal. Tests for rheumatoid factor are negative and synovial fluid complement levels are not depressed.

Radiological signs of sacroiliitis. These begin in the lower parts of the joints with irregularity and marginal sclerosis eventually progressing to fusion. In the lumbar spine there may be 'squaring' of the vertebrae owing to ossification of the anterior longitudinal ligament, syndesmophyte formation, erosion and sclerosis at the anterior corners of the vertebrae and facetal joint changes. Progressive ossification results in the typical 'bamboo spine' (Fig. 15.11). Erosive

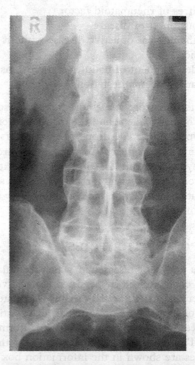

Fig. 15.11   'Bamboo' spine in advanced ankylosing spondylitis with obliteration of the sacroiliac joints.

changes may be seen in the symphysis pubis, the ischial tuberosities and peripheral joints. Osteoporosis and atlanto-axial dislocation can occur.

Radionuclide bone scanning. This may reveal evidence of sacroiliitis or spinal involvement when radiographs are negative but the increased uptake of the bone-seeking isotope is non-specific and reflects bone blood flow and turnover.

Management
The principles are to relieve pain and stiffness, maintain a maximal range of skeletal mobility and avoid the development of deformities. Early in the disease patients should be trained to do regular exercises at home and encouraged to take up active non-contact sports like swimming. Poor bed and chair postures must be avoided.

NSAID are used to relieve symptoms but do not themselves alter the course of the disease. A few patients with spondylitis find phenylbutazone the most effective drug; it can usually be given safely even over prolonged periods provided a daily dose of 300 mg is not exceeded.

Radiotherapy is occasionally indicated if the response to drug therapy is unsatisfactory. It does not affect the course of the disease and earlier regimens of treatment, when excessive radiation was employed, were associated with a tenfold increase in the risk of developing leukaemia.

Local corticosteroid injections can be helpful for plantar fasciitis and the management of other manifestations of enthesopathy. Systemic steroids are sometimes required for treatment of acute iritis.

Hip disease may require surgery and total hip arthroplasty has largely obviated the need for difficult spinal surgery in those with advanced deformity.

Prognosis
75% or more of patients with ankylosing spondylitis are able to remain in employment without significant loss of time from work. Restriction of chest movements does not predispose to pulmonary infection but systemic complications and especially hip involvement carry a worse prognosis.

REITER'S DISEASE

Classically this is the triad of non-specific urethritis, conjunctivitis and arthritis that follows bacterial dysentery or exposure to sexually transmitted infection. Incomplete forms are frequent and include the commonest variety of inflammatory arthritis seen in young

men. When arthritis alone follows sexual exposure or enteric infection the term '*reactive arthritis*' is frequently used. The bacteria implicated in reactive arthritis are listed in the information box below.

ARTHRITOGENIC BACTERIA IMPLICATED IN REACTIVE ARTHRITIS

- Salmonella
- Shigella
- Campylobacter
- Yersinia
- Chlamydia

Epidemiology
1–2% of patients with non-specific urethritis seen at clinics for sexually transmitted diseases have Reiter's disease and there is a similar incidence following outbreaks of shigellosis. A male with HLA-B27 runs a 20% risk of getting the disease following an attack of shigella dysentery. Although predominantly a disease of young men, the apparent 50:1 male to female ratio is spuriously high as urethritis is frequently ignored in women and children.

Clinical features
The onset is typically acute with the simultaneous development of urethritis, conjunctivitis (in about 50%) and an inflammatory oligoarthritis affecting the large or small joints of the lower limbs, 1–3 weeks following sexual exposure or an attack of dysentery. There may be considerable systemic disturbance with fever, weight loss and vasomotor changes in the feet.

Often the onset is more insidious and many patients present with no more than monoarthritis of a knee or an assymetrical inflammatory arthritis of some interphalangeal joints. Symptoms and signs of urethritis or conjunctivitis may have been minimal or forgotten. In such patients heel pain, Achilles tendonitis or plantar fasciitis are valuable clues while the presence of circinate balanitis or the rash of keratoderma blennorrhagica can clinch the diagnosis even in the absence of the classical triad and without an overt history of sexual promiscuity or dysentery. The skin lesions can vary from faint macules, vesicles and pustules on the hands and feet to marked hyperkeratosis with plaque-like lesions spreading to the scalp and trunk. These may be associated with severe nail dystrophy and massive subungual hyperkeratosis (Fig. 15.12).

Ocular involvement is normally limited to mild bilateral conjunctivitis which subsides spontaneously within a month. Acute iritis occurs at the outset in 10% of patients. It is distinguished from simple conjunctivi-

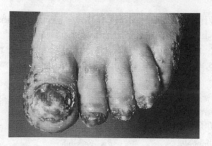

Fig. 15.12 Subungual hyperkeratosis and keratodomia blennorrhagica in Reiter's syndrome.

tis by injection of the ciliary vessels around the cornea, by a constricted, irregular or unreactive pupil and by cells in the anterior chamber on slit lamp examination. Unlike the conjunctivitis it requires urgent treatment. Chronic iritis may lead to glaucoma and blindness.

The urethritis is usually associated with minor dysuria and a clear sterile discharge. Sometimes it is asymptomatic and detected only by finding mucoid threads in the first voided specimen of early morning urine. Occasionally there may be severe dysuria, haematuria and suprapubic discomfort from an associated acute haemorrhagic cystitis and prostatitis.

The arthritis is usually self-limiting with spontaneous remission of symptoms within 2–3 months of onset. There is, however, a recurrence rate of about 15% per annum not necessarily related to further overt exposure to infection. Low back pain and stiffness from sacroiliitis are common and 15–20% of patients develop spondylitis. Iritis occurs in 30% of patients with recurring arthritis. Other extra-articular features are less common and are listed in the information box below.

REITER'S SYNDROME: EXTRA-ARTICULAR FEATURES

- Conjunctivitis
- Iritis
- Urethritis

- Aortic incompetence
- Cardiac conduction defects
- Meningoencephalitis
- Pericarditis/pleurisy
- Peripheral neuropathy

Diagnosis
The ESR is often greatly raised during the acute phase and may remain so long after joint symptoms have settled. Polymorphonuclear leucocytosis and an anaemia of chronic disease are further indications of active systemic disturbance. The synovial fluid has the characteristics of a low viscosity inflammatory effusion with leucocyte counts as high as 50 000/ml but it is

sterile on culture. Giant synovial macrophages can be seen but synovial fluid complement levels are not depressed as they are in seropositive rheumatoid arthritis. Serum tests for rheumatoid factor and antinuclear factor are negative. Tissue typing reveals HLA-B27 in more than 70% of cases.

Radiological examination. Periarticular osteoporosis, reduction of joint space and erosive changes can be seen when there is prolonged or recurrent inflammatory arthritis. The changes are often accompanied by marked periostitis especially in the metatarsals, phalanges and pelvis; there may be large and 'fluffy' calcaneal spurs. Sacroiliitis is indistinguisable from that seen in ankylosing spondylitis but the spinal changes include early isolated bony spurs and paravertebral ossification. These are also seen in psoriasis but not in ankylosing spondylitis.

Management
This is mainly symptomatic and supportive. Rest and NSAID are required during the acute phases together with judicious aspiration of joints and intra-articular or other local steroid injections. Systemic corticosteroids are rarely required. Iritis is a medical emergency requiring topical, subconjunctival or systemic corticosteroids. Severe progressive arthritis and intractable keratoderma blennorrhagica occasionally warrant cytotoxic drug therapy. The non-specific urethritis is usually treated with a short course of tetracycline and there is now some evidence that it reduces the frequency of arthritis in sexually acquired cases.

10% of patients have evidence of active disease 20 years after the onset. Spondylitis, chronic erosive arthritis, recurrent acute arthritis and uveitis are the major causes of long-term morbidity.

PSORIATIC ARTHRITIS

This is a seronegative inflammatory arthritis found in patients with psoriasis, a past or family history of psoriasis or with characteristic changes in the nails.

Epidemiology
Psoriatic arthritis occurs in about 1 out of 1000 of the general population and in 7% of patients with psoriasis. 20% of all patients with seronegative polyarthritis have psoriasis while the prevalence of psoriasis in seropositive rheumatoid arthritis is no higher than that in the general population, suggesting that the association of the skin disease with seronegative arthritis does not arise by chance alone. The onset is usually between the ages of 25–40 years.

Clinical features

Five distinct clinical patterns of psoriatic arthritis are recognised and are listed in the information box below.

CLINICAL PATTERNS OF PSORIATIC ARTHROPATHY

- Asymmetrical oligoarthritis   70%
- Symmetrical seronegative arthritis   15%
- Distal interphalangeal joint arthritis   15%
- Arthritis mutilans   5%
- Sacroiliitis/spondylitis

An inflammatory arthritis affecting the distal interphalangeal joints which are not typically involved in RA is characteristic and almost invariably associated with nail changes (Fig. 15.13) but an asymmetrical or symmetrical seronegative arthritis resembling RA is more common.

Sacroiliitis and spondylitis indistinguishable from classical ankylosing spondylitis can occur alone or in association with any of the clinical patterns of peripheral arthritis.

Extra-articular features are limited to:

1. skin lesions which may be widespread scaling lesions, typically over extensor surfaces, or insignificant and confined to such areas as the scalp, natal cleft and umbilicus where they are easily overlooked;
2. nail changes including pitting, onycholysis, subungual hyperkeratosis and horizontal ridging;
3. iritis.

Diagnosis

The ESR is usually only moderately raised and there may be a mild normochromic normocytic anaemia in active cases. Tests for rheumatoid factor and antinuclear factor are negative. Radiographs showing asymmetrical disease, terminal IP joint involvement and relatively little periarticular osteoporosis may help to distinguish psoriatic arthritis from rheumatoid arthritis. The changes in the axial skeleton resemble those in ankylosing spondylitis.

Management

NSAID are usually all that are required to control symptoms. Gold therapy can be used in persistently symptomatic progressive cases without exacerbation of the psoriasis but the antimalarials, chloroquine and hydroxychloroquine may give rise to exfoliative reactions. Methotrexate and other immunosuppressive drugs are given occasionally in an attempt to control progressive arthritis mutilans or extensive incapacitating skin disease. The retinoid etretinate (30 mg/d) has been shown to be effective in treating the arthritis as well as the skin lesions but it must be avoided in young women because of potential teratogenicity and its use can be complicated by mucocutaneous side-effects, hyperlipidaemia, myalgias and extra-spinal calcification. Photochemotherapy with methoxypsoralen and long-wave ultra violet light (PUVA) is primarily used for patients with severe skin lesions but it can also help some patients with synchronous exacerbations of inflammatory arthritis. Splints and prolonged rest are avoided because of the increased tendency to fibrous and bony ankylosis but intra-articular steroid injections can be used with good effect in persistently active and symptomatic joints.

Prognosis

This is better than for rheumatoid arthritis with the exception of those rare cases with arthritis mutilans.

OTHER SERONEGATIVE SPONDARTHRITIDES

ARTHRITIS AND INFLAMMATORY BOWEL DISEASE

Two patterns of seronegative inflammatory arthritis are associated with ulcerative colitis and Crohn's disease.

Enteropathic synovitis

An acute, often migratory, non-erosive, oligoarthritis occurs in the course of the disorder in 12% of patients with ulcerative colitis and 20% of those with Crohn's disease.

Clinical features

The knees, ankles and other weight-bearing joints are

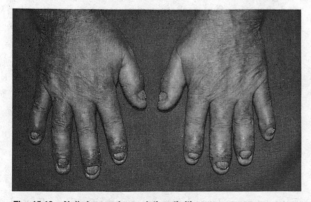

Fig. 15.13   Nail changes in psoriatic arthritis.

most commonly affected but the wrists and small joints of the fingers and toes can also be involved. The arthritis tends to follow exacerbations of the underlying bowel disease sometimes in association with aphthous mouth ulcers, iritis and erythema nodosum. It ceases to be a problem following total colectomy for ulcerative colitis. The higher prevalence in Crohn's disease may reflect the greater difficulty in eradicating the bowel problem.

Sacroiliitis (16%) and ankylosing spondylitis (6%)
These are also seen in the course of these disorders, but they pursue an independent course and often precede the bowel disease.

BEHCET'S SYNDROME

This disease is rare in Western Europe but more common in Japan and Eastern Mediterranean countries where it has an association with HLA-B5.

Clinical features
Major criteria are recurrent aphthous stomatitis, skin lesions, iritis and genital ulceration. Minor criteria are inflammatory arthritis of large joints, intestinal ulceration, meningoencephalitis, epididymitis and thrombophlebitis. In the presence of all four major criteria the syndrome is said to be 'complete'; in the presence of three, 'incomplete'. The arthritis is mono-articular or oligo-articular and non-erosive. It most frequently involves the knees, ankles, wrists and elbows. Occasionally the sacroiliac joints are affected.

Management
Treatment is symptomatic with NSAID; corticosteroids and immunosuppressive therapy are reserved for the more serious systemic manifestations.

WHIPPLE'S DISEASE

This is a rare disorder.

Clinical features
These include diarrhoea, abdominal pain, weight loss, pyrexia, skin pigmentation, malabsorption and arthritis. The pattern of the non-erosive arthritis can resemble the migratory oligo-articular enteropathic arthritis but sometimes it is symmetrical and polyarticular. Joints symptoms, most commonly affecting the knee or ankle, may precede other clinical manifestations by months or years and sacroiliitis and ankylosing spondylitis may occur.

Diagnosis
This is confirmed by demonstrating the presence of para-aminosalicylic acid (PAS) positive macrophages in a small intestinal biopsy.

Management
Treatment is with prolonged antibiotic therapy, usually tetracyline 1 g daily for 1 year. Arthralgias and arthritis settle within a month of starting treatment.

JUVENILE CHRONIC ARTHRITIS

The four main patterns of chronic arthritis that commence in childhood before the age of 16 years are listed in the information box below.

PATTERNS OF JUVENILE CHRONIC POLYARTHRITIS	
Systemic (Still's disease)	10%
Polyarticular	
Seronegative	20%
Seropositive	10%
Pauciarticular	
Young girls (ANF+, HLA DR5)	40%
Older boys (HLA B27)	20%

SYSTEMIC ONSET JUVENILE CHRONIC ARTHRITIS (STILL'S DISEASE)

This pattern of disease is most common between the ages of 1 and 5 years.

Clinical features
Lymphadenopathy, hepato-splenomegaly, pleurisy, pericarditis and a high intermittent fever are associated with myalgias, arthralgias and eventually polyarthritis. Weight loss and retardation of growth may be striking and there is often a characteristic evanescent macular rash which tends to appear when the temperature is raised. Remission of symptoms usually occurs within 6 months but half the children have recurrent attacks and one-quarter go on to develop a severe chronic polyarthritis.

POLYARTICULAR JUVENILE CHRONIC ARTHRITIS

This can occur at any age.

Clinical features
Four or more large joints are commonly first affected

acutely or insidiously. Inflammatory arthritis in the proximity of growing epiphyses may result in growth acceleration or arrest. Early fusion in the cervical spine and mandible gives rise to the short stiff neck and receding chin very characteristic of adults who have had juvenile chronic arthritis. The overall prognosis is good and only 10–15% have severe destructive arthritis.

SEROPOSITIVE POLYARTICULAR DISEASE

The onset is usually after the age of 8 years. The disease resembles severe adult onset rheumatoid arthritis with progressive erosive joint changes in more than half of those affected. Extra-articular features include nodules and vasculitis. Antinuclear factor tests are positive in 75%.

PAUCIARTICULAR JUVENILE CHRONIC ARTHRITIS

This involves four or less joints. At least two distinct subsets can be identified.

1. *Young girls* with mono- or pauci-articular arthritis but seldom any constitutional symptoms. HLA-DR5 and positive tests for antinuclear factor appear to be a marker for chronic iritis which can occur in up to half of this group. Three-monthly slit lamp examinations are required if this complication is to be detected and treated early enough to preserve normal vision.
2. *Older boys* with mono- or pauci-articular arthritis affecting hips, knees or ankles. Sacroiliitis is common and there is frequently a family history of iritis, ankylosing spondylitis or another spondarthritis. 75% of these boys are HLA-B27 positive and in some the disease gradually evolves into ankylosing spondylitis in early adult life.

Differential diagnosis

Diagnosis of acute arthritis in childhood includes bacterial, viral and reactive arthritis as it does in adults and also rheumatic fever, leukaemia and osteomyelitis.

Henoch-Schönlein (anaphylactoid) purpura.

This is a small vessel vasculitis which is associated with abdominal pain and an acute arthritis affecting one or more joints for a few days at a time. The disease frequently follows an upper respiratory infection and usually lasts for less than 3 months. Boys are affected twice as frequently as girls. Non-thrombocytopenic purpura is found characteristically over the buttocks and lower legs and up to half the children affected have angiooedema. Intussusception, rectal bleeding and renal involvement are features of more severe cases.

Management

The principles of management in juvenile chronic arthritis do not differ from those in adult rheumatoid arthritis but special consideration is given to maintaining the child's education and helping parents to develop a sensible, vigilant but not overprotective approach to the child's disease. Bed-rest may be essential during acute phases but care must be taken to avoid development of flexion deformities of the hips and knees by regular prone lying and appropriate lightweight splints. Whenever possible the child should be kept mobile and ambulant and daily physiotherapy is given throughout to maintain a good range of joint movements and muscle strength. Hydrotherapy in a warm pool is particularly useful.

Until recently aspirin was the drug of choice and its use in JCA is an exception to the recommendation that aspirin should not be given to children aged under 12 years because of the risk of Reye's syndrome. Naproxen (5 mg/kg) is safe and effective in children and experience is accumulating with other NSAID. Chloroquine, hydroxychloroquine, gold salts and penicillamine can be used with the same precautions as in adults.

Corticosteroids are reserved for children with severe systemic disease, those with chronic iritis not responding to local therapy and where very active joint disease does not respond to other measures. The use of corticotrophin or alternate day corticosteroids should always be considered because daily doses of prednisolone as low as 3 mg can inhibit growth in children under the age of 5 years. Older children can be taught to give their own injections of corticotrophin if this has to be continued for any length of time. Corticosteroids do not arrest the progression of disease. Immunosuppressive drugs are used only in persistently active disease associated with amyloidosis.

Surgery is usually limited to the rehabilitation of children with deformities. Soft tissue release operations may be helpful in eliminating difficult flexion contractures and osteotomies may be required when joints have been allowed to fuse in poor positions. Total hip arthroplasty can be considered for severely destroyed joints as soon as growth has ceased.

INFECTIVE ARTHRITIS

Septic arthritis can accompany septicaemia at any age. *H. influenzae* is the common causative organism in infancy; staphylococcal and streptococcal infections are usually responsible in older children and adults. Other organisms which may be implicated are gonococci, pneumococci, meningococci, *Escherichia coli*, *Pseudomonas* and *Proteus*. Important predisposing factors include debilitating illnesses, diabetes mellitus, immunodeficiency disorders and immunosuppression. Joint trauma, surgery, penetrating injury and intra-articular injections may lead to bacterial joint infections and may complicate rheumatoid arthritis and other established arthritides.

Clinical features

Characteristically septic arthritis has an abrupt onset with severe pain and swelling of a single joint associated with a swinging fever, severe malaise and a polymorphonuclear leucocytosis. Large joints are most frequently affected and the joint is hot, tender and swollen with an effusion and marked limitation of movement. The diagnosis may be missed when more than one joint is involved, in patients with rheumatoid arthritis or when the presentation is less acute in patients receiving corticosteroids or immunosuppressive drugs.

Diagnosis

It is essential to establish the diagnosis early by joint aspiration and blood culture. The synovial fluid is typically turbid with a high polymorphonuclear cell count ($> 50\,000/mm^3 > 80\%$ polys). Organisms may be easily and immediately identified on Gram stain of a film but special culture techniques are required especially for gonococci and anaerobic organisms. Elevated levels of lactic and succinic acid detectable by gas liquid chromatography suggest bacterial infection.

Radiographs show no more than soft tissue swelling initially. Later there may be periarticular osteoporosis, joint space narrowing, periostitis and articular erosions. In more long-standing infections the joint margins have a peculiar 'rubbed-out' appearance. Radionuclide imaging with gallium shows changes earlier than on plain radiographs and is especially useful in detecting infection in the axial and other deeper inaccessible joints.

Management

In all patients where bacterial infection is suspected treatment should be commenced with high parenteral doses of a broad spectrum antibiotic as soon as joint aspiration and blood cultures have been completed; it is continued until the responsible organism and its sensitivity have been established. Appropriate antibiotics must then be administered for several weeks. Antibiotics readily cross the inflamed synovial membrane and there is no need to inject them intra-articularly.

The joint should be rested and immobilised with a splint and daily joint aspiration undertaken until no more fluid reaccumulates. If the fluid becomes loculated or too thick for aspiration, surgical drainage is required.

Prognosis

The prognosis for recovery without joint damage is directly related to the speed with which antibiotic therapy is instituted.

GONOCOCCAL ARTHRITIS

This is more common in females than males and not infrequently commences at the time of a menstrual period within 2–3 weeks of genital infection.

Clinical features

Joint involvement is usually asymmetrical and polyarticular with an acute or subacute, migratory polyarthralgia or polyarthritis. Tenosynovitis, an 'additive' as opposed to a 'flitting' pattern of joint involvement and a macular, vesicular or pustular rash are important diagnostic clues even in the absence of overt genital gonorrhoea.

Diagnosis

This can be established by cultures from synovial fluid, blood or skin lesions or from the genital tract but organisms are identified in joints in only 20% of cases.

Management

Most patients respond to penicillin, 1 mega unit daily for 2 weeks with dramatic improvement in 3–4 days.

MENINGOCOCCAL INFECTION

This can be associated with:

1. an acute transient polyarthritis that is seen simultaneously with a characteristic petechial rash;
2. a purulent monoarthritis which usually occurs after 5 days or;
3. a flitting polyarthralgia in patients with chronic meningococcaemia.

Penicillin is the treatment of choice.

BRUCELLOSIS

This is associated with polyarthralgia or transient polyarthritis. Much more rarely there may be a septic arthritis or spondylitis. Destructive lesions in one or more contiguous vertebrae lead to severe pain, disc narrowing and marginal proliferation of osteophytes with early bony fusion of vertebrae. Chronic bursitis and osteomyelitis may also occur. Diagnosis is established by blood and synovial fluid cultures coupled with rising antibody titres. Treatment is given on page 131.

TUBERCULOSIS OF JOINTS

This is usually secondary to an established focus in the lungs or kidneys. Articular infection is rarely seen except in malnourished, socially deprived elderly or immigrant groups following the eradication of bovine tuberculosis in Britain. A single large joint is affected in more than three-quarters of all patients.

Clinical features
Joint pain, stiffness, swelling and restriction of movements are associated with anorexia, weight loss and night sweats.

Diagnosis
In the early stages radiographs show only periarticular osteoporosis and soft tissue swelling. Later there is narrowing of the joint space, bony erosion and collapse of subchondral bone with little associated periosteal reaction. The tuberculin skin test is strongly positive and diagnosis can sometimes be made by direct bacteriological examination and culture of synovial fluid. In other patients synovial biopsy is required. After antibiotic control has been established (see p. 367), synovectomy may be required in those with extensive disease.

LEPROSY

This can have a number of osteoarticular manifestations. Joint deformities of the hands and feet are common as a sequel to peripheral nerve involvement and these may be complicated by neuropathic (Charcot) joints. Osteomyelitis may complicate digital ulceration and hypersensitivity reactions may resemble rheumatoid arthritis.

SYPHILITIC ARTHRITIS

Congenital syphilis may be associated with painful para-articular swelling due to epiphyseal involvement soon after birth or painless effusions of the knees (Clutton's joints) in adolescents. *Acquired* secondary syphilis may be associated with a migrating polyar-thralgia resembling rheumatic fever and Charcot (neuropathic) joints are a feature of tabes dorsalis.

LYME ARTHRITIS

This is an intermittent pauciarticular inflammatory arthritis which is preceded by a characteristic rash (erythema chronicum migrans). It is a tick-borne (*Ixodes dammini*) spirochaetal disease (*Borrelia burgdoferi*) which was first described in Lyme, Connecticut. Later manifestations include meningoencephalitis, ocular inflammation and cardiac conduction defects, as well as inflammatory arthritis. The diagnosis is made by serological testing and the disease responds to penicillin or tetracycline.

FUNGAL INFECTIONS

These are rare. Blastomycosis, histoplasmosis and sporotrichosis can be associated with destructive lesions of bones and joints. Histoplasmosis and coccidiomycosis may also be associated with erythema nodosum and a benign polyarthritis.

VIRAL INFECTIONS

A number of viral infections are commonly associated with arthralgia and transient polyarthritis. These include hepatitis B, mumps, chickenpox, infectious mononucleosis, adenoviral, enteroviral, parvoviral and arboviral infections. Hepatitis associated arthritis occurs in up to 30% of patients with hepatitis B. Typically it is associated with fever and rash and precedes the onset of jaundice. Rubella arthritis follows 1–7 days after the rash or 2–6 weeks after vaccination in 30–40% of adults. A symmetrical inflammatory polyarthritis may be associated with symptoms of carpal tunnel compression or tenosynovitis. Joint pain, stiffness and swelling, which may be severe, usually settle in the 1–4 weeks but the condition may persist with intermittent arthralgia for some months. Posterior cervical lymphadenopathy and a high lymphocyte count in the synovial fluid may be helpful in diagnosis.

MISCELLANEOUS DISORDERS OF SYNOVIAL JOINTS

ACROMEGALY

This is associated with a symmetrical arthropathy in 50% of patients. The small joints of the hands, wrists and knees are particularly affected as is the spine. Hypertrophy of synovium and articular cartilage are characteristically associated with periosteal new bone formation, osteophytosis, 'tufting' of the terminal phalanges and premature osteoarthrosis and hypertrophic spondylosis.

AMYLOIDOSIS

This can be associated with carpal tunnel compression and a polyarthritis superficially resembling rheumatoid arthritis. The synovium is infiltrated with amyloid protein and the diagnosis can be made by finding fragments of amyloid tissue in the synovial fluid.

HYPERLIPIDAEMIA

Type II can be associated with a migratory polyarthritis, and widespread xanthomas with tendon deposits. Type IV can be associated with arthralgia and morning stiffness and also hyperuricaemia and gout.

SARCOIDOSIS

Erythema nodosum and hilar lymphadenopathy are frequently associated with a symmetrical non-destructive inflammatory arthritis especially affecting the knees, ankles and wrists. A more specific asymmetrical destructive arthritis affects similar joints especially in blacks and biopsy of the synovium in these shows evidence of noncaseating granulomas. Radiologically there may be 'punched out' cystic bone lesions and also 'cortical erosions' and joint destruction.

SYSTEMIC LUPUS ERYTHEMATOSUS (SLE)

This is a multisystem connective tissue disease characterised by the presence of numerous autoantibodies,

Table 15.13   Immunological abnormalities detectable in the blood of patients with SLE

Antinuclear antibodies	Lymphocytotoxins
Anti-DNA-histone (and LE cells)	Depression of CH_{50} and C3 and C4
Anti-DNA (single strand)	Antibodies against erythrocytes,
Anti-DNA (double strand)	leucocytes and platelets
Anti-RNA	Biological false positive tests for
Anti-Sm	syphilis
Anti-UI-RNP	Circulating anticoagulants (anti-
Anti-Ro/SS-A	cardiolipin antibodies)
Anti-La/SS-B	Anti-thyroid (and other organ
Anti-MA	specific autoantibodies)
Anti-PCNA	Rheumatoid factors
	Cryoglobulins
	Circulating immune complexes

circulating immune complexes and widespread immunologically determined tissue damage.

Epidemiology

SLE affects individuals throughout the world but occurs more frequently in the United States and the Far East. American blacks are particularly susceptible, with a prevalence as high as 1 in 250 among females. The increasing use of sensitive tests for antinuclear antibodies suggest that mild and incomplete cases frequently occur. The onset is most commonly in the 2nd and 3rd decades, with a female/male ratio of 9:1. The sex incidence is more equal in children and the elderly.

Aetiology and pathogenesis

Although the cause of SLE remains obscure, current concepts suggest that this is a multifactoral disorder in which there is profound *disturbance of immune regulation*. A defect of suppressor T lymphocytes is associated with polyclonal B lymphocyte activation and the uncontrolled production of autoantibodies and immune complexes (Tables 15.13 and 15.14).

Table 15.14   Frequency (%) diagnostically useful autoantibodies in connective tissue diseases

	dsDNA	Sm	RNP	Jo-1	PM-Scl	Scl-70	Centromere	XR	Ro	La
SLE	60	20	25	—	—	—	—	—	25	10
MCTD	—	Occ	100	Occ	—	—	—	—	20	Occ
SS	Occ	—	Occ	—	—	—	—	—	75	40
PSS	—	—	Occ	—	—	20	Occ	—	Occ	—
CREST	—	—	—	—	—	—	30	—	—	—
Myositis	—	—	15	25	10	—	—	—	10	—
PBC	Occ	—	—	—	—	—	10	10	5	—
CAH	Occ	—	—	—	—	—	—	25	—	—

SLE Systemic lupus erythematosus
MCTD Mixed connective tissue disease
SS Primary Sjogren's (sicca syndrome)
PSS Progressive systemic sclerosis
CREST Calcinosis, Raynaud's syndrome, oesophageal involvement, sclerodactyly, telangiectasia
PBC Primary biliary cirrhosis
CAH Chronic active hepatitis

Evidence for *genetic factors* in the aetiology of the disease includes:

1. its occurrence in monozygotic twins pairs;
2. a higher than expected prevalence of SLE, other connective tissue diseases, antinuclear antibodies and immune complexes in related family members;
3. inherited deficiency of isolated complement components, notably C2 in some patients;
4. increased prevalence of the histocompatibility antigens HLA-B8 and DR3.

Evidence for the influence of *environmental factors* includes:

1. the provocative effect of sunlight;
2. the induction of lupus erythematosus by drugs;
3. the importance of oestrogens as determinants of disease expression. Exacerbations commonly occur in pregnancy and the puerperium and prevalence is increased in fertile women, those using oral contraceptives and men with Klinefelter's syndrome.

There is evidence of *viral infection* in animal models of SLE but not in humans.

Immunologically-mediated tissue damage results from at least two different mechanisms on SLE:

1. Direct Type II antibody-mediated cytotoxicity. Brain damage and abortion may be a consequence of cytotoxicity by cold reactive antibodies which cross-react with neural and trophoblast tissues.
2. Immune complex (and complement) mediated Type III hypersensitivity. The renal and vascular lesions of SLE appear to be a consequence of deposition of circulating DNA-Anti-DNA and other complexes in tissues.

Clinical features

Arthritis, arthralgia and fever. These are the commonest presenting features. Unlike other types of inflammatory arthritis, symptoms may begin during pregnancy and there may be a past history of spontaneous abortions. The arthritis can be transient and migratory or a more persistent seronegative polyarthritis. Chronic inflammatory arthritis and tenosynovitis may lead to deformities and contractures but erosive changes are very uncommon.

Skin lesions. These are seen in more than two-thirds of patients. In addition to the classical, photosensitive erythematous 'butterfly' rash (Fig. 15.14) across the face, there may be lesions of discoid lupus or

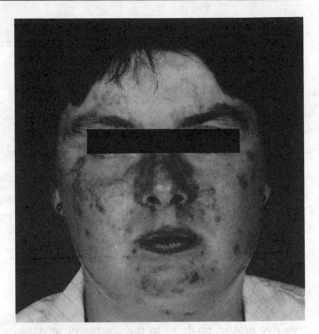

Fig. 15.14   'Butterfly' distribution facial rash in SLE.

a vasculitic rash. The latter may present as purpura or periungual erythema with 'chilblain-like' lesions or digital infarcts. Livedo reticularis and Raynaud's phenomenon are common while bullous eruptions and panniculitis ('lupus profundus') occur more rarely. Alopecia can be a useful diagnostic pointer and is seen in more than 50% of patients. Painful oral or nasopharyngeal ulcers are less common.

Cardiopulmonary features. These include pericarditis, myocarditis and endocarditis, pleurisy, fibrosing alveolitis and acute lupus pneumonitis as well as a 'shrinking lung syndrome' with progressive elevation of the diaphragms and linear scars from recurrent pulmonary infarction. Lung function tests reveal impairment of ventilation and diffusion in these and many patients without overt clinical or radiological evidence of pulmonary involvement. Verrucous (Libman-Sachs) endocarditis may be demonstrated by echocardiography.

Renal involvement. This carries the worst prognosis. It may result in the nephrotic syndrome and renal failure or it may be limited to insignificant proteinuria or the presence of red cells or casts (see p. 574).

Central nervous system involvement. This occurs in up to half the patients. In the majority it is limited to mild psychiatric disturbance or epilepsy but in a few there may be severe depression, dementia, organic psychosis, cranial nerve lesions, hemiplegia, transverse myelitis, chorea, cerebellar ataxia or peripheral neuropathy. The more severe manifestations are associated with a poor prognosis.

Other manifestations. Gastrointestinal symptoms are frequent but non-specific. Abdominal pain can be due to peritonitis, perisplenitis, pancreatitis or vasculitis. Gastric or duodenal perforation may be complications of corticosteroid therapy; colonic or gallbladder perforations are more likely to be a consequence of necrotising arteritis. Lymphadènopathy is found in half the patients and a moderately enlarged spleen in 20–30%. Ocular findings include keratoconjunctivitis sicca, episcleritis, retinal vasculitis and soft exudates.

Diagnosis
The ESR is usually raised in active disease but the C reactive protein rarely so in the absence of infection. Haematological findings may include a normocytic normochromic anaemia of chronic disease, a Coombs' positive haemolytic anaemia, leucopenia, thrombocytopaenia and immunological abnormalities.

Immunological findings
The immunological abnormalities found in SLE are given in Tables 15.13 and 15.14 on page 788.

Antinuclear antibodies (ANF). These can be detected by indirect immunofluorescence in the serum of more than 90% of patients but positive tests are found in many other conditions and these are listed in the information box below. Positive tests in low titre have no clinical significance and are frequently found in normal elderly people. The *LE cell test* is less sensitive, very time consuming and hardly more specific.

ANTINUCLEAR ANTIBODIES: DISEASE ASSOCIATIONS

- SLE
- MCTD
- Polymyositis
- Scleroderma
- Polyarteritis
- Sjogren's syndrome
- Rheumatoid arthritis
- Fibrosing alveolitis
- Chronic liver disease
- Thyroiditis
- Myasthenia gravis
- Leukaemia

Anti-DNA antibodies and immune complexes. Radioimmunoassays for antibodies to undenatured double stranded DNA have much greater specificity but anti-DNA antibodies are present in the serum in significant amounts in only about half the patients at any one time. High levels of anti-DNA antibodies coupled with depressed total haemolytic complement (CH_{50}) activity and low C3 and C4 complement components suggest that there is activation of the classical complement pathway by active immune complex disease. Further evidence for circulating immune complexes may be obtained by finding a cryoprecipitate or by using one of a number of tests for CIq binding. Tissue evidence for immune complex deposition comes from detection of complement components and immunoglobulins by immunofluorescence at the dermoepidermal junction of normal skin (lupus 'band' test) or in organ biopsies.

The lupus anticoagulant. This is an anticardiolipin antibody which may also give rise to false positive biological tests for syphilis. Lupus anticoagulant activity is detected by a prolongation of the partial thromboplastin time (PTTK, APTT) which is not correctable by the addition of normal plasma or by a prolongation of the dilute prothrombin time. Anticardiolipin antibodies are detected by ELISA. High titres are associated with thrombocytopaenia, thrombotic manifestations and in some cases recurrent abortion.

Management
Acute and life threatening manifestations of SLE require systemic corticosteroid therapy, often initially in doses of 40–80 mg prednisolone or equivalent daily. 'Pulse' therapy with methylprednisolone (1 g i.v. on 3 successive days) is occasionally required in patients with proliferative glomerulonephritis and rapidly deteriorating renal function. With remission of disease careful attempts are made to withdraw steroids or maintain patients on very low doses or alternate day regimes of steroid therapy. Articular symptoms and less severe inflammatory manifestations should be managed without corticosteroids whenever possible, but NSAIDs must be used with care in patients with renal disease. Antimalarials are particularly useful in the management of patients with troublesome skin and joint lesions and they can reduce the frequency of severe exacerbations of disease.

Immunosuppressive drugs are reserved for patients with severe diffuse proliferative glomerulonephritis who are not responding adequately to corticosteroids and for those requiring maintenance steroid doses so high as to cause severe side-effects. The combination of plasma exchange and immunosuppressive drug therapy may be useful in some patients with serious steroid resistant exacerbations.

Prognosis

Prognosis for life has improved dramatically over the last 30 years and the 5-year survival should now be better than 90%. Much of this apparent improvement results, however, from the detection of milder cases using highly sensitive immunological tests for diagnostic purposes. Patients with severe renal, neurological or pulmonary involvement have the worst prognosis. Renal biopsy can provide a guide to prognosis. Infection is an important cause of morbidity particularly in patients receiving high doses of corticosteroids and immunosuppressives. Pregnancy is not contraindicated provided the disease is in reasonable remission and renal, cardiac and cerebral functions are intact.

CHRONIC DISCOID LUPUS ERYTHEMATOSUS

This is more common than SLE. The skin lesions are characterised by photosensitivity, erythema, scaling, follicular plugging and telangiectasia. In most patients the disease is limited to the skin. ANF tests are positive but anti-DNA antibodies are not usually found and complement levels are normal. SLE may occasionally supervene.

DRUG-INDUCED SLE

Positive tests for antinuclear factor are frequently encountered in patients receiving procainamide, hydralazine, anti-convulsants, oral contraceptives and phenothiazines. Much more rarely a syndrome resembling SLE develops. Fever, polyarthritis, skin lesions, lymphadenopathy, serositis and pulmonary infiltrates are frequent, but renal disease and neurological manifestations are rare. Complement levels are usually normal and antibodies to double standard DNA absent. Slow acetylators of hydralazine and those with the HLA-DR4 histocompatibility antigen appear to be particularly at risk. Remission usually follows drug withdrawal. Occasionally a short course of corticosteroids is required.

MIXED CONNECTIVE TISSUE DISEASE (MCTD)

This is characterised by overlapping clinical features suggesting systemic lupus erythematosus, progressive systemic sclerosis (see below) and polymyositis in association with very high titres of a circulating antinuclear antibody with specificity for a ribonuclease sensitive extractable nuclear antigen (ENA) identified as a nuclear ribonucleoprotein (nRNP).

Clinical features

Women are affected four times more commonly than men. The onset is usually in the 3rd or 4th decade but may be at any age. Raynaud's phenomenon with 'sausage' swelling of the fingers, skin changes resembling dermatomyositis or scleroderma and a mild inflammatory polyarthritis are typically associated with proximal muscle weakness and tenderness and abnormal oesophageal motility. Diffuse interstitial pulmonary fibrosis is not uncommon but cardiac, renal and central nervous system involvement are very rare. The ESR and muscle enzymes are usually moderately raised. The condition is further characterised by a relatively good prognosis and a good response to low dosage steroid therapy.

PROGRESSIVE SYSTEMIC SCLEROSIS

This is a generalised disorder of connective tissue characterised by fibrosis and degenerative changes in the skin (scleroderma) and many internal organs. Although its aetiology is unknown, it is believed to be at one end of the spectrum of diffuse connective tissue diseases where immunologically determined inflammation is followed by intimal thickening of small blood vessels and excessive production and cross-linking of collagen. Persons with the HLA haplotype A1 B8 DR3 appear to be genetically predisposed, and there is evidence of vascular hypersensitivity to cold and serotonin. Systemic sclerosis is less common than SLE but is seen throughout the world. Women are affected four times more frequently than men.

Clinical features

The onset is most frequently in the 30–50 age group. Severe Raynaud's phenomenon is usually the presenting complaint and may precede other features by months or years.

Skin changes. Initially there is often well demarcated non-pitting oedema and induration associated with 'sausage' swelling and restriction of movement of the fingers. Later the skin becomes shiny with atrophy and ulceration of the finger tips with or without associated calcinosis. The skin of the face, limbs and trunk is variably affected and there may be striking pigmentation and telangiectasia. As scleroderma advances, the face may become taut and 'mask-like' with 'beaking' of the nose and difficulty in opening the mouth. Tightening of skin over bony prominences results in flexion contractures and liability to trauma.

Musculo-skeletal manifestations. These include arthralgia and a mild non-erosive inflammatory arthritis often characterised by 'leathery' crepitus in affected tendon sheaths or joints. Muscle weakness and wasting result from both disuse atrophy and low-grade myositis.

The gastrointestinal tract. This is involved in the majority of patients. Reflux oesophagitis associated with a sliding hiatus hernia is a common problem and loss of oesophageal peristalsis on recumbent barium swallow examination is often detected even in the absence of dysphagia. Dilatation of segments of large and small bowel occur less frequently, causing intermittent abdominal pain, constipation, distension and obstruction; there may be diarrhoea and malabsorption secondary to bacterial overgrowth. Systemic sclerosis may be associated with primary biliary cirrhosis and with Sjogren's syndrome.

Pulmonary fibrosis. This occurs in the majority of patients. In many it is limited to a symptomless defect in gaseous diffusion. In others progressive fibrosis is accompanied by increasing dyspnoea on exertion, a restrictive pattern of impaired lung function and reticulation and 'honeycomb' changes in the lower zone on a chest radiograph. Pulmonary involvement can be complicated by pulmonary hypertension and right ventricular failure, or by alveolar cell or bronchiolar carcinoma. Aspiration pneumonia may be a consequence of oesophageal involvement.

Other manifestations. Cardiac involvement is usually secondary to systemic rather than pulmonary hypertension but pericarditis, cardiomyopathy, heart block and aortic valve lesions can also occur. Renal involvement may develop at any stage of the disease and is an important cause of morbidity and mortality. Cranial or peripheral nerve lesions occur rarely.

THE CRST OR CREST SYNDROME

This comprises a subset of patients whose disease is limited to calcinosis, Raynaud's phenomenon, oesophageal involvement, sclerodactyly and telangiectasia. An anticentromere antinuclear antibody with specificity for a protein of the chromosomal kinetochore is present in the serum (Table 15.14, p. 788).

MORPHOEA AND LINEAR SCLERODERMA

These are localised forms of disease limited to characteristic, well-demarcated, lesions of the skin and subcutaneous connective tissues. Serological findings are similar to those of systemic sclerosis and very occasionally systemic features develop.

EOSINOPHILIC FASCIITIS

This is a scleroderma-like condition characterised by pain, swelling and tenderness of the hands, forearms and feet where induration of the skin and subcutaneous tissues is not associated with Raynaud's phenomenon or systemic sclerosis. Carpal tunnel compression may be an early feature and the onset frequently follows abnormal exercise. Eosinophilia and hyperglobulinaemia are characteristic and the diagnosis is confirmed by finding an inflammatory cell infiltrate with prominent eosinophils in association with marked fibrosis of the subcutaneous fascia. Eosinophilic fasciitis responds to corticosteroids but is usually self-limiting.

PSEUDO-SCLERODERMA

Other conditions which may give rise to induration or brawny oedema of the skin that must be considered in the differential diagnosis of scleroderma include scleredema, scleromyxoedema, amyloidosis and acromegaly.

Diagnosis

The ANF is positive in about 50% of patients with a nucleolar or speckled staining pattern. Antibodies to single stranded RNA and to an extractable nuclear antigen (anti-Scl-70) occur in 20% and may be a marker for pulmonary involvement. Anti-DNA antibodies are not detected and complement levels are normal.

Management

No form of drug therapy has been proved to be effective in arresting the course of systemic sclerosis. Corticosteroids may produce some symptomatic benefit in early disease where inflammatory oedema or associated myositis and/or arthritis are prominent features and penicillamine can interfere with collagen cross linking. Nifedipine and prostacyclin infusions may occasionally be helpful in patients with severe Raynaud's phenomenon.

Attention should be paid to protecting the limbs from cold, the urgent treatment of chest infections and therapy for cardiac, respiratory and renal failure. Articular symptoms should be managed with NSAID. Episodes of steatorrhoea often respond to a short course of a broad spectrum antibiotic.

Prognosis

The outlook appears to be worse in those with late onset disease, widespread skin involvement of the trunk and renal, cardiac or respiratory disease. The overall 5-year survival is about 70%.

POLYMYOSITIS AND DERMATOMYOSITIS

These are diffuse connective tissue disorders in which muscle weakness and inflammatory changes in muscle and skin are the predominant features. They are relatively rare but occur throughout the world in all races and at all ages. The aetiology is obscure but persons with HLA-B8/Dr3 appear to be genetically predisposed.

Viral infection (overt or latent) may be one of the factors which may stimulate or precipitate the autoimmune process responsible for the disease. Skeletal muscle cells appear to be destroyed by sensitised lymphocytes.

Clinical features

It is possible to define five clinical subsets which are listed in the information box below.

MYOSITIS SUBSETS

- Adult polymyositis
- Adult dermatomyositis
- Adult polymyositis with malignancies
- Childhood dermatomyositis
- Polymyositis in other connective tissue diseases

ADULT POLYMYOSITIS

This occurs three times more frequently in women than men. The onset is usually insidious in the 3rd to 5th decade. The patients may experience difficulty in climbing stairs or rising from a low chair and on examination there is weakness of the pelvic and shoulder girdle muscles. Sometimes the onset is more abrupt with rapid progression of muscular weakness. Involvement of pharyngeal, laryngeal and respiratory muscles can lead to dysphagia, dysphonia and respiratory failure within a few days. In the majority of cases progression is less rapid and profound. Spontaneous remissions are followed by some return of muscle strength but there may be atrophy, calcinosis and fibrosis in damaged muscles causing flexion contractures. Muscle pain and tenderness are unusual except in very acute illness. Mild arthralgia or inflammatory arthritis, Raynaud's phenomenon and erythematous rashes on the elbows and knuckles are frequent associated features.

ADULT DERMATOMYOSITIS

This is also more common in women. Acute or subacute muscle weakness is accompanied by periorbital oedema and a characteristic purple 'heliotrope' rash on the upper eyelids. In addition, there may be a photosensitive, erythematous, scaling rash on the face, shoulders, upper arms and chest with red patches over knuckles, elbows and knees. Muscle pain, tenderness and weight loss are common as are arthralgia and mild inflammatory polyarthritis.

INFLAMMATORY MYOSITIS ASSOCIATED WITH MALIGNANCY

This is less common than was previously thought. It is seen only after the age of 40 years. The onset of symptoms is usually insidious and the clinical picture does not differ from that of typical polymyositis or dermatomyositis. The associated carcinoma may not become apparent for 2–3 years. Its resection is sometimes associated with remission of the myositis.

CHILDHOOD DERMATOMYOSITIS

This most commonly affects children between the ages of 4 and 10 years. Muscle weakness is usually accompanied by the typical rash of dermatomyositis. Muscle atrophy, contractures and subcutaneous calcification may be widespread and severe. Recurrent abdominal pain due to vasculitis is also a feature.

Diagnosis

Serum aminotransferases, aldolase and creatinine phosphokinase are usually raised and are useful guides to the activity of the disease. Tests for rheumatoid factor and ANF are often positive and there may be antibodies to an extractable nuclear antigen (PM-Scl, Jo-1, Mi). Electromyography may show characteristic changes which can be very helpful in distinguishing polymyositis from peripheral neuropathy. Muscle biopsy shows fibre necrosis and regeneration in association with an inflammatory cell infiltrate.

Management

Prednisolone, 40–60 mg daily, is used initially to induce a remission. Muscle enzyme levels may fall before clinical improvement is noted. The dose is then gradually reduced whilst continuing to monitor muscle strength and serum enzyme levels. Doses of 10–15 mg prednisolone daily are often needed to maintain remission. Immunosuppressive therapy is occasionally used when there is no response to corticosteroids. The use of splints and physiotherapy to prevent contractures should not be neglected. Prognosis is closely related to the presence or absence of associated malignancy and to the age of onset, being poorer in older patients.

VASCULITIS

A classification of vasculitis is given in the information box below.

A CLASSIFICATION OF SYSTEMIC VASCULITIS

Systemic necrotising vasculitis
Polyarteritis nodosa
Churg Strauss vasculitis
Wegener's granulomatosis

Lymphomatoid granulomatosis

Hypersensitivity vasculitis
Serum sickness, drug reactions
Henoch-Schonlein purpura
Infections
Neoplasms

Vasculitis associated with connective tissue disease
Rheumatoid arthritis
Systemic lupus erythematosus
Progressive systemic sclerosis
Polymyositis

Large vessel arteritis
Giant cell arteritis
Takayasu's disease

Kawasaki's disease

Buerger's disease

Vasculitis which occurs as part of rheumatoid arthritis, systemic lupus erythematosus, progressive systemic sclerosis and childhood dermatomyositis has been described above.

Polyarteritis nodosa, Takayasu's arteritis and cranial arteritis are diffuse connective tissue disorders in which immunologically determined vasculitis is the cause of the pathological changes. Polymyalgia rheumatica is related to cranial arteritis.

POLYMYALGIA RHEUMATICA

This is a relatively common condition in elderly Caucasians, especially women.

Clinical features

The onset is often abrupt with severe pain and stiffness in the neck, back, shoulders, upper arms and thighs, often worse in the morning. There may also be fever, weight loss and depression. Physical signs are usually limited to slight tenderness of the acromio-clavicular or sterno-clavicular joints. Occasionally there may be evidence of a mild inflammatory arthritis in a more peripheral joint. The muscles usually show no evidence of tenderness or atrophy and examination of the peripheral arteries is usually normal. However, up to one-third of patients at some time develop symptoms of cranial arteritis and are at risk of blindness from arteritic involvement of a branch of the ophthalmic artery.

The ESR is markedly raised in the majority of cases and there may be a normochromic normocytic anaemia of chronic disease. Temporal artery biopsy shows evidence of giant cell arteritis in about 40% of cases but the true frequency of arteritis is probably much higher.

Management

The response to corticosteroid therapy is dramatic. The diagnosis must be reviewed if there is no striking remission of symptoms within 4–5 days of starting prednisolone 15 mg once daily. Two to three weeks after starting therapy the dose of prednisolone is gradually reduced over several weeks. Most patients can be maintained in remission with 5–7.5 mg prednisolone daily. High dosage corticosteroids are given initially to patients with cranial arteritis.

Prognosis

The natural history is for remission to occur in 6 months to 2 years although relapses are not uncommon and occasional patients have a more prolonged chronic disease. The need for maintenance corticosteroids should be reviewed by an attempt at gradual steroid withdrawal every 6 months.

METABOLIC AND DEGENERATIVE DISEASES OF CONNECTIVE TISSUES AND JOINTS

CRYSTAL DEPOSITION DISEASES

GOUT

Gout is not a single disease. The term is used to describe a number of disorders in which crystals of monosodium urate monohydrate derived from hyperuricaemic body fluids give rise to inflammatory arthritis, tenosynovitis, bursitis or cellulitis, tophaceous deposits, urolithiasis and renal disease. Hyperuricaemia is a necessary but not a sufficient prerequisite for clinical manifestations of gout.

Epidemiology
Gouty arthritis is predominantly a problem of post-pubertal males and is seldom seen in women before the menopause. Asymptomatic hyperuricaemia is 10 times more common. Serum uric acid concentrates are distributed in the community as a continuous variable and are determined by a number of demographic factors of which age, sex, body bulk and genetic constitution are the most important. Serum uric acid levels are higher in urban than in rural communities and are positively correlated with intelligence, social class, weight, haemoglobin, serum proteins and a high protein diet.

Hyperuricaemia is arbitrarily defined as a serum uric acid level greater than two standard deviations from the mean, i.e. above 0.42 mmol/l in adult males and 0.36 mmol/l in adult females.

Aetiology of gout and hyperuricaemia
Various genetic and environmental factors lead to hyperuricaemia and gout by decreasing the excretion of uric acid and/or increasing its production (Table 15.15).

Diminished renal excretion of uric acid
In more than 75% of patients with gout there appears to be a genetically determined defect in fractional urate excretion which results in an inability to increase uric acid excretion in response to a purine load.

Increased production of uric acid
This is at least partly responsible for hyperuricaemia in 20–25% of gout patients. In the absence of significant renal impairment such patients are hyperexcretors of uric acid. Specific enzyme defects resulting in an increase in de novo purine synthesis should be suspected:

1. in the absence of disorders resulting in increased turnover of purines (Table 15.15);
2. if gout develops at an unusually early age;
3. if there is a family history of gout commencing at an early age;
4. if uric acid lithiasis is the first presenting feature.

Deficiency of hypoxanthine-guanine-phosphoribosyl transferase (HGPRT). The Lesch-Nyhan syndrome is a rare X-linked recessive inborn error of metabolism in which gout and severe over-production of uric acid are associated with choreoathetosis, spasticity, a variable degree of mental deficiency and compulsive self-mutilation. The enzyme defect can be detected in red cell lysates; female carriers can be identified from skin fibroblast cultures or hair root analysis and pre-natal detection can be undertaken using amniotic fluid cells. The elucidation of the mechanism whereby this deficit in the activity of purine salvage enzyme leads to primary purine overproduction has been a key to the understanding of purine metabolism and the development of allopurinol for the treatment and prevention of gout.

Phosphoribosyl pryrophosphate (PRPP) synthetase overactivity. Severe gouty arthritis and uric acid lithiasis is seen from an early age in families with inborn errors of metabolism resulting in increased activity in this enzyme. The defect can be detected in red cell lysates.

Glucose-6-phosphatase deficiency. Children with glycogen storage disease Type I (von Gierke's disease) who survive to adult life develop severe gout and hyperuricaemia as a consequence of impaired uric acid excretion secondary to lactic acidosis and also of

Table 15.15   Factors predisposing to hyperuricaemia and gout

Diminished renal excretion of uric acid		Increased production of uric acid
Renal failure	Lactic acidosis	*Increased turnover of purines*
Drugs	Alcohol	Myeloproliferative disorders, e.g.
Diuretics	Exercise	polycythaemia vera
Pyrazinamide	Starvation	Lymphoproliferative disorders, e.g.
Low doses aspirin	Vomiting	chronic lymphatic leukaemia
Lead poisoning	Toxaemia of pregnancy	Psoriasis—severe, exfoliative
Hyperparathyroidism	Type 1 glycogen storage disease	*Increased purine synthesis de novo*
Myxoedema	Unidentified	HGPRT deficiency
Down's syndrome	inherited defect	PRPP synthetase overactivity
		Glucose-6-phosphatase deficiency
		Idiopathic

increased purine synthesis de novo. The enzyme defect can be detected only in the liver, kidney or intestine.

Idiopathic. The enzyme defect(s) responsible for most cases of gout with increased synthesis of purine de novo remain to be discovered.

Clinical features

Acute gout

The metatarso-phalangeal joint of a great toe is the site of the first attack of acute gouty arthritis in 70% of patients; the ankle, the knee, the small joints of the feet and hands, the wrist and elbow follow in decreasing order of frequency. The onset may be insidious or explosively sudden, often waking the patient from sleep. The affected joint is hot, red and swollen with shiny overlying skin and dilated veins; it is excruciatingly painful and tender. Very acute attacks may be accompanied by fever, leucocytosis and a raised ESR and are occasionally preceded by prodromal symptoms such as anorexia, nausea or a change in mood. If untreated, the attack lasts for days or weeks but it eventually subsides spontaneously. Resolution of the acute attack may be accompanied by local pruritis and desquamation.

Some patients have only a single attack, or suffer another only after an interval of many months or years. More often there is a tendency to have recurrent attacks. These increase in frequency and duration so that eventually one attack may merge into another and the patient remains in a prolonged state of subacute gout. Acute attacks are occasionally polyarticular and tenosynovitis, bursitis or cellulitis may be the presenting feature.

Acute attacks may be precipitated by sudden rises in serum urate following dietary excess, alcohol, severe dietary restriction or diuretic drugs or by sudden falls following initiation of therapy with allopurinol or uricosuric drugs. Acute attacks may also be provoked by trauma, unusual physical exercise, surgery or severe systemic illness.

Chronic gout

First attacks of gouty arthritis are seldom associated with residual disability but recurrent acute attacks are followed by progressive cartilage and bone erosion in association with deposition of tophi and secondary degenerative changes. Severe functional impairment and gross joint deformities may occur in chronic tophaceous gout. Tophi are frequently found in the cartilage of the ear, bursae and tendon sheaths.

Urate urolithiasis

This occurs in about 10% of patients with gout attending British hospital clinics. The incidence is much higher in hot climates. The formation of urate calculi is also favoured by:

1. hyperuricosuria
2. purine overproduction
3. excessive purine ingestion
4. uricosuric drugs and defects in tubular reabsorption of uric acid and
5. low urine pH, e.g. in chronic diarrhoeal diseases or following ileostomy.

Chronic urate nephropathy

This results from a combination of renal tubular obstruction, uric acid calculi, hypertension, glomerulosclerosis and secondary pyelonephritis. It is rare in the absence of well-established chronic gouty arthritis.

Other manifestations

Gout and hyperuricaemia are frequently associated with obesity, type IV hyperlipoproteinaemia, diabetes mellitus, hypertension and ischaemic heart disease. Hyperuricaemia itself does not, however, appear to be a risk factor for vascular disease or diabetes mellitus.

Diagnosis

The serum urate level is usually raised but it is important to appreciate that this does not prove the diagnosis because asymptomatic hyperuricaemia is very common. Whenever possible synovial fluid should be aspirated and examined under polarising light (Fig. 15.15). Acute attacks of gout can occur when the serum urate level is normal. This is usually seen in patients who have received treatment with allopurinol, a uricosuric agent or NSAID with uricosuric side-effects such as azapropazone.

Joint radiographs are seldom useful in establishing

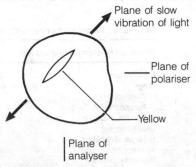

Fig. 15.15 Diagram of needle-shaped crystal of monosodium urate in polymorph from joint fluid of patient with acute gouty arthritis.

the diagnosis. Although they may show characteristic punched-out erosions associated with the soft tissue swelling of urate tophi, occasionally flecked with calcium, the diagnosis will be clinically apparent in such patients and in others the erosions may be indistinguishable from those seen in various forms of inflammatory arthritis.

Management

NSAID are the agents of choice. It is important to start treatment as early as possible, to use adequate doses and to avoid salicylates and diuretics. Patients known to have gout should keep a supply of an NSAID with which they are familiar so that an acute attack can be aborted as soon as the first symptoms are noticed. Indomethacin (50 mg) 6-hourly, azapropazone (600 mg 8-hourly) or naproxen (250 mg t.i.d.) are given until the acute attack subsides. Treatment is then continued with lower doses for 7–10 days. Colchicine is highly effective but causes vomiting and diarrhoea in many patients in the doses that need to be used (1 mg stat followed by 0.5 mg 2-hourly).

Prevention

Prolonged administration of drugs which lower the serum urate level should be considered following the resolution of the acute attack in patients with:

1. recurrent attacks of gouty arthritis
2. tophi or evidence of chronic gouty arthritis
3. associated renal disease
4. gout and markedly raised serum urate.

Allopurinol. This is the drug of choice for long-term prophylaxis because of its convenience and low incidence of side-effects. It lowers the serum urate by inhibiting xanthine oxidase which is responsible for the conversion of xanthine and hypoxanthine to uric acid. Treatment is commenced with 300 mg once daily together with colchicine 0.5 mg b.d. to avert the acute attacks of gouty arthritis which frequently follow initiation of hypouricaemic drug therapy. It is important not to commence treatment with allopurinol until several weeks have elapsed after the last acute attack and to continue concurrent administration of colchicine for several months. The dose of allopurinol may have to be adjusted in the range of 300–900 mg daily to bring the serum urate within the normal range. If renal function is impaired lower doses (100 mg/d) should be used.

Uricosuric agents. These can also be very effective in lowering the serum urate level, reducing the

frequency of acute attacks of gout and decreasing the size of the tophi. Probencid 0.5–1 g b.d. or sulphinpyrazone 100 mg t.d.s. are given with colchicine 0.5 mg b.d. Salicylates must be avoided as they antagonise the uricosuric effects of these drugs. Uricosuric drug therapy is contraindicated:

1. in gout in overproduction of uric acid and gross uricosuria
2. in patients with renal failure (ineffective)
3. in patients with urate urolithiasis.

Diet. There is no need for severe dietary restrictions but excessive purine intake and overindulgence in alcohol should be avoided. Gradual weight loss is encouraged in obese patients and is associated with a fall in serum urate. Severe calorie restriction must be avoided as it causes lactic acidosis and a rise in serum urate.

Surgery. This is occasionally required to deal with a large or ulcerating tophus.

Asymptomatic hyperuricaemia. This does not require prophylactic treatment in the absence of a history, family history or clinical evidence of gout. A search should be made for causes of secondary hyperuricaemia (Table 15.15, p. 795). Obese subjects should lose weight gradually and blood pressure and renal function are monitored annually.

CHONDROCALCINOSIS AND PSEUDO-GOUT
(Pyrophosphate arthropathy: calcium pyrophosphate dihydrate (CPPD) deposition)

In this variety of crystal deposition disorder, calcium pyrophosphate dihydrate (CPPD) crystals are deposited in fibrous and articular cartilage where they are associated with degenerative changes. Shedding of crystals into the joint space provokes an acute attack of synovitis – 'pseudo-gout'. Autopsy and radiological surveys indicate that chondrocalcinosis is a common age-related finding often unassociated with symptoms of articular disease. The menisci and articular cartilage of the knee are the commonest sites.

Aetiology

Chondrocalcinosis and pseudo-gout are clearly not a single disease. The majority of cases are sporadic and no underlying cause can be found. Genetic factors are important in some families. A variety of metabolic disorders clearly predispose to chondrocalcinosis and these are listed in the information box (p. 798).

CHONDROCALCINOSIS (PYROPHOSPHATE ARTHROPATHY)

- Familial
- Sporadic
- Metabolic
  Hyperparathyroidism
  Haemochromatosis
  Hypothyroidism
  Hypomagnesaemia
  Hypophosphatasia
  Gout

No common determinant, comparable to the hyper-uricaemia of gout has been identified but pyrophosphate concentrations are increased in synovial fluids. This, coupled with the association with hypophosphatasias, has suggested that the disease may be a consequence of defective pyrophosphatase activity.

Clinical features

Pyrophosphate arthropathy can mimic many other conditions. Six clinical patterns of disease are described in the information box below.

Diagnosis

Radiographs show CPPD in articular cartilage, the

CHONDROCALCINOSIS — PATTERNS OF CLINICAL DISEASE

Type A: Pseudo-gout
As with gout the affected joint becomes suddenly painful, warm, swollen and tender. The knee is the site of more than half of all attacks, the duration of which can vary from a few days to four weeks. Subacute or 'petit' attacks are not uncommon and there may be polyarticular clustering of acute attacks. Men are affected more frequently than women.

Type B: Pseudo-rheumatoid arthritis
In a few patients there is a subacute inflammatory polyarthritis which may last for several months.

Type C: Pseudo-osteoarthritis with superimposed acute attacks.

Type D: Pseudo-osteoarthritis without acute attacks.
Types C and D account for nearly half the patients. Women are more frequently affected. Prominent involvement of the wrists and MCP joints clearly distinguishes pseudo osteoarthritic chondrocalcinosis from primary generalised osteoarthrosis.

Type E: Asymptomatic
This is the most common.

Type F: Pseudo-neuropathic
Severe destructive changes resembling those of Charcot joints can occur in the knee and shoulder in the absence of any neurological defect.

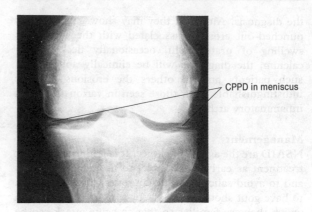

Fig. 15.16   Chondrocalcinosis in calcium pyrophosphate deposition disease.

menisci of the knees, (Fig. 15.16) the labrum of the acetabulum and glenoid cavity, the triangular cartilage of the wrist and the symphysis pubis. Examination of synovial fluid under polarising light microscopy allows CPPD crystals to be distinguished from monosodium urate crystals. X-ray diffraction techniques differentiate CPPD from calcium phosphate and calcium hydroxyapatite seen in synovial fluid in degenerative joint disease.

Management

Joint aspiration and intra-articular injection of corticosteroids are the most effective means for treating acute attacks of pseudo-gout. Colchicine and NSAID are less effective than in classical gout.

OSTEOARTHROSIS

Osteoarthrosis (OA, osteoarthritis, arthrosis or degenerative joint disease) is not a single disease. Rather it is the end-result of a variety of patterns of joint failure. To a greater or lesser extent it is always characterised by both degeneration of articular cartilage and simultaneous proliferation of new bone, cartilage and connective tissue. The proliferative response results in some degree of remodelling of the joint contour. Inflammatory changes in the synovium are usually minor and secondary.

Epidemiology

Radiological and autopsy surveys show a steady rise in degenerative changes in joints from the age of 30. By the age of 65, 80% of people have radiographic evidence of osteoarthrosis although only 25% may have symptoms. Males and females are both affected but OA is more generalised and more severe in older women. Geographical surveys show differences in both the prevalence of OA and the pattern of joint involvement. OA of the hips is much more frequent in Caucasians than in Blacks or Chinese. Cold, damp climates are associated with more symptoms but not with greater radiological prevalence.

Aetiology and pathogenesis

OA is classified as primary if the aetiology is unknown and secondary when degenerative joint changes occur in response to a recognisable local or systemic factor. The causes of secondary osteoarthrosis are listed in the information box below. Developmental abnormalities are believed to be of major importance in the aetiology of OA of the hip in the vast majority of cases. Abnormal surface contacts and weight-bearing alignments lead to increased local mechanical stress and wear. Post-traumatic malalignment and incongruity of joints are well established as important predisposing causes of premature OA.

CAUSES OF SECONDARY OSTEOARTHROSIS

Developmental
Perthes' disease
Slipped capital
femoral epiphysis
Epiphysiolysis
Hip dysplasia
Epiphysial dysplasias
Intra-articular
acetabular labrum

Traumatic
Intra-articular fracture
Meninsectomy
Occupational, e.g. elbows
of pneumatic drill workers
Hypermobility,
e.g. Ehlers-Danlos syndrome
Long leg arthropathy

Metabolic
Alkaptonuria (ochronosis)
Haemochromatosis
Wilson's disease
Chondrocalcinosis

Endocrine
Acromegaly

Inflammatory
Rheumatoid arthritis
Gout
Septic arthritis
Haemophilia

Aseptic necrosis
Corticosteroids
Sickle-cell disease
Caisson sickness
SLE and other
collagenoses

Neuropathic
Tabes dorsalis
Syringomyelia
Diabetes mellitus
Peripheral nerve lesions

Miscellaneous
Paget's disease
Gaucher's disease

Metabolic diseases lead to degeneration of cartilage by very different mechanisms. In alkaptonuria (ochronosis) the genetically determined defect of homogentisic acid oxidase results in the accumulation of a pigmented polymer that binds to collagen rendering it brittle and prone to mechanical degradation. There may be other inborn errors of metabolism where unknown colourless metabolites may induce changes in the biochemical composition of cartilagenous matrix in a similar way and so predispose to OA. Crystal deposition of calcium pyrophosphate dihydrate or hydroxyapatite may alter the properties of cartilage matrix directly and low-grade crystal inflammation may play a part in pathogenesis.

It is uncertain whether the degenerative joint disease seen in acromegaly is a consequence of joint incongruity following cartilage overgrowth or whether the endocrine disturbance results in a mechanically defective matrix. Paget's disease, Gaucher's disease and the various diseases associated with aseptic necrosis result in pathological changes in subchondral bone with consequent altered stresses on the overlying articular cartilage.

Current concepts of the pathogenesis of OA are based on the assumption that whatever the provoking cause, the final pathway of changes in articular cartilage will be identical. Two mechanical hypotheses merit consideration. The first suggests that the initiating event is fatigue fracture of the collagen fibre network which is followed by increased hydration of the articular cartilage with unravelling of the proteoglycans and loss of proteoglycans into the synovial fluid. There is some tentative supportive evidence of augmented neutral protease and collagenolytic activity but collagen may also be lost simply as a result of mechanical attrition.

The alternative hypothesis suggests that the initial lesions are microfractures of the subchondral bone following repetitive loading. Healing of the microfracture leads to significant loss of resilience of the subchondral bone which in turn creates a shear stress gradient in the adjacent articular cartilage. As the process evolves, the cartilage surface becomes fibrillated and deep clefts appear with reduplication and proliferation of chondrocytes within them. Simultaneous proliferative changes commence at the joint margins with formation of osteophytes. Eventually articular cartilage is lost altogether in areas of maximum mechanical stress and the underlying bone becomes hardened and eburnated. Cysts may form but bony alkylosis does not occur.

Clinical features

The joints most frequently involved are those of the spine, hips and knees. The disease is confined to one or only a few joints in the majority of patients. The symptoms are gradual in onset. Pain is at first intermittent and aching and is provoked by the use of the joint and relieved by rest. As the disease progresses, movement in the affected joint becomes increasingly limited, initially as a result of pain and muscular spasm, but later because of capsular fibrosis, osteophyte formation and remodelling of bone. There may be repeated effusions into joints especially after minor twists or injuries. Crepitus may be felt or even heard. Associated muscle wasting is an important factor in the progress of the disease, as in the absence of normal muscular control the joint becomes more prone to injury. Pain arises from trabecular microfractures, traumatic lesions in the capsule and periarticular tissues, and a low grade synovitis. Nocturnal aching may be attributable to hyperaemia of the subchondral bone.

Nodal osteoarthrosis

This is a clinically distinct form of primary generalised OA which occurs predominantly in middle-aged women. Characteristically it affects the terminal interphalangeal (IP) joints of the fingers with the development of gelatinous cysts or bony outgrowths on the dorsal aspect of these joints (Heberden's nodes). The onset is sometimes acute with considerable pain, swelling and inflammation. Although these lesions may be associated with a good deal of deformity they seldom cause disability. Similar lesions may affect the proximal IP joints and the disorder also frequently involves the carpometacarpal joints of the thumbs, the spinal apophyseal joints, the hips and the knees. A strong family history of Heberden's nodes is usual in such patients and though the existence of multigeneration families with the disorder appears to suggest a single autosomal dominant gene, careful family studies reveal polygenic inheritance in both nodal and non-nodal primary generalised osteoarthrosis. Patients with nodal primary generalised osteoarthrosis are also more susceptible to secondary OA, again emphasising the multifactorial aetiology of this disorder.

Diagnosis

The blood count and ESR are characteristically normal. Synovial fluid is viscous and has a low cell count; apatite crystals can rarely be detected. Radiographs show loss of joint space and formation of marginal osteophytes. Subchondral bone sclerosis, bony remodelling and cyst formation are seen in more advanced disease (Fig. 15.17).

Management

Although the pathological changes of osteoarthrosis are irreversible much can be done to alleviate symptoms particularly in the early stages. Periods of rest and avoidance of undue trauma and physical stress to

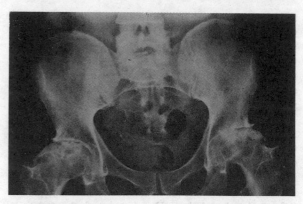

Fig. 15.17   Osteoarthritis showing joint space narrowing and new bone (osteophyte) formation. The changes are most obvious in the hip joint on the right.

affected joints are essential. This may involve such measures as the fitting of rubber heels to reduce jarring and minimise the risk of slipping, the provision of built-up shoes to equalise leg lengths, weight loss in obese patients with OA of the knee or hip and the provision of a suitable walking stick. Occasionally patients are advised to change their occupation, transfer to lighter work or give up unduly strenuous hobbies.

NSAID can be used to relieve pain and stiffness but are often disappointingly ineffective in osteoarthrosis.

Occasional intra-articular or periarticular corticosteroid injections can be helpful especially in the knee. Hydrotherapy may be useful for patients with OA of the hip associated with pain and muscle spasm. Hip or knee arthroplasty may be necessary in patients with advanced disease. Arthrodesis is occasionally considered if the knee is the only joint involved.

MISCELLANEOUS LESIONS OF CONNECTIVE TISSUE

General aspects

Musculo-skeletal aches and pains are extremely common and become more frequent with increasing age. More than one-third of all 'rheumatic' complaints cannot be attributed to defined diseases of the spine, peripheral joints or connective tissues. Many are trivial, self-limiting and cause little disability. Others can be more troublesome. The neck, shoulder girdle, back and gluteal regions are the common sites for many of these complaints. Muscular spasm of reflex origin is a prominent feature and must be differentiated from limitation of movement due to structural damage. Absence of signs of systemic illness and a normal ESR will help to distinguish these *regional rheumatic disorders* from the inflammatory connective tissue diseases.

Certain factors may be of importance in precipitating attacks in susceptible individuals. Exposure to cold and damp has always been suspected as a cause of nonarticular 'rheumatic' complaints. Unaccustomed physical effort, undue fatigue, minor injuries and poor posture have also been incriminated. Any reduction in muscular efficiency will render an individual more prone to sprains of tendons, ligaments and extra-articular soft tissue structures. Loss of resilience and elasticity of the intervertebral discs can occur long before radiological evidence of disc degeneration becomes apparent and the interfacetal joints of the spine may be more exposed to strains and sprains.

Pain arising from deep structures is poorly located and referred diffusely to the overlying skin. Pain may be referred from the cervical intervertebral joints to the occipital region, shoulder girdle and arm. 'Lumbago' and 'sciatic pain' without signs of root pressure can be caused by minor disc injury. More often they appear to be associated with acute or chronic 'sprain syndromes'. Although poor posture, flabby muscles and obesity may be predisposing causes, occupational factors may be of great importance. Absence from work due to 'rheumatic' complaints is much higher among miners, dockers and foundry workers than it is among clerks or employees in light industry. Up to 10% of the population may have abnormally lax joints and ligaments without the stigmata of inherited connective tissue disorders such as the Marfan or Ehlers-Danlos syndromes. Such persons are particularly prone to recurrent sprains, dislocations and arthralgia — the *'hypermobility syndrome'*.

Diffuse muscular pain and stiffness is common in certain infections, particularly of viral origin, such as influenza, rubella and measles. Localised pain occurs in epidemic myalgia (Bornholm disease), while myalgic encephalitis (chronic fatigue syndrome) is characterised by relapsing episodes of prolonged fatigue following physical or mental effort. Many anxious and depressed people complain of aches and pains, particularly in the region of the neck, shoulders or lower back.

Specific lesions

Shoulder pain. This is frequently a consequence of extra-articular traumatic, degenerative or inflammatory lesions of the capsule or 'rotator cuff' of tendons.

Supraspinatus tendinitis. This is characterised by a 'painful arc' on arm abduction which can be abolished by external rotation.

Clinical features
There is localised tenderness over the greater tuberosity of the humerus and a radiograph may show calcification in the supraspinatus tendon. Rupture of calcific material into the subacromial bursa occasionally results in acutely painful 'gout-like' attacks of inflammatory *subcromial bursitis*.

Diagnosis
Fluid aspirated from the bursa beneath the acromion contains crystals of calcium hydroxyapatite.

Management
Local infection of hydrocortisone is used to give symptomatic relief.

Bicipital tendinitis. This can be recognised by pain and tenderness over the bicipital groove aggravated by resisted flexion of the elbow.

Capsulitis (Frozen shoulder). In this common and disabling condition there is severe spontaneous shoulder pain associated initially with capsular tenderness and painful restriction of all shoulder movements and later with painless restriction of movements alone. A frozen shoulder may be a late consequence of a rotator cuff lesion and sometimes follows myocardial infarction, hemiplegia, herpes zoster, breast or thoracic surgery.

Management
Treatment is with analgesics and local corticosteroid injection in the early phase and mobilising exercises after the pain has resolved.

Prognosis
The natural history is for slow but complete recovery, the complete cycle sometimes taking as long as two years.

Shoulder-hand syndrome. In the shoulder-hand syndrome restricted shoulder movements are associated with a painful swollen hand.

Clinical features
The condition is characterised by burning pain, vasomotor changes and severe limitation of movements of the hand. A radiograph of the hand shows patchy osteoporosis after some weeks or months. It may be a sequel to the same disorders that precede a frozen shoulder but epilepsy, barbiturates and antituberculous drugs can also be predisposing factors. Not

infrequently these patients have an hysterical personality.

Management

Treatment is aimed at mobilising the affected limb. Analgesics, a short course of systemic corticosteroids, sympathetic nerve block and physiotherapy each have their advocates in this difficult situation. The prognosis for complete recovery is less certain than in frozen shoulder.

'Tennis elbow'. This appears to follow partial tears of the origin of the extensor muscles at the lateral epicondyle. Local tenderness and pain on active wrist extension are characteristic.

'Golfer's elbow'. This results from similar lesions in the origin of the common flexor tendon at the medial condyle. Local corticosteroid injections relieve both conditions.

DISEASES OF BONE

PHYSIOLOGY

Bone is a specialised form of metabolically active, mineralised connective tissue. It consists of cells of monocyte-macrophage origin (bone forming osteoblasts, bone-resorbing osteoclasts, resting osteocytes) and an organic matrix of type I collagen, proteoglycan and some bone specific glycoproteins. The skeleton contains more than 99% of the body calcium in the form of a crystalline calcium phosphate complex (hydroxyapatite). The tubular mid-sections of long bones (diaphyses), which make up 80% of the skeletal mass, are composed of circumferential lamellae of compact, cortical bone consisting of longitudinally orientated osteons surrounding central Haversian canals which carry the capillaries. Extracellular fluid reaches the bone osteocytes by a radial system of canaliculi and there are lateral vascular communications with the periosteal vessels through Volkmann's canals. The distal ends of the long bones (metaphyses), the vertebrae and the flat bones are composed of more loosely packed cancellous bone. Although it accounts for only 20% of the skeletal mass, the trabecular surface area of this cancellous bone is as large as that of compact bone, rendering it relatively more susceptible to metabolic diseases. It is important to realise that bone is bounded by a number of distinct cellular surfaces — the endosteal, periosteal, Haversian and trabecular envelopes.

The size and shape of bones changes rapidly in the growing phase of infancy as part of the modelling process. The marrow cavity and outer cortex expand due to endosteal resorption and peristeal accretion of bone and bone turnover may be as high as 200% per annum. Following skeletal maturity this is reduced to less than 5% but the rate of endosteal resorption is reduced less than that of periosteal accretion. Thus while the outer diameter of normal older bones is greater than that of younger, the cortex is progressively thinned with advancing years. Deformities and short stature may be a consequence of diseases interfering with the modelling process during the growing period. Examples include metabolic diseases such as rickets, inflammatory diseases such as polyarticular juvenile chronic arthritis, and bone dysplasias such as osteopetrosis.

Modern methods of bone histomorphometry, in which iliac biopsies are taken following double tetracycline labelling, have revealed a second form of bone turnover or remodelling. This occurs throughout life and accounts for more than 95% of turnover in the mature skeleton. Remodelling occurs in 'programmed packages'; the sequence of cellular events is invariably one of activation followed by a period of osteoclastic resorption and then a period of osteoblastic formation along the freshly resorbed trabecular surface. The whole

---

CLASSIFICATION OF DISEASES OF BONE

Infections

Metabolic and endocrine diseases:
Rickets and osteomalacia
Nutritional deficiency, e.g. of calcium
Osteoporosis
Post menopausal
    Associated with endocrine disease, e.g. in
    hypogonadism, Cushing's syndrome and hypopituitarism
    Iatrogenic, e.g. corticosteroid therapy
    Chronic wasting diseases, e.g. rheumatoid arthritis or
    malignancy
    Hereditary diseases, e.g. osteogenesis imperfecta
    Idiopathic juvenile osteoporosis
Hyperparathyroidism

Paget's disease

Disorders of collagen
e.g. Marfan's syndrome

Mucopolysaccharidoses
e.g. Hurler syndrome and Hunter's syndrome

Skeletal dysplasias

Neoplastic disease
Primary, benign or malignant
Secondary malignant

sequence is completed in 4–6 months in healthy adults. Trauma and hyperthyroidism are two of the numerous factors that can activate the remodelling process, while oestrogens suppress it. Fluoride uncouples the remodelling sequence and stimulates osteoblastic activity.

Increased turnover of bone, whatever the cause, is associated with a rise in the plasma alkaline phosphatase and an increase in the urinary excretion of hydroxyproline and the bone specific glycoprotein, osteocalcin.

A classification of bone disease is given in the information box (p. 802).

INFECTIONS

OSTEOMYELITIS

This is most commonly encountered in children under the age of 12.

Clinical features
The onset is abrupt with fever, malaise and severe pain at the site of bone infection. When this is close to a joint there may be a 'sympathetic' effusion and diagnostic confusion with septic arthritis. Isotope scanning and careful delineation of the site of bone tenderness can be helpful in establishing the correct diagnosis but radiographic changes do not occur for some days or weeks.

Staphylococci are the most frequent organisms responsible and in about half the cases haematogenous spread has occurred from a boil or superficial infection. Hypogammaglobulinaemia, malnutrition or debilitating illness may all be predisposing factors. Salmonella can also cause osteomyelitis and this infection is a common complication of sickle-cell anaemia.

Management
An antibiotic, e.g. sodium fusidate must be commenced after taking blood for culture as soon as the diagnosis is suspected, and continued in adequate doses for long enough to eliminate the infection. Delay in starting treatment or inadequate therapy may result in chronic indolent bone infection (Brodie's abscess) with sequestrum formation. Surgical exploration and decompression are required if there is not an immediate response to antibiotics.

Tuberculous osteomyelitis
This has become much less common in Britain since the elimination of bovine tuberculosis but there is evidence of a recent increase in the elderly population and immigrant communities. The spine is affected in 50% of patients.

Clinical features
Typically the infection starts at the margins of vertebral bodies with subsequent invasion of the disc space. Destruction of bone leads to angular kyphosis. A paravertebral 'cold' abscess may form and track to the thigh, chest wall or neck. The hip, knee, ankle or wrist joint may be affected by spread from adjacent bone. Tuberculous dactylitis and sacroiliitis are unusual but characteristic lesions.

Management
The treatment of tuberculosis is described on pages 367–369.

RICKETS AND OSTEOMALACIA

Rickets and osteomalacia are metabolic bone diseases characterised by increased amounts of unmineralised osteoid and a decrease in the rate of bone formation. Vitamin D metabolism is depicted in Fig. 15.18. The

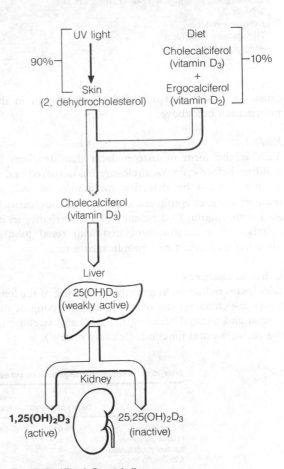

Fig. 15.18 Vitamin D metabolism.

CAUSES OF RICKETS AND OSTEOMALACIA

Vitamin D deficiency
Dietary deficiency
Lack of synthesis in skin

Decreased absorption
  Coeliac disease
  Hepatobiliary disorders
  Pancreatic disease
  Gastric and intestinal surgery

Defective metabolism
  Drugs (anticonvulsants, sedatives, rifampicin)
  Chronic renal failure
    Renal osteodystrophy
    Dialysis bone disease
  Vitamin D dependent rickets

Hypophosphataemia with normal vitamin D
Familial hypophosphataemic rickets
Inherited and acquired renal tubular defects (e.g.
Fanconi syndrome, cadmium poisoning, multiple
myelomatosis)

*Osteomalacia with normal calcium phosphate and
vitamin D*
Hypophosphatasia
Fibrogenesis imperfecta
Aluminium bone disease

---

causes of rickets and osteomalacia are shown in the information box above.

Rickets

This is the form of osteomalacia that develops in children before epiphyseal closure has occurred and it is characterised by defective maturation as well as mineralisation of epiphyseal cartilage. Although associated with vitamin D deficiency or a disturbance in its metabolism it is also associated with renal tubular disorders and inherited hypophosphataemia.

Clinical features

Bone pain, reduction in growth and bowing of the long bones are characteristic of rickets with bossing of the frontal and parietal bones of the skull and swelling of the costochondral junctions ('rickety rosary').

Diagnosis

X-rays show widening of the growth plate with a cupped and ragged metaphysis. Biochemical findings vary according to aetiology (Table 15.16).

Osteomalacia

This is characterised by bone pain, tenderness, skeletal deformity and a proximal myopathy which often results in a waddling gait and difficulty in rising from low seats.

X-rays. These show typical pseudo-fractures (Looser's zones) in the ribs, long bones, pelvis and scapuli in advanced cases.

Biochemical changes. Characteristic changes include a low plasma calcium, phosphate, 25,hydroxyvitamin D and urine calcium with an increase in alkaline phosphatase, but biochemical findings vary with the underlying aetiology (Table 15.16).

Bone biopsy. This shows wide uncalcified osteoid seams.

Management

Most patients with rickets or osteomalacia respond rapidly to vitamin D but the dose and metabolite to be used are determined by the underlying cause. Lack of response to microgram doses should suggest a cause other than simple dietary deficiency and vitamin D resistant types require 10–200 000 IU daily. 1 alpha hydroxyvitamin D must be used in patients with chronic renal failure.

OSTEOPOROSIS

Osteoporosis is defined as a decrease in the absolute amount of bone leading to fractures following minimal trauma. It is by far the commonest form of metabolic bone disease and a major public health problem.

Epidemiology

Bone mass is determined by genetic and environmental factors and reaches a peak before the age of 40 years.

Table 15.16 Biochemical findings in rickets and osteomalacia

	Dietary deficiency	Vitamin D resistant rickets	Renal phosphate depletion	Renal osteodystrophy
Plasma calcium	↓	N	N	↓
Plasma phosphate	↓	↓	↓	↑
Alkaline phosphatase	↑	↑	↑	↑
1,25(OH)$_2$D3	↓	N	↑	↓

Age-related bone loss is greatly accelerated in women after the menopause and women lose approximately 30% of their cortical bone and 50% of their trabecular bone during their lifetime. Colles fractures, femoral neck fractures and vertebral fractures are all related to osteoporosis. 25% of women over the age of 60 suffer vertebral fractures and 30% hip fractures. It has been calculated that four-fifths of the 37 500 femoral neck fractures occurring annually in England and Wales are at least in part attributable to osteoporosis. With a mean hospital stay of 40 days and mortality of 16% the annual cost of these fractures has been estimated at £165 million. There are about a quarter of a million femoral neck fractures in the United States and the cost of treating osteoporosis-related problems is 6 billion dollars annually. Lifetime oestrogen exposure is an important determinant of bone mass but a number of risk factors for osteoporosis have been identified (Table 15.17).

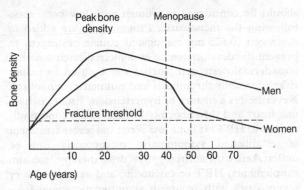

Fig. 15.19   Changes in bone mass with age in men and women. Postmenstrual osteoporosis with increased fracture risk follows reduction in bone mass below fracture threshold in postmenopausal women with low initial peak bone mass.

Table 15.17   Risk factors for osteoporosis

Endogenous	Exogenous
Female	Low calcium intake
Asian/Caucasian	Reduced physical activity
Small stature	Cigarette smoking
Thin physique	Alcohol abuse
Family history	Aluminium antacids
Nulliparity	Surgical menopause
Early menopause	Steroid therapy
Advanced age	

Clinical features

Two types of involutional osteoporosis can be distinguished (Table 15.18). Type I is associated with forearm fractures, back pain and crush vertebral fractures in the post-menopausal period, while Type II which is age related occurs later and is associated with progressive loss of height, thoracic kyphosis and wedge fractures ('Dowager's hump') and hip fractures. Factors which predispose to falls in the elderly are

obviously also important but fractures become much more likely when bone mass has fallen below a notional fracture threshold (Fig. 15.19). Other diseases predispose to osteoporosis by inhibiting bone formation or accelerating the rate of bone loss (Table 15.17).

Diagnosis

Plasma biochemical measurements are usually normal but the alkaline phosphatase may be raised following a recent fracture and the calcium and hydroxyproline: creatinine ratio in the urine is increased after the menopause due to accelerated bone resorption. X-rays show decreases in bone density and a more prominent trabecular pattern as well as the characterisitic wedge and crush fractures in the spine but it has been calculated that at least 40% of bone mineral must be lost before changes are detectable on plain X-ray films. The recent development of single and dual photon absorptiometry and quantitative digital radiography allows measurement of bone mineral at forearm, hip or vertebral sites with an in-vivo precision of about 1%. Skeletal scintigraphy with bone seeking isotopes can help to reveal recent fractures and exclude other pathology. Quantitative histomorphometry on transiliac bone biopsies following tetracycline labelling is only required in difficult cases where osteomalacia and other pathology needs to be excluded.

Management

Effective treatment for established osteoporosis is difficult once bone mass has fallen below the fracture threshold so emphasis is placed on preventing osteoporosis in high-risk subjects (Table 15.17). Physical exercise, ensuring an adequate calcium intake (1500 mg daily) and avoiding cigarette and alcohol abuse are encouraged. Hormone replacement therapy (HRT)

Table 15.18   Involutional osteoporosis

	Type I Menopause related	Type II Age related
Age (years)	50–70	>70
Sex ratio (F:M)	6:1	2:1
Type bone lost	Trabecular	Trabecular/cortical
Fractures	Colles	Hip
	Crush vertebrae	Wedge vertebrae
PTH		
Calcium absorption		
Vitamin D metabolism (25OHD₃ 1,25(OH)2D₃)	Secondary decrease	Primary decrease

should be considered in women with low bone mass following the menopause. Progestogens are added to oestrogen (0.625 mg conjugated equine oestrogen) to prevent the development of endometrial carcinoma and transdermal oestrogen patches can be used to reduce risks of venous thrombosis and pulmonary embolism. Nevertheless a history of hypertension, stroke, ischaemic heart and thromboembolic disease are contraindications to HRT. If bone loss is not too severe treatment of established symptomatic osteoporosis can be undertaken with antiresorptive drug therapy (calcium supplements, HRT or calcitonin) and in selected very severe cases with recurrent symptomatic spinal fractures bone stimulating drug therapy with anabolic steroids and/or fluoride can be attempted.

PAGET'S DISEASE (OSTEITIS DEFORMANS)

This disease which is characterised by softening, enlargement and bowing of bones is uncommon before the age of 40 years but increasingly frequent thereafter. There is increased blood flow through affected bones with resorption followed by excessive osteoblastic bone formation resulting in a high rate of bone turnover, raised levels of plasma alkaline phosphatase and increased urinary excretion of hydroxyproline. This activity is reflected in abnormal isotope bone scans and radiological evidence of localised bone enlargement, altered trabecular pattern and alternating areas of rarefaction and increased density. Recent evidence suggests that Paget's disease may be associated with a paramyxovirus infection of osteoclasts.

Clinical features
Men are more commonly affected and there may be a family history of the disease. Often the condition is symptomless and detected only when radiological examination is made for some other reason. In others there is pain of a deep aching character often aggravated by weight bearing. The pelvis, femur, tibia,

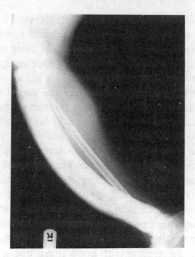

Fig. 15.20   Paget's disease of bone.

lumbar spine and skull are common sites of bone involvement. The increased vascularity may cause warmth of the affected part on palpation; rarely widespread arteriovenous shunting causes high output cardiac failure. Enlargement and deformity of bones develop when the condition is advanced. Bowing of the femur and tibia is characteristic and Paget's disease may predispose to secondary osteoarthrosis of the hip or knee (Fig. 15.20). Fractures may occur spontaneously or after minor trauma but they usually heal normally. Skull involvement may result in headache, progressive enlargement of the cranium and deafness from compression of the auditory nerves. Paraplegia can follow vertebral involvement. Osteogenic sarcoma is an uncommon late complication.

Diagnosis
The serum calcium and phosphate are usually normal with high levels of alkaline phosphatase and increased hydroxyproline excretion during phases of active disease.

Table 15.19   Osteogenesis imperfecta

| Type | Bone fragility | Clinical features | | | Inheritance |
		Blue sclerae	Dental defects	Deafness	
I	Mild late fractures	Yes	Some	Some	Autosomal dominant
II	Extreme lethal perinatal fractures	Yes	Some	—	Sporadic new mutations Autosomal recessive
III	Severe fractures Deformity	Blue at birth Not adults	Some	Some	Autosomal recessive
IV	Short stature Brittle bones	No	Some	Some	Autosomal dominant

Management

Calcitonin is used for severe bone pain not controlled by analgesics. Subcutaneous injection of 100 MRC units of salmon calcitonin 3 times weekly can be continued for 6 months and recommended if pain recurs. Mithramycin and the diphosphonate, etidronate, which reduce bone turnover, are less satisfactory alternatives, but the second generation diphosphonate amidronate (APD) will probably become the drug of choice for patients with bone pain. Confinement to bed may be followed by rapid mobilisation of calcium with hypercalcaemia, hypercalciuria and formation of renal calculi. Such patients should be given a high fluid intake and measures must be taken to lower the serum calcium if it becomes dangerously high. Pain due to secondary degenerative joint disease is treated with NSAID. Hip arthroplasty is occasionally required. Osteogenic sarcoma is treated with early surgery but has a poor prognosis.

DISORDERS OF COLLAGEN AND PROTEOGLYCAN

OSTEOGENESIS IMPERFECTA

This is a collective name for a heterogeneous group of rare inherited disorders of Type I collagen characterised by brittle bones and abnormalities of the skin, tendons, teeth and sclerae. The current classification (Table 15.19) is based on clinical features and patterns of inheritance but current research is revealing a wide range of molecular defects with mutations in the genes coding for the pro alpha 1 (1) and pro alpha 2 (1) collagen chains which do not allow easy prediction of the clinical phenotype.

THE MARFAN SYNDROME

This is another phenotypically heterogeneous dominantly inherited condition in which abnormalities of alpha 2 (1) collagen have been described. Skeletal disproportion (span greater than height) is associated with arachnodactyly, sternal depression, lens dislocation and a high arched palate. Cardiac complications can include mitral valve prolapse, aortic incompetence and dissection of the aorta.

THE EHLERS-DANLOS SYNDROME

This is the name given to a group of conditions in which genetically determined abnormalities of collagen are associated with skin laxity, hypermobility of joints and a range of more serious features including scoliosis, short stature, ocular fragility, skin bruising and visceral vascular catastrophes (Table 15.20). Biochemical defects include a deficiency of Type II collagen (ED Type III), lysyl oxidase deficiency (ED Type V), a defect in procollagen cleavage (ED Type VII), abnormal copper metabolism (ED Type IX) and a defect in fibronectin (ED Type X).

Table 15.20   The Ehlers-Danlos syndromes

| Type | Clinical features | | | | Inheritance |
	Skeletal	Skin extensibility	Bruising	Other	
I	Hypermobility Deformities	Gross	Marked	Pseudotumours	Autosomal dominant
II	Minimal	Mild	Mild	—	Autosomal dominant
III	Hypermobility	Mild	Mild	Dislocations, OA	Autosomal dominant
IV	Digital hypermobility	Thin skin	Gross	Vascular catastrophies	Autosomal dominant Autosomal recessive
V	Minimal	Mild	Mild	—	x-linked
VI	Hypermobility	Moderate	Moderate	Scoliosis, Ocular fragility	Autosomal recessive
VII	Hypermobility	Moderate	Moderate	Short stature	Autosomal dominant Autosomal recessive
VIII	Hypermobility	Mild	Mild	Periodontitis	Autosomal dominant
IX	Hypermobility	Moderate	Moderate	Bowing long bones	x-linked
X	Hypermobility	Mild	Mild	—	x-linked Autosomal dominant

HOMOCYSTINURIA

This is an inborn error of methionine metabolism in which deficiency of the enzyme cystathionine synthetase is associated with mental retardation, venous thromboses, osteoporosis and skeletal features resembling the Marfan syndrome. The diagnosis is made by finding homocystine in the urine and patients respond to treatment with pyridoxine (20–300 mg/d).

MUCOPOLYSACCHARIDOSES

These form a group of inborn errors of glycosaminoglycan metabolism in which lysosomal enzyme defects lead to abnormal substrate accummulation and a wide variety of clinical features (Table 15.21). All are associated with stiff joints and short stature except for the Morquio syndrome which is associated with hypermobility and atlantoaxial subluxation. The diagnoses are confirmed by identification of the urinary metabolites and detection of the enzyme defects in fibroblast cultures. Treatment by enzyme replacement therapy has had limited success in slowing progression in selected cases.

SKELETAL DYSPLASIAS (Table 15.22)

The skeletal dysplasias form a large and heterogeneous group of conditions which cause bone and joint deformity. Those with predominant epiphyseal involvement such as multiple epiphyseal dysplasia may be associated with premature osteoarthrosis. Those with predominant metaphyseal involvement such as achondroplasia are associated with short-limbed dwarfism. There are disorders such as osteogenesis imperfecta, idiopathic juvenile osteoporosis and the hereditary osteolyses in which decreased bone density, fractures and bone loss are prominent features and others, such as osteopetrosis and sclerosteosis where increased bone density occurs.

Skeletal abnormalities are prominent in a number of hereditary disorders of connective tissue such as the Marfan syndrome or neurofibromatosis as well as inborn errors of metabolism such as the mucolipidoses, and homocystinuria. The reader is referred to Fairbank and McKusick's books for details of all these groups of conditions.

Table 15.21   The mucopolysaccharidoses

Type	Name	Clinical features	Inheritance	Urine MPS	Enzyme deficiency
MPS-1 H	Hurler	Cloudy cornea Mental deficiency	Autosomal recessive	Dermatan/heparan sulphate	Alpha-L-iduronidase
MPS-I S	Scheie	Cloudy cornea Stiff joints	Autosomal recessive	Dermatan/heparan sulphate	Alpha-L-iduronidase
MPS-I H/S	Hurler-Scheie	Intermediate phenotype	Autosomal recessive	Dermatan/heparan sulphate	Alpha-L-iduronidase
MPS-II	Hunter	Stiff joints Mild general mental deficiency	x-linked	Dermatan/heparan sulphate	Iduronate sulphatase
MPS-III (a–d)	San Filippo (a–d)	Stiff joints CNS defects	Autosomal recessive	Heparan sulphate	a) Heparan N-sulphatase b) N-acetyl alpha D-glucosaminidase c) Acetyl-CoA alpha glucosaminidase N-acetyltransferase d) N-acetylglucosamine-6-sulphate sulphatase
MPS-IV	Morquio A & B	Cloudy cornea Aortic incompetence Hypermobile joints	Autosomal recessive	Keratan sulphate	a) Galactosamine-6-sulphate sulphatase b) Beta galactosidase
MPS VI	Maroteaux Lamy	Stiff joints Mild severe bone, cornea, heart valve changes	Autosomal recessive	Dermatan sulphate	Arylsulfatase Beta
MPS VII	Sly	Mental retardation Dysostosis Hepatosplenomegaly	Autosomal recessive	Dermatan/heparan sulphate	Beta glucuronidase
MPS VIII	DiFerrante	Short stature Dysostosis	Autosomal recessive	Keratan/heparan sulphate	Glucosamine-6-sulfate sulphatase

Table 15.22   Skeletal dysplasias

Epiphyseal	*Miscellaneous*
Multiple epiphyseal dysplasias	Neurofibromatosis
Chondrodysplasia punctata	Marfan syndrome
Dysplasia epiphysealis hemimelica	Cleido-cranio dysplasias
Hereditary arthroophthalmopathy	Nail-patella syndrome
Metaphyseal	*Increased bone density*
Achondroplasia	Osteopetrosis
Hypochondroplasia	Dysosteosclerosis
Lethal forms short limbed dwarfism	Pycnodysostosis
Chondroectodermal dysplasia	Sclerosteosis
Metaphyseal chondrodysplasias	Diaphyseal dysplasias
Hypophosphatasias	Pachydermperiostitis
Vertebral	*Anarchic bone*
Brachyolmia	Diaphyseal aclasis
	Olliers disease
	Maffucci's disease
Vertebral and Epiphyseal	Meiorheostosis
Spondyloepiphyseal dysplasias	
Vertebral and Metaphyseal	
Spondylometaphyseal dysplasia	
Vertebral, epiphyseal and metaphyseal	
Pseudochondroplasia	
Metatropic dwarfism	
Kniest disease	
Diastrophic dwarfism	
Parastremmatic dwarfism	
Dygve-Melchior-Clauson disease	

NEOPLASTIC DISEASE

Malignant neoplasms of bone can cause diffuse skeletal aches and pains that are not infrequently dismissed as being 'rheumatic'.

Metastases. Resulting from carcinoma of the bronchus, breast or prostate, these are the commonest tumours of bone. Secondary deposits from most primary tumours appear typically as osteolytic on radiological examination and are frequently associated with a rise in serum alkaline phosphatase. Only prostatic metastases are commonly osteosclerotic and associated with a rise in serum acid phosphatase. Metastatic deposits can often be localised by skeletal isotope scans before radiological changes are apparent and widespread bone metastases can occur even in the absence of symptoms. A number of malignancies are hormone dependent and useful remission can sometimes be obtained following hypophysectomy or administration of androgens to patients with metastatic breast cancer, or dienoestrol to those with prostatic metastases. Local radiotherapy and cytotoxic chemotherapy can occasionally be helpful in symptomatic management.

Multiple myeloma (p. 745). This may also present with skeletal aches and pains associated with 'punched-out' osteolytic lesions on radiological examination. Unlike metastatic carcinoma these deposits usually fail to take up bone seeking isotopes and the serum alkaline phosphatase is normal.

Primary bone tumours. These are less common. Ivory *osteomas* are benign tumours which occur most frequently in the vault of the skull and are not usually associated with symptoms. Cancellous osteomas (osteochondromas or exostoses) are slender out-growths of bone which arise from the metaphyses of long bones or from flat bones of the pelvis and saculae. They may give rise to pressure symptoms and most frequently present during adolescence. Diaphyseal aclasis (multiple exostosis) is a rarer disorder inherited as an autosomal dominant and seen in younger children.

Primary osteosarcomas. These occur most frequently in the lower end of the femur, the upper end of the tibia and the upper end of the humerus. They are tumours of young people rarely seen after the age of 20. Swelling with or without vague aching are the presenting symptoms and the bone may be tender and warm. Radiographs show a characteristic increase in radiolucency associated with bone expansion, triangular areas of new bone formation at the periosteal margin and a 'sun-ray' appearance due to new bone formation. Early blood-borne metastases to the lungs are common and the 5-year survival is less than 10% despite treatment with radiotherapy and amputation.

Fibrosarcomas. These are of two types. Endosteal fibrosarcomas arise within bones and give rise to destructive lesions as they grow out. They metastasise to both the local lymph nodes and the lungs and are associated with a poor prognosis despite treatment with radiotherapy or amputation. In contrast periosteal fibrosarcomas seldom invade bone or metastasise to distant sites. Treatment is with local excision, repeated in the event of recurrence.

Benign chondrosarcomas. These arise from cartilage within the long bones or small bones of the fingers. Multiple enchondromatosis is an unusual disorder of childhood in which multiple chondromas give rise to unsightly swellings attached to bones. Malignant change is very rare in chondromas.

Chondrosarcomas. These occur in the long bones, pelvis or scapulae of adults. Pain and swelling are the presenting features and bone radiographs show only loss of bone density associated with some speckled calcification. Amputation is the treatment of choice and the 5-year survival is better than 50%.

Ewing's tumour. This is a highly malignant bone neoplasm which affects children between the ages of 5 and 15. It probably arises from the marrow endothelium and has characteristic radiographic features. Areas of osteolyte bone destruction are surrounded by layers of periosteal new bone formation giving lesions an 'onion skin' appearance. Pain, swelling and tenderness may be associated with fever and leucocytosis so that these tumours can easily be mistaken for osteomyelitis. The 5-year survival is virtually nil despite radiotherapy and amputation.

Giant cell tumours of bone. These may be benign or malignant. They usually occur in young adults and present with pain and swelling of a long bone in the neighbourhood of a joint. Radiographs show a typically eccentric tumour with a 'soap bubble' appearance. With local excision the prognosis is relatively good even for malignant tumours.

Osteoid osteoma. This is a rare cause of severe bone pain which is characteristically worse at night and relieved by NSAID. The condition occurs between the ages of 10 and 30 in any bone except the skull. There may be warmth, swelling and tenderness on palpation and radiographs show some increase in sclerosis with a characteristic area of translucency surrounding a central nidus. Excision of the nidus cures the symptoms and these lesions do not recur.

FURTHER READING

Dieppe P A, Docherty, M, Macfarlane D G, Maddison P J 1985 Rheumatological Medicine. Churchill Livingstone, Edinburgh. Concise British textbook.

Hadler N H 1984 Medical Management of the Regional Musculoskeletal Diseases. Grune and Stratton, New York

Hughes G R V 1986 Connective Tissue Diseases, 3rd Edn. Blackwell Scientific Publications, Oxford. Concise clinical monograph on the diffuse connective tissue diseases. Includes information on clinical applications of immunological tests.

Kelley W N, Harris E D Jnr, Ruddy S, Sledge C B (eds.) 1989 Textbook of Rheumatology, 3rd Edn. Saunders, Philadelphia. Major international textbook with comprehensive basic science and clinical coverage.

Lawrence J S 1971 Rheumatism in Populations. Heinemann, London. Source book of information on epidemiology of rheumatic diseases.

Moll J H, Bird H A, Rushton A (eds.) 1986 Therapeutics in Rheumatology. Chapman Hall Medical, London.

Nordin B E 1984 Metabolic bone and stone diseases, 2nd Edn. Churchill Livingstone, Edinburgh.

Nuki G 1987 Disorders of Purine Metabolism In:

Weatherall D J, Ledingham J G G, Warrell D A (eds.) Textbook of Medicine, 2nd Edn. Oxford University Press, Oxford.

Scott J H S In: Munro J, Edwards C R W (eds.) 1990 Macleod's Clinical examination, 8th Edn. Churchilll Livingstone, Edinburgh. Gives an account of the examination of the locomotor system.

Scott J T 1986 Copeman's Textbook of the Rheumatic Diseases, 6th Edn. Churchill Livingstone, Edinburgh. Standard British textbook. Excellent and comprehensive source of information on all aspects of clinical rheumatology.

Sokoloff L 1985 Osteoarthritis. Clin. Rheum. Dis., 11: 175–449. Good reviews.

Wynne-Davis R, Fairbank T D 1976 Fairbank's atlas of general affections of the skeleton. Churchill Livingstone, Edinburgh. Concise and beautifully illustrated introduction to skeletal dysplasias and other general disorders of bone.

Zvaifler N J (ed.) 1987 Pathogenesis of chronic inflammatory arthritis. Rheum. Clinics North American, 13: 179–410. Current Reviews.

16

Diseases of the Nervous System

Although abnormal brain function which causes disorders of thought, mood or behaviour is often the province of psychiatry, there are areas of overlap where organic disease causes both physical and mental problems. A knowledge of basic anatomy and physiology of the nervous system is essential for it can be applied to clinical examination and lead to often precise localisation of the lesions causing clinical problems. Diagnosis of the nature of such lesions is however seldom possible for examination alone – few clinical signs are due only to one disease – and must be made by analysis of the history, clinical signs and results of investigation.

The history is all-important, and in some disorders (e.g. migraine) is the only method of diagnosis. The time-course of symptoms may give valuable clues (Table 16.1).

Table 16.1 Typical time-course of neurological symptoms

Disorder	Onset	Typical course
Vascular	Acute (seconds-minutes)	Recovery in hours-days
Degenerative	Slow (months-years)	Gradual worsening
Tumour	Slow (weeks-months)	Gradual worsening
Infective	Sub-acute (hours-days)	Worsening-recovering
Demyelination	Sub-acute (days-weeks)	Varying severity, site
Epilepsy	Acute (seconds)	Recurrent attacks (minutes)
Migraine	Acute (minutes)	Recurrent attacks (hours)

THE MOTOR SYSTEM

Movements are achieved by contraction and relaxation of skeletal muscles. The motor unit (Fig. 16.1) is the final common pathway through which spinal, cerebral and cerebellar control systems act to co-ordinate movement. The motor unit comprises a spinal anterior horn cell (or cranial nerve motor neurone), its motor axon and the muscle fibres it supplies. The number of muscle fibres innervated by one axon varies from 10 to 1000 or more in different muscles. The motor axons terminate in specialised end-plates on the muscle surface. Activity in the nerve releases acetyl choline at the end-plate, causing depolarisation of the fibre and activation of the contractile process. Muscle fibres may have different biochemical and contractile characteristics (Table 16.2); most muscles contain a mixture, though one type may predominate.

The activity of motor units is governed by both local spinal reflex activity and by descending pathways from the cerebrum and cerebellum. Spinal reflexes may be monosynaptic as in the stretch reflex or polysynaptic as

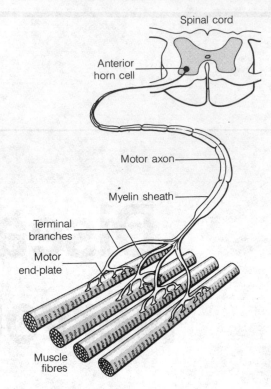

Fig. 16.1 The motor unit.

with flexor withdrawal and extensor plantar responses. The important supraspinal mechanisms involved in movement control are the pyramidal, the extrapyramidal and the cerebellar systems. These descending pathways interact via excitation and inhibition of the motor neurones and also with one another within the brain (Fig. 16.2). Signs of damage to the motor unit (lower motor neurone) are listed in the information box (p. 813).

THE PYRAMIDAL SYSTEM

The neurones of origin of the pyramidal tracts lie in the cerebral cortex just anterior to the central sulcus in the pre-central gyrus or 'motor strip'. Fibres from the pyramidal cells come close together in the internal

Table 16.2 Main types of muscle fibre

Type	Contraction	Fatigue	Enzymes	Nerve activity
I	Slow	Resistant	Oxidative	Tonic
IIa	Fast	Resistant	Glycolytic Oxidative	Phasic
IIb	Fast	Prone	Glycolytic	Phasic

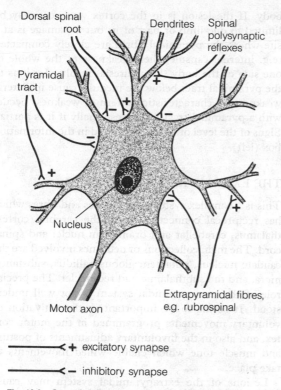

Dorsal spinal root

Dendrites

Spinal polysynaptic reflexes

Pyramidal tract

Nucleus

Motor axon

Extrapyramidal fibres, e.g. rubrospinal

−< + excitatory synapse

−< − inhibitory synapse

Fig. 16.2   Synaptic influences on the activity of motor neurones.

capsule which passes close to the thalamus and basal ganglia deep in the cerebral hemisphere. As it descends the brain stem, the pyramidal tract innervates contralateral cranial nerve motor nuclei and sends fibres to the cerebellum via the middle cerebellar peduncle. At the lower medulla, the tract decussates, most of its fibres crossing over and descending the contralateral side of the spinal cord. As is seen in Fig. 16.2 pyramidal fibres have both excitatory and inhibitory effects on the anterior horn cell. A strict topographical arrangement exists (Fig. 16.3) whereby specific areas of the precentral gyrus control movements of different parts of the contralateral side of the body. The larynx and pharynx are represented at the most inferior end of the

SIGNS OF LESIONS AFFECTING MOTOR UNITS (LOWER MOTOR NEURONE)

- Weakness or paralysis of muscles supplied by affected motor neurone or axons
- Hypotonia
- Reduced or absent tendon reflexes
- Flexor (or absent) plantar response
- Wasting and fasciculation of affected muscle

gyrus, followed by relatively large contiguous areas for movements of the face, mouth and hand. The trunk is represented by a smaller area near the midline, and the foot on the medial aspect of the hemisphere.

In addition to causing weakness and impairment of fine movements, pyramidal tract lesions also cause increased muscle tone of spastic type ('clasp knife'), hyperactivity of stretch (tendon) reflexes and release of polysynaptic spinal reflexes, of which the extensor plantar response is the best example. These changes

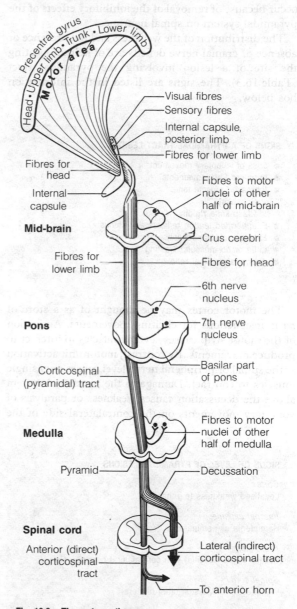

Precentral gyrus

Head · Upper limb · Trunk · Lower limb

Motor area

Visual fibres

Sensory fibres

Internal capsule, posterior limb

Fibres for lower limb

Fibres for head

Internal capsule

Mid-brain

Fibres to motor nuclei of other half of mid-brain

Crus cerebri

Fibres for lower limb

Fibres for head

6th nerve nucleus

Pons

7th nerve nucleus

Corticospinal (pyramidal) tract

Basilar part of pons

Medulla

Fibres to motor nuclei of other half of medulla

Pyramid

Decussation

Spinal cord

Anterior (direct) corticospinal tract

Lateral (indirect) corticospinal tract

To anterior horn

Fig. 16.3   The motor pathways.

Table 16.3   Distribution of weakness in pyramidal tract lesions

	Most affected	Least affected
Upper limb	Shoulder abduction Elbow extension Finger extension Finger abduction	Shoulder adduction Elbow flexion Wrist flexion Finger flexion
Lower limb	Hip flexion Knee flexion Foot dorsiflexion Foot eversion	Hip extension Knee extension Foot plantar flexion Foot inversion

occur because of removal of the inhibitory effects of the pyramidal system on spinal neurones.

The distribution of the weakness and the presence or absence of cranial nerve deficits are of help in locating the site of a lesion involving the pyramidal tract (Table 16.3). The signs are listed in the information box below.

SIGNS OF A PYRAMIDAL TRACT LESION

- Loss of voluntary movements
- Impaired fine movements
- Increased muscle tone
  - Spasticity
  - Clasp knife rigidity
- Exaggerated tendon reflexes and clonus
- Extensor plantar response
- Little or no muscular wasting
- Absent abdominal reflexes

The motor cortex may be thought of as a store of basic instructions for eliciting movements. Activation of the motor strip causes several muscles to interact to produce movements. By contrast, motor unit activation at the spinal or peripheral nerve level causes only single muscles to contract. Damage to the pyramidal system above the decussation causes weakness or paralysis of voluntary movements on the contralateral side of the body. If the lesion is in the cortex weakness may be limited to one limb or part of it; but if damage is at a site where the pyramidal fibres are closely compacted (e.g. internal capsule) then weakness of the whole of one side of the body (hemiparesis) results. Lesions to the pyramidal tract below the medulla cause ipsilateral weakness. A characteristic pattern of weakness occurs with a pyramidal tract lesion, especially if it is partial. Signs of the level of lesions are listed in the information box (left).

THE EXTRAPYRAMIDAL SYSTEM

This is a complex system of neurones and fibres which has reciprocal connections with the cerebral cortex, thalamus, cerebellar and brain-stem nuclei and spinal cord. The main collections of neurones involved are the caudate nucleus, putamen, globus pallidus, substantia nigra, and the subthalamic and red nuclei. The precise role of the extrapyramidal system is not well understood. It seems to be important in the activation of voluntary movements programmed in the motor cortex, and also in the involuntary adjustments of posture and muscle tone which enable willed movements to take place.

Lesions of the extrapyramidal system may cause various problems depending on their site (Table 16.4.).

Table 16.4   Clinical features of extrapyramidal lesions

Signs	Usual site of lesion
Resting tremor	Substantia nigra, red nucleus
Muscular rigidity	Substantia nigra, putamen
Hypokinesis	Substantia nigra, putamen, globus pallidus
Chorea	Caudate nucleus
Hemiballismus	Subthalamic nucleus
Dystonia, athetosis	Putamen

Slowness in initiating movements (hypokinesis) and difficulty with fine tasks are common, but muscular weakness is absent. Tendon reflexes are usually normal and plantar responses are flexor. Muscular tone may be either decreased (as in chorea) or increased in either a smooth fashion ('lead pipe') or have a phasic component as in the cog-wheel rigidity of parkinsonism.

THE CEREBELLUM

The cerebellum is concerned with the control of voluntary movements and the maintenance of posture and balance. It is closely connected to the vestibular system, and receives further proprioceptive input from

---

SIGNS OF LEVEL OF PYRAMIDAL LESIONS

Cortex
Localised weakness (e.g. hand)

Internal capsule
Hemiplegia or hemiparesis

Brain stem
Cranial nerve deficit(s) with contralateral hemiparesis

Spinal cord
Weakness below lesion often bilateral

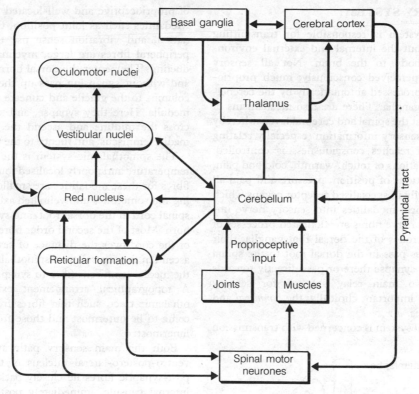

Fig. 16.4   Main connections of the cerebellum.

the spinocerebellar tracts of the spinal cord which send fibres through the inferior cerebellar peduncle. Information about cortical motor instructions is relayed from the pyramidal tracts via the middle cerebellar peduncle to the cerebellum. The chief outputs are through the superior cerebellar peduncle to the ventrolateral thalamus and thence to the cerebral cortex, and also to the spinal motor neurones via the reticular formation, red nucleus and the vestibular nuclei. The midline (vermis) and the anterior lobe are concerned chiefly with maintenance and posture and balance, while the posterolateral lobes are responsible for co-ordination of the limbs. (Fig. 16.4).

The cerebellum may be seen as a feedback computer which compares the intended actions of the motor cortex with the resultant movements of the body, and makes adjustments to the impulses relayed to the spinal motor neurones in order to achieve smooth control of movement and balance. The lateral parts of the cerebellum interconnect with the contralateral thalamus and cerebral cortex, thus controlling movements of the ipsilateral limbs. Clinical features of cerebellar lesions are listed in the information box (right).

CLINICAL FEATURES OF CEREBELLAR LESIONS

Inco-ordination of ipsilateral limbs
Past pointing (dysmetria)
Intension tremor
Decomposition of movements
Impaired alternating movements

Loss of balance
Ataxic, broad based gait
Leaning towards side of lesion

Dysarthria
Slurred indistinct speech
Loss of normal rhythm

Nystagmus
Phasic usually horizontal nystagmus
Maximal on looking to side of lesion

Hypotonia of limbs

Decreased tendon reflexes

Head tremor

Head tilt

THE SENSORY SYSTEM

The sensory system is responsible for transmitting information about the internal and external environment of the body to the brain. Not all sensory information is perceived consciously; much proprioceptive data is processed automatically by the cerebellum and basal ganglia. There are also mechanisms of variable gating at the spinal and cerebral levels whereby the amount of sensory information (especially relating to pain) which reaches consciousness is controlled. Superficial sensations of touch, warmth, cold and pain, and deep sensations of position, pressure and pain all begin peripherally in specialised receptor organs which transduce physical modalities into sensory nerve impulses. Sensory nerve fibres are elongated processes of the bipolar neurones of the dorsal root ganglia; their central processes pass in the dorsal root to the spinal cord and either synapse there or pass directly towards the brain. Two main relay systems for sensory information are important clinically: the *lemniscal* and the *spinothalamic*.

The lemniscal system is concerned with transmission of proprioceptive and well-located touch information. Modalities such as joint position, two-point discrimination, and vibration sense use this pathway. The peripheral fibres are large, myelinated and fast conducting. They enter the dorsal horn of the spinal cord and without synapsing pass up the dorsal (posterior) columns to the gracile and cuneate nuclei in the lower medulla. Here they synapse, and second order fibres cross the midline and ascend the brain stem in the medial lemniscus, and thence to the thalamus Fig. 16.5.

The spinothalamic system is the pathway for pain, temperature and poorly localised touch. The peripheral fibres for these modalities are smaller, slower conducting and sometimes unmyelinated axons. They enter the spinal cord in the dorsal root, and synapse in the dorsal horn. Most of the second order fibres cross the midline of the cord over the distance of several segments and ascend in the contralateral spinothalamic tracts, joining the medial lemniscus fibre to synapse in the thalamus. A topographical arrangement exists in the spinothalamic tract, such that fibres from the lower limb come to lie outermost and those from the upper limb innermost.

Both the main sensory pathways synapse in the ventro-postero-lateral nucleus of the thalamus. The post-synaptic fibres lie closely packed together in the internal capsule, immediately posterior to the pyramidal tract fibres. They project up to the post-central gyrus (primary sensory cortex) in a topographical arrangement, similar to that on the motor strip. Although some appreciation of sensation and pain probably occurs at the thalamus, the sensory cortex is necessary for localisation of sensations from different parts of the body and provides the accuracy needed for two-point discrimination and joint position sense. Further analysis goes on in the adjoining parietal lobe which is responsible for perception of pattern, shape, size, texture and weight.

Collateral fibres from the ascending sensory pathways also make contact with the reticular formation. This is a chain of interconnecting short fibre neurones which lies in the centre of the brain stem and projects up to the midline thalamic nuclei, which in turn send fibres widely over the cortex. These non-specific projections (the reticular activating system) are important for maintaining awareness.

Lesions of the sensory system may cause negative and positive symptoms and signs. Negative symptoms of decreased sensation may be described as 'numbness', but also altered temperature perception may provoke descriptions of 'coldness'. Positive sensory symptoms may be paraesthesiae ('pins and needles'), warmth, burning, or tightness. The symptoms and signs caused

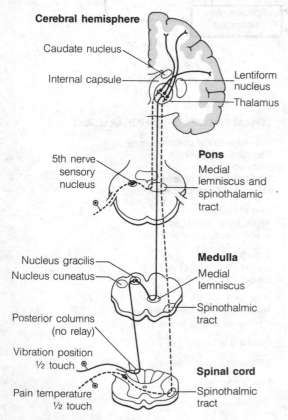

Cerebral hemisphere

Caudate nucleus

Internal capsule

Lentiform nucleus

Thalamus

5th nerve sensory nucleus

Pons

Medial lemniscus and spinothalamic tract

Nucleus gracilis

Nucleus cuneatus

Medulla

Medial lemniscus

Spinothalmic tract

Posterior columns (no relay)

Vibration position ½ touch

Spinal cord

Pain temperature ½ touch

Spinothalmic tract

Fig. 16.5   The sensory pathways.

Table 16.5 Symptoms and signs of sensory lesions

Site	Symptoms	Signs	Associated features
Peripheral nerve (partial)	Numbness paraesthesiae	Reduced sensation in territory of nerve (hyperpathia)	Weakness of muscles supplied by nerve
Many peripheral nerves (polyneuropathy)	Numbness and paraesthesiae hands and feet	'Glove and stocking' reduced sensation impaired vibration at at extremities	Weakness of distal muscles, loss of tendon reflexes
Spinal root (radiculopathy)	Numbness paraesthesiae hypersensitivity 'tightness'	Reduced sensation ± hyperpathia in dermatomal pattern	Weakness of muscles and reduced tendon reflexes of that segment
Posterior column	Numbness 'band-like' sensations, unsteadiness clumsiness	Reduced joint position sense, vibration and 2-point discrim. and touch ipsilaterally normal pain and temp.	Sensory ataxia loss of balance worse with closed eyes (Romberg's Test)
Spinothalamic tract	Numbness, warmth coldness diffuse distrib. contralaterally below lesion	Reduced pain and temp. sensation below and contralateral to lesion normal proprioception and vibration	Area of altered sensation begins several spinal segments below lesion
Brain stem (pons or lower)	Numbness and paraesthesiae face with coldness/warmth opposite limbs and trunk	Ipsilateral facial anaesthesia, with contralateral loss of pain/temperature limbs and trunk	May be lower cranial nerve lesions ipsilat. (v, vi, vii, ix, x, xi, xii)
(above pons)	Contralateral numbness or coldness/warmth face, limbs, trunk	Contralateral reduced pain/temperature on face, limbs, trunk	Ipsilateral upper cranial nerve lesion (iii, iv)
Thalamus	Diffuse deep pain on opposite side of body	Reduced touch, pain and temp. + hyperpathia contralaterally	Pain threshold raised, but more unpleasant
Internal capsule	Contralateral numbness of face, limbs, trunk	Reduced touch, pain, temperature on face, limbs and trunk contralateral side	Hemiparesis or hemianopia if other parts of capsule involved
Sensory cortex	Numbness localised to limb or part of	Loss of position sense, 2-point discrimination and stereognosis	Weakness of affected part if motor cortex involved
Parietal lobe	Difficulty in identifying shape, size, texture spatial disorientation	Impaired recognition of shapes, sizes denial of limbs on affected side	Apraxia for purposeful movements/speech dressing apraxia spatial problems

by lesions at different levels are summarised in Table 16.5. Partial lesions of peripheral nerves or roots tend to cause altered sensation rather than anaesthesia. Because of disturbance of the normal gating of painful stimuli, these lesions are often cause hypersensitivity to painful stimuli, but with reduced sensitivity to well localised touch (hyperpathia).

REFLEX ACTIVITY

Reflexes represent the simplest forms of integrated activity in the nervous system. The functional components of a reflex are listed in the information box (right).

FUNCTIONAL COMPONENTS OF A REFLEX

- A peripheral receptor organ
- A sensory nerve (or autonomic afferent)
- A central neurone or chain of neurones (spinal, cranial or autonomic)
- A motor nerve (or autonomic efferent)
- An effector organ (skeletal/smooth muscle, gland)

The activity of a given reflex may be altered by local or descending neural influences acting on the central neurones (Fig. 16.6). For example, tendon reflexes

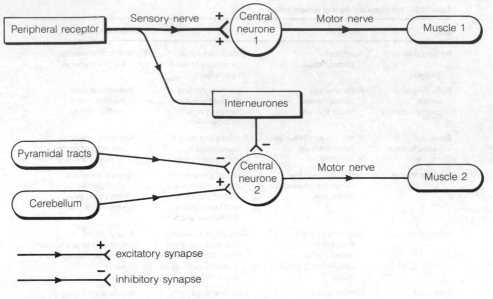

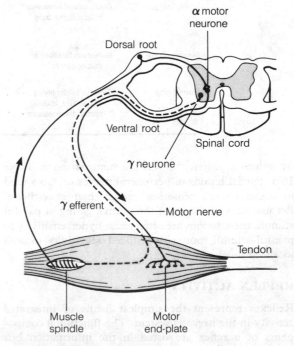

Fig. 16.6   Reflex activity.

become exaggerated when there is damage to the pyramidal tract, or depressed when there is a cerebellar lesion.

Many reflexes involve not only activation of an effector muscle but also relaxation of antagonists. A simple way to look at reflexes is to divide them into monosynaptic (or oligosynaptic) and polysynaptic types.

MONOSYNAPTIC AND OLIGOSYNAPTIC REFLEXES

The best-known example of a monosynaptic reflex is the tendon stretch reflex. This serves to maintain muscle tone and to adjust it during movement. Clinically, the reflex can be tested by applying a sharp stretching force (hammer tap) to a muscle tendon. This activates stretch receptors in the muscle spindle organs which send a synchronised volley of sensory activity up the rapidly conducting large afferent fibres which enter the spinal cord at the dorsal root. The sensory fibres synapse directly on the anterior horn cell, promoting depolarisation by excitatory transmission. The motor-fibre volley passes to the same muscle, causing contraction which is observed as a brief jerk (see Fig. 16.7). The intrafusal fibres of the muscle spindle control the sensitivity of its stretch receptors, and are in turn adjusted by gamma efferent fibres whose activity is controlled by descending influences from the cerebellum, and pyramidal and extrapyramidal systems

(Table 16.6). The tendon reflexes serve as a convenient way for the clinician to test the integrity of the reflex arc components at different spinal levels (Table 16.7), and also to judge changes in the descending (especially pyramidal) systems.

Fig. 16.7   The tendon stretch reflex.

Table 16.6   Lesions affecting tendon reflex activity

Site of lesion	Effect on reflexes
Sensory fibres/roots	Diminished/absent
Motor neurone	Diminished/absent
Motor roots/nerves	Diminished/absent
Cerebellum	Diminished/pendular
Pyramidal tract	Increased ± clonus

Table 16.7   Segmental supply of tendon reflexes

Reflex	Spinal segment
Biceps	Cervical 5/6
Brachioradialis	Cervical 5/6
Triceps	Cervical 7
Finger flexors	Cervical 7/8 Thoracic 1
Quadriceps (knee)	Lumbar 3/4
Hamstrings	Lumbar 5/sacral 1
Gastrocnaemius (ankle)	Sacral 1

Other monosynaptic or oligosynaptic reflexes can be elicited in the cranial nerves. *The jaw jerk* is mediated by stretching the muscles of mastication, the reflex loop passing to and from the pons in the trigeminal nerves. Lesions of the pyramidal tracts above the pons exaggerate the reflex. The *corneal reflex* is oligosynaptic, involving mainly the first division of the trigeminal sensory root as the afferent limb. Fibres enter the pons, descend in the tract of the fifth nerve and synapse in its nucleus from where second-order fibres pass to both facial nuclei to cause bilateral eye closure from contraction of orbicularis oculi. The reflex is diminished by lesions of the first trigeminal sensory division, by damage to the facial nerve and in lesions of the lateral pons and medulla.

POLYSYNAPTIC REFLEXES

These more complex reflexes involve chains of interconnected neurones within the spinal cord which activate several muscle groups to produce co-ordinated movements in response to usually noxious stimuli. The presence and sometimes nature of the reflexes is modified by descending fibre systems, particularly the pyramidal tracts. The *plantar reflex* is an example of polysynaptic activity. After the first year of life, the normal plantar response is flexion of the great toe, with adduction of the other toes. If the pyramidal tract is damaged or rendered temporarily non-functional (e.g.

during an epileptic seizure), the same stimulus causes extension of the great toe and abduction of the other toes – the extensor plantar response. The *flexion withdrawal reflex* may be seen in conjunction with an extensor plantar response. Here a noxious stimulus will cause reflex flexion of the hip and knee to withdraw the foot from the stimulus. Sometimes when the pyramidal tract damage is severe, the ipsilateral flexion reflex is accompanied by extension of the opposite leg – the crossed extensor reflex.

The *abdominal reflexes* are also examples of polysynaptic activity which has protective function. Damage to the pyramidal tract on one side will abolish the reflex on that side; this phenomenon being particularly common in multiple sclerosis. Damage to the peripheral elements of the reflexes (T 8–12 spinal nerves) also abolishes the response, as do obesity, pregnancy, abdominal surgery and muscle laxity.

CONTROL OF THE BLADDER AND SPHINCTERS

BLADDER

The nerve supply to the bladder derives from three sources (Fig. 16.8):

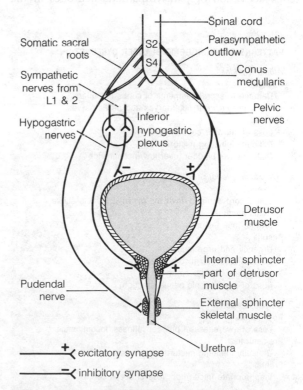

Fig. 16.8   Nerve supply to the bladder and sphincters.

Sympathetic fibres. Coming from spinal segments L1 and 2 these pass via the inferior hypogastric plexus and the hypogastric nerves to the bladder wall and internal sphincteric part of the detrusor muscle. When activated they cause relaxation of the bladder wall but closure of the internal sphincter. These effects are inhibited by alpha-adrenergic blocking drugs such as phenoxybenzamine.

Parasympathetic fibres. These derive from the sacral outflow (S2–4) and pass to the bladder via the pelvic nerves. They effect contraction of the detrusor muscle and opening of the internal sphincter. These cholinergic effects are inhibited by drugs such as atropine and probanthine.

Somatic fibres. These also emerge from spinal segments S2–4 and pass to the skeletal muscle of the external sphincter. The same nerves supply the anal sphincter muscles.

Bladder function

Afferent fibres from the bladder wall pass via the pelvic and hypogastric nerves, and from the sphincters in the pudendal nerves. Distension of the bladder evokes reflex activation of parasympathetic neurones in the sacral 2–4 segments which causes detrusor contraction and sphincter opening to effect automatic bladder emptying. Reciprocal changes in the sympathetic outflow from L1 and 2 aid this process. Awareness of bladder fullness reaches consciousness via the lateral spinothalamic tracts of the spinal cord, eventually reaching the parasagittal part of the post-central gyrus. Voluntary inhibition of the bladder reflex and its release which permits micturition are controlled by the parasagittal part of the frontal cortex, the efferent fibres descending the spinal cord close to the pyramidal tracts. Several patterns of neurogenic bladder dysfunction may occur and these are listed in the information box (left).

RECTUM

The rectum has an excitatory cholinergic input from the parasympathetic sacral outflow, and inhibitory sympathetic supply similar to the bladder. Continence depends largely on skeletal muscle contraction in the puborectalis and pelvic floor muscles supplied by the pudendal nerves which influence the angle of the ano-rectum as well as the internal and external anal sphincters. Damage to the autonomic components causes constipation. Lesions affecting the conus medullaris, the somatic sacral 2–4 roots and the pudendal nerves cause faecal incontinence.

PENILE ERECTION AND EJACULATION

These related functions are under autonomic control via the pelvic nerves (parasympathetic S2–4) and the

---

PATTERNS OF NEUROGENIC BLADDER DYSFUNCTION

Atonic Bladder
Cause
    Damage to sacral segments of conus medullaris
    Damage to sacral roots/nerves and pelvic nerves
Results
    Loss of detrusor contraction
    Difficulty initiating micturition
    Distension of bladder, overflow incontinence

Hypertonic Bladder
Cause
    Spinal-cord damage involving pyramidal tracts above
    conus medullaris
    Frontal lobe lesions
Results
    Urgency and urge incontinence
    Bladder/sphincter inco-ordination
    Incomplete bladder emptying
    (loss of psychogenic penile erection)

Cortical Lesions
Post-central
    Loss of awareness of bladder fullness, incontinence
Pre-central
    Difficulty initiating micturition
Frontal
    Inappropriate micturition, loss of social control

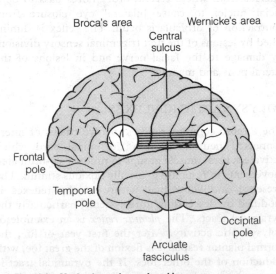

Fig. 16.9 Mechanisms of speech and language.

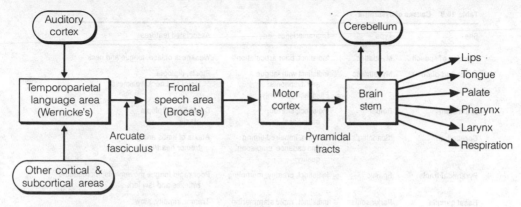

Fig. 16.10   Cortical language areas in the left cerebral hemisphere.

hypogastric nerves (sympathetic L1 and 2). Descending influences from the cerebrum are important for psychogenic erection, but this can occur as a purely reflex phenomenon in response to genital stimulation. Erection is largely parasympathetic in control, and is impaired by drugs which have anticholinergic effects. Sympathetic activity is important for ejaculation, and may be inhibited by alpha-adrenergic blocking drugs.

SPEECH

Speech enables the communication of ideas from person to person by the use of verbal symbols produced by the larynx, pharynx, lips and tongue. A schematic representation of the mechanisms involved in speech and language is shown in Fig. 16.10. The important cortical area for language lies in the dominant hemisphere. This is on the left side for right-handed people; left-handers may have language functions mostly on the right, mostly on the left or shared between both sides. The cortical language areas are shown in Fig. 16.9.

The posterior language (Wernicke's) area in the dominant temporo-parietal region is important in the comprehension of received speech and in the selection of words to express ideas. In simple terms, this area acts like a dictionary. A bundle of subcortical fibres, the arcuate fasciculus, connects it with the anterior speech (Broca's) area in the inferior third frontal convolution. Broca's area is important for the fluency and rhythm of speech and for the maintenance of grammar and syntax.

DYSPHASIA

Dysfunction of the language areas results in dysphasia, where there is disordered use of language with or without impaired comprehension of received speech. Lesions of the anterior speech area cause *expressive dysphasia*, characterised by poor fluency, with reduced output of words, but usually preserved comprehension. By contrast, with damage to the temporo-parietal region, fluency, grammar and articulation are preserved, but the speech lacks correct meaning, with inappropriate letters or words (paraphasias) or entirely new words (neologisms). In addition there is a degree of difficulty with comprehension of heard speech (receptive dysphasia). Lesions in the perisylvian region, damaging the arcuate fasciculus, may have elements of both expressive and receptive difficulty, but are characterised particularly by impaired ability to repeat heard speech; this picture is known as conduction dysphasia. The features of lesions in the different language areas are shown in Table 16.8.

In clinical practice, analysis of speech is carried out

Table 16.8   Characteristics of dysphasias

Site	Output	Fluency	Paraphasias	Comprehension	Repetition
Anterior (Broca)	Reduced	Poor	Absent	Retained	Variable
Posterior (Wernicke)	Normal/increased	Good	Present	Impaired	Variable
Arcuate fasciculus (conduction)	Variable	Variable	Mild	Variable	Impaired
Fronto-parietal (global)	Very reduced	Poor	Jargon	Impaired	Impaired

Table 16.9 Causes of dysarthria

Site	Type	Characteristics	Associated features
Muscles of speech	Myopathic	Indistinct, poor articulation	Weakness of face, tongue and neck
Motor end-plate	Myasthenic	Indistinct with fatigue and dysphonia. Fluctuating severity	Ptosis, diplopia facial and neck weakness
Brain stem	Bulbar	Indistinct, slurred often nasal	Dysphagia, diplopia ataxia
Cerebellum	'Scanning'	Slurring, impaired timing and cadence 'sing-song' quality	Ataxia of limbs and gait tremor head/limbs
Pyramidal tracts	Spastic	Indistinct, breathy, mumbling	Poor rapid tongue movements; increased reflexes and jaw jerk
Basal ganglia	Parkinsonian	Indistinct, rapid stammering, quiet	Tremor, rigidity, slow shuffling gait
Basal ganglia	Dystonic	Strained, slow	Dystonia, athetosis

not only to localise the lesion, but, in the case of a vascular or traumatic insult, to give some idea of prognosis. Global dysphasia carries a poor chance of recovery, while pure forms of anterior or posterior dysphasia are more likely to recover, especially if repetition is preserved.

DYSARTHRIA

When the motor control systems for the muscles of speech, or the muscles themselves are impaired, dysarthria results. The dysarthric patient uses language normally with correct grammar, appropriate words, and retained comprehension; but speech is indistinct or even unintelligible because of weakness, slowness or inco-ordination of the muscles responsible (Table 16.9). The lesion causing dysarthria may be peripheral in the muscles of the face, tongue or pharynx; at their neuromuscular junctions; in the brain stem or the cerebellum, the pyramidal tracts or motor cortex, or in the extrapyramidal system.

DYSPHONIA

When there is impaired air flow, damage or dysfunction of the vocal cords or soft palate, the generation of notes is impaired. Speech may be softer, hoarse or husky. The generation of hard consonants (G or B) is impaired if the soft palate cannot close off the nasopharynx; this gives speech a 'nasal' quality (e.g. 'frog' becomes 'frong'). Severe damage to both vocal cords causes total lack of phonation – aphonia.

VISION

The visual system is frequently involved by intercranial disease because, starting in the eyes and terminating in the occipital cortex, its fibres traverse a wide area of the cerebrum. Light rays are refracted by the media and lens of the eye and an inverted image of the external world is focused on to the retina. Fine adjustment of focus is carried out by the ciliary muscle, under control of the third nerve parasympathetic outflow. The light-sensitive retinal rods and cones convert photic energy into nerve impulses which undergo preliminary integration at the retinal ganglion cells. Fibres from these cells make up the optic nerves which pass back through the optic foraminae towards the optic chiasm. Each optic nerve carries a covering of meninges which may transmit cerebrospinal fluid (CSF) pressure changes to the nerve head in the eye, causing optic disc swelling (papilloedema) if the pressure is elevated. Pathophysiologically, the optic nerve behaves more like cerebral white matter than peripheral nerve.

Because of the image inversion produced by the eye's optics, the temporal visual field is represented on the nasal retina, and the upper field on the lower retina. At the optic chiasm, fibres from the nasal retinae (temporal fields) cross over to the contralateral optic tract, while the temporal retinal fibres (nasal fields) remain uncrossed. The optic tract fibres pass mostly to the lateral geniculate bodies where some synaptic integration takes place. A few fibres leave before the geniculate and pass to the mid-brain to supply the afferent limb of the pupil light reflex. After the geniculate bodies, the optic radiation fibres sweep posteriorly through the temporal and parietal lobes towards the calcarine cortex in the occipital lobe. The vertical arrangement is maintained so that fibres in the parietal lobe come from the upper retinae (lower visual fields) and those in the temporal lobe from the lower retinae (upper fields) (Fig. 16.11). In the occipital lobe further analysis of

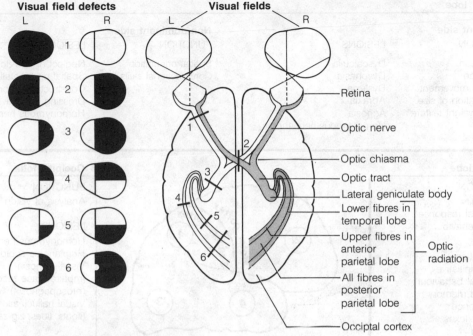

Visual field defects

L   R

Visual fields

L   R

- Retina
- Optic nerve
- Optic chiasma
- Optic tract
- Lateral geniculate body
- Lower fibres in temporal lobe
- Upper fibres in anterior parietal lobe } Optic radiation
- All fibres in posterior parietal lobe
- Occipital cortex

Fig. 16.11   Visual pathways and field defects.

visual information from the contralateral side of the visual field takes place. Cells in the calcarine cortex are synaptically connected so that they detect rectangular shapes, moving edges, and bars or lines in different orientations. Stereoscopic vision is also served in this area by cells activated by corresponding retinal points.

There are a variety of visual defects associated with lesions of the visual pathway which help to localise the site of the disease (Table 16.10).

Clinical features of localised cerebral lesions

Although the brain functions in an integrated fashion, certain cortical areas are allied to specific functions. The effects of lesions at different sites are summarised in Fig. 16.12.

NEUROLOGICAL INVESTIGATIONS

While clinical examination often will lead to accurate

Table 16.10   Clinical manifestations of lesions of the visual pathway

Site	Clinical features
Retina	Partial lesions – patches of visual loss (scotomas). Damage to macula causes severe loss of acuity. Large lesions diminish pupil light reflex
Optic nerve	Partial – scotomas, esp. central or between fixation and blind spot (centrocaecal). Vascular lesions tend to affect upper or lower field of one eye (altitudinal defects). Severe lesions cause blindness and loss of pupil light reflex
Optic chiasm	Midline lesions (e.g. pituitary tumour) damage crossing nasal fibres, causing bitemporal defects. Compression from below affects upper fields first. Lateral compression rare, but causes loss in nasal fields of vision. Large chiasmatic lesions, impair pupil light reflex bilaterally
Optic tract	Impairment of same side of vision in each eye, often assymmetrically (incongruous homonymous hemianopia). Affected fields opposite side to lesion
Optic radiation	Homonymous hemianopia contralateral to lesion. Upper fibres (parietal) – lower quadrantic defects; lower fibres (temporal) – upper quadrantic
Occipital lobe	Contralateral homonymous hemianopia. Small lesions may cause homonymous scotomas, sectorial or altitudinal defects

1 Parietal lobe

Dominant side		Non-dominant side	
FUNCTION	LESIONS	FUNCTION	LESIONS
Calculation	Dyscalculia	Spatial orientation	Neglect of non-dominant
Language	Dysphasia	Constructional skills	Spatial disorientation
Planned movement	Dyslexia		Constructional apraxia
Appreciation of size,	Apraxia		Dressing apraxia
shape, weight texture	Agnosia		Homonymous hemianopia
	Homonymous hemianopia		

2 Frontal lobe

FUNCTION
Personality
Emotional response
Social behaviour

LESIONS
Disinhibition
Lack of initiative
Antisocial behaviour
Impaired memory
Incontinence
Grasp reflexes
Anosmia

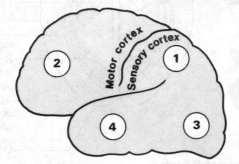

3 Occipital lobe

FUNCTION
Analysis of vision

LESIONS
Homonymous hemianopia
Hemianopic scotomas
Visual agnosia
Impaired face recognition
(prosopagnosia)
Visual hallucinations
(lights, lines, zig-zags)

4 Temporal lobe

Dominant		Non Dominant	
FUNCTION	LESIONS	FUNCTION	LESIONS
Auditory perception	Dysphasia	Auditory perception	Poor non-verbal memory
Speech, language	Dyslexia	Music, tone sequences	Loss of musical skills
Verbal memory	Poor memory	Non-verbal memory	Complex hallucinations
Olfaction	Complex hallucinations	(faces, shapes, music)	Homonymous hemianopia
	(smell, sound, vision)	Olfaction	
	Homonymous hemianopia		

Fig. 16.12 Features of localised cerebral lesions.

localisation of lesions within the nervous system, the precise diagnosis of the nature of such lesions relies firstly on analysis of the history and secondly on methods of investigation. The tests which offer the best diagnostic accuracy are frequently the most invasive and hazardous; as a general rule it is wise to begin investigation with non-invasive screening tests and to select only the most appropriate invasive methods for each case.

RADIOLOGY

Plain radiographs are frequently normal even in the presence of quite advanced cerebral or spinal disease.

Skull films are nevertheless useful for demonstrating sinus disease, fractures, pituitary tumours, bony metastatic deposits and calcified intracranial lesions. Abnormalities most likely to calcify include meningiomas, tuberculomas, oligodengliomas, giant aneurysms and arteriovenous malformations. Chronically raised intracranial pressure may sometimes be inferred from erosion of the clinoid processes of the pituitary fossa. Lateral shift of the calcified normally mid-line pineal gland can provide evidence of a mass lesion.

Plain spine radiographs may show evidence of degenerative bony changes, with reduction of the disc spaces and misalignment, and are particularly helpful after trauma. Oblique views of the cervical spine help delineate narrowing of the intervertebral neural exit foramina. Plain films also aid detection of metastatic or infective lesions affecting the spine, where erosion of the vertebral body, laminae or disc may be evident.

Contrast radiology

If a contrast medium (usually iodine based) is introduced into the cerebral blood vessels or the cerebrospinal fluid surrounding the brain or spinal cord, then normal and abnormal structures can be demonstrated.

Angiography

In conventional cerebral angiography contrast is injected into the carotid or vertebral arteries. Selective catheterisation of the relevant vessel is usually performed via a catheter inserted into the femoral artery in the groin. A series of X-ray films is taken usually in two planes during contrast injection so that arterial, capillary and venous phases can be studied (Fig. 16.13). In modern practice angiography is used mainly to study the extracranial and intracranial vessels, to outline regions of arterial disease, aneurysms and arteriovenous malformations. Conventional angiography carries a small but significant risk of stroke or death, particularly in the elderly and patients with vascular disease, and should be undertaken only if management is likely to be altered by the result.

Digital subtraction angiography (DSA)

This offers a less invasive way of demonstrating cerebral vasculature by computer enhancing techniques. Contrast is injected either by a central venous bolus or a low dose arterial injection. With the venous route (DVI), there is less risk than with conventional angiography, but the image quality especially of intracranial vessels is inferior. Studies of sufficient quality may however be obtained to exclude a major stenosis of the cervical carotid and vertebral arteries (Fig. 16.14).

Myelography and radiculography

It is usually necessary to introduce contrast liquid into the subarachnoid space by lumbar, cervical or cisternal puncture to investigate disorders of the spinal cord or roots. Water-soluble non-ionic contrast media are in routine use. The patient is tilted on a table so that contrast can be manipulated up or down the spinal subarachnoid space, permitting visualisation of the spinal cord (myelography) and lumbo-sacral roots (radiculography). Headache is a common sequel, and occasionally seizures, meningitis and muscle spasms occur. It is likely that Magnetic Resonance Imaging (MRI) will replace many myelographic examinations.

Pneumoencephalography

The injection of air into the lumbar subarachnoid space to outline the cerebral ventricles and CSF spaces is rarely performed. Air-CT meatography is a modern refinement in which small volumes of air are manouevred into the cerebello-pontine angle and CT images taken to outline the internal auditory meatus and the seventh and eighth cranial nerves within it. The technique is used for the detection of small acoustic neuromas.

Computed tomography (CT)

This non-invasive technique has revolutionised investigation of the central nervous system. The method is very sensitive and will show the normal outlines of the brain, cerebral ventricles and CSF spaces, and after intravenous contrast injection, some of the larger blood vessels. CT will demonstrate the vast majority of cerebral haemorrhages, tumours, cysts and abcesses and will readily demonstrate hydrocephalus and cerebral atrophy. Although many cerebral infarcts and subdural haematomas will also be seen, small early lesions may be undetected. Because of interference from bony structures CT is less useful for visualisation of the brain stem, cerebellum and spinal cord, but with modifications of technique, these structure can be demonstrated (Fig. 16.16).

CT is largely non-invasive and carries little risk. Spinal CT scanning is being used increasingly to outline disc protrusions, spinal canal stenosis and intramedullary lesions.

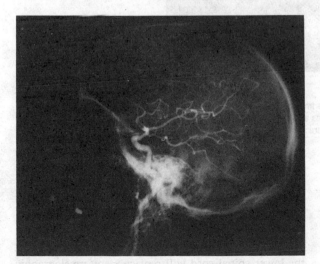

Fig. 16.13   Normal carotid angiogram (lateral view). It shows cervical carotid artery, its bifurcation and internal carotid circulation within the head.

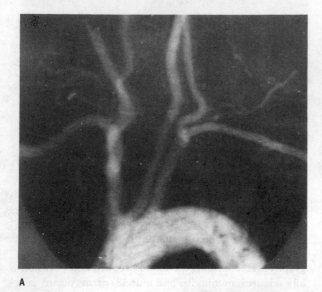

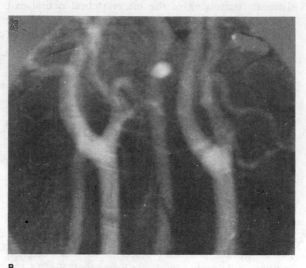

Fig. 16.14   Normal digital venous imaging. A. Aortic arch and great vessels. **B.** Cervical carotid arteries and their bifurcations with vertebral arteries alongside. **C.** Intracranial views of both carotid and vertebral arterial systems.

MAGNETIC RESONANCE IMAGING (MRI)

This technique is a powerful, non-invasive tool for imaging the brain and spinal cord; but machines are as yet very expensive, and MRI is not yet freely available. MRI is particularly sensitive to differences between grey and white matter, and shows areas of demyelination (e.g. in multiple sclerosis) much more readily than CT. MRI is insensitive to compact bone and therefore renders excellent images of the posterior fossa and cranio-vertebral regions. The technique is the investigation of choice for demonstrating lesions in suspected multiple sclerosis, brain-stem tumours and infarcts, and intrinsic lesions in the spinal cord, especially syringomyelia. It is likely that MR images of the lower spinal cord will replace many myelographic examinations as more sophisticated equipment becomes available.

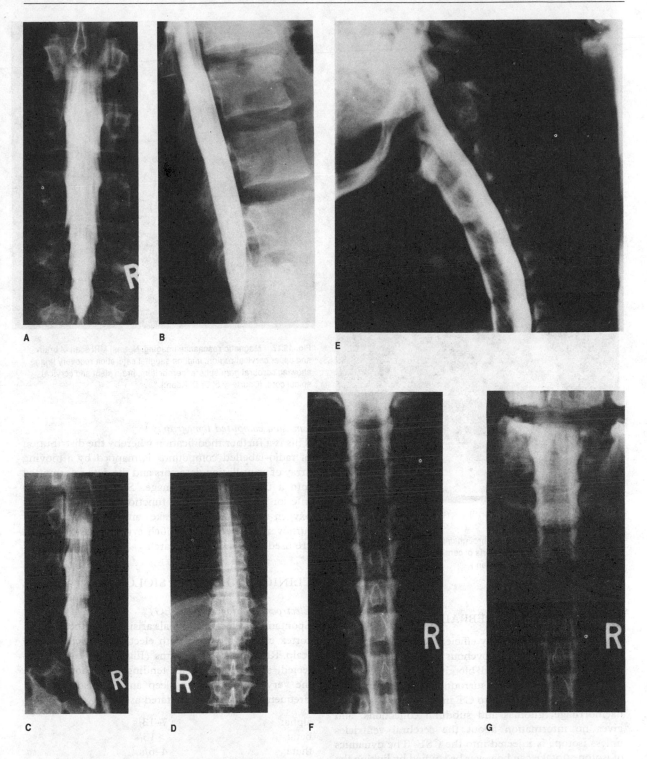

Fig. 16.15   Normal myelogram. Water soluble contrast (iopamidol) introduced by lumbar puncture at L2/3 level. **A.** Anteroposterior view. **B.** Lateral view. **C.** Oblique view. All in the lumbar region demonstrating the lumbo-sacral roots. **D & E.** The dorsal and cervical spinal cord is seen against the positive contrast as a central shadow. **F, G.** The cervical spinal roots can be identified in the posteroanterior views. (Courtesy of Dr D. Kean.)

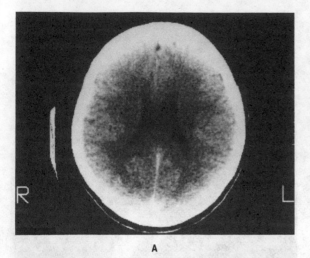

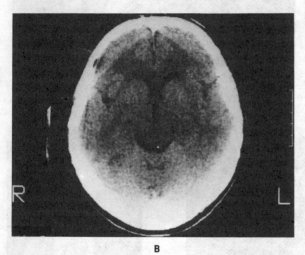

Fig. 16.16   Normal CT scan. A. Through upper part of cerebral hemisphere. **B.** Showing lower parts of cerebral hemisphere and upper brain stem. (Courtesy of Dr. D. Kean.)

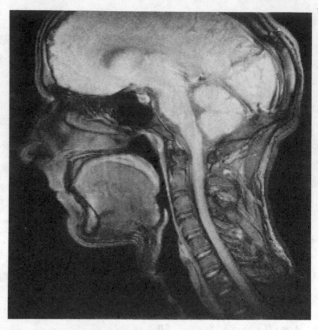

Fig. 16.17   Magnetic resonance imaging. Normal MRI scan of brain and upper cervical region; midline saggital saturation recovery image showing cerebral hemisphere, cerebellum, brain stem and cervical spinal cord. (Courtesy of Dr D. Kean.)

RADIONUCLIDE CEREBRAL SCANNING

This method is reasonably efficient in the detection of meningiomas and arteriovenous malformations, because they have increased blood supply and take up isotope more avidly than surrounding brain. However it is considerably inferior to CT in detecting infarction, haemorrhage, gliomas and subdural collections, and gives no information about the cerebral ventricles unless isotope is injected into the CSF. The dynamics of isotope uptake can however be studied by linking the gamma camera to a computer, and images of regional cerebral blood flow can be thus obtained.

Emission computed tomography

This is a further modification whereby the distribution of radio-labelled compounds is mapped by a moving array of scintillation detectors and the data reformatted into a two-dimensional image. Spacial resolution is inferior to X-ray CT, but functional changes such as oxygen and glucose uptake and neurotransmitter turnover can be studied. Such systems are costly and are used primarily for research.

CLINICAL NEUROPHYSIOLOGY

Electroencephalography (EEG)

Spontaneous electrical signals arising from the cerebral cortex can be recorded with electrodes placed on the scalp. Rhythmical waveforms (Fig. 16.18) can be detected, slower frequencies tending to predominate in the very young, during sleep and in disease states. Frequency bands are annotated as:

alpha:	7–13/s
beta:	>13/s
theta:	4–6/s
delta:	<4/s

In alert adults alpha activity predominates, especially

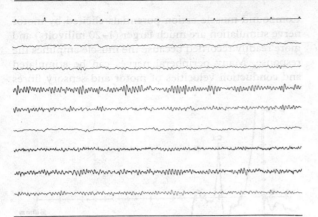

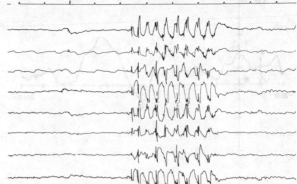

Fig. 16.18 Portion of an 8-channel EEG record taken from a normal adolescent. Four channels running anterior to posterior over the parietal regions are displayed from each side. Top four traces – right side; lower four – left side. Uppermost trace is a 1 second time marker. Note the posteriorly dominant 10/s waves – the alpha rhythm.

Fig. 16.19 Abnormal EEG from a patient suffering from generalised tonic-clonic seizures. This inter-ictal record shows a paroxysm of generalised spike and slow wave activity lasting about 3 seconds, during which the patient showed no clinical abnormality.

when the eyes are shut, and is found best over the posterior quadrants. In disease states (see Table 16.11), slow activity (theta and delta) may be focal or generalised.

The EEG is used mainly for detection and characterisation of epileptic disturbances, but also has a role in other states of altered brain function (e.g. encephalitis) where imaging techniques may be unhelpful. In epilepsy, focal or generalised high voltage fast transients (spikes and sharp waves) are recorded during seizures and sometimes interictally. The chance of detecting such phenomena is improved by hyperventilation, photic flicker, sleep and some drugs. In selected cases of diagnostic difficulty it is possible to record EEG from ambulant patients for 24 hours or longer using a light-weight tape recorder, or to use prolonged video-monitoring of the patient and his EEG simultaneously. It is important to recognise that up to 40% of patients with clinical epilepsy may have a normal routine EEG, and that an abnormal EEG record does not establish a diagnosis of epilepsy in the absence of appropriate history.

Evoked potential recording

The development of electronic signal averaging by computer techniques now permits recording of very small cerebral or spinal event-related potentials. Stimulation by visual, sensory nerve or auditory routes is time-locked to the averager so that a processed signal, relatively free from interference, can be made up from 100–1000 evoked responses. Visually evoked potentials (VEP) are the most useful clinically, and are recorded with an array of scalp electrodes over the occipital region. The dominant response wave from a normal eye is a positive wave peaking at about 100 ms (Fig. 16.20). Lesions of the retina, optic nerve, chiasma, tract, radiation of cortex may all disrupt or delay the response, but demyelinating lesions of the optic nerve often cause marked delay with relatively good preservation of the wave form. A delayed VEP in a patient with clinically normal vision can therefore be of much diagnostic help in multiple sclerosis.

Somato-sensory evoked potentials (SSEP) recorded from the brachial plexus, cervical spine and contralateral parietal area when the median or ulnar nerve is stimulated electrically may similarly help detect lesions in the sensory pathways. Similar responses may be produced over the lumbar and dorsal spine and vertex by posterior tibial nerve stimulation in the leg (Fig. 16.21) SSEP are less useful than VEP for detecting subclinical demyelination, but can be of help in delineating lesions of the brachial plexus, spinal roots and cord.

Table 16.11 EEG changes in disease states

Disorder	EEG pattern
Cerebral tumour	Focal theta/delta
Cerebral abscess	Focal delta
Cerebral infarct	Focal theta/delta
Encephalitis	Theta/delta/sharp waves usually generalised
Metabolic coma (e.g. hypoglycaemia)	Diffuse theta/delta
Sub-dural haematoma	Reduced amplitude over side of lesion
Epilepsy	Focal or generalised spikes, sharp waves, spike-wave complexes

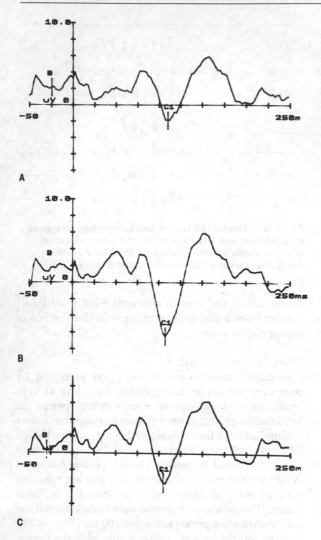

Fig. 16.20   Normal visual evoked responses elicited by reversing chequer-board pattern stimulus to right eye. A. trace – right occipital; **B.** trace – mid occipital; **C.** trace – left occipital recording electrons. 100 individual responses are computer averaged to produce these traces. The major positive (downward) deflection occurs about 110 ms after the stimulus (marked C1) and is called the P100 response.

Auditory evoked potentials (AEP) in response to click stimuli arise largely from the brain stem, and may give evidence of cochlear, acoustic nerve or brain stem disorders.

Electromyography (EMG)
Muscle or nerve action potentials can be detected by surface or needle electrodes. After electrical stimulation of a peripheral nerve trunk, compound action potentials can be recorded over the nerve's course, their normal amplitude varying from 5–30 microvolts.

Compound muscle action potentials elicited by motor nerve stimulation are much larger (1–20 milivolts) and more readily recorded because the muscle amplifies the response. Many peripheral nerves can be stimulated and conduction velocities of motor and sensory fibres

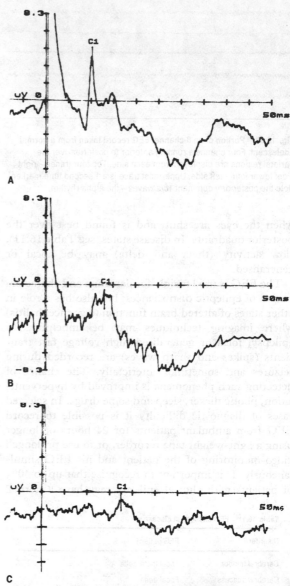

Fig. 16.21   Normal somato-sensory evoked response elicited by electrical stimulation of the median nerve at the wrist. Each trace is a computer average of 500 responses. **A.** trace – recorded at supraclavicular fossa, shows a negative (upward) potential at 10 ms. **B.** trace – recorded from posterior mid-cervical regional shows at C1 a negative response with a latency of 12–13 ms. **C.** trace – recorded from contralateral parietal area shows at C1 a smaller negative response of 17–18 ms latency.

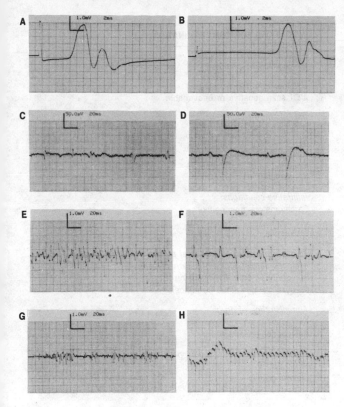

Fig. 16.22 Normal and abnormal electromyographic recordings. A and **B** show compound muscle action potential responses recorded with surface electrodes on the thenar eminence when the median nerve is stimulated at the wrist (**A**) and elbow (**B**). Note the difference in latency; this is used to calculate conduction velocity – usually 50–60 m/s.
C–H show EMG recordings made with a concentric needle electrode. **C** shows small short duration fibrillation potentials, and **D** positive sharp waves, both features seen in acute muscle denervation. **E** shows a normal pattern of motor unit recruitment when a subject makes a strong voluntary muscle contraction. Impaired recruitment of enlarged motor units is seen in chronic denervation (**F**). In myopathy (**G**) recruitment is full but the motor units are reduced in amplitude and duration. **H** shows an example of a high frequency burst of muscle activity recorded from a patient with dystrophia myotonica.

can be measured separately. Velocity and amplitude measurements help gauge the type and severity of polyneuropathies and may define the site of localised nerve compression, as in the carpal tunnel syndrome.

Demyelination of peripheral nerve causes marked reduction in conduction velocity, whereas primary axonal degeneration is associated with reduction of motor and sensory action potential amplitude with little or no reduction in velocity. Concentric needle EMG is used to sample motor units in muscle at rest and during voluntary activity. Primary myopathy is associated with reduction in motor unit amplitude and duration with normal numbers of units activated during effort. Denervation on the other hand, causes spontaneous fibrillation and fasciculation at rest, and a reduced number of normal or enlarged units during activity (Fig. 16.22). Repetitive stimulation of a motor nerve with trains of impulses at 3–15/s may detect a characteristic decremental response in myasthenia gravis, although false negative results are common. In Lambert-Eaton myasthenic syndrome (LEMS), higher frequency stimulation (20–50/s) nearly always produces striking incrementation of the motor response.

BIOCHEMICAL TESTS

Tests of muscle breakdown

Enzymes released from muscle increase in concentration in peripheral blood in muscle disease. The highest enzyme levels are seen in active polymyositis and the more severe forms of muscular dystrophy. Widespread denervation may cause modest enzyme elevations. The enzymes most commonly measured are: creatinine phosphokinase (CPK), aldolase and lactate dehydrogenase (LDH).

Tests for specific disorders

Rare disorders of muscle and nerve metabolism can sometimes be diagnosed by measuring enzymes in blood or muscle. Some examples are listed in the information box below.

RARE DISORDERS OF MUSCLE AND NERVE METABOLISM

Myophosphorylase deficiency (McCardle's disease)
Muscle pain on exercise
Increased glycogen in muscle
Failure of blood lactate to rise on exercise
Reduced concentration of myophosphorylase in muscle

Phosphofructokinase deficiency
Similar to above but reduced phosphofructokinase in muscle

Carnitine-palmityl transferase (CPT) deficiency
Muscle pain after prolonged exercise
Increased lipid in muscle on biopsy
CPT deficient in muscle biopsy specimen

Refsum's disease
Abnormal storage of phytanic acid in peripheral nerve tissue

Hypertrophic polyneuropathy
Retinal pigmentation
Elevated serum phytanic acid level

MUSCLE AND NERVE BIOPSY

Biopsy of skeletal muscle usually provides more helpful information than that of peripheral nerve. Histological examination with light microscopy, enzyme histochemistry and electron microscopy may be helpful in defining which type of muscle or nerve fibre is affected, whether any inflammation is present, and whether any abnormal accumulations (e.g. excess glycogen, lipid, amyloid, mitochondria) are present to suggest a specific defect of metabolism. Peripheral nerve is less easily biopsied without causing deficit. The distal sural nerve at the ankle or the superficial radial nerve at the wrist are the most suitable since the resultant sensory deficit is mild and localised. Partial thickness biopsy causes less sensory deficit. The pathological process, whether primarily affecting axons or myelin, may be evident, and abnormal infiltration (e.g. amyloid) is occasionally seen. The presence of perineural vasculitis is the most therapeutically useful finding, since corticosteroid therapy may be indicated.

TESTS OF THE AUTONOMIC NERVOUS SYSTEM

These are based mostly on measuring cardiovascular responses to the Valsalva manoeuvure, deep breathing, sustained hand grip and changing from lying to standing posture. Pupil cycle time is also relatively easily measured with a slit lamp and stop watch, and gives an indication of parasympathetic function in the oculomotor nerve. Peripheral autonomic abnormalities are seen in patients with diabetes mellitus, alcoholism, and amyloidosis; central forms of disorder occur in some patients with Parkinson's disease and rarer multi-system degenerations.

EXAMINATION OF CEREBROSPINAL FLUID (CSF)

Examination of CSF is undertaken less often now than in the past, because of the development of more accurate and non-invasive techniques for demonstrating cerebral and spinal lesions. Nevertheless, examination of CSF obtained by lumbar (or occasionally cisternal) puncture is still a valuable procedure in certain types of disorder. The indications and contraindications for lumbar puncture are listed in the information boxes (right).

When CSF pressure is raised due to an intracranial mass lesion, shift of the midline structures, or internal hydrocephalus, lumbar puncture may provoke downward shift of the brain stem. The resultant herniation of the medulla and cerebellum at the foramen magnum,

---

INDICATIONS FOR CSF EXAMINATION

Infections
Meningitis, encephalitis

Subarachnoid haemorrhage
If CT scan negative or unavailable

Inflammatory conditions
Multiple sclerosis
Sarcoidosis
Acute polyneuritis
Systemic lupus erythematosis
Neurosyphilis

Infiltrative conditions
Carcinomatous meningitis
Lymphoma
Leukaemia

To confirm raised intracerebral pressure when CT scan excludes danger of brain-stem herniation
Benign intracranial hypertension (BIH)
Cerebral venous sinus thrombosis

Administration of drugs
Antibiotics (meningitis)
Antimitotics (oncology)

Instillation of contrast media or isotopes
Myelography
Cisternography

---

or the pons and temporal lobes at the tentorial hiatus may be fatal. A sample of venous blood should be taken at the same time as CSF so that blood glucose and immunoglobulin levels can be compared with those in CSF. Normally CSF glucose concentration is about 2/3 that of blood. Small vessels are often damaged at lumbar puncture rendering the initial CSF sample blood stained (traumatic tap). Usually the staining clears in subsequent collection tubes, and a mildly traumatic tap will not affect protein or IgG analysis especially if the sample is centrifuged. A clear supernatant distinguishes a traumatic sample from blood staining due to sub-arachnoid haemorrhage, where the fluid is yellow tinged (xanthochromic) due to the presence of bile pigments.

CONDITIONS UNDER WHICH LUMBAR PUNCTURE IS NOT PERFORMED

- Depressed consciousness especially if focal neurological signs

- Papilloedema

Proceed to CT scan initially

Table 16.12   Screening tests for nerve and muscle disorders

Neuropathy	Myopathy
Full blood count, ESR	Full blood count, ESR
Urea, electrolytes, calcium, creatinine	Urea, electrolytes, calcium, phosphate
Serum lipoproteins	Urinary calcium
Liver function tests	Liver function tests
Blood glucose $\pm$ tolerance test	Plasma and urinary corticosteroids
Thyroxine and TSH	Thyroxine and TSH
Plasma protein electrophoresis Urinary Bence-Jones protein Urinary porphyrins	Creatine phosphokinase Lactate dehydrogenase

Blood vitamin assays:
  B$_{12}$, folic acid
  (thiamine, pyridoxine)
  (nicotinamide, vitamin E)
Toxic metals (e.g. Pb, Hg)
  in urine, blood, hair, nails.
Exclude drug intoxication
	Tests of energy metabolism
	  (e.g. lactate production)
	Tissue enzyme assays:
	  myophosphorylase
	  phosphofructokinase
	  acid maltase, carnitine,
	  carnitine-palmitoyl transferase

Serum autoantibodies:
  Antinuclear
  Double-stranded DNA
  Rheumatoid factor
	Serum autoantibodies:
	  Antinuclear
	  Double-stranded DNA
	  Rheumatoid factor
	  Acetylcholine receptor*

Nerve condution/EMG	Nerve conduction/EMG
Nerve biopsy	Muscle biopsy

Exclusion of malignancy and systemic disorders:
  Chest X-ray
  Faecal occult blood
  Abdominal ultrasound scan
	Exclusion of malignancy and systemic disorders:
	  Chest X-ray
	  Faecal occult blood
	  Abdominal ultrasound scan

* Myasthenia

Table 16.13   CSF parameters in health and some common disorders

	Normal	Subarachnoid haemorrhage	Pyogenic meningitis	Tuberculous meningitis	Viral meningitis	Multiple sclerosis
Pressure	50–180 mm CSF	Increased	Normal/ increased	Normal/ increased	Normal	Normal
Colour	Crystal clear	Blood stained xanthochromic	Cloudy	Clear/ cloudy	Clear	Clear
Cell count	0–4/mm³	Increased red blood cells	Polymorphs 1000–50 000	Lymphocytes 50–5000	Lympho. 10–2000	Lympho. 0–100
Glucose	2/3 blood level	Normal	Decreased	Decreased	Normal	Normal
Protein	<500 mg/l	Increased	Increased	Increased	Normal/ increased	Normal/ increased
IgG/total protein %	<13%	–	(Not routinely measured)			Increased
IgG index	<0.45	–	(Not routinely measured)			Increased
Oligoclonal IgG bands	Absent	–	(Not routinely measured)			Present
Microbiology	Sterile	Sterile	Organisms on Gram stain and culture	Organisms on ZN stain and culture	Sometimes viruses	Sterile

DISORDERS AFFECTING THE CRANIAL NERVES

Cranial nerves are often involved singly or in groups by intracranial disease and occasionally by generalised neuropathies or myopathies. Intracranial disease such as cerebral tumour may involve a cranial nerve directly (e.g. acoustic neurinoma) or may cause secondary dysfunction of the nerve by stretching it or compressing it against other structures (e.g. sixth nerve palsy secondary to tentorial herniation of mesial temporal lobe due to raised intracranial pressure).

I OLFACTORY NERVE

Nasal chemoreceptor fibres pass through the cribriform plate in the floor of the anterior cranial fossa and synapse in the olfactory bulb. Second order fibres pass along the olfactory tract, which lies on the floor of the anterior fossa under the frontal lobe, to the olfactory cortex in the anteromedial temporal lobe. Damage to the olfactory system may be bilateral (e.g. trauma and infection) or unilateral (e.g. frontal lobe tumour) (Table 16.14).

Table 16.14   Sites of damage to the olfactory pathway

Site	Example
Nasal mucosa	Upper respiratory infection
Cribriform plate	Head trauma
Olfactory tract	Frontal meningioma
Temporal lobe	Tumour or trauma

II THE OPTIC NERVE

The components of the visual system and the effects of lesions at various sites have been described above (pp. 822–3). Clinical testing of vision is summarised in the information box below.

TESTS OF VISION

Visual acuity
Distance (6 m chart)
Near (reading types)

Fields of vision
Confrontation
Perimetry

Colour vision
Ishihara plates

Pupil reflexes
Light
Accommodation

Ophthalmoscopy

Alterations in the appearance or reaction of the pupils occur for a variety of reasons (Table 16.15).

OPTIC DISC OEDEMA (PAPILLOEDEMA)

Optic disc oedema is recognised by swelling of the disc with blurring of its margins, often hyperaemia of the disc with loss of the normal central cup, and when acute, haemorrhages at the disc margins. The vessels on the disc become curved over its edges, the veins are engorged and cease to pulsate. The unifying mechanism for all forms of optic disc oedema is blockage of axonal transport in the optic nerve with swelling of its axons due to accumulation of sub-cellular organelles, which in turn results in capillary and venous congestion and further swelling of the disc (Fig. 16.23). Common causes of disc oedema are shown in the information box (p. 835).

OPTIC NEURITIS

Aetiology

This is usually an acute inflammatory disorder causing demyelination in the optic nerve near the disc (optic

Table 16.15   Types of pupil abnormality

Defect	Example	Appearance	Direct light response	Consensual response in other eye	Near response
Afferent	Optic neuritis	Normal/large	Impaired	Impaired	Normal
III nerve plasy	Cerebral aneurysm	Large	Impaired	Normal	Impaired
Myotonic (Adie's) pupil	Holmes-Adie syndrome	Small or large	Impaired	Normal	Normal with slow relaxation
Argyll-Robertson	Neurosyphilis	Small irregular	Impaired	Impaired (usually bilateral)	Normal
Horner's syndrome	Cervical sympathetic chain lesion	Small + ptosis	Normal	Normal	Normal

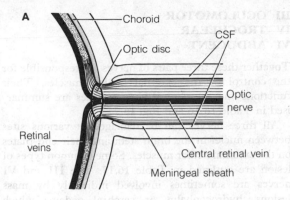

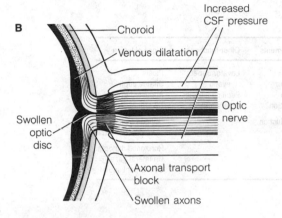

Fig. 16.23 Mechanism of optic disc oedema (papilloedema). **A.** Normal. **B.** Disc oedema (e.g. due to cerebral tumour).

COMMON CAUSES OF OPTIC DISC OEDEMA (PAPILLOEDEMA)

Raised intracranial pressure
Cerebral tumour, abscess
Hydrocephalus, oedema
Haemorrhage, haematoma

Obstruction of ocular venous drainage
Central retinal vein occlusion
Cavernous sinus thrombosis

Systemic disorders affecting retinal vessels
Hypertension
Vasculitis
Hypercapnia

Optic nerve damage
Demyelination (optic neuritis)
Ischaemia
Toxins (e.g. methanol)

Infiltration of optic disc
Sarcoidosis
Glioma
Lymphoma

few weeks, but some patients are left with impaired vision, especially for colour, and occasionally vision fails to improve. Ophthalmoscopy after recovery may show pallor of the optic disc, particularly on its temporal side. Other causes of optic nerve damage are given in the information box below.

CAUSES OF OPTIC NERVE DAMAGE

● Optic neuritis
● Compression in or behind orbit
   e.g. tumour, aneurysm
● Toxins
   Methyl alcohol, cyanide, chloroquine
● Direct trauma
   Head injury
● Increased intraocular pressure
   Glaucoma
● Ischaemia
   Atherosclerosis, giant cell arteritis
● Raised intracranial pressure
   Disc, oedema, secondary ischaemia

neuritis) or more posteriorly (retrobulbar neuritis). Some cases follow an acute viral infection, this form being seen especially in children when the disorder may be bilateral. More often in adults it is part of the spectrum of multiple sclerosis (MS), and more than 50% of patients who have had optic neuritis eventually develop MS.

Clinical features

The onset of symptoms is acute or sub-acute, often with pain in the eye especially on movement, and blurring of central vision. A central scotoma is frequently present, causing marked reduction in visual acuity; the direct pupil light reflex is impaired. If the inflammatory process is close to the optic nerve head, optic disc oedema (papillitis) is seen in the acute phase. The visual evoked potential is diminished and delayed or absent early on, but may return later with a delayed latency or altered waveform. Recovery is usual within a

OPTIC ATROPHY

This is the end result of many processes which damage the optic nerve. There is loss of axons with glial proliferation and decreased vascularity of the nerve head. The disc appears pale white or grey and has clear margins. The causes are listed in the information box below.

COMMON CAUSES OF OPTIC ATROPHY

- Previous optic neuritis, ischaemic or toxic damage
- Previous disc oedema from raised intracranial pressure
- Chronic optic nerve compression
- Chronic glaucoma
- Previous trauma
- Degenerative conditions
  e.g. Friedreich's ataxia

III OCULOMOTOR
IV TROCHLEAR
VI ABDUCENT

Together these three pairs of nerves are responsible for the control of the external ocular muscles. Their functions and the clinical abnormalities are summarised in Table 16.16 and Fig. 16.24.

All three nerves can be damaged at various sites between nuclei in the brain stem and their end-plates on the external ocular muscles. Some common types of lesion are outlined in Table 16.17. The III and VI nerves are sometimes involved indirectly by mass lesions, hydrocephalus or cerebral oedema which

Table 16.16   Cranial nerves III, IV and VI – clinical aspects

Nerve	Name	Muscles	Eye movements	Other functions	Signs of lesion
III	Oculomotor	Superior rectus Inferior rectus Medial rectus Inferior oblique	Elevation Depression Adduction Up/adduction	Levator upper eyelid Pupil constrictor Ciliary muscle	Ptosis Dilated pupil Abducted eye Divergent squint
IV	Trochlear	Superior oblique	Down/adduction	–	Oblique diplopia on down/in gaze
VI	Abducent	Lateral rectus	Abduction	–	Horizontal diplopia On lateral gaze Convergent squint

Table 16.17   Common lesions affecting cranial nerves III, IV and VI

Nerve	Site	Pathology	Clinical associations
III	Midbrain	Infarction Haemorrhage Demyelination	May or may not affect pupil; may be bilateral lesions; contralateral pyramidal signs
III	Circle of Willis	Aneurysm at origin of posterior communicating artery	Pupil involved early, headache over affected eye
III	Cavernous sinus	Int. carotid aneurysm Sinus thrombosis	VI and IV also often involved ± pain and proptosis of eye

III	Orbit	Infarction of nerve,
		  e.g. in diabetes; giant
		  cell arteritis
			Pupil often spared, may be painful or painless

IV	Cavernous sinus	Carotid aneurysm Thrombosis	Seldom involved alone, usually VI and III lesions also
IV	Orbit	Trauma	Dislocation from trochlea
IV	Orbital fissure	Tumour Granuloma	Pain in eye, III and VI likely to be involved ± ophthalmic branch of V
VI	Pons	Infarction Haemorrhage Demyelination	± associated facial weakness contralateral pyramidal signs
VI	Tentorial orifice	Compression Meningioma	May be secondary to raised intracranial pressure as false localising sign
VI	Cavernous sinus	Carotid aneurysm Thrombosis	± III and IV involvement
VI	Orbit	Infarction Tumour	May be secondary to diabetes or giant cell arteritis

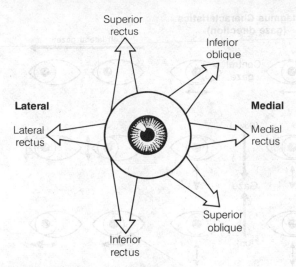

Fig. 16.24   External ocular muscle function.

stretch or compress the nerves against other structures; the cranial nerve palsies are then referred to as 'false-localising signs'.

SQUINT (STRABISMUS)

Squint occurs when the two eyes fail to move in a co-ordinated fashion. Diplopia results unless one eye has very poor vision or the defect has been of long-standing since childhood, when information from one eye becomes suppressed at cortical level (amblyopic eye). Squint may be paralytic or non-paralytic (concomitant).

Paralytic squint. This is due to weakness of one or more of the external ocular muscles because of lesions of the III, IV or VI nerves or of muscles disease (e.g. myasthenia gravis).

Non-paralytic or concomitant squint. This usually has onset in childhood, and is due to failure of

development of normal fixation reflexes. This is commonly due to refractive error or some other ocular defect, and provision of appropriate correcting lenses may prevent the squint form becoming permanent.

NYSTAGMUS

Nystagmus describes a series of rhythmical oscillations of one or both eyes. The movements may be horizontal, vertical or rotatory, and the oscillations may be equal in velocity and amplitude to either side (pendular) or may have a slow phase and a fast phase in opposite directions (phasic or jerk nystagmus) (Fig. 16.25). By convention, the direction of phasic nystagmus is denoted by its fast phase, and the movement is usually exaggerated on gaze to that side. The degree of phasic nystagmus can be graded from 1 to 3 and the causes are shown in Table 16.18.

Internuclear ophthalmoplegia
This curious disorder of eye movement is caused by lesions of the medial longitudinal fasciculus which links the sixth nerve nucleus in the pons with the third nerve nucleus in the midbrain. It causes disconjugation of lateral eye movements, especially during rapid changes of gaze, so that one eye is slow to adduct while the abducting eye shows coarse horizontal nystagmus ('ataxic nystagmus'). The disorder is frequently bilateral. Occasionally failure of full abduction with nystagmus in the adducting eye is seen. Often up-beating vertical nystagmus is present on up-gaze. The commonest cause is multiple sclerosis, but vascular disease, tumour, sarcoidosis and Wernicke's encephalopathy may be responsible.

Other forms of nystagmus

Ocular. Ocular fixation is poor when there is a defect of central vision and may result in nystagmus. The defect is often congenital and sometimes associ-

Table 16.18   Causes of phasic nystagmus

Site of lesion	Clinical features
Cerebellum	Horizontal nystagmus maximal on gaze to side of lesion
Vestibular apparatus or nerve	Horizontal or rotatory nystagmus maximal on gaze opposite to side of lesion (unless irritative lesion in labyrinth)
Mid-brain, superior colliculus	Vertical up-beating nystagmus evoked by upward gaze
Pons-midbrain, medial longitudinal fasciculus	'Ataxic' nystagmus most marked in abducting eye, associated with internuclear ophthalmoplegia, vertical up-beating nystagmus on up-gaze
Lower medulla	Down-beating nystagmus on downward or lateral gaze

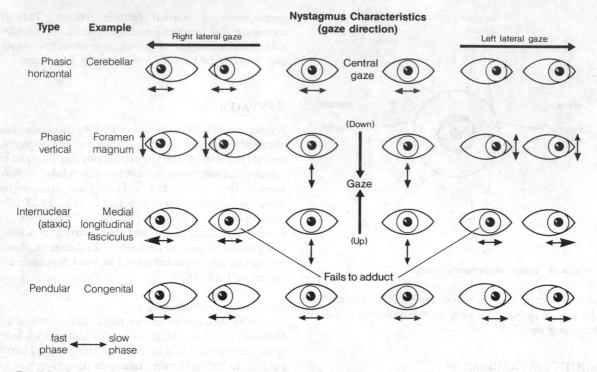

Fig. 16.25 Common types of nystagmus.

ated with head tilt and titubation. The nystagmus is pendular in type to central gaze but may become phasic on lateral gaze, and tends to diminish with convergence. Pendular nystagmus may occur also in diffuse brain-stem disease due to multiple sclerosis or tumours.

Positional. Nystagmus and usually vertigo may occur only in certain head positions. Two types of positional nystagmus are recognised.

Peripheral Type: in benign positional vertigo calcific degeneration in the utricle and saccule of the inner ear causes small particles to fall on to the cupola of the semicircular canals when the head is tilted back below the horizontal and turned with the affected ear lowermost. If the patient is put into this position, after a latent period of a few seconds, vertigo is experienced and rotational nystagmus can be observed. If the position is maintained, the vertigo and nystagmus abate usually within a minute. The condition may follow head injury, ear infection, and viral or vascular damage to the inner ear. Vestibular sedatives such as cinnarizine 15–30 mg t.i.d. or prochlorperazine 5–10 mg t.i.d. help suppress the symptoms which are troublesome when the patient lies down or turns over in bed.

Usually the disorder is self-limiting and settles after a few months.

Central type: lesions of the cerebellum or brain-stem vestibular connections may cause positional nystagmus.

V TRIGEMINAL

The trigeminal nerve has motor and sensory roots. The motor root supplies the muscles of mastication (Table 16.19).

LESIONS OF THE TRIGEMINAL SYSTEM

The cranial motor neurones of the motor root lie in the pons. The principal trigeminal sensory nucleus lies close by and relays common touch and position sense to the contralateral medial lemniscus and thence to the thalamus. Fibres serving pain and temperature descend in the tract of trigeminal nerve to the medulla and upper cervical region, where they synapse and cross the midline to join the spinothalamic tract. Lesions affecting the trigeminal sensory system may thus lie between the pons and the upper cervical spinal cord. Examples of lesions affecting the V nerve are listed in Table 16.20.

Table 16.19   Motor and sensory functions of the trigeminal nerve

Motor	Muscle	Function
	Masseter temporalis	Jaw closure
	Medial and lateral pterygoid	Jaw opening side–side movement

Sensory	Division	Name
	I	Ophthalmic
	II	Maxillary
	III	Mandibular
Areas of sensory supply	Skin of face	
	Cornea	
	Mucosa of sinuses	
	Mucosa of cheek	
	Teeth, gums	
	Typanic membrane	
	Anterior 2/3 of tongue	

TRIGEMINAL NEURALGIA

Aetiology
This condition affects mainly middle-aged and elderly people. Occasionally younger patients suffering from multiple sclerosis develop similar symptoms. It was for many years regarded as idiopathic, but recent evidence suggests that in many patients an aberrant loop of artery is pressing on the trigeminal rootlets as they emerge from the pons.

Clinical features
Paroxysms of sharp lancinating pain radiating into the territory of one or more of the trigeminal sensory divisions are characteristic. The pain is often set off by touching or washing the face, shaving, tooth cleaning, eating, talking and exposure to cold. The II and III divisions are usually affected first, but the condition may spread to involve all three. Paroxysms of pain last only a few seconds, but may be repetitive or be followed by a dull ache. In its early course the disorder may show spontaneous remissions lasting weeks or months.

There are usually no abnormal motor or sensory signs of trigeminal nerve dysfunction, with the exception of finding localised trigger spots which set off pain when touched. If clinical abnormalities are present, the diagnosis is more likely to be of structural disease such as multiple sclerosis, meningioma, aneurysm or neurinoma.

Management
Membrane-stabilising drugs such as carbamazepine or phenytoin should be tried first. With carbamazepine sedative side-effects should be avoided by starting with a small dose (100 mg once daily or b.d.) and increasing gradually to 200–400 mg t.i.d. over the course of 2–3 weeks, aiming for a plasma level of 30–50 µmol/l. Slow introduction is not needed with phenytoin, but patients have differing tolerance within the range 150–500 mg/d; an average dose being 300 mg/d. Plasma level monitoring should be used to achieve about 40–80 µmol/l. Clonazepam 0.5–2 mg t.i.d. is sometimes effective.

Various surgical procedures can be considered if drug treatment proves ineffective, or its side-effects intolerable. These range from injection of the trigeminal ganglion with phenol or alcohol, radiofrequency thermocoagulation of a branch of the ganglion, intracranial section of the trigeminal sensory root, and microvascular decompression procedures. The latter are theoretically the most attractive, but may be too hazardous in an elderly patient. Phenol injection or thermocoagulation can be carried out percutaneously and at low risk, but have the disadvantage of giving only temporary relief lasting weeks or months.

Table 16.20   Lesions affecting the trigeminal system

Site	Example	Clinical features
Pons	Infarction, demyelination	Motor and sensory function impaired corneal and jaw flexes diminished
Medulla	Infarction, syrinx	Loss of pain and temperature sensation on face
Semi-lunar ganglion	Meningioma Aneurysm	All 3 sensory divisions may be involved
Cavernous sinus	Aneurysm Thrombosis	Ophthalmic division affected, corneal reflex impaired
Maxillary sinus	Antral carcinoma	Maxillary division affected
Infratemporal fossa	Nasopharyngeal carcinoma	Mostly mandibular division, sensory and motor involvement

VII FACIAL

The chief function of the facial nerve is the supply of motor fibres to the muscles of facial expression. The facial motor neurones lie in the ventral part of the pontine tegmentum, their fibres looping around the sixth nerve nucleus before emerging from the lateral aspect of the pons. This portion of the nerve enters the internal auditory meatus at the cerebello-pontine angle, along with the acoustic nerve (VIII) and the nervus intermedius. The latter contains parasympathetic fibres concerned with salivation and lacrimation; at the geniculate ganglion it receives sensory fibres for taste on the anterior 2/3 of the tongue from the chorda tympani. A small sensory component serves cutaneous sensation on the external ear. As it passes through the petrous temporal bone, the facial nerve sends a small motor branch to the stapedius muscle (Tables 16.21 and 16.22).

IDIOPATHIC (BELL'S) PALSY

Bell's palsy is a common condition affecting patients of all ages and sex. The cause is unknown; viral infection, vascular damage, trauma, and cold exposure have all been implicated. The site of damage is probably the labyrinthine portion of the facial nerve within the facial canal. Swelling of the nerve at this site has been observed, and may be responsible for the initial loss of nerve impulse conduction leading to facial paralysis.

Clinical features
The onset is subacute with symptoms coming on over a few hours or overnight. There may be pain in the face and around the ear before the patient or their family notice loss of movement on one side of the face. Sometimes patients describe the face as being numb, but objective evidence of loss of sensation (except taste) is lacking. The chorda tympani fibres are often affected so that taste is impaired on the anterior 2/3 of the

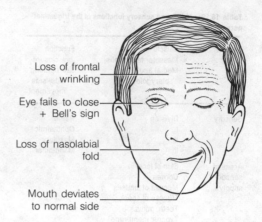

Fig. 16.26 Lesion of facial nerve or nucleus (lower motor neurone).

tongue, and occasionally the tongue tingles on the affected side. Hyperaccusis occurs if the nerve to stapedius is involved. More severe lesions cause loss of salivation and tear secretion.

Examination reveals weakness or paralysis of the

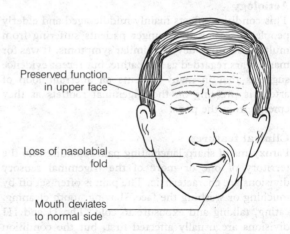

Fig. 16.27 Lesion of precentral area or pyramidal tract (upper motor neurone).

Table 16.21 Functional components of the facial nerve

Component	Connections	Function/supply
Somatic motor	VII nucleus in pons: facial nerve	Muscles of facial expression +stapedius
Visceral efferent parasympathetic	Superior salivary nucleus: nervus intermedius	Lacrimal gland, submandibular and sublingual salivary glands
Special afferent (taste)	Lingual nerve, chorda tympani, geniculate ganglion, nervus intermedius, tractus solitarius	Taste sensation on anterior 2/3 of tongue
Somatic afferent	Geniculate ganglion	Cutaneous sensation to external ear

Table 16.22 Causes of facial weakness

Site	Examples	Clinical features
Cortex	Cerebral infarction Haemorrhage Tumour	Contralateral facial weakness mainly of lower face often associated hemiparesis
Pons (nuclear)	Infarction Demyelination Haemorrhage Tumour	All parts of ipsilateral face weak; often VI nerve affected $\pm$ contralateral hemiparesis
Cerebello-pontine angle	Acoustic neurinoma Meningioma	All parts of face affected + deafness and tinnitus $\pm$ trigeminal nerve
Facial canal (petrous bone)	Bell's palsy Mastoiditis Herpes zoster	All parts of face affected $\pm$ loss of taste, salivation and lacrimation, hyperacusis if stapedius weak
Parotid gland	Tumour Sarcoidosis	Selective weakness of parts of face due to branch involvement
Neuromuscular junction	Myasthenia gravis	Associated ptosis and external ophthalmoplegia, dysphagia, dysarthria, $\pm$ limb weakness
Muscles	Muscular dystrophy Myositis	Limb muscles also weak

facial muscles on one side, with failure of eye closure and visible upward deviation of the eye as this is attempted (Bell's sign). The mouth is drawn over to the normal side and saliva may drool from it. The tongue may appear to deviate to the normal side, but this is usually due to distortion of the mouth and not hypoglossal weakness. A degree of dysarthria often accompanies the facial weakness.

Management
About 70–80% of patients with Bell's palsy recover spontaneously within 2–12 weeks. A short course of dexamethasone 2 mg t.i.d. for 5 days is worthwhile if the patient is seen within 48 hours of the onset. There is some evidence that this reduces oedema of the facial nerve, and may limit damage and speed recovery. The patient should wear a pad over the eye if eye closure is affected, especially during sleep, to protect the cornea.

Surgical decompression of the nerve in the facial canal is advocated by some, but since most patients recover well without interference, and there is no good way of predicting poor outcome during the first few days of the condition (when surgery might be most helpful), the indications for operation are unclear.

Prognosis
Elderly patients with complete facial paralysis tend to have the worst prognosis. Slower or incomplete recovery can be predicted if facial EMG studies show marked reduction in the amplitude of evoked facial muscle action potentials after the first week. Preservation of the response and a measurable blink reflex are good prognostic signs. With a severe palsy, axonal

degeneration occurs and recovery is slower and less complete. Aberrant reinnervation may take place, so that unwanted facial movements occur (e.g. the eye may close when the mouth is moved), sometimes adding to the disfigurement.

CLONAL FACIAL (HEMIFACIAL) SPASM
This disorder presents mostly after middle age.

Clinical features
Symptoms usually start with intermittent twitching around one eye. Over the course of months or years, clonic twitches increase in frequency and severity so that the eye may close for a few seconds at a time, and gradually the movements begin to affect the lower face. The spasms are intermittent, sometimes being more prominent during talking and eating or when the patient is under stress. Occasionally sufferers report transient dulling of hearing on the affected side during a facial spasm – presumably due to stapedius contraction. Examination reveals, in addition to the spasms, mild weakness of the affected musculature.

Investigation
Facial nerve conduction studies are usually normal or show only minor defects of distal conduction and the blink reflex. EMG recording shows bursts of rapid motor unit firing during the spasms, with periods of silence interposed. The pathophysiology is now believed to be due to an aberrant loop of artery irritating the facial nerve as it emerges from the pons – similar to

the mechanism postulated for trigeminal neuralgia (see above).

Management

Treatment with carbamazepine or phenytoin as for trigeminal neuralgia may help reduce the frequency and severity of the spasms, but is often disappointing. If the disorder is severe and disfiguring, posterior fossa exploration and microvascular decompression may be justifiable, but the risks of this in an elderly patient must be balanced against the benign nature of the condition. Injections of botinulinum toxin into the affected muscles may control symptoms for several months, and is becoming an established treatment.

VIII   VESTIBULO-COCHLEAR

The eighth cranial nerve transmits special sensory information from the vestibular system (head position and movement) and the cochlea (hearing). From the sensors in the inner ear the VIII nerve fibres pass through the internal auditory meatus, emerge at the cerebello-pontine angle and enter the brain stem at the ponto-medullary junction where they synapse in the vestibular and cochlear nuclei. Vestibular information is passed to the cerebellum, reticular formation, spinal motor neurones and oculomotor nuclei. Much of this information is involved with reflex control of head, eye and body posture but some of it reaches consciousness by a pathway to the superior temporal lobe. Auditory

signals are relayed to the temporal lobe via the lateral lemniscus (Table 16.23).

VERTIGO

This is an hallucination of movement of either the body (or part of it) or the surroundings. The perceived movement may be of falling or rotating or a sensation that the outside world is spinning; sometimes the vertigo is so intense that the sufferer falls to the gound. Vertigo of labyrinthine origin is often marked, and accompanied by nausea, vomiting, oscillopsia, pallor and occasionally syncope. It is important to establish whether the patient is describing true vertigo, or less precise feelings of imbalance or light headedness; the latter are less likely to be of vestibular origin. Table 16.24 lists the main causes of vertigo together with the site of lesion and relevant clinical features.

DEAFNESS

Deafness is often accompanied by tinnitus, especially when the lesion lies in the cochlea or auditory nerve. Blockage of the external auditory meatus or damage to the ear drum ossicular chain cause *conductive deafness*. Normally hearing through air transmission via the drum and ossicles is more efficient than conduction of vibration by bone; this difference is reversed in conductive deafness. *Sensorineural deafness* is due either to disease of the cochlea or the auditory fibres in

Table 16.23   Components, symptoms and signs of lesions affecting the VIII cranial nerve

Component	Sensors	Parameter	Symptoms of lesion	Signs of lesion
Vestibular	Utricle saccule	Head position	Vertigo Loss of balance Oscillopsia Nausea Vomiting Faintness	Poor balance Nystagmus Positional Vertigo and Nystagmus
	Semi-circular canals	Head movement		
Cochlear	Spiral hair cells	Hearing	Deafness Tinnitus	Sensori-neural Deafness

Table 16.24   Types of lesion causing vertigo

Site of lesion	Example	Clinical features
Labyrinth	Ménière's disease	Vertigo, deafness, tinnitus
VIII nerve	Acoustic neuroma	Deafness, tinnitus, vertigo, trigeminal and cerebellar signs
Vestibular neurones	Vertebral artery ischaemia	Vertigo, ataxia, diplopia, syncope, dysarthria
Cerebellum	Tumour, infarct	Vertigo, ataxia, dysarthria
Temporal lobe	Epilepsy Tumour	Vertigo accompanying seizures

Table 16.25   Common causes of deafness and their features

Type of deafness	Site of lesion	Example	Clinical features
Conductive	External meatus	Wax	Air conduction < bone conduction Weber's test → deaf ear
Conductive	Ear drum	Otitis media	Pain in ear, fever
Conductive	Ossicular chain	Otosclerosis	Progressive deafness; tinnitus
Sensorineural	Cochlea	Ménière's disease	Mid-low tone deafness, loudness recruitment, tinnitus, vertigo
Sensorineural	Cochlea	Noise induced	'Notch' pattern deafness for specific frequencies
Sensorineural	Cochlea	Senile	Deaf mainly for higher frequencies
Sensorineural	VIII nerve	Acoustic neuroma	Deafness, tinnitus, air conduction > bone conduction, Weber's test → normal ear

the VIII nerve and its connections in the brain stem. Both air and bone conduction hearing are affected, and tinnitus is often present. Common causes of deafness and tinnitus are listed in Table 16.25.

MÉNIÈRE'S DISEASE

Aetiology
This is a disorder of the inner ear in which there is excessive pressure and dilatation of the endolymphatic system. This results in damage to both the vestibular and cochlear sense organs. The cause is unknown, although there is some overlap with other functional vasospastic disorders such as migraine.

Clinical symptoms
Symptoms rarely start before middle age; the patient suffers from recurrent bouts of profound vertigo, nausea and vomiting associated with deafness (especially for middle and low frequencies) and tinnitus. Acute attacks may be preceded by discomfort in one ear, and increasing tinnitus and deafness. The attack usually lasts several hours or a day, and is accompanied by prostration, pallor, vomiting, nystagmus and occasionally by syncope. Deafness and tinnitus tend to persist between attacks and sensorineural mid-low frequency hearing loss with loudness recruitment may be found on audiometry. Caloric tests show impaired vestibular function on the affected side.

Management
Bed rest and administration of vestibular sedatives are required during acute attacks. Cinnarizine (15–30 mg t.i.d.) or prochlorperazine (5–10 mg t.i.d.) help suppress vertigo and vomiting. In more severe attacks, intramuscular injection of prochlorperazine 12.5 mg or cyclizine 50 mg may be required. Some authorities also give intravenous diuretics (frusemide 40 mg i.v.) to try

to reduce the endolymphatic pressure. Prophylaxis from recurrent episodes is sometimes effective with vasodilators such as betahistine (8 mg t.i.d.), but if disabling attacks continue or hearing deteriorates progressively, surgical endolymph drainage may be necessary.

VESTIBULAR NEURONITIS

This a common disorder affecting mainly young adults. The aetiology is presumed to be due to viral infection, and it occasionally occurs in small epidemics.

Clinical features
There is usually a degree of systemic illness with fever, malaise, myalgia and gastrointestinal upset, suggesting that enteric viruses may be implicated. Vertigo, often with a marked positional element, accompanies the acute illness and may persist for days or several weeks, and sometimes relapses occur. Nystagmus is present in the acute phase, but there is no disturbance of hearing. Caloric tests may show impaired vestibular function on one or both sides.

Management
Treatment is with bed rest and vestibular sedatives as for Ménière's disease (see above). Recovery in a few weeks is usual, but sometimes symptoms persist with positional vertigo for several months, and there is some overlap with the post-viral fatigue syndrome (myalgic encephalomyelitis).

ACOUSTIC NEUROMA (NEURILEMMOMA)

This is a benign tumour arising from the covering tissues of the VIII nerve. The tumour usually starts in the internal auditory meatus and expands towards the cerebello-pontine angle, where it may involve the V

Table 16.26 Components of the lower cranial nerves IX, X and XI

Nerve	Component	Nucleus	Functional supply
IX	Motor	Nucleus ambiguus	Stylopharyngeus
	Secretory	Inferior salivary nucleus	Parotid gland
	Sensory	Tractus solitarius	Common touch and taste for posterior 1/3 tongue, soft palate, tonsil, eardrum
X	Motor	Nucleus ambiguus	Palate, pharynx and larynx, heart, lungs,
	Parasympathetic	Dorsal vagal nucleus	abdominal viscera
	Sensory	Spinal tract of V	dura, ear, pharynx, soft palate
XI	Motor	Nucleus ambiguus (medullary portion)	Pharynx and larynx via X
		C1–5 anterior horn cells (spinal portion)	Trapezius, sternomastoid

Table 16.27 Causes and features of lesions to cranial nerves IX, X and XI

Site	Causes	Clinical features
IX/X nuclei (medulla)	Infarction Syringobulbia Tumour Demyelination	Nasal voice, palatal weakness, absent gag reflex, impaired sensation posterior 1/3 tongue and pharyngeal wall, laryngeal stridor, bovine cough
Jugular foramen	Glomus tumour Metastatic tumour Meningioma	As above + spinal accessory nerve affected: weakness trapezius and sternomastoid
Diffuse lesions	Polyneuritis Guillain-Barré syndrome Motor neurone disease Myasthenia gravis	Usually bilateral involvement No sensory deficit
Supra-nuclear (cortex, pyramidal tract)	Stroke Cerebral tumour Demyelination Motor neurone disease	Unilateral lesions do not cause persisting deficit (bilateral supply); bilateral lesions cause loss of coordination of pharynx and palate, brisk gag reflex (pseudobulbar palsy)
XI nucleus	As for IX, X	Same functions as IX and X
XI jugular foramen	Glomus tumour, etc.	Weakness of sternomastoid and trapezius
Supra-nuclear IX	Stroke etc., as for IX, X	Slowness and weakness of contralateral trapezius, but ipsilateral sternomastoid

and VII nerves, the cerebellum and the brain stem. Bilateral acoustic neuromas may occur in neurofibromatosis type II.

Clinical features
Early symptoms are unilateral deafness and tinnitus and insidious vertigo. Larger lesions cause facial numbness and weakness, ataxia and features of raised intracranial pressure. Examination reveals unilateral sensorineural deafness, and sometimes phasic nystagmus intially on looking away from the lesion. Later on, as the tumour invades the cerebello-pontine angle, the nystagmus is of cerebellar origin and most marked on gaze towards the lesion. Facial numbness, and weakness, loss of the corneal reflex and onset of cerebellar and pyramidal tract sign are late features.

Investigation
Diagnosis at an early stage rests on demonstration of unilateral sensorineural deafness and impaired caloric vestibular function on the same side. A delayed or absent auditory evoked potential may be helpful at this stage. Plain radiographs or tomograms of the internal auditory meati may show enlargement or erosion of the canal. Larger tumours may be demonstrated by contrast enhanced CT scanning, but for small lesions air-CT meatography or high quality MRI scanning are more reliable.

Management
The results of surgical treatment are optimal when the tumour is still within the internal auditory meatus. Deafness and facial weakness may result, but long-term

prognosis is good if complete removal of the lesion is achieved.

IX GLOSSOPHARYNGEAL
X VAGUS
XI SPINAL ACCESSORY

These nerves are grouped together because they all pass through the jugular foramen at the skull base, and tend to be affected as a group. Their cells or origin lie in the medulla oblongata (XI, X) and the upper cervical cord (XI), their roots emerging adjacent to one another. Their main functional components are shown in Table 16.26.

Isolated lesions of IX and X are very rare, usually they are affected together. Lesions at the jugular foramen tend to affect IX, X and XI simultaneously. Common examples of disorders of these nerves are listed in Table 16.27.

XII HYPOGLOSSAL

The hypoglossal nerve supplies motor fibres to the intrinsic and extrinsic muscles of the tongue. The hypoglossal nuclei lie in the medulla near to the midline beneath the floor of the IV ventricle. The nerves leave

Table 16.28 Causes of lesions of the hypoglossal nerve

Site	Causes
XII nucleus	Infarction
	Syringobulbia
	Tumour
	Motor neurone disease
Skull base	Metastatic tumour
	Meningioma
	Vertebral aneurysm
	Cranio-vertebral anomalies (e.g. basilar impression)
Neck	Trauma
	Surgery (e.g. carotid endarterectomy)

the medulla on its ventral aspect and pass through the hypoglossal canal at the skull base and cross the carotid vessels on their way to the tongue.

BULBAR AND PSEUDOBULBAR PALSY

Lesions of cranial nerves IX, X, XI, and XII often occur together, frequently because of vascular disease affecting the medulla. The resultant palatal, pharyngeal and tongue weakness causing dysphonia, dysphagia and dysarthria is known as 'bulbar palsy'. Bilateral supra-nuclear lesions affecting the pyramidal tracts (e.g. due to diffuse vascular disease, motor neurone disease, multiple sclerosis) cause loss of voluntary palatal and pharyngeal movements, but the gag reflex is preserved. The tongue is small (spastic) and shows poor rapid movement, this resulting in indistinct speech (spastic dysarthria). The jaw jerk is brisk. This state is known as 'pseudobulbar palsy'.

CEREBRAL TUMOURS

Cerebral tumours account for 2% of deaths at all ages. The majority are benign or malignant neoplasms arising from cellular components within the central nervous system, with metastatic tumours from systemic malignancies largely accounting for the remainder. Malignant brain tumours rarely give rise to extracerebral metastases and the clinical features and prognosis depend on the anatomical localisation and histological characteristics of the lesion.

PATHOLOGY

Primary intracerebral tumours are classified by their cell of origin and degree of malignancy, and vary in incidence by age and localisation (Table 16.29). Cerebral metastases usually occur in the white matter

Table 16.29 Malignant intracranial tumours

Histological type	Common site	Malignancy	Age
Glioma (astrocytoma)	Cerebral hemisphere	+-+-++++	Adult
	Cerebellum	+-++	Childhood
		++-+++	Adult
	Brain stem	+-++	Childhood/adolescence
Oligodendroglioma	Cerebral hemisphere	++-+++	Adult
Medulloblastoma	Posterior fossa	+++-+++++	Childhood
Ependymoma	Posterior fossa	+++-+++++	Childhood/adolescence
Microglioma (cerebral lymphoma)	Cerebral hemisphere	++-+++	Adult

+-+++ Relatively benign–highly malignant

Table 16.30 Benign intracranial tumours

Histological type	Common site	Age
Meningioma	Cortical dura Parasagittal Sphenoid ridge Suprasellar Olfactory groove	Adult
Neurofibroma	Acoustic neuroma	Adult
Craniopharyngioma	Suprasellar	Childhood/adolescence
Pituitary adenoma	Pituitary fossa	Adult
Colloid cyst	Third ventricle	Any age

of the cerebral or cerebellar hemispheres and common primary sites are bronchus, breast, and gastrointestinal tract.

Benign intracranial tumours are slow growing but may cause disability and death by impinging on and displacing the intracranial contents. The commoner histological types are listed in Table 16.30. Cerebral lesions resembling tumours also occur in sarcoidosis, cystercercosis, echinococcosis (as hydatid cysts), and schistosomiasis. Tuberculoma is common in Third World countries.

Meningiomas account for about a fifth of intracranial tumours. Intraventricular tumours, including colloid cysts of the third ventricle and choroid plexus papilloma are rare but can cause an acute rise in intracranial pressure and sudden death.

Clinical features
The clinical features of an intracranial tumour relate to the site of the tumour and its rate of expansion. Symptoms and signs are produced by a number of mechanisms which are listed in the information box below.

CLINICAL FEATURES OF CEREBRAL TUMOURS

- Local effects on adjacent cerebral tissue
- Raised intracranial pressure
- Epilepsy
- False localising signs

Local effects
In general the focal disabilities produced by a cerebral tumour are of slow onset and progressive. Tumours may present at an early stage in areas of the brain, such as the brain stem, where structural disturbance quickly results in a neurological deficit. In other regions, including the frontal lobe, the tumour may attain a large size before clinical evidence of a structural lesion is evident. The clinical features of dysfunction in the various lobes of the brain are outlined on page 824 (Fig. 16.12).

Occasionally localised oedema in the brain tissue surrounding a tumour will cause a rapid progression of symptoms and, rarely, haemorrhage into a tumour causes an acute presentation resembling a stroke.

Raised intracranial pressure
This may be caused by the tumour mass, reactive cerebral oedema or obstruction of cerebrospinal fluid pathways. The major features are:

Headache. This is a common but not invariable manifestation of cerebral tumour. Pain may be caused by distortion of or traction on nearby arteries, venous sinuses or meninges which are pain sensitive structures. The localisation of the headache does not generally correlate with the site of the tumour although posterior fossa tumours often cause pain in the occiput or nuchal area.

Headache due to raised intracranial pressure is felt diffusely over the cranium and may be aggravated by manoeuvres which further increase the intracranial pressure, including coughing, bending and straining. Typically the headache is most severe in the morning and may disturb sleep, although as intracranial pressure rises the pain becomes more constant.

Impairment of conscious level. This ranges from listlessness and drowsiness to coma and is related to the level of intracranial pressure. Cerebral tumours occupy space within the rigid skull but compensatory mechanisms involving alteration in the volulme of fluid in cerebrospinal fluid spaces and venous sinuses may delay the development of raised pressure. Benign tumours may thereby attain a large size before causing a rise in intracranial pressure, but raised pressure develops early in rapidly expanding tumours or even acutely if the cerebrospinal circulation is obstructed by, for example, posterior fossa masses or intraventricular tumours. Raised intracranial pressure may also cause personality change including apathy, irritability, withdrawal and inattention.

Papilloedema. This is a significant but not invariable sign of raised intracranial pressure and may develop acutely or insidiously. Swelling of the optic nerve head may be accompanied by haemorrhages in the optic disc, but often causes little subjective visual disturbance. Perimetry may reveal peripheral constriction of the visual field or enlargement of the blind spot, but visual acuity is usually preserved. Rarely acute blurring of vision or transient blindness precipitated by postural change (visual obscurations) may be an early feature and indicates severely raised intracranial pressure. Papilloedema progresses in parallel to the level of intracranial pressure and eventually results in visual failure due to extensive retinal haemorrhage or secondary optic atrophy. Rarely, but significantly, papilloedema may not develop in raised intracranial pressure, particularly if this is of acute onset as may occur in obstruction of cerebrospinal fluid pathways.

Vomiting, bradycardia, arterial hypertension. These develop as the intracranial pressure continues to rise. These features usually parallel the other clinical signs, but sudden vomiting may be an early feature of tumours of the cerebellar hemisphere.

Epilepsy
Infiltration by tumour cells of an area of cerebral cortex often invokes excitatory responses in neighbouring neurones and may result in an epileptic focus. The resulting seizures may be generalised or focal in nature, and the development of focal motor or sensory seizures in adult life should always suggest the possibility of a tumour.

False localising signs
The rise in intracranial pressure may not be uniform within the cerebral substance and sudden alterations in pressure relationships within the skull may lead to displacement of parts of the brain. Downward displacement of the temporal lobes due to a large hemisphere mass may result in stretching of the third and sixth cranial nerves, or pressure on the contralateral cerebral peduncle may result in ipsilateral upper motor neurone

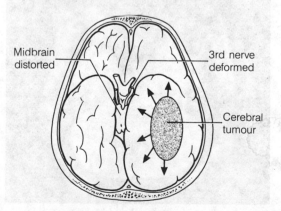

Fig. 16.28 Cerebral tumour of the medial part of the temporal lobe causing distortion of the midbrain, and the third nerve.

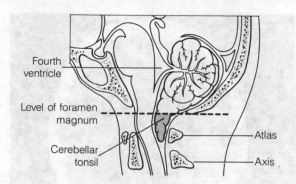

Fig. 16.29 Downward displacement of the cerebellar tonsils below the level of the foramen magnum. The shaded area represents the position of the cerebellum that is displaced.

signs (Fig. 16.28). Another form of displacement is the downward movement of the cerebellar tonsils so that they impact within the foramen magnum thus compressing the medulla (Fig. 16.29). This 'coning' may result in brain-stem haemorrhage or acute obstruction of the cerebrospinal fluid pathways and is often associated with loss of consciousness and paresis of the sixth and third cranial nerves, with dilatation of the pupil on the side of the lesion. The patient may adopt a decerebrate posture and death almost invariably ensues. This type of brain displacement may occur spontaneously in relation to critical levels of intracranial pressure, but is particularly likely to develop if the pressure dynamics are disturbed by lumbar puncture.

Investigation
Investigation for cerebral tumour should be considered in any patient presenting with the recent onset of progressive neurological dysfunction, symptoms or signs suggestive of raised intracranial pressure, or who develops epilepsy over the age of eighteen. Coma as a presenting feature is rare with the exception of intraventricular tumours which may suddenly obstruct cerebrospinal fluid pathways.

CT head scan is the definitive investigation for cerebral tumour, allowing accurate localisation of the lesion and providing some guidance as to the likely histological type (Fig. 16.30). Distortion of intracranial structures and the size of the ventricular system may also be assessed and high definition views or computerised reconstruction of the images may provide accurate evaluation of the extent of the tumour. Plain skull X-rays are rarely of diagnostic value with the exception of pituitary tumours and neoplasms which calcify, such as oligodendroglioma and craniopharyngioma. Chest X-ray is an important investigation and may provide evidence of a pulmonary tumour or other systemic

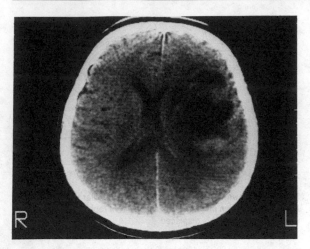

Fig. 16.30   CT scan of cerebral glioma. There is an irregular area of low density in the left cerebral hemisphere with surrounding oedema and shift of midline structures to the right. (Courtesy of Dr R.J. Sellar.)

malignancy. Cerebral angiography provides information on the vascularity of the tumour and may be important if surgery is planned. Magnetic resonance imaging is of particular value in the investigation of tumours of the posterior fossa and brain stem, areas in which the CT scan has a relatively poor resolution (Fig. 16.31).

Management

Medical

The medical management of cerbral tumours can never be anything more than temporary or palliative. Relief of raised intracranial pressure is often required when surgery is not possible or when life is threatened before investigation has revealed the diagnosis. The main therapeutic agent used to lower intracranial pressure is dexamethasone, 4 mg 4 times daily either orally or by injection. A striking improvement in conscious level is often produced and focal disabilities may regress. In severe and acutely raised intracranial pressure 16–20 mg of dexamethasone may be given intravenously or 200 ml of a 20% solution of the osmotic agent mannitol may be infused. These treatments provide only a temporary decrease in intracranial pressure and neurosurgical advice should be urgently considered.

Surgical

Surgery is the mainstay of treatment, although only partial excision may be possible if the tumour is inaccessible or if its exposure is likely to cause

unacceptable brain damage. Tumours may invade areas of the brain where excision of small amounts of tissue is likely to cause major disability. The accurate diagnosis of an intracranial lesion does however have important implications for management and prognosis and biopsy by direct or stereotactic technique should be considered even if the tumour cannot be removed.

Meningiomas and acoustic neuromas offer the best prospects for complete removal without unacceptable damage to surrounding structures. Meningiomas of the olfactory groove, suprasellar area and the convexity of the cerebral hemisphere only rarely recur, while those of the sphenoid ridge can often only be partially excised although recurrence is commonly delayed for many years. Craniopharyngiomas and colloid cysts are technically more difficult to remove in their entirety and, in common with other benign tumours, the possibility of complete excision depends on early diagnosis. Pituitary adenomas can be extirpated and surgery can often be performed by a trans-sphenoidal route, thus avoiding the necessity for a craniotomy. Prolactin or growth hormone secreting tumours may respond to a medical treatment with bromocriptine.

Prognosis

Gliomas can rarely to excised and infiltration may spread beyond the radiologically evident boundaries of the tumour. Recurrence is common even if the mass of the tumour is apparently removed, although survival in some cases may be prolonged for several years. Partial excision may be useful in alleviating raised intracranial pressure, but survival in highly malignant gliomas

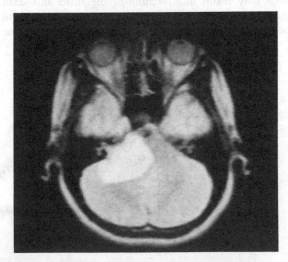

Fig. 16.31   MRI scan showing a large right acoustic neuroma distorting the cerebellum and brain stem. (Courtesy of Dr R. Grant.)

(glioblastoma multiforme) is measured in months even if such a decompressive procedure is attempted.

Ependymomas and medulloblastomas may be excised with minimal residual disability, but often recur with seeding of the tumour via the cerebrospinal fluid. Oligodendrogliomas are often slowly growing and relatively benign in the early stages, but may transform to a more malignant form and behave as gliomas.

Some tumours, including ependymoma and microglioma, are radiosensitive and chemotherapy prolongs survival in medulloblastoma, but the prognosis in malignant glioma is only marginally prolonged by either radiotherapy or chemotherapy.

The prognosis in benign tumours is good provided complete surgical excision can be achieved.

HYDROCEPHALUS

Hydrocephalus (dilatation of the ventricular system) may be due to obstruction of the cerebrospinal fluid circulation or failure of absorption of cerebrospinal fluid by the arachnoid villi, which lie in the parasagittal region (Fig. 16.32). Obstruction may occur anywhere within the ventricular system, but is most common in the narrow channels in the third ventricle, aqueduct and fourth ventricle and may be caused by tumour or a congenital anomaly such as aqueduct stenosis. Impairment of cerebrospinal fluid absorption may follow meningitis, head injury, subarachnoid haemorrhage or sagittal sinus thrombosis.

In 'normal pressure' hydrocephalus the dilatation of the ventricular system is caused by intermittent rises in cerebrospinal fluid pressure, which occur particularly at night. The condition occurs predominantly in old age and the characteristic clinical features are dementia, ataxia of gait and incontinence.

Diversion of the cerebrospinal fluid by means of a shunt procedure between the ventricular system and the peritoneal cavity or right atrium may result in a prompt relief of symptoms in obstructive or communicating hydrocephalus, but the result is less predictable in 'normal pressure' hydrocephalus.

HEADACHE AND FACIAL PAIN

Custom usually restricts the term headache to describe pains in the region of the cranial vault, while pain in the maxillary and mandibular regions may be classified as facial pain. Although the lines of demarcation are often vague, headache and facial pain are considered separately.

HEADACHE

Headache is one of the most common and difficult clinical problems in medicine. In the majority of patients, the cause is trivial and reversible and a careful clinical history and examination often allows a specific diagnosis thereby avoiding unnecessary investigation. Headache may presage serious intracranial disease, but the clinical features of raised intracranial pressure or meningitis can usually be distinguished from those of the more common forms of headache.

Pain in the head may be due to lesions in nearby structures such as the eye and ear causing referred headache, it may be due to meningeal irritation, vascular disturbance, traction and distortion of intracranial structures, or to psychogenic causes. The clinical features of the commoner causes of headaches are listed in Table 16.31. Headache of raised intracranial pressure due to a mass lesion is described on page 846.

BENIGN INTRACRANIAL HYPERTENSION

This is a rare condition, usually occurring in obese

Table 16.31   Clinical features in headache

Cause	Site	Duration	Character	Associations
Tension	Generalised/nuchal	Constant	Dull, tight pressure	Local tenderness, anxiety/depression
Migraine	Unilateral/bitemporal	Episodic	Aching, throbbing	Prostration, nausea, vomiting, photophobia, visual features
Temporal arteritis	Temporal	Constant (nocturnal)	Burning	Scalp tenderness, jaw claudication, malaise
Meningitis	Generalised/nuchal	Acute progressive	Throbbing	Meningism, pyrexia
Raised pressure	Generalised	Progressive	Throbbing	Papilloedema, drowsiness, vomiting

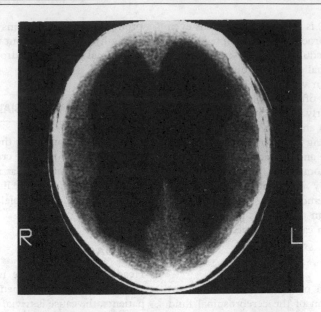

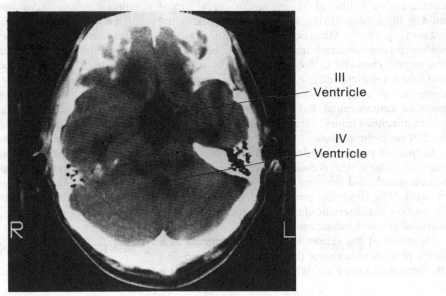

III
Ventricle

IV
Ventricle

Fig. 16.32 CT scan in hydrocephalus. A. There is a marked enlargement of the lateral ventricles. **B.** The lower cut shows enlargement of the third ventricle and a normal fourth ventricle consistent with a diagnosis of aqueduct stenosis. (Courtesy of Dr R.J. Sellar.)

young women, in which raised intracranial pressure develops without a space-occupying lesion. The aetiology is uncertain, although the condition can be precipitated by drugs including tetracycline, steroids, and the oral contraceptive pill.

Management
Treatment involves withdrawal of any precipitating medication and diet; in cases in which chronic papilloedema threatens vision, lumboperitoneal shunt may be necessary.

TENSION HEADACHE

Clinical features

This is the commonest form of headache. The pain is usually constant and may be generalised or predominantly nuchal. The pain is characterised as dull, tight, or like a pressure, and there may be a sensation of a band round the head or pressure at the vertex. In contrast to migraine, the pain may continue for weeks or months without interruption, although the severity may vary, and there is no associated vomiting or photophobia. The patient can usually continue normal activities and the pain may be less noticeable when the patient is occupied. Local tenderness may be present over the skull vault or in the occiput, but this should be distinguished from the acute pain precipitated by skin contact in trigeminal neuralgia.

Stress or anxiety are common precipitants to tension headache and there is sometimes an underlying depressive illness. Anxiety about the headache itself may lead to continued propagation of symptoms, and patients often become convinced of a serious underlying condition. A detailed history followed by a meticulous examination helps not only to clarify the diagnosis but may provide reassurance to the patient. A careful explanation of the symptoms and likely precipitants of tension headache are more likely to be beneficial than analgesics.

Management

Treatment of underlying anxiety of depression may be helpful, but many forms of stress are not amenable to medical intervention.

MIGRAINE

Migraine is characterised by episodic headache, which is typically unilateral and often associated with vomiting and visual disturbance. In many patients, however, the headache is bitemporal and generalised and there may be no associated focal visual or neurological disturbance. The single most characteristic feature is the episodic nature of the headache.

Pathogenesis

There is a decrease in cerebral blood flow at the onset of an attack and relative oligaemia may result in focal disturbance of cortical function, particulary in the occipital and parietal lobes. During the phase of headache, there is dilatation of the extracranial arteries, which may be related to fluctuations in blood 5-hydroxytryptamine levels.

Approximately half of patients who suffer from migraine have an affected relative, suggesting a genetic predisposition. Dietary factors, including chocolate, cheese, and alcohol may precipitate attacks, and episodes may occur more frequently peri-menstrually or in patients taking oral contraceptives. Stress and anxiety may initiate attacks or lead to perpetuation of headache and both stress and migraine headache not uncommonly co-exist.

Clinical features

The condition usually starts after puberty and continues until late middle life. Attacks occur at intervals which vary from a few days to several months, and last for hours to days. Premonitory symptoms occur in some patients in the form of zig-zag lines, flashing coloured lights, or defects in the visual field, and in others dysphasia, hemiparesis or hemianaesthesias may develop in association with the headache. The headache is usually localised to the frontal region and spreads to affect the whole of one side of the head, but may become generalised. The pain is severe and throbbing and may be associated with vomiting, photophobia, pallor, and prostration, which may necessitate the patient taking to bed in a darkened room. Variants are shown in the information box below.

CLASSIFICATION OF PRINCIPAL FORMS OF MIGRAINE

Classical migraine
Visual or sensory symptoms precede or accompany the headache

Common migraine
No visual or sensory features
Headaches, nausea, vomiting, photophobia

Hemiplegic migraine
Prolonged headache lasting hours or days, followed by hemiparesis which recoveres slowly over days

Basilar migraine
Occipital headache preceded by vertigo, diplopia, dysarthria
± visual and sensory symptoms

Management

Dietary or other precipitants to attacks should be avoided, and may sometimes be identified by advising the patient to keep a diary of attacks. The oral contraceptive pill should be stopped if the attacks are frequent or if there is associated focal neurological disturbance.

Acute attacks of common migraine usually respond to soluble aspirin (600–900 mg) or paracetamol (1 g) with or without an antinauseant such as metaclopramide or prochlorperazine. In classical migraine, ergotamine tartrate, 0.5–1.0 mg sublingually, rectally or by inhaler, may abort the headache phase if taken as soon as visual or sensory symptoms are felt. Ergotamine itself causes nausea and vomiting and many patients cannot tolerate it. Excessive use may lead to vasospasm and, paradoxically, headache. No more than 12 mg should be given in a week, and it is contraindicated in pregnancy, ischaemic heart disease and peripheral vascular disorders.

If migraine attacks occur frequently enough to disrupt work and social life (e.g. weekly), then drug prophylaxis is justified. Useful agents are propranolol (40–80 mg t.i.d.), and pizotifen (1.5–3 mg nocte). Antidepressants such as amitriptyline (25–100 mg at night) may also be helpful. All these agents have some blocking activity on 5-HT receptors, and in resistant cases methysergide (1–2 mg t.i.d.) is often effective. This is a potent 5-HT antagonist and can cause retroperitoneal fibrosis with prolonged use; it should be given for courses of only 3 months and renal function should be carefully monitored.

Investigation of headache

The extent and nature of investigations are determined by the history and clinical examination. In the great majority of patients no specific investigation is necessary, other than perhaps an ESR and serology for syphilis. Plain skull X-ray is of little diagnostic value but may provide reassurance in some patients. CT head scan is rarely necessary, but should be considered if raised intracranial pressure is suspected, there are focal neurological signs or if there is diagnostic doubt.

FACIAL PAIN

Common causes of facial pain are listed in Table 16.32. The differentiation between the causes of facial pain depends primarily on the clinical history. The treatment of trigeminal neuralgia is discussed on page 839. Migrainous neuralgia may respond to ergotamine tartrate (see above) or oxygen inhalation, but in many patients prophylactic therapy with lithium carbonate 0.25–2 g daily, methysergide 1–2 mg 3 times daily, or steroids may be necessary. Atypical facial pain often responds to antidepressant medication, while a prosthetic device to correct malocclusion and sometimes surgery are indicated in tempero-mandibular arthritis.

EPILEPSY

Definition

Epilepsy is a group of disorders in which there are recurrent episodes of altered cerebral function associated with paroxysmal excessive and hypersynchronous discharge of cerebral neurones. The clinical accompaniments of these episodes – seizures – vary in manifestation from brief lapses of awareness to prolonged bouts of unconsciousness, limb jerking and incontinence.

Pathophysiology

In health the widely interconnected neurones of the cerebral cortex are held in a state of relative quiescence by inhibitory synaptic influences. Synchronous discharge amongst neighbouring groups of neurones is limited by recurrent and collateral inhibitory circuits. The inhibitory transmitter gamma-aminobutyric acid (GABA) is thought to be particularly important in this role; drugs which block GABA receptors provoke seizures. There are also a large number of excitatory neurotransmitters, of which acetylcholine and the amino acids glutamate and aspartate are examples. Epileptic cerebral cortex exhibits hypersynchronous repetitive discharges involving large groups of neu-

Table 16.32 Common causes of facial pain

Cause	Site	Duration	Character	Associations
Trigeminal neuralgia	Unilateral Maxillary/mandibular	Occurs in bouts	Lancinating	Triggering by touch, chewing, speaking, etc.
Migrainous neuraliga	Unilateral Ocular/cheek/forehead	Occurs in bouts	Severe throbbing (nocturnal)	Lacrimation Nasal blockage
Atypical facial pain	Bilateral/unilateral	Constant	Aching, boring	
Temporomandibular arthritis	Unilateral Angle of jaw Cheek	On chewing	Aching	Malocclusion

Table 16.33   Clinical classification of epilepsy

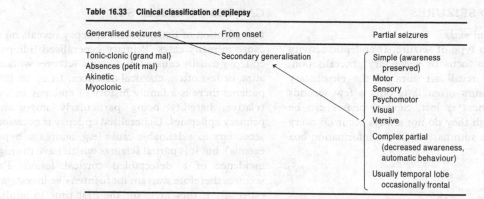

Generalised seizures	From onset		Partial seizures
Tonic-clonic (grand mal)		Secondary generalisation	Simple (awareness preserved)
Absences (petit mal)			Motor
Akinetic			Sensory
Myoclonic			Psychomotor
			Visual
			Versive
			Complex partial (decreased awareness, automatic behaviour)
			Usually temporal lobe occasionally frontal

rones; intracellular recordings show bursts of rapid action potential firing, with reduction of the transmembrane potential (paroxysmal depolarisation shift). It is likely that both reduction in inhibitory systems and excessive excitation play a part in the genesis of seizure activity.

CLASSIFICATION OF EPILEPSY

The chief division of seizure types is between *partial (focal) seizures* in which paroxysmal neuronal activity is limited to one part of the cerebrum, and *generalised seizures* where the electrophysiological abnormality involves large areas of both hemispheres simultaneously and synchronously (Table 16.33). If partial seizures remain localised, the symptomatology is elementary and depends on the cortical area affected; awareness is preserved, and the attack is termed 'simple'. If however, the activity spreads to involve the reticular activating system at the thalamic level, awareness is lost and a 'complex partial seizure' results. Further spread may lead to a secondarily generalised seizure. Some generalised seizures arise without any clear focal onset, such patients appearing to have diffusely impaired cortical inhibitory mechanisms.

PARTIAL SEIZURES

Motor. Epileptic activity arising in the precentral gyrus causes partial motor seizures affecting the contralateral face, arm trunk and leg. Seizures are characterised by rhythmical jerking or sustained spasm of the affected parts. They may remain localised to one part, or may spread to involve the whole side. Some attacks begin in one part (e.g. mouth, thumb, great toe) and spread gradually, this form being called Jacksonian epilepsy. Attacks vary in duration from a few seconds to several hours. More prolonged episodes may leave

paresis of the involved limb for several hours after the seizure ceases (Todd's palsy).

Sensory. Seizures arising in the postcentral gyrus cause tingling or 'electric' sensations in the contralateral face and limbs. A spreading pattern like a Jacksonian seizure may occur.

Versive. A frontal epileptic focus may involve the frontal eye field, causing forced deviation of the eyes to the opposite side. This type of attack often rapidly becomes generalised to a tonic-clonic seizure.

Visual. Occipital epileptic foci cause simple visual hallucination such as balls of light or patterns of colour. Formed visual hallucinations of faces or scenes arise more anteriorly in the temporal lobes.

Psychomotor. Seizures which cause alterations of mood, memory and perception usually arise from the medial temporal lobe. This is a common form of epilepsy, causing both partial and secondary generalised seizures. Occasionally, a similar clinical picture arises from inferior frontal foci. Simple partial temporal lobe attacks may cause disordered perception such as undue familiarity (deja vu) or unreality (jamais vu); complex hallucinations of sound, smell, taste, vision; emotional changes (fear, sexual arousal); visceral sensations (nausea, epigastric discomfort). Complex partial seizures may be preceded by an aura of these phenomena, lasting seconds or minutes, and then awareness is diminished or lost for typically several minutes. During this phase of a complex partial seizure, the sufferer may stare and be unresponsive to questions. Automatic movements (e.g. lip smacking, swallowing, fidgeting with clothes) may occur at this stage, and some patients fall down. If the attack procedes further, a tonic-clonic seizure may ensue.

GENERALISED SEIZURES

Tonic-clonic (grand mal)

This is a common type of seizure. If epileptic activity has spread from a focus by secondary generalisation, the patient may recall an aura of the elementary symptoms. The aura often lasts only a few seconds before consciousness is lost. Several phases can be identified, although they do not always occur on every occasion; they are summarised in the information box below.

PHASES OF A TONIC-CLONIC SEIZURE

Prodromal phase
Hours or days before attack, unease, irritability

Aura
Due to partial onset of seizure last seconds or minutes. e.g. olfactory hallucination, epigastric discomfort, deja-vu, jerking of one limb

Tonic phase
Rapid discharging of motor cortex cells causes tonic contractions of muscles; arms flexed and adducted, legs extended; respiratory muscle spasm causes 'cry' as air expelled; cyanosis; loss of consciousness. Lasts 10–30 s

Clonic phase
Less rapid, gradually slowing discharge of cortical cells; violent jerking of face and limbs; tongue biting, incontinence. Lasts 1–5 min

Post-ictal phase
Deep unconsciousness, flaccid limbs and jaw, loss of corneal reflexes, extensor plantar responses. Lasts a few minutes to several hours. Headache, confusion, aching muscles and sometimes automatic behaviour, occasional violence

---

Classical absences (petit mal)

This is a relatively uncommon form of generalised epilepsy, seen mostly in children. Typical absences are always due to primary generalised (idiopathic) epilepsy; the symptoms start in childhood or adolescence. During an absence attack the child stops activity, stares, may blink or roll up the eyes, and fails to respond to commands. Each attack lasts only a matter of seconds, but many hundred absences may occur in a day. Occasionally, loss of posture occurs and the child falls, but is able to get up again quickly (akinetic attack). The EEG recorded during attacks shows generalised bilaterally synchronous spike and wave complexes at a frequency of 3/s (see Fig. 16.19, p. 829). Attacks may go unnoticed by the patient, and sometimes their family.

CAUSES OF EPILEPSY

Investigation of patients with epilepsy reveals no clear cause in many cases. Primary generalised (idiopathic) epilepsy usually causes tonic-clonic seizures without an aura, or less often, classical absences. In up to 40% of patients there is a family history of epilepsy in a close relative; heredity being particularly important in primary epilepsies. Generalised epilepsy is occasionally secondary to a definable cause (e.g. anorexia, hypocalcaemia), but it is partial seizures which have the highest incidence of a detectabled cortical lesion. Partial seizures therefore warrant more intensive investigation, especially if they arise for the first time in adult life. Common causes of epilepsy are listed in Table 16.34.

FACTORS PRECIPITATING SEIZURES

Sometimes specific trigger factors which set off seizures can be identified. Some are listed in the information box below.

FACTORS WHICH MAY TRIGGER SEIZURES

- Sleep deprivation
- Emotional stress
- Physical and mental exhaustion
- Infections, pyrexia
- Drug or alcohol ingestion, or withdrawal
- Flickering light, visual patterns, proximity to television screens
- Uncommon triggers
  Loud noise
  Hot baths
  Music
  Reading

Clinical features

The most important steps in making a diagnosis of epilepsy are listed in the information box (p. 855). In many patients these two steps are sufficient to establish the diagnosis, or may suggest an alternative (e.g. syncope).

Clinical examination is often unhelpful. Rarely clinical features may suggest a specific diagnosis such as Tuberous Sclerosis or pseudohypoparathyroidism. A good general examination with emphasis on the nervous and cardiovascular systems should be performed. Particular points of note are listed in the information box (p. 855).

Investigations

The investigations which may be undertaken in a

Table 16.34   Common causes of epilepsy

Seizure type	Aetiology	Other factors
Generalised Tonic-clonic Absences Akinetic Myoclonic	Primary (idiopathic)	Family history Seizures more common soon after waking

Generalised
Tonic-clonic
Atypical absences
	Diffuse cerebral damage
	  e.g. encephalitis, anoxia, storage
	  diseases.
	Metabolic
	  e.g. hypocalcaemia, hypoglycaemia, hyponatraemia,
	  porphyria, hypoxia, renal or hepatic failure
	Drugs/toxins
	  e.g. Alcohol withdrawal, tricyclics, phenothiazines, MAOIs[1],
	  amphetamines, lignocaine
		Often associated with
		mental and physical handicaps

Partial
 	
Simple
Complex
Secondarily
generalised
tonic-clonic
	Cerebral trauma
	Birth damage, head injury
	Vascular: infarction, cerebral haemorrhage,
	vascular malformation, cerebral aneurysm
	Cerebral tumours
	Infections
	Meningitis, encephalitis, cerebral abscess, empyema,
	  syphilis, tuberculosis, HIV
	Inflammatory
	  Sarcoidosis, SLE[2], MS
		Partial seizures may occur
		while awake or asleep, sometimes
		only in sleep. Progress from
		partial to generalised may be so
		rapid that seizures appear
		to be generalised

[1]Monoamine oxidase inhibitors.
[2]Systemic lupus erythematosus.

DIAGNOSING EPILEPSY

- Take a detailed history from the patient
- Interview an eye-witness who has observed the attacks

Specific questions
- Events leading up to attack
    Sleep deprivation, drugs, alcohol, near TV screen
- Time of day or night
- Symptoms of aura, duration
- Abnormal movements
    Limb stiffening, jerking, automatisms
- Salivation, cyanosis
- Tongue biting, incontinence
- Post-ictal symptoms
    Limb pains, headache, drowsiness

GENERAL EXAMINATION IN EPILEPSY

- Ausculation of neck and eyes for bruits
- Pulse, blood pressure, heart auscultation
- Head for evidence of trauma
- Skin for lesions of epiloia, neurofibromatosis
- Visual fields, optic fundi
- Limbs for evidence of hemiparesis or hyper-reflexia

---

patient with suspected epilepsy are shown in the information box below.

Electroencephalography (EEG)
The EEG may help establish and characterise the type of epilepsy; interictal records are abnormal in about

---

INVESTIGATIONS IN EPILEPSY

Routine tests
Full blood count, ESR
Blood urea, electrolytes, calcium, glucose
Liver function tests
Serological tests for syphilis
HIV serology in high risk groups
X-rays of chest and skull
Electrocardiogram (ECG)

Special investigations
Electroencephalography (EEG)
    Routine EEG
    Sedated sleep EEG
    24-hour ambulatory EEG/ECG
    Video/EEG monitoring
    EEG with special electrodes (foramen ovale, sphenoidal)
Computed Tomography (CT)
Magnetic Resonance Imaging (MRI)

60% of cases. Details of EEG recording methods, and examples of abnormalities are given on pages 828–829. The yield of diagnostic abnormalities can be increased by prolonging recording time, and including a period of natural or drug induced sleep. In cases of diagnostic difficulty with frequent symptoms, ambulatory EEG recording or video/EEG monitoring may provide helpful information, but are costly and time-consuming. It is important to remember that a normal interictal EEG does not negate a good clinical diagnosis of epilepsy; but nor does an abnormal record establish a diagnosis in the absence of an appropriate history.

Computed tomography (CT)

CT brain scanning does not help establish a diagnosis of epilepsy, but is often useful in defining or excluding a structural cause for seizures. As a general rule, a CT scan should be carried out if:

1. epilepsy starts after the age of 20 years;
2. at any age if seizures have focal features clinically;
3. the EEG shows a focal seizure source;
4. control of seizures is difficult or deteriorates.

CT scanning is not required if a confident diagnosis of primary generalised epilepsy can be made clinically. Examples:

1. tonic-clonic seizures without aura, on waking in morning, in a teenager with a positive family history, EEG shows generalised paroxysms;
2. typical absences in a child of 10, with 3/s spike and wave bursts on EEG.

Management

General

The nature of epilepsy should be explained to patients and their relatives. Many people with epilepsy feel stigmatised by society and may become unnecessarily isolated from work and social life. It should be emphasised that epilepsy is a common disorder which affects just under 1% of the population, and that good or complete control of seizures can be expected in more than 80% of patients.

Immediate care of seizures. Little can or need be done for a person having a major seizure. Some simple guidelines are listed in the information box (right).

Restrictions. Until good control of seizures has been established, work or recreation above ground level, with dangerous machinery or near open fires should be avoided. Patients should take a shallow bath, only when a relative is in the house, and should not lock

---

IMMEDIATE CARE OF SEIZURES

- Move person away from danger (fires, water, machinery)
- After convulsions cease, turn patient into semi-prone position, ensure their airway is clear
- If convulsions continue for more than 5 minutes or begin again, summon medical help
- To try to prevent tongue biting a padded gag or tightly rolled handkerchief may be inserted between the teeth. Metallic or plastic objects and helpers' fingers should not be used. It is often not possible to prevent tongue biting once a seizure has started
- To offset cerebral hypoxia, give oxygen at high concentration, if available

---

the bathroom door. Cycling and swimming should be discouraged until at least six months' freedom from seizures has been achieved, and swimming should always be in the company of someone who is aware of the slight chance of a seizure occurring. Any activity where loss of awareness might be very dangerous (e.g. mountaineering) should be discouraged.

Driving. Legal restrictions apply to vehicle driving. Patients with epilepsy must be free from all types of seizure for two years (on or off medication), or seizures must have been exclusively during sleep for a period of three years before driving may be resumed. The patient should inform the licensing authorities about the onset of seizures, and it is also wise for them to notify their motor insurance company. Vocational drivers are not permitted a heavy goods or public service vehicle licence if any seizure occurs after the age of five years.

Anticonvulsant drug therapy

Traditionally, a single seizure has been regarded as an indication for investigation and assessment, but not for drug treatment unless a second attack follows closely. Prospective studies have shown that the recurrence rate after a first seizure approaches 70% during the first year, most recurrent attacks occurring within a month or two of the first. Further seizures are less likely if a trigger factor is definable (e.g. sleep deprivation, exhaustion). Drug treatment should certainly be considered after two seizures have occurred, and in some cases (very abnormal EEG, strong family history) a single unprovoked seizure is sufficient indication. There is some evidence to uphold the notion that the earlier seizures are brought under control, the more easily will they remain quiescent.

Use of anticonvulsant drugs. Several effective agents are available. Their mode of action is not well understood, but they probably affect both the stability of neuronal membranes and affect neurotransmitter systems by promoting inhibitory activity. Good or total control of seizures can be expected in about 80% of epileptic patients using a single drug in adequate dosage. Dose regimens should be kept as simple as is necessary to maintain therapeutic plasma levels of the drug; the simpler the regimen, the more likely the patient is to comply with it. Some useful guidelines are listed in the information box below.

USE OF ANTICONVULSANT DRUGS

- Begin with a single drug
- With sedative agents (carbamazepine, primidone, clonazepam) begin with a small dose, increasing gradually over 4–6 weeks
- Adjust dose to achieve plasma plateau level in lower part of the therapeutic range for that drug
- If seizures not controlled, increase dose to attain plasma level in upper part of therapeutic range, or until side-effects appear
- If seizures poorly controlled, change to a different drug by gradually reducing dose of initial agent while simultaneously introducing the new one. This usually takes 3–4 weeks
- Try 3 single drugs before resorting to drug combinations, which help in only a minority of cases

---

Measuring plasma anticonvulsant drug levels. Levels of all the major antiepileptic drugs can be measured in blood routinely. Agents which have a long plasma half-life (e.g. phenytoin – 24–36 hours) can adequately be given once a day. Plateau levels taken 4–6 hours after the last dose are preferable to peak samples when measuring drugs with shorter half-lives (carbamazepine and sodium valproate). Plasma level monitoring is particularly useful for phenytoin, because of the marked variation in dose requirements between individuals and the saturation kinetics of the drug which give rise to an exponential dose/blood level relationship. The measurements of plasma levels for carbamazepine and the barbiturates are helpful but not essential; valproate levels are rarely a useful guide to adequate dosage, and serve often only to confirm patient compliance. It is important to recognise that quoted 'therapeutic' ranges are approximations from experience, and need not be adhered to rigidly if the patient is otherwise well.

Efficacy and choice of drug. Overall, generalised tonic-clonic seizures are more readily controlled than partial epilepsy. Although some agents seem more effective in certain types of seizure, with the exception of absence attacks there are no hard and fast rules as to which drug is superior. The choice may lie more in the suitability of a particular drug for a specific patient. For example, phenytoin and carbamazepine are not ideal agents for a young woman wishing to use oral contraception, because the drugs induce liver enzymes which render the contraceptive less effective. Sodium valproate should be avoided in children with progressive cerebral disorders because the risk of fatal hepatic damage is much higher in this group; it is also unsuitable for obese patients since it tends to cause weight gain.

The commonly used drugs, dose ranges, therapeutic levels and side-effects are shown in Table 16.35. A guide to the choice of appropriate drugs is given in Table 16.36.

Withdrawal of anticonvulsant therapy. After a period of complete control of seizures, withdrawal of medication may be considered. How long complete control should be achieved before considering withdrawal is debatable; periods of two to four years are usually required. Childhood onset epilepsy, particularly classical absence seizures, carry the best prognosis for successful drug withdrawal. Seizures which begin in adult life, particularly those with partial features are the most likely to recur. Overall, the recurrence rate of seizures after drug withdrawal is about 35%; some adult patients tend to opt for continuation of therapy for they feel the threat of further attacks greater than continuing with medication. The EEG does not seem to be a good predictor of seizure recurrence, although if the record is still very abnormal drug withdrawal is unwise. Withdrawal should be undertaken slowly, reducing the drug dose gradually over 6–12 months.

STATUS EPILEPTICUS

Status epilepticus exists when a series of seizures occurs without the patient regaining awareness between attacks. Most commonly this refers to recurrent tonic-clonic seizures (major status), this condition being a life-threatening state and therefore a medical emergency. Partial motor status is obvious clinically, but complex partial status and absence status may be difficult to diagnose, because the patient may merely present with a dazed, confused state. Status may be precipitated by abrupt withdrawal of anticonvulsant drugs, major intracranial disasters (e.g. cerebral haemorrhage), and tends to be more common with frontal epileptic foci.

Table 16.35   Major anticonvulsant drugs, doses, therapeutic ranges, side-effects

Drug	Seizure types	Dose range mg/day	Doses per day	Therap. range μmol/l	Side-effects dose related	idiosyn-cratic	long term
Phenytoin	Tonic-clonic Partial	150–600	1–2	40–80	Ataxia Nystagmus Lethargy Tremor Dystonia Confusion	Rashes Lymphad-enopathy Blood dycrasia Liver damage SLE[2]	Gum hyper-trophy Hirsuitism Folate deficiency Osteomalacia Neuropathy
Carbamazepine	Partial Tonic-clonic	200–2000	2–3	20–50	Drowsiness Ataxia Nystagmus Diplopia Headache Hyponatraemia	Rashes Dyspepsia Blood dyscrasia	Not recognised
Sodium Valproate	Tonic-clonic Absences Myoclonus	400–3000	2–3	200–700 Poorly defined	Nausea Anorexia Tremor Drowsiness	Alopecia Thrombo-cytopenia Hepatic necrosis	Weight gain
Primidone	Tonic-clonic Partial	250–1000	2–3	50–150[1]	Nausea Drowsiness Ataxia Nystagmus	SLE[2]	Folate deficiency Osteomalacia Neuropathy
Phenobarbitone	Tonic-clonic Partial	60–180	1–2	50–150	Drowsiness Lethargy Ataxia Nystagmus	Rashes SLE[2]	As primidone
Ethosuximide	Absences (petit mal)	500–1500	2	200–700	Dizziness Insomnia	Nausea Rashes Blood dyscrasia	
Clonazepam	Partial (adjunctive)	1–6	2–3	50–300	Drowsiness irritability		Useful effects decline after a period of weeks

[1]Measured phenobarbitone.
[2]SLE. Systemic lupus erythematosus.

Management
This summarised in the information box (p. 859).

Epilepsy and pregnancy
Reference has already been made to the hepatic enzyme induction caused by carbamazepine, phenytoin and the barbiturates which accelerate metabolism of the oral contraceptives, causing breakthrough bleeding and contraceptive failure. The safest policy is for women taking these drugs to use an alternative contraceptive method, but it is sometimes possible to overcome the problem by giving a higher oestrogen dose (50–80 μg) preparation.

Epilepsy may worsen during pregnancy, particularly during the third trimester when plasma anticonvulsant levels tend to fall. More frequent monitoring of blood levels during pregnancy is therefore advisable. All the major anticonvulsant drugs have been associated with an increased incidence of fetal congenital abnormalities (cleft lip, spina bifida, cardiac defects). The risk is greatest during the first trimester. It is seldom possible to withdraw or change therapy before conception, but carbamazepine may be less teratogenic than the other agents. Occasionally in a well-controlled patient anti-convulsants can be withdrawn before conception, but if seizures have occurred in the preceding year this is

Table 16.36   Guidelines for selection of anticonvulsant drugs

Seizure	Types	Drug preference order
Tonic-clonic	Primary generalised	Valproate Phenytoin Carbamazepine Barbiturates
	Secondary generalised	Phenytoin Carbamazepine Valproate Barbiturates
Partial		Carbamazepine Phenytoin Valproate Barbiturates Benzodiazepines
Classical absences (petit mal)		Valproate Ethosuximide

unwise as the risk to the fetus from uncontrolled maternal seizures is probably greater than the teratogenic effects.

CEREBRAL VASCULAR DISORDERS

Damage to brain tissue due either to cerebral infarction or haemorrhage ('stroke') is the third commonest cause of death in developed countries. Stroke is uncommon below the age of 50 and affects males 1.5 times more often than females. Younger people occasionally sustain a stroke because of trauma to cerebral vessels, inflammatory disorders of arteries, or congenital vascular anomalies. In an average population, the annual

MANAGEMENT OF STATUS EPILEPTICUS

- Maintain airway with oropharyngeal tube; give high-flow oxygen
- Give diazepam i.v. 10–20 mg over 1–3 min. This may cause hypotension and impair respiration; use i.v. only if resuscitation facilities available, otherwise rectal route safer
- Transfer patient to Intensive Care Area; monitor BP, ECG, EEG and blood gases
- Set up i.v. infusion of diazepam 10–50 mg/h. Adjust dose to control seizures
- Give loading dose of phenytoin i.v. 18 mg/kg body weight at a rate no faster than 50 mg/min (omit if patient already taking phenytoin)
- Try chlormethiazole i.v. 0.5–1.2 g/hour by infusion if diazepam fails to control seizures
- If seizures still uncontrolled set up i.v. infusion of thiopentone. This usually necessitates assisted ventilation
- When seizures controlled, determine cause. Check electrolytes, calcium, glucose, urea. Consider urgent CT scan if patient not previously known to have epilepsy. In established epileptic, check plasma anticonvulsant levels

incidence of new strokes is 2 per 1000 people. Stroke is therefore a prominent cause of disability, particularly in the elderly. Pathological studies indicate that 80–85% of strokes are due to cerebral infarction; 15–20% are caused by haemorrhage. The most common vascular disorder underlying stroke is atherosclerosis affecting intracranial and extracranial arteries; less common mechanisms are listed in Table 16.37. Strokes are common in patients with other cardiovascular disorders, particularly ischaemic heart and peripheral

Table 16.37   Vascular disorders causing stroke

	Infarction	Haemorrhage
Atherosclerosis	Extracranial Intracranial	Aneurysms of major arteries (berry aneurysms)
Arteriolar sclerosis	Hypertensive Degenerative Inherited	Small arteriolar aneurysms (hypertensive) Arteriovenous malformations Atheromatous aneurysms
Embolism	From heart From vessels	Infective (mycotic) aneurysms
Arteritis	Infective Giant cell SLE, polyarteritis Granulomatous	Head trauma
Dissection	Traumatic Spontaneous	
Vasospasm	Migraine Subarachnoid haemorrhage Angiography	

Table 16.38   Risk factors for stroke

Major risks	Other risks
Arterial hypertension	High alcohol intake
Cigarette smoking	Positive family history
Diabetes mellitus	Oral contraceptives
Hyperlipidaemia	Trauma
Polycythaemia	
Thrombocythaemia	

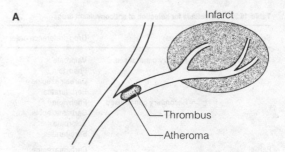

vascular disease. The major risk factors for stroke are listed in Table 16.38.

MECHANISMS OF STROKE

CEREBRAL INFARCTION

Occlusion of a major cerebral artery usually leads to infarction unless, as in some young people, a collateral circulation is well developed. Thrombosis at the site of atheromatous degeneration in a major cerebral vessel is probably the commonest mechanism, but embolism of thrombotic or atheromatous material from the heart or an extracranial artery is also frequent. Thromboemboli of cardiac origin may arise from mural thrombus after myocardial infarction, and are often associated with atrial fibrillation, especially when it is secondary to valvular disease. Cardiac emboli tend to be large and cause occlusion of one of the principal cerebral arteries or a major branch, thereby causing usually major strokes. By contrast, emboli arising from the carotid bifurcation are more often particulate, due to deposition of platelets, and often cause minor or transient cerebral or ocular symptoms.

Once deprived of blood supply cerebral tissue undergoes infarction within a few minutes. Released excitatory amino acids may exacerbate the neuronal damage by promoting calcium influx. The damaged neurones and glia become oedematous after some hours, the resultant cerebral oedema causing more damage by further impairing cerebral blood flow.

CEREBRAL HAEMORRHAGE

About half the strokes caused by cerebral haemorrhage are due to subarachnoid bleeding from rupture of an aneurysm at the the circle of Willis or less commonly from an arteriovenous malformation. In other patients, haemorrhage is mainly into the cerebral substance and is due to rupture of small perforating arteries or arterioles weakened by hypertension or atheromatous degeneration (Fig. 16.34). Intracerebral haemorrhage of this type tends to occur at three distinct sites:

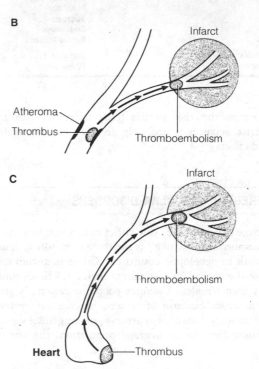

Fig. 16.33   Mechanism of stroke – cerebral infarction. A. Thrombosis at side of atheroma. **B.** Embolism for major artery. **C.** Thromboembolism from cardiac source.

1. the internal capsule – from lenticulo-striate arteries
2. the pons – from perforating branches of the basilar artery
3. the cerebellum.

Subarachnoid haemorrhage may induce secondary arterial spasm and thereby cerebral infarction. Although large cerebral haemorrhages cause severe disability, small bleeds in the deep cerebral white matter may cause only mild and transient defects. Cerebellar haemorrhage can be fatal if secondary compression of the brain stem occurs.

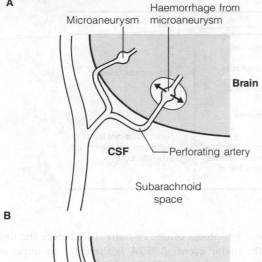

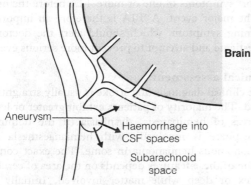

Fig. 16.34   Mechanism of stroke – cerebral haemorrhage. A.
Intracerebral (hypertensive). B. Subarachnoid (aneurysmal).

Clinical features

The clinical classification of a stroke is given in the
information box below.

CLINICAL CLASSIFICATION OF STROKE

● Completed stroke
   Major
   Minor
● Evolving stroke
● Transient ischaemic attack (TIA)

Completed stroke

This is an episode of focal cerebral dysfunction, due
either to cerebral infarction or haemorrhage, with
symptoms lasting longer than 24 hours. Strokes usually
evolve rapidly over a few minutes, and reach maximum
disability within an hour or two. Sometimes a slower

course occurs, the disability advancing gradually over
several hours or days. This is known as an evolving
stroke, or 'stroke in evolution'. Headache is a common
accompaniment to acute stroke and does not help
distinguish infarction from haemorrhage. Epileptic
seizures, vomiting and depressed consciousness may
also occur, the latter usually indicating a severe lesion.
The precise features of a stroke depend on the vascular
territory involved. Fig. 16.35 shows the territories of
the three main cerebral arteries; Table 16.39 sets out
the features of stroke lesions at different sites.

Evolving stroke

In some patients the symptoms worsen gradually or in
a step-wise fashion over a matter of hours or days. This
clinical picture can be due to cerebral tumour or
subdural haematoma, but is more often due to slow
occlusion of a major cerebral vessel such as the internal
carotid or the middle cerebral artery.

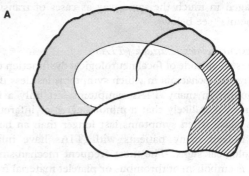

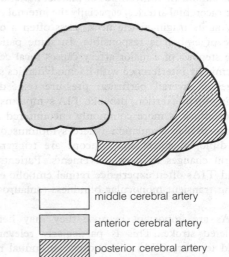

---

	middle cerebral artery
	anterior cerebral artery
	posterior cerebral artery

Fig. 16.35   Supply territories of cerebral arteries. A. Lateral view of
left hemisphere. B. Medial view of right hemisphere.

Table 16.39 Features of stroke in different arterial territories

Main artery	Branch	Clinical features	Side
Internal carotid	Middle Cerebral	Hemiparesis (face and arm > leg) Hemianaesthesia Dysphasia, Dysarthria, Dyspraxia Hemianopia	Opposite side to lesion
	Anterior cerebral	Hemiparesis (leg > arm and face) Incontinence	
Vertebral	Posterior cerebral	Hemianopia, cortical blindness Amnesia Thalamic pain	Nuclear symptoms ipsilat. to lesion: contralat. sensory and pyramidal signs
	Cerebellar Basilar	Ataxia, diplopia, nystagmus, dysarthria, dysphagia, facial weakness/numbness, bilateral sensory symptoms, loss of consciousness	

Minor stroke

Some patients with a completed stroke improve rapidly, with recovery from disability over the course of the first week or two. The rather arbitrary definition of minor strokes is useful because such patients can be managed in much the same way as cases of transient ischaemia (see below).

Transient ischaemic attack (TIA)

This is an episode of focal neurological dysfunction due to cerebral ischaemia in which symptoms last less than 24 hours. In many TIAs symptoms last only a few minutes; it is likely that a minor degree of infarction takes place when symptoms last longer than an hour, and indeed many patients with TIAs have minor neurological signs. The most frequent mechanism of TIA is embolism of thrombus or platelet material from the extracerebral arteries, especially the internal carotid artery at its origin in the neck. Less often a cardiac source of emboli is responsible. In some patients a severe stenosis of a major artery causes focal cerebral ischaemia by interference with haemodynamics so that changes in overall perfusion pressure (e.g. due to standing up or exertion) provoke TIA symptoms. This type of attack is more commonly encountered in the vertebro-basilar circulation where symptoms of vertigo, diplopia, ataxia and syncope are triggered by postural changes or neck movements. Patients with carotid TIAs often experience retinal embolic events, causing transient monocular blindness (amaurosis fugax).

TIAs are important because they may herald a completed stroke. This is particularly relevant for carotid territory TIAs which carry an annual risk of completed stroke of about 5%; vertebrobasilar TIAs are less sinister, but still carry an increased risk. About 25% of patients who have suffered a completed stroke

report symptoms of one or more TIA before the onset of the major event. A TIA is therefore an important warning symptom, which should alert the doctor to investigate and attempt to prevent more serious events.

Clinical assessment

The clinical diagnosis of a stroke is usually straightforward. The majority of patients exhibit greater or lesser degrees of hemiparesis, dysphasia (if the dominant hemisphere is involved), with hemianaesthesia and homonomous hemianopia in some. The exact combination of these features depends on the area of cerebral cortex or deep while matter involved. Initially the paralysed limbs may be flaccid and reflexes can be decreased despite an extensor plantar response. After a few days, tone usually increases and reflexes become hyperactive on the affected side. Ataxia or hemisensory disturbance may dominate the picture with deeply placed small lacunar infarcts. With severe hemisphere damage, flaccid hemiplegia is accompanied by paresis of gaze to the affected side, and consciousness is impaired as cerebral oedema develops. Papilloedema may be present under these circumstances.

Strokes affecting the brain stem are more likely to cause loss of consciousness because of damage to the reticular activating system. The cardinal features of brain-stem stroke are a combination of nuclear signs on the side of the lesion (e.g. oculomotor palsy, palatial weakness) and pyramidal and spinothalamic signs in the contralateral limbs. A characteristic syndrome occurs with infarction of the lateral medulla, due to occlusion of either the posterior-inferior cerebellar artery or the vertebral artery itself; there is ipsilateral ataxia, nystagmus, facial numbness and palatial palsy and sometimes ipsilateral Horner's syndrome; damage to the spinothalamic tract causes impairment of pain and temperature sensation contralateral to the lesion.

In addition to careful assessment of the neurological lesions, general examination should pay special attention to the cardiovascular system, noting blood pressure, cardiac rhythm, peripheral vasculature, arterial bruits and any cardiac murmurs.

Investigations

The more routine tests are given in the information box below.

ROUTINE TESTS IN STROKE PATIENTS

Routine
Full blood count, ESR
Serological tests for syphilis
Blood glucose
Blood urea, electrolytes, proteins
Chest X-ray
ECG

Additional tests in younger patients
Antinuclear factor
Antibodies to double-stranded DNA
Anti-cardiolipin antibodies
Lupus anticoagulant
Cholesterol

CT scanning. With the exception of MRI, CT scanning provides the only reliable method of distinguishing cerebral infarction from haemorrhage. Clinical assessment has been shown to be very unreliable, and if any treatment with anticoagulents or even antiplatelet drugs is planned, CT scanning is essential to exclude cerebral haemorrhage. Occasionally a cerebral tumour presents as a stroke, usually because of haemorrhage into the lesion. Early or very small infarcts may not be detected by CT, but the vast majority of haemorrhages will be. (Examples of typical lesions are shown in Figures 16.36 and 16.37.) Infarcts appear as areas of low density, usually with little or no mass effect unless they are very large. Some contrast enhancement may be present within infarcts, especially after a few weeks when they exhibit increased vascularity.

Angiography. This is not usually indicated during the acute phase of a stroke, unless a specific cause such as arterial dissection is suspected and intervention is likely to result. Angiography may exacerbate the stroke symptoms.

Echocardiography. This is sometimes performed if there is a suggestion of a cardiac source of embolism causing a stroke, and anticoagulation is being con-

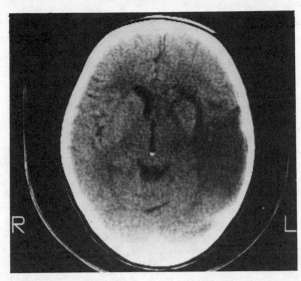

Fig. 16.36   CT scan of cerebral infarction. A large wedge shaped low density lesion is seen in the left temporoparietal area, due to infarction in the territory of the middle cerebral artery. The left lateral ventricle is compressed indicating that there is oedema associated with recent infarction. (Courtesy of Dr D. Kean.)

sidered. In a young patient with an unexplained stroke, echocardiography may demonstrate cardiac thrombus, vegetations or myxoma.

Management

General measures
These are listed in the information box (p. 864).

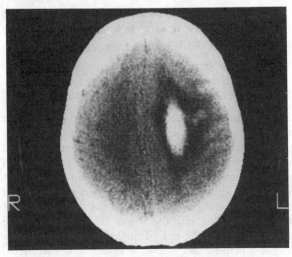

Fig. 16.37   CT scan of intracerebral haemorrhage. A large high-density lesion typical of recent haemorrhage is seen deep in the left hemisphere. The likely site of bleeding is in the internal capsule, in which region hypertensive microaneurysms often rupture. (Courtesy of Dr D. Kean.)

MANAGEMENT OF ACUTE STROKE — GENERAL MEASURES

Careful nursing
Regular turning of patient to avoid pressure sores; skin kept dry and clean

Care of airway
Oropharyngeal tube with regular suction of secretions if patient unconscious

Fluid balance
Nasogastric feeding if patient cannot swallow; bladder catheterisation if incontinence

Physiotherapy
Start immediately to prevent joint contractures; to clear chest secretions; to promote recovery of strength and coordination

Speech and occupational therapy
Start once acute stage over to assess functional problems and to encourage recovery of skills

Specific measures

Blood pressure. Many patients show a reactive rise in blood pressure in the acute phase of a stroke. This is a compensatory change attempting to maintain cerebral blood flow; hypotensive agents should not be used at this stage unless there are features of accelerated hypertension or end signs of end-organ involvement are present. If treatment is necessary, this should be gentle to avoid a sudden lowering of cerebral perfusion pressure, which can exacerbate infarction.

Anticoagulation. There is usually no indication for the use of anticoagulants in acute stroke. The only positive indications are:

1. if there is a clear persisting embolic source (e.g. atrial fibrillation; dissection of carotid artery) or
2. features of stroke are evolving over hours or days.

In both instances, cerebral haemorrhage or tumour must be ruled out by urgent CT scanning before anticoagulation is started. Initial treatment should be with an intravenous infusion of heparin; oral warfarin may be instituted at the same time, and the heparin withdrawn after 3–4 days. When there is an established cerebral infarct, anticoagulation carries a risk of causing bleeding into the lesion. This risk has to be weighed against the risk of further progression of the stroke due to further emboli or extension of thrombus.

Oedema-reducing agents. Osmotic agents (i.v. mannitol 20%, 200 ml) and potent steroids (dexamethasone 4 mg i.v. q.i.d.) may help reduce mortality in patients with severe strokes and secondary cerebral oedema by limiting brain swelling and brain-stem compression. They are not indicated for an uncomplicated stroke, and their use in severe stroke is debatable because they have not been shown to prevent disability.

Vasodilating agents. There is no good evidence to support the use of vasodilators in acute stroke. Inhibitors of the excitatory amino acids are currently under trial, but have not yet been evaluated.

Surgery. Carotid arterial surgery carries a high risk during the first month after cerebral infarction, and early surgical treatment of carotid occlusion has not been shown to be of benefit. Neurosurgical evacuation of a cerebral haematoma is sometimes indicated if the patient continues to deteriorate, and the lesion is easily accessible. In cerebellar haemorrhage with secondary brain-stem compression, urgent surgical drainage of the haematoma may be life saving.

Continuing management

Rehabilitation. About 30% of stroke patients will die as a direct result of the acute lesion. Of the survivors, most will recover some useful function over periods ranging from 1 to 12 months. At this stage, active help from enthusiastic physiotherapists, speech and occupational therapists is invaluable. The risk of further strokes is 5–10% per annum and so if risk factors can be identified, they should be corrected as far as possible. Aspirin 300 mg/day reduces the risk of further stroke and death by about 25%, but carries a small increase in the risk of cerebral haemorrhage. Patients who make a good functional recovery should be managed along the lines described for TIA in the information box (p. 865).

Management of TIA

Risk factors. These should be identified and corrected. Hypertension, smoking and diabetes are the most important. Hyperlipidaemia and polycythaemia are also worth treatment in younger patients.

Antiplatelet agents. Aspirin 300 mg/day reduces the risk of stroke by 25% and of death by 30%. If patients are intolerant of 300 mg of aspirin, lower doses (75–150 mg/d) may be tried, or dipyridamole 100 mg t.i.d. given instead. There is as yet no good evidence to confirm their value in these doses however.

Anticoagulants. The use of oral anticoagulants in TIA has not been subjected to modern randomised

CLINICAL ASSESSMENT OF TIA AND MINOR STROKE

History
Vascular territory involved
Duration of symptoms
Associated cardiac, peripheral vascular or retinal symptoms
Other possible diagnoses (epilepsy, migraine, hypoglycaemia)

Examination
Hypertension
Diabetes mellitus
Hyperlipidaemia
Arterial disease (peripheral pulses, carotid or subclavian bruits)
Cardiac disease (arrhythmias, murmurs)
Previous CNS damage (weakness, sensory loss, inco-ordination, reflex, changes)
Ocular involvement (retinal emboli, arterial disease)

Investigation
Routine tests as for stroke (p. 863)
Special tests
  Vertebral/basilar TIA
    Lying/standing blood pressure
    24-hour ECG monitoring
    X-rays of cervical spine
  Carotid TIA
    CT brain scan
    Carotid Doppler ultrasound scanning
    Arteriography (DVI or formal angiography)*

*Only if carotid surgery is contemplated

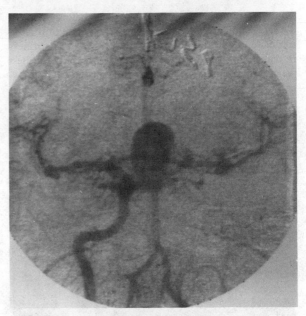

Fig. 16.38 Digital venous imaging (DIV) – intracranial view demonstrating a large saccular aneurysm arising from the basilar artery. Smaller aneurysms are also seen on the middle cerebral arteries. (Courtesy of Dr D. Kean.)

clinical trials. These drugs carry more risk than aspirin, and are usually given only if there is a definable cardiac source of thromboemboli. They are occasionally useful when TIAs fail to come under control with antiplatelet agents, and arterial surgery is not possible.

Arterial surgery. Carotid endarterectomy by an experienced surgeon lowers the risk of further TIA and stroke. In order to be effective there must be a suitable stenosis at the origin of the internal carotid artery on the symptomatic side, and the patient must be fit for operation. Totally occluded vessels cannot be treated in this way, and by-pass procedures have not been shown to improve outlook. Carotid endarterectomy carries an operative risk of stroke or death in up to 10% of cases, and this has to be weighed against that of spontaneous stroke (5% per annum). Patients with frequent TIAs associated with tight carotid stenosis should probably be offered surgery especially if symptoms continue despite aspirin.

SUBARACHNOID HAEMORRHAGE

Subarachnoid haemorrhage (SAH) accounts for about 8% of all strokes. In more than 50% of cases, SAH is due to rupture of an aneurysm of one of the major cerebral arteries or their branches at the circle of Willis. Figure 16.38 shows the common sites of aneurysm formation, usually at the branch points of the arteries. Other causes of SAH are listed in the information box below.

CAUSES OF SAH

Ruptured aneurysm
Arteriovenous malformations
Extension of intracerebral haemorrhage
Haemorrhage into cerebral infarct
Haemorrhage into cerebral tumour
Rupture of atheromatous vessel
Rupture of mycotic aneurysm
Clotting disorders, anticoagulation

Clinical features

SAH often occurs during exertion (e.g. straining, sexual intercourse) when blood pressure is increased. There is usually sudden severe headache which radiates occipitally; neck pain and stiffness often follow. Consciousness may be lost and sometimes a tonic-clonic seizure is provoked. Some patients experience small warning headaches a few days before a major SAH. Examination reveals a variable degree of unconsciousness, photophobia and irritability. Neck stiffness is usually present, but may be absent in the earliest stages. Kernig's sign tends to develop later. Fundoscopy may show subhyaloid haemorrhages and sometimes optic disc oedema. Focal neurological signs may be present because of bleeding into the brain substance or from cerebral ischaemia consequent on arterial spasm. In severe cases, signs of decerebration with extensor posturing and extensor plantar responses are seen. A bruit may be audible over the head or eyes if bleeding is from an arteriovenous malformation.

Investigation

CT scanning. This is the investigation of choice; it will demonstrate the presence of subarachnoid blood in about 90% of cases (Fig. 16.39).

Lumbar puncture. This should be carried out if SAH is suspected and if the scan fails to show bleeding. This will show uniformly blood-stained CSF; after 3–4 hours the supernatant becomes xanthochromic. A lumbar puncture is unnecessary and hazardous if CT scan shows definite subarachnoid blood.

Management

If SAH is proven, urgent transfer to a neurological unit for cerebral angiopathy is usually indicated, unless the patient is deeply comatose. Surgical clipping of the aneurysm is usually feasible. The majority of second haemorrhages occur about 14 days after the initial SAH, and surgery should ideally be performed before this time. If the patient is alert and fit, operation within the first few days is successful, but in some patients surgery is delayed the allow arterial spasm to settle.

Other features of cerebral aneurysms and arteriovenous malformations

Cerebral aneurysms may present in ways other than SAH and some of these are listed in Table 16.40. For features of arteriovenous malformations see the information box below.

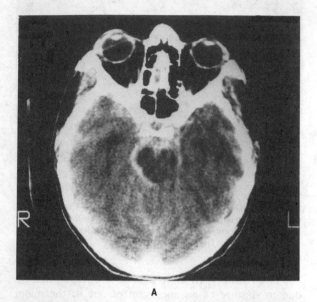

A

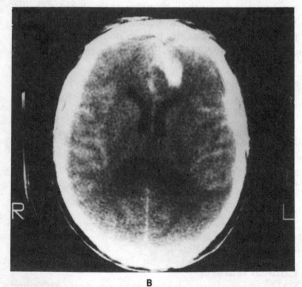

B

Fig. 16.39 CT scan of subarachnoid haemorrhage. A. Extensive blood (high density) in the basal cisterns, outlining the brain stem. **B.** There is a small intracerebral component to the haemorrhage in the left frontal lobe making it likely that the source of bleeding is from a ruptured aneurysm at the junction of the anterior cerebral and the anterior communicating arteries. (Courtesy of Dr D. Kean.)

ARTERIOVENOUS MALFORMATIONS

Clinical features
Subarachnoid haemorrhage
Epilepsy
Headache
Vascular steal episodes (like TIAs)
Tinnitus, vascular noises in head

Investigation
CT scan with contrast enhancement
Cerebral arteriography

Management
Surgical resection (not always possible)
Stereotactic radiotherapy (reduces risk of haemorrhage)
Anticonvulsants if epilepsy present

Table 16.40 Other presentations of cerebral arterial aneurysms

Mechanism	Vessel	Lesion
Compression of cranial nerves	Carotid aneurysm in cavernous sinus	IV, III, VI palsies
	Internal carotid/posterior communicating aneurysm	III nerve palsy
	Anterior communicating artery aneurysm	Optic nerve/chiasm lesions
Compression of cerebral tissue	Middle cerebral artery	Epilepsy, hemiparesis
	Basilar artery	Diplopia, ataxia, tetraparesis

OTHER VASCULAR DISORDERS

GIANT CELL ARTERITIS

Giant cell or temporal arteritis is an inflammatory disease of medium sized arteries, in which there is disruption of the elastic layers, intimal thickening and infiltration of the media by chronic inflammatory and giant cells. Affected vessels may become occluded. The pathological process is of unknown cause, but may have an autoimmune basis since it occurs more frequently in patients with other autoimmune disorders such as thyroid disease or rheumatoid arthritis. The external carotid artery and its branches are particularly susceptible, and the ophthalmic, vertebral and subclavian vessels are often involved. Less commonly, the internal carotid, coronary and mesenteric arteries are affected. The disorder affects mainly people over the age of 60.

Clinical features

These are listed in the information box below.

CLINICAL FEATURES OF GIANT CELL ARTERITIS

- Headache, scalp tenderness
- Malaise, anorexia, weight loss
- Fever
- Arthralgia
- Muscle tenderness and stiffness (not weakness)
- Visual impairment
- Arm and jaw claudication
- Brain-stem ischaemia/infarction (ataxia, diplopia, dysarthria, syncope)
- Cerebral hemisphere infarction

Examination may reveal thickened and tender temporal arteries. Visual impairment is usually due to anterior ischaemic optic neuropathy from occlusion of the posterior ciliary arteries. The diagnosis should be suspected in any elderly patient with visual impairment, especially if headache and malaise are present.

Investigation

The erythrocyte sedimentation rate (ESR) is usually, elevated above 50 mm/hour and may be more than twice this level. Temporal artery biopsy may prove the diagnosis but is not always positive, and treatment should be started immediately if clinical suspicion is strong, since the risk of further visual loss is high.

Management

Treatment is with high dose steroids (prednisolone 60–100 mg/d) initially, reducing the dose gradually over the first few weeks to a maintenance level of 10–20 mg/day as guided by the ESR response. The symptoms improve dramatically within a day or two of starting steroids, but visual failure is usually permanent. If clinical suspicion is high, and the ESR elevated, steroids should be started immediately; temporal artery biopsy may be delayed for 48 hours before histological resolution is likely to take place. Maintenance therapy is required for at least a year, and sometimes for the rest of the patient's life.

CEREBRAL VENOUS THROMBOSIS

Thrombosis of cerebral veins and venous sinuses is uncommon. The causes are listed in the information box below.

CAUSES OF CEREBRAL VENOUS THROMBOSIS

Predisposing causes	Local causes
Polycythaemia	Paranasal sinusitis
Dehydration	Facial skin infection
Hypotension	Otitis media, mastoiditis
Pregnancy	Meningitis, subdural
Oral contraceptives	empyema
	Skull fracture
	Penetrating head and
	eye wounds

Cortical vein thrombosis

This causes local cerebral dysfunction (epilepsy, hemiparesis, dysphasia) though the area involved may enlarge if spreading thrombophlebitis occurs.

Cerebral venous sinus thrombosis

Clinical features

These vary in their manifestation depending on the sinus involved. They are listed in the information box below.

CLINICAL FEATURES OF CEREBRAL VENOUS SINUS THROMBOSIS

Cavernous sinus
Proptosis, ptosis, headache, external and internal ophthalmoplegia, papilloedema, reduced sensation in trigeminal first division.
Often bilateral, patient ill and febrile

Superior sagittal sinus
Headache, papilloedema, seizures
May involve veins of both hemispheres causing advancing motor and sensory deficits

Transverse sinus
Hemiparesis, seizures, papilloedema.
May spread to jugular foramen to involve cranial nerves IX, X, XI

Investigation

CT scanning may show evidence of sinus occlusion but is often normal. There may be evidence of cerebral oedema with small ventricles, and low density changes at sites of cortical infarction. Angiography shows impaired filling of veins and sinuses. CSF is under increased pressure, may be xanthochromic with excess of red and white blood cells and have an increased protein content.

Management

Appropriate broad spectrum antibiotics should be given intravenously, and any infected site (paranasal sinus, middle ear, facial abscess) must be drained. Cerebral oedema may respond to dexamethasone 4 mg t.i.d. The use of anticoagulants is controversial but may be helpful in limiting the spread of thrombosis early in the disorder.

MOVEMENT DISORDERS

This is a varied group of conditions in which there are abnormal involuntary movements, and in some cases impaired voluntary movements, without loss of muscle strength. The extrapyramidal system (p. 814) and particularly the basal ganglia are believed to be the main sites of dysfunction although the pathophysiology is often poorly understood. The main types of disorder and their likely site of damage are listed in Table 16.41.

Table 16.41   Movement disorders and putative sites of causative lesions

Movement disorder		Sites of lesion
Tremor		Substantia nigra
Hypokinesis	} Parkinsonism	Corpus striatum
Rigidity		
Chorea		Caudate nucleus
Athetosis	}	Putamen
Dystonia		Corpus striatum
Hemiballismus		Sub-thalamic nucleus

PARKINSONISM

In his essay on 'The Shaking Palsy', James Parkinson described the three main components of the syndrome that bears his name:

Tremor
Muscular Rigidity
Hypokinesis

Hypokinesis or bradykinesia describes slowness in initiating and repeating voluntary movements, despite normal muscular strength. These features are described in more detail below. The pathophysiological mechanism which links the various forms of Parkinsonism is either defective release or impaired postsynaptic response to the neurotransmitter dopamine in the corpus striatum. The causes of Parkinsonism are listed in Table 16.42.

IDIOPATHIC PARKINSONISM (PARKINSON'S DISEASE)

Parkinson's disease has an overall prevalence of about 1/1000 of the general population, but it is more common in the elderly, the prevalence rising to 1% of those over 60 years.

Aetiology

The cause of the disease is unknown. Genetic factors are not important in typical cases, and there is no good evidence for a viral mechanism. The discovery that methyl-phenyl-tetrahydropyridine (MPTP) caused severe Parkinsonism in drug addicts has provoked the theory that the idiopathic disease might be due to an environmental toxin. There is some evidence to suggest that Parkinsonism is more common in country areas frequently sprayed with herbicides, some of which (e.g. paraquat) have chemical similarity to MPTP.

Table 16.42   Causes of Parkinsonism

Mechanism	Example
Impaired release of dopamine	
Idiopathic	Parkinson's disease
Drugs depleting dopamine stores	Reserpine, tetrabenazine
Toxins damaging dopaminergic neurones	Methyl-phenyl-tetrahydropyridine
	Manganese
Viral infection	Encephalitis lethargica
	Japanese 'B' encephalitis
Trauma	Repeated head injury 'punch drunk' syndrome
Blockade of striatal dopamine receptors	Phenothiazines
	Butyrophenones
Damage to striatal neurones	Viral infection
	Multisystem atrophy
Miscellaneous	Wilson's disease
	Huntington's disease
	Cerebral tumour
	Neurosyphilis

Pathology

There is depletion of pigmented neurones in substantia nigra, hyaline material (Lewy bodies) in nigral cells, atrophic changes in the substantia nigra and depletion of neurones in locus caeruleus.

Clinical features

Both sexes are affected equally. The onset of the disease is usually after the age of 50 years, the incidence increasing with advancing age. Occasionally symptoms start in the third or fourth decades. Classical features of tremor, rigidity and hypokinesis may be absent initially, when non-specific symptoms of tiredness, aching limbs, mental slowness, depression and small handwriting (micrographia) may be noticed.

Tremor. Tremor at rest, affecting one or both hands is often the reason for referral. Tremor may also affect the legs, mouth and tongue; head tremor is rare. Tremor may remain the predominant symptom for some years.

Hypokinesis. This may develop gradually. Many patients have difficulty in initiating rapid fine movements and slowness of gait, and difficulty with tasks such as fastening buttons or writing.

Rigidity of muscular tone. This causes stiffness, and flexed posture. As the disease advances, speech becomes softer and indistinct; postural balance reflexes tend to decline so that falls occur.

There are a number of abnormalities on neurological examination and these are listed in the information box (right).

PHYSICAL ABNORMALITIES IN PARKINSONISM

General
  Expressionless face
  Greasy skin
  Soft, rapid, indistinct speech
  Flexed posture

Gait
  Slow to start walking
  Shortened stride
  Rapid small steps, tendency to run (festination)
  Reduced arm swinging
  Impaired balance on turning

Tremor
Resting 4–6 Hz
  Usually first in fingers/thumb
  Coarse, complex movements, flexion/extension of fingers
  Abduction/adduction of thumb
  Supination/pronation of forearm
  May affect arms, legs, feet, jaw, tongue
  Intermittent, present at rest and when distracted
  Diminishes on action
Postural 8–10 Hz
  Less obvious, faster, finer amplitude
  Present on action or posture, persists with movement

Rigidity
Limbs
  Cogwheel type, mostly upper limbs, phasic element to stiffness in all directions of movement
  Plastic (lead pipe) type, mostly legs and trunk
Trunk
  Flexed, stooped posture

Hypokinesis
  Slowness initiating movements
  Impaired fine movements, especially of fingers
  Poor precision of repetitive movements

The features of Parkinsonism may be unilateral initially, but gradually bilateral involvement is the rule. Muscle strength and reflexes remain normal; plantar responses are flexor. Facial reflexes may be enhanced despite paucity of facial expression, thus tapping the forehead causes repetitive blinking (glabellar tap sign). Eye movements may show impaired upgaze and convergence. Sensation is normal and intellectual faculties are not markedly affected although many patients become depressed, and some show mild cognitive impairment as the disease advances.

Investigation

Usually a diagnosis of Parkinson's disease can be made on clinical grounds; detailed investigation is not required in a typical patient. Some exceptions are listed in the information box below.

TESTS IN PARKINSONISM

Serological tests for syphilis
All patients

CT-brain scanning
Patients under age 50
Signs entirely unilateral
Atypical signs (e.g. pyramidal)

Tests to exclude Wilson's disease
Young patients (2nd to 4th decade)
  Serum caeruloplasmin
  Serum copper
  Urine copper
  Liver function

Management

Any identifiable cause should be treated. Drug induced Parkinsonism may respond to withdrawal of the causative drug, but the features may persist for many months and in some cases are permanent. It is possible that such patients have idiopathic disease that has been unmasked by the drug.

Drug therapy

Anticholinergic agents. These have a useful effect on tremor and rigidity, but do not help hypokinesis. They can be prescribed early in the disease before hypokinesis is a problem, but should be avoided in the elderly (over age 65) because they cause confusion and hallucinations. Other side-effects include dry mouth, blurred vision, difficulty with micturition and constipation. Many anticholinergics are available; benzhexol (1–5 mg t.i.d.) and orphenadrine (50–100 mg t.i.d) are in common use.

Amantidine. This has a mild usually short-lived effect on hypokinesis, but may be used early in the disease before more potent treatment is needed. It acts by potentiating the action of endogenous dopamine. A dose of 100 mg b.d. or t.i.d. is adequate. Side-effects include livedo reticularis and oedema due to vasodilatation, confusion and seizures.

L-DOPA containing agents. The introduction of levodopa (L-DOPA) was a dramatic step in the management of Parkinson's disease. The rationale for this treatment relies on the fact that the enzymic step converting the precursor DOPA to dopamine is dependent on the concentration of available substrate. Thus, although the number of dopamine releasing terminals in the striatum is diminished in Parkinson's disease, it is possible to overdrive the remaining neurons to produce more dopamine by administering DOPA. More than 90% of orally administered L-DOPA is decarboxylated peripherally in the gastrointestinal tract and blood vessels to dopamine, and only a small proportion reaches the brain. This peripheral conversion is responsible for the high incidence of side-effects (nausea, vomiting, vasodilatation) encountered when L-DOPA was used alone. The problem is largely overcome by giving along with the L-DOPA a peripherally acting decarboxylase inhibitor. This combination therapy permits a much lower dose of L-DOPA to be used and markedly reduces the incidence of side-effects. Two combination preparations are available:

L-DOPA + carbidopa (4:1 and 10:1 ratios available)
L-DOPA + benserazide (4:1 combination)

Each preparation is formulated in doses of 50, 100 and 250 mg of L-DOPA. Initial treatment should be with the 50 mg strength b.d. or t.i.d., increasing gradually over 2–4 weeks to 100 mg t.i.d. The therapeutic effect increases gradually over the first 4–8 weeks even when the dose is held steady. Tremor, rigidity and especially hypokinesis are improved. Nausea and vomiting are uncommon, but can be offset with a peripheral dopamine antagonist such as domperidone 10 mg. Dose related side-effects are mainly involuntary movements particularly orofacial dyskinesias, limb and axial dystonias, and occasionally depression, hallucinations and delusions. The L-DOPA dose may be increased gradually up to 800–1000 mg/day, but higher doses often induce troublesome involuntary movements.

Table 16.43 Therapeutic strategy in Parkinson's disease

Stage	Features	Drugs
Early		Under age 65
	Tremor	Anticholinergics
	Rigidity	Amantidine
		Over age 65
		Avoid Anticholinergics
		Amantidine
Moderate		
	Tremor	L-DOPA combinations
	Rigidity	Anticholinergics
	Hypokinesis	In younger patients consider low dose bromocriptine + L-DOPA combination
Severe		
	Tremor	Frequent small doses of L-DOPA combination (1.5–3 hourly)
	Rigidity	$\pm$ selegiline 10 mg/d
	Hypokinesis	$\pm$ low dose bromocriptine 15–30 mg/d
	Dyskinesias	
	Fluctuations	

Late deterioration in response to L-DOPA therapy occurs after 3–5 years in 1/3 to 1/2 of patients. Usually this manifests as fluctuations in response at different times of the day (the 'on-off' effect). In simplest form this is end of dose deterioration due to progression of the disease and loss of capacity to store dopamine. More complex fluctuations are unpredictable changes in response hour to hour with periods of hypokinesis, tremor and dystonia alternating with dyskinesia and agitation. End of dose deterioration can often be improved by dividing the L-DOPA into smaller but more frequent doses (e.g. 50–100 mg every 1.5 to 3 hours). Individual doses may be potentiated and prolonged by the addition of the selective type B monamine oxidase inhibitor selegiline 5 mg b.d. In more difficult cases the combination of low doses of a dopamine receptor agonist bromocriptine to frequent small doses of L-DOPA can be beneficial.

Dopamine receptor agonists. Although a number of drugs which stimulate striatal postsynaptic dopamine receptors have been tried clinically, only bromocriptine is readily available. The drug is very costly, and when used alone is less well tolerated and less impressive in controlling Parkinsonism than L-DOPA. Dyskinesias and fluctuations in response are less likely with bromocriptine, but the incidence of side-effects (nausea, vomiting, mental changes) is higher. Initially 1–2.5 mg bromocriptine is given with food, and the dose increased slowly to 2.5 mg t.i.d. over the first week. Nausea can be suppressed with domperidone 10 mg with each dose if necessary. The dose can then be built up slowly over several months to 60 mg daily or more, depending on response and tolerance.

There may be a case for using bromocriptine alone or in low dose combination with L-DOPA in young patients who will require treatment for many years.

The management of Parkinsonism depends on the stage of the disease and the therapeutic approach is summarised in Table 16.43.

Surgery
Stereotactic thalamotomy is only performed occasionally because of the good response to medication, but is worth considering in patients with severe unilateral tremor which fails to respond to drugs. It is too early to judge whether implantation of fetal mid-brain or adrenal cells into the basal ganglia of Parkinsonian patients will prove of long-term value.

Physiotherapy and speech therapy
Patients at all stages of Parkinson's disease benefit from physiotherapy which helps reduce rigidity and corrects abnormal posture. Speech therapy is indicated for more severe cases where dysarthria and dysphonia interfere with communication.

Prognosis
The outlook for patients with idiopathic Parkinsonism is variable, and depends partly on the age of onset. If symptoms start in middle life, the disease is usually slowly progressive and likely to shorten life-span because of the complications of immobility and tendency to falling. Onset after the age of 70 is unlikely to shorten life or to become severe. L-DOPA itself may accelerate the loss of nigral neurones, so treatment should probably be withheld until symptoms are significant and the dose kept low enough to relieve major symptoms without inducing dyskinesias.

Table 16.44   Wilson's disease (Hepato-lenticular degeneration)

Pathophysiology
Autosomal recessive inherited deficiency of copper carrying protein (caeruloplasmin) in blood
Deposition of copper in liver, eyes and brain

Clinical features
Presentation in adolescence and childhood
Tremor, choreoathetosis, dystonia
Parkinsonism, dementia
Cirrhosis of liver

Diagnosis
Extrapyramidal syndrome in young person
Copper deposits at corneo-scleral junction (Kayser–Fleischer rings)
Low blood copper level
Low serum caeruloplasmin
Raised urinary copper excretion
Abnormal liver function tests

Management
Oral penicillamine 250–500 mg t.i.d.–q.i.d. (or oral EDTA)

Prognosis
Improvement of neurological features if treated early. Life-long treatment required.
Hepatic and haematological side-effects may limit treatment doses

Table 16.45   Kernicterus

Pathophysiology
Damage to basal ganglia and cortex by high levels of unconjugated bilirubin in premature infants with haemolytic disease

Clinical features
Early
Convulsions, opisthotonus, rigidity, coma

Later
Athetosis, choreoathetosis, deafness, mental subnormality, spasticity

Prevention
Avoidance of rhesus incompatibility
Prompt exchange transfusion of severely jaundiced neonates

Table 16.46   Chorea

Definition
Repetitive jerky, semi-purposive movements of limbs, face and trunk

Site of lesion
Mainly in caudate nucleus

Causes
Inherited
  Huntington's disease
Infection
  Encephalitis; acute rheumatism
Metabolic
  Hypoparathyroidism
  Hyperthyroidism
  Pregnancy, oral contraception
Vascular
  Polycythaemia, SLE
Drugs
  L-DOPA, phenothiazines

Management
Dopamine receptor antagonists: phenothiazines, butyrophenones, e.g. haloperidol 0.5–1.5 mg t.i.d.
Dopamine depleting agents: tetrabenazine, reserpine, e.g. tetrabenazine 25–50 mg t.i.d.
GABA enhancing agents: sodium valproate, e.g. 200–1000 mg t.i.d.

OTHER MOVEMENT DISORDERS

Other movement disorders are summarised in Tables 16.44–51.

Table 16.47   Specific types of chorea

Huntington's disease

Inheritance
Autosomal dominant

Age of onset
Middle adult life

Clinical features
Chorea
Progressive Dementia
Seizures
Parkinsonism (juvenile cases)

Diagnosis
Clinical features
Family history (may be absent)
Caudate nucleus atrophy on CT scan
Earlier diagnosis becoming likely with gene linkage probes

Management
Symptomatic only; chorea responds to tetrabenazine (25–50 mg t.i.d.) or dopamine antagonists (haloperidol 0.5–1.5 mg t.i.d.)
Long-term institutional care needed as dementia progresses

Table 16.48   Rheumatic chorea (Sydenham's Chorea)

Aetiology
Sequel to streptococcal infection
Affects children and adolescents mostly females

Clinical features
Chorea, emotional lability

Investigation
Elevated antistreptolysin titres

Management
Sedation, rest
Dopamine antagonists (e.g. haloperidol 0.5–1.5 mg t.i.d.)
Penicillin to eradicate infection (phenoxymethyl–penicillin 250–500 mg t.i.d.)

Prognosis
Recovery within a few weeks
Relapses may occur in pregnancy

Table 16.49   Hemiballismus

Definition
Wild flailing proximal movements of arm and leg on one side

Cause
Usually vascular lesion of contralateral subthalamic nucleus. Typically hypertensive elderly patients

Management
Tetrabenazine (25–50 mg t.i.d.) or dopamine antagonists (e.g. haloperidol, 0.5–1.5 mg t.i.d.). Stereotactic thalamotomy if persistent

Prognosis
Movements usually cease after a few weeks. Patients may become exhausted if untreated

Table 16.50   Athetosis and dystonia

Athetosis
Slow writhing distal movements affecting fingers, hands, toes, feet

Dystonia
Sustained abnormal posture of limbs, neck and trunk

Causes
Lesions of basal ganglia, especially putamen
Kernicterus, birth injury, hypoxia, encephalitis, vascular lesions
Idiopathic forms, some familial

Management
Often very difficult
Anticholinergic drugs, large doses, e.g. benzhexol built slowly up to 100 mg/d
Baclofen (5–20 mg t.i.d.), benzodiaepines (e.g. diazepam 2–10 mg t.i.d.), L-DOPA
(e.g. Madopar '125' 2–6 doses/d) and sodium valproate (200–1000 mg/t.i.d.) may
help. Stereotactic surgery if unilateral

MULTIPLE SCLEROSIS

Multiple sclerosis affects 1 in 2000 of the population in Britain and is one of the commonest causes of long-term disability.

Aetiology

The cause of the disease is unknown. Epidemiological evidence suggest an environmental influence on causation: the prevalence varies in relationship to latitude with low prevalence in the tropics and high prevalence in the temperate zones of both northern and southern hemispheres. Migration before the age of 15 between areas of contrasting prevalence affects the risk of developing the disorder and children born in Britain of immigrants from areas of low prevalence have the same risk of developing the condition as the indigenous population.

A genetic influence on susceptibility is suggested by a tenfold increase in risk in first degree relatives and the higher concordance for multiple sclerosis in monozygotic twins in comparison with dizygotic twins. HLA tissue-typing has demonstrated an increased prevalence of haplotypes A3, B7, Dw2 and DR2 in affected patients in Britain, but different haplotypes have been associated with an increased risk for multiple sclerosis in other countries. An immune mechanism is suggested by increased levels of activated T lymphocytes in the CSF, and increased immunoglobulin synthesis within the central nervous system. There are increased levels of antibody to some viruses, including measles virus, in the CSF but this may be an epiphenomenon.

The relative importance of environmental, genetic and immunological factors is unresolved: multiple sclerosis is likely to be multifactorial in origin.

Pathology

The acute lesion is the plaque, a circumscribed area of demyelination with swelling of axis cylinders and patchy infiltration of inflammatory cells. Gliosis follows and the chronic lesion is a scar with a shrunken greyish appearance, most commonly occurring in the

Table 16.51   Miscellaneous movement disorders

Type	Characteristics	Pathophysiology	Treatment
Spasmodic torticollis	Dystonia of neck movements. Head turns to one side for prolonged periods	Unknown	Anticholingergics Tetrabenazine (25–50 mg t.i.d.) Benzodiazepines Botulinum toxin injections Surgery
Tardive dyskinesia	Facial grimacing chewing and tongue movements. Usually elderly	Altered dopamine receptor sensitivity following phenothiazine or butyrophenone drugs	Withdraw drug. Substitute a selective alternative, e.g. sulpiride (200–400 mg b.d.) tetrabenazine (25–50 mg t.i.d.)
Tics	*Simple* Repeated stereotyped brief face and limb co-ordinated movements	*Unknown* Presumed basal ganglia in origin. Common in childhood	Behaviour therapy. Sulpiride (200–400 mg b.d.) Pimozide (1–4 mg t.i.d.)
	Complex Multiple tics vocalisation often obscene (coprolalia) and rude gestures (Giles de la Tourette syndrome)	*Unknown* Presumed to have basal ganglia origin	Pimozide (1–4 mg t.i.d.) Sulpiride (200–400 mg b.d.) Haloperidol (0.5–1.5 mg t.i.d.)

Table 16.52 Common presentations in multiple sclerosis

Mode of onset	Frequency
Weakness or loss of control of one or more limbs	50%
Visual symptoms (including optic neuritis)	30%
Sensory symptoms	10%
Miscellaneous	10%

periventricular region, the optic nerves and the subpial regions of the spinal cord.

Clinical features

Characteristically the clinical course involves relapsing and remitting neurological dysfunction, mainly affecting the optic nerves, brain stem, cerebellum and spinal cord. The first manifestation may occur at any age, but onset before puberty or after the age of 60 is rare. There is no typical clinical history, but some types of presentation are more frequent and suggestive symptoms may develop in the course of the illness (see Table 16.52 and the information box below).

SUGGESTIVE SYMPTOMS IN MULTIPLE SCLEROSIS

- Tingling in spine or limbs on neck flexion (Lhermitte's phenomenon)
- Exacerbation of symptoms by exercise or rise in body temperature
- Trigeminal neuralgia under the age of 50
- Recurrent facial palsy

The symptoms and signs of the first attack usually recover within 1–3 months and after a variable interval there may be a recurrence, in many cases within 2 years. Frequent relapses with incomplete recovery indicate a poor prognosis and in many patients a phase of progressive deterioration supersedes the phase of relapse and remission. In a minority of patients there may be an interval of years or even decades between attacks and in some, particularly if optic neuritis is the initial manifestation, there is no recurrence. In the middle aged, multiple sclerosis may present with a spastic paraparesis, which may be only slowly progressive.

The physical signs depend on the localisation of areas of demyelination, and reflect the common pathological sites of plaques, with some physical signs occurring frequently and others rarely. Common physical signs are listed in the information box (right). No sign is specific to multiple sclerosis and diagnosis depends on the identification of combinations of signs,

---

COMMON PHYSICAL SIGNS IN MULTIPLE SCLEROSIS

- Upper motor neurone signs
- Optic atrophy, afferent pupillary defect, impaired colour vision, internuclear ophthalmoplegia
- Nystagmus, dysarthria, ataxia
- Peripheral impairment of position sense, light touch sensation

---

for example optic atrophy and paraparesis, or mixed cerebellar and pyramidal signs in the limbs. Sensory signs are almost invariable at some time in the course of the disease, but are usually less prominent than sensory symptoms. Some patients become euphoric and, although significant intellectual impairment is unusual, mild impairment of memory is common.

Investigation

The diagnosis of multiple sclerosis depends clinically on the demonstration of lesions occurring at different times and at different sites in the central nervous system. Investigation is aimed at providing evidence for an inflammatory disorder and for multiple sites of neurological involvement (see the information box below).

INVESTIGATIONS IN MULTIPLE SCLEROSIS

Evoked potentials	Immunoglobulin content
Visual	Protein electrophoresis
Auditory	(oligoclonal bands)
Somatosensory	
	Myelogram
CSF examination	
Cell count	*CT/MRI scan*

There is no specific test for multiple sclerosis and, although abnormalities may be revealed by any of these investigations, interpretation depends on the rest of the clinical picture. Visual evoked potentials can detect clinically silent lesions in up to 70% of patients, but auditory and somatosensory evoked potentials are less frequently of diagnostic value. The CSF may show a lymphocytic pleocytosis in the acute phase and persistent elevation of gammaglobulin or oligoclonal bands of IgG in 70–90% of patients between attacks. CT scan may show plaques, but MRI scan is the most sensitive technique for imaging lesions in multiple sclerosis and is positive in over 95% of definite cases (Fig. 16.40). Oligoclonal bands occur in a range of other disorders and the MRI appearances in multiple sclerosis cannot

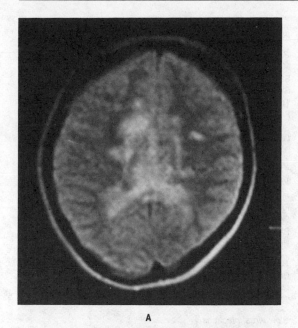

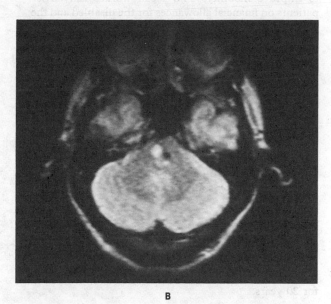

A   B

Fig. 16.40   MRI scan in multiple sclerosis. A. Shows multiple areas of high signal in a periventricular distribution and separate areas of high signal in the white matter of both cerebral hemispheres. **B.** Shows areas of high signal in the brain stem.

be distinguished from those of cerebrovascular disease or cerebral vasculitis. Diagnosis depends on the clinical history and examination, taken in combination with the investigative findings.

It is important to exclude potentially curable conditions such as syphilis, vitamin B_{12} deficiency and spinal cord compression.

Management

There is no curative treatment but much can be done to support the patient during the course of the illness. Management is aimed at specific therapy for the underlying condition and symptomatic treatment of complications.

Corticosteroids may promote more rapid and complete recovery in acute exacerbations. Intramuscular adrenocorticotrophic hormone (ACTH) has no advantage over dexamethasone given orally in a dosage of 2 mg 3 times daily for 10 days, but intravenous methylprednisolone 500 mg daily for 5 days is of particular benefit in individual patients and is currently under trial. Prolonged administration of steroids does not alter the long-term prognosis and immunosuppressant agents, including azathioprine, are of little benefit. Gluten-free diet, linoleic acid supplements or hyperbaric oxygen therapy are not of benefit.

The treatment of complications of multiple sclerosis are summarised in Table 16.53.

Table 16.53   Treatment of complications of multiple sclerosis

Complication	Treatment
Spasticity	Baclofen 15–100 mg*
	Diazepam 2–15 mg*
	Dantrolene 25–400 mg*
	Chemical neuronectomy
	Physiotherapy
Ataxia	Isoniazid 600–1200 mg*
	Clonazepam 2–8 mg*
Dysaesthesia	Carbamazepine 200–1800 mg*
	Phenytoin 200–400 mg daily
	Tricyclic antidepressant
Urinary symptoms	
Failure to store urine	Propantheline 30–90 mg*
	Oxybutynin 10–20 mg*
	Imipramine 25 mg t.i.d.
Failure to empty bladder	Bethanecol 30–120 mg*
	Baclofen 15–100 mg*
	Intermittent self-catheterisation

*In divided dosage.

Of prime importance is the encouragement and support of patients and their relatives. A frank discussion of the diagnosis and prognosis is necessary and may dispel fears, which are often ill-founded. Periods of physiotherapy may improve functional capacity in those patients who become disabled and assessment by the occupational therapist will provide guidance in the provision of aids within the home and to improve mobility. The social worker can advise patients on financial allowances for the disabled and the provision of social services support.

The care of the bladder is particularly important. Infections should be treated with an appropriate antibiotic. Incontinence, urgency and frequency may be treated pharmacologically, by external drainage or by urinary catheter, which may be passed intermittently by the patient rather than left permanently indwelling. The choice of treatment is difficult to make clinically and urodynamic assessment may be necessary in patients with troublesome symptoms. Sexual dysfunction is a source of anxiety in many patients and may be relieved by skilled counselling.

Prognosis

The outlook cannot be predicted with confidence in any individual patient and, although approximately 5% of patients die within 5 years of onset, a rather larger proportion remain well and retain unlimited mobility for 20 years.

INFECTIONS OF THE NERVOUS SYSTEM

The major infections of the nervous system are listed in the information box (right).

VIRAL INFECTIONS

VIRAL MENINGITIS

Viral infection is the commonest cause of meningitis, and usually results in a benign and self-limiting illness requiring no specific therapy. Virus (aseptic) meningitis is usually a much less serious illness than bacterial meningitis unless there is associated encephalitis which is rare. The majority of patients suffering from this condition have a transient self-limiting illness and never reach medical attention. A number of viruses can cause meningitis, the commonest being echoviruses and the mumps virus. Causes of meningitis and encephalitis are listed in the information box (p. 877).

Clinical features

Viral meningitis usually occurs in isolation without clinical evidence of parenchymal involvement of the nervous system. Causative organisms include arena, echo, and Coxsackie viruses, but in the majority of patients no specific virus is isolated. The condition occurs mainly in children or young adults, with the acute onset of headache and irritability and the rapid development of meningeal irritation. There may be a

---

INFECTIONS OF THE NERVOUS SYSTEM*

Bacterial infections
Meningitis
Suppurative encephalitis
Brain abscess
Tuberculosis
Paravertebral (epidural) abscess
Neurosyphilis
Leprosy (peripheral nerves)
Diphtheria (peripheral nerves)
Tetanus (motor cells)

Virus infections
Meningitis
Encephalitis
Poliomyelitis
Rabies
Human immunodeficiency virus (HIV) infection

Post-viral infections
Demyelinating encephalitis (also post-vaccine)
Guillain-Barré syndrome (also post-vaccine)
??Chronic fatigue syndrome (myalgic encephalomyelitis)

Slow virus infections
Creutzfeldt-Jakob disease
Kuru
Sub-acute sclerosing panencephalitis
Progressive multifocal leucoencephalopathy

Protozoal infections
Malaria
Toxoplasmosis (immunosuppressed)
Trypanosomiasis
Amoebic abscess

Helminth infections
Schistosomiasis (spinal cord)
Cysticercosis
Hydatid disease
Strongyloidiasis

Fungal infections
Cryptococcal meningitis (immunosuppressed)
Candida meningitis or brain abscess

*A number of these infections are not included in this chapter. They can be found in Chapter 5 Diseases due to Infection.

---

high pyrexia, but focal neurological signs are uncommon.

Meningeal irritation ('meningism') may occur in bacterial, viral, and fungal infections and in a range of non-infectious conditions including subarachnoid haemorrhage, malignant disease, and connective tissue disorders such as sarcoidosis and systemic lupus erythematosus. Careful interpretation of CSF indices is essential to accurate diagnosis (Table 16.54).

Investigation

The CSF contains an excess of lymphocytes, but

Table 16.54 Cerebrospinal fluid indices in meningitis

Condition	Cell:		Glucose	Protein	Gram stain
	Type	Count			
Viral	Lymphocytes	10–2000	normal	normal	–
Bacterial	Polymorphs	1000–50 000	low	normal/elevated	+
Tuberculous	Polym/Lymph/mixed	50–5000	low	elevated	often –
Fungal	Lymphocytes	50–500	low	elevated	±
Malignant	Lymphocytes	0–100	low	normal/elevated	–

CAUSES OF VIRAL MENINGITIS AND ENCEPHALITIS

Enteroviruses,
(Echoviruses, coxsackieviruses, polioviruses)
Herpes simplex virus
Mumps virus
Influenza virus
Japanese encephalitis virus
Arboviruses
    Togaviruses (e.g. yellow fever)
    Bunyaviruses (e.g. sandfly fevers)
Rabies virus
Human immunodeficiency virus
Lymphocytic choriomeningitis virus (arenavirus)

Table 16.55 Viruses causing encephalitis transmitted by mosquitos and ticks

Infection	Vector	Endemic in
Yellow fever	Mosquito	Africa and South America
Japanese encephalitis		South East Asia
Ross river fever		Australia
California encephalitis		North America
Omsk haemorrhagic fever	Tick	Russia
Louping ill		North Britain

---

normal glucose and protein levels. There is no specific treatment and the condition is usually benign and self-limiting.

Management
The patient should be treated symptomatically in a quiet environment. Recovery usually occurs within days, although a lymphocytic pleocytosis may persist in the CSF.

Meningitis may also occur as a complication of a viral infection primarily involving other organs; for example in mumps, measles, infectious mononucleosis, herpes zoster and hepatitis. Complete recovery is the rule without specific therapy.

VIRAL ENCEPHALITIS

A range of viruses cause encephalitis but there is no recognisable combination of symptoms and signs specific to virus type. Only a minority of patients have a history of recent viral infection and viral isolation is often unrewarding. The development of effective therapy for some forms of encephalitis therefore enhances the importance of clinical diagnosis. The

viruses which are transmitted by mosquitoes and ticks are shown in Table 16.55.

Pathology
Inflammation can occur in the cortex, white matter, basal ganglia and brain stem and the distribution of lesions varies with the type of virus. Inclusion bodies are often present in the neurones and glial cells and there is an infiltration of polymorphonuclear cells in the perivascular space. There is neuronal degeneration and diffuse glial proliferation, often associated with cerebral oedema.

Clinical features
Viral encephalitis presents with acute onset of headache, often accompanied by fever. Disturbance of consciousness ranging from drowsiness to deep coma supervenes early and may advance dramatically. Meningism occurs in 75% of patients and there may be a variety of focal signs such as aphasia, hemiplegia, tetraplegia, or cranial nerve palsies. Epilepsy and raised intracranial pressure commonly develop as the condition progresses. Rabies presents a distinct clinical picture and is described on page 880.

Acute encephalitic illness may occur in HIV infection, occasionally at the time of infection, but more commonly as a manifestation of AIDS.

Encephalitis lethargica occurred in epidemic form in the 1920s and was presumed to be of viral aetiology although this has never been established. Parkinsonism may be a late sequel of this disease.

In *herpes encephalitis* signs of temporal lobe dysfunction may be detected and confusional states, which may be misdiagnosed as a psychosis, develop.

Investigation

The differential diagnosis of viral encephalitis is summarised in the information box below.

DIFFERENTIAL DIAGNOSIS OF VIRAL ENCEPHALITIS

- Acute metabolic encephalopathy
- Cerebral tumour
- Stroke
- Bacterial meningitis/abscess
- Tuberculous meningitis

Approximately half of all patients suspected on admission as suffering from viral encephalitis have other diseases. The investigations listed in the information box below are indicated in suspected viral encephalitis:

CSF examination may be hazardous and should be preceded by a CT scan, which will exclude a structural lesion and may provide evidence of reactive oedema. The cerebrospinal fluid is usually lymphocytic, but polymorphonuclear cells may predominate in the early stages and occasionally the fluid is normal. The protein content may be elevated, but the glucose is normal. The electroencephalogram is usually abnormal with diffuse slow-wave activity, but is non-specific unless there are periodic discharges to suggest herpes simplex encephalitis. Serological tests and culture may identify the causative virus, but are usually available too late to influence treatment.

INVESTIGATIONS IN VIRAL ENCEPHALITIS

- Full blood count/ metabolic screen
- Viral studies
- CT scan (MRI scan)
- CSF examination
- Electroencephalogram

Management

Patients suffering from viral encephalitis require skilled nursing care and careful monitoring of fluid balance and nutritional state. Anticonvulsant treatment is often necessary and raised intracranial pressure is treated with dexamethasone 4 mg 6-hourly. Herpes simplex virus encephalitis may respond to acyclovir 10 mg/kg intravenously 3 times daily. This medication is relatively safe and should be given to all patients suspected of suffering from viral encephalitis as specific diagnosis is often impossible.

Even with optimum treatment mortality is 10–30% and a significant proportion of survivors have residual epilepsy or cognitive impairment.

Brain-stem encephalitis

Clinical features

This presents with dysarthria, diplopia or cranial nerve palsies.

Investigation

The CSF is lymphocytic with a normal glucose. The causative agent is presumed to be viral, although listeria meningitis may cause a similar syndrome and require specific treatment with ampicillin 500 mg 4 times daily.

POLIOMYELITIS

Aetiology and pathology

The disease is caused by one of three related polio viruses which comprise a subdivision of the group of enteroviruses. It is much less common following the widespread use of oral vaccines but is still a major problem in developing countries. Infection usually occurs through the nasopharynx.

The virus is liable to affect the grey matter of the spinal cord, brain stem and cortex and has a particular propensity to damage anterior horn cells especially those within the lumbar segments. There is often accompanying infiltration of the meninges with lymphocytes.

Clinical features

Figure 16.41 illustrates the various features of the infection. The incubation period is 7–14 days. At the onset there is usually mild fever and headache which improves after a few days. Many patients do not progress beyond this stage. In other instances, after a period of well-being lasting approximately a week, there is recurrence of pyrexia and headache accompanied by neck stiffness and signs of meningeal irritation. Paralysis may occur later and is of variable extent. Weakness of one muscle group may progress to widespread paresis. Respiratory failure may supervene if intercostal muscles are paralysed or the medullary motor nuclei are involved.

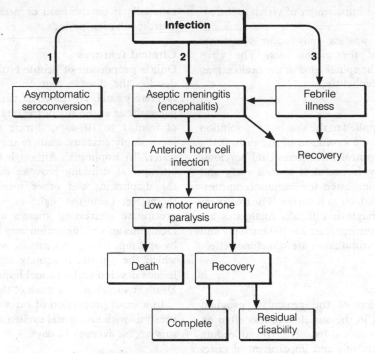

Fig. 16.41 Poliomyelitis – possible consequences of infection.

Investigation

The CSF shows a lymphocytic pleocytosis, a rise in protein and a normal sugar content.

Management

In the early stages bed rest is imperative. At the onset of respiratory difficulties a tracheostomy and intermittent positive pressure ventilation are required. Subsequent treatment is by physiotherapy and orthopaedic measures.

Prognosis

Epidemics vary widely in their incidence of abortive and non-paralytic cases and in mortality rate. Death occurs from respiratory paralysis. Muscle weakness is maximal at the end of the first week and gradual recovery may then take place for several months. Any muscle showing no signs of recovery by the end of a month will not regain useful function. It is difficult to make a more definitive prediction about the extent of permanent disability until 3–6 months after the onset. Second attacks are very rare but occasional patients show late deterioration in muscle bulk and power many years after the initial infection.

Prevention

This is by immunisation.

HERPES ZOSTER (SHINGLES)

Herpes zoster is the result of reactivation of the varicella/zoster virus which has lain dormant in a posterior nerve root ganglion following chickenpox earlier in life. Reactivation may be apparently spontaneous (as usually occurs in the middle-aged or elderly) or be due to immunosuppression as in patients with malignant disease or AIDS. Chickenpox may be contracted from a patient with shingles but the reverse does not occur.

Clinical features

The first symptom is usually severe continuous pain in the distribution of the affected nerve root. After 3 or 4 days the skin in the affected area becomes reddened and vesicles appear which dry up over 5 or 6 days leaving small scars. The pain of zoster usually subsides as the eruption fades, but occasionally, especially in old people, it may be followed by a persistent and intractable neuralgia.

Any dorsal root ganglion may be infected, most commonly those supplying the trunk where two or three adjacent dermatomes on one side only are often involved. Infection of the trigeminal ganglion usually involves the ophthalmic division; the vesicles appear on the cornea and may lead to corneal ulceration with the danger of scarring and impairment of vision (ophthalmic herpes).

Segmental muscle wasting may occur sometimes from involvement of the motor root. The virus occasionally invades the spinal cord or the brain giving rise to myelitis or encephalitis.

Management
Idoxuridine may be applied to the skin in a 5% solution in the early stages of the evolution of the rash; 0.1% drops are used for corneal infections. Oral acyclovir 200 mg 5 times daily is useful if started early and systemic acyclovir is indicated for immunocompromised patients or when infection is severe. The treatment of post-herpetic neuralgia is difficult. Analgesics are often unhelpful, but amitriptyline 25–100 mg daily and transcutaneous nerve stimulation are sometimes effective.

Ramsay-Hunt syndrome
Herpes zoster infection of the geniculate ganglion presents with vesicles in the auricle and less often on the palate. The facial nerve is usually involved leading to ipsilateral facial paralysis and impairment of taste. Oral acyclovir 200 mg 5 times daily may be of benefit if started early.

RABIES
Rabies is caused by a rhabdovirus which infects the central nervous tissue and salivary glands of a wide range of mammals, and is usually conveyed, by saliva, through bites or licks on abrasions or on intact mucous membranes. Man is most frequently infected from dogs. In Europe the maintenance host is the fox and in recent years the zoonosis has spread from Poland westwards through Germany and France (Table 16.56).

The incubation period, during which the virus is spreading centripetally along axons to the brain, varies in man from a minimum of 9 days to many months but is usually between 4 and 8 weeks. Severe bites,

Table 16.56 Sources of infection in rabies

Area	Source	Transmission
World-wide	Dogs, other canines, cats	Bite, lick
	Cattle, etc. (to farmers)	Hand into mouth
	Other mammals	Bite, tick
	Man (undiagnosed)	Corneal graft
North America	Skunks and racoons	Bite, lick
Central and South America	Vampire bats	Bite
	Cave dwelling bats	Salivary aerosols

especially if on the head or neck are associated with short incubation periods.

Clinical features
Only a proportion of people bitten by a rabid animal develop the disease, but once manifest it is almost invariably fatal. At the onset there may be fever, and paraesthesia at the site of the bite. A prodromal period of from 1 to 10 days, during which the patient is increasingly anxious, leads to the characteristic fear of water, 'hydrophobia'. Although the patient is thirsty, attempts at drinking provoke violent contractions of the diaphragm and other inspiratory muscles and thereafter, even the sight or sound of water may precipitate distressing spasms and attacks of panic. Delusions and hallucination may develop accompanied by spitting, biting and mania, with lucid intervals in which the patient is acutely anxious. Cranial nerve lesions develop and terminal hyperpyrexia is common. Death ensues, within a week of the onset of symptoms.

In a small proportion of cases there is an ascending paralysis without mental excitement and these patients survive, on average 12 days.

Investigation
During life the diagnosis is usually made on clinical grounds but rapid immunofluorescent techniques can detect antigen in corneal impression smears or skin biopsies.

Management
A few patients with rabies have survived. All received some post-exposure prophylaxis, and needed intensive care with facilities to control cardiac and respiratory failure. Otherwise, only palliative treatment is possible once symptoms have appeared. The patient should be heavily sedated with diazepam 10 mg 4–6 hourly, supplemented by chlorpromazine 50–100 mg, if necessary. Nutrition and fluids should be given intravenously or through a gastrostomy.

Prevention
Pre-exposure prophylaxis is required by those who by profession handle potentially infected animals, those who work with rabies virus in laboratories and those who live at special risk in rabies endemic areas. Protection is afforded by two intradermal injections of 0.1 ml human diploid cell strain vaccine, or two intramuscular injections of 1 ml, givin 4 weeks apart, followed by yearly boosters.

Post-exposure prophylaxis
The wounds should be thoroughly cleaned, preferably

with a quaternary ammonium detergent or soap; damaged tissues should be excised and the wound left unsutured. Rabies can usually be prevented if treatment is started within a day or two of biting. Delayed treatment may still be of value. For maximum protection hyperimmune serum and vaccine are required.

The safest antirabies antiserum is human rabies immune globulin, the dose is 20 i.u/kg body weight. Half is infiltrated around the bite and half is given intramuscularly at a different site from the vaccine. The dose of hyperimmune animal serum is 40 i.u./kg; hypersensitivity reactions, including anaphylaxis are common.

The safest vaccine, free of complications, is human diploid cell strain vaccine; 1.0 ml is given intramuscularly on days 0, 3, 7, 14, 30 and 90. In developing countries, where human rabies globulin may not be obtainable, 0.1 ml of vaccine should be given intradermally into 8 sites on day 1, with single boosters on days 7 and 28. Where human products are not available and when risk of rabies is slight (licks on the skin, or minor bites of covered arms or legs) it may be justifiable to delay starting treatment up to 5 days while observing the biting animal or awaiting examination of its brain rather than use the older vaccine.

The biting animal should be confined, if possible. If it is healthy after 5 days, it does not have rabies and treatment is stopped. If it dies, escapes or is killed, the brain is examined by immunofluorescence for Negri bodies. If positive treatment is continued.

Control of spread
Human rabies is an infrequent disease even in endemic areas. Its fearful manifestations, however, justify stringent attempts being made to limit its spread and prevent its importation into uninfected countries, such as Britain. Measures to control rabies are listed in the information box below.

CONTROL OF RABIES

- License and vaccinate domestic dogs
- Kill stray dogs
- Monitor reservoir hosts
- Control and quarantine imported animals
- Vaccinate at-risk animals and man

JAPANESE ENCEPHALITIS

This arbovirus is transmitted to man by the bites of infected culicine mosquitoes which have fed on in-

fected animals or birds, notably nestling herons. Pigs and other domestic animals are important sources of infection acting chiefly as amplifiers of the virus brought to them by mosquitoes. The virus is widespread in the Pacific Islands from Japan to Guam in the Phillipines, Taiwan, Borneo, Malaysia and Singapore and is spreading slowly west across the Indian subcontinent. Devastating epidemics, with a high mortality rate, have occurred. In endemic areas, serological surveys indicate a high incidence of subclinical infection and only sporadic cases may be encountered. Inflammatory and degenerative changes are found in the brain.

Clinical features
Many infections are sub-clinical. Overt disease may occur at any age, although children are particularly susceptible. Typical clinical features of encephalitis (p. 877) develop quickly and last from a few days to 2 weeks or longer and convalescence is prolonged. The CSF is under raised pressure and an increase of cells and protein appears within several days. Persistant neurological damage is common. The mortality in overt disease varies from 15 to 40%.

Investigation
The virus has only rarely been recovered from the blood or CSF but in fatal cases may sometimes be obtained from the brain. A rise in antibody titre is the usual basis for diagnosis.

Management
There is no specific treatment. Skilled nursing for the patient in coma may be life-saving.

Prevention
The elimination of breeding places of the vector mosquitoes, the control of piggeries, and the use of insecticides, where practicable, should be instituted. A vaccine, made in Japan and available in Britain, is safe and effective.

SLOW VIRUS INFECTIONS

A number of neurological diseases develop many months or even years after infection with transmissible agents which are known or presumed to be viruses.

KURU

This is a disease which occurs only in the members of a cannibalistic New Guinea tribe and is probably transmitted by eating the brains of dead tribal members. There is degeneration of grey matter, most marked in the cerebellum, causing a progressive ataxia.

CREUTZFELDT-JAKOB DISEASE

This is a sub-acute encephalopathy characterised by pre-senile dementia, myloclonus and motor neurone signs. The cause is not known but it may be a virus as infection can be transmitted from man to chimpanzees and also from man to man by corneal grafting.

SUBACUTE SCLEROSING PANENCEPHALITIS

This is a rare, chronic, progressive and eventually fatal neurological disease caused by the measles virus, presumably as a result of an inability of the nervous system to eradicate the virus. It occurs in children and adolescents, usually many years after the primary virus infection. The onset is insidious with intellectual deterioration, apathy and clumsiness followed by myoclonic jerks, rigidity and dementia. The EEG is distinctive showing bursts of triphasic slow waves.

Investigation
The CSF may show a mild lymphocytic pleocytosis and the electroencephalogram is distinctive with periodic bursts of triphasic waves.

Management
Although there is persistent measles specific IgG in serum and CSF, antiviral therapy is ineffective and death ensues within years.

PROGRESSIVE MULTIFOCAL LEUCO-ENCEPHALOPATHY

This is a rare condition which usually occurs as a complication of reticulosis, leukaemia, or carcinomatosis, but may also develop in previously fit individuals. A papovavirus, SV40, has been identified as the causative organism and pathologically there is widespread demyelination of the white matter within the cerebral hemispheres. CT scan shows areas of low density in the white matter and associated clinical signs include dementia, hemiparesis and dysphasia which progress rapidly, leading to death within weeks or months.

POST-VIRAL SYNDROMES

ACUTE DEMYELINATING ENCEPHALOMYELITIS

This occurs about a week after diseases such as measles and chickenpox or following vaccination, and is probably immunologically mediated. There are areas of perivenous demyelination widely disseminated throughout the brain and spinal cord.

Clinical features
Headache, vomiting, pyrexia, confusion and meningism are presenting features and fits or coma may develop. Flaccid paralysis and extensor plantar responses are common and cerebellar signs may be present, particularly when the disorder follows chickenpox.

Investigation
The CSF may be normal or show a small increase in mononuclear cells and protein.

POST-INFECTIVE POLYNEURITIS

This condition, commonly referred to as the Guillain-Barré syndrome, can rarely develop during or immediately after a virus infection, usually of the upper respiratory tract. (See pp. 896–897)

MYALGIC ENCEPHALOMYELITIS

This is also known as the post-viral syndrome or chronic fatigue syndrome. Enteroviruses have been postulated as a possible cause. The syndrome not infrequently occurs following infectious mononucleosis. It is most commonly seen in teenagers and young adults especially those with more demanding occupations or preparing for examinations.

Clinical features
It is an ill-defined condition with a range of symptoms including malaise, fatigue, myalgia, headache and exhaustion. There are no abnormal physical signs and investigation is negative.

Investigation
There is no specific test for the syndrome but serum antibodies to Coxsackie-B or Epstein-Barr viruses may be present.

Management
Although a proportion of affected individuals respond to antidepressant medication, many patients become

Table 16.57   Bacterial meningitis

	Common	Less common
Neonate	Gram-negative bacilli (*E. coli*, Proteus, etc.) Group B streptococci	Listeria monocytogenes
Pre-school child	Haemophilus influenzae Neisseria meningitidis Streptococcus pneumoniae	Mycobacterium tuberculosis
Older child and adult	Neisseria meningitidis Streptococcus pneumoniae	Listeria monocytogenes Mycobacterium tuberculosis Cryptococcus neoformans (Immunosuppressed) Staphylococcus aureus (skull fracture)

chronically disabled and all that can be offered is sympathy and moral support.

BACTERIAL INFECTIONS

MENINGITIS

Bacterial meningitis is usually secondary to a bacteraemic illness although infection may result from direct spread from an adjacent focus of infection in the ear, skull fracture or sinus. Any bacterium can cause meningitis but some are more frequent causes than others (Table 16.57). Bacterial meningitis has become less common but the mortality and morbidity remain high despite the availability of an increasing range of antibiotics. An important factor in determining prognosis is early diagnosis and the prompt initiation of appropriate therapy.

Pathology
The pia arachnoid is congested and infiltrated with inflammatory cells. A thin layer of pus forms and this may later organise to form adhesions. These may cause obstruction to the free flow of CSF leading to hydrocephalus, or may damage the cranial nerves at the base of the brain. The CSF pressure rises rapidly, the protein content increases and there is cellular reaction which varies in type and severity according to the nature of the inflammation and the causative organism. Pneumococcal meningitis is often associated with a very purulent CSF and a high mortality especially in older adults.

Clinical features
Headache, drowsiness, fever and neck stiffness are the usual presenting features of bacterial meningitis. Neck stiffness can be elicited by passive flexion of the neck which is resisted as a result of muscle spasm. In severe bacterial meningitis the patient is usually comatose and there may be focal neurological signs. In pneumococcal and haemophilus infections there may be otitis media. Pneumococcal meningitis is often associated with pneumonia especially in older patients and alcoholics. It is common in patients without functioning spleens.

Neisseria meningitides
The meningococcus is the commonest cause of bacterial meningitis in Britain where any increasing proportion of meningococci have become sulphonamide-resistant; fortunately, all strains remain sensitive to penicillin. Spread is by air-borne route and epidemics occur, particularly in cramped living conditions or when the climate is hot and dry, e.g. Africa. The organism invades through the nasopharynx producing bacteraemia which is usually associated with pyogenic meningitis. Complications of meningococcal septicaemia are listed in the information box below.

COMPLICATIONS OF MENINGOCOCCAL SEPTICAEMIA

- Meningitis
- Shock
- Intravascular coagulation
- Renal failure
- Peripheral gangrene
- Arthritis (septic or reactive)
- Pericarditis (septic or reactive)

Chronic meningococcaemia is a rare condition in which the patient can be unwell for weeks or even months with recurrent fever, sweating, joint pains and transient rash. It usually occurs in the middle-aged and elderly.

Listeria monocytogenes
This has recently emerged as an increasing cause of meningitis in the immunosuppressed, diabetics, alco-

Table 16.58 Chemotherapy of bacterial meningitis

	Drug of choice	Alternative agents
Meningococcal	Benzylpenicillin	Chloramphenicol Cefuroxime
Pneumococcal	Benzylpenicillin	Chloramphenicol Cefuroxime
H. influenzae	Chloramphenicol	Cefuroxime
Neonatal Gram-negative bacilli Group B streptococci	Cefotaxime Gentamicin + ampicillin	Gentamicin + ampicillin Chloramphenicol
L. monocytogenes	Gentamicin + ampicillin	Co-trimoxazole Rifampicin
C. neoformans	Amphotericin + flucytozine	Fluconazole
M. tuberculosis	Rifampicin + Isoniazid + Pyrazinamide + Streptomycin	

holics and pregnant women. It can also cause meningitis in the neonatal period.

Diagnosis
In bacterial meningitis the CSF is cloudy (turbid) due to the presence of many neutrophils (often more than 1000 cells mm^3), the protein content is significantly elevated and the glucose reduced. Gram film may reveal the identity of the causative organism but this is by no means always so even after the results of culture are available. Blood cultures may be positive.

Management
The choice of antibiotic depends on the infecting organism. Tables 16.58 and 16.59 give guidance as to the preferred antibiotic:

1. if the organism has not been identified
2. if the organism is known.

The dose of the various antibiotics which must be given intravenously depends on the age and weight of the patient.

Table 16.59 Treatment of pyogenic meningitis. Cause unknown

Neonate
Gentamicin + ampicillin
or
Third generation cephalosporin (e.g. cefotaxime)

Pre-school child
Chloramphenicol
or
Cefuroxime

Older child and adult
Chloramphenicol
or
Cefuroxime

Prevention of meningococcal infection
Household and other close contacts of patients with meningococcal infections, especially children, should be given 2 days of rifampicin. The dose for adults is 600 mg twice a day. Children under one year are given 5 mg/kg 12-hourly and those over 12 months 10 mg/kg 12 hourly. Vaccines are available for the prevention of disease caused by meningococci of Groups A and C but not Group B which is the commonest serogroup isolated in many countries including Britain.

TUBERCULOUS MENINGITIS
Pathology
The condition occurs most commonly shortly after a primary infection in childhood or as part of miliary tuberculosis. The usual local source of infection is a caseous focus in the meninges or brain substance adjacent to the CSF pathway.

The brain is covered by a greenish, gelatinous exudate especially around the base, and numerous scattered tubercles are found on the meninges.

Clinical features
The clinical features are listed in the information box below.

CLINICAL FEATURES OF TUBERCULOUS MENINGITIS

Children	*Adults*
Lassitude	Malaise
Loss of interest in toys	Headache
Unwillingness to talk	Vomiting
Anorexia	Low-grade fever
Constipation	
Headache	

Investigation
The CSF is under increased pressure. It is usually clear but, when allowed to stand, a fine clot may form. The fluid contains up to 400 cells/mm^3, predominantly lymphocytes. There is a rise in protein and a marked fall in glucose. Detection of the tubercle bacillus in a smear of the centrifuged deposit from the CSF may be difficult. The CSF should be cultured on appropriate media but as the result will not be known for up to 6 weeks, treatment must be started without waiting for confirmation.

Management
Chemotherapy should be started as soon as the diagnosis is made using one of the regimens described

on page 884, together with pyrazinamide. All patients should also receive prednisolone, 10 mg 4 times daily. Surgical methods for ensuring ventricular drainage must be adopted if obstructive hydrocephalus develops. Skilled nursing is essential during the acute state of the illness and measures must be taken to maintain adequate hydration and nutrition.

The intensive regime of drug treatment should be continued for 8 weeks and followed by a continuation phase.

Prognosis

Untreated tuberculous meningitis is fatal in a few weeks but complete recovery is the rule with modern treatment if it is started before the appearance of focal signs or stupor. When treatment is started at a later stage the recovery rate is 60% or less and the survivors may be mentally deficient, epileptic, deaf, blind or show some other permanent neurological deficit.

TETANUS

This disease results from infection with *Clostridium tetani*, which exists as a commensal in the gut of man and domestic animals and is found in the soil. Infection enters the body through wounds, often trivial, such as those caused by a splinter, a nail in the boot or a garden fork or following septic infection such as a dirty abrasion. Tetanus is rare in Britain and occurs mostly in gardeners and farmers. By contrast the disease is common in many developing countries where dust contains spores derived from animal and human excreta. If childbirth takes place in an unhygienic environment *Tetanus neonatorum* may result from infection of the umbilical stump or the mother may develop the disease.

In circumstances unfavourable to the growth of the organism, spores are formed and these may remain dormant for years in the soil. Spores germinate and bacilli multiply only in the anaerobic conditions which occur in areas of tissue necrosis or if the oxygen tension is low as a result of the presence of other organisms, particularly aerobic ones. The bacilli remain localised but produce an exotoxin with an affinity for motor nerve endings and motor nerve cells. The anterior horn cells are affected after the exotoxin has passed into the blood stream and their involvement results in rigidity and convulsions. Symptoms first appear from 2 days to several weeks after injury–the shorter the incubation period, the more severe the attacks and the outcome may well be fatal with an incubation period of only a few days.

Clinical features

Much the most important early symptom is trismus – spasm of the masseter muscles which causes difficulty in opening the mouth and in masticating, hence the name 'lock-jaw'. This tonic rigidity spreads to involve the muscles of the face, neck and trunk. Contraction of the frontalis and the muscles at the angles of the mouth gives rise to the 'risus sardonicus'. There is rigidity of the muscles at the neck and trunk of varying degree. The back is usually slightly arched and there is a board-like abdominal wall.

In the more severe cases violent spasms lasting for a few seconds to 3 to 4 minutes occur spontaneously or may be induced by stimuli such as moving the patient, or making a noise. These convulsions are painful, exhausting and of very serious significance especially if they appear soon after the onset of symptoms. They gradually increase in frequency and severity for about 1 week and the patient may die from exhaustion, asphyxia or aspiration pneumonia. In less severe illness convulsions may not commence for about a week after the first sign of rigidity and in very mild infections they may never appear. Autonomic involvement may cause cardiovascular complications such as hypertension.

Rarely the only manifestation of the disease may be 'local tetanus' – stiffness or spasm of the muscles near the infected wound – and the prognosis is good if treatment is commenced at this stage.

Investigation

The diagnosis is made on clinical grounds. It is rarely possible to isolate the infecting organism from the original locus of entry. Spasm of the masseters due to dental abscess, septic throat or other causes is painful, in contradistinction to tetanus. Conditions which can mimic tetanus include hysteria and phenothiazine overdosage.

Tetanus is still one of the major killers of adults, children and neonates in the tropics where the mortality rate can be nearly 100% in the newborn and around 40% in others.

Management

This should be begun as soon as possible. The essentials are shown in the information box (p. 886).

Prevention

Active immunisation must be given. Contaminated injuries are treated by debridement. The immediate danger of tetanus can be greatly reduced by the injection of 1200 mg of penicillin followed by a 7-day course of oral penicillin. When the risk of tetanus is judged to be present, an injection of 250 units of human

TREATMENT OF TETANUS

Neutralise absorbed toxin
i.v. injection of 3000 i.u. of antitoxin

Prevent further toxin production
Debridement of wound
Benzylpenicillin 600 mg 6-hrly i.v.
(metronidazole if allergic to penicillin)

Control spasms
Nurse in a quiet room
Avoid unnecessary stimuli
i.v. diazepam – if spasms continue paralyse patient and ventilate

General measures
Maintain hydration and nutrition
Treat secondary infections

tetanus antitoxin should be given and an intramuscular injection of toxoid which should be repeated 1 month and 6 months later. For those already protected only a booster dose of toxoid is required.

LYME DISEASE

This is caused by the spirochaete *Borrelia burgdorferi*, which is transmitted by the bite of a tick.

Clinical features

Patients may present with arthritis, carditis or neurological signs and in the majority there is a characteristic skin condition, erythema chronicum nigrans. Neurological presentations include cranial nerve palsies, chronic lymphocytic meningitis, motor or sensory radiculitis, encephalitis and myelitis.

Investigation

The diagnosis rests on the history and clinical findings and may be confirmed by a serological test.

Management

Early cases are given tetracycline 250 mg 4 times daily or erythromycin 250 mg 4 times daily. Late cases and in particular those with neurological involvement require parenteral therapy with a cephalosporin, for example cefotaxime 1 g twice daily.

NEUROSYPHILIS

Neurosyphilis may present as an acute or chronic process and may involve singly or in combination the meninges, blood vessels and parenchyma of the brain and spinal cord. The clinical manifestations are diverse and, although the condition is now rare, early diagnosis and treatment remain important.

Clinical features

The clinical and pathological features of the three most common presentations are summarised in Table 16.60.

Neurological examination reveals signs appropriate to the anatomical localisation of lesions. Pupillary abnormalities, described by Argyll Robertson may accompany any neurosyphilitic syndrome. The pupils are small and irregular, and react to convergence but not directly to light. Delusions of grandeur suggest general paresis of the insane, but more commonly there is simply progressive dememtia. The combination of physical signs in tabes dorsalis are characteristic. Argyll Robertson pupils are found in 90% of patients and there is depression of tendon reflexes, hypotonia, distal impairment of deep pain sensation in the legs resulting in perforating painless ulcers and Charcot joints, and

Table 16.60 Clinical and pathological features of neurosyphilis

Type	Pathology	Clinical features
Meningovascular (5 years)*	Endarteritis obliterans Meningeal exudate Granuloma (gumma)	Stroke Cranial nerve palsies Seizures/mass lesion
General paralysis of the insane (5–15 years)*	Degeneration in cerebral cortex/cerebral atrophy Thickened meninges	Dementia Tremor Bilateral upper motor signs
Tabes dorsalis (5–20 years)*	Degeneration of sensory neurones Wasting of dorsal columns Optic atrophy	Lightning pains Sensory ataxia Visual failure Abdominal crises Incontinence Trophic changes

*Interval from primary infection.

impairment of pin-prick sensation over the nose, perineum and distal lower limbs.

The clinical syndromes outlined above may occur in combination giving rise to mixed pictures, which may mimic many other neurological disorders.

Investigation

Routine screening for syphilis is warranted in the great majority of neurological patients. Serological tests (p. 189) are positive in the serum in most patients, but CSF examination is essential if neurological involvement is suspected. Active disease is suggested by an elevated cell count, usually lymphocytic, and the protein content may be elevated to 0.5–1.0 g/l with an increased gammaglobulin fraction. Serological tests in the CSF are usually positive, but progressive disease can occur with negative CSF serology.

Management

The essential part of the treatment of neurosyphilis of all types is the injection of procaine penicillin 600 mg–1.2 g daily for 3 weeks (p. 189). Further courses of penicillin must be given if symptoms are not relieved, or the condition continues to advance, or the CSF continues to show signs of active disease. The cell count returns to normal within 3 months of completion of treatment, but the elevated protein takes longer to subside, and some serological tests may never revert to normal. Evidence of clinical progression at any time is an indication for renewed treatment.

OTHER FORMS OF MENINGITIS

Fungal meningitis (cryptococcosis p. 150)

This usually occurs in patients who are immunosuppressed or have a focus of fungal infection. It is a recognised complication of HIV infection (p. 103). The CSF findings are similar to those of tuberculous meningitis, but the diagnosis can be confirmed by microscopy of specific serological tests.

Malignant meningitis

The cerebrospinal fluid may contain reactive lymphocytes with a low CSF glucose and the diagnosis depends on cytological examination, which may be enhanced by cytospin techniques.

Sarcoidosis or connective tissue disorder

The distinction between meningitis in these conditions and infectious conditions can be difficult and often rests on the recognition of the systemic features of these disorders.

In somea areas meningitis may be caused by spirochaetes (leptospirosis p. 140), Lyme disease (p. 886), syphilis (p. 187), Rickettsia (typhus fever p. 118) or protozoa (amoebiasis p. 155).

CEREBRAL ABSCESS

Bacteria may be introduced into the cerebral substance through penetrating injury, direct spread from sinuses or the middle ear, or through embolism from systemic infection, most commonly subacute bacterial endocarditis or pulmonary abscess. The site of abscess formation and likely causative organism are related to the source of infection (Table 16.61).

Table 16.61   Site, source and organism in cerebral abscess

Site of abscess	Source of infection	Likely organism
Frontal	Frontal sinusitis	Streptococcus
Temporal	Otitis media	Streptococcus Bacteroides Proteus
Cerebellar	Otitis media	Streptococcus Bacteroides Proteus
Parietal	Embolic	Streptococcus Bacteroides Proteus
Any site	Trauma	Staphylococcus

Initial infection leads to local suppuration followed by loculation of pus within a surrounding wall of gliosis, which in chronic abscess may form a tough capsule. Multiple abscesses occur particularly with metastatic spread.

Clinical features

Cerebral abscess may present acutely with fever, headache, meningism and drowsiness, but more commonly presents over days or weeks as a cerebral mass lesion with little or no evidence of infection. Epilepsy, raised intracranial pressure and focal hemisphere signs occur alone or in combination and distinction from a cerebral tumour may be impossible on clinical grounds.

Investigation

Lumbar puncture is potentially hazardous in raised intracranial pressure and CT scan should always precede lumbar puncture if focal neurological signs are present. The CT scan shows single or multiple low density areas which enhance peripherally with contrast to provide a ring appearance with central low density

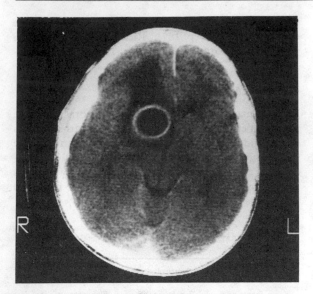

Fig. 16.42 CT scan in cerebral abscess (after contrast enhancement). There is ring enhancement of a lesion deep in the right cerebral hemisphere with surrounding cerebral oedema and shift of midline structures to the left. (Courtesy of Dr R.J. Sellar.)

and surrounding cerebral oedema (Fig. 16.42). Plain skull X-ray may provide evidence of sinusitis and there may be an elevated white cell count and ESR in patients with active local infection.

Management
Antimicrobial therapy should be recommended once the diagnosis is made and the likely source of infection should guide the choice of antibiotic (Table 16.61). The presence of a capsule may lead to a persistent focus of infection despite antibiotics and in these patients surgical treatment by repeated burrhole aspiration or excision of abscess may be necessary. Anticonvulsants are often necessary as there is a high incidence of epilepsy, which may develop acutely or in the recovery phase.

Prognosis
The mortality rate remains at 10–20% despite an improvement in available surgical and medical treatments and in some patients this is related to delay in diagnosis and initiation of treatment.

SUBDURAL EMPYEMA

This is less common than cerebral abscess and occurs as a complication of frontal sinusitis, osteomyelitis of the skull vault, or middle ear disease. A collection of pus in the subdural space spreads over the surface of the hemisphere causing underlying cortical oedema or thrombophlebitis.

Clinical features
Epilepsy and progressive hemiparesis are common presentations.

Investigations
The diagnosis rests on plain skull X-ray, to provide evidence of a focus of infection, and CT head scan. This may show a subdural collection with underlying cerebral oedema but may be normal. The diagnosis is often dependent on suspicion of subdural empyema in patients with a local focus of infection.

Management
Pus is aspirated via a burrhole and appropriate parenteral antibiotic treatment commenced. Any local source of infection must be treated to prevent reinfection.

SPINAL EPIDURAL ABSCESS

Clinical features
The characteristic clinical features are pain in a root distribution and progressive transverse myelitis with paraparesis, sensory impairment and sphincter dysfunction. Infection is usually metastatic, but a primary source of infection is easily overlooked

Investigation
Plain X-rays of the spine may show osteomyelitis and urgent neurosurgical intervention, preceded by myelography, is essential to prevent complete and irreversible paraplegia.

Management
Decompressive laminectomy relieves the pressure on the dura and allows the abscess to be drained and organisms to be cultured. The patient must be given appropriate intravenous antibiotics.

DISEASES OF THE SPINAL CORD

COMPRESSION OF THE SPINAL CORD

Acute spinal cord compression is one of the commonest neurological emergencies encountered in clinical practice. Early diagnosis is essential to allow appropriate management and may prevent persistent and disabling neurological deficit. Pressure on the spinal cord may

Table 16.62   Causes of spinal cord compression

Site	Frequency	Causes
Vertebral (extradural)	80%	Trauma Intervertebral disc Secondary carcinoma Breast Prostate Bronchus Myeloma Tuberculosis
Meninges (Intradural extramedullary)	15%	Tumours Meningioma Neurofibroma Ependymoma Metastasis Lymphoma Leukaemia Epidural abscess
Spinal cord (intradural intramedullary)	5%	Tumours Glioma Ependymoma Metastasis

arise from lesions of the vertebral column, the spinal meninges, or the spinal cord and common causes are listed in Table 16.62.

A space-occupying lesion within the spinal canal may involve nerve tissue directly by pressure or indirectly by interfering with the blood supply. Oedema from venous obstruction impairs neuronal function, and ischaemia from arterial obstruction leads to necrosis of the spinal cord. The earlier stages are reversible, but severely damaged neurones do not recover, enhancing the importance of early diagnosis and treatment.

Clinical features

The onset of symptoms of spinal cord compression is usually slow but can be acute with trauma or metastases, especially if there is arterial occlusion. The symptoms are

1. pain, localised over the spine or in a root distribution, which may be aggravated by coughing, sneezing or straining;
2. paraesthesia, numbness, or cold sensations, especially in the lower limbs, which spread proximally often to a level on the trunk;
3. heaviness, weakness or stiffness of the limbs, most commonly the legs;
4. urgency or hesitancy of micturition, leading eventually to urinary retention.

Pain and sensory symptoms occur early, while weakness and sphincter dysfunction are usually late manifestations.

The signs on examination vary according to the level

of cord compression and the structures involved. There may be tenderness to percussion over the spine, if there is vertebral disease and this may be associated with a local kyphosis. Involvement of the roots at the level of compression may give dermatomal sensory impairment and lower motor signs at the corresponding level. Interruption of fibres in the spinal cord causes sensory loss and upper motor neurone signs below the level of the lesion, and there is often disturbance of sphincter function.

The distribution of these signs varies with the level of the lesion:

1. above the fifth cervical segment – upper motor neurone signs and sensory loss in all four limbs;
2. between fifth cervical and first thoracic – lower motor neurone signs and segmental sensory loss in the arms and upper motor neurone signs in the legs;
3. thoracic cord – spastic paraplegia with a sensory level on the trunk;
4. lumbosacral cord and cauda equina – lower motor neurone signs and segmental sensory loss in the legs. (The spinal cord ends at approximately the T12/L1 spinal level and spinal lesions below this level can only cause lower motor neurone signs).

The *Brown-Sequard syndrome* results if damage is confined to one side of the cord. On the side of the lesion there is a band of hyperaesthesia with below it loss of proprioceptive sense and upper motor neurone signs. On the other side there is loss of spinothalamic sensation (pain, temperature) as fibres of that tract decussate soon after entering the cord.

Investigation

Patients with a short history of progressive spinal cord compression should be investigated urgently. Investigations necessary are listed in the information box below.

INVESTIGATION FOR SPINAL CORD COMPRESSION

- Plain X-rays of the spine
- Chest X-ray
- Myelogram
- Spinal CT scan

Plain X-rays may show bony destruction and soft-tissue abnormalities and are an essential part of investigation (Fig. 16.43). Routine investigations, including chest X-ray, may provide evidence of systemic disease. Myelography localises the lesion and, with CT

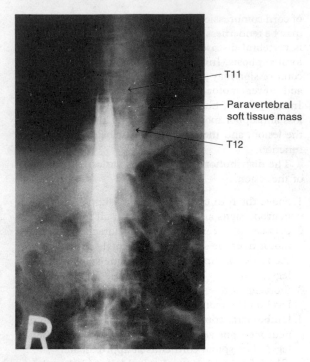

T11

Paravertebral
soft tissue mass

T12

Fig. 16.43 Myelogram in malignant spinal cord compression. The
column of contrast medium is obstructed at the level of T11/T12. There
is partial collapse of the body of the T11 vertebra with loss of the
pedicle and a paravertebral soft tissue mass at this level on the left
side. (Courtesy of Dr R.J. Sellar.)

in suitable cases, defines the extent of compression and
associated soft-tissue abnormality. The CSF should be
taken for analysis at the time of myelography, and in
cases of spinal block shows a normal cell count, very
elevated protein and xanthochromia (Froin's syndrome). Acute deterioration may develop after myelography and it is preferable to alert neurosurgeons
before such procedures are undertaken.

Management
The treatment and prognosis depend on the nature of
the underlying lesion. Benign tumours should be
surgically excised and a good functional recovery can
be expected, unless a marked neurological deficit has
developed before diagnosis. Extradural compression
due to malignancy is the commonest cause of spinal
cord compression and has a poor prognosis. Surgical
decompression may be appropriate in some patients,
but has a similar prognosis to needle biopsy, to
establish the histological nature of the tumour, followed by radiotherapy. Traumatic lesions of the
vertebral column require specialised treatment in a
neurosurgical centre.

PARAPLEGIA

This may result from many causes such as tumours,
trauma and other forms of spinal compression, multiple
sclerosis, subacute combined degeneration of the cord
and, in India, lathyrism.

Management
This must be directed to the cause but management of
the paraplegia itself is most important if complications,
which may in themselves lead to death, are to be
avoided. Pressure sores, urinary infections, renal
calculi, faecal impaction and contractures can all be
prevented.

Skin. Pressure sores are liable to develop because of
the loss of sensation, diminished blood supply and
immobility. The patient must be turned every 2–4
hours to a position which avoids pressure on bony
prominences such as the sacrum and heels. The skin
must be kept dry and clean and the patient nursed, if
possible, on a specially designed mattress or bed.

If pressure sores develop, the patient must not lie on
the affected side and scrupulous asepsis must be
observed. Skin grafting may be necessary and it is
important to maintain nutrition.

Bladder. Aseptic intermittent catheterisation must
be performed if retention occurs. An indwelling
catheter is not desirable as it predisposes to infection,
reduces bladder capacity and promotes calculus formation. Many paraplegic patients are able to establish
automatic bladder emptying, often assisted by manual
compression of the lower abdomen; in others intermittent self-catheterisation or a urinary diversion procedure may be necessary. Urinary infection should be
treated promptly and an adequate fluid intake encouraged.

Bowel. Constipation must be prevented by suitable
diet and laxatives. Enemas or manual evacuation may
be necessary if the faeces become hard and impacted.

Paralysis. Spasticity can lead to the development
of flexor spasm and contractures in the limbs which
may be prevented by regular passive movement of the
limbs and by nursing the patient in postures that
discourage flexion of the joints. A cradle to remove the
weight of the bedclothes from the lower limbs may help
prevent reflex stimulation and foot-drop deformity. In
severe spasticity, without hope of recovery, flexor
spasms can be relieved by intrathecal injection of
phenol in glycerine or by section of the anterior nerve
roots.

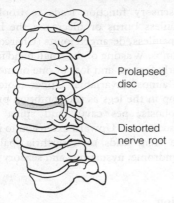

Fig. 16.44   C4/5 vertebral level. A lateral disc protrusion compressing the C5 root.

Prolapsed disc

Distorted nerve root

Rehabilitation. A great deal can be done by rehabilitation when the cause of paralysis is not progressive. Patients may learn to walk with calipers or to use a wheelchair. Many achieve independence, may follow suitable occupations, and take part in a variety of recreational activities.

CERVICAL SPONDYLOSIS

Degenerative change in the cervical spine is a common radiological finding in the middle-aged and elderly. Degeneration of the intervertebral discs and secondary osteoarthrosis (cervical spondylosis) is often asymptomatic, but may be associated with neurological dysfunction. The C5/6, C6/7, and C4/5 vertebral levels and C6, C7 and C5 roots respectively are most commonly affected (Fig. 16.44).

CERVICAL RADICULOPATHY

Compression of a nerve root occurs when a disc prolapses laterally and may develop acutely or more gradually due to osteophytic encroachment of the intervertebral foramina.

Clinical features
The patient complains of pain in the neck which may radiate in the distribution of the nerve root. The neck is held rigidly and neck movements may exacerbate pain. Paraesthesia and sensory loss may be found in the affected segment and there may be lower motor neurone signs, including weakness, wasting and reflex impairment (Table 16.63).

Investigation
Plain X-rays, including lateral and oblique views,

Table 16.63   Physical signs in cervical root compression

Root	Muscle weakness	Sensory loss	Reflex
C5	Biceps, deltoid, spinati	Upper lateral arm	Biceps
C6	Brachioradialis	Lower lateral arm, thumb, index finger	Supinator
C7	Triceps, finger and wrist extensors	Middle finger	Triceps

should be obtained to confirm the presence of degenerative changes and to exclude other conditions, including destructive lesions. Electrophysiological studies rarely add to the clinical examination, but may be necessary if there is diagnostic doubt.

Management
Conservative treatment with analgesics and a cervical collar results in resolution of symptoms in the great majority of patients. In chronic nerve root compression cervical myelography may be indicated in the few patients who require surgery in the form of foraminotomy or disc excision.

CERVICAL MYELOPATHY

Dorsomedial herniation of a disc and the development of transverse bony bars or posterior osteophytes may result, alone or in combination, in pressure on the spinal cord or the anterior spinal artery, which supplies the anterior two-thirds of the cord.

Clinical features
The onset of symptoms is usually insidious and painless, although acute deterioration may occur after trauma, especially hyperextension injury. Upper motor neurone signs develop in the limbs, with spasticity of the legs usually appearing before the arms are involved. Dermatomal sensory loss is common in the upper limbs, while pain, temperature and joint position sense may be impaired in the legs. The neurological deficit usually progresses gradually and disturbance of control of micturition is a late feature.

Investigation
Plain X-rays confirm the presence of degenerative changes and myelography may be indicated if surgical treatment is being considered. MRI scan has the advantage of being non-invasive and is a sensitive technique for demonstrating disordered anatomy and may also show areas of high signal within the spinal cord at the level of compression. Imaging of the cervical spine should be considered if there is diagnostic doubt or prior to surgery.

Management

Surgical procedures, including laminectomy and anterior discectomy, may arrest progression in disability but do not usually result in neurological improvement and carry a significant risk, particularly in the elderly. The judgement as to when surgery should be undertaken may be difficult. Manipulation of the cervical spine is of no proven benefit and may precipitate acute neurological deterioration.

Prognosis

The prognosis in cervical myelopathy is unpredictable. In many patients the condition stabilises or even improves without intervention, but if progressive disability does develop surgical decompression may be essential.

SYRINGOMYELIA

In this condition cavities filled with fluid and surrounded by glial cells develop near the centre of the spinal cord and may communicate with the central canal. The expanding cavity disrupts second-order spinothalamic neurones, may extend laterally to damage the anterior horn cells, and may compress the long fibre tracts.

Aetiology

The most frequent cause is blockage of the exit foramina of the fourth ventricle. Cerebrospinal fluid cannot escape into the subarachnoid space and the pressure rise within the closed ventricular system is communicated to the central canal of the cord, which expands along irregular paths of least resistance. In the majority of patients obstruction to the flow of CSF is due to congenital herniation of the cerebellar tonsils through the foramen magnum (Chiari Type I malformation) and in others to basal arachnoiditis or, rarely, following trauma. Following disturbed CSF dynamics hydrocephalus may occur in association and, rarely, extension of the cavities caudally produces brain-stem dysfunction (syringobulbia).

Clinical features

Patients usually present in the third or fouth decade and symptoms are of insidious onset and slowly progressive. Pain in the neck or shoulder is common and patients may seek advice because of sensory loss in the upper limbs. The most characteristic physical sign is dissociated sensory loss (loss or depression of pain and temperature sensation with preservation of other sensory modalities), which has an upper and lower level in a mantle or hemi-cape distribution. Loss or protective sensory function leads to trophic lesions such as painless burns or ulcers on the hands, and sometimes painless, deranged joints (Charcot joints) in the upper limbs. Wasting of the small hand muscles is a common early feature and loss of one or more reflexes in the arm almost invariable. Upper motor neurone signs develop in the legs as the condition progresses.

Kyphoscoliosis, pes cavus and spina bifida are common associations. Upward extension to involve the lower brain stem leads to dysarthria, palatal palsy, Horner's syndrome, nystagmus and sensory loss on the face.

Investigation

Plain X-rays may demonstrate congenital anomalies around the foramen magnum or expansion of the cervical canal. The most sensitive and least invasive investigation for syringomyelia is magnetic resonance imaging (Fig. 16.45), although myelography, often combined with CT scan, allows accurate diagnosis in the great majority of patients.

Management

Surgical decompression of the foramen magnum or the syrinx itself may arrest progression of the neurological deficit and often alleviates pain. The results of surgery are however often disappointing and in some patients

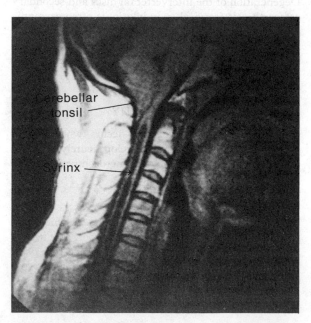

Fig. 16.45 Sagittal MRI scan showing a syrinx extending the length of the cervical cord. There is associated displacement of the crebellar tonsils (Arnold-Chiari-Type 1) downward. (Courtes6y of Dr R. Grant.)

the condition continues to progress and worsens if the brain stem is involved.

LUMBAR DISC HERNIATION

Low back pain, 'lumbago', is the commonest medical cause of inability to work, but in the great majority of patients is due to abnormalities of joints and ligaments in the lumbar spine rather than herniation of an intervertebral disc. Pain in the distribution of the lumbar or sacral roots is more often due to disc protrusion, but is also a feature of other rare but important disorders including spinal tumour, malignant disease in the pelvis and tuberculosis of the vertebral bodies.

Acute lumbar disc herniation is often precipitated by trauma, usually by lifting heavy weights while the spine is flexed. The nucleus pulposus may bulge or rupture the annulus fibrosus, giving rise to pressure on nerve endings in the spinal ligaments, changes in the vertebral joints, or pressure on the nerve roots.

Clinical features

The onset may be sudden, often following trauma to the back, or gradual and repeated episodes of low back pain may precede sciatica by months or years. Constant aching pain is felt in the lumbar region and may radiate to the buttock, thigh, calf and foot. Pain is exacerbated by coughing or straining and may be relieved by lying flat.

The altered mechanics of the lumbar spine results in loss of lumbar lordosis and there may be spasm of the paraspinal musculature. Root pressure is suggested by limitation of flexion of the thigh on the affected side if the straight leg is raised (Lasegue's sign). If the third or fourth lumbar roots are involved Lasegue's sign may be negative, but pain in the back may be induced by hyperextension of the hip (femoral nerve stretch test). The roots most fequently affected are S1, L5 and L4 and the signs of root pressure at these levels are summarised in Table 16.64.

Investigation

Plain X-rays of the lumbar spine. These may show no abnormality in acute disc herniation or there may be narrowing of the disc space. There may be degenerative changes including osteophyte formation at the margins of the vertebral bodies in chronic low back pain, and plain X-rays also exclude other conditions such as malignant infiltration of a vertebral body.

Myelography. This is required if there is diagnostic doubt or for purposes of localisation before operation. It is unlikely to be of diagnostic value unless there is clinical evidence of root compression and is rarely indicated if pain is the only clinical feature.

MRI scan. Using external coils, this has the potential to supersede myelography and has the great advantage of being non-invasive.

Management

The initial treatment in all patients is bed rest on a firm mattress, if necessary supported by wooden boards. Provided rest is absolute, with prohibition from sitting up or leaving the bed for toilet purposes, pain and neurological signs, if present, resolve in over 95% of patients. Bed rest should be continued for 2–4 weeks and on recovery the patients should be instructed in back strengthening exercises and advised to avoid physical manoeuvres likely to strain the lumbar spine.

Injections of local anaesthetic or steroids may be a useful adjunct to bed rest if symptoms are due to ligamentous or joint dysfunction.

In a few patients with clinical evidence of nerve root compression, surgery may have to be considered if there is no response to conservative treatment or if progressive neurological deficits develop. Central disc prolapse with bilateral symptoms and signs and disturbance of sphincter function requires urgent surgical decompression.

LUMBAR CANAL STENOSIS (OR CAUDA EQUINA CLAUDICATION)

This is due to a congenital narrowing of the lumbar spinal canal, exacerbated by the degenerative changes which commonly occur with age.

Table 16.64 Physical signs in lumbar root compression

Spinal level	Root	Sensory loss	Weakness	Reflex
L5/S1	S1	Sole and lateral foot	Eversion of foot	Ankle
L4/L5	L5	Outer calf and dorsum foot	Dorsiflexion of hallux/toes	Hamstring
L3/L4	L4	Inner calf	Inversion of foot	Knee

Clinical features

Characteristically the patients, who are usually elderly, develop exercise induced weakness and paraesthesia distally in the legs. These systems progress rapidly with continued exertion until the patient can no longer walk, but are quickly relieved by a short period of rest. Physical examination is usually normal at rest, with preservation of peripheral pulses, but weakness or reflex loss may be detected if the patient is examined immediately after exercise.

Investigation

Plain X-rays of the lumbar spine show narrowing of the lumbar canal, which may be confirmed by myelography or CT scan.

Management

Extensive lumbar laminectomy results in an often complete relief of symptoms and recovery of normal exercise tolerance.

DISORDERS OF PERIPHERAL NERVES

Peripheral nerves are made up of axons, which represent elongated processes originating from neurones in the anterior horn cells of the spinal cord and dorsal root ganglia. These are enveloped in a series of Schwann cells which form the fatty myelin sheath. Pathological processes may affect cell bodies, the myelin sheath, or the connective tissue and blood vessels of peripheral nerves. Although these processes cannot be clinically distinguished, a knowledge of the pathological nature of a neuropathy is helpful in assessing prognosis and deciding on treatment. The clinical classification of peripheral nerve lesions comprises involvement of one or more individual peripheral nerves or a generalised polyneuropathy.

MONONEUROPATHY

The most frequent causes of damage to a single nerve are entrapment, particularly in fibro-osseous tunnels, trauma and diabetes mellitus.

ENTRAPMENT NEUROPATHIES

Clinical features

The diagnosis of these conditions rests on the often characteristic clinical history and a careful evaluation of the physical signs (Tables 16.65, 16.66).

Table 16.65 Symptoms in entrapment neuropathy

Nerve	Symptoms
Median (Carpal tunnel syndrome)	Pain and paraesthesia on palmar aspect of hands and fingers, waking the patient from sleep. Pain may extend to arm and shoulder
Ulnar	Paraesthesia on lateral border of hand, wasting and weakness of hand muscles
Radial	Weakness of extension of wrist and fingers, often precipitated by sleeping in abnormal posture, e.g. arm over back of chair
Peroneal	Foot drop, trauma to head of fibula
Meralgia paraesthetica	Tingling and dysaethesia on lateral border of the thigh (Lateral cutaneous nerve of the thigh)

Management

Lateral popliteal nerve palsies and radial nerve palsies are commonly due to local trauma and complete recovery in 6–8 weeks can be expected without intervention. Meralgia paraesthetica often develops in relation to weight loss or gain and may respond to appropriate dietary advice and reassurance. Carpal tunnel syndrome and ulnar nerve palsy may remit if patients are advised to avoid activities involving repetitive wrist movement or pressure on the elbows. Precipitating causes including diabetes mellitus and hypothyroidism should be excluded. Persistent symptoms may respond to nocturnal splinting of joints, but in some patients decompression of the carpal tunnel or transposition of the ulnar nerve may be necessary. In these electrophysiological investigation is advisable pre-operatively in order to confirm the diagnosis and site of compression.

MONONEURITIS MULTIPLEX

In this condition, multiple peripheral or spinal nerve lesions occur serially or concurrently. Pathologically there is ischaemia of the peripheral nerves due to vasculitis of the vasa nervorum, which renders the nerves susceptible to mechanical compression. Common causes are: polyarteritis nodosa, rheumatoid arthritis, diabetes mellitus, sarcoidosis and leprosy.

BRACHIAL PLEXUS LESIONS

Trauma is the commonest cause of damage to the brachial plexus, and frequently involves forced separation of head and shoulder or excessive abduction of the arm. Other causes include neoplasia in the cervical lymph nodes or pulmonary apex, compression at the thoracic outlet, and damage due to radiotherapy of the axillary area.

Table 16.66   Signs in entrapment neuropathy

Nerve	Muscle weakness/wasting	Area of sensory loss
Median (at wrist)	Abductor pollicis brevis	Lateral palm and thumb, index, middle, and half ring finger
Ulnar (at elbow)	All small hand muscles, excluding abductor pollicis brevis	Medial palm and little, and half ring finger
Radial	Wrist and finger extensors Supinator	Dorsum of thumb
Peroneal	Dorsiflexion and eversion of foot	Nil or dorsum of foot
Meralgia paraesthetica	Nil	Lateral border of thigh

Table 16.67   Physical signs in brachial plexus lesions

Site	Root	Affected muscles	Sensory loss
Upper plexus (Erb–Duchenne)	C5 (C6)	Biceps, deltoid, spinati, rhomboids, brachioradialis (triceps, serratus ant.)	Patch over deltoid
Lower lexus (Dejerine–Klumpke)	T1 (C8)	All small hand muscles, claw hand (ulnar wrist flexors)	Ulnar border hand/forearm
Thoracic outlet syndrome	C8/T1	Small hand muscles, ulnar forearm	Ulnar border hand/forearm (upper arm)

Clinical features

The clinical signs depend on the anatomical site of damage (Table 16.67). There may be associated vascular symptoms in thoracic outlet syndrome including blanching and cyanosis of the fingers, and physical signs including asymmetry of radial pulses and a subclavian bruit.

Management

Regular passive movements of the affected limb prevent contractures while nerve fibres are regenerating. Splinting is ineffective, except in Erb's paralysis, and surgery is rarely indicated. Minor symptoms due to thoracic outlet syndrome often settle with rest and physiotherapy, but surgical treatment of underlying congenital anomalies such as cervical rib or fibrous band may be necessary if neurological signs progress.

Prognosis

The prognosis for recovery in traumatic lesions is dependent on the site and severity of neuronal damage and may be assessed electrophysiologically.

NEURALGIC AMYOTROPHY

Clinical features

This presents with severe pain over one shoulder and sometimes follows infection, inoculation or operation. Within days paralysis develops in the painful muscles, most commonly deltoid, spinati and serratus anterior

and is rapidly followed by muscle wasting. There may be a patch of sensory loss over the deltoid and occasionally more extensive involvement of the muscles of the upper arm.

Prognosis

Pain usually subsides within 1–2 weeks and complete recovery of paralysis and wasting can be expected in 3–6 months in the great majority of patients.

CHRONIC POLYNEUROPATHY

There are numerous causes of peripheral neuropathy (Table 16.68), but classification by clinical type (motor, sensory, or mixed) and by whether axons or myelin are predominantly affected (as judged by electrophysiological studies) allows a narrowing of diagnostic possibilities in the individual patient.

Clinical features

When the causal lesion lies in the nerve cell body, the first manifestations are at the distal end of the longest nerves. This gives rise to the typical picture of a generalised polyneuropathy with distal paraesthesia usually affecting the feet and then later the hands, which progresses proximally up the limbs. These sensory symptoms are associated with diminution of superficial sensation in a 'glove' and 'stocking' distribution. There is distal weakness with diminished or absent tendon reflexes.

Table 16.68   Causes of peripheral neuropathy

Genetic
Hereditary motor and sensory neuropathy (Charcot–Marie–Tooth disease)
   Type I: demyelinating
   Type II: axinal
   Type III: congenital

Metabolic
Diabetes mellitus
Renal and hepatic failure
Paraproteinaemia
Amyloidosis
Acute intermittent porphyria
Hypothyroidism

Toxins
Alcohol
Heavy metals
Organic solvents
Drugs, e.g. amiodarone, vincristine, hydrallazine, phenytoin

Connective tissue disorders
Polyarteritis nodosa
Rheumatoid arthritis
Systemic lupus erythematosus

Deficiency states
Deficiency of vitamins A, B_2, B_6, B_{12}, and E
Folate deficiency

Infections
Leprosy
Diphtheria
Typhoid
HIV

Malignant disease
Carcinoma of bronchus and other malignant tumours, including lymphoma and myeloma

Investigation

The clinical features localise the lesion to the peripheral nerves. A careful clinical history, including details of family history, drug intake and potential exposure to toxins is essential. Routine screening for a metabolic disorder should be undertaken and the possibility of diabetes mellitus must be excluded. Nerve conduction studies may be necessary if there is diagnostic doubt or if the condition is progressive. These studies confirm the presence of a neuropathy and provide an estimation of the nerve conduction velocity, which indicates whether the axons or myelin are primarily affected. In some cases and in particular those in which a vasculitic aetiology is suspected sural nerve biopsy may be indicated.

Management

No cause is found in the majority of patients with peripheral neuropathy and in many patients no treatment is necessary as the condition may stabilise or progress only slowly. Empirical treatment with steroids may be attempted if there is a progressive neurological deficit, but this is usually disappointing.

Exposure to drugs or toxins should be avoided if a causal link is suspected and in metabolic neuropathy appropriate treatment should be initiated without delay. Deficiency states require appropriate vitamin supplements and absolute abstention is essential in chronic alcoholism.

No specific therapy is available for hereditary neuropathies, but advice from physiotherapists and occupational therapists is important in helping patients to maintain their functional capacity and this also applies to other forms of chronic neuropathy.

ACUTE POLYNEUROPATHY

Guillain-Barré syndrome or acute inflammatory poly-neuropathy develops 1–4 weeks after viral infection in 70% of patients and more rarely follows surgery or immunisation. Pathologically there is demyelination of spinal roots or peripheral nerves, which is almost certainly immunologically mediated.

Clinical features

The characteristic clinical feature is muscle weakness, which is more marked proximally than distally and progresses, often rapidly. Distal paraesthesia ascending proximally is common and bilateral facial weakness develops in 50% of patients. The most striking findings on examination are diffuse weakness and widespread loss of reflexes. In the majority of patients muscle weakness progresses for 1–3 weeks, but occasionally rapid deterioration with respiratory failure develops within hours.

Investigation

The protein content of the CSF is raised at some stage of the illness but may be normal in the first 10 days. There is usually no rise in cells and a lymphocytosis of greater than $50/mm^3$ should raise the possibility of an alternative diagnosis. Electrophysiological studies are usually normal in the early stages of Guillain-Barré syndrome, but may be helpful if there is diagnostic doubt. Acute porphyria (p. 556) may cause a neuropathy similar to Guillain-Barré syndrome but may be excluded by urinary porphyrin estimation. Serum lead should be measured if there are only motor signs.

Management

During the phase of deterioration regular monitoring of respiratory function is essential. Respiratory failure may develop with little prior clinical warning and the development of dyspnoea or a drop in vital capacity below 1 litre may indicate the urgent necessity for intubation and positive pressure ventilation. Steroid therapy is ineffective, but plasma exchange shortens the

Table 16.69   Diagnostic features in muscular dystrophy

Dystrophy	Inheritance	Age at onset	Muscles affected
Duchenne	X-linked recessive	3–10	Proximal legs and arms, then general
Limb girdle	Autosomal recessive	10–30	Pelvic girdle, shoulder girdle or both
Facio-scapulo-humoral	Autosomal dominant	10–40	Facial, shoulder girdle, serratus anterior
Dystrophia myotonica	Autosomal dominant	Any age (20–60)	Temporalis, facial, sternomastoid, distal limbs, myotonia

duration of ventilation and improves the prognosis provided treatment is started within 14 days of the onset of symptoms.

Prognosis

Overall 80% of patients recover completely within 3–6 months, 10% die, and 10% are left with residual neurological disability which can be severe.

DISEASES OF MUSCLE

The voluntary muscles are subject to a range of disorders, which result in a limited spectrum of symptoms and physical signs. These are listed in the information box below.

DISORDERS OF VOLUNTARY MUSCLES

- Muscular dystrophy
- Metabolic and endocrine myopathy
- Inflammatory myopathy
- Congenital myopathy
- Toxic myopathy
- Disorders of the neuromuscular junction

Diagnosis is largely clinical, depending on a recognition of the distribution of affected muscles, the identification of associated signs and symptoms, and, in many patients, a thorough family history.

MUSCULAR DYSTROPHY

Progressive muscular dystrophy is a group of hereditary disorders characterised by progressive degeneration of a group of muscles without involvement of the nervous system.

Clinical features

The wasting and weakness are symmetrical, there is no fasciculation, tendon reflexes are preserved until a late stage and there is no sensory loss. Differential diagnosis depends on the age onset, distribution of affected muscles, and type of inheritance (Table 16.69).

Investigation

The diagnosis of muscular dystrophy can be confirmed by electromyography and muscle biopsy. Creatinine kinase is markedly elevated in Duchenne muscular dystrophy, but is normal or only moderately elevated in the other types.

Dystrophia myotonica may be diagnosed by the distribution of muscle weakness and other features including myotonia (slow relaxation of muscle), cataract, ptosis, frontal baldness and gonadal atrophy.

Management

There is no specific therapy for these conditions, although advice from the physiotherapist and occupational therapist may help the patient to cope with disability. Genetic counselling is an important component of management. Recombinant DNA linkage analysis in combination with creatine kinase estimation has allowed increasing accuracy in the identification of femal carriers in some families at risk from Duchenne dystrophy and prenatal diagnosis of these conditions may be possible. In dystrophia myotonica affected patients have usually reproduced by the time of diagnosis, but other potentially affected family members should receive counselling.

Most patients with Duchenne dystrophy die within ten years of diagnosis, while the life-span in limb girdle and facio-scapulo-humeral dystrophies is unaffected. Premature death due to respiratory or cardiac failure is the usual outcome in dystrophia myotonica.

METABOLIC AND ENDOCRINE MYOPATHY

Muscle weakness may develop in a range of metabolic and endocrine disorders and is usually reversible. The causes are listed in the information box (p. 898).

METABOLIC AND ENDOCRINE CAUSES OF MUSCLE WEAKNESS	
Acute muscle weakness	*Proximal myopathy*
Hypokalaemia	Hyperthyroidism
Hyperkalaemia	Hypothyroidism
Hypocalcaemia	Cushing's syndrome
Hypercalcaemia	Addison's disease

Clinical features

The weakness is often acute and generalised in metabolic disorders, while a proximal myopathy predominantly affecting the pelvic girdle is a feature of some endocrine disorders, and may develop without other manifestations of hormonal disturbance. An awareness of the possibility of these conditions is the most important factor in diagnosis. Hypo and hyperkalaemia may occur in familial periodic paralysis, which is a dominantly inherited condition characterised by attacks of profound weakness lasting for several hours and often precipitated by exertion.

Muscle pain on exercise is the characteristic feature of myophosphorylase deficiency (McArdle's syndrome) and a number of other rare recessively inherited disorders of metabolism (p. 831).

INFLAMMATORY MYOPATHY OR POLYMYOSITIS (see p. 793)

CONGENITAL MYOPATHY

This is rare and presents in infancy with muscular weakness and limpness. Serum enzymes may be normal or slightly elevated and the electromyogram is usually myopathic. The syndrome may be caused by a number of specific conditions which have a variable inheritance, and are defined by the type of structural abnormality present in skeletal muscle fibres. Most patients have a slowly progressive disease and there is no specific therapy.

TOXIC MYOPATHY

A wide variety of drugs may cause disorders of muscle, including carbenoxolone, thiazide diuretics and steroids. Alcohol may cause a spectrum of muscle disease varying from a mild, proximal weakness to severe muscle necrosis. Avoidance of the offending agent usually results in recovery of muscle function.

Penicillamine rarely causes a myasthenic syndrome, which may persist on drug withdrawal.

DISORDERS OF THE NEUROMUSCULAR JUNCTION

MYASTHENIA GRAVIS

This condition is characterised by progressive failure to sustain a maintained or repeated contraction of striated muscle.

Aetiology and pathology

Nicotinic receptors of acetylcholine in the post-junctional membrane of neuromuscular junctions are blocked or lysed by a complement mediated autoimmune reaction between receptor protein and anti-acetylcholine-receptor antibody. The antibody is produced by B lymphocytes defectively controlled by T lymphocytes because of a disorder of the thymus gland. About 15% of patients, mainly of late onset, have an encapsulated or locally invasive thymoma. The majority, including all young individuals, have one of a number of thymic abnormalities, the most characteristic being germinal centres in the medulla of the gland. The latter group has a marked personal and familial relationship with other autoimmune diseases (p. 39), and many have inherited an immunoreactive gene which is linked to some of the HLA haplotypes; in a North European population these are HLA-B8 and DRw3. Inheritance of this gene is not obligatory for myasthenia and nothing is known about possible triggering factors for the spontaneous disease. Penicillamine may be one such breaker of immunological tolerance.

Clinical features

The disease usually appears between the ages of 15 and 50 years and females are more often affected than males. It tends to run a remitting course especially during the early years. Relapses may be precipitated by emotional disturbances, infections, pregnancy and severe muscular effort.

The cardinal symptom is abnormal fatigue of the muscles; movement although initially strong rapidly weakens. Intensification of symptoms towards the end of the day or following vigorous exercise is characteristic.

The first symptoms are usually intermittent ptosis or diplopia but weakness of chewing, swallowing, speaking or of moving the limbs also occurs. Any muscle of a limb may be affected, most commonly those of the shoulder girdle, so that the patient is unable to undertake work above the level of the shoulder, such as combing the hair, without frequent rests. Respiratory muscles may be involved and respiratory failure is a not uncommon cause of death. Asphyxia occurs readily as the cough may be too weak to clear foreign bodies from the airways. Muscle atrophy may occur in long-standing cases. There are no signs of involvement of the central nervous system.

Investigation
Recommended investigations are listed in the information box below.

INVESTIGATION OF MYASTHENIA GRAVIS

- Tensilon test
- Autoantibody screen (including skeletal muscle antibody)
- Thyroid function tests
- Anti-acetylcholine receptor antibody titre
- PA and lateral chest X-ray/CT scan of thorax
- EMG

The intravenous injection of a short-acting anticholinesterase, edrophonium hydrochloride, is a valuable diagnostic aid (the Tensilon test). An initial dose of 2 mg is injected and a further 8 mg given half a minute later if there are no undesirable side-effects. Improvement in muscle power occurs within 30 seconds and usually persists for 2 or 3 minutes.

Screening for other autoimmune disorders, particularly thyroid disease, is necessary and elevated acetylcholine receptor antibody is found in 80% of cases, although much less frequently in ocular myasthenia. Positive skeletal muscle antibodies suggest the presence of thymoma and all patients should undergo radiological investigation to exclude this condition. EMG with repetitive stimulation may show a characteristic decremental response.

Management
The principles of treatment are:

1. to maximise the activity of acetylcholine at the remaining receptors in the neuromuscular junctions
2. to limit or abolish the immunological attack on motor endplates.

The duration of action of acetylcholine is greatly prolonged by inhibiting its hydrolysing enzyme, acetylcholinesterase. The most commonly used anticholinesterase drug is pyridostigmine, which is given orally in a dosage of 60–120 mg at intervals determined by supervised trial (2–8 hours). Side-effects, including diarrhoea, colic and other autonomic symptoms, may be controlled by propantheline (15 mg as required).

Overdosage of anticholinesterase drugs may cause a cholinergic crisis due to depolarisation block of motor endplates, with muscular fasciculation, paralysis, pallor, sweating, excessive salivation and persistently small pupils. This may be distinguished from severe weakness due to exacerbation of myasthenia (myasthenic crisis) by the clinical features and if necessary by the injection of a small dose of edrophonium hydrochloride. Sudden weakness from either cause may require intermittent positive pressure ventilation to save life and early intubation before a crisis has developed will normally remove the need for tracheostomy.

The immunological disorder is treated by various procedures which are listed in the information box below.

IMMUNOLOGICAL TREATMENT OF MYASTHENIA

Thymectomy
Should be performed as soon as feasible in any patient with myasthenia not confined to extraocular muscles, unless the disease has been established for more than seven years; the indication for surgery is the stage of myasthenia gravis, not the presence of thymoma.

Plasma exchange
Removing antibody from the blood, may give marked improvement but, as this is usually brief, such therapy is normally reserved for myasthenic crisis or for preoperative preparation.

Corticosteroid treatment
May cause improvement but this is commonly preceded by marked exacerbation of myasthenic symptoms and should be initiated in hospital. It is usually necessary to continue treatment for months or years, with the possibility of adverse effects, and steroids are not recommended for first-line management.

Other immunosuppressant treatment
e.g. azathioprine 2.5 mg/kg daily, may be of value in reducing the dosage of steroids necessary to control symptoms and in some cases may allow steroids to be withdrawn.

Prognosis
Prognosis is variable. Remissions sometimes occur spontaneously. When myasthenic affection is confined to the eye muscles prognosis for life is normal and disability slight. Rapid progression of the disease more than 5 years after its onset is uncommon. Thymectomy, perhaps followed by high dosage steroid treatment, often leads to marked improvement so that disability is minimal and life expectancy normal. When the disease is associated with a thymoma, even if this is removed, the outlook is markedly worse.

DEGENERATIVE DISORDERS

MOTOR NEURONE DISEASE

This is a progressive disorder of unknown cause, in which there is degeneration of spinal and cranial motor neurones and pyramidal neurones in the motor cortex. About 5% of cases are familial. A variety of possible causes including viral infection, trauma, exposure to toxins, and electric shock have been suggested, but no sound evidence exists to support any of these in typical cases. The prevalence of the disease is about 5 per 100 000; males are affected more often than females.

Clinical features

These are listed in the information boxes below.

CLINICAL FEATURES OF MOTOR NEURONE DISEASE

Age of onset
Usually after age 50 years occasional cases in 30–50 years group

Course
Symptoms often begin focally in one part and spread gradually but relentlessly to become widespread

Death
Usually within 3–5 years of onset from respiratory failure/infection immobility and inability to swallow

Signs
Wasting and fasciculation of muscles, weakness of muscles of limbs, tongue, face and palate (dysarthria, dysphagia)
External ocular muscles and sphincters usually remain intact
Pyramidal tract involvement causes spasticity, exaggerated tendon reflexes, extensor plantar responses
No objective sensory deficits
No intellectual impairment

Investigation

In many patients the clinical features are diagnostic. Electromyography helps confirm the presence of fasciculation and denervation, and is particularly helpful when pyramidal features predominate. Sensory nerve conduction is normal and motor studies show loss of axons with only modest reduction in conduction velocity. Myelography and CT brain scanning are sometimes necessary to exclude local spinal or cerebral disease when clinical abnormalities are localised. CSF examination is usually normal, a mild elevation of protein concentration may be found. Treatable disorders such as diabetes mellitus, syphilis, sarcoidosis, and spinal disorders should be excluded.

PATTERNS OF INVOLVEMENT

Progressive muscular atrophy
Predominantly spinal motor neurones affected
Weakness and wasting of distal limb muscles at first
Fasciculation in muscles
Tendon reflexes may be absent

Progressive bulbar palsy
Early involvement of tongue palate and pharyngeal muscles.
Wasting and fasciculation of tongue: dysarthria/dysphagia.
May be pyramidal signs as well

Amyotrophic lateral sclerosis
Combination of distal and proximal muscle wasting and weakness, fasciculation.
Spasticity, exaggerated reflexes, extensor plantars.
Bulbar and pseudobulbar palsy follow eventually.
Pyramidal tract features may predominate

Management

No treatment alters the progress of this disease. Mental and physical support, with help from occupational and speech therapists and physiotherapists, is essential to keep the patient's quality of life as good as possible. Mechanical aids such as splints, walking aids, wheelchairs and communication devices all help to maintain morale of both the patient and their carers.

Prognosis

Motor neurone disease is progressive, most patients dying within 3–5 years of the onset of symptoms. Younger patients and those with early bulbar symptoms tend to show a more rapid course, whereas older patients and those with mainly peripheral involvement may survive 10 years. Death is usually from respiratory infection and failure, and the complications of immobility. Relief of distress in the terminal stages warrants the use of opiates and sedative drugs.

SPINAL MUSCULAR ATROPHIES

These are a group of genetically determined disorders affecting spinal motor and cranial motor neurones characterised by proximal and distal wasting, fasciculation and weakness of muscles. Involvement is usually symmetrical, but occasional localised forms occur. With the exception of the infantile form, progression is slow and the prognosis better than in motor neurone disease, from which they can usually be distinguished by the age of onset and rate of progress. Examples are given in Table 16.70.

Table 16.70   Types of spinal muscular atrophy

Type	Onset	Inheritance	Features	Prognosis
Werdnig–Hoffman	Infancy	Autosomal recessive	Severe muscle wasting/weakness	Poor
Kugelberg–Welander	Childhood Adolescence	Autosomal recessive	Proximal weakness and wasting. EMG shows denervation	Slowly progressive disability
Distal forms	Early adult life	Autosomal dominant	Distal weakness and wasting of hands and feet	Good, seldom disabling
Bulbospinal	Adult life males only	X-linked	Facial and bulbar weakness, proximal limb weakness	Good

Table 16.71   Types of hereditary ataxias

Type	Inheritance	Onset	Clinical features
Friedreich's ataxia	Autosomal recessive	8–16 years	Ataxia, nystagmus, dysarthria, spasticity, areflexia, prorioceptive impairment, diabetes mellitus, optic atrophy, cardiac abnormalities. Chairbound by age 20 usually
Ataxia telangectasia	Autosomal recessive	Childhood	Progressive ataxia, athetosis, telengectases on conjuctivae, impaired DNA repair, immunodeficiency, tendency to malignancies
Olivo-ponto-cerebellar atrophy	Autosomal dominant	Adult life	Slowly progressive ataxia, spasticity, dysarthria, extra-pyramidal features, optic atrophy, deafness, pyramidal signs
Hereditary spastic paraplegia	Autosomal dominant	Adult life	Slowly progressive spasticity affecting legs > arms, extensor plantar responses, sensory signs minimal or absent

HEREDITARY ATAXIAS

This is a group of inherited disorders in which degenerative changes occur in the cerebellum, brain stem, pyramidal tracts, spinocerebellar tracts and optic nerves. Onset may be in childhood or in middle adult life. Most childhood forms are of recessive inheritance, while the late onset disorders are usually autosomal dominant. Clinically, combinations of cerebellar, pyramidal, sensory and extra-pyramidal features may occur. Recognition and classification of the disorders is important to give a prognosis and accurate genetic counselling. Patterns of involvement are listed in Table 16.71.

NEUROFIBROMATOSIS (VON RECKLINGHAUSEN'S DISEASE)

This is a genetic disorder of autosomal dominant inheritance probably due to an abnormal gene on chromosome 22. Multiple fibromatous tumours develop from the neurilemmal sheaths of peripheral and cranial nerves. Most of the lesions are benign but sarcomatous change occasionally occurs. Cerebral gliomas, meningiomas, endocrine tumours (e.g. phaeochromocytoma), intellectual subnormality and epilepsy may be associated with the cutaneous manifestations.

Table 16.72   Types of neurofibromatosis

Type I Peripheral form > 70% of cases	Multiple cutaneous neurofibromas, 'soft' papillomas, cafe-au-lait patches, axillary freckling, iris fibromas, plexiform neurofibromas, spinal neurofibromas, aqueduct stenosis, scoliosis, endocrine tumours
Type II Central form	Few or no cutaneous lesions, bilateral acoustic neuromas, cerebral and optic nerve gliomas, meningiomas, spinal neurofibromas

Two genetically distinct forms of neurofibromatosis are now recognised (Table 16.72).

The peripheral form is readily recognised by the cutaneous lesions which gradually increase in number throughout life. Investigation and treatment is only indicated if there are symptoms of cerebral or spinal involvement, or if malignant change is suspected. Because the central form may have no cutaneous signs, a family history of cerebral or spinal lesions should be noted with care.

DISORDERS OF SLEEP

Normal sleep is thought to be under control of the reticular activating system in the upper brain stem and diencephalon. During overnight sleep, a series of repeated cycles of EEG patterns can be recorded. As drowsiness occurs, alpha rhythm disappears (stage I) and the EEG gradually becomes dominated by deepening slow activity which reaches delta frequencies in stages III and IV. After 60–80 minutes this slow-wave pattern, is replaced by a short spell of low amplitude EEG background on which are superimposed rapid eye movements (REM). After a few minutes of REM sleep, another slow-wave spell starts and the cycle repeats several times throughout the night. The REM periods tend to become longer as the sleep period progresses. Dreaming takes place during REM sleep; it is accompanied by muscle relaxation, penile erection and loss of tendon reflexes. REM sleep seems to be the most important part of the sleep cycle for refreshing cognitive processes; deprivation of REM sleep causes tiredness, irritability and impaired judgment.

Disorders of slow-wave sleep

Sleep talking and sleep walking. Automatic behaviour not recalled by the sufferer may take place during light sleep. Such phenomena are common in normal children. Sleep walking is uncommon in adults.

Night terrors. These occur as sudden arousals from deep (stage III and IV) slow-wave sleep. They are more common in children, but may affect adults. The sufferer wakes in a state of agitation, screaming and fearful. Occasionally violent behaviour occurs. The agitation may last many minutes.

Disorders of REM sleep

Nightmares. These are frightening dreams from which the sufferer wakes in a state of fear or agitation. Most normal people have experienced such phenomena.

Sleep paralysis. This may occur in otherwise normal people, but is more commonly reported by those with the narcoleptic tetrad (see below). The person wakes in the night or morning and is aware of their surroundings, but is unable to move or speak for seconds or minutes. This probably represents dissociation between the inhibitory part of the REM sleep system and the waking role of the reticular formation.

Hypnagogic hallucinations. These also sometimes affect normal people but are more common in narcolepsy/cataplexy. Frightening hallucinations are experienced soon after falling asleep, or just before waking.

Narcolepsy. This is abnormal. Sufferers experience recurrent bouts of irresistible sleep during which the EEG often shows direct entry into REM sleep. Sufferers tend to fall asleep when unstimulated or carrying out monotonous activity (bathing, eating, driving). The periods of sleep are usually short and the person can be woken relatively easily. They usually feel refreshed after waking. Paradoxically, overnight sleep is often fitful.

Cataplexy. This probably represents spontaneous activation of the REM sleep spinal inhibitory mechanism. Attacks are set off by surprise, emotion, laughter, fear and embarrassment. Muscle tone is lost in the limbs, face and trunk so that the sufferer sinks to the ground and is unable to move for seconds or minutes. Consciousness is not impaired and the EEG remains normal during attacks. Examination during an attack reveals loss of tendon reflexes and sometimes extensor plantar responses.

Narcolepsy, cataplexy, sleep paralysis and hypnagogic hallucinations may occur together in the same patient (Gélineau's tetrad); most often, narcolepsy and cataplexy occur together. The disorder has strong HLA association with DRW 2 and is sometimes familial.

Management

Narcoleptic attacks are treated by stimulant drugs such as dexamphetamine (5–10 mg t.i.d.). Cataplexy responds to tricyclic antidepressants particularly Clomipramine (25–50 mg t.i.d.).

NUTRITIONAL NEUROLOGICAL DISEASES

Vitamin deficiency due to malabsorption or malnutrition can cause lesions in a number of sites in the nervous system. The neurological and other features of vitamin deficiency are summarised in Table 16.73.

ALCOHOLISM

The commonest cause of vitamin deficiency in Britain is chronic alcoholism in which the clinical effects of vitamin deficiency may be complicated by the neurotoxic effect of alcohol itself, including cerebellar degeneration, dementia, peripheral neuropathy and myopathy.

Central pontine myelinolysis occurs in alcoholics and following over-rapid correction of hyponatraemia.

Table 16.73 Clinical features of vitamin deficiency

Vitamin deficiency	Neurological features	Systemic features
B₁₂	Confusion/dementia Subacute combined degeneration of the cord Peripheral neuropathy Optic atrophy	Megaloblastic anaemia Glossitis
Folic acid	Dementia Myelopathy Peripheral neuropathy	Megaloblastic anaemia
Thiamine	Beriberi Polyneuropathy *Korsakoff's psychosis* Memory impairment Confabulation *Wernicke's encephalopathy* Confusion/nystagmus Ophthalmoplegia	Cardiomyopathy Hypothermia
Vitamin E	Myelopathy Ataxia Peripheral neuropathy	Other features of malabsorption
Nicotinic acid	Mania/dementia Diplopia/dysarthria Ataxia	Diarrhoea Cutaneous lesions Glossitis
Pyridoxine	Peripheral neuropathy	

There is widespread destruction of myelin in the pons, resulting in tetraparesis, dysphagia and anarthria, and death.

VITAMIN B₁₂ DEFICIENCY

Vitamin B₁₂ deficiency may cause cognitive impairment, neuropathy, optic atrophy and subacute combined degeneration of the cord. This is characterised by demyelination of the corticospinal tracts and posterior columns of the spinal cord, and is usually associated with a peripheral neuropathy.

Clinical features

The physical signs include glove and stocking impairment of superficial sensation, impairment of joint position and vibration sense in the legs, exaggerated knee reflexes, extensor plantar responses and commonly absent ankle jerks.

Management

Vitamin B₁₂ deficiency is treated with hydroxycobalamin 1 mg daily for 5 days, followed by maintenance therapy of 1 mg 3-monthly.

Prognosis

Prognosis for recovery of the sensory signs and ataxia is good if treatment is initiated at an early stage, but dementia and spasticity often persist. Neurological

complications of Vitamin B₁₂ deficiency can occur without haematological evidence of deficiency.

PERIPHERAL NEUROPATHY

Thiamin, nicotinic acid and pyridoxine deficiency may cause a symmetrical, mixed sensory-motor neuropathy. In many instances, particularly in alcoholics and in the burning feet syndrome in the elderly, there are combined deficiencies of these vitamins. If treated early, nutritional polyneuropathy responds well to a mixed diet and generous doses of the vitamin B complex.

LATHYRISM

The consumption of peas, a common constituent of Indian diets, may produce an acute or slowly progressive spastic paraplegia if the pulses include *Lathyrus sativus* which contains a neurotoxin.

PARANEOPLASTIC NEUROLOGICAL SYNDROMES

These syndromes arise at a distance from a primary carcinoma in the absence of metastases. Neural disturbance may occur at any stage during the develop-

Table 16.74 Paraneoplastic neurological syndromes

Disorder	Clinical features	Investigations
Peripheral neuropathy	Sensori-motor neuropathy	EMG Elevated CSF protein
Myopathy/myositis	Proximal muscle weakness	Myopathic EMG
Myasthenic syndrome	Generalised weakness Dry mouth Potentiation of tendon reflexes	Incremental EMG response
Cerebellar degeneration	Ataxia, nystagmus often rapidly progressive	CT scan
Encephalopathy	Progressive dementia Brain stem signs	CT scan
Myelitis	Motor neuropathy Spinal cord dysfunction	(Myelogram)

ment of the primary lesion and may antedate the symptoms directly attributable to the carcinoma by weeks or months. They may affect singly or in combination muscles and peripheral nerves as well as central neural structures and the brain.

Clinical features

The syndromes are most conveniently categorised anatomically, although over 50% of cases present with a mixed neuromyopathy.

Management

The treatment of the paraneoplastic syndrome is that of the primary lesion. Improvement and occasionally complete remission of a myasthenic-myopathic syndrome may occur with removal of the primary tumour but this is by no means invariable. In most instances the response of the neurological complications is unpredictable.

FURTHER READING

Asbury A K, McKhann G M, McDonald W I (eds) 1986 Diseases of the Nervous System. Heinemann medical books, London. A comprehensive up-to-date textbook with many expert contributors; presented in 2 volumes. Suitable for post-graduate and specialist study

Bannister Sir Roger 1985 Brain's Clinical neurology, 6th Edn. Oxford University Press, Oxford. Eminently suitable for undergraduates, this book is popularly known as 'little Brain'

Brain Lord, Walton Sir John 1985 Diseases of the Nervous System, 9th Edn. Oxford University Press, Oxford. A comprehensive text primarily for postgraduate students

Cull R E 1990 In: Munro J Edwards C R (eds) Macleod's Clinical Examination, 8th edn. Churchill Livingstone, Edinburgh. Contains an account of the examination of the nervous system designed to be read in conjunction with this chapter

Jennett W B, Galbraith S 1983 An Introduction to Neurosurgery, 4th Edn. Heinemann, London. A succinct and clearly written introduction to surgical neurology

Matthews W B 1982 Diseases of the Nervous System, 4th Edn. Blackwell Scientific Publications, Oxford. A concise, readable account of neurological disorders intended for undergraduates

Ross Russell R W, Wiles C M 1985 Integrated clinical science: neurology. Heinemann, London. An up-to-date account of common neurological disorders, with an approach based on the pathophysiology. Written for undergraduates, but of a level suitable for postgraduate study. Well illustrated

Weller R D, Swash M, McLellan D L, Scholtz C L 1983 Clinical neuropathology. Springer Verlag, Berlin. A valuable short account of pathological processes related to clinical neurology. It includes clear accounts of biochemical disorders of the nervous system.

17

Diseases of the Skin

Large community studies in the UK and USA have revealed that between 20 and 30% of the population has a skin disease requiring attention, but only one in five of these will seek medical help. In spite of this some 10% of those who go to their family doctors do so with skin problems, but self medication is much more common than treatment prescribed by doctors.

Skin diseases can harm affected individuals in a number of ways as shown in the information box below.

THE 4 Ds

Death
Rare but still seen (e.g. angioedema, metastatic skin cancer and widespread blistering)

Discomfort
Most often itching or pain (e.g. eczema and post-herpetic neuralgia)

Disfigurement
Leading to embarassment and withdrawal from society (e.g. birth marks, acne vulgaris and psoriasis)

Disability
Leading to loss of work and wages (e.g. dermatitis of the hands and feet)

Although there are reputed to be over 2000 skin conditions this Chapter covers only those which are commonly seen in general practice and the general medical clinic, and those which are skin markers of systemic disease. Infections and infestations of the skin are dealt with in Chapter 5 and connective tissue disorders, which often involve the skin, are described in Chapter 15.

Every clinician has ample opportunity to look at the skin, when listening to or examining a patient. This Chapter will explain the significance of what he or she sees; there is no branch of medicine more dependent on clinical acumen and experience and less dependent on the laboratory.

THE STRUCTURE AND FUNCTION OF THE SKIN

The skin of an adult weighs an average of 4 kg and covers an area of 2 m². It has three layers: the outer *epidermis*, an avascular epithelium, which is firmly attached to, and supported by, connective tissue in the underlying *dermis*; beneath the dermis a layer of loose connective tissue, the *hypodermis*, which often contains abundant fat (Fig. 17.1).

Keratinocytes make up about 90% of the epidermal cells, their main function being to synthesise insoluble proteins, keratins. Keratinocytes are generated by division of cells in the basal layers of the epidermis and move outwards, die in the granular layer and become the flattened dead cells in the most superficial horny layer, finally being shed at the surface. In normal skin this process takes about 4 weeks but in some conditions (e.g. psoriasis) it is greatly accelerated.

Two types of dendritic cell make up the remaining 10% of the epidermal cells.

1. The *Langerhans cell*, is a modified macrophage

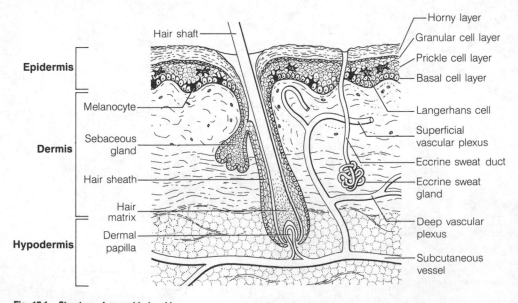

Fig. 17.1   Structure of normal hairy skin.

Table 17.1 Functions of the skin

Function	Structure/cell involved
Protection against	
Chemicals, particles	Horny layer
Ultraviolet radiation	Melanocytes
Antigens, haptens	Langerhans cells, lymphocytes mononuclear phagocytes, mast cells
Microbes	Horny layer, Langerhans cells mononuclear phagocytes, mast cells
Preservation of a balanced internal environment	
Prevents loss of water, electrolytes and macromolecules	Horny layer
Shock absorber	
Strong, yet elastic and compliant covering	Dermis and subcutaneous fat
Sensation	Specialist nerve endings
Calorie reserve	Subcutaneous fat
Vitamin D synthesis	Keratinocytes
Temperature regulation	Blood vessels Eccrine sweat glands
Lubrication and waterproofing	Sebaceous glands
Protection and prising	Nails
Body odour	Apocrine sweat glands
Psycho-social	Hair, nails

circulating between the epidermis and the local lymph nodes whose prime function is presentation of antigen to T lymphocytes in, for example, an allergic contact dermatitis reaction. The Langerhans cell may also play a part in immunosurveillance of viral and tumour antigens.

2. *Melanocytes* are found mainly in the basal layer; they are the only epidermal cell capable of synthesising melanin which they transfer to surrounding keratinocytes.

The dermis is vascular and supports the epidermis structurally and nutritionally. It is separated from the epidermis by a basement membrane zone and has three components: cells (many fibroblasts and a few mononuclear phagocytes, lymphocytes, Langerhans cells and mast cells), fibres (collagen, reticulin and elastin) and an amorphous ground substance (mostly the glycosaminoglycans hyaluronic acid and dermatan sulphate). The dermis also supports hair, sweat and sebaceous glands, cutaneous muscles and nerves, and blood and lymphatic vessels.

The functions of the skin are summarised in Table 17.1.

DIAGNOSIS OF SKIN DISORDERS

The key to successful treatment is accurate diagnosis.

This requires a careful history, thorough examination of the skin, hair and nails and the judicious use of the laboratory. Often it is best to have a quick look at the skin before obtaining a full history as this should prompt the right questions.

HISTORY

The principles of a general medical history should be followed with emphasis on the events surrounding the onset of the skin lesions and on the progression of the disease. A careful inquiry into drugs, a past or family history of skin disorders, and details of the occupation and any hobbies are important. The more difficult the diagnosis – the more important the history.

EXAMINATION

To examine the skin properly the lighting must be uniform and bright, the patient undressed (if necessary) and make-up and dressings removed. The signs to note are shown in the information box (p. 908).

A *magnifying lens* is essential; rashes and lesions cannot often be diagnosed at arms length. A lens or glass slide can also be pressed on lesions to determine if they are vascular and to unmask their true colour.

The terminology commonly used in skin diseases is given in Table 17.2.

SIGNS TO NOTE

● Distribution of rash. Is it symmetrical or asymmetrical? Is it dermatomal? Are any areas spared?
● Morphology of lesions. Appreciation of the definitions in Table 17.2 will save much time in describing lesions. The colour, surface contour, geometric shape, texture, temperature and even smell of lesions often warrant further description
● Configuration of lesions. Are the lesions discrete, confluent, grouped, circinate or linear?

INVESTIGATION

Biopsy

This is performed, either with a special 'punch biopsy' instrument or a scalpel. Select an early and typical lesion, if possible one on a non-exposed site and where a good scar may be anticipated (avoid the upper back, shoulder tips and presternal area, where keloids commonly develop, and the lower legs of obese women). Use 1% xylocaine for local anaesthesia. Remove the specimen, avoiding crushing, and place in formol-saline. The wound is sutured; firm compression for a few minutes stops oozing. Fine sutures are used on the face. Stitches on the head are usually removed in 4–5 days, from the anterior trunk and arms in 7 days and from the back and legs in 10 days.

ECZEMA

The terms eczema and dermatitis are now used synonymously. They refer to a distinctive reaction pattern of the skin showing a combination of signs which depends on the duration of the rash and the type of eczema (see below).

Aetiology

There are two groups of eczema: exogenous (or contact) and endogenous (or constitutional). While overlap between the two groups is common, distinction between them is critical for treatment because avoidance of incriminating contactants takes precedence over other measures in the management of contact eczema. Table 17.3 shows the basic classification.

EXOGENOUS

IRRITANT CONTACT ECZEMA

Detergents, alkalis, acids, solvents and abrasive dusts

Table 17.2   Terminology of skin lesions

Primary lesions	
Papule	Small solid elevation of skin, less than 0.5 cm in diameter
Plaque	Elevated area of skin greater than 2 cm in diameter but without substantial depth
Macule	Small flat area of altered colour or texture
Vesicle	Circumscribed elevation of skin, less than 0.5 cm in diameter, and containing fluid
Bulla	Circumscribed elevation of skin over 0.5 cm in diameter and containing fluid
Pustule	A visible accumulation of pus in the skin
Abscess	A localised collection of pus in a cavity, more than 1 cm in diameter
Wheal	An elevated white compressible, evanescent area produced by dermal oedema
Angioedema	A diffuse swelling of oedema which extends to the subcutaneous tissue
Nodule	A solid mass in the skin, usually greater than 0.5 cm in diameter
Papilloma	A nipple-like mass projecting from the skin
Petechiae	Pinhead-sized macules of blood in the skin
Purpura	A larger macule or papule of blood in the skin
Ecchymosis	A larger extravasation of blood into the skin
Haematoma	A swelling from gross bleeding
Burrow	A linear or curvilinear papule, caused by a burrowing scabies mite
Comedo	A plug of keratin and sebum wedged in a dilated pilosebaceous orifice
Telangiectasia	The visible dilation of small cutaneous blood vessels
Secondary lesions (which evolve from primary lesions)	
Scale	A flake arising from the horny layer
Crust	Looks like a scale, but is composed of dried blood or tissue fluid
Ulcer	An area of skin from which the whole of the epidermis and at least the upper part of the dermis has been lost
Excoriation	An ulcer or erosion produced by scratching
Erosion	An area of skin denuded by a complete or partial loss of the epidermis
Fissure	A slit in the skin
Sinus	A cavity or channel that permits the escape of pus or fluid
Scar	The result of healing, in which normal structures are permanently replaced by fibrous tissue
Atrophy	Thinning of skin due to diminution of the epidermis, dermis subcutaneous fat
Stria	A streak-like, linear, atrophic, pink, purple or white lesion of the skin due to changes in the connective tissue

are common causes. There is a wide range of susceptibility to weak irritants. Irritant contact eczema accounts for the majority of industrial cases and work loss. The elderly, those with fair and dry skin and those with an atopic background (personal or family history of asthma, hay fever or eczema) are especially vulnerable. Napkin eczema in babies is common and due to irritant ammoniacal urine and faeces.

Table 17.3 The classification of eczema

Exogenous	Irritant
	Allergic
Endogenous	Atopic
	Seborrhoeic
	Discoid
	Asteatotic
	Gravitational
	Neurodermatitis
	Pompholyx

ALLERGIC CONTACT ECZEMA

This is due to a delayed hypersensitivity reaction (p. 38) following contact with antigens or haptens. Previous exposure to the allergen is required for sensitisation and the reaction is specific to the allergen or closely related chemicals. Common allergens and their origin are listed in Table 17.4.

Table 17.4 Some common allergens

Allergen	Present in
Nickel	Jewellery, jean studs, bra clips
Dichromate	Cement, leather, matches
Rubber chemicals	Clothing, shoes, tyres
Colophony	Sticking plaster, collodion
Paraphenylenediamine	Hair dye, clothing
Balsam of Peru	Perfumes, citrus fruits
Neomycin Benzocaine	Topical applications
Parabens	Preservative in cosmetics and creams
Wool alcohols	Lanolin, cosmetics, creams
Epoxy resin	Resin adhesives

ENDOGENOUS

ATOPIC ECZEMA

Atopy is a genetic predisposition to form excessive IgE antibodies to inhaled, injected and ingested antigens and to develop one or more of a group of diseases which include asthma, hay fever, urticaria, food and other allergies and this distinctive form of eczema. About 15% of the population have at least one atopic manifestation.

SEBORRHOEIC ECZEMA

The name is a poor one because the condition is un-related to seborrhoea but it is used so often that it cannot be discarded. Its cause remains unknown though the yeast-like fungus, *Pityrosporum orbiculare*, appears to be a perpetuating factor. The condition often runs in families but the precise mode of inheritance is unclear.

The causes of the other endogenous forms of eczema are ill-understood though asteatotic eczema occurs most often on the lower limbs of the elderly, especially when the skin is dry; low humidity caused by central heating, overwashing and diuretics are contributory factors. Gravitational eczema is often, though not always, associated with venous insufficiency. Pompholyx, sometimes provoked by heat or emotional upset, may occur in nickel-sensitive patients after they ingest small amounts of nickel in food.

Pathology

In the acute stage oedema of the epidermis (spongiosis) progresses to the formation of intra-epidermal vesicles, which may enlarge and rupture. In the chronic stage there is less oedema and vesication but more thickening of the epidermis (acanthosis); this is accompanied by a variable degree of vasodilation and T helper lymphocytic infiltration in the upper dermis.

Clinical features

General

The reaction is similar in all types but varies according to the duration of the rash. The signs of acute eczema and chronic eczema are listed in the information boxes below.

ACUTE ECZEMA

- Redness and swelling, usually with ill-defined margin
- Papules, vesicles and more rarely large blisters
- Exudation and cracking
- Scaling

CHRONIC ECZEMA

- May show all of the above features, though it is usually less vesicular and exudative
- Thickening. Lichenification, a dry leathery thickening with increased skin markings, is secondary to rubbing and scratching and is most often seen in atopic eczema
- Fissures and scratch marks
- Pigmentation

SPECIFIC

IRRITANT CONTACT ECZEMA

Strong irritants elicit an acute reaction on the site of contact whereas weak irritants most often cause chronic eczema, especially of the hands, after prolonged exposure.

ALLERGIC CONTACT ECZEMA

The eczema reaction occurs wherever the allergen contacts the skin and sensitisation persists indefinitely. It is important to determine the original site of the rash before secondary spread obscures the picture, as this often provides the best clue to the contactant. There are many easily recognisable patterns, e.g. eczema of the earlobes, wrists and back due to contact with nickel in costume jewellery, watches and bra clips; eczema of the hands and wrists due to rubber gloves. Oedema of the lax skin of the eyelids and genitalia is a frequent concomitant of allergic contact eczema (Fig. 17.2).

ATOPIC ECZEMA

The cardinal feature of atopic eczema is itch and scratching may account for most of the signs.

Actopic eczema usually begins before the age of six months but, paradoxically, seldom presents during the neonatal period. The rash remits spontaneously in at least two-thirds of children before the age of ten. The distribution and character of the rash vary with age as shown in the information box below.

DISTRIBUTION AND CHARACTER OF RASH

● Infancy – the eczema is often acute and involves the face and trunk. The napkin area is frequently spared
● Childhood – the rash settles on the backs of the knees, fronts of the elbows, wrists and ankles (Fig. 17.3)
● Adults – the face and trunk are once more involved, lichenification is common

---

SEBORRHOEIC ECZEMA

The three common patterns involving seborrhoeic eczema are shown in the information box below. This type is associated with a tendency to dandruff.

PATTERNS OF SEBORRHOEIC ECZEMA

● Scalp, ears, face and eyebrows
● Presternal and interscapular skin
● Flexures of axillae, umbilicus, breasts and groin

DISCOID ECZEMA

This common form of eczema is seen most often on the limbs of elderly males. The lesions are more discrete than those of other types of eczema and are usually multiple, coin-shaped, vesicular and crusted.

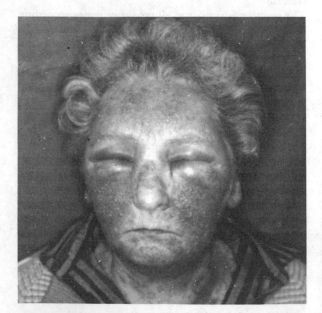

Fig. 17.2 Allergic contact eczema. This was caused by the application of an antihistamine cream. The acute eczematous reaction, associated with bilateral periorbital oedema, are typical.

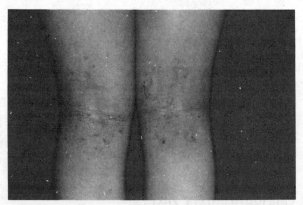

Fig. 17.3 Subacute eczema. In this case it involved the backs of the knees of a teenager; the patient also had asthma.

ASTEATOTIC ECZEMA

This is frequently seen in the hospitalised elderly. It occurs most often on the lower legs as a rippled or 'crazy paving' pattern of fine fissuring on an erythematous background.

GRAVITATIONAL (STASIS) ECZEMA

This occurs on the lower legs and is often associated with signs of venous insufficiency (oedema, red or bluish discolouration, loss of hair, induration, haemosiderin pigmentation and ulceration).

POMPHOLYX (DYSHIDROTIC ECZEMA)

This describes a form of eczema in which bouts of recurrent vesicles or bullae affect the palms, fingers and soles.

Complications of eczema

All types of eczema may be complicated, and often worsened by the conditions listed in the information box below.

COMPLICATIONS

- Superinfection – most often with bacteria (*Staph. aureus*) but also with yeasts (*Candida albicans*) and viruses (atopic eczema patients are especially prone to papilloma virus, herpes simplex and molluscum contagiosum infections). Superinfection is encouraged by the use of local steroids
- Reaction to local medicaments
- Psychological factors – anxiety states are common and compensation neuroses may dominate the picture in cases of industrial dermatitis

---

Investigations

Patch testing to allergens. This is used in suspected cases of allergic contact eczema. Patch testing to irritants (which cause reactions in everybody) is not advised.

Standard dilutions of the test substance are applied to the back under aluminium discs and the patches secured in place for 48 hours. The sites are inspected for eczematous reactions 1 hour after removal and after a further 48 hours.

Prick testing. This is used for a few patients with stubborn atopic eczema if food or inhalant allergens are suspected as exacerbating factors. It detects immediate (IgE mediated) hypersensitivity. Commercially prepared dilute antigens and a control are placed as single drops on the volar aspect of forearm. Prick the skin through the drop (using a fresh sterile needle for each test and without drawing blood) and remove the drop with a tissue. After 10 minutes inspect the sites for wheal and flare reactions and measure positive responses. The radio allergosorbent technique (RAST) is a blood test which answers the same questions as prick testing but is more expensive.

Both patch and prick testing should be carried out only by trained personnel.

Culture. This is for bacterial yeast and fungal pathogens where superinfection is suspected.

Management

General

The main points are listed in the information box below.

GENERAL (FOR ALL TYPES OF ECZEMA)

- Explanation, reassurance and encouragement
- Avoidance of contact with irritants
- The careful use of topical steroids

Lotions and creams are preferable in acute eczema and ointments in chronic cases; they are usually applied twice daily. Only 1% hydrocortisone should be used on the face and in infancy. Even in adults it is seldom necessary to prescribe more than 200 g of a mildly potent steroid (e.g. 1% hydrocortisone), 50 g of a moderatley potent steroid (e.g. 0.05% clobetasone butyrate) or 30 g of a potent steroid (e.g. 0.1% betamethasone valerate) per week. Very potent topical steroids (e.g. 0.05% clobetasol proprionate) should not be used long-term. The side-effects of strong or extensive local steroid therapy should always be borne in mind in patients applying these preparations for years on end. They include skin thinning (with striae, fragility and purpura), enhanced or disguised infections and systemic absorption (causing suppression of the pituitary-adrenal axis and even Cushingoid features).

Bland emollients (e.g. emulsifying ointment) are used regularly either directly on the skin or in the bath. Emollient soap substitutes (e.g. aqueous cream) are also helpful. Sedative antihistamines (e.g. trimeprazine tartrate) are of value if sleep is interrupted.

Specific measures (for certain types of eczema) additional to general treatment

Irritant contact eczema. This is treated by using protective clothing, especially gloves and barrier creams which allow the skin to be cleaned easily.

Allergic contact eczema. As for irritant contact eczema but a change of job is often unavoidable.

Atopic eczema. Some advise that cow's milk and eggs should be avoided for the first six months of life by children with atopic parents. After this the role of diet is debatable. Similarly, the place for gamma-linolenic acid as a dietary supplement remains controversial. Routine inoculations are allowed during quiescent phases of eczema though children who are allergic to eggs should not be inoculated against measles, influenza and yellow fever. Systemic antibiotic treatment (e.g. erythromycin or flucloxacillin) is indicated for treating bacterial superinfection which is usually due to *staphylococcus aureus*.

Seborrhoeic eczema. Local antiseptic steroid or antifungal steroid combinations (e.g. vioform-hydrocortisone and miconazole nitrate-hydrocortisone) are often helpful.

Gravitational eczema. Local steroids (see above) should be applied only to eczematous areas and not to ulcers. Neomycin should be avoided as sensitisation is common in this setting. Treatment of this type of eczema should also include the elimination of oedema by leg elevation and graded compression bandages.

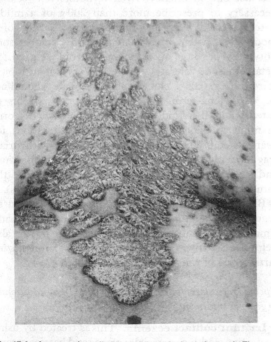

Fig. 17.4 Large and small plaques of psoriasis on the trunk. The sharply demarcated edges and the silvery scaling are typical.

PSORIASIS

Psoriasis is a non-infectious, inflammatory disease of the skin, characterised by well-defined erythematous plaques with large, adherent, silvery scales (Fig. 17.4).

The main abnormality in psoriasis is increased epidermal proliferation due to excessive division of cells in the basal layers and a shorter cell cycle time. The transit time of keratinocytes through the epidermis is shortened and the epidermal turnover time falls from 28 to 5 or 6 days.

1–3% of most populations has psoriasis. It is commonest in Europe and North America. It may start at any age but is rare under 10 years and often seen between 15 and 40 years. The course of disease is unpredictable but is usually chronic with exacerbations and remissions.

Aetiology

Basic defect
This remains unknown but the following factors are involved:

Genetic. There is frequently a genetic predisposition. A child with one affected parent has a 25% chance of developing the disease and this rises to 60% if both parents are affected. If non-psoriatic parents have a child with psoriasis the risk for subsequent children is about 20%. Inheritance may be polygenic or autosomal dominant with incomplete penetrance. There is a strong association between the disease and HLA–CW6 and those antigens of the major histocompatibility complex linked with CW6.

Biochemical. It is not known if biochemical abnormalities are the cause or result of increased epidermal proliferation. There are increased levels of prostaglandins, leukotrienes and hydroxyeicosatetraenoic (HETE) acids. These may cause both the increased cellular proliferation seen in psoriasis and the inflammatory changes. Increased activity of phospholipase A_2, the rate limiting enzyme in this cascade, appears to be primarily responsible for these changes.

Decreased cAMP and increased cGMP are found in lesions, and beta-blockers and lithium may exacerbate psoriasis by inhibiting cAMP formation. Polyamines are elevated in lesional skin, due to increased activity of ornithine decarboxylase, and may be intimately associated with cellular proliferation. Plasminogen activator is greatly increased in the lesions of psoriasis and its level parallels the epidermal mitotic rate.

Finally, the level of calmodulin, the specific receptor protein for calcium, is greatly raised in lesions and falls with successful treatment. The calcium-calmodulin complex may regulate epidermal cell proliferation by influencing phospholipase A_2 and phosphodiesterase (catalyses cAMP to AMP).

Immunopathological. Many immunological abnormalities have been found but their role is uncertain. Immune complexes to epidermal antigens have been detected in damaged skin and may activate complement, thereby attracting neutrophils to the area. The dermal mononuclear infiltrate is mainly of T lymphocytes, most of which are of the helper type. The beneficial effect of cyclosporin A in psoriasis may be due to its anti-T helper cell effect.

Dermal. There is substantial evidence to suggest that the increased epidermal cell proliferation of psoriasis is related to the increased replication and metabolism of dermal fibroblasts. Both dermal and epidermal abnormalities appear to be necessary for the sustenance of psoriasis.

Given the basic defect, an individual may not inevitably develop psoriasis but certain precipitating factors make this more likely.

Precipitating factors
Although there appears to be no obvious precipitating factor in about 70% of exacerbations of psoriasis the factors shown in the information box (right) are responsible for the minority of flare-ups.

Pathology
The histology of psoriasis is depicted in Figure 17.5.

FACTORS CAUSING FLARE-UPS

Trauma
When the condition is erupting lesions appear in areas of skin damage such as scratches or surgical wounds (Köbner phenomenon)

Infection
Beta-haemolytic streptococcal throat infections often precede guttate psoriasis

Sunlight
Although ultraviolet radiation is usually therapeutic, 10% of psoriatics become worse

Drugs
Antimalarials, beta-blockers and lithium may worsen psoriasis and the rash may 'rebound' after treatment with systemic steroids or potent local steroids

Emotion
Anxiety seems to precipitate some exacerbations

Clinical features

Common patterns of psoriasis

Plaque pattern. This is the most common type. Individual lesions are well demarcated and range from a few millimetres to several centimetres in diameter (Fig. 17.4, p. 912). The lesions are red with dry, silvery-white scaling, which may be obvious only after scraping the surface. The elbows, knees, lower back and scalp are most commonly involved.

Guttate psoriasis. This is usually seen in children and adolescents and may be the first sign of psoriasis. The rash often appears rapidly and individual lesions are small (seldom greater than 1 cm in diameter) and scaly. Bouts of guttate psoriasis usually clear in a few

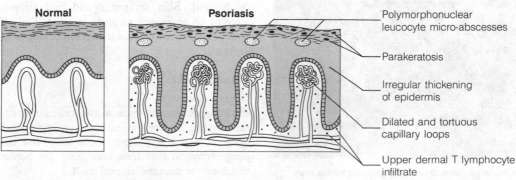

Normal   **Psoriasis**

Polymorphonuclear leucocyte micro-abscesses

Parakeratosis

Irregular thickening of epidermis

Dilated and tortuous capillary loops

Upper dermal T lymphocyte infiltrate

Fig. 17.5   The histology of psoriasis.

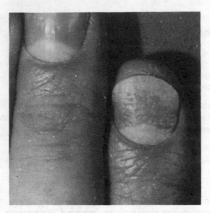

Fig. 17.6 **Coarse pitting of the nail and separation of the nail from the nail bed (onycholysis).** These are both classical features of psoriasis.

months, but patients may develop the plaque pattern later.

Scalp. This site is often involved, presumably due to repeated trauma from brushing and combing. Areas of marked scaling are interspersed with normal skin producing a lumpiness which is more easily felt than seen. Significant hair loss occurs only if there is gross involvement.

Nails. Involvement of the nails is common with 'thimble pitting', onycholysis (separation of the nail from the nail bed) (Fig. 17.6) and subungual hyper-keratosis. It often reflects the severity of the psoriasis elsewhere.

Flexures. Psoriasis involving the natal cleft, sub-mammary and axillary folds is not scaly but red, glistening and symmetrical (Fig. 17.7).

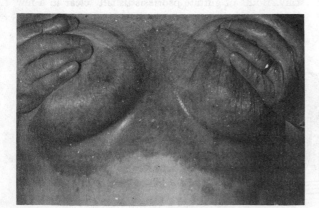

Fig. 17.7 **Flexural psoriasis. Showing the glistening but not scaly rash.**

Palms. Psoriasis here is often difficult to recognise as individual plaques may be poorly demarcated and barely erythematous.

Less common patterns

These are included in the information box below.

LESS COMMON PATTERNS IN PSORIASIS

Napkin psoriasis
May give the first hint of a psoriatic tendency in an infant

Localised pustular psoriasis
Most often involves the palms and soles. The eruption consists of numerous small sterile pustules lying on an erythematous base which leave brown macules or scaling in their wake. Some regard this as a separate disease entity

Erythrodermic psoriasis
The skin becomes universally red and scaly. Shivering compensates for the considerable heat loss. This unpleasant variant may be initiated by the irritant effect of tar or dithranol or the withdrawal of systemic or potent topical steroids

---

Complications

Psoriatic arthropathy is a possible complication. Arthritis occurs in about 5% of psoriatics. Distal arthritis involves the terminal interphalangeal joints of the toes and fingers, especially those with marked nail changes. Other patterns include involvement of a single large joint, a variety which mimics rheumatoid arthritis and which may be destructive, and one involving the sacro-iliac joints and lumbar spine (associated with HLA B27). Tests for rheumatoid factor are usually negative in true psoriatic arthropathy and nodules are absent.

Investigations

Few are indicated. Biopsy is seldom necessary because the clinical picture is usually characteristic. Throat swabbing for beta-haemolytic streptococci should be performed in guttate psoriasis and an ASO titre may be helpful. Skin scrapings and nail clippings may have to be examined to exclude tinea. Radiology and tests for rheumatoid factor are important in assessing arthritis.

Management

General measures

Explanation, reassurance and instruction are vital and must relate to the patient's or parent's intelligence. Both doctor and patient must keep the disease in perspective, so that treatment does not become more troublesome than the disease itself.

Physical and mental rest help to support the specific

management of acute flare-ups of psoriasis. Concomitant depression and anxiety should be treated.

Local measures

Coal tar preparations. Crude coal tar and its distillation products have been used to treat psoriasis for many years. Their main mode of action is probably by inhibiting DNA synthesis.

Many products are available; in general the messier, less refined, preparations (e.g. 100% strong coal tar solution and 4% tar paste) are more effective than the more refined and cleaner proprietary ointments. They are applied to the patches of psoriasis once or twice daily. Surprisingly, no increase in skin cancer has been found in patients treated for years with tar preparations. Salicylic acid (1-2%), sometimes added to tar preparations to remove scaling, is useful in the management of scalp psoriasis.

Dithranol. This also inhibits DNA synthesis. Although it is irritant and more tricky to use than coal tar, its use has become widespread. The most popular regimen is short contact therapy in which the cream is applied to lesions for no longer than 30 minutes and then washed off. Initially 0.1% dithranol cream is used but, depending on the response, the strength may be increased stepwise to 2% over a few weeks. Dithranol stains normal skin purple-brown but the discolouration peels off after a few days.

Eruptive and unstable patches of psoriasis are unsuitable for treatment with coal tar or dithranol and those with limited experience of their use should select test patches of psoriasis for initial treatment. Coal tar preparations and dithranol are best avoided on the face, genitalia and body folds because they are irritating.

Topical steroids. These are liked by patients and some doctors because they are clean and effective initially. However, there are few indications for their long-term use as on their withdrawal, psoriasis may relapse rapidly or even change to an unstable phase which is more difficult to manage than previously. Their use should be limited as shown in the information box below.

LIMITATIONS ON USE OF TOPICAL STEROIDS
- The face, ears, genitalia and flexures where tar and dithranol are seldom tolerated
- Patients who cannot use tar or dithranol because of allergic or irritant reactions
- Unresponsive psoriasis of the scalp, palms and soles

Only mild steroids should be used on the face but moderately potent ones are suitable for elsewhere. Tar-steroid combinations are a useful stepping stone to pure tar preparations, while steroid-antifungal combinations are helpful for flexural psoriasis.

Ultraviolet radiation. Most patients improve with natural sunlight and many clear their psoriasis by sunbathing during holiday periods. During the winter 6-8-week courses of medium-wave ultraviolet radiation (UVB) given in specialist centres 2-3 times weekly are often helpful. In the majority of patients sunbeds (emitting long-wave ultraviolet waves – UVA) are not beneficial. Combination therapies with UVB, coal tar preparations and dithranol are used to clear psoriasis more quickly than can be achieved by monotherapies.

Systemic treatment. This will be considered by a dermatologist if extensive psoriasis fails to respond to the local measures outlined above. The most commonly used systemic treatments are photochemotherapy with PUVA (psoralen + UVA), retinoids (etretinate and etretin) and methotrexate. All of these treatments have potential side-effects and patients receiving them require regular, specialist supervision. The use of cyclosporin A in the treatment of severe psoriasis is being evaluated at present.

ACNE VULGARIS

This disorder of the pilosebaceous apparatus affects many teenagers. Its prevalence is similar in both sexes but the peak age of severity in females is 16-17 years and in males 17-19 years. Acne clears by the age of 23-25 years in 90% of patients but some 5% of women and 1% of men still need treatment in their thirties or even forties.

Aetiology
Many factors, rather than a single one, combine to cause chronic inflammation of blocked pilo-sebaceous follicles (Fig. 17.8).

Sebum excretion is increased, but this alone need not cause acne: for example, patients with acromegaly or Parkinson's disease have high sebum excretion rates but no acne. The sebum excretion rate may remain high after acne has healed. The sebum of patients with acne contains an excess of free fatty acids.

Hormones are another factor and androgens from the testes, ovaries and adrenals are the main hormones which stimulate sebum excretion. In acne the sebaceous

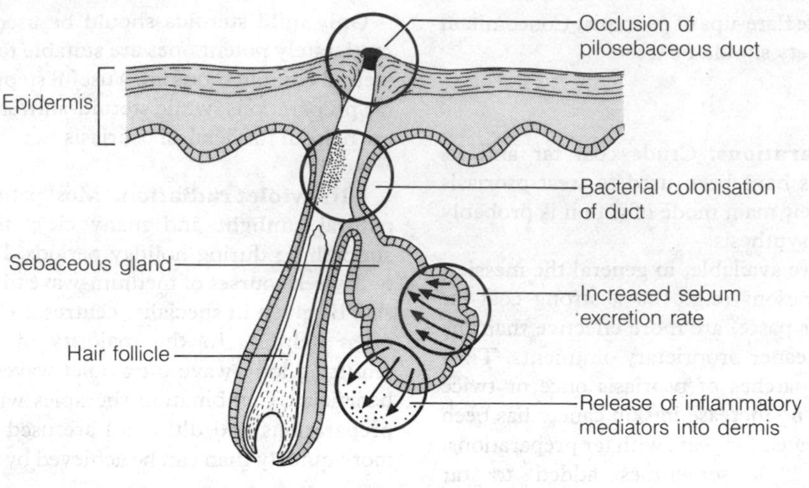

Epidermis

Sebaceous gland

Hair follicle

Occlusion of
pilosebaceous duct

Bacterial colonisation
of duct

Increased sebum
excretion rate

Release of inflammatory
mediators into dermis

Fig. 17.8   The pathogenesis of acne.

glands appear to be unduly sensitive to normal levels of these hormones.

Increased and abnormal keratinisation at the exit of the pilosebaceous follicle obstructs the flow of sebum. Fluid retention swells keratin and accounts for premenstrual flares. Bacteria play a pathogenic role. *Proprionobacterium acnes* is a normal skin commensal. It colonises the pilosebaceous ducts, breaks down triglycerides in the sebum to free fatty acids and sparks off the inflammatory process.

Acne is often familial. The inheritance pattern is probably polygenic.

Clinical features

Lesions are limited to the face, shoulders, upper chest and back. Seborrhoea (greasy skin) is often present. Open comedones (blackheads) due to plugging by keratin and sebum of the pilosebaceous orifice, or closed comedones (whiteheads) due to accretions of sebum and keratin deeper in the pilosebaceous ducts, are always evident. Inflammatory papules, nodules and cysts occur (Fig. 17.9), with one or two types of lesion predominating. Scarring may follow.

There are less common variants of acne: conglobate acne is severe with many abscesses and cysts, often connected by intercommunicating sinuses; scarring is severe. Acne fulminans is a type of conglobate acne accompanied by fever, joint pains and a high erythrocyte sedimentation rate (ESR). Excoriated acne manifests as discrete denuded areas caused by picking and is seen most often in early teenage girls. Infantile acne is rare and is due to transplacental stimulation of the infant's adrenals. It may last up to three years and may be the forerunner of severe acne in adolescence.

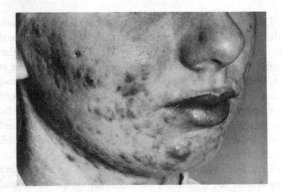

Fig. 17.9   Cystic acne in a teenager.

Exogenous acne may be caused by tars, chlorinated hydrocarbons, oils and oily cosmetics; comedones dominate the clinical picture. Drug induced acne may result from treatment with corticosteroids, androgenic steroids, lithium, oral contraceptives, and anticonvulsant therapy. Acne associated with virilisation may be due to an androgen secreting tumour of the adrenals, ovaries or testes.

Investigations

None are usually necessary though swabs may be needed to exclude a pyogenic infection, an anaerobic infection or Gram-negative folliculitis. Full endocrinological assessment is required for the investigation of acne associated with virilisation to exclude an androgen secreting tumour.

Management

Comedo-papular acne is managed by local treatment

alone; pustular-cystic and scarring acne require local and systemic treatment.

Local measures

Regular washing with soap and water is essential. Antibacterial skin cleansers containing chlorhexidine such as Hibiscrub are also useful. Preparations containing benzoyl peroxide and retinoic acid such as Panoxyl 5 Gel, are the cornerstone of local treatment and many proprietary products are available. They are irritant and drying and although some care is required to gauge an appropriate and regular regimen of application, most are applied once daily at nightime. Courses of ultraviolet B are often helpful but their beneficial effect is usually short-lived.

Systemic measures

Antibiotics are used initially. They should not be used for less than 3 months and may even be necessary for 2 or 3 years. Oxytetracycline (up to 250 mg 4 times daily), minocycline (50 mg twice daily) and erythromycin (up to 250 mg 4 times daily) are suitable doses for adults with moderate acne, but larger doses may be required. Patients taking long-term antibiotics should be reviewed regularly for side-effects which fortunately are rare, though they include potentially dangerous benign intracranial hypertension (with tetracyclines).

Isotretinoin (13-cis-retinoic acid) is a recent and very valuable addition to the list of drugs used for treating severe acne. It reduces sebum excretion dramatically and is given in a four-month course. Although sebum excretion eventually rebounds to its former level after the drug is stopped, the acne does not usually recur. Minor side-effects, especially drying of the skin and mucous membranes, are common but well tolerated. Rarely, abnormalities of liver function occur and limit treatment. The main problem is that the drug is highly teratogenic and females requiring it must have a negative pregnancy test before treatment and take an oral contraceptive for at least a month before the course of isotretinoin, during the course and for 3 months after. Pregnancy tests at monthly reviews are also advisable.

Hormonal treatment in the form of a combined antiandrogen (cyproterone acetate)/oestrogen pill, taken in courses as an oral contraceptive, is available in many countries and may help women with persistent acne resistant to treatment with antibiotics. Monitoring is as for any female on an oral contraceptive.

Physical measures

Cysts can be incised and drained under local anaesthetic. Intralesional injections of triamcinolone acetonide (0.1–0.2 ml of a 10 mg/ml solution) hastens the resolution of stubborn cysts.

SKIN TUMOURS

The increasing number of patients over 70 years old is parallelled by an increasing incidence of skin tumours. Only the most common benign tumours and a few malignant ones will be described in this section.

BENIGN

MELANOCYTIC NAEVI

Melanocytic naevi (moles) are localised benign proliferations of melanocytes. Their cause is unknown but they are often familial. With the exception of congenital melanocytic naevi (which are present at birth or appear shortly after birth), most melanocytic naevi appear in early childhood, at adolescence and during pregnancy or oestrogen therapy. New lesions appear less often after the age of 20.

Clinical features

Acquired melanocytic naevi are classified according to the microscopic location of the clumps of melanocytes in the skin. The *junctional* type shows these clumps at the epidermal-dermal junction, the *intradermal* type within the dermis and the *compound* type at both of the above sites. There is a reasonable correlation between their clinical and histological appearance. Junctional naevi are usually circular and macular; their colour ranges from mid to dark brown and may vary within a single lesion. Compound and intradermal naevi are similar to one another in appearance; both are nodules of up to 1 cm in diameter though intradermal naevi are usually less pigmented than compound naevi. Their surface may be smooth, cerebriform or even hyperkeratotic and papillomatous and they are often hairy.

Clinically and histologically atypical naevi, so-called dysplastic naevi, may run in some families in which cases of malignant melanoma are seen. These profuse, large, and irregularly pigmented naevi are most obvious on the trunk. Their edges are irregular and they vary greatly in size, often being over 1 cm in diameter. Some are pinkish and an inflamed halo may surround them.

Except in the larger congenital melanocytic naevi, where the risk of subsequent malignancy has been estimated as high as 3–6% depending on their size, a rare but very important complication of melanocytic naevi is malignant change. It should be considered if the changes listed in the information box (p. 918) occur.

CHANGES IN MELANOCYTIC NAEVUS

- Itch
- Enlargement
- Increased or decreased pigmentation
- Asymmetry
- Irregularity of surface or edge
- Inflammation
- Ulceration
- Bleeding

Such lesions should be examined carefully remembering the 'ABCDE' features of malignant melanoma listed in the information box below.

ABCDE FEATURES

Asymmetry
Border irregular
Colour irregular
Diameter often greater than 0.5 cm
Elevation irregular

Management

Excision and histological examination is needed when malignancy is suspected or is a significant risk, for example in a large congenital melanocytic naevus, when a naevus becomes repeatedly inflamed or traumatised and when a naevus is deemed ugly.

SEBORRHOEIC KERATOSIS (BASAL CELL PAPILLOMA)

These common benign epidermal tumours are unrelated to sebaceous glands. Their appearance is usually unexplained but multiple lesions may be inherited as an autosomal dominant. Occasionally they appear in the wake of an inflammatory dermatosis and, very rarely, a sudden eruption of multiple itchy lesions may be associated with an internal tumour.

Clinical features

They appear usually after the age of 50 years but flat inconspicuous lesions may be visible earlier. They are most commonly found on the trunk and face. The sexes are equally affected. The lesions vary in colour from yellow to dark brown and have a distinctive, raised and 'stuck-on' appearance. They are sometimes pedunculated. Their surface may have greasy scaling and scattered pinpoint keratin plugs. They become more profuse with age but remain benign.

Investigation

Biopsy is necessary only in dubious cases.

Management

They may be left alone but unsightly or easily traumatised lesions are easily removed by curettage under local anaesthetic or by cryotherapy.

VIRAL WARTS

Most people have warts at some time of their life, usually before the age of 20. Genital warts occur during the sexually active years. They result from infection with the DNA human papillomavirus of which over 50 subtypes are now recognised. Different subtypes are responsible for several clinical variants. Transmission is by contact with the virus either in living skin or in fragments of shed skin, and is encouraged by trauma and moisture (e.g. at swimming pools, amongst butchers, fishmongers, etc). Genital warts are spread by intercourse and perianal warts may reflect homosexual activity.

Clinical features

Common warts appear initially as smooth skin-coloured papules. As they enlarge their surfaces become irregular and hyperkeratotic producing the typical 'warty' appearance. They usually occur on the hands but may

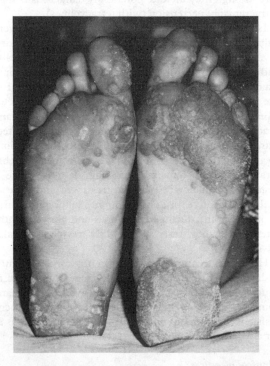

Fig. 17.10 Extensive plantar warts. In this case they appeared in a patient receiving immunosuppressive treatment after a renal transplant.

also often be seen on the face and genitalia; warts are frequently multiple. Plantar warts ('verrucae') are characterised by a rough surface, protruding only slightly from the skin and surrounded by a horny collar. On paring, oozing capillary loops distinguish plantar warts from corns. Often multiple, plantar warts may be painful. Other variants of warts include mosaic warts (mosaic-like plaques of tightly packed individual warts), plane warts (smooth, flat-topped papules seen most commonly on the face and backs of hands), facial warts (often filiform and hyperkeratotic) and anogenital warts (may be papillomatous and even cauliflowerlike).

Most viral warts in the healthy will eventually resolve spontaneously but this may take years. In immuno-compromised patients warts persist and spread (Fig. 17.10); 70% of renal allograft recipients will have warts five years after transplantation.

Management

Warts may be treated in many different ways. Common warts in children should be managed with wart paints containing salicylic acid. Stubborn lesions should be treated with liquid nitrogen cryotherapy or removed by curettage. Anogenital warts are treated with either cryotherapy or podophyllin paint (applied initially for only 2 hours and avoided in pregnancy). Facial warts are most easily treated with cryotherapy or electro-desiccation. Plane warts are often best left alone.

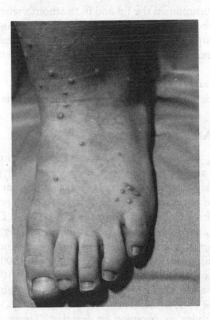

Fig. 17.11 Multiple lesions of molluscum contagiosum. These are shown here on the ankle and forefoot of an atopic child.

MOLLUSCUM CONTAGIOSUM ('WATER WARTS')

This common and easily recognised pox virus infection usually affects children, atopic or immunocompromised adults. Spread is by direct contact or by infected towelling, clothing, etc. The incubation period is from 2–6 weeks.

Clinical features

Individual lesions are shiny, white and hemispherical and grow slowly up to about 0.5 cm in diameter. Their characteristic unbilicated look is due to a central punctum which may contain a cheesy core. Multiple lesions are common (Fig. 17.11). Like warts many lesions will clear spontaneously often after brief local inflammation.

Management

No treatment may be best in some children but cryo-therapy or rapid expression is tolerated well by others, especially if performed by an experienced operator.

ACTINIC KERATOSIS

These discrete, rough-surfaced lesions occur on light exposed areas. They are caused by cumulative sun exposure. Whites living near the equator are most at risk and invariably develop them though they also affect the middle-aged and elderly in temperate climates. Actinic keratoses are not seen in Blacks.

Clinical features

The multiple pink or grey hyperkeratotic lesions seldom exceed 1 cm in diameter and are most common on the backs of the hands, the face and bald scalp. Many resolve spontaneously. Transition to squamous cell carcinoma, although rare, should be suspected if a lesion enlarges, ulcerates or bleeds.

Management

Cryotherapy with liquid nitrogen is effective though multiple lesions may be treated with 5% 5-fluorouracil cream under specialist guidance. Lesions which do not respond to treatment should be regarded with suspicion and biopsied.

MALIGNANT

BASAL CELL CARCINOMA

This is the most common form of skin cancer and is usually found on the face of the middle-aged or elderly. The tumour invades locally but, rarely metastasises.

'Rodent ulcer' is a term commonly used for slowly expanding ulcerative basal cell carcinoma. The malignant cells resemble basal keratinocytes.

Aetiology

Cumulative sun exposure is the most important factor in their development and these tumours are more common in Whites living near the equator. They may also occur in scars following vaccination, trauma or X-irradiation.

Clinical features

The most common type is the nodulo-ulcerative form. The earliest lesion is a small glistening, skin coloured papule, often with fine telangiectatic vessels on the surface, which slowly enlarges (Fig. 17.12). Central necrosis may occur which leaves an ulcer surrounded by a rolled pearly edge. Without treatment lesions may reach 1–2 cm in diameter over 5 to 10 years. Slow but relentless growth causes local tissue destruction. Sometimes this type of tumour becomes cystic or pigmented. The cicatricial variant of basal cell carcinoma is a slowly expanding yellow or grey, waxy plaque with an ill-defined edge. Fibrosis often follows ulceration and crusting and the lesion may appear as an enlarging scar. The superficial (multifocal) variant is seen most often on the trunk; it appears as a slowly enlarging pink or brown scaly plaque with a fine 'whipcord' edge. If left it may grow to 10 cm in diameter.

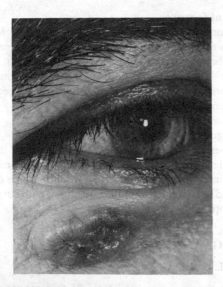

Fig. 17.12 A slowly growing pearly nodule. This appeared below the eye of a middle-aged patient who had spent many years working in the tropics. The telangiectasia and early central ulceration are typical.

Management

Excision, with a half centimetre of normal skin, is the treatment of choice for most patients. Lesions with an ill-defined edge are best excised by specialist surgeons. Radiotherapy is effective and should be reserved for biopsy proven lesions when surgery is contra-indicated. The cure rate for all types of basal cell carcinoma is over 95% but regular follow-up for at least three years is required to detect local recurrence.

SQUAMOUS CELL CARCINOMA

Aetiology

These malignant tumours of keratinocytes often arise in skin damaged by long-term ultraviolet radiation but also by X-rays and infra-red rays. Patients with certain rare genetic disorders, with defective DNA repair mechanisms, such as xeroderma pigmentosum also develop multiple basal and squamous cell carcinomas. The integration of human papilloma virus DNA detected in some squamous cell carcinomas suggests an oncogenic potential for certain types of this group of viruses; immunosuppression and ultraviolet radiation appear to be important contributory factors.

Clinical features

Squamous cell carcinoma usually presents as a keratotic nodule, though anaplastic lesions may be seen as an ulcer with a granulating base and indurated edge. The tumour is common on the lip and in the mouth where it may be preceded by leukoplakia. Those arising in actinic keratoses seldom metastasise but all tumours should be treated promptly to prevent nodal spread.

Management

Treatment is similar to that for basal cell carcinoma.

MALIGNANT MELANOMA

Malignant melanoma attracts a disproportionate amount of attention because it is so lethal and prevention, early diagnosis and treatment are by far the best ways of combating its dangers. It is rarely seen in Blacks but its incidence in Whites in the UK and USA is doubling, approximately every 10 years. Sunlight is the most important cause. There is a higher incidence in Whites living near the equator (over 40 per 100 000 per annum) than those living in temperate zones (5–10 per 100 000 per annum). The tumour is rare before puberty and in areas of low incidence (including the UK) the tumour is twice as common in females. Those with blond or red hair, fair skin which tans poorly, many freckles and melanocytic naevi, dysplastic melanocytic naevi and a family or personal history of a previous melanoma have an increased risk of developing the tumour.

Clinical features

Two-thirds of invasive melanomas are preceded by a superficial and radial growth phase characterised by an expanding, irregularly pigmented macule or plaque. Its margin is usually irregular with reniform projections and nodules. *Lentigo maligna* (in situ changes of malignancy only) and *lentigo maligna melanoma* occur most often on the exposed skin of the elderly. A speckled macular lentigo maligna may have been present for many years before a nodule of invasive melanoma appears within it (Fig. 17.13). The in situ

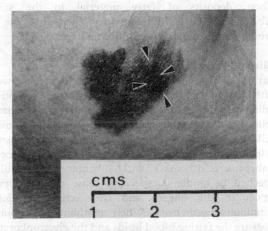

Fig. 17.13 Lentigo maligna melanoma; a slowly expanding pigmented lesion on the cheek of an elderly lady. The irregular shades of brown and irregular edge spell malignancy. An area (outlined by arrows) has recently become palpable and indicates dermal invasion by the tumour cells.

phase of *superficial spreading melanoma*, the most common type in Whites, seldom lasts for longer than 2 years, usually shows much colour variation and is often palpable. *Acral lentiginous melanoma* occurs on the palms and soles and is the most common type in the Chinese and Japanese. *Nodular melanoma* develops as a pigmented nodule with no preceding in situ phase. All changing pigmented lesions deserve careful examination remembering the 'ABCDE' features of malignant melanoma (p. 918). About 30–50% of melanomas appear to develop in a preceding melanocytic naevus (p. 917). A change in any naevus should raise suspicion of malignant transformation.

True *amelanotic melanomas* occur but are rare; flecks of pigmentaion can usually be seen with a lens. *Subungual melanomas* present as painless, expanding areas of pigmentation under a nail and usually involve the nail fold.

The clinical stages of malignant melanoma are shown in the information box below.

CLINICAL STAGES OF MALIGNANT MELANOMA

- Stage I: primary lesion only
- Stage II: regional nodal disease
- Stage III: distant disease (nodal or visceral)

The diagnosis should be established by local excision biopsy of the suspected lesion. Incisional biopsies are not recommended as a routine but may be unavoidable with some doubtful lesions and at certain sites.

Management

Only surgical excision is effective. A 3-cm clearance is recommended for tumours greater than 1 mm thick. Direct closure, without grafting, may be possible. Tumours less than 1 mm thick are removed with a 1 cm clearance; direct closure is nearly always possible. Elective (prophylactic) local node dissection may benefit some patients with tumours of intermediate depth (2.0–3.5 mm). Palpable local nodes in Stage II patients should always be removed by radical block dissection. Chemotherapy, rarely curative, is palliative in 25% of patients with Stage III melanoma.

Prevention and early diagnosis are best achieved by education of those at highest risk who live or holiday in sunny climates. Successful campaigns have focused on regular self-examination and the ways in which sun exposure can be reduced by avoidance, clothing and sunscreen preparations. Public awareness and compliance has been encouraged by imaginative and gimmicky slogans like the Australian 'Slip, Slap and Slop' advice (slip on the shirt, slap on the hat and slop on the sunscreen).

Prognosis

The prognosis of patients with a malignant melanoma can be determined with reasonable accuracy. Those with clinical Stage III disease fare least well (less than 10% survive 2 years), patients with Stage II disease have a 20–30% chance and those with Stage I disease a 60–70% chance of surviving 5 years. The thickness of the tumour (measured microscopically by Breslow's method) is a reliable predictor of the prognosis for patients with Stage I disease. The prognosis is excellent for those with tumours less than 1 mm thick (over 90% survive 5 years), but becomes less good with thicker tumours. The 5-year survival of patients with tumours greater than 3.5 mm thick is about 50%. In general females fare better than males and tumours at certain sites (e.g. lower leg) are less aggressive.

THE SKIN AND SYSTEMIC DISEASE

Skin reactions can be linked with an underlying systemic disease in a number of ways as shown below in Table 17.5.

Only common or important associations will be discussed below.

GENODERMATOSES

NEUROFIBROMATOSIS (p. 901)

Clinical features
The skin markers include scattered and discrete light brown (café au lait) macules, axillary freckling and a variable number of cutaneous neurofibromata. The tumours may be small and superficial or large and deep

Table 17.5   Skin reactions in systemic disease

Part of a multisystem disease
Genodermatoses (e.g. neurofibromatosis and tuberous sclerosis)
Xanthomas
Amyloidosis (p. 575)
Porphyria
Sarcoidosis (p. 409)

A non-specific and not invariable reaction pattern to a systemic disease
Urticaria
Erythema multiforme
Annular erythemas
Erythema nodosum
Pyoderma gangrenosum
Sweet's syndrome
Generalised pruritus

A sign of internal malignancy
Dermatomyositis (p. 793)
Generalised pruritus
Acanthosis nigricans
Superficial thrombophlebitis

A sign of internal organ failure
Liver
    Generalised pruritus, pigmentation, spider naevi and palmar erythema
Kidney
    Generalised pruritus and pigmentation
Pancreas (Diabetes mellitus)
    Necrobiosis lipoidica

A result of a common genetic link with the systemic disorder
Dermatitis herpetiformis and gluten sensitive enteropathy
Psoriasis and some types of arthropathy

The cause of the systemic disease
Exfoliative dermatitis causing high output Cardiac failure

A result of treatment of the systemic disease
Drug eruptions

TUBEROUS SCLEROSIS
This is an autosomal dominant condition with hamartomas affecting many systems.

Clinical features
The classic triad of features is mental retardation, epilepsy and skin lesions but not all are invariably present. The skin signs include small white oval (ash leaf) macules, pink or yellowish papules on the centre of the face (adenoma sebaceum), peri and subungual fibromata and connective tissue naevi (cobblestone-like plaques at the base of the spine, sometimes called shagreen patches).

XANTHOMAS

These deposits of fatty material in the skin, subcutaneous fat and tendons may be the first clue to primary or secondary hyperlipidaemia (p. 697).

Clinical features
Various clinical patterns are seen which correlate well with the underlying cause. They include eruptive yellow papules on the buttocks (eruptive xanthomas), yellowish macules or plaques (plane xanthomas), small yellow-grey plaques around the eyes (xanthelasma palpebrarum), nodules over the elbows and knees (tuberous xanthomas) and subcutaneous nodules attached to tendons, especially those on the dorsal aspect of the fingers and the Achilles tendons (tendinous xanthomas). When xanthomas are found measure the fasting blood lipids and the electrophoretic pattern of plasma lipoproteins must be measured though abnormalities will not always be found.

AMYLOIDOSIS (p. 575)

Skin lesions are uncommon in systemic amyloidosis secondary to rheumatoid arthritis or other chronic inflammatory diseases.

Clinical features
Deposits of amyloid in the skin, appearing often as waxy plaques around the eyes, are prominent in *primary systemic amyloidosis* and in amyloid associated with multiple myeloma. 'Pinch purpura', due to amyloid infiltration of blood vessels, may also be a striking feature.

PORPHYRIA
Clinical features
Skin lesions do not occur in *acute intermittent porphyria*.

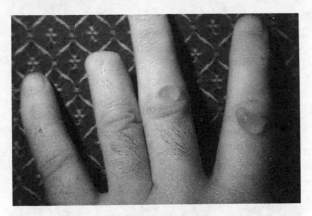

Fig. 17.14 Recent skin fragility and blistering on the backs of fingers of a 45-year-old male. The signs, although trivial, are highly suggestive of cutaneous hepatic porphyria. The urine of this patient, with alcoholic liver damage, contained excessive uroporphyrins.

This is characterised by attacks of abdominal pain, neuropsychiatric symptoms and the passage of dark urine. Attacks may be triggered by drugs, especially barbiturates, oestrogens, griseofulvin and sulphonamides.

Fragility, blistering (Fig. 17.14), hairiness and scarring of exposed skin are features of *cutaneous hepatic porphyria*. The condition is most common in patients with alcoholic liver damage

The autosomal dominantly inherited *variegate porphyria* is common in South Africa. The features include the systemic symptoms and drug provocation of acute intermittent porphyria and the skin signs of hepatic cutaneous porphyria

SARCOIDOSIS

Skin lesions are seen in about one third of patients with systemic sarcoidosis.

Clinical features

They include erythema nodosum (p. 924), granulomatous deposits in longstanding scars, dusky infiltrated plaques on the nose and fingers (lupus pernio) and scattered brownish-red, violaceous or hypopigmented papules or nodules which vary in number, size and distribution.

URTICARIA

This common reaction pattern may be due to a particular food or food additive, a drug or, more rarely, an underlying systemic disease.

Aetiology

The final common pathway for all types of urticaria is the release of mediators which cause increased capillary permeability and the accumulation of fluid in the surrounding tissue. Histamine released from mast cells is important in most cases but kinins or serotonin may play a part in the deeper, more persistent, types of physical urticaria.

Many types of urticaria do not have an immunological or allergic basis. Amongst these are the physical urticarias which may be induced by heat, sweating, cold, pressure, sun exposure and even contact with water; their pathogenesis is diverse. Urticaria of sudden onset, widespread distribution and lasting only for a few days may be a manifestation of a type I allergic reaction, even associated with a serum sickness-like reaction (p. 37) and the history often reveals a clear-cut cause such as a particular food or drug.

Hereditary angioedema is a rare but important condition, inherited as an autosomal dominant. It is due to a functional deficiency of the inhibitor of the activated first component of the complement system.

Clinical features

Urticaria describes an eruption of itchy wheals, sometimes accompanied by deeper and more diffuse swelling (angioedema) which is seldom itchy. By definition the wheals are evanescent and individual lesions are seldom present for longer than 12 hours; however, they may recur for a few days, weeks or even years.

The most serious complications of acute urticaria are anaphylactic shock: pallor, sweating, hypotension and collapse which may be preceded by headache, bronchospasm, nausea and vomiting and angioedema, causing obstruction of the respiratory tract.

Investigation

A good history and examination will usually be more helpful in investigation than laboratory tests. First a physical cause should be excluded. If none is obvious an underlying systemic condition should be considered including viral infections such as early viral hepatitis, infectious mononucleosis and primary HIV infection, but also systemic lupus erythematosus and thyrotoxicosis. Drugs, especially salicylates which are histamine releasers, should then come under suspicion. Occasionally exacerbations may coincide with ingestion of a particular food and specially kept food diaries may help to identify causative items. Additives such as tartrazine, salicylates and yeasts have received much attention. Finally laboratory tests should be performed to confirm underlying systemic disease, to check the complement systemic in suspected familiar angioedema and to look for an eosinophilia which might be a clue to parasitosis.

Management

Any obvious cause should be avoided and underlying systemic conditions should be treated. The majority of acute and subacute cases respond well to the new generation of non-sedative antihistamines, e.g. terfenadine 60–120 mg twice daily, but different anti-histamine combinations may have to be tried in chronic cases. Calamine lotion is as good as any local treatment. Potential airway obstruction is an emergency and is treated with adrenaline (1 in 1000), 0.5 ml given slowly subcutaneously or intramuscularly followed by intra-venous chlorpheniramine (10 mg) and intravenous hydrocortisone (100 mg). If treatment is given early enough tracheostomy should be avoidable. The management of anaphylactic shock is similar and described on page 37.

ERYTHEMA MULTIFORME

As its name implies this is a reaction pattern of multiform erythematous lesions. The precipitating factor may not be found in some cases but attacks are provoked by the factors listed in the information box below.

PRECIPITATING FACTORS

- Herpes simplex infections
- Other viral (e.g. (orf) and mycoplasma infections
- Bacterial infections
- Drugs (especially sulphonamides, penicillins and barbiturates)
- Internal malignancy or its treatment with radiotherapy

Clinical features

The multiform erythematous lesions may be urticarial-like and some have obvious 'bull's eye' or 'target' lesions. Blisters may be seen in the centre or around the edges of the lesions. In some cases blisters dominate the picture; the Stevens-Johnson syndrome is severe bullous erythema multiforme with emphasis on mucosal involvement including the mouth, eyes and genitals with accompanying constitutional disturbance.

Management

Severe cases are usually managed with tapering courses of systemic steroids after treatment, if possible, of the primary cause.

ERYTHEMA NODOSUM

This characteristic reaction pattern is due to a vasculitis in the deep dermis and subcutaneous fat.

Erythema nodosum may be provoked by factors listed in the information box below.

PROVOKING FACTORS

Infections
Bacteria (streptococci, tuberculosis, brucellosis and leprosy), viruses, mycoplasma, rickettsia, chlamydia and fungi

Drugs
E.g. sulphonamides and oral contraceptives

Systemic disease
E.g. sarcoidosis, ulcerative colitis and Crohn's disease

Clinical features

Painful, palpable, dusky blue-red nodules are most commonly seen on the lower legs. Malaise, fever and joint pains are common. The lesions resolve slowly over a month leaving bruise-like marks in their wake.

Management

The underlying cause should be determined and treated. Bed rest and oral, non-steroidal anti-inflammatory drugs or potassium iodide may hasten resolution. Tapering systemic steroid courses may be required in stubborn cases.

ACANTHOSIS NIGRICANS

Clinical features

This is a velvety thickening and pigmentation of the major flexures. Sometimes it may be associated with obesity or insulin resistant diabetes but, if not, the chances are high of an underlying carcinoma, usually within the abdomen.

GENERALISED PRURITUS

This is a symptom with many causes, rather than a disease in its own right. It may be due to a skin disorder (e.g. eczema, scabies, lichen planus) or to an internal cause such as those listed in the information box below.

INTERNAL CAUSES

- Liver disease. Itching signals biliary obstruction
- Chronic renal failure
- Iron deficiency
- Polycythaemia. The itching is often triggered by a hot bath
- Thyroid disease. Both hypothyroidism and hyperthyroidism
- Internal malignancy – especially Hodgkin's disease and other lymphomas

NECROBIOSIS LIPOIDICA

This condition is important because of its association with diabetes mellitus. Less than 1% of diabetics have necrobiosis, but more than 85% of patients with necrobiosis will have or will develop diabetes.

Clinical features

Typically the lesions appear as shiny, atrophic and slightly yellow plaques on the shins (Fig. 17.15). Underlying telangiectasia is easily seen. Minor knocks may precipitate slow-healing ulcers.

Management

No treatment is effective.

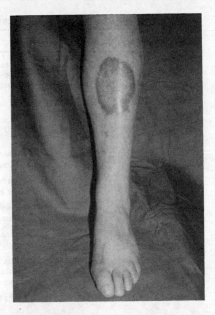

Fig. 17.15   Necrobiosis lipoidica; a shiny, atrophic plaque on the shin of a patient with insulin dependent diabetes mellitus.

DRUG ERUPTIONS

Cutaneous drug reactions are common and almost any drug can cause them. Drug reactions may reasonably be included in the differential diagnosis of most skin diseases. Although the mechanisms are poorly understood, drug eruptions may be classified as shown in Table 17.6.

Table 17.6   Drug eruptions and their mechanisms

Mechanism	Example
Non Immunological (non allergic)	
Unwarranted pharmacological effect	Striae due to corticosteroids, Mouth ulcers due to methotrexate
Drug overdosage or failure to metabolise or excrete the drug	Morphine rashes in patients with liver disease
Drug interaction	Warfarin toxicity when co-administered with aspirins or phenylbutazone
Idiosyncratic reaction (odd reactions which may be genetically determined and are peculiar to an individual)	Drug induced variegate porphyria
Phototoxic reaction	Chlorpromazine induced light reactions
Altered skin ecology	Tetracyclines causing vaginal candidiasis
Exacerbation of pre-existing skin condition	Lithium and beta-blocker worsening of psoriasis
Immunological (allergic)	
Immediate hypersensitivity	Penicillin induced urticaria
Immune complex reaction	Drug induced vasculitis or erythema multiforme
Delayed hypersensitivity	Drug induced exfoliative dermatitis or photoallergic reactions

Table 17.7   Drug eruptions and some drugs which may cause them

Name of reaction pattern	Clinical features	Drugs which commonly cause reaction
Toxic erythema	Erythematous plaques Morbilliform, sometimes with urticarial or erythema multiforme-like elements	Antibiotics (especially ampicillin) Sulphonamides, thiazide diuretics phenylbutazone PAS
Urticaria	See text (p. 923)	Salicylates and antibiotics
Allergic vasculitis	Painful, palpable purpura followed by necrotic ulcers	Sulphonamides, phenylbutazone, indomethacin, phenytoin and oral contraceptives
Erythema multiforme	Target-like lesions and bullae on the extensor aspects of the limbs	Sulphonamides, phenylbutazone and barbiturates
Purpura	Widespread purpura not due to thrombocytopenia or a coagulation defect	Thiazides, sulphonamides, phenylbutazone sulphonylurea, barbiturates and quinine
Bullous eruptions	May be associated with above eruptions. May occur at pressure sites in drug induced coma	Barbiturates
Exofoliative dermatitis	Universal redness and scaling, shivering	Phenylbutazone, para-aminosalicylic acid (PAS), isoniazid and gold
Fixed drug eruptions	Round, erythematous, and sometimes bullous, plaques develop at the same site every time the drug is given. Pigmentation left in wake	Tetracyclines, quinine, sulphonamides and barbiturates
Acneiform eruptions	Rash resembles acne (see text)	Lithium, oral contraceptive, androgenic or glucocorticoid steroids. Antituberculosis and anti-convulsant drugs
Toxic epidermal necrolysis	Rash resembles that of scaled skin (Fig. 7.16)	Barbiturates, phenytoin, phenylbutazone and penicillin
Hair loss	Diffuse	Cytotoxic agents, etretinate, anticoagulants, antithyroid drugs and oral contraceptives
Hypertrichosis		Diazoxide, minoxidil and cyclosporin A
Photosensitivity	Rash limited to exposed skin	Thiazides, tetracyclines, phenothiazines, sulphonamides, nalidixic acid and psoralens
Pigmentation	Irregular melanin pigmentation on face Slate-grey colour of exposed skin Diffuse yellow colouration of skin Streaky depigmentation of hair	Oral contraceptives Phenothiazines Mepacrine Chloroquine

Clinical features

The most common types of drug eruptions and their cause are listed in Table 17.7. It is important not to forget the possibility of a drug eruption when faced with

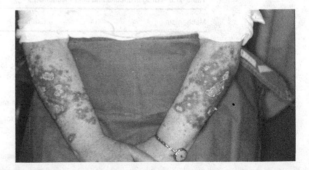

Fig. 17.17   Drug eruption; a weird but symmetrical erythematous scaly rash on the fore arms of a patient who had recently been prescribed a sulphonylurea. The rash persisted until the drug was withdrawn.

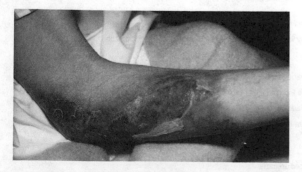

Fig. 17.16   Toxic epidermal necrolysis. In this case it was due to a barbiturate.

a rash which is atypical of a known skin disease. Further clues to make the diagnosis are included in the information box (p. 927).

DIAGNOSTIC CLUES

- Past history of reaction to suspected drug
- Introduction of suspected drug a few days before onset of rash
- Recent prescription of a drug (e.g. penicillins, sulphonamides, thiazides, allopurinol, phenylbutazone etc) commonly associated with rashes
- A symmetrical eruption which may fit with a well-recognised pattern caused by one of the current drugs (Fig. 17.17)

Investigations

There are no specific investigations, which help. Prick tests and in vitro tests for allergy are too unreliable for routine use. Readministration, as a diagnostic test, is usually unwise unless the reaction is mild and there is no suitable alternative drug.

Management

The first step is to withdraw the suspected drug(s) which may not be easy, or even possible, if there is no alternative available. The decision will depend on many factors including the severity and nature of the drug reaction, its potential reversibility and the probability that the drug caused the reaction. Supportive treatment with antihistamines or a tailored course of systemic steroids may be indicated depending on the type of skin reaction. The emergency treatment of anaphylactic shock is described on page 37.

FURTHER READING

Fundamental texts
Burton J L 1985 Essentials of Dermatology, 2nd Edn, pp. 260. Churchill Livingstone, Edinburgh
HunterJ A A, Savin D S, Dahl M V 1989 Clinical Dermatology. Blackwell Scientific Publications, Oxford

Reference books
Fitzpatrick T B, Eisen A Z, Wolff K, Freedberg I M, Austen K F Dermatology in General Medicine 3rd Edn. McGraw Hill Book Company, New York
Rook A, Wilkinson D S, Ebling F J G, Champion R H, Burton J L 1986 Textbook of Dermatology 4th Edn. Blackwell Scientific Publications, Oxford

18

Psychiatry

Diagnosis in psychiatry is mainly based on recognised patterns of subjective symptoms which are volunteered by the patient or elicited during a clinical interview. With the exception of the organic psychiatric disorders there are no objective markers of disease, such as radiological or laboratory abnormalities, by which diagnosis can be confirmed. In this context psychiatry differs from other branches of medicine where diseases have come to be classified in terms of their aetiology, such as an infective agent, biochemical abnormality or structural lesion. The symptoms of mental disorders involve abnormalities of behaviour, mood, perception, thinking and intellectual function. Some of these abnormalities impair judgement or contact with reality so that patients become a danger to themselves or other people. This is recognised in law and the Mental Health Act gives doctors the authority to treat patients against their will in exceptional cases. However the great majority of patients with psychiatric disorders are managed in general practitioners' surgeries or hospital outpatient clinics in much the same way as patients with any other medical condition. In 1985 only 7% of those who required inpatient treatment were admitted to hospital in England under the provisions of the Mental Health Act.

The number of inpatients in psychiatric hospitals has decreased sharply during the last two decades. In part this has been due to improved methods of treatment but it is also a result of government policy to treat patients in the community and to avoid hospital admission whenever possible. Long-stay patients have been moved out of hospital into community facilities such as hostels or group homes although the development of these facilities has not kept pace with plans for hospital closure. The overall result is that psychiatrists spend more time working in the community and have had opportunities to work more closely with their colleagues in general practice and other hospital specialties.

EPIDEMIOLOGY

Epidemiology is concerned with the study of disease in relation to the population in which it occurs, particularly its variation between subgroups and its association with environmental factors. Prevalence rates provide an estimate of how common a particular disease is in a given population; these rates can be expressed for a particular time (point prevalence) or for a given period (period prevalence). One month and life-time prevalence figures for psychiatric disorders from a large American study are shown in Table 18.1.

Table 18.1   Prevalence rates of psychiatric disorders (%) (from Regier et al, 1988)

	1 month	Lifetime
Any psychiatric disorder	15.4	32.2
Affective disorders	5.1	8.3
Mania	0.4	0.8
Major depression	2.2	5.8
Dysthymia	3.3	3.3
Anxiety disorders	7.3	14.6
Phobia	6.2	12.5
Panic	0.5	1.6
Obsessive compulsive	1.3	2.5
Schizophrenia	0.7	1.5
Substance use disorders	3.8	16.4
Alcohol abuse	2.8	13.3
Drug abuse	1.3	5.9
Somatisation disorder	0.1	0.1
Antisocial personality disorder	0.5	2.5
Severe cognitive impairment	1.3	1.3

These figures are probably representative of other Western countries. In the United Kingdom the prevalence of psychiatric illness in different populations can be summarised as shown in the information box below.

PREVALENCE OF PSYCHIATRIC ILLNESS IN DIFFERENT POPULATIONS IN PERCENTAGES

- Community   15–20%
- General practice attenders   30%
- General hospital outpatients   20–30%
- General hospital inpatients   25–40%

The average general practitioner can expect to be consulted by one in seven of his patients because of psychiatric disorder during one year. The spectrum of illness treated in primary care differs from that treated by psychiatrists in outpatient clinics. General practitioners see a greater proportion of patients with neurotic illnesses and relatively few with psychotic illnesses; their patients are less severely ill than those attending a psychiatrist. There is considerable variation between general practitioners in their ability to identify psychiatric illness. Cases are likely to be missed especially if psychiatric illness is associated with physical illness or presents with somatic complaints.

Psychiatric disorders are commoner in inner city areas than in rural communities, and among women than men although the sex distribution becomes more even if personality disorders and alcohol abuse are taken into account.

CLASSIFICATION OF PSYCHIATRIC DISORDERS

Psychiatric disorders have traditionally been classified into two main groups, *organic* and *functional*. In the *organic* disorders a known physical aetiology can be established, the symptoms resulting from coarse brain disease, as in dementia, or from metabolic upset or circulating toxins as in acute confusional states. In the *functional* disorders, which constitute the large majority of psychiatric illnesses, no such physical factors can be demonstrated. This distinction is still useful in clinical practice although its theoretical basis is becoming weaker as evidence accumulates to demonstrate the presence of neurotransmitter disturbance at synaptic level in schizophrenia and the affective disorders which have been classified as functional disorders.

Another traditional distinction which has become eroded is the separation of the functional disorders into psychotic or neurotic, depending on the presence of certain 'psychotic' symptoms. These are abnormal beliefs (delusions), abnormal perceptions (hallucinations and illusions) and certain disturbances in the pattern of thinking. Neurotic symptoms, in contrast, are mainly exaggerations of emotions such as anxiety and depression which are universally experienced. Psychotic illnesses were often regarded as being associated with lack of insight while patients with neurotic disorders were considered to have insight into their condition. Although this is true as a generalisation there are important caveats. Many psychotic patients have a lot of insight into their illness while some neurotic patients are strikingly lacking in understanding. Insight varies from time to time and its presence is not an all-or-none phenomenon, rather a matter of degree. Nor is it true to say that all psychotic illnesses are severe while neurotic illnesses are mild.

The usefulness of the psychotic-neurotic distinction continues to be argued by psychiatrists. The term neurosis has been abandoned by the American Psychiatric Association's classification (DSM-III) but is still applied in clinical practice and will be retained in this chapter.

A classification which accords well with clinical practice involves a hierarchical model in which certain symptoms are given greater significance and therefore take precedence over others. Thus the presence of definite cognitive impairment justifies the diagnosis of an organic disorder regardless of what other symptoms may be present. Next in the hierarchy comes schizophrenia, symptoms of which take diagnostic precedence over conditions lower in the hierarchy, namely affective disorders, neurotic (or non-psychotic) disorders and personality disorders. Thus if a patient has symptoms of schizophrenia and agoraphobia the diagnosis of schizophrenia is made. Other conditions such as alcoholism, drug dependence and eating disorders do not fit neatly into this model and have to be classified separately. These are shown in the information box (left).

CLASSIFICATION OF PSYCHIATRIC DISORDERS

Organic
Acute e.g. confusional state
Chronic e.g. dementia

Schizophrenia

Affective Disorders
Depression
Mania

Neurotic disorders
Anxiety disorders
  Generalised anxiety
  Phobias
  Panic attacks
Obsessive compulsive disorder
Hysteria
Hypochondriasis
Factitious disorders

Personality disorders

Others
  Alcoholism
  Drug dependence
  Eating disorders
    Anorexia nervosa
    Bulimia nervosa
    Obesity
  Psychosexual disorders

AETIOLOGICAL FACTORS

The causes of most psychiatric disorders are unknown yet there is considerable information concerning the range of factors which are regarded as important aetiologically. Causation is nearly always multifactorial and the aetiological factors should be regarded as having *predisposing*, *precipitating* or *maintaining effects*. The classification of these factors is shown in the information box (p. 932).

Genetic factors

There is a genetic contribution to several psychiatric disorders, including schizophrenia and depressive illness. The evidence is derived from various observations: a higher prevalence of the disorder among first degree relatives than in the general population; a higher

CLASSIFICATION OF AETIOLOGICAL FACTORS

Predisposing
Increase susceptibility to psychiatric disorder
Established in utero or in childhood
Operate throughout patient's lifetime (e.g. genetic factors, congenital defects, chronic physical illness, disturbed family background)

Precipitating
Trigger an episode of illness
Determine its time of onset (e.g. stressful life events, acute physical illness)

Maintaining
Delay recovery from illness (e.g. lack of social support, chronic physical illness)

concordance rate in monozygotic than in dizygotic twins, even if the monozygotic twins have been reared apart; a higher prevalence rate for children of mentally ill parents who are brought up by healthy adoptive parents. Some disorders are due to single gene transmission. These include Huntington's chorea (autosomal dominant) and some uncommon causes of mental retardation.

Family background
Many patients with psychiatric disorder report an unhappy childhood background and it seems likely that a traumatic upbringing predisposes to future mental illness. Important factors are loss of a parent in childhood, either due to death or separation, parental disharmony and physical, especially sexual, abuse. In later life the family environment can adversely influence the course of an illness if parents are emotionally over-involved and express critical or hostile attitudes towards the patient.

Physical illness
Chronic physical ill-health predisposes to psychiatric disorder. There is an especially well-established link between brain injury and subsequent schizophrenic and depressive illness. Physical illness of acute onset can give rise to psychiatric disorder due either to its effect on cerebral anatomy and physiology or to its emotional significance and implications for the patient's future well-being.

Stressful life events
A wide range of stressful life events can precipitate episodes of illness in vulnerable people. These events usually involve a sense of loss and include death of a close relative, marital breakdown, redundancy, retirement and major financial crisis.

Social network
Many psychiatrically ill patients are socially isolated. The lack of a network of people with whom they can interact socially often appears to be a contributory factor in their illness. Particularly important is the lack of a close, confiding relationship.

THE CLINICAL INTERVIEW

Wherever the interview is conducted, interviewers should introduce themselves to a newly referred patient and explain the purpose of the interview. Patients should be allowed to describe their problems in their own words but the doctor must be in charge and guide the course of the interview by appropriate prompting and interjections. If possible the doctor should ask to see a reliable informant who should be interviewed separately. There are several aims to be borne in mind during the interview and these are listed in the information boxes below and on page 933.

AIMS OF INTERVIEW

● Establish rapport with patient
● Elicit symptoms and history
● Examine mental state
● Facilitate cathartic effect by allowing patient to ventilate symptoms and associated problems

MENTAL STATE EXAMINATION

Several aspects of the patient's current mental state will have become apparent while the history is being recorded. However it is always necessary to proceed to ask about current symptoms. The sequence of questions should be flexible depending on which aspects of the mental state seem most important. These aspects are listed in the information box (p. 933).

General appearance and behaviour
Describe succinctly the patient's appearance, dress and general tidiness. Is there a normal relationship with the examiner or is there avoidance of eye contact or uncooperative behaviour? Note any abnormalities of alertness and motor behaviour. For example is there restlessness or retardation? Does the patient pace repeatedly up and down the interview room?

TOPICS COVERED DURING INTERVIEW

Reason for referral
Why the patient has been referred and by whom.

Presenting complaints
The patient should be asked to describe briefly the symptoms for which help is requested.

History of present illness
The patient should then be asked to describe the course of the illness from the time when symptoms were first noticed. The interviewer needs to ask direct questions to determine the nature, duration and severity of symptoms and factors associated with them.

Family history
Description of parents and siblings, the patient's relationship with them and a record of mental illness in relatives.

Personal history
Major landmarks in childhood, schooling, higher education, occupational history, sexual development, relationships, marriage, children, current social circumstances and forensic problems.

Previous medical and psychiatric history
An enquiry into previous health, accidents and operations; use of alcohol, tobacco and other drugs. Direct questions may be needed concerning previous psychiatric history since this may not be volunteered, for example 'have you ever been treated for depression or nerves?' or 'have you ever suffered a nervous breakdown?'

Previous personality
This refers to the characteristic patterns of behaviour and thinking which determine a person's adjustment to the environment — including attitudes, moral values, interests, quality of relationships with other people and reactions to stress. Personality attributes are usually developed by adolescence and are then stable throughout the person's life, and should be assessed independently of symptoms of psychiatric illness. However certain personality types predispose to illness; an individual's personality will also influence the nature of the symptoms if psychiatric illness develops and the emotional reaction if physical illness occurs. Several questionnaires are available for quantifying personality, the best known in Britain being the Eysenck Personality Questionnaire which measures extraversion, neuroticism and psychoticism as dimensions. For clinical purposes the most useful information can be obtained from a personality description given by one or more reliable informants who have known the patient well for many years.

ASPECTS OF MENTAL STATE TO BE EXAMINED

- General appearance and behaviour
- Speech
- Mood
- Thought content
- Abnormal beliefs
- Abnormal perceptions
- Cognitive function

Speech

Speed and fluency of speech should be noted. Is there retardation of speech or difficulty finding words? Does the patient speak excessively rapidly so that it appears speech is generated under pressure and it is difficult to interrupt the flow? Are there rapid changes in the topic of the conversation? Is it difficult to follow the patient's train of thought?

Mood

Does the patient appear anxious, depressed or elated? These can be judged by facial expression, mannerisms, posture and other motor movements. The patient's subjective mood should be elicited by asking for a description of current spirits. Some patients find it difficult to describe their mood in terms of anxiety or depression; questions which help elicit their mood include inquiries as to whether they have lost the ability to enjoy themselves or derive pleasure from life (anhedonia) or whether they have lost interest in themselves and those around them. People who are depressed should be asked about feelings of low self esteem, guilt and worthlessness. It is also important to determine how they see their future. They should be asked about suicidal ideation, for example 'do you ever feel that life is not worth living?'. Patients who reply positively need to be asked whether they have suicidal thoughts and active plans for putting an end to their lives.

Elated patients should be asked about feelings of grandiosity and general well being. Manic patients may be irritable with the examiner who does not share their view of themselves. However irritability is seen in other disorders of mood, not only mania.

Thought content

Patients should be asked about their main preoccupations and this is best done by simply asking them to describe what is on their mind at present or what are their main worries. It can then be elicited whether the preoccupations are appropriate to the circumstances or whether they are indicative of psychological disorder. Is there evidence of phobic symptoms? A phobia is defined as an abnormal fear of an object or situation, the fear being sufficiently intense as to lead to avoidance of the particular stimulus. Are there any obsessional symptoms? These are defined as thoughts, impulses or actions which enter the patient's mind repeatedly against his resistance but which nevertheless are recognised as his own thoughts. They are often associated with behavioural rituals such as repeated hand washing or checking.

Abnormal beliefs

It is necessary to establish whether the patient has any delusional beliefs. These are abnormal beliefs which are held with conviction and which cannot be argued away but which are out of keeping with the patient's social, cultural and educational background. They may be paranoid, grandiose or depressive in nature. Leading questions are often necessary to elicit delusional beliefs, for example, whether the patient believes anything unusual is going on or, if paranoid delusions are suspected, whether there are beliefs that people have malevolent intent. Primary delusions arise suddenly, often on the basis of a normal perception which is interpreted by the patient in a morbid manner. Thus the patient may see special significance in a particular arrangement of furniture in the room and conclude that there is a conspiracy organised by a secret political agency. Primary delusions of this type are characteristic of schizophrenia. Secondary delusions are those which occur due to some other psychological disorder such as a mood disturbance and they are commonly encountered in severe depression when they tend to involve gloomy themes of guilt, wickedness and punishment. When the mood is abnormally elated, as in mania, the delusions are typically grandiose.

Abnormal perceptions

The patient may report unusual sensory experiences but more often these have to be elicited by direct questions such as 'have you had any strange experiences recently?' or 'do you ever hear people talking about you even though there is no one near you at the time?'. The main abnormalities of perception are depersonalisation, illusions and hallucinations. Depersonalisation refers to an unpleasant subjective feeling in which the patient's body is perceived as if it is changed, lifeless or unreal. It is often accompanied by a sensation that the external world seems changed in that it appears grey, unreal or two dimensional; this phenomenon is known as derealisation.

Illusions are abnormal perceptions of normal external stimuli. They occur most commonly in the auditory and visual modalities. Sounds appear distorted, muffled or louder than usual. Objects may be seen as larger (macropsia) or smaller (micropsia) than normal, distorted in shape or more vividly coloured. Hallucinations are sensory perceptions which occur in the absence of external stimuli. They can also occur in any sensory modality. It is important to establish whether the patient perceives the sensation as emanating from within the mind or from the outside world. It is also important to establish the degree of insight into the experience. Hallucinations which arise from within the patient's mind and whose origins the patient recognises are known as pseudohallucinations. Auditory hallucinations are characteristic of schizophrenia and affective psychoses. Visual, olfactory, gustatory and tactile hallucinations usually indicate organic mental disorder.

Cognitive function

Intellectual abilities need to be assessed, particularly with regard to the possibility of mental handicap or dementia. They can be gauged from the history of the patient's educational background and attainments but can also be assessed during the interview from the patient's fluency, vocabulary and grasp of the interviewer's questions.

The level of consciousness should be noted. Does the patient remain alert throughout the interview or is there a tendency to drift off and lose the ability to concentrate on what is being asked? Concentration can be assessed more thoroughly by asking the patient to perform a simple repetitive task, such as subtracting 7 from 100 serially or repeating the months of the years backwards. Memory should be assessed under several headings. Recall of recent and distant events is determined by the patient's ability to describe details of personal history, dating back to childhood. It is also important to determine the ability to recall events occurring during the last few days and weeks. Registration is determined by presenting the patient with simple new information such as a name and address and then asking for this to be repeated immediately. The ability to consolidate and recall the information is checked by asking for the information to be repeated five minutes later, during which time the patient's attention should be diverted to other tasks. Memory is also assessed by checking on orientation. Does the patient know the exact location (orientation in place) and what day, date, month and year it is now (orientation in time)? Orientation in person refers to the patient's ability to describe details of personal identity, that is name, date of birth, marital state, address and other intimate details. Loss of personal orientation does not usually occur in organic brain disorders but is a feature of psychogenic amnesia. The patient should be asked to describe recent current affairs; this gives an indication of general intelligence and interest in external events.

It is useful to record patients' understanding of their problems, particularly whether they regard themselves as being ill or not. Finally doctors should note their own response to the patient. Did they feel sympathetic or warm towards the patient or were they made to feel irritable, frustrated or angry?

TREATMENTS USED IN PSYCHIATRY

Some of the treatment approaches in psychiatry are unfamiliar in other branches of medicine so they will be reviewed here before the clinical syndromes are discussed. The doctor is often the co-ordinating member of a multi-disciplinary team and needs to liaise closely with other professionals such as nurses, occupational therapists, social workers and psychologists, any one of whom may be responsible for a particular aspect of treatment.

PSYCHOLOGICAL

Psychotherapy

This is based on a continuing relationship between patient and doctor in which the patient confides his symptoms and the doctor uses his understanding of the patient in a therapeutic manner. There are two main types, supportive and interpretive. Supportive psychotherapy underlies all other treatments in psychiatry. Indeed it is a crucial element in treatment throughout clinical medicine, much more so than many doctors realise. It involves a process of empathic listening during which the doctor encourages patients to describe their symptoms, express their feelings and reflect on associated problems in their lives. A single interview conducted sympathetically often has a healthy cathartic effect, but usually the doctor has to see patients at regular intervals over a long period and to be prepared for them to become dependent. The doctor should give an explanation of symptoms, advice, practical guidance and reassurance when indicated. Supportive psychotherapy does not aim at any fundamental psychological change but when successful it fosters a therapeutic alliance and improves compliance with other forms of treatment. In patients with incurable and chronic conditions it forms a vital source of emotional support over many years.

Interpretive psychotherapy, in contrast, attempts a radical restructuring of the patient's psychological conflicts and behaviour. It is based on one of the several schools of psychoanalytic theory and should only be conducted by professionals with special training. At the basis of all types of interpretive psychotherapy lies the assumption that the presenting symptoms result from unacceptable memories or impulses which have been repressed so that they exist only in the patient's unconscious mind. Treatment aims at bringing these memories or impulses into patients' consciousness by allowing them to associate freely or to describe the content of dreams which the therapist can interpret, and help them understand and modify their behaviour as a result. An important element in treatment is an analysis of the transference, a term which refers to the patients' attitudes and feelings towards the doctor. The transference is thought to reflect the patients' feelings towards other people during their development, particularly their parents. Patients suitable for this type of treatment have to be highly motivated and are usually suffering from anxiety, depression or certain types of personality disorders especially when these conditions are associated with disturbed interpersonal relationships. Treatment is contraindicated for those who have psychotic symptoms, paranoid traits, alcohol or drug abuse or who act out in an antisocial manner. Interpretive psychotherapy is conducted during regular sessions of an hour's duration at least once a week and lasts for several months or even years. It can be conducted on an individual or group basis; its principles are also applied in marital and family therapy.

Behaviour therapy

Behaviour therapy is derived from the psychological principles of learning theory which state that many psychiatric disorders result from maladaptive patterns of learned behaviour. Treatment is aimed specifically at relief of symptoms. It is not thought necessary to modify or even understand aetiological factors from the patients' previous experiences. A behavioural analysis is essential before treatment is planned. This involves a detailed account of the symptoms, their severity, frequency and duration together with an assessment of factors which trigger and maintain them. Several types of behaviour therapy have been evolved:

Systematic desensitisation. This is used in the treatment of phobias and other anxiety-related disorders. Its key elements are listed in the information box below.

KEY ELEMENTS OF SYSTEMATIC DESENSITISATION

- Training the patient to relax
- Constucting a hierarchy of anxiety-provoking situations
- Introducing the patient, while fully relaxed, to anxiety provoking stimuli from the hierarchy, working from the least to the most distressing. This can be done in imagination or in real life.

Flooding. This is also used in the treatment of phobias. It involves introducing the patient to the most stressful stimulus from the start and keeping him in contact with it until his anxiety subsides to normal levels. It stems from observations that anxiety eventually diminishes if avoidance of the anxiety provoking stimulus is prevented. To allow this to occur each session should last at least one hour, sometimes considerably longer.

Response prevention. This is used to treat the compulsive rituals which are characteristic of obsessional neurosis. The patient is exposed to stimuli which induce compulsive behaviour (e.g. checking or hand washing) but is prevented from carrying out the rituals.

Modelling. In this a therapist demonstrates normal behaviour in the presence of the stimulus. It is a useful supplement to response prevention. It is also used as a basis for social skills training.

Operant conditioning. This uses a system of positive and negative reinforcements to alter particular aspects of behaviour. Positive reinforcements (or rewards) are given following desired behaviour while negative reinforcements (or punishments) are used following undesired behaviour. Operant conditioning forms the basis of token economy systems used to reduce behavioural problems in chronic schizophrenia and mental handicap.

Bell and pad training. This is used in the treatment of enuresis. A special pad is placed under the patient's bed sheet. It contains an electrical circuit which is completed when wetted by urine, thereby sounding an alarm bell which wakes the patient. Micturition is interrupted and the patient gets up to complete emptying his bladder. After repeated training the patient learns to respond to sensations of bladder distension and wakens before micturition occurs.

Cognitive therapy
This approach is based on the assumption that some psychiatric disorders are due to a negative pattern of thinking which is an enduring characteristic. In depression a negative triad has been described, the three components of which are:

1. devaluation of the self
2. negative view of current life experiences
3. negative view of the future.

Cognitive therapy aims at modifying patterns of thinking in a positive way; it is assumed that improvements in mood and behaviour will follow. The treatment has been used for depression, anxiety and eating disorders. The therapist has to identify the negative thoughts and help the patient see the connection between them and his mood or behaviour. The patient is encouraged to monitor the negative thoughts and to analyse them logically. The final step is to substitute positive patterns of thinking which are more in keeping with reality.

PHYSICAL TREATMENTS

Drugs
Drugs used to treat psychiatric disorders are known collectively as psychotropics. They are classified according to their main mode of action (Table 18.2).

Table 18.2   Classification of psychotropic drugs

Action	Main groups	Clinical use
Antipsychotic	Phenothiazines	Schizophrenia
	Butyrophenones	Mania
	Thioxanthenes	Acute confusion
	Benzamides	
Antidepressant	Tricyclics and related drugs	Depressive illness
		Obsessive compulsive disorder
	Tetracyclics	Depressive illness
	Monoamine oxidase inhibitors	Depressive illness
		Phobic disorders
Mood stabilising	Lithium	Prophylaxis of manic depression
		Acute mania
	Carbamazepine	Prophylaxis of manic depression
Anti-anxiety	Benzodiazepines	Anxiety disorders
		Insomnia
		Alcohol withdrawal
	Beta-adrenoceptor blockers	Anxiety (somatic symptoms)

Antipsychotics

The essential mechanism of these drugs, which are also known as neuroleptics, is their ability to block central dopamine receptors; this explains their antipsychotic effect. They are used to treat acute schizophrenia and mania and to prevent relapse in chronic schizophrenia. They are also useful in the management of disturbed behaviour due to acute confusional states. In low doses they are used to treat anxiety. The drugs have many unwanted side-effects so the indications for their use should be reviewed regularly. Weight gain due to increased appetite is common and may cause the patient to refuse further treatment. Side-effects related to dopamine blockade include parkinsonism, akathisia, acute dystonia, tardive dyskinesia, gynaecomastia and galactorrhoea. The drugs also possess anticholinergic properties which cause dry mouth, blurred vision, constipation, urinary retention and impotence. In the elderly postural hypotension and hypothermia can occur. Hypersensitivity reactions include cholestatic jaundice, blood dyscrasias and photosensitive dermatitis. Ocular complications which can occur in long-term treatment are opacities in the cornea and lens; retinitis pigmentosa has been described with thioridazine. Commonly used anti-psychotics are shown in Table 18.3.

Table 18.3   Antipsychotic drugs

Group	Drug	Usual dose
Phenothiazines	Chlorpromazine	100–1500 mg daily
	Thioridazine	50–800 mg daily
	Trifluoperazine	5–30 mg daily
	Fluphenazine	20–100 mg fortnightly
Butyrophenones	Haloperidol	5–30 mg daily
Thioxanthenes	Flupenthixol	40–200 mg fortnightly
Diphenylbutylpiperidines	Pimozide	4–30 mg daily
Benzamides	Sulpiride	600–1800 mg daily

Antidepressants

Commonly used antidepressants are shown Table 18.4.

Tricyclic antidepressants are the drugs of first choice in the treatment of depressive illness. They inhibit the re-uptake of amines (noradrenaline and 5-hydroxy-tryptamine) at synaptic clefts and this action has been used to support the hypothesis that affective disorders result from a deficiency of these amines which serve as neurotransmitters in the central nervous system. There is a delay of two to three weeks between the start of treatment and onset of therapeutic effect. Side-effects can be particularly troublesome during this period; they include anticholinergic effects, postural hypotension and cardio-toxicity. The recently introduced

Table 18.4   Antidepressant drugs

Group	Drug	Usual dose
Tricyclics	Amitriptyline	75–150 mg daily
	Imipramine	75–150 mg daily
	Dothiepin	75–150 mg daily
	Clomipramine	75–150 mg daily
5-HT reuptake inhibitors	Fluoxetine	20 mg daily
	Fluvoxamine	100–200 mg daily
Tetracyclics	Mianserin	30–90 mg daily
Monoamine oxidase inhibitors	Phenelzine	60–90 mg daily
	Tranylcypromine	20–40 mg daily

drugs, fluoxetine and fluvoxamine, are selective inhibitors of 5-hydroxytryptamine reuptake. They are less cardiotoxic and less sedative than tricyclics but can cause headache, nausea and anorexia.

The tetracyclic drug mianserin is an alpha 2 adrenoceptor antagonist but has no effect on amine uptake. It has fewer side-effects than the tricyclics but can cause intolerable sedation and rarely leucopaenia.

The monoamine oxidase inhibitors (MAOIs) increase the availability of neurotransmitters at synaptic clefts by inhibiting metabolism of noradrenaline and 5-HT. They are less effective than tricyclics for severe depressive illness but are equally effective for milder illness, particularly when depression is associated with anxiety and phobic symptoms. They also have a place in the management of primary phobic disorders. Monoamine oxidase inhibitors have acquired notoriety because of their interaction with various drugs such as amphetamines and opiates, and foods rich in tyramine such as cheese, pickled herrings, game and red wine. Amines accumulate in the systemic circulation causing a hypertensive crisis and fatalities have occurred from cerebral haemorrhage. These interactions have resulted in considerable anxiety about prescribing the drugs. However they are relatively safe if the offending foods are avoided and MAOIs are not used as often as they should. Patients taking MAOIs should be given a card listing all the substances to be avoided.

Mood stabilising drugs

Lithium carbonate is the main drug used in the prophylaxis of affective disorders and should be given to patients who have had two or more episodes of illness requiring drug therapy within two years. It is more effective in bipolar illness (mania and depression) than in unipolar illness. Lithium is also used for acute mania and in combination with a tricyclic or MAOI for resistant depression. It has a narrow therapeutic range so regular blood monitoring is required to maintain a serum level of 0.5–1.0 mmol/litre. This is usually achieved with a daily dose of 800–1200 mg. Toxic effects include nausea, vomiting, tremor and convulsions. With long-term treatment weight gain, hypothyroidism, nephrogenic diabetes insipidus and renal failure can occur. Thyroid and renal function should be checked before treatment is started and every six months thereafter. Lithium has a significant teratogenic effect and should never be prescribed during the first trimester of pregnancy.

Recently carbamazepine, an established anticonvulsant drug, has been used successfully as prophylaxis in manic depression for patients who have not responded to lithium. The dose is 400–1200 mg daily although it is usual to start with a lower dose and increase it gradually. Common side-effects are drowsiness, ataxia, headache, rashes, nausea and vomiting.

Anti-anxiety drugs
Examples of commonly used anti-anxiety drugs are shown in Table 18.5.

Table 18.5 Anti-anxiety drugs

Group	Drug	Usual dose
Benzodiazepines	Diazepam	2–30 mg daily
	Chlordiazepoxide	5–30 mg daily
	Nitrazepam	5–10 mg at night
	Temazepam	10–20 mg at night
Beta-adrenoceptor blockers	Propranolol	20–80 mg daily

Benzodiazepines have been widely used for the treatment of insomnia and anxiety-related disorders but they have been shown to cause dependence and withdrawal symptoms in many patients who have taken them for six weeks or more. These symptoms occur especially with short-acting benzodiazepines and if medication is stopped abruptly. They are listed in the information box below.

BENZODIAZEPINE WITHDRAWAL SYMPTOMS

- Anxiety
- Heightened sensory perception
- Hallucinations
- Epileptic fits
- Ataxia
- Paranoid delusions

In view of problems of dependence psychological methods of anxiety management should be considered first in the treatment of anxiety but if benzodiazepines are prescribed they should be given in short courses, no more than 3 weeks, to help with limited periods of stress, and the dose should be tailed off gradually thereafter. They have superseded chlormethiazole in the management of alcohol withdrawal.

Beta-adrenoceptor blockers such as propranolol have a limited role in the treatment of anxiety where somatic symptoms are prominent.

Electroconvulsive therapy (ECT)
Electroconvulsive therapy has been used in psychiatry for 50 years. It involves the administration of high voltage, brief, direct current impulses to the head while the patient is anaesthetised and paralysed by muscle relaxants. Electrodes can be placed bilaterally or unilaterally over the non-dominant hemisphere. The main use of ECT is for depressive illness but it is sometimes used in mania and acute schizophrenia. Indications are listed in the information box below.

INDICATIONS FOR ECT IN DEPRESSIVE ILLNESS

- Severe depression with paranoid or nihilistic delusions
- High suicidal risk where quick response is needed
- Failure to respond to a tricyclic and an alternative antidepressant
- Depressive stupor when food and fluid intake is inadequate
- Elderly or physically ill when tricyclic antidepressants may be unsafe
- Inability to tolerate side-effects of antidepressants

Up to 12 applications may be needed to produce optimal results. There has been a decline in its use following the introduction of psychotropic drugs but it remains the most effective treatment for severe depression with psychotic symptoms. ECT is safe and side-effects are few. Headache and a brief period of confusion often occur during the immediate post-ictal period. There may be amnesia for events occurring a few hours before (retrograde) and after (anterograde) ECT. Permanent anterograde amnesia has been claimed to occur but this has not been confirmed. If it does occur it is mild and infrequent.

Psychosurgery
This treatment has been rendered virtually obsolete by antidepressant drug therapy. It is now carried out for a small number of patients with severe, resistant depression and should only be undertaken at specialised centres. The operation consists of making discrete bilateral lesions to interrupt the frontolimbic pathways.

CLINICAL SYNDROMES

ORGANIC PSYCHIATRIC DISORDERS

This group of disorders results from pathological lesions within the brain or acting on the brain from a focus elsewhere in the body. According to their extent and rapidity of onset they can be classified as generalised or focal; acute or chronic.

ACUTE GENERALISED REACTIONS

These are usually referred to as acute confusional states; the term delirium is used to describe acute confusion associated with motor overactivity and behavioural disturbance. The characteristic features of acute confusional states are:

Impairment of consciousness. This sign, often overlooked, is fundamentally important. It covers a spectrum of impairment from a barely detectable dulling of alertness to deep coma. The patient appears drowsy and lethargic; the level of consciousness often fluctuates so that lucid periods alternate with drowsy spells. Consciousness is characteristically most impaired during the evening when there is decreased environmental stimulation. Clinical testing reveals impaired attention and concentration.

Memory disturbance. All aspects of memory-registration, retention and recall are affected. One of the earliest manifestations is disorientation in time and place, resulting from an inability to register the sequence of events and to learn new surroundings. Disorientation in place is particularly evident if the patient has recently been moved to unfamiliar surroundings, e.g. from home to hospital. Learning of other new information is impaired and there is faulty recall of past events, this being most marked for events in the previous few weeks.

Perceptual disturbance. In mild forms normal perceptions are distorted. Objects may be seen as larger (macropsia) or smaller (micropsia) than they are. They may be perceived as distorted in shape or be misinterpreted (illusions). Hallucinations are the most striking perceptual disturbance. Generalised organic reactions are characteristically associated with visual and tactile perceptual disturbances. Focal lesions in the temporal lobe can cause disturbances in taste and smell.

Thinking. There is subjective difficulty in thinking clearly. Speed of thought is slowed, mental fatigue soon occurs and the pattern of thinking becomes muddled. The patient has difficulty grasping the essential features of his environment so that events are misinterpreted and secondary delusional ideas develop, often of paranoid nature.

Psychomotor changes. Mental and motor activity is retarded. There is little spontaneity, speech is sparse and responses to questions are slow in forthcoming. However in some cases the reverse is true. The patient appears agitated and restless and there may be extensive hyperactivity to a dangerous degree. This clinical picture is termed delirium and is associated with toxic reactions to alcohol and other drugs.

Emotional changes. Anxiety, irritability and depression may accompany the other features. In severe cases the emotional response becomes apathetic.

Causes of acute confusional states
The aetiology has to be determined from the history, physical examination and special investigations. The main causes can be grouped and are listed in the information box (p. 940).

Management
The underlying cause must be determined; this usually involves admission to hospital where appropriate investigations are available. Once the cause is established specific treatment is given for the underlying lesion. Supportive measures are also necessary. The patient should be nursed in a well-lit room; frequent changes of nurses should be avoided so that rapport can be built up. Intravenous therapy may be required to correct fluid and electrolyte imbalance. Sedative drugs should not be given unless the patient's behaviour is disruptive; chlorpromazine (50–100 mg 3 times daily) or haloperidol (5–10 mg 3 times daily) are the drugs of choice except in delirium tremens when benzodiazepines (e.g. diazepam 10–20 mg 4 times daily) are preferred.

CAUSES OF ACUTE CONFUSIONAL STATES

Intra-cranial
Trauma
Vascular
  Transient ischaemic attack
  Cerebral haemorrhage
  Cerebral thrombosis
  Subarachnoid haemorrhage
  Subdural haemorrhage
Epilepsy
  Post-ictal state
Infection
  Encephalitis
  Cerebral abscess
  Meningitis
  AIDS
Tumour
  Primary or secondary lesion

Extra-cranial
Infections
  Exanthemata
  Septicaemia
  Pneumonia
  Urinary infection
Toxic
  Alcohol
  Many therapeutic drugs (e.g. anticholinergics, beta-blockers, L-Dopa, isoniazid)
Endocrine
  Hyperthyroidism
  Hypothyroidism
  Hypoglycaemia
  Addisonian crisis
  Hypopituitarism
Metabolic
  Uraemia
  Liver failure
  Remote effects of carcinoma
  Electrolyte imbalance
  Porphyria
Hypoxia
  Respiratory failure
  Cardiac failure
  Acute heart block
  Carbon monoxide poisoning

CHRONIC GENERALISED REACTIONS

These are collectively described under the term dementia which is defined as a clinical syndrome characterised by a loss of previously acquired intellectual function in the absence of impairment of consciousness. The dementias are predominantly associated with the elderly but in some disorders, notably Alzheimer's disease, Pick's disease and Huntington's chorea, the onset of symptoms occurs in middle life. These conditions, known collectively as pre-senile dementias, have a strong familial disposition, Huntington's chorea being transmitted by an autosomal dominant gene. The key features of dementia are:

Loss of general intelligence. There is impairment of abstract thinking, judgement and problem solving ability. Thinking is slow and inflexible and the ability to reason logically is reduced.

Memory impairment. Minor degrees of forgetfulness are often the first signs of dementia and are noticed initially by relatives. Events of the recent past cannot be recalled so patients forget where they have left personal possessions and where they have been. Gas taps, electric lights and switches may be left on. People's names are forgotten, especially those who are newly introduced, and appointments are missed. Patients cannot learn to find their way around in new situations. Consequently they readily lose their way and eventually this applies even in familiar surroundings. Declining memory may lead to secondary delusions. For example patients who forget where they have left important personal possessions may believe people are breaking into their homes and robbing them.

Personality change. There is a decline in personal manners and social awareness. Behaviour becomes rude, tactless and generally insensitive to the feelings of other people. Disinhibited behaviour may lead to episodes of aggression, sexual indiscretions or infringements of the law such as theft. These personality changes are often described as 'coarsening' in that they reflect exaggerations of the less desirable aspects of the patient's character which have previously been kept under restraint. Eventually there is a deterioration in personal appearance and hygiene. Urinary and faecal incontinence are common but appear to cause the patient little embarrassment. There is also a loss of volition and a general decline in interest. Patients may sit for hours without initiating any form of purposeful activity.

Emotional changes. Mood changes may be prominent during the early stages and cause some difficulty in differentiating dementia from affective disorders. Depression, anxiety or irritability may dominate the clinical picture. They appear to depend on some degree of insight into failing intellectual powers. Rapid changes of mood, emotional lability, are also common. In advanced dementia the emotional reaction becomes blunted and patients appear incapable of responding to emotionally charged events in their environment.

Causes of dementia
These are shown in the information box (p. 941).

CAUSES OF DEMENTIA

Degenerative
Senile dementia
Alzheimer's disease
Pick's disease
Huntington's chorea
Creutzfeldt-Jakob disease
Parkinson's disease

Vascular
Cerebrovascular disease
Cerebral emboli

Normal pressure Hydrocephalus
Primary
Secondary to head injury, subarachnoid haemorrhage
or meningitis

Trauma
Post-traumatic dementia; boxer's encephalopathy

Space-occupying lesions
Cerebral tumour
Subdural haematoma

Infections
AIDS
Cerebral syphilis
Viral encephalitis

Endocrine
Hypothyroidism
Hypoglycaemia
Hypopituitarism

Metabolic
Liver failure
Renal failure
Remote effects of carcinoma

Toxic
Alcohol
Chronic barbiturate ingestion
Heavy metals

Anoxia
Cardiac failure
Heart block
Cardiac arrest
Respiratory failure
Carbon monoxide poisoning

Vitamin deficiency
B_{12}, folic acid

Assessment and management

Diagnostic assessment is directed at confirming the diagnosis of dementia, determining its severity by assessing the degree of disability and establishing the underlying cause. The history should be provided by a reliable informant who has known the patient for many years. Careful enquiry should be made concerning any

family history of pre-senile dementia. Physical examination should be undertaken especially with the reversible cause of dementia in mind and particular attention needs to be given to detecting focal neurological signs. Several laboratory and radiological investigations (Figs 18.1 & 18.2) are required and are listed in the information box below. Newer techniques can diagnose more subtle abnormalities (Fig. 18.3).

INVESTIGATIONS FOR DEMENTIA

- Full blood count
- Urea and electrolytes
- Liver function tests
- Thyroid function tests
- Syphilitic serology
- HIV antibodies
- Chest X-ray
- CT brain scan

Detailed assessment of intelligence should be carried out by a clinical psychologist. There are several available tests, the most widely used being the Wechsler Adult Intelligence Scale (WAIS). This provides an intelligence quotient (IQ) which expresses an individual's test score as a percentage of the mean scores obtained by samples of the population on whom the tests were standardised. The WAIS comprises 11 subtests, 6 of which are concerned with words or numbers and whose scores are combined to give a verbal IQ; 5 other subtests are concerned with spatial

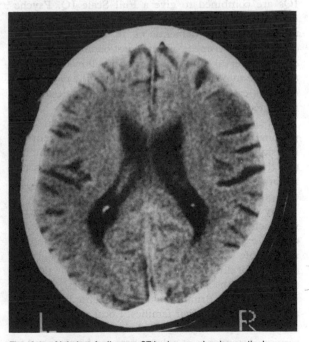

Fig. 18.1 Alzheimer's disease: CT brain scan showing cortical atrophy, widened sulci and enlarged lateral ventricles.

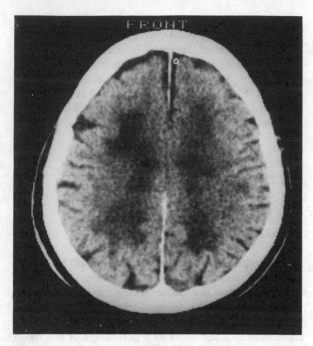

Fig. 18.2 Cerebrovascular dementia: CT brain scan showing multiple, diffuse areas of cerebral infarction.

ability, such as recognising patterns, and are combined to give a Performance IQ. The Verbal and Performance IQs are combined to give a Full Scale IQ. Psychometric testing has several functions; it is useful when the diagnosis of dementia is in doubt, it gives a quantified assessment of deterioration and repeat tests after an interval of at least six months allow the rapidity of change to be determined. Other specific psychological tests can be employed when localised lesions are suspected.

A behavioural assessment, conducted by an occupational therapist, indicates whether the patient has lost skills such as cooking, dressing, spatial orientation and the ability to handle money. These are important factors when considering whether independent living is still possible.

Any reversible cause should be treated appropriately in which case a varying degree of functional recovery can be expected. In the majority of cases, where no remediable condition can be found, management should be directed at providing the best possible support for the patients and their families. Approximately half of Britain's elderly demented are maintained at home by their families. Local authority social services can provide domestic help and a meals delivery service. Attendance at a day centre can be arranged for patients whose relatives cannot cope with full-time

supervision. For the more severely demented and for those without family support admission to residential homes for the elderly is necessary while for those with heavy nursing requirements hospital admission becomes inevitable.

Drugs should be avoided unless there are specific indications. Demented patients are highly sensitive to sedative drugs; if medication is needed to treat episodes of confusion or excitement a small dose of a phenothiazine can be given, for example thioridazine 25 mg 3 times daily.

FOCAL ORGANIC DISORDERS

These arise from discrete cerebral lesions which affect specific cerebral functions although in practice it is common for there to be some evidence of damage elsewhere in the brain.

In psychiatry the most significant disorder is the amnesic syndrome caused by thiamine deficiency. When this has an abrupt onset the patient becomes acutely confused; mental state examination reveals drowsiness, disorientation in time and place and an impaired ability to recall recent events or to register new information. Physical examination reveals a horizontal nystagmus, evidence of external ocular palsies, ataxia and peripheral neuropathy. This syndrome, known as Wernicke's encephalopathy, results from damage to the mammillary bodies, dorso-medial nuclei of the thalamus and adjacent areas of grey matter. In those who die in the acute stage microscopic examination of the brain shows hyperaemia, petechial haemorrhages and astrocytic proliferation. Wernicke's encephalopathy in Western countries is nearly always due to poor nutrition associated with chronic alcoholism; other causes are prolonged vomiting, diarrhoea and severe starvation.

Immediate treament with thiamine 50 mg intravenously is essential to minimise permanent damage. Fluid replacement may also be required and intramuscular thiamine should be given daily until an adequate diet can be resumed. It is usual to give this with other vitamins in the form of Parentrovite which is available as paired ampoules for injection, either as intravenous high potency, intramuscular high potency or intramuscular maintenance. One of the ampoules contains thiamine, riboflavin and pyridoxine and the other nicotinamide and ascorbic acid. Two to four pairs of high potency intravenous ampoules are given 4–8 hourly for 2 days followed by high potency intramuscular injections daily for 5–7 days.

When recovery is incomplete a chronic amnesic syndrome develops, this being known as Korsakoff's psychosis. Characteristically the patient is fully conscious but has a profound impairment of memory recall and new learning ability. A striking feature is a tendency to confabulate which has been defined as a falsification of memory in clear consciousness. For example if the patient is asked to describe his activities during the previous week he will reply by reporting events which have taken place many years previously. Confabulation probably results from an inability to distinguish the temporal sequence of past events. Other cognitive functions remain intact in the Korsakoff syndrome but the memory disturbance is often so profound that the patient is incapable of living independently and institutional care is required.

Amnesia also occurs in bilateral lesions of the hippocampus and hippocampal gyrus which are situated on the inferomedial aspect of the temporal lobe. The conditions chiefly responsible are herpes simplex encephalitis and cerebrovascular disease localised to the posterior cerebral arteries. The clinical picture is similar to that of Korsakoff's psychosis except that confabulation does not occur.

Other deficits associated with focal brain lesions include expressive and receptive aphasias, apraxias and agnosias. These are described in detail in the chapter on neurology.

SCHIZOPHRENIA

In terms of its disabilities and chronicity schizophrenia is the most serious of all psychiatric illnesses. It affects 1% of the adult population at some time in their lives and, when uniform diagnostic criteria are used, the prevalence is similar throughout the world. Descriptions of schizophrenia in medical literature are sparse until the nineteenth century. Then the German psychiatrist Emil Kraepelin, distinguished two major groups of insanity, manic depression which nearly always had a favourable outcome and dementia praecox which usually ran a chronic course. The term schizophrenia replaced dementia praecox after its introduction by Eugen Bleuler in 1911.

Aetiology

Genetic factors
There is no doubt that schizophrenia can be transmitted genetically. Relatives of a schizophrenic have a risk of developing schizophrenia much higher than the general population risk of 1% and this increases with the degree of genetic proximity. Siblings of a schizophrenic have an 8% risk of developing the illness,

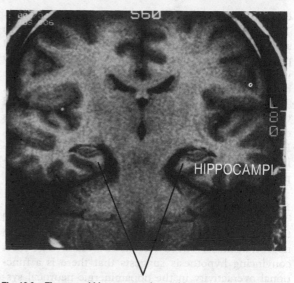

Fig. 18.3 The normal hippocampus imaged by a new magnetic resonance technique which reveals damage in the region with severe amnesia. (Reprinted by permission from *Nature* Vol 341, No 6237, cover photo. Copyright © Macmillan Magazines Ltd.)

children have a 12% chance but when both parents are affected this increases to 35% or more. Twin studies have provided further support. The risk for dizygotic twins is approximately the same as for non-twin siblings whereas for monozygotic twins it is of the order of 45–60%. This high risk for identical twins prevails even if the twins have been reared apart. Similarly adoption studies have shown that the increased risk for children of a schizophrenic parent continues in those cases where the children have been adopted at birth and brought up by healthy parents.

Psychological factors
No convincing evidence has been found to support the various hypotheses that abnormal family relationships have a causal influence on schizophrenia. However it is established that the family environment can influence the course of the illness. An atmosphere in which there are high levels of emotional expression appears harmful to schizophrenics and contributes to relapses of the illness. It is therefore advisable for patients to avoid returning to a family who are critical or who are emotionally over-involved and they do better in an emotionally neutral atmosphere which can be provided in a hostel or group home.

Psychological stress plays a part in precipitating episodes of the illness. It has been shown that schizophrenics are likely to have been exposed to a variety of adverse life events in the three weeks leading up to the onset of acute symptoms.

Cerebral disease

The introduction of the computed tomography (CT) scan has shown that up to one-third of chronically ill patients have evidence of brain damage, particularly ventricular enlargement. This brain damage may have been sustained at birth or acquired in early childhood. The schizophrenia syndrome can also be associated with a wide range of cerebral pathology which becomes evident in adult life including temporal lobe epilepsy, Huntington's chorea, cerebral tumour and demyelinating diseases. This is known as symptomatic schizophrenia.

Neurotransmitter disturbance

The final pathway by which the various aetiological factors cause schizophrenia may be by interfering with neurotransmitter substances in the brain. The most convincing hypothesis suggests that there is a functional overactivity in the dopaminergic neuronal systems in the mesolimbic and mesocortical areas. Drugs which stimulate central dopamine receptors, such as amphetamines and L-DOPA, are known to induce symptoms identical to those seen in paranoid schizophrenia. On the other hand drugs which are effective in the treatment of schizophrenia are known to block dopamine receptors. There is also evidence from postmortem studies that the brains of schizophrenics have an increased number of dopamine receptors.

Clinical features

The term schizophrenia describes a clinical syndrome based on abnormalities reported in the patient's history and observed during mental state examination. The concept of schizophrenia varies slightly from one country to another and some psychiatrists attach particular diagnostic importance to the chronic duration of symptoms and onset before the age of 45. However there is less debate about the characteristic mental state abnormalities. These appear to result from a breakdown in the normal ability to distinguish between experiences arising from the inner self and those coming from the outside world. This phenomenon is aptly described as a dissolution of ego boundaries. The most striking features are the *first rank symptoms* delineated by Kurt Schneider. He believed that a diagnosis of schizophrenia should be made if one or more of these symptoms is present and if the patient is not suffering from structural brain disease or a confusional state. The symptoms of first-rank importance are given in the information box (right).

In the *acute stages* of schizophrenia approximately *two-thirds* of patients have at least one first-rank symptom. The patient may have other symptoms

---

FIRST-RANK SYMPTOMS OF SCHIZOPHRENIA

Thought insertion
The experience of having thoughts put into one's mind by another person, or of thinking someone else's thoughts.

Thought broadcasting
The sensation that one's thoughts are known to other people, sometimes described as a feeling that thoughts are being transmitted by telepathy or radio waves.

Passivity feelings
Emotions, bodily movements or specific sensations which are perceived as being caused and controlled by an external object or another person.

Auditory hallucinations
Voices discussing the patient in the third person.

Auditory hallucinations
One or more voices keeping up a running commentary on the patient's thoughts or actions.

Auditory hallucinations
The experience of hearing one's own thoughts being spoken out loud, this is also known as 'thought echoing'.

Delusional perceptions
A primary delusion which arises from a normal perception which is given delusional significance: e.g. a man who saw a woman lighting a cigarette immediately realised this meant he was to be the next king of England.

---

which are of lower diagnostic significance but which in combination give rise to the diagnosis. These other symptoms are listed in the information box below.

OTHER SYMPTOMS OF SCHIZOPHRENIA

Catatonia
Motor abnormalities of two extreme types, excitable overactivity on the one hand and bizarre posturing with abnormal muscle tone (waxy flexibility) on the other

Thought disorder
A loosening of association between concepts so that thinking lacks a logical flow and appears incoherent to other people

Neologisms
Newly made-up words

Delusions
Of a grandiose, paranoid, sexual or religious nature

Hallucinations
Visual, tactile, olfactory or gustatory

Affective change
The patient may appear bewildered or perplexed by his various strange experiences. There may also be incongruity of affect in which the patient laughs without appropriate stimulus or in response to events which would not be expected to elicit a jocular reaction.

The features described in the information boxes (p. 944) are known as the *positive symptoms* of schizophrenia and some of them are usually present during the acute illness. If there are recurrent episodes, or if recovery is incomplete, the clinical picture can change so that it becomes dominated by *negative symptoms*. These symptoms are listed in the information box below.

NEGATIVE SYMPTOMS

Social withdrawal
The patient avoids interacting with other people, appears unable to motivate himself to work and cannot cope with daily living activities. He loses interest in himself and other people. His manner is generally apathetic.

Poverty of speech
Speech is sparse, conversation is not initiated and answers to questions are monosyllabic or empty. The poverty of speech reflects the poverty of thinking.

Flatness of affect
The patient's mood has a dull, monotonous quality. There is a loss of the normal day-to-day variation in mood and there is little or no response to emotionally charged external events.

Course and prognosis

The four patterns of outcome which have been distinguished are listed in the information box below.

OUTCOME

- 20%   make a full recovery from the acute illness and have no relapses
- 35%   recover completely but have repeated relapses with full recovery each time
- 35%   have recurrent acute episodes with incomplete recovery each time. They are left with negative symptoms which become more disabling after each relapse
- 10%   have a rapid downhill course from the outset and have persistent positive and negative symptoms

---

Several factors have been identified which influence the prognosis and these are listed in the information box (right).

Management

Hospital admission is necessary for a first episode of acute schizophrenia to permit a full physical and psychiatric assessment and to allow medication to be increased quickly to suppress symptoms.

PROGNOSTIC FACTORS IN SCHIZOPHRENIA

Good Prognosis
Acute onset of symptoms
Obvious precipitating factor
Prominent affective symptoms
Catatonic symptoms
No family history of schizophrenia
Normal personality
Stable work record
Calm family environment

Poor prognosis
Insidious onset of symptoms
No precipitating factor
No affective symptoms
No catatonic symptoms
Family history of schizophrenia
Schizoid personality
Poor work record
Highly emotional family environment

Neuroleptic drugs (Table 18.3 p. 937)
These are the mainstay of treatment and the choice is often governed by individual preference. However there are significant differences between the drugs. Thioridazine has fewer extrapyramidal side-effects, chlorpromazine can be given intramuscularly as well as orally while trifluoperazine is less sedative than the other two. Haloperidol has fewer cardiotoxic effects. A conventional regime would be to start with chlorpromazine 100 mg 3 times daily building up gradually to a maximum of 1500 mg daily or until symptoms are abolished. Higher doses are required initially if the patient is aggressive or agitated, for example chlorpromazine 200 mg intramuscularly 3 or 4 times daily. In patients who do not respond well to one drug, improvement can occur after switching to an equivalent dose of another preparation. When symptoms have improved it is usual to reduce the dose or to change to one of the long-acting intramuscular neuroleptics which need only be given once every two weeks (e.g. fluphenazine 20–100 mg fortnightly or flupenthixol 40–200 mg fortnightly). Depot injections improve compliance with treatment as many patients forget or cannot be bothered to take oral drugs every day once they are better. Dosage should be kept as low as possible to avoid recurrent psychotic symptoms. Parkinsonism is a troublesome side-effect and many patients require anti-Parkinsonian drugs as well. (e.g. procyclidine 5 mg 3 times daily). Other extra-pyramidal side-effects include akathisia (an unpleasant, irresistible sensation of motor restlessness), dystonias (acute muscular spasms) and tardive dyskinesia (persis-

tent movements predominantly affecting the tongue and other facial muscles).

The duration of drug treatment is controversial. When the features of the illness and the patient's premorbid adjustment suggest a favourable prognosis it is usual to tail off medication gradually after 12 months and to stop it completely unless there are signs of relapse. When the prognosis is poor most psychiatrists continue maintenance medication indefinitely.

Social measures

These become increasingly important as the patient recovers. Schizophrenics do best in an environment which has a regular, predictable routine. Positive symptoms are exacerbated in highly-charged emotional situations while negative symptoms are induced in environments which are understimulating, such as was often the case in mental hospital wards for the chronically ill. Considerable efforts are now made to discharge the patient from hospital after a brief admission lasting only a few weeks. If the home environment is not suitable accommodation can be provided in a hostel or group home. Alternatively if these facilities are unavailable family therapy conducted along behavioural lines can be arranged to help modify the family's behaviour towards the patient. The specific aims are to reduce the level of emotional expression and face-to-face contact thereby creating a more neutral atmosphere which is less harmful to the patient.

Those who are unable to return to their previous employment can regain occupational skills at special rehabilitation centres. Preparation for this facility can be made by regular occupational therapy during the hospital admission.

AFFECTIVE DISORDERS

The fundamental abnormality of an affective disorder is a disturbance of mood, either depression or mania. Depression is by far the commoner; most patients who have manic symptoms are also prone to depressive episodes but the reverse does not apply. In a few cases depressive and manic symptoms occur simultaneously or in rapid succession (mixed affective state).

There are many ways of classifying affective illnesses, none of which is entirely satisfactory. The simplest classification divides them into *primary* and *secondary* disorders.

Primary affective disorders. These are not secondary to any other psychiatric or physical illness but may be precipitated by a wide range of environmental factors. They are often recurrent; if recurrences always take a depressive form the term *unipolar* disorder is used; if the recurrences are both manic and depressive the term *bipolar* is used.

Secondary affective disorders. These follow another psychiatric (alcoholism, schizophrenia) or physical illness. In the latter case the mood change is usually due to the emotional impact of the illness but in some patients it is due to anatomical or physiological changes in the brain and may be the presenting feature of the underlying physical illness. These are described as organic or symptomatic affective disorders.

Epidemiology

Community studies have shown that the prevalence rate for depression, defined by strict operational criteria, is approximately 6–8% for women and 3–5% for men. Depression is commoner in the lower social classes and among inner city dwellers. Women in their child-bearing years are especially vulnerable.

Bipolar disorder is less common, having a prevalence rate of 1%. There is no difference in prevalence between the sexes nor between social classes.

Aetiological factors

Genetics. There is convincing evidence from adoption and twin studies of a genetic contribution to bipolar disorders although the mode of inheritance is not clear. The genetic basis of unipolar depression has not been established with such certainty.

Environment. Many environmental factors have been implicated but the three most consistently involved are loss of a parent in childhood, lack of social support and recent adverse life events. For women a profile of vulnerability factors has been defined and is given in the information box below.

VULNERABILITY FACTORS FOR AFFECTIVE DISORDERS

- Loss of mother before age of 11
- Three or more children under 14 living at home
- Lack of confiding relationship
- Lack of full-time or part-time employment

These factors do not in themselves cause depression but increase the likelihood that depression will follow major life events involving a loss of some kind.

Physical illness. All physical illnesses can be followed by depression, especially those like cancer and heart disease which carry serious implications. There is considerable interest in the role of viral illnesses in causing depression. Prolonged mood change can follow glandular fever or influenza. Some doctors believe a chronic fatigue syndrome (myalgic encephalomyelitis–ME) can be caused by Coxsackie or other viral infections.

Depression, or less often mania can be the presenting feature of endocrine diseases such as Cushing's syndrome, Addison's disease and hypothyroidism. Mood change can also be associated with drug therapy, for example corticosteroids, beta-adrenoceptor blockers and other anti-hypertensive drugs (e.g. alphamethyl dopa).

Personality. Some depressives have personality characteristics which are thought to predispose to the illness. These involve a negative attitude to oneself, the outside world and the future; the term cognitive triad has been applied to these attitudes. The personality most typically associated with bipolar illness is a cyclothymic one.

Clinical features of depression

The most fundamental symptom, although not always the most prominent, is *depression of mood*. This varies considerably in severity from one patient to another and even within the individual from time to time. There is no clear separation between the mood change of a clinically depressed patient and everyday unhappiness. Mood varies on a continuum and the diagnosis of depressive illness is made depending on the presence of associated features. There may be a diurnal variation of mood, depression being most distressing early in the morning or at the end of the day. Accompanying psychological symptoms are loss of pleasure in life (anhedonia), loss of interest in oneself and others, low self-esteem, self-blame and hopelessness. Suicidal thinking is common. In mild depression this consists of a passive wish to be dead but in more severe cases there are active thoughts of suicide and the patient may have made detailed plans as to how he will end his life. Severe depression may also be accompanied by feelings of guilt and worthlessness which are delusional in nature.

Somatic symptoms may dominate the clinical picture and are the symptoms with which depressed patients usually present to a general practitioner or physician. These symptoms are listed in the information box (right).

The diagnosis of a depressive illness is based on the presence of mood disturbance together with some of the associated features. The criteria in the information box below are those currently proposed by the American Psychiatric Association for the diagnosis of a major depressive episode.

At least five of the symptoms listed in the information box below, including at least one of the first two, must be present nearly every day over a two-week period. To justify the diagnosis of a major depressive episode it is also necessary to establish that the symptoms are not associated with a bereavement reaction, organic lesion or other psychotic disorder. The terms minor depressive episode or dysthymic disorder are applied to depressive symptoms which are not sufficiently severe to warrant the diagnosis of major depression.

Management

Outpatient management is appropriate in most cases. Admission is necessary when there is a strong risk of suicide or when social supports are inadequate. Compulsory admission under the Mental Health Act is required for suicidal patients who do not accept voluntary treatment.

Antidepressant drugs (see Table 18.4 p. 937). These relieve depressive symptoms in approximately

---

SOMATIC SYMPTOMS OF DEPRESSION

- Sleep disturbance (initial insomnia, early morning wakening or hypersomnia)
- Fatigue
- Headache
- Other pains (e.g. chest pain, abdominal pain)
- Anorexia
- Weight change
- Constipation
- Reduced libido
- Poor concentration
- Psychomotor retardation

DIAGNOSTIC CRITERIA FOR DEPRESSION

- Depressed mood most of the day
- Markedly diminished interest in almost all activities most of the day
- Significant weight loss or weight gain (at least 5% in one month)
- Insomnia or hypersomnia
- Fatigue or loss of energy
- Feelings of worthlessness or excessive guilt
- Diminished ability to think or concentrate, or indecisiveness
- Recurrent thoughts of death or suicide; a suicide attempt or a specific plan for suicide.

two-thirds of patients. A tricyclic drug is the first choice of treatment. It needs to be given in adequate doses for at least 6 weeks (e.g. amitriptyline 75–150 mg at night) and then, if symptoms have responded it should be continued at a lower dose for at least 6 months to prevent relapse. Patients should be advised that there may be a delay of 2 to 3 weeks between starting treatment and therapeutic improvement. If response to a tricyclic is poor one of the other drugs such as a monoamine oxidase inhibitor, MAOI, (e.g. phenelzine 15 mg 4 times daily) or mianserin (30–90 mg at night) should be tried. Some psychiatrists use an MAOI as a first choice drug when depression is accompanied by prominent anxiety or phobic symptoms or if there is hypersomnia or hyperphagia.

Cognitive therapy (see p. 936). This has been used successfully in combination with antidepressants and is indicated especially for patients whose depression seems to be perpetuated by a negative pattern of thinking.

Electroconvulsive therapy (ECT). This is indicated when the risk of suicide is so great that one cannot wait for the delayed therapeutic effect of antidepressant drugs. ECT should also be given to patients in depressive stupor, when there are psychotic symptoms or when medication has been ineffective. In approximately 10% of cases depression does not respond to drugs used singly or to ECT. These patients should be treated with *combined antidepressants*, the most popular combination being lithium and a tricyclic or MAOI.

Clinical features of mania
The psychological features of mania are the exact opposite of those of depression. There is a sense of wellbeing which may be evident as elation or even ecstasy. Confidence and self-esteem are high; patients may have grandiose ideas which have little substance but upon which they may act. Thus they may embark on ruinous business ventures or put themselves at risk through reckless behaviour. The grandiose beliefs may involve delusional ideas of being especially gifted or connected to well-known people such as royalty or entertainers. They feel highly energetic, thoughts come rapidly and speech is so fast that it appears to be generated under pressure. Thoughts jump from one topic to another with only chance connections between them (flight of ideas). There may be rhyming speech.

Motor activity is increased. Appetite is enhanced at first although in established mania the patient has no time to eat so weight falls and physical health suffers. The hours of sleep are reduced; typically patients wake after a few hours feeling full of energy and wanting to get on with work or leisure activities. Sexual promiscuity may occur with consequent risk of exposure to venereal disease.

Management
Neuroleptic drugs, either haloperidol (10–30 mg daily) or a phenothiazine (chlorpromazine 100–1500 mg daily) suppress the features of mania in nearly all cases. ECT is useful when symptoms are resistant to medication.

Lithium carbonate is indicated as prophylactic treatment for patients who have had two or more episodes of affective illness, either depression or mania, requiring medical treatment within the previous two years. Before starting lithium patients should be screened for thyroid (serum thyroxine, TSH and thyroid antibodies) and renal (plasma urea and creatinine) disease. Serum lithium should be kept within the therapeutic range of 0.5–1.0 mmol/litre. This is usually achieved with a daily dose of lithium carbonate of 800–1200 mg. Lithium levels should be measured every 3 or 4 months and thyroid and renal function should be assessed 6-monthly.

It is not known how long lithium should be continued but, given that recurrent affective illnesses are largely constitutional, there is much to be said for continuing lithium indefinitely if relapses are prevented or attenuated. Recently carbamazepine (400–1200 mg daily) has been used as an alternative prophylaxis for patients who do not respond to lithium.

NEUROTIC DISORDERS

ANXIETY DISORDERS

GENERALISED ANXIETY

Anxiety is a universal experience which has an important protective function in the face of danger. It becomes morbid when symptoms are out of proportion to external circumstances or if they persist long after a threatening situation has been averted. However there is no clear distinction between the features of normal and pathological anxiety. Symptoms of anxiety are prominent in other psychiatric disorders, such as depressive illness and schizophrenia, so it is important to look for features of these conditions before making a diagnosis of anxiety disorder. Several physical illnesses

PHYSICAL ILLNESSES WHICH MIMIC ANXIETY DISORDER

- Hyperthyroidism
- Phaeochromocytoma
- Hypoglycaemia
- Paroxysmal atrial arrhythmias
- Alcohol withdrawal
- Temporal lobe epilepsy

can present with anxiety and are listed in the information box above.

These need to be considered in the differential diagnosis but special investigations are necessary only when there are suggestive features in the history or clinical examination.

If operational criteria are used generalised anxiety disorder has a prevalence of between 2.0 and 5.0%, with women being more susceptible than men.

Aetiological factors

Genetic studies indicate there is a small genetic contribution. Many patients appear to have personality traits of high anxiety and poor tolerance of stress but perhaps the most important factors are unexpected life events which the patient cannot handle. Sometimes these are relatively minor events, within the range of everyday experience. A particular pattern of anxiety, known as post-traumatic stress disorder, follows the major traumatic events involved in sudden, unexpected disasters such as floods, accidents and terrorist activity.

Clinical features

These are conveniently divided into two groups, psychological and somatic and are shown in the information box below.

SYMPTOMS OF ANXIETY DISORDER

Psychological	Somatic
Apprehension	Tremor
Fears of impending disaster	Sweating
	Palpitations
Irritability	Chest pain
Depersonalisation	Breathlessness
	Headache
	Dizziness
	Diarrhoea
	Frequency of micturition
	Initial insomnia
	Poor concentration

Any of these can form the main presenting symptom; if somatic symptoms predominate the patient is likely to regard himself as physically ill, a view which is often shared initially by his doctor.

The post-traumatic stress syndrome is characterised

by recurrent bouts of severe anxiety accompanied by vivid reminiscences (or 'flashbacks') of the initial trauma which has usually been exceptionally catastrophic. In addition to the episodes of anxiety the patient manifests emotional blunting, withdrawal and avoidance of any situation similar to that in which the original trauma occurred.

PHOBIC DISORDERS

A phobia is an abnormal fear which is brought on by a particular object or situation and which leads to avoidance of the provoking stimulus. Community surveys of phobic disorders have shown a prevalence of 6–8% but only a small proportion of these are sufficiently distressing to need treatment. Phobias have been classified as shown in the information box below.

CLASSIFICATION OF PHOBIAS

Agoraphobia
A fear of open spaces and meeting places

Social phobia
A fear of social gatherings, eating in public etc.

Specific animal phobias
A fear of mice, cats, spiders, snakes etc.

Miscellaneous specific phobias
A fear of heights, thunder, flying etc.

Aetiology

Few clear aetiological factors have been identified. Most phobias are commoner in women and a genetic contribution is probably important. Psychologists have explained phobias in terms of learning theory as being due to conditioning following exposure to a traumatic event in childhood. However it is unusual to uncover specific traumas when taking a history from a phobic patient.

Clinical features

These vary according to the type of phobia but the key elements are the psychological and somatic symptoms of anxiety together with avoidance. Agoraphobia is the most disabling because of the extensive range of provoking situations. Agoraphobic symptoms can be brought on in open spaces, crowded shopping centres, supermarkets, cinemas, churches and public transport. Symptoms become progressively more severe when the patient ventures further away from home, particularly when unaccompanied. Thus there is an increasing restriction in life-style so that in extreme cases the patient is virtually house-bound. Social phobias are triggered by situations which involve personal interaction in public, such as eating or speaking in front of others. This type of phobia is particularly disruptive to social life and to the careers of people whose work involves public engagements. Animal and other specific phobias are less disruptive. The patient is often able to modify his behaviour without much difficulty so that daily activities are hardly affected. However some specific phobias, such as of flying, may be sufficiently handicapping to require treatment.

PANIC DISORDER

This consists of recurrent attacks of severe anxiety which are sudden and unpredictable. Although they are not related to particular situations they may lead to secondary agoraphobic symptoms. Panic disorder has a prevalence of less than 1%. Little is known about its aetiology; some psychiatrists regard it as a variant of depressive illness.

Clinical features

The key feature is a sudden attack of intense anxiety. Physical symptoms are prominent, especially palpitations, chest pain and breathlessness, and the patient often fears he is about to die. The attack lasts from a few minutes to as long as two hours. In-between attacks the patient is free of anxiety although secondary avoidance behaviour may be prominent.

Management of the anxiety disorders

Explanation and reassurance are essential in the management of all forms of anxiety. The nature of the symptoms should be explained and the patients reassured that they form part of a recognised illness. Reassurance is also needed to allay fears of physical illness if this can be done after appropriate examination and investigation. Specific relaxation techniques should be taught to those who do not respond to reassurance and are always required for patients with panic attacks. For phobic disorders relaxation should be accompanied by graded exposure (densensitisation) or flooding.

Drugs

Drugs have a limited role. Benzodiazepines are prescribed less often than previously because of the risk of dependence but they are useful in treating anxiety when symptoms can be expected to last no more than a few weeks. Diazepam can be given in doses of 2–10 mg 3 times daily but should be reduced and tailed off after 3 weeks otherwise dependence may occur. A beta-adrenoceptor blocking drug, such as propranolol 20–80 mg daily, can help when the peripheral somatic symptoms of anxiety are prominent. Antidepressant drugs, either a tricyclic (amitriptyline 50–150 mg at night) or MAOI (phenelzine 15 mg 4 times daily), are the most effective drugs in managing anxiety and should be used for generalised anxiety when symptoms do not respond to psychological approaches. They can be given in conjunction with behaviour therapy for phobic disorders and appear to be very effective for panic attacks.

OBSESSIVE COMPULSIVE DISORDER

An obsessional symptom is an unwanted thought or impulse which enters the subject's mind repeatedly despite his conscious resistance. These symptoms can occur in schizophrenia and depression but when they are primary phenomena a diagnosis of obsessive compulsive disorder is made. This has a prevalence of approximately 1–3% but many people with the condition do not request treatment.

Aetiology

Genetic factors are important, as is the previous personality which is usually characterised by traits of perfectionism, rigidity and conscientiousness. Organic brain disease has been implicated in the light of the occurrence of obsessional symptoms after outbreaks of encephalitis lethargica. However in the great majority of cases seen in current practice there is no evidence of cerebral disease.

Clinical features

Obsessional symptoms are recognised as coming from the subject's own mind. Common themes include repeated thoughts of becoming aggressive or fears of contamination with dirt or chemical substances. These thoughts are often followed by rituals which are patterns of behaviour developed to relieve the anxiety generated by the original obsession. The rituals involve repeated checking, handwashing or changing of clothes. The condition tends to follow a relapsing course so patients may experience distress over many years.

Management

Behaviour therapy is the preferred treatment. This should be carried out under specialist supervision and is most effective when the obsessional rituals are prominent. It consists of repeated exposure to the contaminated objects followed by prevention of the ritualistic behaviour (response prevention). Some patients are helped further if they can observe a therapist modelling normal behaviour in the presence of contamination. Treatment should be given over several sessions and relatives need to be enlisted as co-therapists to prevent recurrence of symptoms in the home environment. Obsessional thoughts not accompanied by rituals are more difficult to treat but some success has been claimed for various psychological techniques designed to interrupt the patient's pattern of thinking (thought stopping).

Additional benefit can be derived if medication is combined with behaviour therapy; clomipramine (50–150 mg daily) is the drug of choice in this condition.

HYSTERIA

This is one of the most controversial concepts in psychiatry. Controversy has occurred because of the high rate of organic disease in patients previously diagnosed as having hysteria and also because of the multiple uses of the term which has been used to describe symptoms, a personality type, an epidemic phenomenon and clinical syndromes. Nevertheless doctors continue to find it a useful concept, particularly if it is regarded as a first stage in diagnosis and as an indication that other psychiatric or neurological disorders may be present.

Hysteria is best used to define a syndrome characterised by a loss or distortion of neurological function not fully explained by organic disease.

Aetiology

The condition is considered to result from unconscious psychological processes, implying that the patient lacks insight into the nature of the symptoms. In psychoanalytic terms hysteria has been seen as a maladaptive way of coping with an unresolved psychological conflict, that is by becoming ill. The patient thus derives primary gain by relieving the conflict and secondary gain by obtaining sympathy and attention from others or by avoiding everyday responsibilities. It is certainly the case that hysteria is more commonly diagnosed in women and children, groups who often lack an effective means of verbal communication because of an inferior social position.

The role of organic neurological disease is unclear. Although, by definition, the symptoms of hysteria are not themselves caused by organic disease, there is coexisting disease of the nervous system in up to 50% of cases. Organic disease may facilitate hysterical mechanisms and provide a model for symptoms, thus explaining the occurrence of pseudoseizures in patients with epilepsy.

Clinical features

The two main variants of hysteria are conversion disorder and dissociation disorder. In conversion disorder the symptoms mimic lesions in the motor or sensory nervous system and in classical cases there is apparent unconcern (belle indifference) even in the face of gross physical disability. However this is not always present and it should not be relied upon for diagnostic purposes. The presentations of conversion disorder are given in the information box below.

COMMON PRESENTATIONS OF CONVERSION DISORDER

- Gait disturbance
- Loss of function in limbs
- Aphonia
- Pseudoseizures
- Sensory loss
- Blindness

Dissociation disorder involves impairment of higher mental functions especially memory and general intelligence.

Hysterical amnesia usually develops acutely. The memory loss is patchy and inconsistent; a characteristic feature is a loss of personal identity so that the patient is unable to recall his name, address or other personal and family details. Memory loss of this degree does not occur in organic disease unless there is gross dementia. Hysterical amnesia is occasionally accompanied by a tendency to travel aimlessly many miles from familiar surroundings; this is known as a hysterical fugue. When global intelligence is affected the cognitive deficits are variable and the patient's behaviour is not in keeping with the apparent degree of dementia.

Another syndrome sometimes described under the general rubric of hysteria is *Briquet's syndrome* or *somatisation disorder*. This is a chronic condition, almost entirely confined to women, which begins before the age of 30 and whose cardinal features are multiple and recurrent somatic complaints in many organ systems for which medical attention is sought.

Management

A full physical and psychiatric assessment should be completed to determine whether other disorders are present. Once the doctor is satisfied that relevant organic disease has been excluded no further investigations should be undertaken and therapeutic effort should be directed towards restoring optimal function. Many patients resist the idea that their symptoms are not entirely somatic. Confrontation is best avoided and initial management should concentrate on simple explanation and reassurance that the symptoms conform to a recognised pattern and will get better with treatment. This involves identifying those factors which appear to have precipitated the symptoms and helping the patient to cope with them more adaptively. Secondary reinforcing factors in the patient's social network must be corrected and physical treatment, for example physiotherapy, should be arranged to provide an acceptable framework for recovery. Little is to be gained by debating how much insight the patient really has into his condition. Acute symptoms respond well to treatment. In resistant cases recovery can be helped by abreaction under the influence of hypnosis or small intravenous doses of amylobarbitone (250–500 mg given over 5 minutes). During abreaction the patient is encouraged to describe, in a cathartic manner, the emotional trauma which provoked the symptoms while the doctor makes use of the patient's enhanced suggestibility to predict symptom relief.

HYPOCHONDRIASIS

This refers to a morbid preoccupation with symptoms and a fear of disease, either physical or psychological. As it is usually applied it refers to physical symptoms and health. Hypochondriacal complaints commonly occur in anxiety and depressive disorders but occasionally they are primary phenomena and persist for many years, being unresponsive to conventional methods of treatment. The symptoms are predominantly neurotic. In a small proportion of cases conviction of disease assumes psychotic intensity, the best known example being the conviction of parasitic infestation ('delusional parasitosis') which leads patients to consult dermatologists. Pimozide (2–12 mg daily) has been claimed to be effective for this syndrome.

FACTITIOUS DISORDERS

This is a group of disorders in which symptoms and signs are deliberately induced. There are definite objective signs or laboratory abnormalities but these have been secretly fabricated in the absence of an underlying disease process. For example the patient may present with recurrent episodes of hypoglycaemia brought on by surreptitious injection of insulin. Other presentations include ulcerating skin lesions (dermatitis artefacta), pyrexia of unknown origin, hyperthyroidism and anaemia. The patients do not admit to feigning illness and many have a great capacity for deception. The only apparent goals are to deceive others and to

adopt the sick role. Their behaviour can best be understood in terms of the attractions which the sick role conveys; only when they are ill do they receive attention or sympathy from other people. The typical patient is a young woman with marked dependency traits who is employed in nursing or one of the other professions allied to medicine.

Munchausen's syndrome

This is another form of factitious disorder which is seen more commonly in men who present with dramatic symptoms of a medical emergency such as a myocardial infarction or intra-abdominal catastrophe. The patient fabricates a convincing history and may persuade an inexperienced doctor to undertake complicated investigations or exploratory surgery. If suspicions are aroused it may be possible to trace the patient's history showing that he has presented similarly at several other hospitals, often changing his name many times in the process. When confronted with the factitious nature of his symptoms the patient discharges himself angrily, only to present again at another hospital shortly afterwards. This condition is named after the German Baron von Munchausen who was legendary for his inventive lying. Treatment is strikingly ineffective but it is important to recognise the syndrome to avoid unnecessary investigations.

PERSONALITY DISORDERS

Psychiatrists often disagree about this concept which refers to a pattern of enduring traits and behaviour which is maladaptive and which causes significant harm to the individual or those around him. The traits of personality disorder are exaggerations of those characteristics which are recognised in many normal members of society. They are usually well developed by late adolescence and persist relatively unchanged throughout life. The diagnosis of a particular type of personality disorder is made separately from a diagnosis of psychiatric illness. This recognises that an individual with a disordered personality may or may not experience discrete episodes of psychiatric illness.

Aetiological factors are not well understood. Many come from deprived families and have been subjected to physical and emotional abuse in childhood. Personality disorders tend to run in families but the relative influence of genetic and environmental factors is not clear.

Personality disorders are usually grouped according to particular traits which tend to go together.

ANTISOCIAL PERSONALITY

Also known as psychopathic personality this refers to recurrent delinquent behaviour with repeated offences against the law, aggression, impulsiveness and lack of feeling for other people. Antisocial personalities have an unstable record with regard to work, marriage and personal relationships. They often serve prison sentences but there is a high rate of re-offending.

PARANOID PERSONALITY

These individuals are very sensitive to criticism and humiliations. They are excessively keen on establishing what they regard as their personal rights and defend them forcefully. They have an exaggerated sense of their own importance so they readily perceive a slight from others where none is intended. If things go wrong for them they blame other people. This is apparent if such people become medically ill when they may accuse their doctor of negligence or bad practice. Relatives of paranoid personalities have a higher than average rate of paranoid psychoses.

DEPENDENT PERSONALITY

These people are indecisive and have difficulty coping with daily responsibilities. They demand constant support from other people and may enter into unsuitable relationships merely to avoid being left to fend for themselves. They tend to comply passively with the wishes of authority figures.

HISTRIONIC PERSONALITY

This term, sometimes called hysterical personality, is usually applied to women who display traits of egocentricity, emotional shallowness, vanity and dramatisation. Relationships are established quickly but do not last. Although they behave in a sexual provocative manner they are usually frigid and afraid of mature sexuality. The concept has been criticised as a caricature of femininity derived by male doctors. It does have some relationship with a tendency to develop hysterical conversion symptoms but most patients with hysteria have normal personalities.

SCHIZOID PERSONALITY

People with this personality type are socially withdrawn, preferring solitary pursuits which are often of an eccentric nature. They appear aloof to other people but in fact are usually socially phobic. This personality type may contribute to the development of schizophre-nia in which case the prognosis is worse than for schizophrenics with normal personalities.

OBSESSIONAL PERSONALITY

Minor obsessional traits of orderliness, cleanliness and punctuality are advantageous to most who possess them and essential for success in certain occupations, including medicine. They become handicapping when they lead to slowness, inflexibility and indecisiveness. Obsessional people are often insecure and like their lives to be as routine and predictable as possible. They may develop a florid obsessional neurosis under stress and are also prone to depressive illnesses during which their obsessional traits become more pronounced.

Management
By their nature personality disorders cannot be cured but some individuals can be helped to make necessary changes so that their behaviour is less distressing to themselves or other people. Various psychological treatments have been used and success has been claimed for behaviour therapy and interpretive psycho-therapy. Some experts believe group therapy is especially helpful.

It is important to remember that people with personality disorders can develop other psychiatric illnesses, the features of which are coloured by underlying personality. These illnesses respond to conventional treatment but often remain undetected.

OTHER DISORDERS

ALCOHOLISM

Alcohol consumption in the United Kingdom has risen greatly since the Second World War and this has been accompanied by increases in the social, psychological and physical problems due to alcohol. The term alcoholism is now used in a broad sense to describe a pattern of drinking which is harmful to the individual or to his family. The more restricted term, alcohol dependence, has the criteria listed in the information box (p. 954).

National statistics indicate that morbidity related to alcohol closely correlates with mean per capita consumption. Men are more likely to have alcohol-related problems than women, although the gap is closing. *Approximately one-quarter of male patients in general hospital medical wards have a current or previous alcohol problem.*

CRITERIA OF ALCOHOL DEPENDENCE

- Narrowing of the drinking repertoire
- Priority of drinking over other activities
- Tolerance of effects of alcohol
- Repeated withdrawal symptoms
- Relief of withdrawal symptoms by further drinking
- Subjective compulsion to drink
- Reinstatement of drinking behaviour after abstinence

Aetiology

Although genetic factors make a small contribution to the development of alcohol abuse cultural factors are much more important. Alcohol problems are rare among Muslims and Jews and common in countries which have large alcohol-producing industries, for example France, Italy and Portugal. In the United Kingdom problems are commoner among Scots and Irish. Availability of alcohol is important as shown by high rates among those employed in the drink trade. Doctors previously held a high position in the occupational league table but are now only just above the average. There is a close correlation between consumption and the price of alcohol relative to average earnings. The cheaper the relative price the higher the consumption with the effect that a larger proportion of the population will develop alcohol related problems.

No consistent predisposing personality profile has been identified. Most people with alcohol problems are distinguished from the rest of the community simply by the fact that they drink more. The majority of alcoholics do not have an underlying psychiatric illness but in a few it appears that heavy drinking has developed in an attempt to relieve the unpleasant symptoms of an anxiety state, depression or schizophrenia.

PROBLEMS CAUSED BY ALCOHOL

Many patients' alcohol problems are not detected by their doctors. A high index of suspicion is important particularly in cases where there are repeated consultations for vague symptoms or minor accidents. If in doubt a drinking history should be taken in which the patient is asked to describe a typical week's drinking. Consumption should be quantified in terms of units of alcohol; one unit contains approximately 9 g alcohol and is the equivalent of half a pint of beer, a single measure of spirits or a glass of table wine. Current opinion suggests that drinking becomes hazardous at levels above 21 units weekly for men and 14 units weekly for women. Laboratory tests are useful in confirming alcohol abuse. Mean corpuscular volume (MCV) or gamma-glutamyl transpeptidase (gamma GT) are raised in approximately 50% of problem drinkers. Their low sensitivity makes them unsuitable for population screening but they are useful for monitoring treatment response in individual cases where their values were elevated originally.

Social problems

These include absenteeism from work, unemployment, marital tensions, child abuse, financial difficulties and problems with the law, including violence and traffic offences.

Psychological problems

Depression. This is common and is usually reactive to the numerous social problems which heavy drinking creates. Alcohol also has a direct depressant effect. Attempted suicide and completed suicide are much commoner in alcoholics than in the rest of society.

Morbid jealousy. This is a syndrome characterised by delusions of sexual infidelity. It is usually seen in alcoholics of sensitive or paranoid disposition whose sexual relationship has deteriorated because of impotence or rejection by the partner. The alcoholic suspects and accuses his partner of having a relationship with another person and goes to extreme lengths to obtain corroborative evidence, such as repeatedly searching the partner's personal possessions or employing a private detective to follow them. Accusations lead to violence and sometimes murder. Morbid jealousy can also occur in schizophrenia, depressive illness and paranoid personality disorder.

Withdrawal symptoms. These indicate physical dependence. The earliest manifestation is a subjective sensation of tension on waking in the morning. This may be accompanied by a tremor which makes it difficult to shave or hold a cup of tea. Another alcoholic drink relieves these symptoms, thus establishing a pattern of morning drinking. Less common but more serious withdrawal symptoms are epilepsy and delirium tremens, the latter having the features of a severe confusional state characterised by impaired consciousness, visual hallucinations, memory disturbance and seizures. Alcoholic hallucinosis also occurs following relative or absolute withdrawal. Its essential features are auditory hallucinations occurring in clear consciousness; the hallucinations take the form of derogatory or persecutory voices which discuss the individual in the third person or comment directly to him. They are similar to the auditory hallucinations reported by schizophrenics.

Vitamin deficiencies. These occur in alcoholics who have a severely impoverished diet. The most important is thiamine (B1) deficiency which leads to the acute phenomena of Wernicke's encephalopathy or the chronic features of Korsakoff's syndrome (p. 14).

Direct toxic effects on the brain. These cause the familiar features of drunkenness. In very heavy drinkers there are periods of amnesia (alcoholic blackouts) for events which occurred during bouts of intoxication. When alcoholism has been established for several years cortical atrophy can occur and the clinical picture of dementia develops.

Indirect effects on behaviour. These can result from head injury, hypoglycaemia and porto-systemic encephalopathy.

Physical problems
These are protean and can affect virtually any organ in the body, giving rise to the comment that alcohol has replaced syphilis as the great mimic of disease. The diseases are grouped together in Table 18.6 and are discussed in detail in their respective sections.

Management
Straightforward advice about the harmful effects of alcohol and safe levels of consumption is often all that is needed. In more serious cases patients may have to be advised to alter leisure activities or change jobs if these are contributing to the problem. Supportive psychotherapy is often crucial in helping the patient effect the necessary changes in life style. Interpretive psychotherapy, either individual or group, can help patients who have recurrent relapses. Treatment of this type is available at specialised centres and is also provided by voluntary organisations such as Alcoholics Anonymous (AA).

Drugs
Drugs are used at various stages in treatment. Benzodiazepines are the drugs of choice for withdrawal symptoms and can be given safely in large doses (e.g. diazepam 20 mg 4 times daily) provided they are tailed off over a period of 5–7 days as symptoms subside. It is usual to give high dose vitamins during withdrawal treatment because of the possibility of thiamine deficiency. These are given in the form of 2–4 pairs of high potency intravenous ampoules of Parentrovite ®

Table 18.6 Physical effects of alcohol abuse

System	Consequences
Cardiovascular	Cardiomyopathy
	Hypertension
Gastro-intestinal	Oro-pharyngeal cancer
	Oesophageal cancer
	Gastritis
	Mallory-Weiss syndrome
	Pancreatitis
	Malabsorption
Liver	Fatty change
	Acute hepatitis
	Cirrhosis
	Primary liver cancer
Neurological	Cerebral haemorrhage
	Peripheral neuropathy
	Dementia
	Wernicke-Korsakoff syndrome
	Cerebellar degeneration
Musculo-skeletal	Myopathy
	Gout
Respiratory	Pneumonia
	Tuberculosis
Endocrine and reproductive	Hypoglycaemia
	Hypogonadism
	Pseudo-Cushing's syndrome
	Infertility
	Foetal alcohol syndrome
Skin	Spider naevi
	Palmar erythema
	Acne rosacea

4–8 hourly for 2 days followed by high potency intramuscular injections for 5–7 days. Only rarely are antidepressants required; the depressive symptoms, if present, usually resolve with abstinence. Phenothiazines (e.g. chlorpromazine 100 mg 3 times daily) are required for alcoholic hallucinosis. Disulfiram (200–400 mg daily) can be given as a deterrent to patients who have difficulty resisting sudden impulses to drink after becoming abstinent. The drug blocks the metabolism of alcohol, causing acetaldehyde to accumulate in the body. When alcohol is consumed by someone taking the drug there follows an unpleasant reaction consisting of headache, flushing, nausea and laboured breathing. Knowledge that this reaction will occur can provide an insurance against drinking and even remove craving. Disulfiram should always be seen as an adjunct to other treatments, especially supportive psychotherapy.

DRUG ABUSE

Dependence on illegal and prescribed drugs has become a major problem in Western countries during the last two decades. In the United Kingdom there are now

50 000–100 000 opiate addicts and 2% of the population regularly take benzodiazepines. Many of the aetiological factors which apply to alcohol abuse are also relevant to drug dependence. The main factors are cultural pressures, particularly within a peer group, and availability of a drug. In the case of some drugs availability has been increased by medical over-prescribing but there has also been a relative decline in price.

BENZODIAZEPINES

More people are dependent on benzodiazepines than on any other group of drugs. They are effective anti-anxiety drugs if given in short courses but tolerance occurs after 6 weeks of daily consumption. Withdrawal symptoms can then occur if the drug is stopped abruptly. These include anxiety, increased sensory perception, epileptic fits and psychotic experiences. Withdrawal symptoms are particularly likely to occur with short-acting drugs such as lorazepam. Benzodiazepine dependence nearly always occurs because the drugs have been prescribed for the wrong reasons or because repeat prescriptions have been issued for several months.

CANNABIS

Cannabis, derived from the plant Cannabis sativa, is usually smoked mixed with tobacco. It quickly produces a sensation of relaxation and well-being; psychological dependence is common but tolerance and withdrawal symptoms are unusual. It is probably the commonest illegal drug taken in the United Kingdom and is often the only drug with which young people experiment. The extent of its use cannot be estimated reliably.

A toxic confusional state occurs after heavy consumption and acute psychotic episodes are well recognised. Long-term consequences of regular consumption are also being recognised. One of the first effects to be described was the 'amotivational syndrome', characterised by apathy and slothfulness. Cerebral atrophy has also been described and recent reports suggest that chronic consumption can lead to a schizophrenia-like illness.

BARBITURATES

These are now rarely prescribed, having been replaced as hypnotics by benzodiazepines. However they are still taken by some people who manage to obtain them indirectly from doctors. They soon cause dependence and sudden withdrawal is very likely to cause epileptic fits. Barbiturates are dangerous in overdose because of their depressant effect on respiration.

OPIATES

Morphine, heroin and codeine are the main drugs in this group, with heroin having become especially prominent recently. Heroin, which is taken orally, intravenously or by inhalation, gives a rapid, intensely pleasurable experience, often accompanied by heightened sexual arousal. Physical dependence occurs within a few weeks of regular high-dose injection, with the result that the dose is escalated and the addict's life becomes increasingly centred around obtaining and taking the drug. Intravenous users are prone to bacterial infections, hepatitis B and human immuno-deficiency virus (HIV) infection through needle contamination. Accidental overdose is common. The withdrawal syndrome, which can start within 12 hours in some people, can present with intense craving, rhinorrhoea, lacrimation, yawning, perspiration, shivering, piloerection, vomiting, diarrhoea and abdominal cramps. Examination shows a tachycardia, hypertension, mydriasis and facial flushing.

AMPHETAMINES

These have a stimulating central effect and are taken to produce increased energy, elevated mood and greater capacity for concentration. There is also a suppression of appetite which accounts for their use in obesity. Amphetamines are taken orally or intravenously. Physical dependence is unusual but withdrawal of the drug results in rebound depression, anxiety and fatigue. Chronic ingestion can cause a syndrome identical to paranoid schizophrenia.

COCAINE

Cocaine is becoming increasingly popular, taken by sniffing or 'snorting' the powder into the nostrils through a tube. Absorption occurs through the nasal mucous membranes and gives a rapid stimulating effect similar to amphetamine. A toxic psychosis occurs with high levels of consumption, and tactile hallucinations (formication) may be prominent. Chronic cocaine sniffing can cause ulceration of the nasal muscoa.

HALLUCINOGENIC DRUGS

Lysergic acid diethylamide (LSD) and psilocybin (magic mushroom) are currently the most commonly used hallucinogens. Perceptual changes occur within

40 minutes of oral ingestion. Vision is affected most often; the subject experiences heightened visual awareness of objects, especially colours. Images may be distorted in shape or size and true hallucinations occur. These can be terrifying in nature, the experience then being referred to as a 'bad trip'. There may also be distorted perception of time, sounds and tactile sensations. Flashback experiences can occur several months after the last dose; during these the psychotic experiences of LSD are experienced again with their original intensity. A chronic psychotic illness has also been reported after regular LSD use.

ORGANIC SOLVENTS

The inhalation of organic solvents has become popular in some adolescent groups. These substances produce acute intoxication characterised by euphoria, excitement, dizziness and a floating sensation. Further inhalation leads to loss of consciousness; death can occur from the direct toxic effect of the solvent or from asphyxiation if the substance is inhaled from a plastic bag.

Management of drug abuse

The first step in management is usually aimed at helping the patient withdraw from the drug. When there are signs of severe physical dependence withdrawal is best undertaken in hospital and this also enables physical complications, such as infections, to be treated. Decreasing doses of the relevant drug are given over a period of 1–3 weeks, the dose being titrated against objective withdrawal symptoms. Oral methadone is used for opiate dependence. In some cases complete withdrawal is not successful and the patient functions better if maintained on regular doses of oral methadone as an outpatient. This decision should only be undertaken by a specialist and the long-term supervision requires the patient to attend a specially designated drug treatment centre. The withdrawal period may need to be extended to several months for some drugs, for example benzodiazepines.

Long-term support is necessary if patients are to remain drug free. Many doctors can achieve good results if they strike up a rapport with the patient. Complicated or relapsing patients should be referred to specialist centres. Support can also be provided by self-help groups and voluntary bodies such as Narcotics Anonymous.

EATING DISORDERS

ANOREXIA NERVOSA

This disorder, which sometimes causes extreme emaciation, typically develops during adolescence and predominantly affects girls. Only 5–10% of cases occur in males; occasionally the condition develops in older women. There is a higher prevalence in the upper social classes and the girls are often hard-working, perfectionist and ambitious. One survey found a prevalence of 1% in girls at an independent school with another 5% showing some features of the condition. Theories about aetiology are speculative. Current social pressures to maintain a slim figure are thought to have caused a recent increased incidence. Some girls have a history of obesity and embark on an extreme course of dieting after being teased about their fatness. Anorexia has also been regarded as an attempt to remain pre-pubertal by girls who have fears of sexual maturation. In other cases anorexia appears a non-specific response to family crises which often involve the parental relationship. Hormonal changes have been suggested as aetiologically important. However the endocrine abnormalities nearly always revert to normal following restoration of weight and are probably secondary to the effects of weight loss.

Clinical features

These are listed in the information box below.

> **ESSENTIAL DIAGNOSTIC CRITERIA FOR ANOREXIA NERVOSA**
>
> - Weight loss of at least 25% of original body weight (or weight 25% below norm for age and height)
> - Avoidance of high calorie foods
> - Distortion of body image so that the patient regards herself as fat even when grossly underweight
> - Amenorrhoea for at least three months

In boys loss of sexual interest replaces amenorrhoea as a diagnostic criterion. Other features include a striking indifference to the weight loss and a denial of problems. Emaciation may be disguised by wearing loosely fitting clothes and hiding heavy objects in the clothing when weight is checked on scales. Subjects are often physically overactive; they may use laxatives or induce vomiting secretly after meals. Although they avoid carbohydrates and fats they are often preoccupied with food and enjoy making elaborate meals for their families. Other physical signs include a downy, lanugo hair on the trunk and limbs, hypotension, bradycardia and peripheral cyanosis. Psychosexual immaturity is often prominent.

Management

The first objective is to restore normal body weight which is most likely to be achieved if a trusting relationship can be established with the patient from the first interview. Treatment is best undertaken in hospital unless the condition is mild; the patient is confined to bed and a controlled diet is given to achieve a weight gain of approximately 1 kg weekly. The patient is supervised during meals and for 1 hour subsequently to ensure vomiting does not occur. A series of target weights should be set and the patient is allowed increasing privileges and independence as each target is achieved. The final target should be within the normal range for the patient's age and height. Psychotherapy is an essential part of management. Individual therapy allows the patient to acquire insight into her condition and associated problems. Family therapy is also necessary to help resolve tensions which are nearly always evident by the time the patient presents for treatment.

The short-term prognosis is good if this programme is followed but the long-term outlook is less favourable. Approximately 20% make a full recovery, 20% remain chronically ill and 60% have recurring episodes of anorexia. Death occurs from suicide or physical complications in 5% of cases.

BULIMIA NERVOSA

This is a recently described disorder which may be related to anorexia nervosa. It is almost exclusively confined to women and the age of onset is slightly older than for anorexia. Prevalence has been estimated at 1% of women in their early twenties.

Clinical features

These are listed in the information box below.

DIAGNOSTIC CRITERIA FOR BULIMIA NERVOSA

- Recurrent bouts of binge-eating
- Lack of self-control over eating during binges
- Self-induced vomiting, purgation or dieting after binges
- Weight maintained within normal limits

The binges occur at least twice weekly and involve rich foods such as cakes, chocolates and dairy products; over 20 000 calories may be consumed during the day of a binge. Despite this intake weight is strictly maintained within the normal range and menstruation is often regular. Physical complications from vomiting and purgation include erosion of dental enamel, hypokalaemia and metabolic alkalosis. Electrolyte and fluid disturbances can be sufficiently severe to cause cardiac arrhythmias or renal damage. A curious bilateral enlargement of the parotid glands is seen in some patients.

Management

Most treatment can be undertaken on an outpatient basis. Cognitive behaviour therapy is the currently preferred approach, the central component being self-monitoring of eating behaviour. The patient is asked to keep a full eating diary, together with a record of emotions and circumstances associated with binges. A series of tasks is set which are directed at helping the patient cope more appropriately with provoking stimuli, thereby reducing the frequency and severity of binges. Treatment may need to be continued for several months; short-term results are encouraging but the long-term prognosis of the condition is not known.

OBESITY

This is the commonest form of eating disorder but it is rarely seen as a presenting problem in psychiatric practice. It results from an excess of fat and is defined in terms of a high body mass index (BMI). This is weight in kilograms divided by the square of height in metres. The normal range of BMI is 19–25 and on these figures one-third of the British population is obese. Obesity results from excessive intake of food and insufficient excercise but constitutional and cultural factors are important in its aetiology and maintenance. There is no consistent association between obesity and psychiatric illness or personality traits but many obese people find the condition highly embarrassing. Mild and moderate obesity can be helped by advice on healthy eating and exercise, supplemented by a behavioural programme. Severe obesity (BMI over 40) may require surgical intervention such as gastric banding or gastrojejunostomy.

PSYCHOSEXUAL DISORDERS

SEXUAL DYSFUNCTIONS

These are the commonest sexual complaints which doctors see in practice. They include low sexual interest and various difficulties experienced during intercourse which reduce mutual satisfaction. Many sexual problems stem from ignorance and fear, often dating back to an excessively prudish upbringing which has caused inhibition in relation to sexual topics. Sexual dysfunction can occur transiently as a symptom of an anxiety disorder or depressive illness or it may be a manifestation of a relationship problem. Physical health has an important influence and needs careful assessment. Sexual interest and performance are impaired during any debilitating illness. Endocrine, cardiovascular and neurological disorders should be especially considered; for example impotence may be a presenting feature of diabetes, peripheral vascular disease or multiple sclerosis. Finally an alcohol and drug history should be taken. Any drug which has a depressant effect on the central nervous system can impair sexual function as also can drugs which act on the peripheral autonomic system (e.g. alphamethyl dopa, phenothiazines, tricyclic antidepressants).

Impotence

This is the commonest problem among men. It involves complete or partial erectile failure with normal sexual desire. It is often transient and improves with reassurance. If persistent it can be helped by a behavioural programme in which the partner's co-operation is essential. The couple are instructed to carry out a graded series of mutually pleasurable sexual activities but intercourse is completely banned until an erection can be confidently maintained. Successful results have also been obtained by injecting papaverine into the corpora cavernosa and this treatment is now preferred in many clinics.

Premature ejaculation

This is defined as ejaculation prior to penetration or, if penetration occurs, before the partner can achieve orgasm. It is often associated with high levels of anxiety which appear to perpetuate the condition. Successful treatment is based on behavioural techniques derived from the work of Masters and Johnson.

Vaginismus

This is due to spasm of the pelvic muscles which prevents full penetration. It results from intense fear of penetration on the part of the woman and a conditioned reflex is established resulting in pelvic spasm even at the thought of intercourse. Treatment consists of instructing the patient in relaxation exercises followed by insertion of vaginal dilators of increasing size, initially by the doctor, then the patient and finally the partner.

Female orgasmic dysfunction

Most cases result from ignorance of sexual technique on the part of patient or her partner. Counselling is usually effective in overcoming the problem. Approximately 10% of women appear physiologically incapable of orgasm due to absence of the bulbo-cavernosus reflex.

SEXUAL DEVIATIONS

Sexual deviations involve obtaining sexual arousal from inanimate objects or unwilling partners. Examples include exhibitionism (genital exposure in public), fetishism (arousal from female clothing), transvestism (arousal by dressing in clothes of opposite sex) and paedophilia (sexual arousal with children).

TRANS-SEXUALISM

This rare condition results from a disturbance of gender identity. The patient, usually a man, is convinced he should have been born female and strongly identifies with feminine psychology. He wishes to live his life as a woman and may request medical help to do so. Trans-sexuals should be referred to special clinics where hormone therapy may be given to develop the secondary sexual characteristics of the opposite sex. Surgical treatment can be undertaken to reassign external genitalia if the patient can successfully adopt the life-style of the opposite sex for at least 12 months.

SPECIAL ASPECTS OF PSYCHIATRY

PSYCHIATRIC PROBLEMS IN THE GENERAL HOSPITAL

There are several reasons why psychiatric illness is commoner in patients attending general hospitals than in the community.

PSYCHOLOGICAL REACTIONS TO PHYSICAL ILLNESS

Most physical illnesses cause some psychological upset which is usually minor in degree and brief in duration. Sick people modify their lifestyle according to the severity of their illness; mood changes are common but are not distressing nor do they interfere with adjustment to the illness. More pronounced mood changes can cause significant distress. They usually resolve with recovery from the physical illness and they are best regarded as adjustment disorders. Anxiety is the commonest re-action within the first few days following the onset of physical symptoms; depression is a later development. Explanation and reassurance help allay the emotional distress; specific psychiatric intervention is not necess-ary. In a minority of patients a depressed mood persists for weeks or months after physical recovery and is accompanied by the characteristic symptoms of loss of interest, low self-esteem, sleep disturbance and weight change. The diagnosis of a secondary depressive illness is then warranted and treatment with antidepressant medication is required. Physically ill patients tolerate antidepressant drugs poorly. Lower doses than usual should be used initially and if side-effects to tricyclics are troublesome one of the newer drugs like mianserin (30–90 mg at night) can be given. Close collaboration between physician and psychiatrist is essential for optimal management. Nowhere is this more important than in the care of the elderly who are prone to multiple problems, physical, psychological and social.

Depression can prolong functional disability follow-ing physical illness, thereby delaying return to work and resumption of leisure activities. In other cases recovery is delayed even though there is no evidence of depression. These patients remain incapacitated and adopt a lifestyle of invalidism or abnormal illness behaviour. The explanation can be found by examining the patient's social environment when various factors prolonging the disability may be uncovered. The patient may be avoiding returning to an unsatisfactory job, may be gaining attention from an otherwise unsympathetic partner or may be exaggerating symptoms for financial gain if compensation is involved.

Anxiety, depression or mania may be the presenting symptoms of various underlying physical illnesses. In these cases the psychological symptoms result from disturbances of neurotransmitter function or interrup-tion of anatomical pathways in the brain. Physical examination is essential in patients presenting with a new episode of psychiatric illness and suspicion of underlying physical pathology should be aroused partic-ularly in the circumstances listed in the information box below.

These symptomatic psychiatric disorders can occur in the conditions listed in the information box below.

POINTERS TO AN ORGANIC CAUSE FOR PSYCHIATRIC DISORDER

- Late age of onset of psychiatric illness
- No previous history of psychiatric illness
- No family history of psychiatric illness
- No apparent psychological precipitant

ORGANIC CAUSES OF AFFECTIVE DISORDERS

Neurological	Herpes simplex
Cerebrovascular	Brucellosis
disease	Typhoid
Cerebral tumour	Toxoplasmosis
Multiple sclerosis	
Parkinson's disease	*Collagen disease*
Huntington's chorea	Systemic lupus
Alzheimer's disease	erythematosus
Epilepsy	
	Malignant disease
Endocrine	
Hypothyroidism	*Drugs*
Hyperthyroidism	Reserpine,
Cushing's syndrome	phenothiazines
Addison's disease	Methyldopa, oral
Hyperparathyroidism	contraceptives
	Corticosteroids,
Infections	phenylbutazone
Glandular fever	

SOMATIC PRESENTATION OF PSYCHIATRIC ILLNESS

Somatic symptoms such as fatigue, dizziness, headache and other pains are commonly experienced during periods of emotional stress. This becomes a medical problem when the symptoms are attributed to physical illness for which the patient requests medical attention. Many patients with psychiatric illness present in this manner to their general practitioner or hospital specialist. This phenomenon, known as somatisation, results in considerable misdiagnosis because the somatic presentation misleads the doctor into suspecting physical illness and distracts attention from underlying psychiatric problems. Not only does the patient have somatic symptoms but sometimes there is also a concern about a specific physical illness such as cancer, heart disease, AIDS or myalgic encephalomyelitis.

Among patients attending general hospital medical clinics at least one-fifth have no significant organic disease to account for their symptoms but have a psychiatric illness which is only detected when specific questions are asked.

Most have a depressive illness or one of the anxiety disorders (generalised anxiety, panic attacks or phobic disorder). The symptoms may have an abrupt onset in which case the history is short and a good response can be expected to conventional treatment. In a small proportion there is a longer history of complaints and disability; these patients are often diagnosed as having hypochondriasis, Briquet's syndrome or hysteria and are less easy to treat.

Aetiology

The presenting somatic complaints are often amplifications of normal physiological sensations or muscular aches which everyone experiences. During episodes of depression or anxiety these sensations are exaggerated, and interpreted in a morbid manner, thus becoming the focus for medical complaint. A family history or previous personal history of a particular physical illness may influence the location of symptoms as well as their interpretation. Although somatisation is a universal phenomenon it is commoner in Third World cultures and in immigrants from those countries into Britain. The social stigma of being psychiatrically ill probably accounts for the higher prevalence of somatisation in these immigrant groups. Many patients selectively emphasise somatic symptoms when they visit their doctor because they believe there is more medical interest in physical illness. Their pattern of somatisation is subsequently reinforced if special investigations are arranged, particularly if these yield equivocal results.

PUERPERAL MENTAL DISORDERS

There is a sharp increase in psychiatric illness following childbirth. Three different syndromes have been defined according to their severity and time of onset although there is some overlap between them.

POST-NATAL BLUES

These occur in 50–60% of women following delivery. Symptoms are evident by the third post-natal day, reach a peak on the fifth day and subside rapidly during the next ten days. The predominant features are tearfulness, irritability, lability of mood, anxiety about the baby and poor concentration. These symptoms are unexpected and bewildering to a new mother and consequently cause considerable distress. Prompt recognition and reassurance by nursing staff nearly always succeed in alleviating this distress.

A hormonal basis has been suspected in view of the rapid changes in progesterone and oestrogen levels which follow childbirth. However no consistent association has yet been found between hormonal changes and symptoms of the 'blues'.

POST-NATAL DEPRESSION

This is the most important psychiatric disorder following childbirth in terms of its frequency and disabilities. Within 6 weeks of delivery 10–15% of mothers have developed a new episode of depressive illness. In addition to the usual features of depression there may be excessive concern about the baby's health, fears of harming the baby, guilt about maternal deficiencies and marital tensions including loss of sexual interest. Diagnosis may be missed at a routine post-natal examination because attention is concentrated on the baby's welfare and on possible gynaecological complications. Furthermore women are embarrassed by admitting to feeling depressed after what is expected to be a joyful event in their lives.

Post-natal depression can last for several months if it is not treated. Once symptoms are recognised support and counselling should be arranged; counselling from a health visitor has been shown to have a significant effect in hastening recovery. Antidepressant drugs are required in severe cases (see p. 937).

Post-natal depression probably occurs as a result of various social and psychological changes following childbirth including giving up work, financial hardship, altered status, marital friction and the sheer exhaustion of broken nights.

PUERPERAL PSYCHOSES

These occur following approximately 0.2% of deliveries. Although they are infrequent they are severe and have a devastating effect on the mother's bonding with her child and on other family relationships.

The psychosis can take the form of affective (manic depressive) or schizophrenic illness. The former predominate with liability of mood being a characteristic feature. Perplexity and disorientation are relatively more common than in psychoses unrelated to childbirth. In the majority of cases symptoms develop during the first fortnight after delivery. Transfer to a psychiatric ward is nearly always necessary and in some hospitals there are mother and baby units which allow the baby to be admitted with the mother. The theoretical advantage of this arrangement is that it enables mother-child bonding to develop without interruption. However some mothers are so disturbed that they cannot relate adequately to their baby. Alternative arrangements should then be made for the baby's care until the mother's mental state has improved sufficiently for her to care for the child.

Neuroleptic or antidepressant drugs are prescribed depending on the nature of the psychosis. ECT is given for severe psychotic depression if it is accompanied by stupor, refusal to eat and drink, or suicidal risk.

The aetiology of puerperal psychosis is not understood. There is an increased risk of psychotic illness among first-degree relatives and an increased personal risk of psychosis not related to childbirth. Despite the intuitive appeal of a hormonal aetiology no distinct hormonal changes have been discovered. A psychological contribution is suggested by observations that puerperal psychoses are commoner in unmarried women, after a first child and following Caesarian section. These factors are probably important because of the increased stress associated with them.

The short-term outcome is nearly always good but there is at least a 20% risk of recurrent illness after a subsequent birth. If there have been previous episodes of affective illness unrelated to childbirth the risk of puerperal psychosis rises to 40%.

Psychotropic drugs in pregnancy and the puerperium
Certain precautions need to be observed when prescribing psychotropic drugs in pregnancy and the puerperium because of possible teratogenic effects during the first trimester, withdrawal symptoms following delivery and toxic effects on the baby of drugs excreted in breast milk. Lithium is the most dangerous drug concerned. It has definite teratogenic effects and should not be prescribed at all during the first trimester. If a woman taking prophylactic lithium wishes to become pregnant the drug should be stopped gradually beforehand and contraception continued until the drug is completely withdrawn. If pregnancy occurs while taking lithium the drug must be stopped immediately. Lithium is excreted in breast milk and can cause toxicity in the newborn baby. It should therefore be avoided in the puerperium if breast-feeding is practised.

Benzodiazepines also have a weak teratogenic effect. They can cause over-sedation (floppy-baby syndrome) or withdrawal symptoms in the neonate immediately following delivery if taken beforehand so they should be avoided in pregnancy and during lactation.

Tricyclic antidepressants, phenothiazines and butyrophenones do not appear to have teratogenic effects so they can be given during pregnancy if indicated clinically. They are excreted in breast milk in very small amounts; breast-feeding is therefore not contraindicated if the mother is taking these drugs.

GYNAECOLOGICAL DISORDERS

Several gynaecological disorders have been associated with psychiatric morbidity but there are few definite conclusions. A specific menstrual mood disorder has been described. This condition, also known as the premenstrual syndrome, is characterised by depression, irritability, tension, poor concentration and a general bloated sensation; it occurs a few days before the onset of menstruation and subsides rapidly once menstruation begins. In women with affective disorders symptoms are accentuated premenstrually but never clear completely so they continue throughout the cycle. No consistent hormonal abnormalities have been found to account for menstrual mood disorder. Symptomatic improvement may be achieved by giving progesterone or diuretics.

Therapeutic abortion, hysterectomy and the menopause may be followed by psychiatric illness in some women but for the majority there are no significant psychological complications.

ATTEMPTED SUICIDE

There was a steady increase in hospital admissions for suicide attempts from the early 1960s so that by the end of the 1970s there were over 100 000 admissions annually in Britain. Since then there has been a slight decrease but attempted suicide is still one of the commonest reasons for acute medical admissions. The term attempted suicide is potentially misleading in that the majority of patients are not unequivocally trying to kill themselves. However, alternative terms such as parasuicide and deliberate, non-fatal self-harm have not been widely accepted and attempted suicide can be retained provided it is realised that it does not inevitably involve fatal intent.

Most suicide attempts are due to drug overdose, either prescribed or non-prescribed. Less common methods include wrist slashing, asphyxiation, drowning, hanging, jumping from a height or in front of a moving vehicle, and using firearms. Methods which carry a high chance of being fatal are more likely to be associated with serious psychiatric illness.

Suicide attempts are commoner in women than in men and in young adults than in the elderly. In contrast completed suicide is commoner in men and in the elderly although there has recently been an increased rate of suicide in young adults. There is a higher incidence of suicide attempts among the lower socio-economic groups, particularly those living in crowded, socially deprived urban areas. They often have a deprived family background due to early loss of a parent through death or separation. There are also links with alcohol abuse, child abuse, unemployment and recently broken relationships.

A thorough psychiatric and social assessment must be carried out in all cases. In most hospitals this involves an interview with a psychiatrist. This need not always be the case because it is now recognised that junior physicians, nurses and social workers can assess these patients competently if properly trained and supervised. The assessment should be undertaken after emergency medical treatment has been completed. In patients who have taken drug overdoses it is important that sufficient time has elapsed to allow the toxic effects of the drug to wear off. Topics to be covered when assessing a patient are listed in the information box below.

ASSESSMENT OF PATIENTS AFTER ATTEMPTED SUICIDE

- Explanation of the attempt
- Degree of suicidal intent
- Presence of psychiatric illness
- Current suicidal risk
- Previous suicide attempts
- Family and personal history
- Social support available to patient
- Patient's usual ability to cope with stress
- Further management

The patient should be asked about events occurring immediately before the act and whether the attempt had been planned beforehand. In some cases there will be clear evidence that suicide was intended; the patient may have recently made a will, disposed of treasured possessions, gone to considerable effort to avoid discovery or have left an explicit suicide note. All these help explain the motivation behind the attempt. The interviewer needs to assess the severity of any current symptoms of psychiatric illness and to assess what personal and social supports are available if the patient were to leave hospital.

The majority of patients have depressive and anxiety symptoms which are reactive to an acute life crisis superimposed on a background of chronic social and personal difficulties. They do not require psychotropic medication or specialised psychiatric treatment. They need emotional support and practical advice to help them cope with the crisis which has precipitated the attempt. A social worker may be the most appropriate person to provide this help. Admission to a psychiatric ward is necessary for patients who have a major psychiatric illness, who remain intent on suicide or who require temporary respite from intolerable domestic circumstances. Admission should also be arranged when further information is needed to clarify the patient's mental state.

Approximately 20% make a repeat attempt during the following twelve months and 1% succeed in killing themselves. Factors which are known to be associated with an increased risk of suicide after a suicide attempt are listed in the information box below.

RISK FACTORS FOR SUICIDE AFTER A SUICIDE ATTEMPT

- Psychiatric illness (depressive illness, alcoholism, schizophrenia)
- Age over 45
- Male sex
- Living alone
- Unemployed
- Recently bereaved, divorced or separated
- Chronic physical ill-health
- Drug or alcohol abuse
- Violent method used (e.g. hanging, jumping)
- Suicide note written
- History of previous attempts

PSYCHIATRIC EMERGENCIES

These can occur in the community or in hospital wards but one of the commonest locations where doctors encounter psychiatric emergencies is in the accident and emergency department of a general hospital. They require urgent action because the patient's behaviour is potentially dangerous to himself or other people; the behaviour disturbance may be aggression, extreme overactivity or suicidal activity.

Rapid assessment is required. Two main decisions need to be taken. First, is the behaviour disturbance due to psychiatric illness? If not, the patient may have to be dealt with by the police. If the patient is psychiatrically ill, the second decision is whether it is an organic or functional illness. A full history and mental state examination will be out of the question. As much information as possible should be obtained from informants. This should include enquiries about recent mood change, paranoid ideas or other psychiatric symptoms. There may be a history of previous psychiatric illness, recent physical illness, head injury or drug abuse. When assessing the patient's mental state the key elements are evidence of cognitive impairment, paranoid delusions, and aggressive or suicidal intent. It is also important to understand any triggering events which have precipitated the emergency.

Many aggressive and overactive patients are frightened because their behaviour is determined by paranoid experiences. They can be calmed by a confident, non-threatening approach. It is helpful if they feel the doctor understands what has brought on their distress. If there is a high risk of violence the patient must be restrained. This should not be attempted until sufficient staff are present to overpower the patient safely. The police need to be involved if the patient is armed or causing actual physical harm. Once restraints have been imposed it is likely that sedation will be required. Haloperidol is the

Table 18.7   Important provisions of the Mental Health Act, 1983 (England and Wales)

Purpose	Section	Duration	Signatures required	Appeal
Emergency admission	4	72 hours	One doctor plus relative or social worker	None
Assessment and Treatment	2	28 days	Two doctors (one approved) plus nearest relative or social worker	To Tribunal within 14 days of admission
Treatment	3	6 months	Two doctors (one approved) plus nearest relative or social worker	To Tribunal within first 6 months and once during each subsequent period for which detention renewed
Emergency detention of patient in hospital	5 (2)	72 hours	Doctor in charge	None
Emergency detention of patient in hospital	5 (4)	6 hours	Nurse (RMN status)	None
Assessment of persons in public places thought to be mentally ill and in need of safety	136	72 hours	Police officer	None

Table 18.8   Important provisions of Mental Health (Scotland) Act, 1984

Purpose	Section	Duration	Signature required	Appeal
Emergency admission	24	72 hours	One doctor; consent of relative or mental health officer if practicable	None
Short-term detention and treatment	26	28 days (further to Section 24 or 25 (i))	Approved doctor in addition to recommendation under Section 24 or 25 (i); consent of nearest relative or mental health officer if practicable	To Sheriff or Mental Welfare Commission
Non-urgent admission	18	6 months	Two doctors (one approved); nearest relative or mental health officer; Sheriff's approval	To Mental Welfare Commission; to Sheriff if detention extended after 6 months
Emergency detention of patient in hospital	25(i)	72 hours	Doctor in charge	None
Emergency detention of patient in hospital	25(ii)	2 hours	Nurse (RMN status)	None
Detention of person in public place thought to be mentally ill and in need of safety	118	72 hours	Police officer	None

drug of choice. It can be given intravenously or intramuscularly at an initial dose of 10–20 mg; this can be repeated if necessary until the patient is calmed. A decision can then be taken about the next stage in management depending on the nature of the underlying psychiatric disorder.

LEGAL ASPECTS OF PSYCHIATRY

Psychiatry has closer links with the law than most other branches of medicine because psychiatric illness sometimes impairs judgement to the extent that the patient is not considered fully responsible for his actions. A doctor may therefore be required to prepare a report if one of his patients is considered psychiatrically ill and has been charged with committing an offence. This may need to concentrate on whether the patient is able to understand the charge brought against him, fit to plead, able to instruct a lawyer, able to follow proceedings in court and can understand the verdict. The report should describe the patient's background and mental state at the time of the assessment together with an opinion of the patient's mental state at the time the offence was committed. A summary should comment on the patient's criminal responsibility and make recommendations for future management if it is thought more appropriate for the patient to be treated in a medical context rather than be sent to prison. This may involve a probation order conditional on regular psychiatric outpatient attendance.

All doctors in clinical practice need to be familiar with the legal aspects of admitting psychiatrically ill patients to hospital against their will or detaining them in hospital after admission. It should be reiterated here that these regulations apply only to a small minority, less than 10% of psychiatric inpatients.

The law in England and Wales is governed by the Mental Health Act, 1983. This is principally concerned with the grounds for detaining patients in hospital or placing them under guardianship. Application for compulsory admission to hospital can only be made when the patient, who is suffering from mental disorder, is not willing to be admitted voluntarily and ought to be detained in the interests of his own health or safety or with a view to the protection of other persons. The definition of mental disorder includes mental illness, mental impairment and psychopathic disorder, the latter resulting in abnormally aggressive or seriously irresponsible conduct. The Act introduced significant changes to improve patients' rights by allowing appeal against detention under certain sections of the Act. Appeals are heard by a Mental Health Review Tribunal. This consists of three members, a Circuit Judge or equivalent who acts as President of the Tribunal, a medical representative and a lay representative. Table 18.7 summarises the most important sections of the Act with which doctors need to be familiar.

Similar legislation for Scotland was passed by the Mental Health (Scotland) Act, 1984. Reasons for hospital admission and detention are similar to those for England and Wales except that psychopathic disorder is not included. Appeals in Scotland can be made to the Mental Welfare Commission or to the Sheriff. The most important sections of this Act are summarised in Table 18.8.

FURTHER READING

American Psychiatric Association 1987 Diagnostic and Statistical Manual of Mental Disorders, 3rd Edn.–revised. APA, Washington

Bancroft J 1989 Human Sexuality and its problems, 2nd Edn. Churchill Livingstone, Edinburgh

Goldberg D, Benjamin S, Creed F 1987 Psychiatry in medical practice. Tavistock, London

Institute of Psychiatry, London 1987 Notes on eliciting and recording clinical information, 2nd. Edn. Oxford University Press, Oxford

Kendell R E, Zealley A K (eds) 1988 Companion to psychiatric studies, 4th Edn. Churchill Livingstone, Edinburgh

Leff J P, Isaacs A D 1981 Psychiatric examination in clinical practice, 2nd Edn. Blackwell, Oxford

Lishman W A 1987 Organic psychiatry, 2nd Edn. Blackwell, Oxford

Regier D A, Boyd J H, Burke J D, et al 1988 One-month prevalence of mental disorders in the United States. Archives of General Psychiatry 45: 977–986

Silverstone T, Turner P 1988 Drug treatment in psychiatry, 4th Edn. Routledge, London

19

Acute Poisoning

Acute poisoning is a common and urgent medical problem in all developed, and many developing, countries of the world. In Britain it accounts for 15–20% of all acute medical emergency admissions to hospital. The different types of acute poisoning, and their relative frequency in patients above the age of 12, are shown in Table 19.1. In young children, particu-

Table 19.1   Types of acute poisoning and their relative importance as causes of admission to hospital in patients above the age of 12

Type		Admissions to hospital (% of total)
Accidental		10
Intentional	True attempted suicide	10
	Self-poisoning (parasuicide)	80
	Homicide	rare

larly below the age of five, they are virtually all accidental, whereas in older age groups the great majority are intentional and self-inflicted but not suicidal. For this reason, the terms self-poisoning or para-suicide are used to distinguish this major type. This is defined as a conscious impulsive action designed

Discharges (including deaths) × 1000

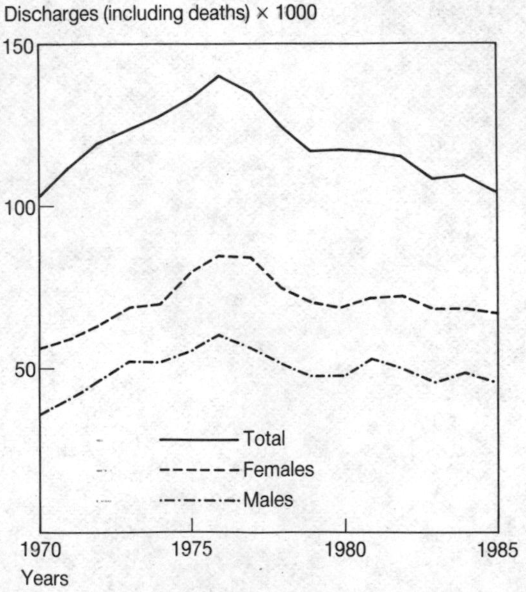

Fig. 19.1   Estimated total discharges and deaths due to the adverse effects of medicinal agents and chiefly non-medicinal substances. (Scotland, England and Wales 1970–85.) (Sources: Common Services Agency, Information Services Division. SCOTTISH HOSPITAL IN-PATIENT STATISTICS. Department of Health and Social Security and Office of Population Censuses and Surveys. Hospital In-Patient Enquiry. Welsh Office. HOSPITAL ACTIVITY ANALYSIS: MEDICAL STATISTICS.)

to secure redress of an intolerable situation with, often, strong manipulative motives. Criminal homicidal poisoning by comparison is rare.

This chapter deals with the clinical features, diagnosis, treatment and prevention of acute poisoning. Food poisoning is discussed on page 127. Brief reference is made to industrial and agricultural poisons.

EPIDEMIOLOGY

The trends in yearly admission to hospital for acute poisoning in the United Kingdom are shown in Figure 19.1. There was a dramatic and progressive increase in incidence until about 1976, since when there has been a relative decline in the frequency of admission. This may be partly due to changes in admission policy across the country during these recent years. As a result many symptomless children and up to 40% of adults reaching Accident and Emergency Departments are discharged and a further 30% are treated at home by their general practitioners. Many patients are thought not to seek medical advice and recover in their own homes. Despite this the number of patients admitted with acute poisoning remains well in excess of 100 000 each year and the true incidence of poisoning in the community is much higher.

SOCIAL PATTERNS

Acute poisoning is more common in females than in males in all age groups, the composite ratio of females to males being about 1.4:1.0. The major rise in incidence has been among patients in the second and third decades reaching levels that are now many times higher than amongst the middle-aged and elderly. The increase has been particularly marked in patients of lower social class. The rate of self-poisoning in males is more than eight times higher in the unskilled lowest social class group than in men from the professional highest social class. Divorcees have substantially higher rates than the single, married or widowed and a large proportion of patients are unemployed, have social problems such as alcoholism, criminal records, debt or a history of family violence. Up to 50% of those who self-poison have done so before, and 20% will attempt it again within twelve months. These figures for repetition are remarkably consistent from year to year in different centres in the UK, as is the frequency with which suicide follows self-poisoning. This is the case particularly in the above high-risk groups, in whom the incidence of subsequent suicide is about 1% per annum. A broadly similar picture occurs in other

European countries and in the United States there are 2.3 million acute poisonings every year.

CHANGING PATTERN OF POISONINGS

Drugs have always been the most frequent agents taken by adults and, after household products, are the commonest substances ingested by children. At least 30% of self-poisoning episodes involve more than one drug and alcohol will be taken together with the drug by 60% of males and 40% of females. In adults more than 60% ingest drugs that have been prescribed for themselves or a close relative and so the pattern of acute poisoning closely reflects prescribing habits. It is not surprising, therefore, that the major groups of drugs involved in acute poisoning at the present time are benzodiazepines, tricyclic and related antidepressant drugs and analgesics, which include paracetamol, nonsteroidal anti-inflammatory drugs and opiate analogues. The changing fashions are shown in Figure 19.2.

MORTALITY STATISTICS

In all European countries and also in those with predominant populations from European sources, such as in North America and Australasia, suicide is commoner in the elderly over 60 years and more common in all age groups in males than in females. Figure 19.3 shows the relevant pattern in England and Wales. There are large national differences which have persisted throughout this century with few changes in the rank order of countries for which statistics are available. In the United States and Australia studies of suicide rates in immigrant populations from different countries have demonstrated variations in the population similar to those of the country of origin suggesting that these variations are true national characteristics.

Since 1960 the suicide rate for young adults has increased in both sexes in more countries than it has decreased and, among the elderly, similar trends are appearing. In Britain more than 80% of deaths due to poisoning occur outside hospital and so it is important that hospital statistics should not be considered alone in an estimate of the physical consequences of poisoning in the community. In hospital, for example, there has been a dramatic fall in mortality due to this cause over the last 40 years. In 1945 up to 25% of patients admitted with acute barbiturate poisoning died. The mortality from that cause has now been reduced to 0.45% and less than 1% for all poisonings. Even in severely ill patients less

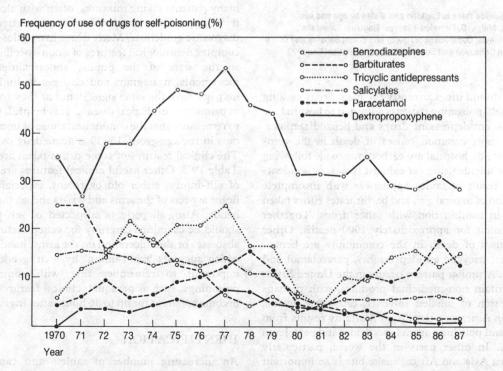

Fig. 19.2   The changing pattern of drugs involved in self-poisoning in Scotland (1970–87). (Source: Common Services Agency. Information Services Division. SCOTTISH HOSPITAL IN-PATIENT STATISTICS.)

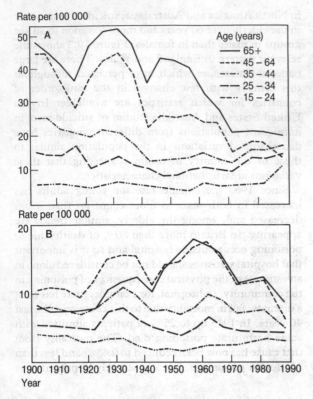

Fig. 19.3   Suicide rates in England and Wales by age and sex (1900–88). A. Males. **B.** Females. (Source: Registrar General's statistical reviews. Department of Health and Social Security and Office of Population Censuses and Surveys. Hospital In-Patient Enquiry.)

than 2% should die. Currently the main drugs causing death of self-poisoning patients admitted to hospital are analgesics, antidepressant drugs and benzodiazepines. The two most common causes of death in the community outside hospital are carbon monoxide following deliberate suicide using car exhaust fumes, or accidentally as a result of faulty appliances with incomplete combustion of natural gas, and barbiturates either taken alone or in combination with other drugs. Together these account for approximately 1900 deaths. Other major causes of death in the community are benzodiazepines, tricyclic antidepressants, paracetamol and salicylate. A similar pattern occurs in the United States but in Britain non-medicinal products, with perhaps the exception of inhaled solvents, cause few deaths, whereas in America a significant mortality results from cleaning and polishing agents, pesticides and petroleum distillates. In other parts of the world, particularly India, East Asia and Africa, snake bite is an important cause of mortality, accounting for over 30 000 deaths every year.

DIAGNOSIS

Information can be obtained immediately, on a 24-hour basis, regarding the ingredients of a substance and the approximately fatal dose of a poison from any one of the five centres in the British Isles providing the National Poisons Information Services. The telephone numbers are shown in Table 19.2.

Table 19.2   Telephone numbers of National Poisons Information Service (UK and Republic of Ireland)

London	071 635 9191
Edinburgh	031 229 2477
Cardiff	0222 709901
Belfast	02322 40503
Dublin	0001 379966

CLINICAL FEATURES

The clinical features of most poisons are non-specific, but the diagnosis is seldom in doubt as the circumstantial evidence is often strong and many patients, or their relatives or friends, give a clear history of it. When this information is lacking difficulties arise, particularly when the patient is unconscious. The range of substances involved in acute poisoning is so great, with many patients taking mixtures, often with alcohol, that it is impossible to provide comprehensive clinical diagnostic guidelines. Many drugs in overdose produce complex neurological features of a non-specific type and so the state of the pupils, abnormalities of eye movements, nystagmus and changes in limb reflexes may not have the same significance as they would have in primary neurological disease. It is helpful, therefore, to remember that the commonest cause of unconsciousness in the age group 15–35 is acute drug overdosage. The clinical features of some drugs taken are listed in Table 19.3. Other useful clinical features are evidence of self-injury, either old or recent, especially on the flexor aspects of the arms and wrists and on the face and hands. Also, all patients suspected of self-poisoning should be examined carefully for venepuncture marks, abscesses or skin ulceration on the arms, hands and feet which suggests 'main-lining' by a drug addict. It is important to remember that with some serious poisonings, such as paraquat, clinical features may not become apparent for up to 36 hours after ingestion

IDENTIFICATION

An increasing number of tablets and capsules are marked with a code letter and number and others can be recognised by their characteristic appearance. When in

Table 19.3 Clinical features of drugs or poisons

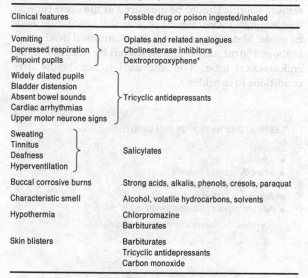

Clinical features	Possible drug or poison ingested/inhaled
Vomiting Depressed respiration Pinpoint pupils	Opiates and related analogues Cholinesterase inhibitors Dextropropoxyphene*
Widely dilated pupils Bladder distension Absent bowel sounds Cardiac arrhythmias Upper motor neurone signs	Tricyclic antidepressants
Sweating Tinnitus Deafness Hyperventilation	Salicylates
Buccal corrosive burns	Strong acids, alkalis, phenols, cresols, paraquat
Characteristic smell	Alcohol, volatile hydrocarbons, solvents
Hypothermia	Chlorpromazine Barbiturates
Skin blisters	Barbiturates Tricyclic antidepressants Carbon monoxide

* Especially likely to cause respiratory arrest, particularly if taken with alcohol or sedatives. Administration of specific opiate antagonist naloxone (0.4–2.0 mg i.v.) may be both therapeutic and diagnostic.

doubt, however, more precise identification may be obtained from hospital pharmacists and information services. The only conclusive identification is, however, toxicological analysis of urine, gastric aspirate or plasma and simple rapid screening methods are available for approximately 90% of common poisonings. It is important that the correct specimens are sent for analysis when the poison has been taken orally. Samples of vomitus or gastric aspirate, taken in the first few hours following ingestion, are ideal for diagnostic confirmation. Urine is a good alternative and often more appropriate than blood as the concentration of toxic substances or related metabolites is almost always much higher in urine than in serum or plasma. The appropriate samples are 50 ml gastric content or urine, with no added preservative, and 10 ml whole blood. Although these analyses can be carried out the results seldom influence treatment, but may be of value for medico-legal purposes. *Important common exceptions are salicylate or paracetamol overdoses in which rapid and accurate measurement of the blood levels is vital for the correct management of the poisoning.*

ASSESSMENT OF SEVERITY

The individual variation in response to drugs is very wide, depending on differences in tissue tolerance, drug interaction and the ability of an individual patient to metabolise the toxic substance. It is, therefore,

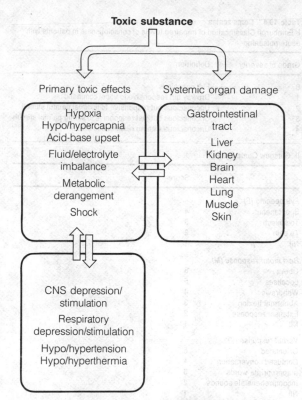

Fig. 19.4 Main ways in which a toxic substance may cause organ damage with resultant functional disturbance.

dangerous to allow efforts to identify and quantify the poisoning by laboratory means to delay emergency supportive treatment. In general, therefore, the severity of any poisoning must be judged on the basis of clinical assessment. This initial evaluation is of paramount importance, not only for determining the patients' condition from which their progress may be appraised, but also for deciding upon the treatment required.

Poisonous substances may give rise to *primary toxic effects*, which may result in *organ damage* of a non-specific or specific type (Fig. 19.4). The ensuing organ damage may then lead to respiratory or metabolic disturbance, or a combination of these, hence to a variety of clinical features. Initial physical examination, therefore, should be directed to determining the magnitude of disturbance of these vital functions and although it must be rapid, it must also be sufficiently comprehensive to detect any coincident disease which may influence the treatment given.

NEUROLOGICAL ASSESSMENT

In overdoses of hypnotic, sedative and psychotropic drugs, estimation of the level of consciousness is the

Table 19.4   Coma scales
I Edinburgh Classification of impaired levels of consciousness in patients with acute poisoning

Grade of severity	Definition
0	Full conscious
1	Drowsy but responsive to vocal command
2	Unconscious but responsive to minimal painful stimuli
3	Unconscious but just responsive to strong painful stimuli
4	Unconscious with no response to stimuli

II Glasgow Coma Scale

	Score
Eye opening (E)	
Spontaneous	4
To speech	3
To pain	2
Nil	1
Best motor response (M)	
Obeys	6
Localises	5
Withdraws	4
Abnormal flexion	3
Extensor response	2
Nil	1
Verbal response (V)	
Orientated	5
Confused conversation	4
Inappropriate words	3
Incomprehensible sounds	2
Nil	1

Coma Score = E + M + V
Minimum   = 3
Maximum   = 15

most important initial part of the neurological assessment. In acute poisoning drug effects may produce such complex neurological abnormalities that this is most effectively done using a simple grading of coma. In the Edinburgh classification the response of the patient to a standard painful stimulus is assessed. An alternative is to use the more complicated Glasgow coma scale (Table 19.4). In addition depression of respiratory, circulatory and metabolic function must also be assessed.

RESPIRATORY FUNCTION

A practical and simple screening measurement of respiratory function is measurement of the respiratory minute volume using a Wright spirometer. If the minute volume is less than four litres significant respiratory depression should be assumed and arterial blood gas analysis undertaken immediately. Accurate monitoring of the respiratory rate is a valuable part of the assessment of respiratory efficiency in poisoned patients. A consistent very high respiratory rate may result in a high minute volume even if only the dead

space is ventilated. Both the respiratory rate and the minute volume should be measured at the same time so that a rough measurement of alveolar ventilation may be made. Note that, although the anatomical dead space is about 150 ml, this is almost halved by insertion of an endotracheal tube. The information box below lists conditions to consider.

RESPIRATORY RATE > 20 PER MINUTE

Consider
- Acidosis
- Acute pulmonary oedema
- Pneumonia (inhalation/hypostatic)
- Pulmonary embolism
- Adult respiratory distress syndrome (p. 353)*

 * Develops 12–24 hours after initial poisoning.

CARDIOVASCULAR FUNCTION

Clinical assessment of circulatory function in acute poisoning is often difficult since the typical features of shock may not be apparent in the presence of central nervous depression and hypothermia. True shock occurs in less than 10% of all cases of acute poisoning but when it does occur it poses a severe threat to the patient's recovery. In practice it is reasonable to assume that shock exists if the systolic blood pressure falls below 90 mm of mercury in patients over the age of 50 and below 80 mm mercury in younger patients. The procedures for dealing with shocked patients are listed in the information box below.

TREATMENT FOR ALL 'SHOCKED' PATIENTS

- Core/peripheral temperature deficit measured (low reading rectal thermometer) as guide to adequacy of tissue perfusion
- Fluid intake and urine output measured (indwelling urinary catheter attached to urimeter) as guide to renal perfusion
- Continuous ECG monitoring to detect cardiac arrhythmias

Depression of metabolism is a common feature of many types of overdosage. Moderate hypothermia is present when the rectal temperature is 30–36°C and below 30°C this is potentially life-threatening as the body temperature in these circumstances tends to fall progressively unless active reheating is given. Hypothermia is a significant finding as it contributes to shock, acidosis and hypoxia. In severely poisoned patients electrolyte balance should be monitored by appropriate biochemical testing.

Table 19.5 Poisonings for which there are specific drug therapies

Poisoning	Antidote	
Cholinesterase inhibitors (organophosphorus insecticides)	Pralidoxime mesylate Obidoxime Atropine	see p. 979
Cyanide	Dicobalt edetate Sodium nitrite Sodium thiosulphate	see p. 976
Gold, mercury arsenic copper, zinc	Dimercaprol 2.5–5 mg/kg body weight by deep i.m. injection every 4 hours for 2 days; 2.5 mg/kg body weight twice daily for 7–14 days	
	Penicillamine 250 mgm–2 g daily orally in divided doses	
Iron	Desferrioxamine	see p. 978
Lead (inorganic)	Sodium calcium edetate 50–75 mg/kg body weight by slow i.v. injection daily for 5 days (each 2 g being diluted with 250 ml isotonic saline)	
	Penicillamine	see above
Opiates and analogues	Naloxone	see p. 978
Paracetamol	Methionine N-acetylcysteine	see p. 979
Thallium	Prussian blue 10 g twice daily until urinary excretion of thallium < 0.5 mg per 24 hours	

GENERAL PRINCIPLES OF TREATMENT

Specific antidotes are available in only about 2% of acute poisonings (Table 19.5). Some of these cause significant side-effects and therefore they should be used only where the patient has serious and possibly life-threatening poisoning. Treatment in the great majority of cases, therefore, is dependent on the application of basic but good quality modern intensive therapy on a background of careful clinical assessment, coupled with a sound knowledge of the poison involved. Although the mortality in hospital is low, there are many 'near misses' in those who subsequently recover and so patients with significant poisoning should be regarded as genuine medical emergencies.

EMERGENCY MEASURES

These are listed in the information boxes right.

Prevention of absorption of the poison

Patients with inhalant poisoning must be removed to fresh air as quickly as possible, but rescuers should, under no circumstances, expose themselves to toxic gases without care for their own safety and, if necessary, use appropriate breathing apparatus. When a liquid or solid poisoning capable of cutaneous absorption is in

---

ESTABLISHMENT AND MAINTENANCE OF A CLEAR AIRWAY

- Remove dentures, debris and secretions from the mouth and fauces.
- If patient drowsy but has good cough and gag reflex, nurse semi-prone and if possible insert oropharyngeal airway. The neck should be extended.
- If more deeply unconscious and gag reflex in doubt, insert cuffed endotracheal tube. In this case the neck should be slightly flexed.
- Keep airway patent by regular aspiration of secretions.
- Tracheostomy should be considered only if endotracheal intubation is required for longer than 7–10 days.

MAINTENANCE OF RESPIRATION

- If Pa_{O_2} is < 10 but > 8 kPa and the Pa_{CO_2} is between 5.3 and 6.6 kPa, high-flow oxygen (6–8 l per minute) should be given. In patients with suspected or known chronic obstructive airways disease use initially 24% Ventimask with an oxygen flow rate of 4 litres per minute. Provided the Pa_{CO_2} has not risen after 30 minutes, higher concentrations of oxygen may be given.
- In the presence of more serious impairment of ventilation as indicated by a rising Pa_{CO_2} administer high-flow oxygen using an Ambu bag as an emergency measure whilst arranging intubation and more formal mechanical ventilation (p. 351).

MAINTENANCE OF CIRCULATION

'Shocked' patients:
Correct hypoxia
Correct acidosis
Elevate foot of bed
If no response, institute further measures (p. 282)

In serious cardiac arrhythmias
Correct hypoxia
Correct acidosis
Administer anti-arrhythmic drugs* (p. 273)

Intensive cardio-respiratory resuscitation may be required (p. 272)

* Particular attention must be given to the pharmacological actions of the poisoning to avoid adverse reactions to the anti-arrhythmic therapy.

---

contact with the patient's clothes these must be removed and any poison on the skin washed off carefully with soap and water. Care should also be taken during these procedures to avoid personal contamination. When the poison has been swallowed measures to limit further absorption of ingested poisons include the following.

Oral adsorbents

The role of these substances, of which activated charcoal is the safest, is debatable. However, activated charcoal given with water can be usefully used when emesis and gastric aspiration and lavage are contra-indicated, and also as an adjunct to these procedures. In the case of emesis, the vomiting should be over before the charcoal is given. The effective ratio of charcoal to estimated amount of poison to be adsorbed is of the order of 10:1. It is therefore most useful when the poison ingested is toxic in small doses such as tricyclic antidepressants.

Induction of emesis

The oral administration of syrup of ipecacuanha pediatric BPC has gained popularity in the treatment of poisoned patients as a means of effective gastric emptying. It should be used only in conscious patients within four hours of ingestion of a potentially toxic dose of poison. Exceptions to this are salicylate, tricyclic antidepressants and other anticholinergic drugs, where useful recoveries are obtained up to 12 hours following ingestion. It is contraindicated in poisoning with petroleum distillates as vomiting of these carries a high risk of aspiration into the lungs. Also it should not be used following ingestion of corrosive substances. The effective dosage regimen is 10 ml in children aged 6–18 months, 15 ml in older children and 30 ml in adults. This should be followed by a drink of 200 ml water. The dosage may be repeated after 20 minutes if emesis has not occurred. This is the treatment of choice in young children in whom gastric emptying is indicated, but its use should be reserved for hospital practice in view of the danger of aspiration pneumonia.

Gastric aspiration and lavage

The indications and contraindications for gastric aspiration and lavage are the same as those for induction of emesis, but with some important exceptions:

1. Gastric aspiration and lavage is indicated in unconscious patients irrespective of the time after ingestion since a toxic dose has clearly been taken and in these patients gastric motility and, therefore, emptying may be considerably impaired.
2. The procedure should only be done in these patients if an endotracheal tube has been inserted.
3. When corrosive poisons have been ingested there is a substantial risk of perforation of the oesophagus or stomach during the procedure and, on the whole, it is best avoided in these patients. In some corrosive poisonings such as paraquat, however, the danger of systemic toxicity is high and in such cases cautious lavage is indicated.

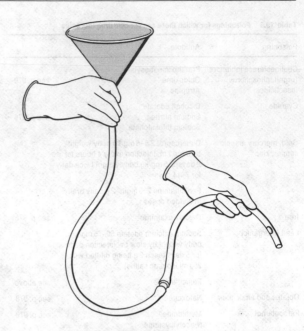

Fig. 19.5   Apparatus for gastric lavage.

4. In patients with chronic alcoholism special care must also be taken to avoid rupture of possible oesophageal varices.

The technique of gastric aspiration and lavage is described in the information box (p. 975).

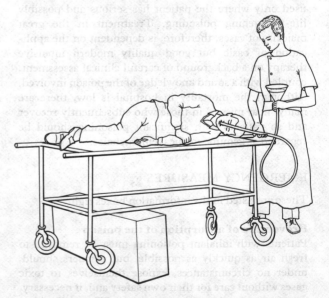

Fig. 19.6   Position of patient for gastric emesis and gastric aspiration and lavage.

TECHNIQUE OF GASTRIC ASPIRATION AND LAVAGE

- Proceed only if there is a good cough reflex or if a cuffed endotracheal tube has been inserted.
- Place the patient recumbent in the left lateral position.
- Pass a lubricated large bore soft rubber Jacques tube (30 English gauge). The position of the tube may be checked by aspiration of gastric content or by blowing a small amount of air down the tube and auscultating over the epigastrium.
- Aspirate by lowering the free end of the tube, to which a large funnel is attached, below the level of the patient. If required for toxicological analysis, collect 50 ml of the fluid aspirated or of the first lavage cycle.
- Lavage is carried out by pouring 300 ml portions of warm water slowly down the tube and syphoning as for aspiration until the recovered fluid is clear. Care should be taken to empty the stomach as far as possible after each lavage.
- Tubes and other apparatus should be carefully cleaned and sterilised after each procedure.

Other methods of elimination of poisons

If considerable absorption has occurred the patient may be gravely ill; hence measures to enhance elimination of the poison may be required. These can be carried out only in hospital because of the technical skill and special apparatus required. They include forced diuresis (p. 980), peritoneal dialysis, hemodialysis and hemoperfusion. In recent years attempts have been made to develop safer ways of increasing removal of toxic substances from the body. The most effective of these is hemoperfusion whereby heparinised blood from the patient is passed through a column containing granules of activated charcoal coated with synthetic acrylic hydrogel or, alternatively, ion exchange resins. This method may be life-saving for some severe poisonings, such as those due to medium and short-acting barbiturates, glutethimide, methacholine and meprobamate, for which previous techniques of elimination were inadequate. It is indicated, however, only in seriously ill patients in whom intensive supportive therapy fails.

Additional supportive therapy

Hypothermia is common in severely poisoned patients. In moderate cases (p. 972) the aim of treatment is to prevent further heat loss by nursing the patient covered in a space blanket in a humid but warm room between 26 and 29°C. In severe hypothermia, where the above treatment is ineffective, active heating is required. This may provoke serious cardiac arrhythmias and irreversible peripheral circulatory failure and so should be done with caution, especially in elderly patients. Reheating may be achieved by heating the inspired air by passing administered oxygen through a Water's

canister or, by immersing one forearm in water at 43°C in addition to the above measures. Intravenous fluids should be brought to warm room temperature prior to infusion. Acid-base disturbances should be corrected and fluid and electrolyte balance achieved by appropriate replacement therapy. Epileptiform convulsions should be treated with intravenous diazepam (p. 859).

Table 19.6 Psychiatric disposal of patients admitted with acute poisoning related to the depth of coma (Edinburgh classification) at the time of admission

Psychiatric disposal	Grade of coma		
	0–2 (%)	3 (%)	4 (%)
In-patient care	20	31	28
Out-patient care	36	38	34
Other (e.g. GP, social care)	44	31	38

PSYCHIATRIC ASSESSMENT

It is important to recognise that the management of poisoned patients, particularly the very large majority who are suffering from self-poisoning, is incomplete without early and adequate psychiatric assessment and management. It is established that the size of the overdose bears little relation to the severity of the underlying psychological or sociological upset (Table 19.6). Ideally the psychiatrist should become involved as quickly as possible before the circumstances of the poisoning are obscured or rationalised. In reality, however, the numbers of patients presenting with acute poisoning are now so great that it has become necessary to try to be more selective in the patients actually admitted to hospital for this reason.

The recognition of patients who have genuine suicidal tendencies, or may be in need of other help in association with their poisoning, is difficult in practice, particularly for young and inexperienced doctors in Accident and Emergency Departments. There is no problem if the patient is significantly poisoned as all of these require admission for physical as well as psychiatric assessment. The difficulty arises when the patient shows only minimal signs of acute poisoning and, from the history, there is little likelihood of any physical signs appearing later. The risk of repetition and possibly suicide remains and the decision for admission or not has to be made. The information box (p. 976) gives some of the main indications for admission irrespective of the physical condition of the patient. Where there is any doubt, however, it is wise for the patient to come into hospital.

INDICATIONS FOR ADMISSION OF PATIENTS WITH ACUTE POISONING IRRESPECTIVE OF THEIR PHYSICAL CONDITION

- A verbal or written statement of suicidal intent or suspicion of this
- A diagnosis or suspicion of accompanying psychiatric illness, especially depression
- Evidence of self-injury
- History of previous self-poisoning
- If living alone, especially if the self-poisoning occurs at night or during main holiday periods
- If it is not possible for the patient to stay with relatives or reliable friends
- If adequate assessment cannot be made

NOTES ON CLINICAL FEATURES AND TREATMENT OF POISONING AND ENVENOMATION BY SPECIFIC AGENTS
(including common insect stings and poisoning by marine animals, mushrooms, scorpions, snakes, spiders, ticks and vegetables)

The following descriptions are directed primarily towards adults. For children, appropriate adjustments in doses of drugs suggested in treatment regimens would require to be made.

Amphetamine group. *Clinical features.* Alertness, excitement, tremor and insomnia are common. Confusion, aggressiveness, hallucinations and even homicidal tendencies may occur. Initial excitement may give way to lethargy and depression. Brisk reflexes, tachycardia and hypertension occur and nausea, vomiting, diarrhoea and abdominal colic may be severe. In heavy overdosage convulsions and deep unconsciousness are characteristic.

Treatment (1) General measures. (2) Droperidol (5–15 mg) or haloperidol (5–10 mg) by slow intravenous injection are the recommended treatments. Alternatively, chlorpromazine 100 mg intramuscularly. (3) In severe poisoning, forced diuresis using intravenous ammonium chloride to make the urine acid.

Barbiturates. *Clinical features.* Absorption is unpredictable but drowsiness and coma develop rapidly. The duration of cerebral depression varies greatly with the type of barbiturate taken, the dose and the tolerance of the patient. In general a large dose of short- or medium-acting barbiturate causes more severe poisoning than long-acting phenobarbitone. Changes in the pupils and limb reflexes are very variable and are unreliable guides to the severity of the poisoning. Withdrawal features such as restlessness, insomnia, delirium and convulsions may occur. Ventilatory depression and hypotension may be severe. Hypothermia is common and if severe may be associated with renal failure. Bullous lesions occur in 6% of patients with acute barbiturate overdosage especially with short- or medium-acting drugs.

Treatment. (1) General measures with particular emphasis on respiratory and cardiovascular support. (2) When these measures fail, haemodialysis for phenobarbitone and barbitone, and charcoal haemoperfusion for short- and medium-acting barbiturates.

Benzodiazepines. *Clinical features.* Drowsiness, ataxia, dizziness, hypotension and ventilatory depression may all occur, but the toxic effects are usually surprisingly mild.

Treatment. General supportive treatment is adequate in almost all cases.

Beta-adrenoceptor antagonists. *Clinical features.* Bradycardia and hypotension with low output cardiac failure. Bronchospasm. Cardio-respiratory arrest may occur. Drowsiness, delirium, fits and hallucinations. Hypoglycaemia.

Treatment. (1) Gastric aspiration and lavage if appropriate and intensive supportive measures. (2) When bradycardia is severe, atropine 0.6–3 mg intravenously (50 µg/kg in children), followed if necessary by isoprenaline 2 mg diluted in 500 ml normal saline or 5% dextrose at a rate of 20–40 drops per minute depending on the response. A cardiac pacemaker should be inserted. (3) If significant hypotension occurs, the inotropic action of glucagon is beneficial – 50–150 µg/kg intravenously over 1 minute, followed by an infusion of 1–5 mg/h. In severe cases dobutamine infusion 2.5–20 µg/kg/min may be effective. (4) For bronchospasm, salbutamol by nebuliser. Intravenous salbutamol or aminophylline may be required. (5) Intravenous glucose for hypoglycaemia.

Cocaine. This is now a common drug of abuse. Acute toxicity may arise following inhalation, ingestion or injection. *Clinical features.* Euphoria, excitement, restlessness, feeling of great power, vomiting, pyrexia, mydriasis, delirium, tremor, convulsions, hyperrflexia. Hypertension, hypotension, tachycardia, ventricular arrhythmias, cardiac failure. Hyperventilation and respiratory failure.

Treatment. Symptomatic and supportive measures. *Note.* Avoid beta-blockers to treat hypertension or sinus tachycardia as these cardiac effects tend to be transient and beta-blockade may cause cardiac failure.

Corrosives. *Clinical features.* Stains and burns of the mouth, lips and fauces. Abdominal pain, shock and hepatic or renal damage.

Treatment. (1) General measures. (2) Gastric lavage is contraindicated in severe poisoning. (3) Neutralise acid or alkali. Milk by mouth is often the most effective available treatment. (4) Analgesics, blood transfusion and correction of acid-base balance all may be required.

Cyanides and hydrocyanic acid. *Clinical features.* Odour of bitter almonds with shallow breathing; pink colour of skin and mucosa; widely dilated pupils and shock.

Treatment. This is very urgent. (1) General measures. (2) Cobalt edetate 600 mg in 20 ml intravenously over 1 minute. (3) If no recovery in the next minute, repeat 300 mg cobalt edetate. (4) If no response to cobalt edetate, give 10 ml i.v. of 3% sodium nitrite solution, followed by 25 ml i.v. of 50% sodium thiosulphate solution. (5) If ingested, gastric lavage with 50% sodium thiosulphate. (6) Correct acidosis with i.v. sodium bicarbonate.

Dextropropoxyphene. See opium alkaloids.

Digoxin. (p. 276).

Dinitro-ortho-cresol weedkillers. *Clinical features.* These may develop very rapidly. Yellow skin and burns of the lips and mouth. Anxiety, restlessness, fatigue, convulsions and coma. Tachypnoea, pulmonary oedema, hyperpyrexia and intense sweating are common. Acute renal and liver failure may result.

Treatment. (1) Wash exposed skin. (2) Sedation with chlorpromazine 100 mg intramuscularly. (3) General measures. (4) Tepid sponging to reduce temperature.

Domestic bleach. *Clinical features.* Local irritation if on contact with skin. If inhaled, cough and possible pulmonary oedema. If ingested, burning sensation of mouth and fauces, nausea and vomiting.

Treatment. (1) Gastric lavage with 2.5% sodium thiosulphate or alternatively with milk. If severely ill sodium thiosulphate (1%) 250 ml intravenously.

Ethanol. See blood levels page 989.

Fish and other marine animals. Poisonous fish are numerous and widely distributed around the world. In some areas they are a common source of poisoning.

CIGUATERA POISONING. This is common, particularly in the Indo-Pacific and the Caribbean. It occurs sporadically after eating reef-dwelling fishes, which are popular items of diet. It is impossible to identify fish which are poisonous from others which are not and the toxins responsible are unaffected by all forms of preparation and cooking. Ciguatoxin is the cause of poisoning and the primary source is thought to be an alga (*Gambierdiscus toxicus*) eaten by herbivorous fish such as parrot fish and surgeon fish. Ultimately carnivorous fish such as barracuda also become poisonous.

Clinical features. The onset of symptoms is usually 1–6 hours after eating toxic fish, but may vary from a few minutes to 30 hours. Numbness and paraesthesiae of the lips, tongue and throat are common, followed by abdominal pain, diarrhoea, headache, arthralgia and myalgia. In 20% of patients, dyspnoea, hypotension and paresis occur.

Treatment. Principally symptomatic with bed-rest and analgesics. Most patients recover after about 3 days, and sometimes arthralgia and myalgia may be prolonged.

SCROMBOID FISH POISONING. The flesh of scromboid fish, such as mackerel, tuna, bonito and skipjack, has a high free histidine content. Many bacteria decarboxylate histidine to histamine and, if fish become contaminated by these organisms, large amounts of histamine accumulate in the flesh.

Clinical features. Flushing, headache, dizziness, abdominal cramps and symptoms of gastroenteritis occur. These usually develop 30 minutes after ingestion and the upset lasts for about 4 hours.

Treatment. Symptomatic.

SHELLFISH POISONING. Paralytic shellfish poisoning results from eating filter-feeding shellfish such as mussels, clams, oysters and scallops contaminated by the toxic protozoa, *Gonyaulax catanella* and *G. tamarensis*. The neurotoxin involved is called saxitoxin. These protozoa tend to colour the sea when present in numbers and fishing communities are well aware that it is dangerous to eat molluscs when the tide is red, blue or green. Food poisoning due to infected shellfish is described on page 127

Clinical features. Circumoral paraesthesia, a 'floating' feeling, headache, nausea, vomiting and diarrhoea are common with, in severe cases, weakness, dysarthria and respiratory depression.

Treatment. (1) Gastric aspiration and lavage. (2) Symptomatic and supportive therapy. A less severe, but similar, poisoning results from eating shellfish contaminated by another dinoflagellate, *Gymnodinium breve*. The resultant illness is self-limiting, requiring only symptomatic treatment.

TETRODOTOXIC POISONING. This is generally known as 'puffer fish poisoning'. These fish are found in all warm and tropical seas. In Japan the detoxicated puffer fish ('fugu') is a popular delicacy. The mortality is as high as 50% because tetrodotoxin is one of the most powerful neurotoxins known.

Clinical features. Early symptoms are circumoral paraesthesiae, malaise, hypotension, dizziness and a feeling of 'floating in air'. In severe poisoning, ataxia, dysphagia and profound descending neuromuscular paralysis develop.

Treatment is symptomatic as there is no known antidote.

VENOMOUS MARINE ANIMALS. Serious illness from venomous marine creatures is rare in temperate waters. Poisoning by sea snakes is described under snake bites.

VENOMOUS FISH. Although many species occur, only two major groups are of real significance, the sting-rays and scorpion fishes. All sting-rays inhabit warm or tropical coastal waters with the exception of one fresh water variety in South America. These fish will sting only if stood upon by mistake. Scorpion fish include the zebra fishes, the true scorpion fishes and the stone fishes. The spines of these fish are their offensive weapons and they are all capable of aggressive stinging. The stone fishes are particularly poisonous and zebra fishes are becoming popular for domestic aquaria.

Clinical features. Immediate intense pain and swelling at the site of the sting. Severe tissue necrosis may occur and systemic features include nausea, vomiting and diarrhoea. Cardiac arrhythmias may occur.

Treatment. (1) Analgesics and local anaesthesia if pain severe. (2) Careful cleansing of the wound and surgical removal of the sting sheath if it has been retained. (3) The venoms are heat-labile and if possible the wound should be immersed in water as hot as can be borne for 1 hour. (4) In the case of stone fish antivenoms are available.

VENOMOUS MOLLUSCS. Only two members of this very large species are venomous to man. These are the cone shells and the octopuses. The cone shells are not uncommon causes of poisoning as the colourful shells are eagerly collected. These predatory gastropods catch their prey by shooting out a dart-like tooth attached to a muscular venom gland. The only octopuses of importance are the small blue ringed octopuses of Australia which have toxic saliva and this may flow into wounds made by the beak of the octopus.

Clinical features. There is a local inflammatory response with generalised paraesthesia. This is rapidly followed by muscular paresis which in severe poisoning may result in respiratory failure. Fatalities have occurred.

Treatment. Symptomatic and supportive therapy.

VENOMOUS COELENTERATA. These include the hydroids, jellyfish, sea anemones and corals. Although many of these animals may cause painful and at times disfiguring stings, few fatalities have resulted. The most important are the Portuguese man-of-war (*Physalia physalis*), sea wasps (*Cubomedusae*) and the true jellyfishes *Chironex fleckeri* and *Chiropsalmus quadrigatus*. Some authors suggest that only *Chironex* should be considered truly lethal. The precise toxins are not yet fully identified but haemolytic, dermatonecrotic and cardiotoxic substances have all been isolated.

Clinical features. All species cause intense pain at the site of envenomation and large wheals appear which may become necrotic, leading to extensive scar formation. Severe abdominal and generalised pains may result. In severe poisoning the patient rapidly loses consciousness with cyanosis and hypotension. Death may occur quickly or be delayed for some hours.

Treatment. (1) Analgesics and local anaesthesia if pain severe. (2) Any tentacles must be carefully removed with adhesive tape. The bare hand should not be used as the tentacles may still be capable of causing stings for many hours after removal from the water. Vinegar can be used to inactivate adhering tentacles, but alcohol solutions should not be used as this may stimulate further stinging. (3) Antivenom for sea-wasp stings is available.

At certain seasons 'Irukandji stings' affect bathers in the sea off N.E. Australia. They are caused by minute *Carybdeid* (simple sea-wasps). Acute poisoning develops in a few minutes characterised by violent abdominal and generalised pains, vomiting and prostration. After a few days of acute illness, full recovery always occurs.

Insect stings. Stings from ants, wasps, hornets and bees result only in local pain and swelling, unless the sting is on the mouth or tongue when local oedema may cause respiratory distress. Occasionally deaths may result from very extensive stings or more commonly due to severe anaphylaxis in individuals previously sensitised particularly to bee stings.

Clinical features. (1) Local pain and oedema. (2) Severe cases may become shocked; local tissue necrosis, acute haemolysis and acute nephritis may occur.

Treatment. Bee stings are acid and wasp, hornet and ant stings are alkaline. Local application is soothing, e.g. bicarbonate for bee, vinegar for wasp; systemic antihistamines may be helpful. The barbed bee stings should be removed as soon as possible as the gland attached continues to release venom. In severe sensitivity reactions, subcutaneous adrenaline (0.5 ml) and hydrocortisone (100 mg) intravenously may be life-saving. Allergic patients should carry adrenaline for immediate self-injection. In some, desensitisation has proved helpful.

See also scorpion, spider and tick.

Iron salts. *Clinical features.* These are more severe in children but this poisoning is potentially dangerous at all ages. It occurs in four stages. The predominant initial features are epigastric pain, nausea and vomiting. Haematemesis is frequent and may cause shock. Respiration and pulse are rapid. These symptoms may settle after a few hours and there may then be a quiescent period lasting for up to several days, suggesting that all is well, but then frequent black and offensive stools may be passed, followed by acute encephalopathy and circulatory failure. Most deaths occur in this second stage, but even if the patient survives, acute liver and renal failure may develop later and both carry a high mortality. Particularly in children 2–6 weeks after ingestion stricture formation may occur in the upper gastrointestinal tract, especially in the pyloric antrum, with vomiting and other features of high intestinal obstruction. A serum iron concentration > 90 µmol/l indicates the need for treatment.

Treatment. Speed is essential. (1) An intramuscular injection of 2 g desferrioxamine is given immediately (1 g in a child). (2) Gastric lavage is performed following which 5 g desferrioxamine is left in the stomach. (3) This is followed by an intravenous infusion of desferrioxamine in saline, dextrose or blood. The amounts should not exceed 15 mg/kg body weight/hour up to a maximum of 80 mg/kg in 24 hours. (4) Full supportive treatment for convulsions, shock, acidosis, blood loss and electrolyte disturbance.

Lithium carbonate/citrate. *Clinical features.* Nausea, vomiting, apathy and sluggishness. Coarse tremor, hypertonicity, vertigo, dysarthria, muscular rigidity and twitching, ataxia, convulsions. Hepatic dysfunction. ECG changes including first degree AV block, prolongation of QRS and QT intervals.

Treatment. (1) Gastric emesis or lavage, if appropriate. (2) Supportive therapy. (3) Peritoneal or haemodialysis if plasma level > 5 mmol/l. Haemodialysis is the more effective. Continue dialysis till plasma lithium level is < 1 mmol/l. *Note.* Forced diuresis is ineffective.

Mushrooms. Serious poisoning is uncommon in Britain. Considering the many types of fungi, a relatively small number are poisonous. The difficulty is that identification of these harmful species is not easy and often dangerous mushrooms grow in the same places as edible varieties. The commonest types of mushroom poisoning result from eating species containing heat-labile toxins, many of which have not been identified. These cause acute and sometimes severe abdominal colic with diarrhoea, nausea and vomiting developing about

two hours after ingestion. Occasionally the features are those of muscarine toxicity with parasympathetic stimulation which can be counteracted with atropine 0.6–2.0 mg in the adult. If the patient is excited or disorientated, atropine should not be given and chlorpromazine prescribed instead. The Common Ink Cap (*Coprinus atramentarius*) contains coprine which has a disulfiram-like action and, if taken with alcohol, provokes acute vomiting.

A trend amongst adolescents has been to ingest 'Magic' mushrooms (*Psilocybe semilanceate*) and *Panaeolus foenisecii* containing psilocybin and psilocin, which are hallucinogens. The amount required to obtain a 'trip' varies greatly from individual to individual and so some develop acute toxic effects. Acute gastroenteritis may result with visual hallucinations lasting up to 6 hours. Occasionally the symptoms last for several days and acute psychiatric upset has been reported continuing for weeks.

DEATH CAP (AMANITA PHALLOIDES). This mushroom accounts for 90% of all deaths due to mushroom poisoning in Britain. It contains two types of toxin; phallotoxins, which cause severe gastroenteritis within 6–12 hours of ingestion, and amatoxins, which also may cause gastric upset, but the major effect is delayed and results in liver and renal tubular damage. These toxins are heat-stable and may survive cooking.

Clinical features. After an initial delay of 6–12 hours and occasionally as long as 24 hours, acute and usually severe gastroenteritis with abdominal colic. The patient may then seem to improve before the onset of liver and renal damage.

Treatment. (1) If possible the mushrooms eaten should be identified, ideally by an expert in mushrooms. It is useful to remember that the later the onset of abdominal symptoms, the more likely it is to be a serious poisoning. (2) Gastric aspiration and lavage. (3) Careful medical care for liver and renal failure if these develop. Haemodialysis and haemoperfusion are ineffective in removing the toxins but the former may be required for renal failure and the latter for liver failure.

Other species of mushroom which produce similar toxic effects to *A. phalloides* are the North American *Deadly Agaric* (*A. verna*), *A. virosa* and some types of *Galerina*.

Non-steroidal anti-inflammatory drugs (NSAID) (p. 773). *Clinical features.* This is a varied group of compounds but the toxic effects in overdosage are relatively similar. Nausea, vomiting, abdominal pain and gastrointestinal hemorrhage; headache, tinnitus, hyperventilation, restlessness, agitation disorientation, hyperreflexia, nystagmus and convulsions; drowsiness, coma and respiratory depression may occur. Haematuria, proteinuria and acute renal failure; hepatic dysfunction; respiratory alkalosis, metabolic acidosis and hyperglycaemia.

Treatment. (1) Gastric lavage following which leave 50–100 g activated charcoal in the stomach. (2) Oral activated charcoal 50 g every 4 hours. (3) Diazepam 5–10 mg intravenously for convulsions. (4) Cimetidine 200 mg intravenously every 4–6 hours. (5) General supportive treatment.

Opium alkaloids (dextropropoxyphene). *Clinical features.* Pinpoint pupils, pallor, nausea and vomiting, depressed respiration and coma are characteristic. These effects are potentiated by alcohol and the combination may cause sudden respiratory and cardiac arrest which may occur even in previously healthy young people.

Treatment. (1) General measures. (2) If ingested gastric lavage with very dilute potassium permanganate – 1 in 10 000. (3) Naloxone 0.4 mg intravenously and 0.8 mg repeated intravenously 3 minutes later, if required. In heavy overdosage larger quantities may be necessary. The patient should be kept under close observation and naloxone repeated if required.

Organophosphorus compounds. *Clinical features.* These insecticides are very toxic. Being cholinesterase inhibitors, the symptoms and rationale of treatment are explained by excess cholinergic activity. Clinical features include constricted pupils; cold perspiration; salivation, nausea, vomiting and diarrhoea; twitching, which may go on to convulsions; bradycardia; bronchospasm, intense bronchorrhoea and pulmonary oedema.

Treatment. (1) Remove contaminated clothing and wash skin, but take care to wear protective gloves. (2) General measures including meticulous care of the airway. (3) Atropine 2 mg intravenously, but if cyanosis is present this must first be corrected by oxygen therapy. The atropine is repeated at 5–10 minute intervals to achieve full atropinisation and this is maintained for at least 2–3 days. (4) Pralidoxime should be given in addition to atropine in a dose of 30 mg/kg intravenously at a rate not exceeding 500 mg per minute and repeated every 30 minutes as necessary. More recently obidoxime 3 mg/kg body weight by intramuscular injection has been reported to be more effective than pralidoxime as it has a faster action and crosses the blood-brain barrier. When these cholinesterase reactivators take effect the dosage of atropine should be reduced to avoid atropine toxicity.

Paracetamol (acetaminophen). *Clinical features.* Nausea and vomiting initially, but at first symptoms are often non-specific. After about 36 hours in severe poisoning (plasma paracetamol levels above the 'treatment' line shown in Fig. 19.7) more serious toxic effects may develop including hypotension, hypothermia, metabolic acidosis, hypoglycaemia, hypoprothrombinaemia, renal failure and delirium. The main

danger, however, is acute liver failure which tends to develop several days after ingestion and carries a high mortality. As a result of many studies it has been found that single plasma paracetamol levels taken after 4 hours following ingestion of the paracetamol (Fig. 19.7) provide good prognostic indicators for the development of liver toxicity and it is on these that the decision to give specific antidote therapy is made. Emergency measurement of blood levels is essential, therefore, in the assessment of the severity of this poisoning.

Treatment. (1) General measures. (2) In patients in whom specific treatment is indicated (Fig. 19.7) to prevent or reduce acute liver damage two alternative treatments are available, (a) oral methionine or (b) intravenous N-acetylcysteine. The drugs are both sulphydryl (SH) group donors and increase hepatic glutathione availability. Both must be given within 10 hours of ingestion of the paracetamol if liver damage is to be prevented and they are ineffective after 16 hours. The regimen for oral methionine is 2.5 g stat, then 2.5 g every 4 hours for a further 3 doses, the total dose being 10 g methionine over 12 hours. In the case of N-acetylcysteine an initial dose of 150 mg/kg in 200 ml 5% glucose is given intravenously over 15 minutes, followed by an infusion of 50 mg/kg in 500 ml 5% glucose in 4, 8 and 8 hours (total 300 mg/kg in 20 hours). (3) Intravenous glucose may be required to correct hypoglycaemia. (4) The best investigation to assess impending acute liver failure is the prothrombin time ratio. If this rises above 3.0 full medical prophylaxis to combat hepatic encephalopathy must be started. (5) Charcoal haemoperfusion for fulminant liver failure. (6) Haemodialysis for acute renal failure.

Paraffin and petroleum distillates. *Clinical features.* Pallor; vomiting and diarrhoea; cough and dyspnoea.

Treatment. (1) Do not wash out stomach (p. 974). (2) Antibiotics if aspiration has occurred. (3) General measures.

Paraquat dichloride. This herbicide is very toxic in the concentrated liquid form supplied to farmers and horticulturists. A granular preparation is available for domestic use.

Clinical features. These may be divided into local and systemic effects.

Local: contact with the eyes results in severe corneal and conjunctival inflammation. On the skin, acute irritation and even blistering may occur. If inhaled, epistaxis and severe pharyngitis/laryngitis. Following ingestion, burning sensation in the mouth, oesophagus, and abdomen. Ulceration of the lips, tongue and pharynx. These features may be absent at first but develop gradually over several hours and are usually at a peak within 24 hours.

Systemic: usually follow ingestion and involve multiple organ failure. Nausea, sweating and vomiting. Tremors and convulsions may occur. Some days after ingestion (even up to a week) dyspnoea with pulmonary oedema due to a relentless proliferative alveolitis and bronchitis. Myocardial and renal failure may accompany these changes but often resolve spontaneously or respond to supportive treatment. Methaemoglobinaemia occurs rarely. Death is usually from respiratory failure.

Treatment. (1) Immediate emesis and gastric lavage leaving 250 ml of a 30% solution of Fuller's Earth, or 7% Bentonite, in the stomach. Repeat doses of Fuller's Earth (or Bentonite) every 4 hours for the following 48 hours. This should be accompanied by regular doses of magnesium (or sodium) sulphate orally to prevent the above adsorbent material causing intestinal obstruction. (2) Supportive treatment with special emphasis on fluid and electrolyte balance. (3) Haemoperfusion or haemodialysis may be of value if started

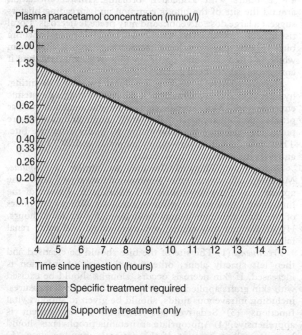

Plasma paracetamol concentration (mmol/l)

2.64
2.00
1.33
0.62
0.53
0.40
0.33
0.26
0.20
0.13

4 5 6 7 8 9 10 11 12 13 14 15

Time since ingestion (hours)

▓ Specific treatment required

▨ Supportive treatment only

Fig. 19.7 Graph for prediction of hepatic toxicity in acute paracetamol poisoning in relation to plasma paracetamol concentrations as an indication for the use of specific protective treatment.

early in mild or moderately severe poisoning, but do not prevent a fatal outcome in severe cases. (4) Methylene blue 1–2 mg/kg body weight (0.1 ml of a 1% solution/kg body weight) slowly intravenously if methaemoglobinaemia occurs.

Salicylates. *Clinical features.* Young children are much more susceptible to the toxic effects of salicylates than adults, particularly to the complex and altering metabolic disturbances which occur. Coma is common in children, in contrast to adults in whom coma is seen only in very severe poisoning. In adults, plasma salicylate levels above 3.6 mmol/l (50 mg/100 ml) indicate moderate or severe poisoning. In this situation, characteristic features are tinnitus, deafness and blurring of vision. Restlessness, sweating and increased metabolic rate also occur. Hyperventilation results in respiratory alkalosis. There may be vomiting and this, together with hyperventilation and profuse sweating, often results in severe dehydration. Hypokalaemia is common. The initial respiratory alkalosis is frequently followed by a metabolic acidosis, which may be severe, especially in children. Despite these formidable fluid, electrolyte and acid-base disturbances the patients may seem less ill than they really are. Marked acidosis should be regarded as a very serious feature as it may herald sudden respiratory or cardiac arrest.

Treatment. (1) General measures, but gastric aspiration and lavage should be done in all patients when practicable. (2) In moderate or severe poisoning *forced alkaline diuresis* should be given. The following should be mixed together and given intravenously at a rate of 2 litres hourly for 3 hours:

Saline (0.9%) .... 0.5 litre
Glucose (5%) .... 1 litre
Sodium bicarbonate (1.26%) .... 0.5 litre
Potassium chloride .... 3 g

If this regimen of diuresis cannot be given because of renal or cardiac impairment, peritoneal dialysis or haemodialysis are effective. Careful monitoring of fluid replacement, electrolyte and acid-base status must be carried out during this treatment.

Scorpion stings. Many genera of scorpions are found in the tropics and subtropics. Stings can cause dangerous poisoning. In Mexico, for example, 1000 deaths occur per year. Paired poison glands are situated in the terminal segment of the jointed tail.

Clinical features. (1) Intense local pain occurs immediately around the single puncture site, followed by erythema, swelling and sometimes ecchymosis. (2) Severe systemic features may follow, especially in children, such as sweating, salivation, nausea, vomiting and respiratory depression. Disseminated intravascular coagulation may occur, and in Trinidad, acute but usually reversible pancreatitis is a feature of stings from the scorpion, *Tityus trinitatis.*

Treatment. (1) A firm pressure bandage should be applied to limit the spread of the neurotoxic venom. (2) Analgesics and general supportive therapy. (3) In children, antivenom (5 ml i.m.) should be given if available. (4) Specific treatment of disseminated intravascular coagulation, if present.

Snake bite. In Britain there is only one indigenous poisonous snake, the adder (*Vipera berus*) which seldom causes significant poisoning. Serious snake bites may still occur as dangerous snakes are kept in zoos and by amateurs, often in less than ideal circumstances. There are three families of medically important venomous snakes. All have fangs at the front of their mouths whereby they inject venom from the parotid glands. The *Elapidae* (cobras, mambas, kraits, tiger snakes, and coral snakes) are found in all parts of the world except Europe. They have short fangs and are land snakes, the venom of which produce neurotoxic features. Local tissue necrosis may occur, a feature characteristic of venom of Asian cobras and the African spitting cobra. The *Hydrophidae* (sea snakes), which abound in the Asian-Pacific coastal waters, also have short fangs and characteristic flattened tails. The venom of these snakes is myotoxic. The *Viperidae*, which have long erectile fangs, are divided into *Viperinae* (true vipers) such as the European adder, Russell's viper and Carpet viper. These occur in all parts of the world except America and the Asian-Pacific area. The second sub-group is the *Crotalidae* (pit vipers) such as rattlesnakes, Fer-de-lance and Malayan pit viper which have a small heat-sensitive pit between eye and nostrils. The venom of the *Viperidae* is vasculo-toxic.

At least 50% of people bitten by snakes suffer few or no toxic effects as little or no venom has been injected. By contrast, if the dose of venom is high mortality without effective treatment is 10% in *Elapidae* poisoning within 5–20 hours of the bites, 10% for sea snakes within 15 hours and 1–15% in *Viperidae* within 2 days. In the early stages snake bite is very unpredictable and all patients must be carefully monitored for at least 12 hours.

First aid measures. Firm pressure bandaging of the bite area and immobilisation of the part substantially delays spread of the venom. Patients are often very apprehensive and should be reassured and sedated if necessary.

Clinical features. Local pain and fang marks are very variable and of no help in diagnosis.

Viperidae. Local swelling starts almost immediately. This is also a feature of poisoning in bites by Asian cobras and the African spitting cobra, but may not develop for up to 2 hours. Early signs of systemic poisoning, which may develop within 15 minutes of the bite include vomiting, hypotension and signs of abnormal bleeding from or into any site. Later signs include increase in local swelling which may become massive over 48–72 hours with associated bruising. Blister formation around the site of the bite is common and spreading blisters suggest a large dose of venom and may precede necrosis. Local tissue necrosis with an offensive putrid smell is typical of cobra bites. Shock may occur and haemorrhage into a vital organ which is often fatal may occur up to a week after the bite if antivenom has not been given.

Elapidae. There is seldom any local swelling. Vomiting, hypotension and a polymorph leucocytosis suggest systemic envenomation. More specific signs of muscle weakness such as ptosis, glossopharyngeal palsy and cough indicate severe poisoning and may be delayed for 10 hours after the bite. There is a danger of respiratory paralysis and ECG changes and rises in cardiac enzymes occur.

Hydrophidae. The early features are similar to *Elapidae.* More specific signs are generalised myalgia, with the appearance of myoglobinuria 3–5 hours later. Paresis of the limbs may follow with respiratory paralysis within a few hours of the bite, although it may be delayed for up to 60 hours. Hyperkalaemia may result in cardiac arrest and acute renal failure may occur.

Treatment. (1) The site of the bite should be cleansed and then left strictly alone; otherwise the risk of infection is increased. If skin necrosis occurs, sloughs should be excised with skin grafts applied as appropriate. (2) General measures, including intravenous fluids, should be given to support vital functions. (3) Sedatives are required if the patient is apprehensive. (4) Appropriate antitetanus prophylaxis should be given taking account of the patient's immune state. (5) Antivenoms should be given only if there is clear evidence of systemic poisoning. Some local effects, however, especially necrosis, may be avoided or minimised if antivenom is given within 4 hours of the bite. This is the case in bites by Asian cobras, African spitting cobras, puff adders and rattlesnakes. In *V. berus* bites, the only poisonous snake in Britain, adult patients may have prolonged and painful local swelling which can be effectively treated by Zagreb antivenom if given within the first few hours. All antivenoms may cause severe allergic reactions which may be fatal. Appropriate precautions, therefore, are mandatory. The potency of the antivenom should be checked by first making sure that it is clear and has no opacities. Depending on the severity of poisoning, 20–100 ml antivenom is diluted in 2–3 volumes of isotonic saline. This is then given by slow intravenous infusion (15 drops per minute). Adrenaline (1:1000 solution) must be immediately available. If a reaction occurs the drip is stopped temporarily and 0.5 ml adrenaline injected intramuscularly. Provided the adrenaline is given at the first sign of anaphylaxis, it is rapidly effective and the drip can be restarted with care. Several injections of adrenaline may be indicated. There is marked variation in the requirements of different patients for antivenom. Therefore it is important to give sufficient antivenom to counteract the toxic effects of the poisoning and children require the same doses of antivenom as adults. This is especially important in neurotoxic poisoning.

Spider bite. Only a few genera of spiders are harmful to man. *Lactrodectus* species are found only in warm climates. The Black Widow Spider (*L. mactans*) is the most dangerous and occurs only in the tropics. The Funnel Web Spider (*Atrax robustus*) also quite often causes venomous bites. These spiders are shy, inhabiting dark corners of sheds, basements and foundations of houses and outside privies. Death may occur in up to 6% of cases, especially in young children.

Clinical features. (1) Burning of the bite site. (2) After about 1 hour, generalised muscular pain, which may simulate an acute abdomen, nausea and vomiting. (3) Pyrexia, sweating and shock.

Treatment. (1) 10–20 ml calcium gluconate (10%) by slow intravenous injection. (2) Analgesics. (3) If severe systemic toxicity give specific antivenom if available.

In the South States of America, Central and South America, the Brown Recluse Spider (*Loxosceles reclusa*) and related species may be found in houses and outbuildings. The spider often crawls into clothing and bed-clothes. Poisoning is relatively uncommon but important as it results in necrosis at the site of the bite, which is slow to heal. Fever, vomiting and rashes may occur and occasionally haemolysis and thrombocytopenia. Analgesics should be given as required and antihistamines and corticosteroids are considered helpful.

Theophylline. *Clinical features.* Nausea, vomiting, abdominal discomfort, gastrointestinal haemorrhage, diarrhoea, hyperventilation, thirst, polyuria, hypokalemia and agitation are common. The development of cardiac arrhythmias, hypotension, metabolic acidosis and convulsions indicates severe poisoning with a poor prognosis, especially in elderly patients.

Treatment. (1) General supportive measures. (2) Gastric aspiration and lavage. (3) Intravenous diazepam (5–10 mg) to control convulsions. (4) Charcoal haemoperfusion if severe poisoning (plasma level > 60 mg/l).

Tick bite. Tick paralysis is due to venom in the saliva of certain hard ticks. If such a tick remains attached to the skin for some days there is increasing and spreading paralysis with a danger of respiratory failure and mechanical ventilation may be required. If the tick is removed in time the patient recovers.

Tricyclic antidepressants. *Clinical features.* These features appear 1–2 hours after ingestion, but seldom last longer than 18–24 hours. Dry mouth, dilated pupils, urinary retention and absent bowel sounds are common. Varying degrees of loss of consciousness result but deep coma is not common. Hallucinations and loquacity occur. Cardiac arrhythmias may be severe, especially in children, and hypotension may result. Torticollis and ataxia may be pronounced in children, but at all ages brisk reflexes are common and tonic-clonic movements occur. Ventilatory depression, on occasions, is severe. Several newer antidepressants have been introduced in recent years and are claimed to be less toxic in overdosage. This is only relative and serious poisoning may still occur with clinical features similar to those of the tricyclics.

Treatment. (1) General measures. (2) Gastric lavage is effective up to 12 hours after ingestion. (3) Supportive therapy is all that is required in the great majority of patients but, if inadequate, physostigmine salicylate (1–3 mg) by slow intravenous injection will abolish the central nervous system effects and some of the cardiac complications. If necessary, the injection may be repeated after 10 minutes. (4) Cardiac arrhythmias may respond to 40 mEq sodium bicarbonate by rapid intravenous infusion over 20 minutes. If this is ineffective, appropriate antiarrhythmics should be given.

Vegetable toxins. The harmful effects of the ingestion of various bush teas (p. 535) are mentioned elsewhere.

EPIDEMIC DROPSY (ARGEMONE POISONING). This is seen mainly in India and in Indian communities elsewhere when curried dishes are prepared with mustard oil contaminated by extracts from the seeds of the poppy weed, *Argemone mexicana*, which contain the toxin, sanguinarine. This substance interferes with the oxidation of pyruvic acid, which accumulates and causes dilatation of capillaries and small arterioles. Haemangiomas may develop.

Clinical features. Nausea, vomiting, diarrhoea and fever occur followed by the development of peripheral oedema and cardiac failure. There is erythematous mottling of the skin and raised haemangiomas may appear. Severe glaucoma may result.

Treatment. All contaminated mustard oil must be identified and further exposure avoided. Supportive therapy for cardiac failure is effective, but the response may be slow.

VOMITING SICKNESS OF JAMAICA (ACKEE POISONING). The unripe fruit of the common West Indian and South American tree, *Blighia sapida*, contains a water-soluble toxin, capable of blocking gluconeogenesis in the liver. If eaten, especially by undernourished children, severe and prolonged hypoglycaemia may result. Vomiting, loss of consciousness and convulsions are common. Continuous intravenous infusion of glucose should be started as soon as possible. Without treatment the mortality is high.

Industrial and agricultural poisoning

Lead, cyanide (p. 976), mercury, beryllium (p. 406) and cadmium are potential causes of industrial poisoning. In agriculture many highly toxic weedkillers, including paraquat and the dinitro-ortho-cresol group, and organophosphorus insecticides have been developed in recent years. They have been responsible for only a small number of cases of acute poisoning in Britain owing to effective legislation for controlling their use. In some countries, however, they have caused many deaths.

Prevention of acute poisoning. An indication of the size and complexity of the problem has been given in the introduction to this chapter. The scope for preventive action is clear.

About 60% of patients consult their doctors in the month prior to taking the overdosage and many do so within a week of their action. Also a considerable number poison themselves again after discharge from hospital or during active treatment for psychiatric conditions such as depression. There can be no doubt, therefore, that doctors can make a very important contribution to the prevention of poisoning by learning to recognise the danger signs of imminent overdosage and take the appropriate preventive action. General practitioners are particularly well placed for this purpose as not only can they assess the personality concerned, but also the social and family circumstances which are often the main cause of the problem. For example, it has become apparent that some poisoning incidents in young children occur as an expression of abuse by their parents. Improvements are required in the social services in order that their response to such difficulties should be more immediate and effective.

At all ages a major predisposing factor is the ready availability of medicaments and toxic household products. In the prevention of poisoning in children, the best method is to keep all medicines in a locked cupboard. Poisoning by household preparations is also common in children under the age of 5 years and is likely to continue as long as these articles are stored in places accessible to inquisitive toddlers. A potentially very dangerous practice is the storage of toxic chemicals such as weedkillers in old lemonade or beer bottles.

Another important factor in acute poisoning is that many tablets and capsules are supplied in a variety of attractive colours and shapes, often similar to popular sweets and therefore very appealing to children. The danger is increased by parents who, often with the best intentions, encourage their children to take medicines by suggesting that the tablets are in fact sweets. Also, many potent and dangerous drugs are dispensed as pleasant elixirs and syrups with an increased danger of overdosage in the unwitting youngster. An effective measure has been the development of drug containers which children find difficult to open. An increasing number of drugs are also being supplied in individual wrapping, a useful deterrent for patients inclined to impulsive self-poisoning. These measures may add substantially to the price of production of drugs, but when one considers the cost of hospital and social care, the additional expense is justified on that basis alone.

There have been various attempts in the field of health education with the aid of schools, national press and television to make the general public aware of the need for preventive measures, but these campaigns are often of limited duration and quickly lose their impact. The medical profession as a whole has not played a very direct role in these educational exercises and much more could be done in this regard. In Britain, poison information services answer questions only from members of the medical profession, but experience in other countries suggests that the scope of these services could be widened with benefit to the community. In the Unites States, for example, poison control centres have provided information and advice direct to the general public and fulfilled a valuable educational role whereby, for example, parents have become more aware of the importance of keeping drugs and household products out of the reach of toddlers. As a result in many parts of the United States, the incidence of childhood poisoning has fallen substantially.

The major cause of acute poisoning incidents is intentional self-poisoning which, as has been stated, is usually of an impulsive and conscious type. The availability of drugs is particularly relevant in this group. Patients should therefore be constantly encouraged to dispose of unused drugs from previous prescriptions and it follows that doctors should make every effort to prescribe numbers of tablets carefully calculated for the immediate needs of the patients. Also, sedative and psychotropic drugs should be prescribed only when there is a clear and genuine medical indication. In the recent past the numbers of prescriptions in Britain for these types of drugs rose in a most dramatic way and there is no reason to suspect that serious psychiatric illness had undergone any major increase in the same time. This suggests that much prescribing of sedative and antidepressant drugs was inappropriate and was given often for psychosocial problems rather than significant psychiatric disorder. On the other hand, patients who are significantly depresse'· must be kept under careful observation when therapy is commenced because the antidepressant may cause partial improvement, but also make these patients capable of taking active measures towards self-destruction.

Considering the large number of people involved and the vast range of possible toxic substances used in industry, accidental industrial poisoning is uncommon in Britain. This is largely due to the vigilance and initiative of industrial medical officers and to the effectiveness of legislation which regulates the safe storage, transport and use of potentially toxic substances. Also, many essential processes in industry involving the use of dangerous poisons have been made safer by the introduction of automatic mechanical techniques which avoid exposure of workers to the risk.

Inevitably, the management of patients with acute poisoning rests with the medical profession and the social services, and it is easy to criticise their apparent inability to improve the situation. The basic problem, however, lies within the community. Until a more responsible attitude emerges with a willingness to be more supportive towards the emotional problems of individuals, there seems little doubt that acute self-poisoning will continue to be an expression of a plea for help to correct a situation which for the individual has become intolerable.

FURTHER READING

Practical manuals for rapid consultation in an emergency:

Dreisbach R H 1987 Handbook of poisoning, 12th Edn. Lange Medical, Los Altos

Haddad L M, Winchester J F 1983 Clinical management of poisoning and drug overdose. Saunders, Philadelphia

Henry J, Volans G 1985 ABC of poisoning: part 1 drugs. British Medical Association, London

Hodgson E 1988 Dictionary of Toxicology. Macmillan, New York

Polson C J, Green M A, Lee M R 1983 Clinical toxicology. 3rd Edn. Pitman, London

Proudfoot A T 1982 Diagnosis and management of acute poisoning. Blackwell Scientific Publications, Oxford

Standing Medical Advisory Committees 1985 Hospital treatment of acute treatment of acute poisoning. HMSO, London

Vale J A, Meredith T J (eds) 1981 Poisoning: diagnosis and treatment. MTP Press, Lancaster

Vale J A, Meredith T J 1985 A concise guide to the management of poisoning, 3rd Edn. Churchill Livingstone, Edinburgh, London, Melbourne, New York

Specialist sources written primarily for the postgraduate, but suitable for reference by the undergraduate:

Clayton G D, Clayton F E (eds) 1981–82 Patty's Industrial hygiene and toxicology, 3rd Edn, vols 2A, 2B & 2C. Toxicology. Wiley, New York

Cooper M R, Johnson A W 1984 Poisonous plants in Britain and their effects on animals and man. HMSO, London

Department of Health and Social Security 1983 Pesticide poisoning. HMSO, London

Frohne D, Pfander H J 1984 A colour atlas of poisonous plants. Wolfe Scientific, London

Gilman G A, Goodman L S, Gilman A (eds) 1980 The Pharmacological basis of therapeutics, 6th Edn. Macmillan, New York

Habermehl G G 1981 Venomous animals and their toxins. Springer Verlag, Berlin

Hayes W J 1982 Pesticides studied in man. Williams and Wilkins, Baltimore

Sax N L 1984 Dangerous properties of industrial materials, 6th Edn. Van Nostrand Reinhold, New York

20

Appendices

Contents

DIETS

The diet sheets that follow have been constructed to illustrate the quantitative and qualitative aspects of diets required for the treatment of obesity and diabetes mellitus. The quantities given in a standard diet sheet will obviously require some modification in relation to the size, age, sex, and occupation of the patient. In the dietetic treatment of most diseases it is unnecessary to weigh accurately the amounts of the different foods eaten. Under these circumstances sufficient accuracy will be secured by the use of household measures as illustrated in Diet 1 and by the terms 'small', 'medium' or 'large' helping for meat, fish or chicken. A small helping weighs approximately 30–60 g (1 to 2 oz), a medium helping 60–90 g (2 to 3 oz) and a large helping 120 g (4 oz) or more.

The qualitative content of the diet, i.e. the actual food consumed, will vary widely. The examples detailed here are suitable for persons whose food habits are those of the Western world. If they are to be effective therapeutically, diet prescriptions must be carefully adapted to take account of national, cultural and local eating habits.

1. LOW ENERGY (CALORIE) DIET

Suitable for adults with obesity with or without diabetes.

Approximately: Protein 60 g. Carbohydrate 100 g. Fat 40 g. Energy 1000 kcal (4184 kJ)

Early morning	Cup of tea, milk from allowance, if desired.
Breakfast	1 egg or 30 g (1 oz) grilled lean bacon (2 rashers) *or* cold ham *or* breakfast fish. 20 g ($\frac{2}{3}$ oz) white or brown bread, *or* exchange, with margarine or butter from allowance. Tea or coffee, with milk from allowance.
Mid-morning	Tea or coffee, with milk from allowance, or 'free' drink from Group A3. 1 cream cracker or water biscuit.
Mid-day meal	Clear soup, tomato juice or grapefruit, if desired. Small helping, 60 g (2 oz) lean meat, ham, poultry, game or offal *or* 90 g (3 oz) white fish (steamed, baked or grilled) *or* 2 eggs *or* 45 g (1½ oz) cheese. Salad or vegetables from Group A1 as desired. 40 g (1½ oz) bread (white or brown) *or* exchange, with margarine or butter from allowance if desired. 1 portion of fruit from bread exchange list below. Tea or coffee with milk from allowance.
Mid-afternoon	20 g ($\frac{2}{3}$ oz) white or brown bread, *or* exchange, with margarine or butter from allowance.
Evening meal	Clear soup, meat or yeast extracts, tomato juice or grapefruit, if desired. Small helping, 60 g (2 oz) lean meat, ham, poultry, game or offal *or* 90 g (3 oz) white fish (steamed, baked or grilled) *or* 1 egg *or* 45 g (1½ oz) cheese. Salad or vegetables from Group A1 as desired. 40 g (1½ oz) bread (white or brown) *or* exchange, with margarine or butter from allowance if desired. 1 portion of fruit from list below. Tea or coffee with milk from allowance.
Before bed	Tea or coffee with milk from allowance. 1 cream cracker or water biscuit.
Allowance for day:	200 ml ($\frac{1}{3}$ pint) milk semi-skimmed or skimmed. 15 g ($\frac{1}{2}$ oz) margarine or butter.

Exchanges for 20 g ($\frac{2}{3}$ oz) bread ($\frac{1}{2}$ slice from a large cut loaf):

2 cream crackers	1 potato (the size of a hen's egg)
1½ of any crispbread	1 portion of fruit (from list below)
2 water biscuits	
1 oatcake	

Exchanges for 40 g (1½ oz) bread (1 slice from a large cut loaf):

4 cream crackers	2 potatoes
3 Ryvita	4 water biscuits
2 oatcakes	

Fruit list: 1 medium apple, 1 orange, 1 pear, 1 small banana, 10 grapes.

Group A: foods which may be taken as desired

1. *Vegetables*

Artichoke, asparagus, aubergine, French beans, runner beans, broccoli, Brussels sprouts, cabbage, carrots, cauliflower, celeriac, celery, chicory, courgette, cucumber, endive, leeks, lettuce, mushrooms, mustard and cress, onions, parsley, pumpkin, radishes, salsify, seakale, spinach, swede, tomatoes, turnip tops, vegetable marrow, watercress.

2. *Fruits* (stewed without sugar, or raw)

Any fruit fresh, frozen or canned in natural fruit juice, but *not* avocado, dried fruit or fruit canned in syrup.

3. *Drinks*

Water, soda water, tea or coffee (without milk or sugar) lemon juice, tomato juice, diabetic fruit squash, diet cola, clear soup (chicken or beef cubes may be used).

4. *Miscellaneous*

Saccharine or any proprietary sweetening agents (except sorbitol) salt, pepper, mustard, vinegar, herbs, spices, gelatine. Flavourings and colourings may be used.

Group B: foods to be avoided

All fried foods.
Sugar (brown or white), glucose, sorbitol.
Sweets, toffees, chocolates, cornflour, custard powder.
Jam, marmalade, lemon curd, syrup, honey, treacle.
Tinned, frozen or bottled fruits.
Dried fruits, e.g. dates, figs, prunes, apricots, sultanas, currants, raisins, bananas, grapes.
Cakes, buns, pastries, pies, steamed or milk puddings.
Sweets or chocolate biscuits, scones.
Cereals, e.g. rice, sago, macaroni, barley, spaghetti.
Breakfast cereal, porridge.
Ice cream, fresh or synthetic cream. Table jelly.
Evaporated or condensed milk.
Peas, parsnips, beetroot, sweetcorn, haricot beans, butterbeans, broad beans, lentils.

Nuts.

Salad cream, salad dressing, mayonnaise.

Tomato and brown sauce or any thickened sauce.

Sweet pickles and chutney.

Thickened soups, gravies.

Alcoholic drinks, e.g. beer, wine, sherry, spirits.

Sweetened fruit juices, fruit squash, Coca Cola and other sweet, fizzy, 'soft drinks'.

Starch-reduced products, 'diabetic' foodstuffs.

Sausages.

All foods must be served without thickened gravies and sauces. All foods may be baked, grilled, boiled or steamed – *but not fried.*

2. WEIGHT-MAINTENANCE DIABETIC DIET

Method of constructing a diet restricted in carbohydrate containing approximately 1800 kcal (7560 kJ) with 230 g carbohydrate, 72 g protein and 66 g fat suitable for adults with diabetic mellitus.

Use is made of the Atwater calorie conversion factors of 4, 4 and 9 kcal/g for carbohydrate, protein and fat respectively. Each *carbohydrate exchange* contains approximately 10 g carbohydrate. 1.5 g protein and 0.3 fat. Calorie value is about 50 (equivalent to 20 g bread).

Each *protein exchange* contains approximately 7 g protein and 5 g fat. Calorie value is about 70 (equivalent to 30 g meat).

Each *fat exchange* contains approximately 12 g fat and almost no carbohydrate or protein. Calorie value is about 110 (equivalent to ½ oz butter). One pint of milk contains approximately 30 g carbohydrate, 18 g protein and 24 g fat. Calorie value is about 400.

In practice, for quick construction of a diabetic diet it is usually only necessary to work in terms of grams of carbohydrate and total calories. Thus, a diet prescription for 230 g carbohydrate, 1800 kcal would be calculated as follows:

1. The daily intake of carbohydrate (230 g) represents 23 carbohydrate exchanges.

2. The daily allowance of milk is decided, either on the basis of the patient's food habits or special requirements. In this example it is 400 ml (⅔ pint), which contains 2 carbohydrate exchanges, leaving 21 for distribution throughout the day.

3. The daily allowance of protein is then decided. Four protein exchanges will provide 280 kcal.

4. The calories allocated so far amount to 1590; a further 220 kcal are needed to bring the total up to approximately 1800 kcal. This must be provided by fat. As one fat exchange provides 110 kcal, two are needed.

Exchanges	Grams of carbohydrate	kcal
400 ml (⅔ pint) milk = 2 carbohydrate exchanges	20	260
21 carbohydrate exchanges	210	1050
4 protein exchanges	—	280
Total	230	1590
2 fat exchanges	—	220
Grand total	230	1810

5. Finally, the exchanges (23 carbohydrate, 4 protein, and 2 fat) are distributed throughout the day according to the eating habits and daily routine of the patient.

Useful CHO exchanges

Each item on this list = 1 CHO exchange (10 g CHO): ½ slice bread from a large loaf, 1 large digestive biscuit, 2 cream crackers, 8 tablespoons natural unsweetened orange juice or grapefruit juice, 1 medium-sized eating apple or orange, 10 grapes, 1 small banana, ⅓ pint milk, 1 teacup cooked porridge, 1 teacup of cream or tinned soup, ⅔ teacup cornflakes, 1 small packet of crisps, one small potato.

3. UNMEASURED DIABETIC DIET

Patients who are unable to measure their diet or for whom this is unnecessary, are given a list of foods which are grouped into three categories.

I. *Foods to be avoided altogether:*

1. Sugar, glucose, jam, marmalade, honey, syrup, treacle, tinned fruits, sweets, chocolate, lemonade, glucose drinks, proprietary milk preparations and similar foods which are sweetened with sugar.

2. Cakes, sweet biscuits, chocolate biscuits, pies, puddings, thick sauces.

3. Alcoholic drinks unless permission has been given by the doctor.

II. *Foods to be eaten in moderation only:*

1. Breads of all kinds (including so-called 'slimming' and 'starch-reduced' breads, brown or white, plain or toasted).

2. Rolls, scones, biscuits and crispbreads.

3. Potatoes, peas and baked beans.

4. Breakfast cereals and porridge.

5. All fresh or dried fruit, tinned fruit in natural juice.

6. Macaroni, spaghetti, custard and foods with much flour.

7. Thick soups.

8. Diabetic foods.

9. Milk.

10. Meat, fish, eggs and cheese.

III. *Foods to be eaten as desired:*

1. Clear soups or meat extracts, tomato or lemon juice.

2. Tea or coffee.

3. Cabbage, Brussels sprouts, broccoli, cauliflower, spinach, turnip, runner or French beans, onions, leeks or mushrooms, lettuce, cucumber, tomatoes, spring onions, radishes, mustard and cress, asparagus, parsley, rhubarb, gooseberries, lemons, blackberries, grapefruit.

4. Herbs, spices, salt, pepper and mustard.

5. Saccharine and aspartame and other preparations for sweetening.

6. Sugar-free squashes and fizzy drinks.

IV. *For overweight diabetics butter, margarine, fatty and dried foods must be restricted.*

4. FAT-MODIFIED DIET

Low in saturated fats and cholesterol with increased amounts of polyunsaturated fat.

For people with elevated plasma cholesterol.

Foods to be avoided:

Butter and hydrogenated margarines. Use polyunsaturated margarine, e.g. 'Flora'.

Lard, suet, shortenings and cakes, biscuits and pastries made with these.

Fatty meat and visible fat on meat, meat pies, sausages and luncheon meats.

Whole milk and cream.

Chocolate, ice cream (except water ices). Cheese, except low fat cottage cheese.

Coconut and coconut oil.

Eggs – no more than 1 to 2 egg yolks per week, including that used in cooking.

Organ meats – liver, kidneys and brain.

Shellfish and fish roes.

Fried foods unless fried in polyunsaturated oil (like sunflower or corn oil).

Potato crisps and most nuts.

Gravy unless made with polyunsaturated oil, and tinned soups.

Salad dressing unless made with polyunsaturated oil.

Use:

Polyunsaturated margarine instead of butter.

Polyunsaturated oil, e.g. sunflower or corn oil in place of lard.

Bread, pasta, rice, oatmeal, breakfast cereals

Vegetables and fruit

Poultry (without skin)

Fish (grilled or steamed)

Legumes

Skimmed or ½ cream milk

Jam, marmalade, honey, marmite

Tea and coffee

Alcoholic drinks (in moderation)

FURTHER READING ABOUT DIETETICS AND ADDITIONAL DIETS:

Thomas, Briony (ed) 1988 Manual of Dietetic Practice. Blackwell Scientific, Oxford.

NOTES ON INTERNATIONAL SYSTEM OF UNITS (SI UNITS)

Examples of basic SI units

Length	metre (m)
Mass	kilogram (kg)
Amount of substance	mole (mol)
Energy	joule (J)
Pressure	pascal (pa)

Examples of decimal multiples and submultiples of SI units

Factor	Name	Symbol
10^6	mega-	M
10^3	kilo-	k
10^{-1}	deci-	d
10^{-2}	centi-	c
10^{-3}	milli-	m
10^{-6}	micro-	μ
10^{-9}	nano-	n
10^{-12}	pico-	p
10^{-15}	femto-	f

Volume. The basic SI unit of volume is the cubic metre (1000 litre). Because of its convenience the litre is used as the unit of volume in laboratory work.

Amount of substance ('molar') concentration (e.g. mol/l, μmol/l) is used for substances of defined chemical composition. It replaces equivalent concentrations (mEq/l), which is not part of the SI system. For univalent ions such as sodium, potassium, chloride and bicarbonate the numerical value is unchanged. For divalent ions such as calcium and magnesium the numerical value is halved.

Mass concentration (e.g. g/l, μg/l) is used for all protein measurements, for substances which do not have a sufficiently well defined composition and for serum vitamin B_{12} and folate measurements. The numerical value in SI units will change by a factor of 10 in those instances previously expressed in terms of 100 ml.

Haemoglobin is an exception. It is generally expressed in terms of g/dl although the International Committee for standardisation in Haematology recommended in 1982 that the unit for haemoglobin should be g/l.

SI units are not employed for enzymes nor usually for immunoglobulins.

BIOCHEMICAL VALUES

Reference ranges are largely those used in the Department of Clinical Chemistry, the Royal Infirmary, University of Edinburgh. These can vary from laboratory to laboratory, depending on the assay method used and other factors; this is especially the case for the enzyme assays. Although the SI system of units is widely used in the UK, *units* of measurement can vary and lead to laboratory differences.

No details are given of the collection requirements which may be critical to obtaining a meaningful result.

Unless otherwise stated, reference ranges apply to adults; values in children may be different.

The values quoted for blood, except for Table 20.1, refer to plasma or serum. As far as possible, routine analyses are carried out on plasma, but serum is preferred for some analyses, especially certain hormones and electrophoretic studies.

Table 20.1   Arterial blood analysis

Analysis	Reference range	Units
Base excess	−4 to +4	mmol/l
Bicarbonate	21−27.5	mmol/l
Hydrogen ion	36−44	nmol/l
Pa_{CO_2}	4.4−6.1	kPa
Pa_{O_2}	12−15	kPa
Oxygen saturation	Normally >97	%

Table 20.2   Cerebrospinal fluid

Analysis	Reference range	Units
Cells	5 (all mononuclear)	cells/mm³
Chloride	120−170	mmol/l
Glucose	2.5−4.0	mmol/l
Immunoglobulin G	20−50	mg/l
Total protein	100−400	mg/l

Table 20.3   Reference values in venous plasma for the more common analytes in adults

Analysis	Reference range	Units
α_1-Antitrypsin	1.7−3.2	g/l
Alanine aminotransferase (ALT)	10−40	U/l
Albumin	36−47	g/l
Alkaline phosphatase	40−100	U/l
Amylase	50−300	U/l
Aspartate aminotransferase (AST)	10−35	U/l
Bilirubin (total)	2−17	µmol/l
Calcium	2.12−2.62	mmol/l
Carboxyhaemoglobin	Not normally detectable Up to 1.5% in non-smokers	%
Ceruloplasmin	50−600	mg/l
Chloride	95−107	mmol/l
Cholesterol (total)	3.6−6.7	mmol/l
HDL-Cholesterol	0.5−1.6 (M) 0.6−1.9 (F)	
Copper	13−24	µmol/l
Creatine kinase (MB isoenzyme)	Normally <5% of total CK	
Creatine kinase (total)	30−200 (M) 30−150 (F)	U/l

Table 20.3   (continued)

Analysis	Reference range	Units
Ethanol	Not normally detectable 65−87 (marked intoxication) 87−109 (stupor) >109 (coma)	mmol/l
Creatinine	55−150	µmol/l
Ferritin	15−350 (M) 8−300 (F)	µg/l
Gamma-glutamyl transferase (GGT)	10−55 (M) 5−35 (F)	U/l
Glucose (fasting)	3.6−5.8	mmol/l
Glycated haemoglobin (HbA₁)	4.5−8	%
Immunoglobulin A	0.5−4.0	g/l
Immunoglobulin G	5.0−13.0	g/l
Immunoglobulin M	0.3−2.2 (M) 0.4−2.5 (F)	g/l
Iron	14−32 (M) 10−28 (F)	µmol/l
Iron binding capacity	45−72	µmol/l
Lactate	0.4−1.4	mmol/l
Lactate dehydrogenase (urea-stable)	100−300	U/l
Lead	<1.8	µmol/l
Magnesium	0.75−1.0	mmol/l
Osmolality	280−290	mmol/kg
Phosphate (fasting)	0.8−1.4	mmol/l
Potassium	3.3−4.7	mmol/l
Protein (total)	60−80	g/l
Sodium	132−144	mmol/l
Total CO_2	24−30	mmol/l
Transferrin	2.0−4.0	g/l
Triglycerides (fasting)	0.6−1.7	mmol/l
Urate	0.12−0.42 (M) 0.12−0.36 (F)	mmol/l
Urea	2.5−6.6	mmol/l
Zinc	9−29	µmol/l

Notes:
1. Values quoted are for venous plasma, but would also apply to serum.
2. For the definition of diabetes mellitus or impaired glucose tolerance, the following apply (WHO criteria for venous plasma):

	Glucose (mmol/l) (fasting)	Glucose (mmol/l) (2 h post 75 g glucose)
Diabetes mellitus	>8.0	>11.0
Impaired glucose tolerance	<8.0	>8.0 but <11.0

Table 20.4 Reference values for the more common analytes in urine

Analysis	Reference range	Units
Albumin	<3.5	mg/mmol creatinine
Calcium	1.2–3.7	mmol/24 h
	(low calcium diet)	
	Up to 12	
	(normal diet)	
Copper	Up to 0.6	µmol/24 h
Cortisol	9–50	µmol/mol creatinine
Creatinine	10–20	mmol/24 h
5-Hydroxyindole-3-acetic acid (5-HIAA)	10–45	µmol/24 h
Metadrenalines	Up to 7	µmol/24 h
Oxalate	50–140	µmol/24 h
Phosphate	15–50	mmol/24 h
Porphyrins:		nmol/24 h
Coproporphyrins	150–230	
Uroporphyrins	Up to 40	
Potassium	25–100	mmol/24 h
Protein	Up to 100	mg/24 h
Sodium	100–200	mmol/24 h
Urate	1.2–3.0	mmol/24 h
Urea	170–600	mmol/24 h

Notes:

1. The urinary output of electrolytes such as sodium and potassium is normally a reflection of intake. This can vary widely, especially on a cultural, worldwide basis. The values quoted are more appropriate to a 'Western' diet.
2. Albumin excretion, which is insufficient to be dipstick positive, yet is abnormal, is known as microalbuminuria. In diabetic patients, this is a predictor of future diabetic nephropathy. Analysis is best carried out on an early morning urine to overcome postural effects on albumin excretion.

Table 20.5 Concentrations of therapeutic drugs in blood

Drug	Sample time	Therapeutic range	Units
Anticonvulsant drugs:			
Carbamazepine	Just before next dose	17–51	µmol/l
Phenobarbitone	Not critical	65–170	µmol/l
Phenytoin	Not critical	40–80	µmol/l
Valproate	Just before next dose	300–600	µmol/l
Antibiotics:			
Amikacin	Peak: 1 h after i.v. dose	15–30	mg/l
	Trough: pre-dose	5–10	
Gentamycin	Peak: 1 h after i.v. dose	8–12	mg/l
Tobramycin	Trough: pre-dose		
Netilmycin		<2	
Streptomycin	Peak: 1 h after i.v. dose	15–40	mg/l
	Trough: pre-dose	<5	
Vancomycin	Peak: 1 h after i.v. dose	30–40	mg/l
	Trough: pre-dose	5–10	
Others:			
Cyclosporin	Just before next dose	70–300	nmol/l
Digoxin	6–18 h after last dose	1.0–2.6	nmol/l
Lithium	12–18 h after last dose	0.6–1.0	mmol/l
Quinidine	Just before next dose	2–5	mg/l
Salicylate	Just before next dose	Up to 250	mg/l
Theophylline	Just before next dose	55–110	µmol/l

Notes:

1. Care should be taken in comparing values between different laboratories. This is especially important since drug measurement units can be different. In the above table, both SI *and* non-SI units feature.
2. Drug pharmacokinetics are dependent on the *individual*. For within-individual comparison, it is advisable to sample at the same relative time(s) in relation to drug administration.

Table 20.6 Tumour markers

Tumour marker	Application
α_1-Fetoprotein	Hepatoma, teratoma
Acid phosphatase (prostatic isoenzyme)	Prostate
CA 15.3	Breast
CA 125	Ovary
Calcitonin	Medullary carcinoma of thyroid
Carcinoembryonic antigen (CEA)	Colon, GI
Human chorionic gonadotrophin	Choriocarcinoma, testicular tumours, hepatoma
Prostatic-specific antigen	Prostate

Notes:

1. Tumour markers have little place in diagnosis, the exception being HCG in the detection of choriocarcinoma. For this reason, reference ranges have not been given.
2. Measurements are useful in monitoring disease progress and in the diagnosis of recurrence.

Table 20.7 Gastrointestinal, pancreatic and liver data

Test	Reference range	Units	Comments
Faecal fat	<18	mmol/24 h	Average over 5 day collection
Stool weight (wet)	<200	g/24 h	
Xylose excretion (5 g test)	>15% excreted at 2 h (urine)	%	Use blood xylose test if plasma (urea) >8.3 mmol/l
	>35% excreted at 5 h (urine)		
	>0.3 (blood concentration at 2 h)	mmol/l	
Secretin stimulation (pancreatic exocrine function)	>2 (juice volume)	ml/kg/h	
	>10 (HCO_3^- output)	mmol/h	
	>80 (HCO_3^- concentration)	mmol/l	
Liver copper	<50	µg/g dry weight	
	>250 (Wilson's disease)		
Liver iron	40–60	µg/100 mg dry weight	
	>1000 (haemochromatosis)		

Miscellaneous

1. Sweat

Sweat $[Cl]^-$ is *normally* <60 mmol/l (equivocal range 50–70 mmol/l).
In cystic fibrosis (CF) high values are obtained.

2. Ascites and pleural effusions

Transudates: total protein <30 g/l
Exudates: total protein >30 g/l.

Table 20.8   Hormones

Hormone	Reference range	Units	Comments
Adrenocorticotrophic hormone (ACTH)	10–80 (at 08:00) <10 (at 22:00)	ng/l	Nycthemeral rhythm, so sampling time is critical. Avoid stress
Cortisol	160–565 (at 08:00) <205 (at 22:00)	nmol/l	Nycthemeral rhythm, so sampling time is critical. Avoid stress
Follicle-stimulating hormone (FSH) (Male)	1.5–9.0	U/l	
Follicle-stimulating hormone (FSH) (Female)	3.0–15 (early follicular) Up to 20 (mid-cycle) 30–115 (post-menopausal)	U/l	
Gastrin	60–200	pg/ml	Collect after overnight fasting
Growth hormone (GH)	Very variable, usually less than 2, but may be up to 50 with stress	mU/l	Avoid stress Stimulation and suppression tests required
Insulin	5–25 (variable)	mU/l	Inappropriate levels in relation to glucose should be assessed
Luteinizing hormone (LH) (Female)	2.5–9.0 (early follicular) Up to 30 (mid-cycle) 30–115 (post-menopausal)	U/l	
Luteinizing hormone (LH) (Male)	1.5–9.0	U/l	
Oestradiol-17β (Female)	110–180 (early follicular) 550–1650 (mid-cycle) 370–770 (luteal) <100 (post-menopausal)	pmol/l	
Oestradiol-17β (Male)	<200	pmol/l	
Parathyroid hormone (PTH)	10–55	ng/l	
Progesterone (Male)	<2.0	nmol/l	
Progesterone (Female)	<2.0 (follicular) >15 (Mid luteal) <2.0 (post-menopausal)	nmol/l	
Prolactin (PRL)	60–390	mU/l	Avoid stress
Testosterone (Male)	10–30	nmol/l	
Testosterone (Female)	0.8–2.8	nmol/l	
Thyroid stimulating hormone (TSH)	0.3–5.0	mU/l	
Thyroxine (free) (free T$_4$)	9–23	pmol/l	Reference range may change in pregnancy
Tri-iodothyronine (T$_3$)	1.1–2.8 (under 65) 0.5–2.2 (over 65)	nmol/l	
TSH receptor antibodies (TRAb)	<7	U/l	

Notes:
1. A number of hormones are unstable and collection details are critical to obtaining a meaningful result. Refer to the local handbook.
2. Values in the table are only a guideline; hormone levels can often only be meaningfully understood in relation to factors such as sex (e.g. testosterone), age (e.g. FSH in women), time of day (e.g. cortisol), or regulatory factors (e.g. insulin and glucose, PTH and [Ca^{2+}]). Also, reference ranges may be critically method-dependent.

HAEMATOLOGICAL VALUES

Table 20.9   Haematological values

	SI units	Other units
Bleeding time (Ivy)	Up to 11 min	
Body fluid (total)		50% (obese) – 70% (lean) of body weight
Intracellular		30–40% of body weight
Extracellular		20–30% of body weight
Blood volume		
Red cell mass, men	30 ± 5 ml/kg	
women	25 ± 5 ml/kg	
Plasma volume (both sexes)	45 ± 5 ml/kg	
Total blood volume, men	75 ± 10 ml/kg	
women	70 ± 10 ml/kg	
Erythrocyte sedimentation rate (Westergren)		0–6 mm in 1 h normal
(Figures given are for patients under		7–20 mm in 1 h doubtful
60 years of age. Higher values in older		>20 mm in 1 h abnormal
persons are not necessarily abnormal)		
Fibrinogen	1.5–4.0 g/l	150–400 mg/dl
*Folate – serum	2–20 µg/l	2–20 ng/ml
– red cell	>100 µg/l	>100 ng/ml
Haemoglobin – men	130–180 g/l	13–18 g/dl
– women	115–165 g/l	11.5–16.5 g/dl
Haptoglobin	0.3–2.0 g/l	30–200 mg/dl
Leucocytes – adults	$4.0–11.0 \times 10^9$/l	4000–11 000/µl
		$4.0–11.0 \times 10^3$/mm³
Differential white cell count		
Neutrophil granulocytes	$2.5–7.5 \times 10^9$/l	40–75%
Lymphocytes	$1.0–3.5 \times 10^9$/l	20–45%
Monocytes	$0.2–0.8 \times 10^9$/l	2–10%
Eosinophil granulocytes	$0.04–0.4 \times 10^9$/l	1–6%
Basophil granulocytes	$0.01–0.1 \times 10^9$/l	0–1%
Mean corpuscular haemoglobin (MCH)	27–32 pg	27–32 µµg
Mean corpuscular haemoglobin concentration (MCHC)	30–35 g/dl	30–35%
Mean corpuscular volume (MCV)	78–98 fl	78–98 µ³ or µm³
Packed cell volume (PCV) or		
haematocrit – men	0.40–0.54	40–54%
– women	0.35–0.47	35–47%
Platelets	$150–400 \times 10^9$/l	150 000–4000 000/µl or /mm³
Prothrombin time	11–15 s	
Red cell count – men	$4.5–6.5 \times 10^{12}$/l	$4.5–6.5 \times 10^6$/µl or mm³
– women	$3.8–5.8 \times 10^{12}$/l	$3.8–5.8 \times 10^6$/µl or mm³
Red cell life span (mean)	120 days	
Red cell life span $T_{\frac{1}{2}}$ (^{51}Cr)	25–35 days	
Reticulocytes (adults)	$10–100 \times 10^9$/l	0.2–2%
*Vitamin B_{12} (in serum as cyanocobalamin)	160–925 ng/l	160–925 pg/ml or µµg/ml

*Also measured by radioassay; normal range of reference values should be obtained from the laboratory carrying out the estimation.

DRUG NOMENCLATURE AND PRESCRIPTION

In this book the names that have been given for drugs have almost invariably been those approved for use in Britain. These are devised or selected by the British Pharmacopoeia Commission and published by the Health Ministers at regular intervals. It must be realised, however, than many countries have their national non-proprietary names, and that the World Health Organization also has its own list. Usually these various names are similar, but there are significant differences; for example, paracetamol (BP) is listed as acetaminophen in the United States Pharmacopeia. Proprietary names are given in this book only in exceptional circumstances, but can usually be found in the British National Formulary, the Data Sheet Compendium and as an addendum to some textbooks. There may be many totally different names for the same substance and this can cause confusion. Doctors must also be prepared to interpret the jargon used by addicts about drugs of dependence and their effects.

Abbreviations used in relationship to the administration of drugs are i.m. (intramuscular injection), i.v. (intravenous injection), s.c. (subcutaneous injection), b.d. (twice daily) and t.i.d. (thrice daily). The dosage given is a guide for use in adults of average build and should be checked against that in a national formulary or in the manufacturer's instructions. It is particularly important to confirm that a dosage given in mg/kg body weight is, indeed, correct, and great care must be taken to ensure that no error occurs in the quantity of a drug prescribed for an infant or child.

Some drugs, e.g. in the chemotherapy of malignant disease, are prescribed in weight of drug per square metre of body surface. With the use of a nomogram, the body surface area can be calculated from the height in centimetres and the weight in kilograms.

Patient compliance (i.e. the taking of medicines as prescribed) is improved if instructions are simple and specific, especially for the elderly. Polypharmacy should be avoided if possible, one reason being the danger of interaction between drugs. Some (e.g. rifampicin) induce liver enzymes which may increase the metabolism of concurrently administered preparations (e.g. corticosteroids, oral contraceptives, oral anticoagulants, oral hypoglycaemic drugs, dapsone and phenytoin). Conversely elimination of compounds metabolised in the liver by oxidation (e.g. oral anticoagulants, phenytoin and diazepam) can be prolonged by the action of other drugs (e.g. cimetidine). All drugs, whenever possible, should be avoided during the early months of pregnancy.

STANDARD REFERENCE BOOKS

British National Formulary 1990 The British Medical Association and The Pharmaceutical Society of Great Britain.

Martindale – the extra pharmacopoeia 1989 29th edn. Pharmaceutical Press, London.

FURTHER READING ABOUT DRUGS

Avery G S (ed.) 1987 Drug treatment, 3rd edn. Churchill Livingstone, Edinburgh.

Index